ESSENTIALS OF PHARMACOLOGY

ESSENTIALS OF PHARMACOLOGY

Cedric M. Smith, MD
Professor, Department of Pharmacology and Toxicology
School of Medicine and Biomedical Sciences
State University of New York
Buffalo, New York

Alan M. Reynard, PhD
Professor, Department of Pharmacology and Toxicology
School of Medicine and Biomedical Sciences
State University of New York
Buffalo, New York

W.B. SAUNDERS COMPANY
A Division of Harcourt Brace & Company
Philadelphia London Toronto Montreal Sydney Tokyo

W.B. SAUNDERS COMPANY
A Division of Harcourt Brace & Company

The Curtis Center
Independence Square West
Philadelphia, Pennsylvania 19106

Library of Congress Cataloging-in-Publication Data

Essentials of pharmacology / [edited by] Cedric M. Smith, Alan M. Reynard. — 1st ed.

p. cm.

ISBN 0-7216-5531-9

1. Pharmacology. I. Smith, Cedric M. II. Reynard, Alan M.
[DNLM: 1. Pharmacology. 2. Drug Therapy. QV 4 1995]

RM300.E833 1995 615'.1—dc20

DNLM/DLC 94-11096

ESSENTIALS OF PHARMACOLOGY ISBN 0-7216-5531-9

Printed in the United States of America

Last digit is the print number: 9 8 7 6 5 4 3 2 1

PREFACE

Understanding what drugs are, what effects they produce, and how these effects occur—pharmacology—is essential in the education of every medical professional. This book provides a succinct, accurate, up-to-date, clinically relevant introduction to the essentials of drug action on which rational therapeutics is based.

This *Essentials* textbook draws heavily on the experience of the editors and authors in preparing Smith and Reynard's *Textbook of Pharmacology* (1992). Although shorter and more succinct than the *Textbook*, the content continues to focus on meeting the ". . . essential knowledge in pharmacology which every medical student . . . must have" as this was identified by a committee of the Association of Medical School Pharmacology Chairmen. The topics include the mechanisms of action of drugs on molecular, cellular, and organ systems, and how they are absorbed, distributed in the body, metabolized, and excreted. In addition, it emphasizes the agents commonly prescribed in the diagnosis and treatment of disease, as well as the substances involved in poisoning and toxic reactions. Essential topics not commonly addressed in other more traditional books include drug effects on sensory systems, adverse drug reactions and interactions, and the use of drugs in special populations of children and the elderly. Inasmuch as pharmacology and therapeutics are rapidly advancing fields, we have devoted an entire chapter to print and computer-based information resources that will assist the readers in making rational therapeutic decisions as practitioners. **Nevertheless, since this book is neither a therapeutic manual nor a comprehensive reference source, all readers about to prescribe a drug are urged to consult the latest and most accurate information for dose and dosage regimens.**

The authors and editors have aimed to make the text readable and useful in the teaching and learning of pharmacology as the basis of therapeutics. In line with this objective, the references in most chapters have been limited to recent articles or reviews judged to be useful to those with an interest in more detailed information.

We acknowledge the important contributions of Rachel Byron Moore of bioGraphics, Inc., for many of the figures taken from the *Textbook of Pharmacology* and William Pudlack for drawings of chemical structures. We wish to thank Ronald Rubin, Ph.D., chairman of this pharmacology department, for his encouragement; Larry McGrew our editor for sustained support and helpful suggestions; and our many colleagues for their helpful reviews and suggestions. Lastly, we acknowledge our indebtedness to the pioneering efforts of the authors of previous textbooks of pharmacology.

CEDRIC M. SMITH
ALAN M. REYNARD

CONTRIBUTORS

Margaret A. Acara, Ph.D., Professor, Department of Pharmacology and Toxicology, School of Medicine and Biomedical Sciences, State University of New York at Buffalo, Buffalo, New York

Ann M. Arvin, M.D., Professor, Department of Pediatrics, Stanford University School of Medicine; Chief, Infectious Diseases Section, Lucile Packard Children's Hospital at Stanford, Stanford, California

Thomas R. Beam, Jr., A.B., M.D., deceased, Professor, Department of Medicine; Associate Professor, Department of Microbiology, State University of New York at Buffalo; Associate Chief of Staff for Education, Buffalo Veterans Administration Medical Center, Buffalo, New York

Joseph R. Bertino, M.D., Professor of Pharmacology and Medicine, Cornell University School of Medicine; Member and Program Chairman, Molecular Pharmacology and Therapeutics, Memorial Sloan-Kettering Cancer Center, New York, New York

Richard E. Bettigole, M.D., Associate Professor, Department of Medicine; Clinical Associate Professor, Department of Pathology, School of Medicine and Biomedical Sciences, State University of New York at Buffalo, Buffalo, New York

Katherine R. Bonson, Ph.D., Instructor, Department of Pharmacology and Toxicology, School of Medicine and Biomedical Sciences, State University of New York at Buffalo, Buffalo, New York

Oliver M. Brown, Ph.D., Associate Professor, Department of Pharmacology, College of Medicine, State University of New York — Health Sciences Center at Syracuse, Syracuse, New York

Alexander C. Brownie, Ph.D., D.Sc., Professor, Department of Biochemistry; Research Professor of Pathology; Research Professor of Medicine, School of Medicine and Biomedical Sciences, State University of New York at Buffalo, Buffalo, New York

Edward A. Carr, Jr., M.D., Emeritus Professor, Department of Pharmacology and Toxicology; Emeritus Professor, Department of Medicine, School of Medicine and Biomedical Sciences, State University of New York at Buffalo, Buffalo, New York

David B. Case, M.D., Clinical Associate Professor, Department of Medicine, Cornell University Medical College; Associate Attending Physician, The New York Hospital — Cornell University Medical Center, New York, New York

Arthur W. K. Chan, Ph.D., Research Professor, Department of Pharmacology and Toxicology, School of Medicine and Biomedical Sciences, State University of New York at Buffalo; Senior Research Scientist, Research Institute on Addictions, Buffalo, New York

Robert M. Cooper, Pharm.D., Associate Professor, Department of Pharmacy; Associate Dean, School of Pharmacy, State University of New York at Buffalo, Buffalo, New York

Roger K. Cunningham, Ph.D., Associate Professor, Department of Microbiology, School of Medicine and Biomedical Sciences, State University of New York at Buffalo, Buffalo, New York

Paul J. Davis, M.D., Professor and Chairman, Department of Medicine, Albany Medical College; Physician-in-Chief, Albany Medical Center Hospital, Albany, New York

Jill G. Dolgin, Pharm.D., A.B.A.T., Clinical Assistant Professor of Pharmacy; Adjunct Clinical Assistant Professor in Departments of Pediatrics and Emergency Medicine, School of Medicine and Biomedical Sciences, State University of New York at Buffalo; Administrative Director, Western New York Regional Poison Control Center, Children's Hospital of Buffalo, Buffalo, New York

Eli R. Farhi, M.D., Ph.D., Assistant Professor, Department of Medicine, State University of New York at Buffalo; Chief, Cardiology Section, Buffalo Veterans Administration Medical Center, Buffalo, New York

Peter K. Gessner, Ph.D., Professor, Department of Pharmacology and Toxicology, School of Medicine and Biomedical Sciences, State University of New York at Buffalo, Buffalo, New York

Linda A. Hershey, M.D., Ph.D., Associate Professor, Departments of Neurology and of Pharmacology and Toxicology, State University of New York at Buffalo; Chief of Neurology Service, Buffalo Department of Veterans Affairs Medical Center, Buffalo, New York

Peter J. Horvath, Ph.D., F.A.C.N., C.N.S., Associate Professor, Nutrition Program, State University of New York at Buffalo; Research Staff, Buffalo General Hospital, Buffalo, New York

Joseph L. Izzo, Jr., M.D., Professor, Departments of Medicine and of Pharmacology and Toxicology; Chief, Division of Clinical Pharmacology, State University of New York at Buffalo; Chairman, Department of Medicine, Millard Fillmore Hospital, Buffalo, New York

William Kennedy, Ph.D., Vice President, Drug Regulatory Affairs, Zeneca Pharmaceuticals, Wilmington, Delaware

Paul R. Knight, III, M.D., Ph.D., Professor and Chairman, Department of Anesthesiology, State University of New York at Buffalo; Professor and Chairman, Buffalo General Hospital, Children's Hospital, Erie County Medical Center, Millard Fillmore Hospital, Roswell Park Cancer Institute, Buffalo Veterans Administration Medical Center, Buffalo, New York

Paul J. Kostyniak, Ph.D., D.A.B.T., Associate Professor, Department of Pharmacology and Toxicology, School of Medicine and Biomedical Sciences; Director, Toxicology Research Center, State University of New York at Buffalo, Buffalo, New York

M. Peter Lance, M.D., Associate Professor, Department of Medicine, Division of Gastroenterology, School of Medicine and Biomedical Sciences, State University of New York at Buffalo, Buffalo, New York

Claire M. Lathers, Ph.D., F.C.P., President and Dean; Professor, Department of Pharmacology, Albany College of Pharmacy, Union University, Albany, New York

Suzanne G. Laychock, Ph.D., Professor, Department of Pharmacology and Toxicology, School of Medicine and Biomedical Sciences, State University of New York at Buffalo, Buffalo, New York

James B. Lee, M.D., Professor, Department of Medicine, School of Medicine and Biomedical Sciences, State University of New York at Buffalo; Attending Physician, Erie County Medical Center, Buffalo, New York

Steven C. Lee, A.B., Research Assistant in Medicine, School of Medicine and Biomedical Sciences, State University of New York at Buffalo, Buffalo, New York

Mark J. Lema, M.D., Ph.D., Associate Professor and Vice Chairman for Academic Affairs, Department of Anesthesiology, School of Medicine and Biomedical Sciences, State University of New York at Buffalo; Chairman, Department of Anesthesiology and Pain Medicine, Roswell Park Cancer Institute, Buffalo, New York

Alan J. Lesse, M.D., Associate Professor, Departments of Medicine and of Pharmacology and Toxicology, State University of New York at Buffalo; Department of Veterans Affairs, Buffalo Veterans Administration Medical Center, Buffalo, New York

Lynnette K. Nieman, M.D., Senior Investigator; Clinical Director, National Institute of Child Health and Human Development, National Institutes of Health, Bethesda, Maryland

James R. Olson, Ph.D., Professor, Department of Pharmacology and Toxicology, School of Medicine and Biomedical Sciences, State University of New York at Buffalo, Buffalo, New York

Alan M. Reynard, Ph.D., Professor, Department of Pharmacology and Toxicology, School of Medicine and Biomedical Sciences, State University of New York at Buffalo, Buffalo, New York

Luther K. Robinson, Jr., M.D., Associate Professor, Department of Pediatrics, School of Medicine and Biomedical Sciences, State University of New York at Buffalo; Director, Clinical Genetics; Medical Director, Teratology Information Service, Children's Hospital of Buffalo, Buffalo, New York

Jerome A. Roth, Ph.D., Professor, Department of Pharmacology and Toxicology, School of Medicine and Biomedical Sciences, State University of New York at Buffalo, Buffalo, New York

Laurie S. Sadler, M.D., Clinical Assistant Professor, Department of Pediatrics, School of Medicine and Biomedical Sciences, State University of New York at Buffalo; Associate Director, Clinical Genetics; Clinical Director, Craniofacial Center of Western New York, Children's Hospital of Buffalo, Buffalo, New York

Robert Scheig, M.D., Professor, Department of Medicine, School of Medicine and Biomedical Sciences, State University of New York at Buffalo; Chief of Medicine, Buffalo General Hospital, Buffalo, New York

Steven M. Simasko, Ph.D., Assistant Professor, Department of Veterinary and Comparative Anatomy, Pharmacology, and Physiology, College of Veterinary Medicine, Washington State University, Pullman, Washington

F. Estelle R. Simons, M.D., F.R.C.P.C., Professor and Deputy Chairman, Department of Pediatrics & Child Health, Faculty of Medicine, University of Manitoba; Head, Section of Allergy & Clinical Immunology, Health Sciences Centre, Winnipeg, Manitoba, Canada

Keith J. Simons, B.Sc.(Pharm), M.Sc., Ph.D., Professor, Faculty of Pharmacy, University of Manitoba, Winnipeg, Manitoba, Canada

Cedric M. Smith, M.D., Professor, Department of Pharmacology and Toxicology, School of Medicine and Biomedical Sciences, State University of New York at Buffalo, Buffalo, New York

Stephen W. Spaulding, M.D., C.M., Professor, Department of Medicine, School of Medicine and Biomedical Sciences, State University of New York at Buffalo; Associate Chief of Staff for Research, Buffalo Veterans Administration Medical Center, Buffalo, New York

David A. Stempel, M.D., Clinical Associate Professor, Department of Pediatrics, University of Washington, Attending Physician, Virginia Mason Hospital, Children's Hospital and Medical Center, Seattle, Washington

Ronald S. Swerdloff, M.D., Professor of Medicine, University of California at Los Angeles, School of Medicine, Los Angeles; Chief, Division of Endocrinology, Harbor – University of California at Los Angeles Medical Center, Torrance, California

Kathleen M. Tornatore, Pharm.D., B.S.Pharm., Assistant Professor, Department of Pharmacy Practice, School of Pharmacy, State University of New York at Buffalo, Buffalo, New York

David J. Triggle, B.Sc., Ph.D., Dean, School of Pharmacy, State University of New York at Buffalo, Buffalo, New York

Elizabeth A. Vande Waa, Ph.D., Instructor; Clinical Assistant Professor, University of South Alabama, Mobile, Alabama

Ravi Vemulapalli, M.D., Department of Medicine, Division of Gastroenterology, School of Medicine and Biomedical Sciences, State University of New York at Buffalo, Buffalo, New York

Christina Wang, M.D., Professor, Department of Medicine, University of California at Los Angeles, School of Medicine, Los Angeles; Director, Clinical Study Center, Harbor – University of California at Los Angeles Medical Center, Torrance, California

Alan Winkelstein, M.D., Professor, Department of Medicine, University of Pittsburgh School of Medicine; Medical Director and Vice President, Central Blood Bank, Pittsburgh, Pennsylvania

Jerrold C. Winter, Ph.D., Professor, Department of Pharmacology and Toxicology, School of Medicine and Biomedical Sciences, State University of New York at Buffalo, Buffalo, New York

CONTENTS

PART I

GENERAL PRINCIPLES

Introduction to Pharmacology: Receptors; Dose-Effect Relationships, Interactions, and Therapeutic Index; Drug Absorption, Distribution, and Termination of Action

1

Jerrold C. Winter

RECEPTORS

Introduction

Pharmacology Defined

Pharmacology is concerned with all facets of the interaction of chemicals with biological systems. When such interactions are applied to the cure or amelioration of disease, the chemicals are usually called *drugs*. This chapter gives a rational basis for the classification of that body of facts and details that composes medical pharmacology. This classification is accomplished by providing a basic pharmacological vocabulary and by presenting the fundamental principles that govern encounters between drugs and living tissues.

Receptor Theory

Receptor theory serves as a unifying concept for the explanation of the effects of chemicals on biological systems, whether these chemicals are of exogenous (pharmacological) or endogenous (physiological) origin. A modern statement of the receptor theorem is that of Goldstein, Aronow, and Kalman (1974): in general, a drug produces a particular effect by combining chemically with some specific molecular constituent (receptor) of the biological system upon which it acts. The function of the receptor molecule in the biological system is thereby modified to produce a measurable effect.

Binding Forces in the Drug-Receptor Complex

If drugs and receptors interact via chemical forces, then our understanding of drug-receptor interactions is limited by our knowledge of such forces. Today, we are reasonably confident that the range of known chemical bonds is adequate to allow the rationalization of all known drug-receptor interactions.

• Covalent Bonds

The sharing of valence electrons between two atoms constitutes a covalent bond. Because of their considerable bond energy, which ranges from 50–150 kcal/mol, covalent bonds are usually irreversible at body temperature in the absence of a catalyst. Examples of covalent bonds include the interaction of an alkylating agent with a cancer cell, monoaminoxidase inhibitors that act irreversibly, and certain organophosphorus insecticides that form covalent bonds with the enzyme cholinesterase. However, the formation of covalent bonds between a drug and its receptor is relatively uncommon in pharmacology.

• Noncovalent Bonds

In the absence of covalent bonds, a reversible interaction occurs between drugs and receptors. Nonetheless, the interaction must be of sufficient duration and stability to initiate the chain of events that leads to a pharmacological effect. These reversible chemical bonds are of several types, and more than one type would be expected to act at the same time. In general, the precise contribution of individual bond types is not known. However, the structural features of a drug provide insight into the nature of the bonds that it is likely to form with receptors.

• IONIC BONDS. Ions are chemical entities that carry a net negative or positive charge. A physiologically significant example is provided by acetylcholine, which permanently carries a positive charge by virtue of its belonging to the quaternary ammonium group. Any model of the interaction between acetylcholine and its receptors must include ionic bonds. The strength of such bonds has been variously estimated at between 5 and 10 kcal/mol—highly significant in initiating biological effects but readily reversible at body temperature. Ionic bonds are coulombic in nature; thus, their force diminishes with the square of the distance between interacting groups. Although some drugs are, like acetylcholine, permanently charged, many more are weak acids and bases that are ionized to varying degrees at the pH levels that are found in biological fluids (see Ionization of Drugs, page 14).

• HYDROGEN BONDS. A number of relatively weak interactions between drugs and receptors are caused by nonuniformities in electron distribution within molecules. The best known of these is the hydrogen bond. First described in detail by Linus Pauling, hydrogen bonds arise between hydrogen atoms that are covalently linked to highly electronegative atoms, such as oxygen, nitrogen, and fluorine. For example, in the water molecule, a shift of electrons away from hydrogen and toward oxygen yields a polar molecule; we can imagine the oxygen atom as having a fractional negative charge that is balanced by the relative positive nature of the hydrogen atoms. In the presence of other water molecules, interactions occur between these electron-rich and electron-poor areas. Hydrogen bonding accounts for the high boiling point of water relative to that of comparable molecules in which such bonds cannot form. Their energy is about 2 - 5 kcal/mol.

In addition to hydrogen bonds, *other coulombic forces of attraction* arise between any molecules that are not fully symmetrical in their distribution of electrons. Thus, complementary areas of electron excess and deficiency attract one another in what are called dipole-dipole interactions. The energy of these interactions is comparable to that of hydrogen bonds.

• **VAN DER WAALS BONDS.** Van der Waals bonds are caused by the mutual interaction of the electrons and nuclei of adjacent molecules. The strength of the attraction is critically dependent upon the distance between the molecules. The maximal force occurs when the molecules are separated by their so-called *van der Waals radii.* If they come closer, strong repulsive forces occur between the electron shells. As the molecules separate beyond the van der Waals radii, the force diminishes as the seventh power of the distance. Van der Waals bonds are relatively weak and contribute about 0.5 kcal/mol. Groups such as benzene rings, with their homogeneous distributions of electron density, are likely contributors to van der Waals interactions.

• **THE HYDROPHOBIC EFFECT.** The formation of hydrogen bonds between water molecules confers sufficient stability that liquid water can be regarded as highly structured. When any solute is dissolved in water, that structure is disturbed. If nonpolar groups are added to water, they will arrange themselves to minimize disturbance of the hydrogen-bonded water structure. Thus, in an aqueous medium, the hydrophobic groups of receptors and drugs may be forced into close contact. The increased stability provided by the most appropriate arrangement of nonpolar groups in aqueous media gives rise to a weak noncovalent bond, the hydrophobic bond. In the polar world of hydrogen-bonded water, nonpolar groups are more likely to be found together than apart.

Stereocomplementarity

Although a single covalent bond is adequate to maintain contact between drugs and receptors, the low energy conferred by noncovalent bonds requires that larger numbers of bonds be formed. The fact that the force of coulombic interactions diminishes as the square of the distance between interacting groups suggests that interacting groups must have structures that permit close approximation of their surfaces. Even more dramatic is the decrease of van der Waals forces as the seventh power of the distance. These factors lead directly to a consideration of the three-dimensional structure of drugs and receptors.

In its common tetravalent state, carbon forms four sp-hybridized bonds with adjacent atoms. The carbon atom can be imagined to be at the center of a tetrahedron with the four bonds directed toward the corners. An interchange of any two groups yields a second structure, nonsuperimposable with the first; such isomers are referred to as *enantiomorphs.*

• The Lock and Key Analogy

The German chemist and enzymologist Emil Fischer (1894) applied Pasteur's concept to the subject of enzyme-substrate interactions. He compared the action of two different enzymes, emulsin from bitter almonds and maltase from yeast, on enantiomeric methylglucosides. He found that emulsin hydrolyzed the one form but not the other, whereas maltase had an opposite action. In 1894, Fischer wrote the following:

> *[the enzymes'] specific effect on the glucosides might thus be explained by assuming that the intimate contact between the molecules necessary for the release of the chemical reaction is possible only with similar geometrical configurations. To use a picture, I would say that the enzyme and the substrate must fit together like lock and key. . . .*

Fischer's lock and key analogy has had great influence upon the course of modern pharmacology.

• Structure-Activity Relationships

Imagine that you have been presented with a lock and an elaborately notched and grooved key and asked to determine the features essential to opening the lock. If you were to proceed to cut a set of keys that incorporates every feature of the original key in isolation and in every possible combination with each of the other features, and to test each key in the lock, you would soon know which features were essential and which were not. Within limits, much the same approach can be taken with drugs.

Morphine provides an interesting example of what may be learned from studies of structure-activity relationships. The pharmacological properties of opium, of which morphine is a major active principle, have been known for several thousand years.

The structure of morphine is shown here. Immediate questions are whether simpler forms might be more or less efficacious, might be agonists or antagonists, might be more or less toxic, and so on. In fact, thousands of morphine congeners have been examined for their pain-relieving properties, and it has been found that drugs such as meperidine and methadone are efficacious for this purpose. Such findings suggest that the essential features for analgesic activity are an electron-rich area (the benzene ring) joined by a three-carbon bridge to a tertiary amino group.

• The Stereoselectivity of Receptors

By identifying the structural and geometric features of a molecule that produce a specific pharmacological effect, we may not only get a new drug but also learn much about the structure of the receptor upon which it acts. For example, humans have physiological receptors that, when occupied by various chemicals, lead to the sensation of sweetness. Saccharin is an intensely sweet substance that a simple molecular modification renders tasteless. Examination of the structures of saccharin and *N*-methylsaccharin suggests complementary structural features in the "sweetness" receptor.

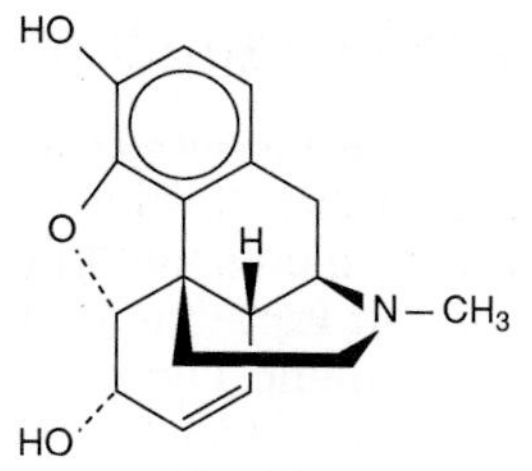

Morphine

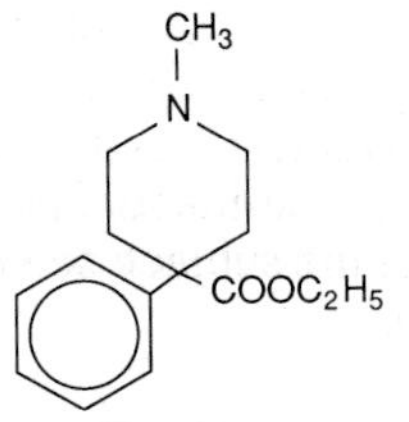

Meperidine

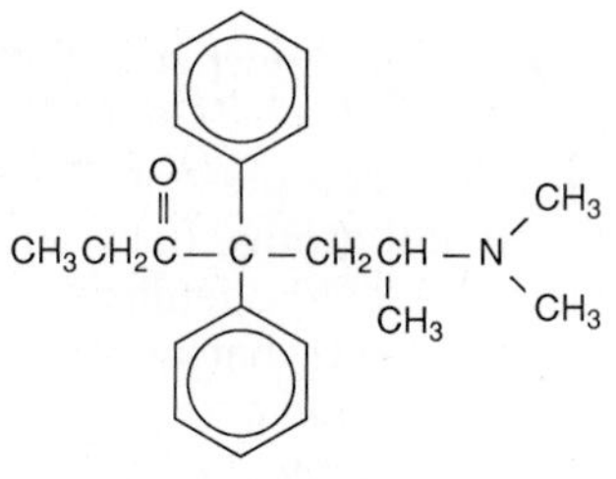

Methadone

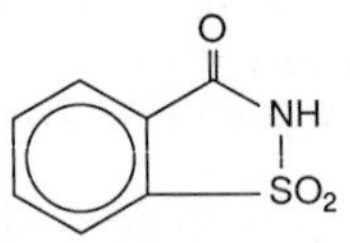

Saccharin

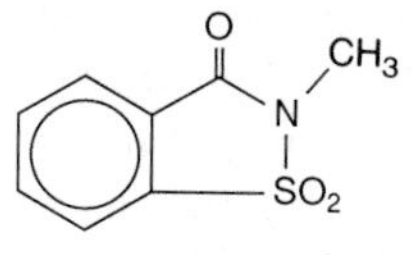

N-methylsaccharin

• Chirality

Many drugs contain an asymmetrical carbon atom, and if there is any validity to our lock and key analogy, at least some optical isomers should interact quite differently with receptors. Indeed, this is certainly the case with the optical isomers levorphanol and dextrorphan; the former is comparable to morphine in its properties, whereas the latter is inactive as an analgesic. (In modern terminology, a center of asymmetry is sometimes called a *chiral center* or *center of chirality* from the Greek *kheir* [hand].)

• Racemic Mixtures as Therapeutic Agents

Despite obvious examples of stereospecificity in drug action, therapeutic agents often are available only as the racemate, an optically inactive equimolar mixture of optical isomers. Although racemic mixtures are commonly regarded as single drugs, this is not true. The two components may have similar or quite different receptor specificities; they may interact or they may exert quite independent pharmacological effects. It has been recognized that the use of racemates hopelessly confounds pharmacokinetic investigations.

Pharmacologic Effects not Mediated by Specific Receptors

Although the majority of the pharmacological effects considered in this book are best accounted for in terms of an interaction between a drug and a macromolecular receptor, there are exceptions. For example, some diuretics work by changes that they effect in osmolality rather than by interaction with a specific receptor. They are filtered in the kidney but are not reabsorbed, which leads to a decrease in back-diffusion of water and a resultant diuresis. Drugs such as ammonium chloride and sodium bicarbonate may be used to alter the pH level of bodily fluids. In toxicology, chelating agents are used to bind toxic heavy metal ions. In cancer chemotherapy, a group of so-called unnatural analogs substitutes for biologically essential chemicals, with resulting cell death. Although we do not understand the way in which drugs such as general anesthetics work, some believe that they have a nonspecific effect on lipid membranes. In none of these instances can we properly speak of a macromolecular receptor. Exceptions such as these do not detract from the utility of the receptor concept, but each is noted in subsequent chapters.

DOSE-EFFECT RELATIONSHIPS, INTERACTIONS, AND THERAPEUTIC INDEX

Introduction

The receptor concept proposed by Ehrlich and by Langley in the early 1900s had little immediate impact upon pharmacology. Textbooks at that time were little more than compilations of verbal descriptions of the effects of drugs. A quantitative and analytical base was needed. In the years following World War I, Alfred Joseph Clark provided that base. Clark (1937) assumed that the interaction between drug and receptor was analogous to the adsorption of gases by a metal surface, *ie, a reversible reaction governed by the law of mass action.*

Beginning with the assumption that drugs and receptors interact in a reversible chemical reaction governed by the law of mass action, the nature of the relationship between the dose of a drug and its effects can be predicted. Prediction and reality are often quite similar: when pharmacological effect is plotted versus the logarithm of the dose, a sigmoid curve results. Such dose-effect curves provide the basis for the terms "affinity" and "intrinsic activity" (i.a.) in isolated systems and for the terms "potency" and "efficacy" in patients.

Drug-Receptor Interactions and the Law of Mass Action

The interaction between drugs and receptors can be represented by the following equation:

$$[R] + [X] \quad [RX]$$

where [R] is the concentration of free receptors, [X] is the concentration of drug in the vicinity of the receptors, and [RX] is the concentration of the drug-receptor complex. The law of mass action states that the velocity of a chemical reaction is proportional to the active masses of the reacting substances. Thus, the dissociation constant, K_X, of the drug-receptor complex is given by the following equation:

$$K_X = [R]\,[X]/[RX] \qquad (1)$$

If we now assume that we can account for all the receptors as being either free or bound, then the concentration of free receptors, [R], is equal to the total concentration of receptors, [RT], minus that fraction occupied by drug, [RX], or

$$[R] = [RT] - [RX]$$

Substituting into equation 1, we obtain

$$K_X = ([RT] - [RX])\,[X]/[RX],$$

$$K_X[RX] = [RT]\,[X] - [RX]\,[X],$$

$$[RX]\,(K_X + [X]) = [RT]\,[X], \text{ and}$$

$$[RX]/[RT] = [X]/(K_X + [X]) \qquad (2)$$

Thus, the fraction of all receptors that is combined with drug is a function of the concentration of drug in the vicinity of the receptor and of the dissociation constant of the drug-receptor complex.

The Occupancy Assumption

Equation 2 assumes practical importance if we make what is generally called the *occupancy assumption* regarding the interaction of drugs with receptors. Specifically, we assume that (1) the magnitude of the pharmacological effect, E, is directly proportional to [RX], the concentration of the drug-receptor complex, and (2) the maximal pharmacological effect, E_{max}, occurs when all receptors are occupied by drug. Equation 2 may now be rewritten as follows:

$$E/E_{max} = [X]/(K_X + [X]) \qquad (3)$$

Although Clark himself expressed reservations about the validity of the occupancy assumption, equation 3 has been found over the years to be in accordance with a remarkable variety of pharmacological observations.

Graphical Representation

In pharmacology it is conventional to plot E or E/E_{max} versus dose expressed on a log scale. Figure 1-1 shows the effects of acetylcholine as determined by Clark in the 1920s. With such data it is possible to estimate K_X directly. Thus, when

$$E/E_{max} = \tfrac{1}{2} = [X]/(K_X + [X]),$$

$$K_X = [X]$$

It must be kept in mind that this estimate of K_X is valid only to the extent that our assumptions regarding the interaction between drugs and receptors are valid. Later, we consider a few of the modifications of Clark's theory that have been necessitated by pharmacological fact. For more advanced treatments of the subject, see Black and Leff (1983) and Kenakin (1993).

Drug-Receptor Versus Enzyme-Substrate Interactions

Recalling that Fischer's lock and key analogy (1894) was based upon enzyme-substrate interactions, it should not surprise us that there are many analogies between enzyme-substrate and drug-receptor interactions. However, in biochemistry it is conventional to rearrange equation 3.

$$E/E_{max} = [X]/(K_x + [X])$$

$$E = [X]E_{max}/(K_X + [X])$$

$$1/E = (K_X + [X])/[X]E_{max}$$

$$1/E = (K_X/E_{max})\,(1/[X]) + 1/E_{max} \qquad (4)$$

As seen in Figure 1-2, the so-called *double-reciprocal* or *Lineweaver-Burke plot* yields a straight line with slope = K_X/E_{max} and intercept = $1/E_{max}$.

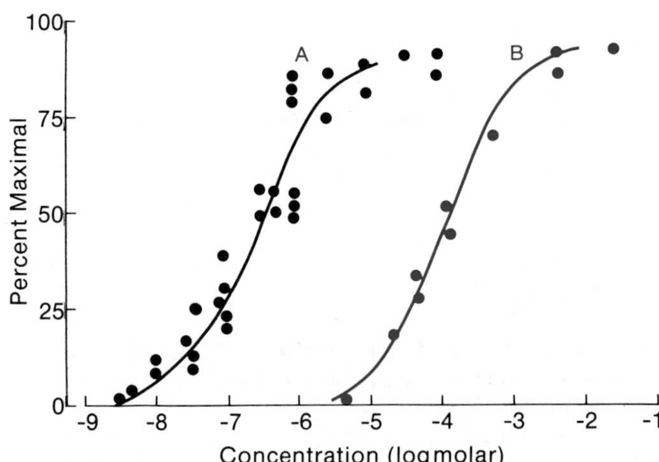

FIGURE 1-1. Dose-response relationships for acetylcholine. (*A*) Inhibition of isometric response of frog ventricle. (*B*) Contraction of frog rectus abdominis. Abscissa: log molar concentration. Ordinate: percent of maximal response. (Redrawn from Clark AJ: General Pharmacology. Vol 4 of Handbuch der experimentation Pharmakologie, 66. Berlin: Springer-Verlag, 1937.)

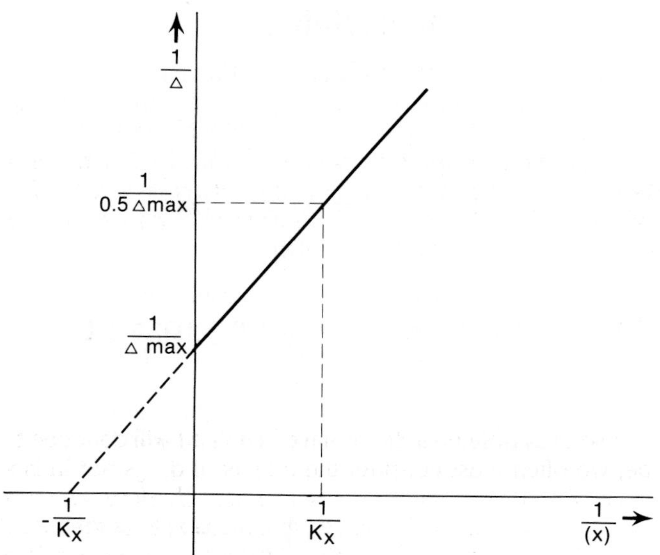

FIGURE 1-2. The double-reciprocal or Lineweaver-Burke plot.

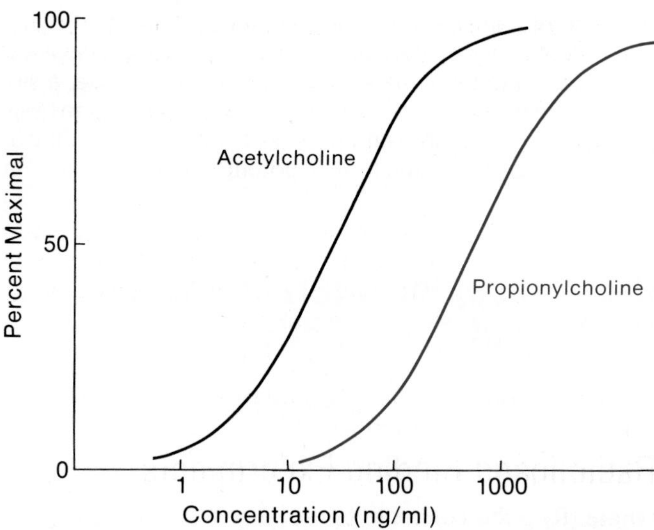

FIGURE 1-3. Dose-response relationships for acetylcholine and propionylcholine in causing contraction of isolated guinea pig ileum. Abscissa: drug concentration expressed on a log scale. Ordinate: percent of maximal response. (Redrawn from Burgen AS, Mitchell JF [eds]: Gaddum's Pharmacology. 6th ed, 3. New York: Oxford University Press, 1968, by permission of the Oxford University Press.)

The Dose-Effect Relationship in Isolated Systems

Much of what is presumed to be known about drug-receptor interactions has been derived from experiments using "isolated systems." For example, a classic experiment involves removing a piece of smooth muscle from the ileum of a guinea pig, suspending the tissue in a bathing solution, and observing contractions or relaxations of the muscle in response to drugs added to the bath. In an isolated system we assume that a direct relationship exists between the calculated drug concentrations in the bath and the concentration to which the relevant receptors are exposed.

Affinity

Figure 1-3 shows the contractile effects of acetylcholine and propionylcholine on a piece of guinea pig ileum. Two features of the figure are obvious: both drugs produce the same maximal effect, but a higher concentration of propionylcholine is required for any given degree of contraction. According to the occupancy assumption, fewer receptors are occupied by propionylcholine than by acetylcholine when the two drugs are present in equal concentrations. In this situation, we say that acetylcholine has a higher affinity for the receptor than does propionylcholine. Affinity is a measure of the probability that a drug molecule will interact with its receptor to form the drug-receptor complex. Affinity is inversely proportional to K_X, the dissociation constant of the drug-receptor complex.

Intrinsic Activity

If mere occupancy of a receptor were sufficient to produce a pharmacological effect, then all drugs acting upon a common receptor would produce the same maximal effect. The data in Figure 1-4 indicate that this is not always the case. A group of drugs acting upon a common receptor produces clearly different maximal effects. To explain observations such as this, the Dutch pharmacologist E. J. Ariens proposed that a drug must not only have affinity for a receptor but must also possess a second property that he called *intrinsic activity*.

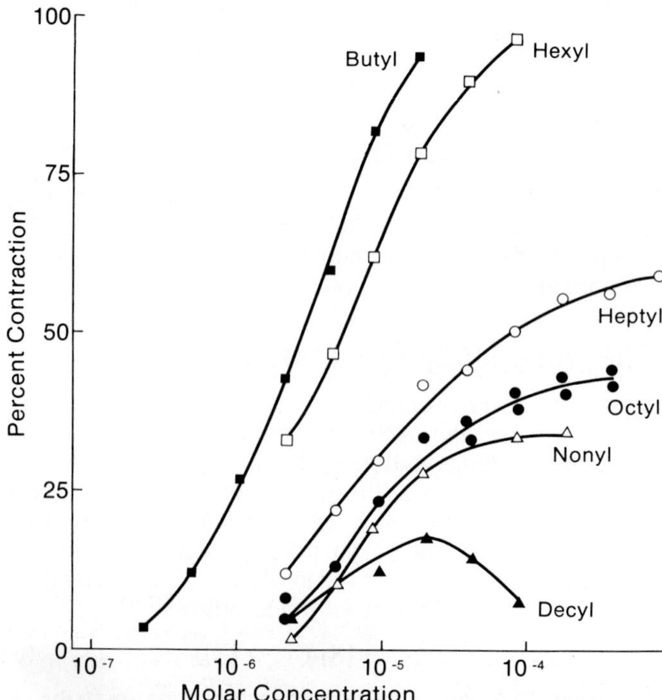

FIGURE 1-4. Dose-response relationships for a homologous series of compounds presumed to act upon a common receptor. Abscissa: percent of maximal response. Ordinate: molar concentration plotted on a log scale. (Redrawn from Stephenson RP: A modification of receptor theory. Br J Pharmacol 11:379-393, 1956.)

Intrinsic activity is a measure of the biological effectiveness of a drug-receptor complex. It is a proportionality constant, here termed k_{ia}, that relates the quantity of complex formed to the magnitude of the pharmacological effect produced. Thus, E is proportional to [RX] or

$$E = k_{ia}[RX]$$

For example, if we imagine two drugs, one with an intrinsic activity of 1 [a **full agonist**] and the other with an intrinsic activity of 0.5 [a **partial agonist**], the pharmacological effects we can expect from the two drugs are given by

$$E_A = 1[RX] \text{ and}$$

$$E_B = 0.5[RX]$$

Radioligand Binding Experiments

Our knowledge of drug-receptor interactions has been aided enormously by the development of techniques to label specific receptors with radioactive substances. The binding agent, a ligand, may be a naturally occurring substance, *eg*, norepinephrine, or any of a variety of drugs that have had a radioactive atom incorporated into their structures; tritium is the most commonly used radioisotope. The receptors to be labeled are contained in tissue or cell preparations.

In a manner analogous to the preceding discussion of drug-receptor interactions, we may represent a reversible ligand-receptor interaction as

$$[L] + [R] \rightleftharpoons [LR]$$

where [L] is the concentration of free ligand, [R] is the concentration of free receptors, and [LR] is the concentration of the ligand-receptor complex. At equilibrium, the dissociation binding constant $[K_D]$ of the ligand-receptor complex is given by the following equation:

$$K_D = [L][R]/[LR] \quad (5)$$

Because the number of receptors in any tissue or cell preparation is finite, we expect the ligand-receptor interaction to be saturable. Thus, the total number of receptors of a specific type $[R_T]$ is equal to the sum of the free and bound receptors, *ie*,

$$[LR] + [R] = [R_T]$$

$$[R] = [R_T] - [LR]$$

Substitution for [R] in equation 5 yields the following:

$$K_D = [L]([R_T] - [LR])/[LR]$$

$$K_D[LR] = [L][R_T] - [L][LR])$$

$$[LR](K_D + [L]) = [L][R_T]$$

$$[LR] = [L][R_T]/(K_D + [L])$$

If it is now assumed that the maximum number of binding sites, B_{max}, corresponds to R_T, and if we now designate [LR], the concentration of bound ligand, as B and designate [L], the concentration of free ligand, as F, we obtain

$$B = B_{max}F/(F + K_D)$$

$$BF + BK_D = B_{max}F$$

$$B + B/F(K_D) = B_{max}$$

$$B/F(K_D) = B_{max} - B$$

$$B/F = (B_{max} - B)/K_D$$

$$B/F = (-1/K_D)B + B_{max}/K_D \quad (6)$$

Equation 6 is the Scatchard equation, which provides a convenient graphical transformation of binding data. The plot of B/F versus B yields a straight line whose slope is $-1/K_D$ and whose x-intercept is B_{max}.

The Dose-Effect Relationship in Intact Organisms

As useful as isolated systems have been and will continue to be, we often must consider the effects of drugs not in isolated bits of tissue but in the whole animal. Here we must deal with the effects of drugs in what we refer to as the *intact organism* or, when the intact organism in question is a human being, the *patient*. In this situation, no direct relationship can be assumed to exist between drug dose and concentration of drug at receptors.

Potency

Figure 1-5 depicts the dose-effect relationship in human subjects for two opioid analgesics, morphine and dihydrocodeine. They have comparable maximal effects in providing pain relief, but their dose-response curves are at different points on the dose axis. We say that the drugs differ in potency; the lower the dose required to produce a given degree of analgesia, the higher the potency of the drug. Thus, morphine is more potent than dihydrocodeine.

Dose-effect curves for drugs of differing potencies in intact organisms can be deceptively similar to those for drugs of differing affinities in isolated systems. However, there are a number of reasons why we should expect no constant relationship between a drug's affinity for an isolated receptor and its potency in a patient. Most of these

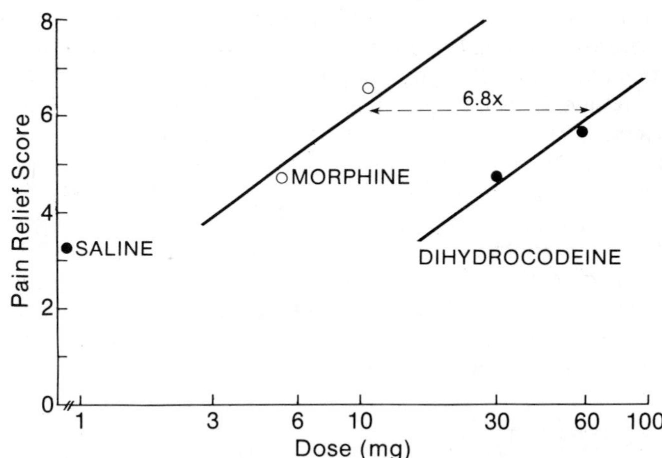

FIGURE 1-5. Dose-response relationships for morphine and dihydrocodeine in relieving pain in human subjects. Abscissa: dose plotted on a log scale. Ordinate: pain relief expressed in arbitrary units. (Redrawn from Goldstein A, Aronow L, Kalman SM: Principles of Drug Action: The Basis of Pharmacology, 2nd ed, 388. New York: John Wiley & Sons, copyright © 1974, John Wiley & Sons.)

have to do with the absorption, distribution, metabolism, and excretion of drugs. For example, a drug that is poorly absorbed following oral administration is far less potent than one that is readily absorbed, even if the two drugs have equal affinities for a common receptor.

It is conventional to express potency in producing a given therapeutic effect in terms of milligrams of drug per kilogram of body weight (mg/kg) or milligrams per patient to produce that effect. For example, only micrograms per kilogram of a "high-potency" antipsychotic drug may be effective, whereas hundreds of milligrams of a "low-potency" drug are needed for the same effect.

Efficacy

The ability of a drug to produce a desired therapeutic effect is called *efficacy*. The two drugs shown in Figure 1–5 are approximately equally efficacious; despite their obvious differences in potency, both produce the same maximal therapeutic effect. In Figure 1–6, two analgesic drugs, oxycodone and nefopam, that differ in their efficacies are shown. The property of efficacy has legal as well as therapeutic importance. The 1962 Kefauver-Harris amendments to the Federal Food, Drug, and Cosmetics Act require *proof of efficacy* of a drug before it can be marketed. Before that time only *evidence of safety* was needed.

Potency Versus Efficacy

Consistent usage of the terms "potency" and "efficacy" as they are defined in this chapter is recommended. However, confusion may arise when either the speaker or listener attaches to potency the common English definition of potent as "the capability of causing strong physiological or chemical effects, as medicines or alcoholic beverages." Occasionally, the intent of the misuse of these terms is to deceive, *eg*, a salesperson may impute greater efficacy to a drug that is merely more potent. More often the misuse of the terms is caused by simple ignorance. For example, heroin is approximately three times as potent as morphine. This has at various times been misinterpreted to the general public as meaning that heroin is three times as effective as morphine in the relief of pain and that pain-sufferers are being denied a dramatically more effective analgesic because of the unapproved status of heroin in the United States. In fact, heroin and morphine are of approximately equal efficacy.

Few drugs are of such low potency that the sheer physical bulk of the administered drug presents a problem. Thus, potency *per se* is rarely of clinical significance.

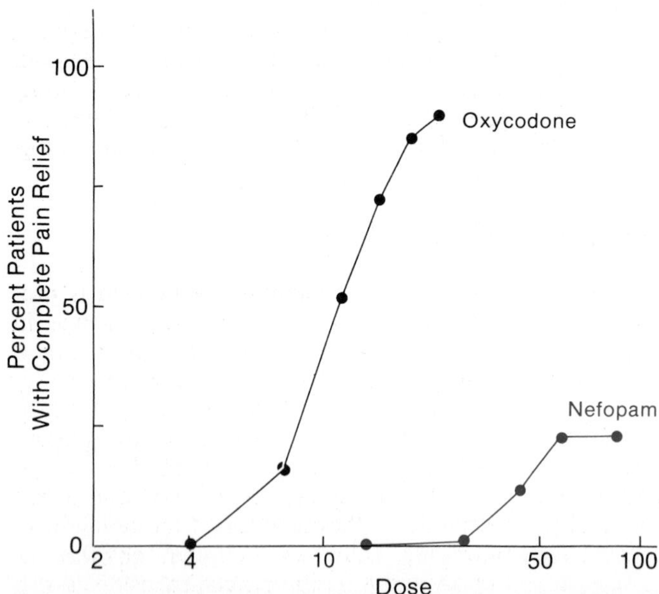

FIGURE 1–6. Dose-response relationships for oxycodone and another analgesic (nefopam) in relieving pain in human subjects. Abscissa: dose plotted on a log scale. Ordinate: percent of patients responding with complete relief of pain. (Redrawn from Tigerstedt I, Tammisto T, Leander P: Comparison of the analgesic dose-effect relationships of nefopam and oxycodone in postoperative pain. Acta Anaesthesiol Scand 23:555–560, 1979.)

Drug Interactions: Summation, Potentiation, and Antagonism

Pharmacology was defined earlier in this chapter as dealing with the interactions of chemicals with biological systems. However, concomitant with actions on biological systems, two drugs may interact with each other. "Drug interaction" is the term applied to this phenomenon. Although the possible mechanisms by which drug interactions may arise are quite varied, the consequences of such interactions are rather simply categorized. Two drugs may interact in a variety of ways to produce a change in the effects of one or the other or both. When the effects are additive or supra-additive, the terms "summation" and "potentiation" are used. The phenomenon in which the effects of two drugs are less than predicted from their effects individually is called *antagonism*. The previously introduced concepts of affinity and intrinsic activity, together with a consideration of possible bonds formed between drugs and receptors, provide a rational basis for the several types of antagonism that have been observed.

Summation or Additivity

When the effects of two drugs given at the same time are exactly as would have been predicted from the sum of their effects when given alone, we speak of *summation* or, alternatively, *additivity*. In effect, summation occurs only when drugs do not interact. Although summation is conceptually simple, this phenomenon is less common than one might expect, and it should never be assumed to occur.

Potentiation

The observation that the effects of two drugs are greater than would have been predicted from their effects in isolation is called *potentiation* or, alternatively, *synergism*. A classic example of potentiation is provided by the sympathomimetic effects of tyramine in the presence of a monoamine oxidase (MAO) inhibitor. Tyramine acts on presynaptic storage sites to release norepinephrine, which then causes an increase in blood pressure. Because MAO is a major regulator of the presynaptic stores, inhibition of the enzyme causes more norepinephrine to be available for release by tyramine. In addition, there is evidence that MAO inhibitors decrease the metabolic inactivation of tyramine. Thus, patients treated with an MAO inhibitor for depression must be warned not to eat foods that are high in tyramine (*eg*, aged cheese).

Antagonism

The phenomenon in which the effects of two drugs are less than predicted from their effects when given alone is called *antagonism*. The term "pharmacological antagonism" usually refers to diminution of a drug's effects at a common receptor site. Clearly, the effects of a drug may be diminished in a number of other ways. In principle, any antidote may be regarded as an antagonist. Examples include diminution of absorption of a toxin by its adsorption on activated charcoal and the inactivation of heavy metals by chelating agents. In addition, a drug that produces a pharmacologically opposite effect but at a different site may be regarded as an antagonist. For example, norepinephrine and acetylcholine are mutually antagonistic in terms of heart rate by effects at pharmacologically distinct sites in the sinoatrial node. Similarly, histamine and norepinephrine produce opposite effects on blood pressure through their effects on independent adrenergic and histaminergic receptors on smooth muscle of blood vessels. The phenomenon in which two drugs are antagonistic because of opposing effects arising at distinct sites is sometimes called *physiological antagonism*.

Although both physiological antagonism and the use of agents such as activated charcoal are of clinical significance, they are not representative of true pharmacological antagonism. This term is reserved for the phenomenon in which two drugs interact either directly or indirectly with a common receptor to produce a diminished total effect. The concepts of affinity and intrinsic activity allow us to rationalize such interactions.

An *agonist* is a drug that has affinity for a receptor and intrinsic activity at that receptor. In contrast, an *antagonist* is a drug that has affinity for the receptor but is devoid of intrinsic activity; formation of the antagonist-receptor complex does not directly produce a pharmacological response. Several types of antagonist-receptor interaction are known and provide the basis for subtypes of *pharmacological antagonism*.

Types of Pharmacological Antagonism

Surmountable Antagonism

The interaction of closely related analogs provides an illustration of surmountable antagonism (Fig. 1 – 7). The agonist succinylcholine has both an affinity for the receptor and intrinsic activity at the receptor, as evidenced by the dose-related contraction of frog muscle that it produces. In the presence of a specific antagonist the agonist is still able to cause contraction, but a higher concentration of the agonist is required for any given degree of contraction. We may assume that the antagonist functions by virtue of its affinity for the acetylcholine receptor together with its lack of intrinsic activity at that receptor. Furthermore, we may assume that the relationship of agonist and antagonist at the receptor is strictly competitive; at any instant the proportion of receptors occupied by the agonist and by the antagonist is a function of the concentrations of each of the two agents in the vicinity of the receptor. Hence, the effects of the antagonist may be reversed simply by increasing the concentration of agonist to a sufficient degree.

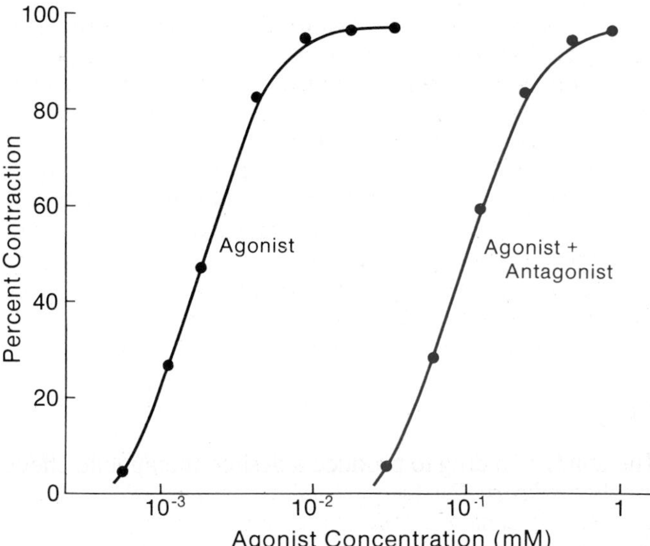

FIGURE 1 – 7. Surmountable antagonism. The dose-response relationship for succinylcholine alone and in the presence of its ethyl analog. Abscissa: molar concentration expressed on a log scale. Ordinate: percent of maximal contraction of frog rectus abdominis. (Data from Ariens EJ, Simonis AM, Van Rossum JM: *In* Ariens EJ [ed]: Molecular Pharmacology: The Mode of Action of Biologically Active Compounds. Vol 1, 151. New York: Academic Press, 1964.)

The terms "reversible antagonism" and "competitive antagonism" are sometimes regarded as being synonymous with surmountable antagonism. However, because "reversible" and "competitive" have had associated with them a variety of mechanistic implications, the purely phenomenological term "surmountable" is preferred.

Insurmountable Antagonism

A classic example of insurmountable antagonism is provided by the interaction of epinephrine and dibenamine. In Figure 1 – 8 it is seen that epinephrine causes contraction of an isolated strip of cat spleen. However, in the presence of *N*-(2-chloroethyl)dibenzylamine hydrochloride (DIBENAMINE HYDROCHLORIDE), the maximal possible degree of contraction is reduced. This type of interaction may be rationalized on the basis of the occupancy assumption and of the irreversible inactivation of the receptor by the antagonist. Thus, if *N*-(2-chloroethyl)dibenzylamine hydrochloride interacts with the epinephrine receptor in such a fashion that it is removed from the pool of receptors available to epinephrine, the occupancy assumption predicts that the maximal effect will be reduced.

The terms "irreversible antagonism" and "noncompetitive antagonism" are sometimes regarded as being synony-

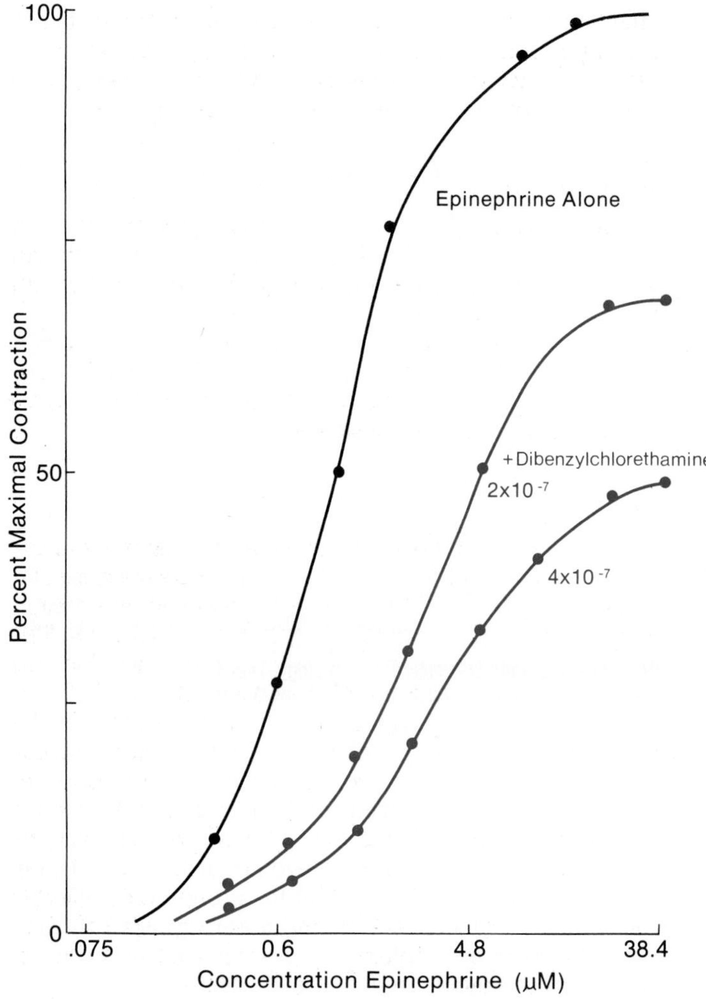

FIGURE 1-8. Insurmountable antagonism. The dose-response relationship for epinephrine alone and in the presence of DIBENAMINE. Abscissa: concentration plotted on a log scale. Ordinate: percent of maximal contraction of isolated cat spleen. (Redrawn from Bickerton RK: The response of isolated strips of cat spleen to sympathomimetic drugs and their antagonists. J Pharmacol Exp Ther 142:99-110, 1963, © by American Society for Pharmacology and Experimental Therapeutics.)

mous with insurmountable antagonism. However, it is once again desirable to avoid unwarranted mechanistic implications. Hence, the purely phenomenological term "surmountable" is preferred.

Partial Agonists

So far we have assumed that an agonist produces the maximal possible effect, *ie*, its intrinsic activity is 1.0. On the other hand, antagonists have been assumed to produce no agonistic effects (*ie*, their intrinsic activity is 0.0). Such drugs are sometimes called *full agonists* (intrinsic activity = 1.0) and *pure antagonists* (intrinsic activity = 0.0), respectively. These qualifying terms are used because, as seen in Figure 1-4, some drugs—those with intermediate intrinsic activities between 0.0 and 1.0—produce less than full agonistic effects, hence the term "partial agonist." In addition, consideration of Figures 1-9 and 1-10 reveals that such drugs not only are partial agonists but also may sometimes serve as *partial antagonists* as well.

For simplicity's sake, the drugs shown in Figure 1-9 are assumed to bind reversibly to a common receptor. They are further assumed to have equal affinity for the receptor and intrinsic activities of 1.0 and 0.25, respectively. Thus, drug A produces 100% of the maximal response when given alone, and drug B produces 25% of the maximal response. However, when both are present at the same time in maximally effective concentrations, the modified occupancy assumption predicts that less than the maximal effect results. The

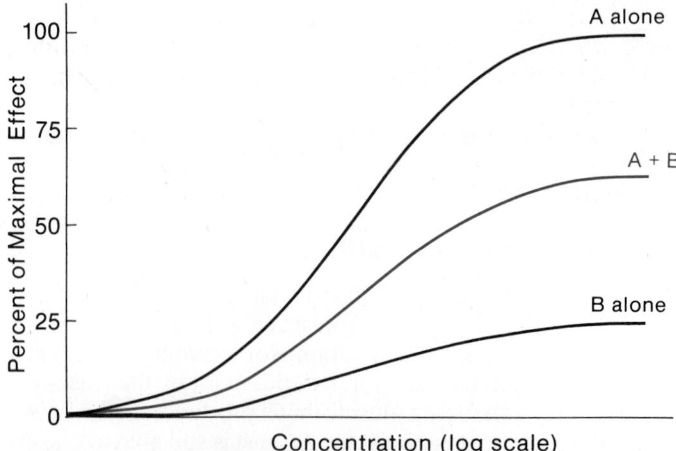

FIGURE 1-9. Hypothetical dose-response relationships for a full agonist (drug A), a mixed agonist/antagonist (drug B), and the two drugs in combination. Abscissa: concentration expressed on a log scale. Ordinate: percent of maximal effect.

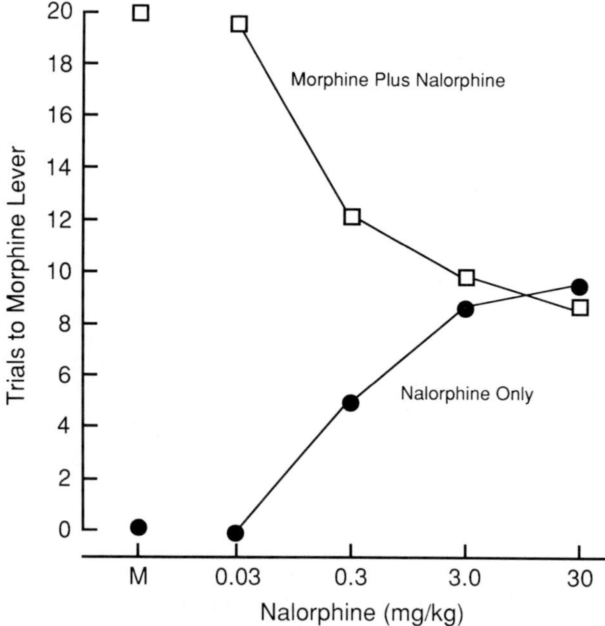

FIGURE 1-10. The effects of a partial agonist alone and in combination with a full agonist. Rats were trained to discriminate the effects of 3.0 mg of morphine from those of saline solution. *Closed circles:* nalorphine alone. *Open squares:* nalorphine in the presence of 3.0 mg of morphine. Ordinate: trials to the morphine lever as morphine-appropriate responses. Abscissa: dose of nalorphine. (Redrawn from Holtzman SG: Discriminative stimulus properties of opioid agonists and antagonists. *In* Cooper SJ [ed]: Theory in Psychopharmacology. Vol 2. London: Academic Press, 1983.)

reason is that one half of the receptors would be occupied by drug A, which yields 50% of the maximal effect, and one half of the receptors would be occupied by drug B, which contributes 12.5% of the maximal effect. The sum of the two is a 62.5% response. In this situation, drug B partially antagonizes drug A.

Figure 1-10 provides experimental evidence in support of the preceding interpretation of the action of partial agonists. The data shown were obtained in drug interaction experiments in rats trained to discriminate between saline solution and 3 mg/kg morphine. When a range of doses of nalorphine is given, partial agonist activity is evident. However, when nalorphine is administered in combination with a fully effective dose of morphine, antagonism of morphine is observed.

As is discussed in detail in Chapter 14, considerable clinical significance is attached to partial agonists of the opioid, narcotic analgesic type. When opioid-mixed agonists/antagonists and some partial agonists are administered alone, they are effective pain relievers; when given in the presence of a complete opioid agonist, however, they may result in antagonistic effects.

The Therapeutic Index

A goal of pharmacological science is to discover drugs that possess efficacy but produce no adverse effects. That goal is but rarely achieved; undesired effects occur with all drugs at some dose. The relationship between adverse and beneficial effects is expressed by the therapeutic index. The response of an individual patient to a drug is influenced not only by the essential features of the drug but also by factors peculiar to the patient, especially genetic and immunological ones.

Selectivity

A drug is often classified in terms of its most prominent effect or the first effect attributed to it. Such descriptions should not obscure the fact that every drug produces multiple effects. Selectivity refers to the degree to which a drug acts upon a given site relative to all possible sites of interaction (Albert, 1979). Thus, a drug is characterized adequately only when its full spectrum of activities — pharmacological, therapeutic, and toxic — is considered.

Therapeutic Index

A simple means to provide a quantitative assessment of the relative benefits and risks of a drug is to divide the dose that produces toxic effects by the dose that produces the desired therapeutic effect. Thus, for a drug that induces sleep in 50% of the treated population at a dose of 1.5 mg/kg and induces death at a dose of 1500 mg/kg, we get a ratio of 1500/1.5, and the drug is said to have a therapeutic index of 1000. The 50%-effective dose is often chosen for reference because this represents the most reliable portion of the dose-response curve. For the therapeutic effect, the 50%-effective dose is called the *ED50* (the median effective dose), and for the median toxic effect, the *TD50.* Thus, in our example, the therapeutic index = TD50/ED50. Where the toxic effect is lethal, the TD50 is alternatively designated the *LD50* (*eg,* the LD50 is a commonly determined measure of toxicity in experimental animals).

Multiple Therapeutic Indices

Textbooks of pharmacology can be searched in vain for a table listing the therapeutic indices for a series of drugs; such a table does not exist. The reason is simple: no drug has a single toxic effect, and many drugs have more than one therapeutic effect. Every drug, then, has not one but many possible therapeutic indices, each one of which considers a specific therapeutic effect, a specific toxic effect, and, perhaps, each of these factors in a specific patient population. For example, Figure 1-11 shows a therapeutic and a toxic effect of digitoxin. It is obvious that such data do not permit neat, single-value expressions of a therapeutic index for digitoxin. In this light we see the therapeutic index not as a single, unchanging number but as a more general expression of the relation between the good (desirable) and the bad (undesirable) effects of drugs. Other terms expressing relationships between desirable and toxic effects are the benefit/risk ratio and the margin of safety.

Heterogeneity of the Patient Population

Students are familiar with the practice of "grading on a curve"; the frequency of occurrence of specific numerical

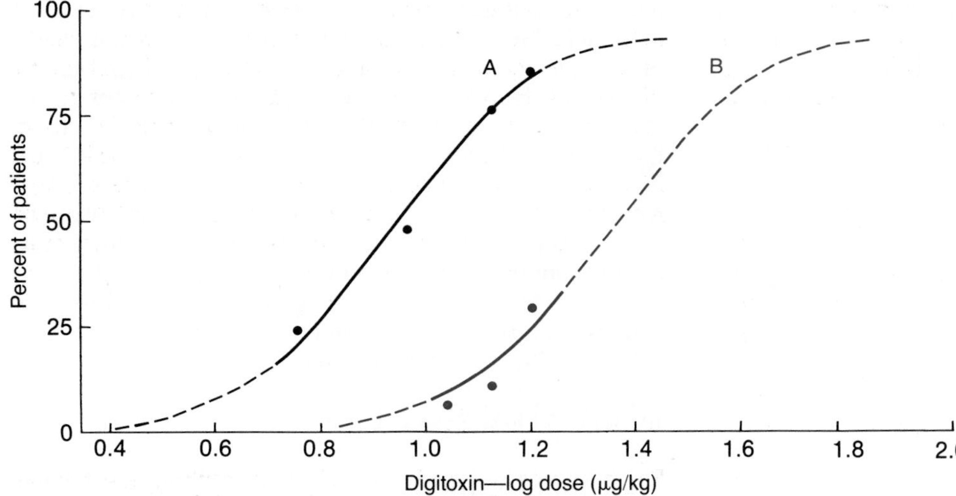

FIGURE 1–11. Therapeutic index. Dose-response relationships for a therapeutic effect (*A*) and a toxic effect of vomiting (*B*) of digitoxin in patients with auricular fibrillation. Abscissa: dose expressed on a log scale. Ordinate: percent of patients responding. (Redrawn from Marsh DF: Outline of Fundamental Pharmacology, 28, 1951. Courtesy of Charles C Thomas, Publisher, Springfield, Illinois.)

values is plotted against the range of possible values, and letter grades are assigned to various parts of the distribution. If a smooth line connecting the points is bell-shaped, the data are said to follow a *normal* or *gaussian distribution.* In nature it is often observed that a normal distribution is more closely approximated when a logarithmic rather than an arithmetic scale is employed; the data are then said to be *log-normally distributed.*

As shown in Figure 1–12, dose-response curves that have been considered so far may be regarded as cumulative frequency curves for a log-normally distributed population. The practical consequence is that the response of isolated tissues to drugs is proportional to the logarithm of drug concentration (*eg*, Fig. 1–1). Furthermore, it is often observed that the data that express the pharmacological response of subjects within a patient population are normalized when dose is expressed on a log scale (*eg*, Fig. 1–5). However, therapeutically significant exceptions are known in which sensitivity to drugs follows neither a normal nor a log-normal distribution.

Pharmacogenetics

The variation in drug sensitivity within a population is assumed to be largely genetic in origin. Often, these sources of variation are sufficiently subtle that no subpopulations can

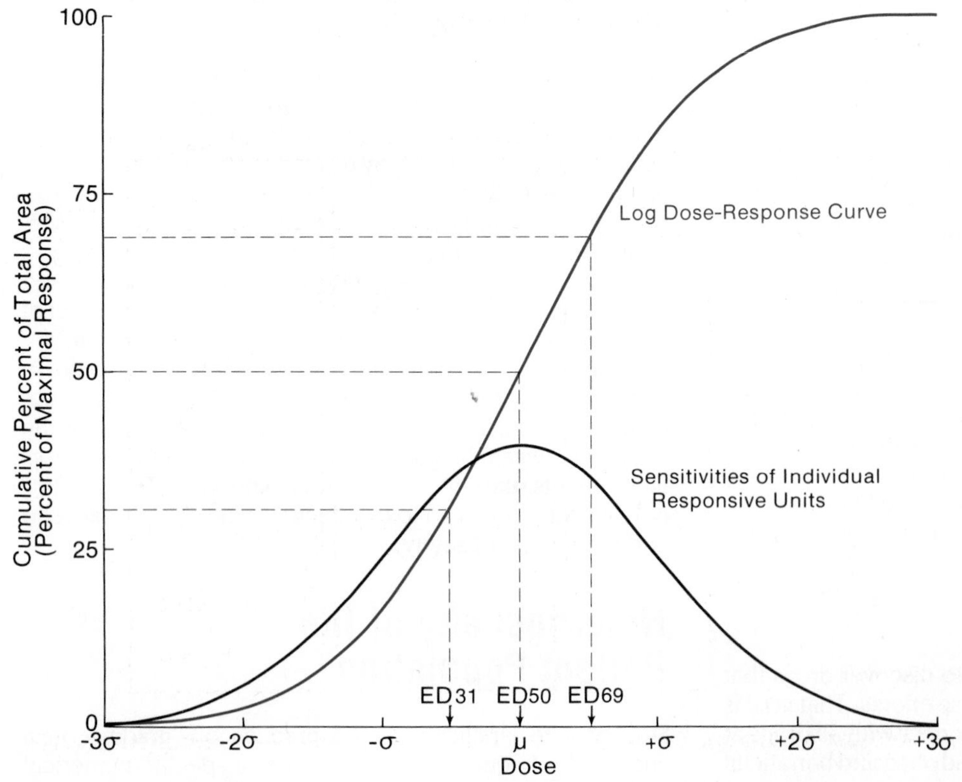

FIGURE 1–12. Log dose-response curve as a cumulative normal frequency distribution of sensitivities of the individual responsive units. (Reprinted with permission of Macmillan Publishing Company from Biostatistics by Avram Goldstein. Copyright © 1964 Avram Goldstein.)

be discerned, and the sensitivity distribution is represented adequately by a log-normal curve. Pharmacogenetics is concerned, in general, with genetic influences upon drug sensitivity and, in particular, with those instances in which distinct subpopulations can be identified.

Drug Allergy

A particularly important form of nonhomogeneous sensitivity to drug effects is mediated by the immune systems of the body. The manifestations of drug allergy range from mild skin irritation to lethal anaphylactic shock. Drug allergy is discussed in detail in Chapter 50.

DRUG ABSORPTION, DISTRIBUTION, AND TERMINATION OF ACTION

Introduction

The movement of a drug from its site of application into the blood is called *drug absorption.* In general, the process may involve diffusion or active transport, and the barriers to that movement are largely lipid in nature. For this reason, the degree of solubility of a drug in lipid is an important factor in its absorption. The lipid solubility of many drugs, so-called weak acids and bases, is influenced by the pH levels of the aqueous media that they encounter. Drug absorption also may be influenced by the way in which the drug is formulated. Thus, when it is therapeutically indicated, a low rate of release and a prolonged period of absorption may be achieved.

In some therapeutic situations, drugs are applied directly to the sites at which they are to act. For example, an antibiotic-containing ointment may be spread over a break in the skin. More often, the receptors to which drugs are directed are located at a distance from the site of application of the drug. For example, the acetylsalicylic acid contained in a swallowed aspirin tablet must somehow make its way to the brain and to the tissues of the head if a headache is to be relieved. The two general processes involved are *absorption, the movement of a drug into the blood from its site of application*, and *distribution, the movement of a drug from the blood to its site(s) of action or storage.*

Physiological Factors in Drug Absorption

For purposes of considering drug absorption, the human body may be regarded as a series of water-filled sacks made of fat, or put another way, a series of aqueous media separated by lipid barriers. Figure 1–13 provides a general scheme.

Consider again an aspirin tablet taken by mouth. The solid tablet must dissolve in the aqueous environment of the stomach and small intestine, *ie*, water solubility is required. Aspirin molecules in solution then encounter a lipid barrier to absorption, the epithelial lining of the gastrointestinal (GI) tract. Because there is no active transport system for aspirin, passage of the drug through that barrier requires lipid solubility. Having passed the epithelial barrier, drug molecules again encounter an aqueous medium, the extracellular fluid, which in turn bathes the endothelial barrier presented by the capillary wall. In fact, capillary walls in the peripheral circulation are so porous that even lipid-insoluble materials can pass through into the blood. At this point, molecules of acetylsalicylic acid have passed from the mouth to the blood; they have been absorbed.

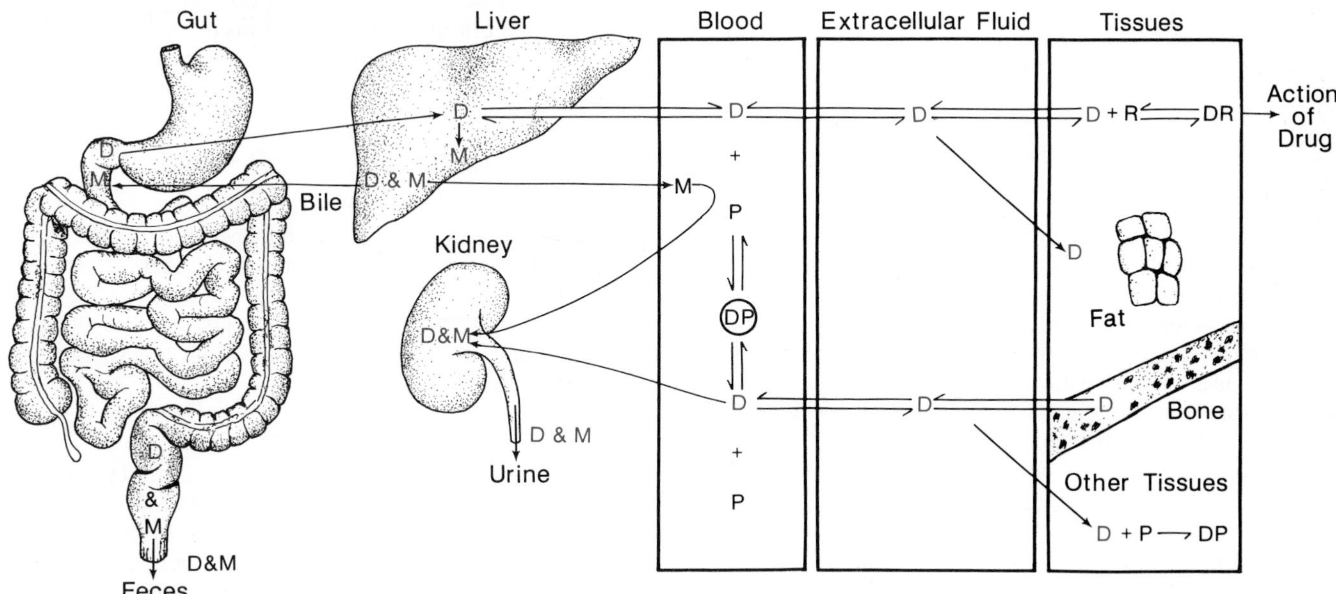

FIGURE 1–13. Schematic representation of what may happen to a drug, D, in the body. (M = metabolites; P = plasma protein; R = receptor.) (Courtesy of DS Riggs.)

Physicochemical Factors in Drug Absorption

The influence of physicochemical factors on drug absorption depends to a significant degree upon the site to which the drug is applied. For drugs that must cross the skin or the epithelial lining of the GI tract, lipid solubility is of great importance. For drugs placed in the vicinity of the peripheral capillary beds of muscles or other tissues, lipid solubility is of minor importance; even the majority of ionized species cross with ease. Indeed, the capillary wall is of sufficient porosity that even drugs with molecular weights as great as 60,000 may be absorbed by passive diffusion.

• Lipid-Water Partition Coefficient

A measure of the distribution of a drug between a lipid and an aqueous phase is provided by the *lipid-water partition coefficient*. Thus, a coefficient of 1 means that a drug is as soluble in a nonpolar solvent, such as *n*-heptane, as it is in water, a polar solvent. Highly lipid-soluble materials, such as the barbiturate thiopental, have coefficients much greater than 1 and readily cross lipid barriers. In contrast, materials that are quite insoluble in both polar and nonpolar media are pharmacologically inert. For example, barium sulfate is a highly toxic material if absorbed, but because of its poor solubility it can be introduced into the GI tract as a contrast medium in radiography without hazard.

• Ionization of Drugs

In general, the ionized form of a drug is less lipid-soluble and more water-soluble than is the nonionized form. The degree to which many drugs are ionized is influenced by the hydrogen ion content (pH) of any aqueous medium in which they are placed. In a limited but significant number of instances in pharmacology and toxicology, the distribution of a drug between its ionized and nonionized forms can be influenced by manipulation of the pH of bodily fluids. Such drugs are referred to as *weak acids* and *weak bases*.

• Dissociation of Weak Acids and Weak Bases

Most are accustomed to regarding as acids those substances that yield hydrogen ions (protons) upon dissociation, and as bases those substances that yield hydroxyl ions. In considering drugs as acids and bases, we define an acid as a substance that in its uncharged form is a proton donor. A base, in contrast, is a substance that in its uncharged form is a proton acceptor. Thus, both acids and bases may exist in a proton donor and in a proton acceptor form.

The dissociation of an acid is given by

$$AH \rightleftharpoons A^- + H^+$$

and of a base by

$$BH^+ \rightleftharpoons B + H^+$$

For each, the proton donor or acid form is written on the left.

A distinction also must be made between "strong" acids and bases and "weak" acids and bases. The degree of dissociation of a strong acid like hydrochloric acid or of a strong base like sodium hydroxide is not influenced by the pH changes normally encountered in physiological systems. Thus, weak acids and bases are defined as those whose dissociation can be altered by pH differences compatible with the function of biological systems.

THE HENDERSON-HASSELBALCH EQUATION. Problems regarding the influence of pH upon weak acids and bases may be solved using the *Henderson-Hasselbalch equation*, which is derived as follows:

$$\text{acid} \rightleftharpoons \text{base} + H^+$$

The acid dissociation constant is expressed as

$$K_a \rightleftharpoons [\text{base}]\,[H^+]/[\text{acid}]$$

Thus,

$$H^+ = K_a\,\{[\text{acid}]/[\text{base}]\}$$

$$pH = pK_a - \log\,[\text{acid/base}]$$

$$pH - pk_a = \log\,[\text{base/acid}]$$

When $pH = pK_a$, $\log\,[\text{base}]/[\text{acid}] = 0$. Because antilog $0 = 1$, the ratio of the concentrations of base to acid is unity, *ie*, equal concentrations of each.

THE INTUITIVE APPROACH. Although the Henderson-Hasselbalch equation may be used directly to solve problems involving weak acids and weak bases, many students prefer an alternative procedure. Simply write the equation for the acid dissociation of the weak acid or base and apply the *principle of Le Chatelier*: if the conditions of a system, originally in equilibrium, are changed, the equilibrium shifts in such a direction as to tend to restore the original conditions. For example, a weak acid

$$AH \rightleftharpoons A^- + H^+$$

when $pH = pK_a$, $[AH] = [A^-]$ (our initial equilibrium). However, when $pH < pK_a$, *ie*, when the concentration of H^+ is greater at equilibrium, the reaction shifts to the left and AH is greater than A^-. The numerical value of the ratio is given by the antilog of the absolute value of the difference between pH and pK_a, *ie*,

$$AH/A^- = \text{antilog}\ \ |pH - pK_a|$$

Similarly, when $pH > pK_a$, *ie*, when the concentration of H^+ is less at equilibrium, the reaction shifts to the right, and A^- is greater than AH. The ratio of A^-/AH is then

$$A^-/AH = \text{antilog}\ \ |pH - pK_a|$$

The same reasoning applies to weak bases, but the starting equilibrium is given by

$$BH^+ = B + H^+$$

When pH is less than pK_a, the equilibrium is shifted to the left, and $BH^+ > B$. Conversely, when pH is greater than pK_a, $B > BH^+$. Again, the numerical values of the ratios are given by the antilog of the absolute differences between pH and pK_a.

Consideration of these facts makes it clear that the consequences of a shift in pH away from equilibrium conditions are opposite for weak acids and weak bases. Thus, at a pH less than pK_a, the nonionized, more lipid-soluble form of a weak acid is favored, whereas it is the ionized, less lipid-soluble form of a weak base that is present in excess.

However, it must be kept in mind that the degree of ionization is but one factor in absorption. For example, a drug whose lipid-soluble form is favored in the acidic conditions of the stomach may nonetheless be absorbed almost entirely in the small intestine because of the much greater absorptive area of the latter organ.

Control of the Rate of Absorption in Poisoning and in Therapeutics

Rate of Perfusion

Rate of perfusion is a factor in drug absorption. When a person is bitten on the hand by a poisonous snake, it is prudent to apply a tourniquet to the affected limb. The pertinent pharmacological principle is that the rate of absorption of a drug from its site of injection is proportional to the rate of blood flow past that site. In contrast to the physical application of a tourniquet, a pharmacological means to control blood flow is provided by vasoconstricting substances. Thus, for example, local anesthetic agents often are administered in combination with epinephrine. Local constriction of arterial vessels by epinephrine diminishes blood flow in the area, diminishes the amount of anesthetic absorbed, and thus diminishes the risk of systemic toxic effects.

Drug Formulation

Often, adequate therapeutic effects are critically dependent upon maintenance of appropriate blood and tissue levels of a drug. Because it is sometimes inconvenient or impractical to administer drugs on a schedule best suited to ensuring adequate blood levels, means of extending the period of absorption of drugs have been sought. In general, these attempts have taken two forms: (1) *chemical alteration* of the drug itself and (2) the use of a *supporting medium*. An example of the former is provided by haloperidol. Intramuscular injection of the decanoate ester of the antipsychotic drug haloperidol provides a drug depot. Slow hydrolysis of the ester and release of the active drug permits a 4-week dosing interval.

An alternative approach to sustained absorption of drugs is to place the drug in a medium from which it will diffuse slowly. A common site of application is the skin. Figure 1–14 shows a skin patch that was designed to deliver nitroglycerine over a period of 24 hours.

Drug Distribution

Upon reaching the general circulation, either by direct injection or following absorption from another site, a drug is distributed throughout the body. The rate at which the drug leaves the blood and reaches extravascular locations and receptors is dependent upon a number of pharmacological and physiological factors. In general, capillary walls are sufficiently porous that lipid solubility is not a limiting factor in the passage of drugs into extracellular water. The capillaries of the brain are an exception; drugs with low lipid solubility and the ionized forms of drugs can cross the blood-brain barrier only slowly if at all.

Once a drug is absorbed into the general circulation, it can be expected to reach every cell in the body. This fact is often brought to our attention by the occurrence of adverse effects in tissues far removed from the intended site of therapeutic action. However, before a drug can act upon specific drug receptors, it must exit the blood. (An exception to this statement would be drugs intended to act upon receptors on the luminal side of blood vessels or on cells or proteins of the blood.) The factors that were considered earlier with respect to drug absorption again are of importance.

General Factors

- **CONCENTRATION GRADIENT.** The rate at which a drug leaves the circulation is proportional to the concentration gradient of unbound drug from plasma to extracellular water.
- **BLOOD FLOW.** The quantity of drug that enters a given tissue is proportional to the rate of blood flow through that tissue.
- **PHYSICOCHEMICAL FACTORS.** For drugs with molecular weights less than about 60,000, the capillary wall presents no barrier to the passage of drugs, even if their lipid solubility is inherently low or they are in the ionized state. Capillaries of the central nervous system (CNS) are an exception (see The Blood-Brain Barrier).

Binding of Drugs to Plasma Proteins

Albumin is the principal protein of plasma in terms of drug binding. The molecular weight of plasma albumin is approximately 69,000. At a pH of 7.4, albumin is capable of interact-

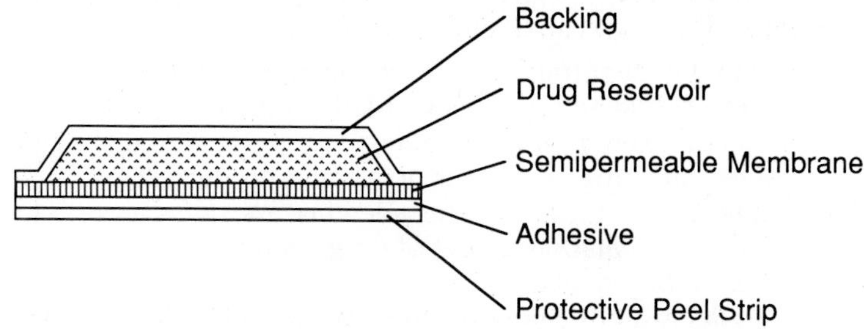

FIGURE 1–14. A cross-sectional diagram of a transdermal drug administration system for nitroglycerine. The trade-marked system, TRANSDERM-NITRO, is depicted. It consists of four layers. Proceeding from the top, externally visible surface toward the bottom surface that is attached to the skin: the backing layer of aluminized plastic that is impermeable to nitroglycerin; the drug reservoir containing nitroglycerin adsorbed on lactose, colloidal silicon dioxide, and silicone medical fluid; an ethylene/vinyl acetate copolymer semipermeable membrane that is permeable to nitroglycerin; and a silicone adhesive surface covered until use by a protective peel strip.

ing with both anions and cations. The interaction between drugs and albumin is characterized in the same way as the drug-receptor interaction discussed previously:

$$X + P \rightleftharpoons XP$$

Although the interaction is nearly always reversible, the half-life of the complex may range from less than a second to more than a year. Because the molecular weight of the complex exceeds 69,000, it cannot cross the capillary wall. While bound to plasma protein, a drug does not contribute to the concentration gradient, cannot be filtered by the kidney, and in general is pharmacologically inert. It should be noted, however, that the reversible binding of a drug to plasma protein may function as a reservoir that slowly releases the active agent.

Relative Permeabilities of Capillary Beds

All capillary beds, with the exception of those found in the CNS, are sufficiently "leaky" to permit the passage of most unbound drug molecules even in the ionized state. Nonetheless, there are differences. The relative order of rates of permeability is generally taken to be as follows:

liver > kidney > muscle = fetus (placental) > > brain

Without reliable evidence to the contrary, the existence of a "placental barrier" to drug distribution should never be assumed; drugs administered to pregnant women should be expected to reach the embryo or fetus.

The Blood-Brain Barrier

Capillaries in the CNS differ from all other capillaries in that cerebral endothelial cells have tight junctions between them. This is the morphological basis for what is termed the *blood-brain barrier.* In a few areas of the brain, the barrier is absent. These areas include the lateral nuclei of the hypothalamus, the area postrema of the fourth ventricle, the pineal body, and the posterior lobe of the hypophysis.

The blood-brain barrier has the properties of a lipid barrier without pores. The consequences for drug distribution are that agents with inherently low lipid solubility as well as ionized forms of drugs are unable to exit the circulation and enter the extracellular water of the brain. It must be noted, however, that for highly lipid-soluble drugs there is, in effect, no blood-brain barrier.

Termination of Drug Action

It is to be expected that the effects of a drug upon the body diminish with the passage of time. Any mechanism that diminishes drug concentration at its receptors contributes to termination of drug action. Principal among these mechanisms are drug excretion, which may occur via several different routes, and drug metabolism to inactive products. Significant interactions may occur between disease states and the rates of drug metabolism and of drug excretion.

Earlier in this chapter, we assumed that most pharmacological effects are the consequence of a reversible interaction between a drug and its receptor and that the magnitude of the effect is proportional to the concentration of the drug-receptor complex. Thus, any process that diminishes the concentration of a drug in the vicinity of its receptor will contribute to the termination of the effects of the drug. Three major contributing factors must be considered: (1) drug redistribution or storage, (2) drug excretion, and (3) drug metabolism.

• Drug Redistribution or Storage

A prime example of the consequences of redistribution is provided by the short-acting barbiturate thiopental sodium. The nonionized form of this drug is highly lipid-soluble. When administered intravenously, the drug rapidly crosses the blood-brain barrier and produces anesthesia. However, as more thiopental enters poorly perfused tissues, such as subcutaneous *fat,* the blood levels of thiopental decline, and a new equilibrium is established. As this slow loss to fat tissues occurs, the thiopental concentration gradient between the blood and the brain soon favors passage from the brain to the blood, and anesthesia is reversed.

• It should be noted that body fat is not an unfillable sink and that with continuous administration of thiopental, a new equilibrium is achieved in which anesthetic levels of the drug are maintained in the blood for an extended period of time. Other examples include fat-soluble agents, such as the insecticide chlorophenothane (DDT) and the psychoactive drug tetrahydrocannabinol, which are detectable in the body long after a single exposure or administration.

• The binding of drugs to *plasma proteins* is a form of drug storage in that bound drug is pharmacologically inert. Disease states such as hypoalbuminemia, in which the concentration of plasma protein is severely depressed, may contribute to elevated blood levels of drugs that are normally bound extensively to plasma protein.

• *Bone* may provide a storage site for drugs as well as for toxic agents. When administered to children during the period of enamel formation, tetracyclines may be deposited in the bone and produce permanent discolorations of the teeth. Of more profound toxicological consequence is the deposition in bone of strontium 90 (^{90}Sr), a product of nuclear fission reactions. A high-energy beta emitter with a half-life of 28 years, ^{90}Sr is a significant radiation hazard, primarily because of its ability to mimic calcium in bone.

• Drug Excretion

Elimination of a drug from the body is an obvious means to terminate its pharmacological actions. Indeed, the effects of some drugs are diminished as a direct function of their rate of excretion. The major routes of excretion are considered briefly here.

• **RENAL EXCRETION.** This is the major route by which drugs exit the body. Nearly all unbound drugs enter the glomerular filtrate. However, net renal excretion depends upon a complex interplay between active or passive reabsorption and tubular secretion. This is discussed in greater detail in Chapter 35.

In general, the rate of renal excretion of a drug is a function of its pharmacological properties and of its concentration in the blood together with the rate of urine production.

The presence of impaired renal function necessitates a re-evaluation of drug dosages that are deemed appropriate for normal individuals.

The renal excretion of some weak acids and bases can be influenced significantly by alteration of the pH level of the urine. This is illustrated in Figure 1–15. Acidification of the urine results in an increase in the rate of urinary excretion of nicotine, a weak base. The explanation is that a more acidic environment favors formation of the ionized, less lipid-soluble form of nicotine with a resultant decline in the amount that is passively reabsorbed following filtration. Conversely, renal excretion of weak acids is favored by more alkaline conditions.

• **BILIARY EXCRETION.** Drugs present in the liver may be secreted along with bile into the duodenum. However, like the bile acids, drugs thus excreted may be reabsorbed along the length of the gut. Thus, net biliary excretion depends upon the rate of subsequent reabsorption through the enterohepatic circulation.

• **EXCRETION BY THE LUNGS.** Detectable quantities of many drugs appear in expired air. Of greatest importance are the anesthetic gases (see Chapter 11). Successful anesthesia by inhalation depends upon the passage of the gas from inspired air to the blood and thence to the brain and to other sites of action. Reversal of this process results in recovery from anesthesia.

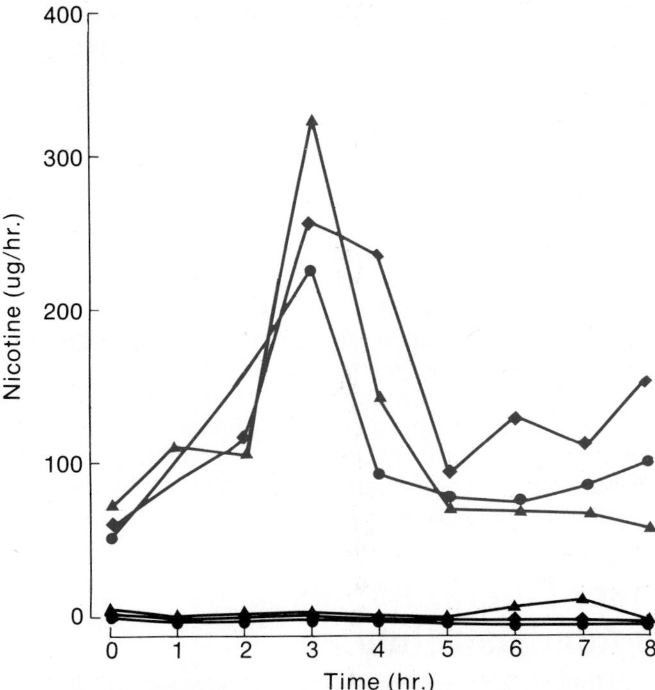

FIGURE 1–15. The effect of urinary pH on the excretion of nicotine during the smoking of a cigarette (*circles*) or during the chewing of gum that contains 2 mg (*triangles*) or 4 mg (*squares*) of nicotine. The top graphs are for a urinary pH of 4.7–5.3, and the bottom graphs are for a urinary pH of 7.4–8.0. Abscissa: time in hours. Ordinate: micrograms of nicotine excreted per hour. (Redrawn from Feyerabend G, Russell MAH: Effect of urinary pH and nicotine excretion rate on plasma nicotine during cigarette smoking and chewing nicotine gum. Br J Clin Pharmacol 5:295, 1978, by permission of Blackwell Scientific Publications, Ltd.)

With the exception of the gaseous anesthetics, excretion of drugs by the lungs does not represent a major means of termination of drug action. However, analysis of the concentration of ethanol in expired air provides a noninvasive, widely used means to assess blood levels and, by inference, degree of intoxication with the drug.

• **EXCRETION IN OTHER FLUIDS.** All drugs, especially those with a high degree of water solubility, are excreted in tears, sweat, and breast milk. Loss of drugs in these fluids is not a significant factor in the termination of drug action. However, there is concern that toxic effects may arise in breast-fed infants. For this reason, all medications taken by nursing women should be regarded as potential hazards to their babies.

Drug Metabolism

Although some drugs are excreted unchanged, most undergo some degree of metabolic alteration in the body. Although drug metabolism occurs at many sites throughout the body, the most significant area quantitatively is the liver. In general, the product of metabolism is more water-soluble, hence more readily excreted through the kidney, and less active pharmacologically than the parent drug.

A few drugs are converted metabolically from inactive to active forms. The classic example of such activation was provided by Gerhard Domagk. He found that sulfamidochrysoidine (PRONTOSIL), inactive against streptococci *in vitro*, was an effective antistreptococcal agent *in vivo*. The active metabolic product of Prontosil was later shown to be sulfanilamide. For his discoveries, Domagk received the Nobel Prize in Medicine for 1939.

Drug metabolism is discussed in detail in Chapter 4.

REFERENCES

INTRODUCTION TO PHARMACOLOGY: RECEPTORS

Albert A: Selective Toxicity, The Physico-Chemical Basis of Therapy, 6th ed. London: Chapman & Hall, 1979.

Fischer E: Einfluss der Configuration auf die Wirkung der Enzyme. Ber Dtsch Chem Gies 27:2985–2993, 1894.

Goldstein A, Aronow L, Kalman SM: Principles of Drug Action: The Basis of Pharmacology, 2nd ed. New York: John Wiley & Sons, 1974.

Pratt WB, Taylor P: Principles of Drug Action. The Basis of Pharmacology, 3rd ed. [Revised edition of Goldstein A, Kalman SM, Aronow L, 2nd ed, 1973, 1974.] New York: Churchill Livingstone, 1990.

DOSE-EFFECT RELATIONSHIPS, INTERACTIONS, AND THERAPEUTIC INDEX

Albert A: Selective Toxicity, The Physico-chemical Basis of Therapy, 6th ed. London: Chapman & Hall: 1979.

Black JW, Leff P: Operational models of pharmacological agonism. Proc R Soc Lond [Biol] 220:141–162, 1983.

Clark AJ: General Pharmacology. Vol 4 of Handbuch der experimentellen Pharmakologie. Berlin: Springer-Verlag, 1937.

Holtzman SG: Discriminative stimulus properties of opioid agonists and antagonists. *In* Cooper SJ (ed): Theory in Psychopharmacology, 1–45. Vol 2. London: Academic Press, 1983.

Kenakin T: Pharmacologic Analysis of Drug Receptor Interaction, 2nd ed. New York: Raven Press, 1993.

2 Routes of Administration

Jerrold C. Winter

INTRODUCTION

Drugs may be introduced into the body in a variety of ways. Among the more common methods of administration are by having the patient swallow the drug and by injecting the drug. The route of administration that is chosen may have a profound effect upon the speed and efficiency with which the drug acts. In addition, adverse effects due both to the drug itself and to the medium of administration are influenced by route. For example, the risk of viral and bacterial infection is maximized when drugs are administered intravenously.

The relative importance of the various physiological and physicochemical factors outlined in Chapter 1 may be profoundly influenced by the way in which a drug is introduced into the body. Traditionally, the so-called routes of administration have been divided into two major classes: enteral, which refers to the intestine, and parenteral, which means other than the intestine. As is demonstrated in this chapter, a purely dichotomous classification of the possible routes of drug administration is simplistic and may be misleading.

THE GASTROINTESTINAL TRACT

For the purposes of this discussion, the gastrointestinal (GI) tract is assumed to run from the mouth to the rectum. A major advantage of administering drugs through the GI tract is that the concomitant risk of viral and bacterial infection is minimized. The precise route that a drug follows from the GI tract to the general circulation is influenced significantly by the sites within the GI tract from which the drug is absorbed.

Oral Administration

Drugs placed in the mouth and swallowed are said to have been taken "by mouth" or in Latin, *per os*. Hence, the abbreviation "p.o." refers to the oral route. It should be noted that swallowing the drug is implicit in oral administration. Drugs that are simply placed in the mouth and held there are absorbed in a significantly different fashion (see Sublingual Administration). Although the stomach is not usually regarded as a major organ of absorption, significant amounts of small, lipid-soluble molecules may be absorbed across the stomach wall when a drug is swallowed. Ascorbic acid is an example. The acidic conditions typical of the stomach favor the occurrence of the uncharged, lipid-soluble, proton-donor form of ascorbic acid.

First-Pass Effect

Drugs absorbed from the small intestine following oral administration enter the hepatic portal circulation and thus may be acted upon by hepatic enzymes prior to their reaching the general circulation. The alteration of a drug by liver enzymes is commonly referred to as the *first-pass effect.* Occasionally, the inactivation of drugs in the first-pass effect is of such magnitude that an alternative route of administration is required. Although the first-pass effect specifically refers to hepatic inactivation, the concept is sometimes extended to include gastric and intestinal inactivation as well.

Other Enteral Routes of Administration

Sublingual Administration

Drugs placed in the mouth and held beneath the tongue are said to be administered sublingually. The mucosal lining of the oral cavity presents a lipid barrier to absorption. However, for drugs with high lipid solubility, the sublingual route is appropriate. For example, when nitroglycerin tablets are placed beneath the tongue, plasma levels of the drug quickly rise to levels that are adequate for the relief of the chest pain of angina pectoris. In addition, absorption is not through the hepatic portal circulation; therefore, the first-pass effect is avoided. For example, morphine recently has been formulated for what has been called *buccal administration* (in Latin, *bucca* means cheek). Absorption of the drug, which is placed between the cheek and the gum, is prolonged, and the first-pass effect can be avoided.

Rectal Administration

The mucosal lining of the rectum provides a relatively convenient site for drug administration. The principles involved are similar to those described previously for the oral mucosa. The first-pass effect is avoided to a significant degree, but the exact extent to which it is avoided depends on the area of the rectal mucosa from which the drug is absorbed. The inferior and middle rectal veins drain directly into the general circulation, but the superior rectal vein enters the hepatic portal circulation. Rectal administration of drugs is often employed in infants and young children, in patients unable to take drugs by mouth, and in patients in whom protracted vomiting makes oral administration ineffective.

DRUG ADMINISTRATION BY INJECTION

Although humans have taken crude drugs by mouth throughout history, administration by injection was made possible only in the past century by the invention of the hypodermic needle. With the availability of thin, hollow needles, drugs could be deposited in various tissues as well as into the general circulation. Such routes are commonly referred to as *parenteral.*

Injection Into the Blood

By direct injection of drugs into the general circulation, all barriers to absorption are bypassed. The onset of drug action is rapid, and between-patient variability associated with absorption is reduced to a minimum. Unfortunately, these advantages are offset to a significant degree by an increased probability of adverse effects, including infection (discussed later in this chapter).

Intravenous Administration

The close control of plasma levels made possible by intravenous (IV) administration is such that an IV line is established routinely in many emergency and inpatient situations. In addition, discrete IV injection is often performed when rapid onset of drug action is essential or in patients in whom a drug is especially irritating to tissue when it is given by other parenteral routes.

Intra-arterial Administration

This route is chosen much less commonly than the IV route. Its use is restricted almost entirely to regional perfusion of an area with a particularly toxic agent, a situation that is not uncommon in cancer chemotherapy, and to diagnostic procedures. In the latter case, a radiopaque material is injected intra-arterially to permit visualization of the vascular system of the brain, heart, or another organ.

Injection Into Other Sites

In addition to direct placement of drugs in the general circulation, injections into muscle or beneath the skin are common. In contrast to IV or intra-arterial administration, injection into other sites does not allow all barriers to absorption to be bypassed and, as a result, considerable variation in the magnitude and time of onset of drug effects is to be expected. Contrary to popular belief, the rate and efficiency of drug absorption following intramuscular (IM) or subcutaneous injection may be greater than, equal to, or less than that following oral administration, depending on the drug under consideration.

Subcutaneous Injection

Because the drug has direct access to skin capillaries, absorption is usually quick and efficient. However, the rate of absorption is proportional to blood flow in the area of injection. A number of drugs are specifically formulated for subcutaneous (SC) injection.

Intramuscular Injection

A large muscle such as the deltoid or gluteus maximus is usually chosen as the site for IM injection. As is the case with SC administration, blood flow in the area of injection is a major factor in rate of absorption. Ready access to muscle capillaries is generally assumed, but current studies indicate that this is not necessarily the case. Thus, for example, in grossly obese patients, injections that are presumed to be IM may in fact be intralipomatous. Because of the relatively low rate of perfusion of fat by the blood, a lower rate of absorption is predicted from fat than from muscle. In addition, there is some evidence that rate of drug absorption may be influenced by the particular muscle chosen for injection. However, the clinical consequences of these and other variables are poorly defined. For example, massage or muscle activity can sometimes significantly increase the rate of absorption.

It was noted previously that drugs are not necessarily more rapidly or more efficiently absorbed following IM injection than when given by mouth. The clearest example of this fact is provided by some of the benzodiazepines, such as diazepam and chlordiazepoxide. The most likely explanation is poor solubility in water coupled with drug-induced irritation at the site of injection. This interpretation is supported by reports by patients of significant pain at the site of injection.

Epidural and Intrathecal Administration

Induction of spinal anesthesia by injection of drugs in the vicinity of the spinal cord has a long history. However, the discovery of opiate receptors in the spinal cord has led to a greatly expanded use of the epidural and intrathecal routes in the treatment of pain. For example, one anticipated advantage of the intrathecal administration of morphine is that sufficient doses are so low that only insignificant amounts of the drug reach other areas of the central nervous system.

OTHER ROUTES OF ADMINISTRATION

The Respiratory Tract

A number of drugs are used for their local effects upon the lungs. For example, an acute asthmatic attack may be treated with the inhalation of an aerosol spray that contains a β-adrenergic agonist. However, because of their large surface area and proximity to the pulmonary circulation, the lungs also provide an efficient means for drug absorption. Lipid-soluble, readily volatilized drugs rapidly reach pharmacologically significant levels in the blood after their introduction into the lungs. The anesthetic gases represent the most common class of therapeutic agents administered as *gases* by inhalation (see Chapter 11). In addition, however, a number of drugs that are used primarily in nonmedical settings for their pleasurable effects may be inhaled after volatilization. Included in the latter group are the free-base forms of nicotine, tetrahydrocannabinol, phencyclidine, cocaine, and heroin. As is the case with nicotine-containing cigarettes, significant pathological effects on lung tissue may be caused by tars and other substances inhaled together with the desired pharmacological agent.

The Skin

Although the stratum corneum provides an effective barrier to the absorption of many drugs, it has long been known that systemic toxic effects may arise following the exposure of large areas of the skin to agents such as the organophosphate insecticides. In the past decade, therapeutic use has been made of the ability of lipid-soluble drugs to reach capillaries beneath the skin. When drugs are administered in this way, the route of administration is referred to as *transdermal, transcutaneous*, or *percutaneous.* Drugs available at present for transdermal delivery include nitroglycerin, scopolamine, clonidine, and some β-adrenergic antagonists.

COMPARATIVE ADVANTAGES OF ENTERAL, PARENTERAL, AND OTHER ROUTES OF ADMINISTRATION

No single method of drug administration is ideal for all drugs in all circumstances. Because of the chemical and pharmacological properties of some drugs, certain methods of administration are ineffective, inefficient, or hazardous. Examples include insulin and other readily digested drugs for which a parenteral route is required; in contrast, a number of drugs are not available in parenteral form and must be given by mouth. When the use of a specific route of administration is contraindicated, that fact will be specified in the prescribing information provided by the manufacturer.

In many instances, drugs are available in a variety of formulations that provide the clinician with opportunity to employ several different routes of administration. Selection of the most appropriate route must take into account a number of factors, some general in nature and others specific to an individual patient.

Compliance or Adherence

It is often assumed that once a drug is prescribed, it will be taken faithfully as directed. Studies of patient compliance with prescribed directions have found this expectation to be unrealistic in a significant proportion of the patient population. It should be noted that "noncompliance" includes not only the patient's failure to take a medication in the prescribed dose or at prescribed times but also the taking of a medication in excess.

A low rate of compliance is particularly likely when (1) the patient's thought processes are impaired by mental retardation, dementia, or psychiatric illness; (2) the patient is physically impaired by paralysis, arthritis, or other conditions; (3) the drug provides no readily perceived beneficial effect, for example as in the prophylactic use of antibiotics; (4) the drug must be taken frequently or at odd times during the day or night (once a day at the same time each day is preferable when possible); and (5) the immediate adverse effects of the drug make the patient feel worse despite a beneficial therapeutic effect. Factor 5 is illustrated by some antihypertensive agents currently in use and, most dramatically, by a number of drugs used in the treatment of cancer.

The probability of patient compliance with a prescribed drug regimen is enhanced by systematic education of the patient with respect to the expected benefits of a given drug as well as the adverse effects that may be expected. Too often it is erroneously assumed either that the patient is already aware of the relevant facts regarding her or his pharmacological treatment or that the patient is incapable of understanding simple explanations and instructions.

In those instances when adequate compliance is deemed unlikely, the drug may be administered by mouth in the presence of a health professional, or more commonly, the drug may be administered by injection. An example of the latter case is provided by the outpatient maintenance of schizophrenic patients in which a slowly absorbed form, or "depot" preparation, of an antipsychotic drug is injected intramuscularly or subcutaneously at 2-week or longer intervals. Conversely, when the probability of compliance is high, the oral route of administration is unsurpassed in terms of convenience and safety.

Risk of Infection

The degree to which barriers to absorption are bypassed is correlated positively with the risk of bacterial or viral infection. Thus, the oral route rarely presents a hazard in this regard, whereas IV administration requires strict adherence to sterile technique. Extensive information regarding infection following parenteral administration has been provided unintentionally by some groups of drug abusers in that a SC or IV route is often employed; unsterile drugs, syringes, and needles are also commonly used; and there is a tradition of sharing among users.

In addition to the possibility of infection at or in close proximity to the site of injection, bacterial endocarditis and viral hepatitis have long been recognized as possible hazards of IV drug use. More recently, transfer of the human immunodeficiency virus and the subsequent development of the acquired immunodeficiency syndrome have been demonstrated.

Efficiency of Absorption

Multiple factors contribute to variation in rate and extent of drug absorption among individuals. The degree of variation is influenced by the route of administration that is chosen. It is reasonable to assume that variation is greatest for drugs taken by the oral route and that variation in absorption is reduced to zero by IV administration.

For drugs taken by mouth, sources of intrapatient and interpatient variability include pH in the stomach and intestine, gastric emptying time, and the presence or absence of food in the GI tract. Manufacturers' prescribing information usually stipulates the most appropriate relationships among eating, drinking, and taking specific drugs (see Chapter 50 regarding food and drug interactions). This information should be diligently passed on to the patient, because this is a common source of uncertainty, confusion, and anxiety.

It previously was noted that IM injection of drugs does not eliminate variability in absorption. Gauge and length of the needle chosen, depth of injection, site of injection, and ratio of fat to muscle are all significant factors in absorption rate.

BOX 2–1
HAZARDS PECULIAR TO INTRAVENOUS ADMINISTRATION

In addition to the risk of infection associated with the IV route, other potential hazards must be considered. These may be summarized as follows:

1. Once the drug is injected, its distribution cannot be altered significantly.
2. IV injection is sometimes associated with cardiac, vascular, or circulatory disturbances that may be fatal. Although such effects are presumed to be more common when highly adulterated drugs of abuse are used, there is some risk even under the best of conditions. The probability of occurrence of such reactions appears to be related, among other factors, to the rapidity of injection. IV injections should be given slowly, preferably over a period of 1 minute or more.
3. Anaphylactoid reactions may be especially severe (see Chapter 50). As with all such reactions, death may occur within a few minutes.
4. Inadvertent injection of air may result in air embolism in the pulmonary or other vasculature.

3 Tolerance, Physical Dependence, and Drug Abuse

Jerrold C. Winter

Chronic administration of drugs may lead to **tolerance**, a state of diminished responsiveness to the drug, and to **physical dependence**, a state in which continued presence of the drug in the body is required for normal function. Tolerance and physical dependence may accompany the use of therapeutic agents as well as the abuse of drugs. The **withdrawal syndrome** characteristic of physical dependence upon various drugs may range from a barely detectable set of signs and symptoms to a potentially fatal condition. Important variables include the specific drug of dependence, its dose, the frequency and duration of use, and the route of administration. Every physician must be aware of the various types of physical dependence and their medical implications.

DEFINITION OF TERMS

• Tolerance

Drug tolerance refers to a state of diminished responsiveness to a drug as a consequence of prior exposure. This phenomenon is sometimes called *acquired tolerance* to distinguish it from *innate tolerance.* The latter term refers to a relative insensitivity to drug action, which is independent of prior exposure.

In its simplest form, drug tolerance is reflected in a parallel shift of the dose-response curve to the right. The degree of drug tolerance, *ie*, the extent to which the dose-response curve is shifted, is quite variable and depends on the effect being measured and on the specific drug. For example, the degree of tolerance to a drug such as ethanol (a factor of about 2) is modest, whereas the dose-response curves for opiates may shift by a log unit or more.

The phenomenon in which tolerance to one drug confers tolerance to another is called **cross-tolerance**. Depending upon the specific mechanism by which tolerance arises, cross-tolerance may or may not reflect similar therapeutic effects (see Cross-tolerance as an Indication of Action Upon a Common Receptor). However, it is not unusual for drugs of a given class, *eg*, opioid analgesics, to display cross-tolerance.

• Physical Dependence

The phenomenon in which, as a consequence of prior exposure to a drug, the continued presence of that drug in the body is required for normal function is called *physical dependence.* Physical dependence is defined in terms of the signs and symptoms that occur following termination of the drug of dependence. Collectively, the signs and symptoms following cessation of drug administration make up the **abstinence syndrome** or the **withdrawal syndrome**. Proof of physical dependence on a given drug is provided by the ability of that drug to relieve the abstinence syndrome. Drug tolerance is correlated generally with physical dependence, and it is commonly assumed that drug tolerance is a necessary prerequisite for the development of physical dependence. However, the converse is not true; physical dependence need not accompany drug tolerance.

As noted previously, tolerance to one drug of a pharmacological class often confers tolerance to others of the same class. A similar phenomenon, **cross-physical dependence**, is observed with respect to physical dependence. Thus, termination of the abstinence syndrome is afforded not only by the primary drug of dependence but also by other drugs of the same class.

• Drug (Substance) Abuse

Drug tolerance and physical dependence are pharmacological phenomena whose parameters may be expressed fully in scientific terms. In contrast, "drug abuse" is commonly defined as the use, usually by self-administration, of any drug in a manner that deviates from the approved medical or social patterns within a given culture. Although drug tolerance and physical dependence may be elements in some forms of drug abuse, they are neither necessary nor sufficient conditions for drug abuse. For example, patients treated with opiates for the relief of pain often display both tolerance and physical dependence; such patients are not drug abusers (see also Chapter 49).

ORIGINS OF DRUG TOLERANCE

Events responsible for drug tolerance may be divided into two categories. First are those that reduce the effective concentration of drug at receptor sites; in general these occur at a distance from the receptor. For example, a drug-induced increase in the rate of its own metabolism results in less of the drug's reaching its pharmacological receptors. Second are those adaptive changes that take place either at the receptor or in systems closely connected with the drug's action; this condition is referred to as **cellular tolerance**.

Dispositional and Metabolic Tolerance

Any process that results in fewer drug molecules reaching their receptors contributes to tolerance. Thus, for example, tolerance would be expected to arise as a consequence of changes in absorption, metabolism, excretion, or rate of passage across membranes. Of these possible mechanisms, clear evidence has been obtained only for altered metabolism following chronic exposure to drugs. Tolerance as a result of metabolic changes is called **metabolic tolerance** or **pharmacokinetic tolerance**.

Metabolic tolerance is observed for any drug able to induce the synthesis of enzymes responsible for its inactivation. The best-documented site of origin of metabolic tolerance is the hepatic microsomal enzyme system. If the enzymes thus induced are responsible for the inactivation of other drugs, cross-tolerance is observed. The example that follows shows the effects of chronic exposure of humans to high doses of pentobarbital (600 – 1200 mg/day) on the rate of metabolism of antipyrine, a drug often used as an indicator of the activity of hepatic mixed-function oxidase. (This is discussed further in Chapter 4.)

Group	N	Antipyrine Half-Life
Control	61	12.5 hours
		($P < 0.001$)
Barbiturate	8	5.3 hours

Cellular Tolerance

For many drugs acting upon the central nervous system (CNS), it is not possible to explain drug tolerance in terms of metabolic adaptation. Either blood levels of the drug are unchanged in the tolerant state, or changes in blood levels are inadequate to explain the degree of tolerance observed. In such situations, it is commonly assumed that adaptation has occurred either at the receptor site or in the transduction system that links receptor occupation with pharmacological effect. Tolerance in the presence of unchanged concentrations of drug in the vicinity of its receptor is called **cellular tolerance** or **pharmacodynamic tolerance**.

Behavioral Tolerance

Behavioral tolerance is a form of cellular tolerance that arises as a consequence of adaptive behavioral mechanisms. It develops most commonly when a drug-induced effect has adverse consequences; behavioral tolerance then tends to be specific for that effect. For example, a physician-alcoholic may become quite adept at masking the ataxic effects of ethanol, but other actions of the drug would remain unaltered.

Cross-tolerance as an Indication of Action Upon a Common Receptor

Although it is certainly true that a group of drugs acting on a common receptor may exhibit cross-tolerance, it is not safe to assume that drugs cross-tolerant to one another act upon a common receptor. For example, barbiturates may induce hepatic enzymes responsible for the metabolism of drugs acting on diverse receptors in the CNS.

Tachyphylaxis (Acute Tolerance)

Because of the influence of dose and frequency of administration upon tolerance, it is seldom possible to define precisely for a given drug the time course over which tolerance develops. Thus, in a clinical setting, tolerance may be apparent only after several weeks of treatment with divided oral doses or may arise much more quickly following continuous intravenous administration. Nonetheless, it generally is observed that the development of tolerance is a relatively slow process, perhaps, as in metabolic tolerance, corresponding to the rate of synthesis of metabolic enzymes.

In those exceptional instances in which tolerance develops rapidly, the term "acute tolerance" or "tachyphylaxis" (rapid protection) is used. A classic example is provided by the sympathomimetic agent tyramine. Closely spaced infusions of tyramine are at first followed by a pronounced pressor effect, which is then quickly decreased in magnitude. Tyramine tachyphylaxis is attributed to rapid depletion by tyramine of presynaptic stores of norepinephrine. Acute tolerance is manifested by many sedative-hypnotics, such as ethanol and benzodiazepines (see Chapters 25 and 48).

BOX 3–1
TYPES OF PHYSICAL DEPENDENCE

It was stated previously that physical dependence is defined in terms of the signs and symptoms that occur following termination of the drug of dependence, and that these signs and symptoms are collectively termed the abstinence or withdrawal syndrome. Based upon observation of their respective withdrawal syndromes, several types of physical dependence are evident.

- **Depressant-type physical dependence.** This form of physical dependence is also call the **ethanol-barbiturate type**. Convulsions are a prominent component of this type of physical dependence; mainly because of this reason, individuals with untreated withdrawal have a significant mortality rate. Although sufficient subtle differences exist between depressants to suggest subtypes of depressant-type physical dependence, the withdrawal syndrome from dependence on ethanol is suppressed significantly by barbiturates and by benzodiazepines (see Chapters 25, 48, and 49 for details).
- **Opiate-type physical dependence.** This, the second major form of physical dependence, is also called **dependence of the narcotic-analgesic type**. The classic reference drug for opiate dependence is morphine. The withdrawal syndrome is characterized by autonomic hyperactivity. Cross-physical dependence, as manifested by suppression of the abstinence syndrome, is exhibited by a large number of drugs that share morphine's pharmacological activities (see Chapter 49 for details).
- **Other forms of physical dependence.** Dependence of the depressant and opiate types has long been recognized. In addition, it is clear now that a variety of nondepressant, nonopiate drugs can induce other forms of physical dependence. Indeed, it can be argued that chronic administration of every drug induces adaptive changes that are evident upon termination of drug treatment.

Whether physical dependence is judged to be present is largely a matter of what is considered acceptable as a withdrawal syndrome. For example, clonidine is a widely used antihypertensive agent that, upon abrupt termination of administration, is associated with rebound hypertension. Likewise, withdrawal of caffeine is associated with headache; of nicotine, with anxiety; and of cocaine, with depression. Most authorities now accept these more subtle signs of abstinence syndromes as indications of true physical dependence.

RATIONAL TREATMENT OF WITHDRAWAL SYNDROMES

It has been noted that the various types of physical dependence are differentiated by the characteristics of their withdrawal syndromes and that cross-physical dependence is defined by the ability of one drug to relieve the withdrawal syndrome of another. Thus, reinstitution of the primary drug of dependence or substitution of a drug that exhibits cross-physical dependence to it represents rational drug therapy. Often, the choice of a specific agent is influenced by local, regional, or national customs. For example, although those experiencing withdrawal from ethanol are seldom treated in a medical setting with ethanol, drugs as diverse as barbiturates, benzodiazepines, and chloral hydrate are often employed. Although there are a number of factors that influence the decision to provide pharmacological treatment for a specific withdrawal syndrome, the primary consideration is the hazard to the patient (see Chapter 49 for details regarding specific drugs of dependence).

Drug Metabolism

4

Jerome A. Roth

FUNCTION AND CONSEQUENCES OF METABOLISM OF DRUGS

The actions of drugs are dependent upon their sufficient lipid solubility to be absorbed across cellular membranes and upon their distribution in an active form to their ultimate receptors. The activity and duration of action of drugs are regulated *in vivo* by a number of factors, including the rate at which the drugs are metabolically inactivated by various enzyme systems. A number of different and specific enzymatic processes throughout the body are responsible for the degradation and subsequent inactivation of drugs and other toxic agents. Although many of these processes function in the homeostatic regulation of endogenous substances, they can also serve to catabolize a variety of pharmacologically and toxicologically active agents. The usual end result of these catabolic processes is the conversion of lipid-soluble xenobiotics to metabolic products that are pharmacologically inactive and more water-soluble; this increased solubility in water facilitates their elimination in the urine or bile. (There are some important exceptions to this general rule, such as pharmacologically active metabolites, that also are addressed.)

The majority of foreign substances that are taken into the body, regardless of the route of administration, are converted into metabolites that are excreted more rapidly than the original agent. During periods of impaired drug metabolism, elimination of drugs can be greatly reduced and, if not appropriately detected and subsequently prevented, can lead to excessive drug levels and subsequent toxic manifestations. Thus, the activity of the enzyme systems involved in drug metabolism can greatly influence the biochemical or pharmacological activity and toxic characteristics of any foreign substance taken into the body.

Before the different biochemical systems that are involved in the inactivation of drugs are described, it must be understood how drug metabolism influences the regulation and the pharmacological properties of drugs.

• Duration of Drug Action

For many drugs, the duration of action is inversely proportional to the rate at which they are metabolically inactivated. The more rapidly a drug is converted into inactive metabolites, the shorter the duration of its stay in the body and thus the briefer its actions; conversely, the slower its rate of degradation, the longer its duration of action. Although these appear to be obvious relationships, they are extremely important because the dosing regimens of many drugs are based primarily on these factors. Thus, factors that influence the activity of the drug-metabolizing enzyme systems subsequently alter the duration of drug action as well as the rate at which the drug might accumulate. The variability in the duration of action of many drugs within the human population is the result, in large part, of the individual differences in the levels of the drug-metabolizing enzyme systems.

The relationship between drug metabolism and duration of drug action has been investigated extensively and is exemplified by the drug hexobarbital. As demonstrated in Table 4 – 1, there is an inverse relationship between the rate of hepatic metabolism of hexobarbital and sleeping time in the various animal species listed. As indicated, the more rapidly hexobarbital is metabolically inactivated, the shorter the duration of its action. These data reveal that the duration of action of hexobarbital is regulated by the rate at which it is enzymatically degraded.

Although this relationship holds true for many drugs, it is important to stress that duration of drug action also can be

TABLE 4–1. Species Differences in Metabolism of Hexobarbital*

Species (n)	Sleeping Time (minutes)†	Hexobarbital Half-Life (minutes)†	Enzyme Activity (μg/g · hour)†
Mice (12)	12 ± 8	19 ± 7	598 ±184
Rabbits (9)	49 ± 12	60 ± 11	196 ± 28
Rats (10)	90 ± 15	140 ± 54	134 ± 51
Dogs (8)	315 ± 105	260 ± 20	36 ± 30

*Dose of barbiturate, 100 mg kg^{-1} (50 mg kg^{-1} in dogs).

†Data are given in mean ± standard deviation.

influenced by a number of other factors, such as transport and redistribution of a drug from one compartment in the body to another. Similarly, drug metabolism does not necessarily lead to the formation of inactive catabolites; thus, duration of drug action may not always be related directly to its rate of degradation. Therefore, it often is difficult to predict *a priori* which factor will be the primary determinant regulating the duration of drug action.

• Drug Interactions

It is not an uncommon medical practice to prescribe more than one medication at a time to treat multiple symptoms or ailments of a patient. Therefore, there is a real potential hazard for any two drugs to influence each other not only at the pharmacologically active site but also at the site of the enzyme system involved in drug detoxification. In regard to the latter interaction, there are two major mechanisms and a number of minor ones by which one drug can alter the rate of metabolism and, ultimately, the inactivation of another drug.

BOX 4–1
SITES OF INTERACTIONS OF ONE DRUG WITH ANOTHER

I. Receptor
II. Metabolic enzymes
   A. Competition for binding to metabolizing enzyme
   B. Induction of increased levels of metabolizing enzyme
   C. Inactivation of metabolizing enzyme(s) (*eg*, inactivation of certain forms of P-450 enzymes by erythromycin or chloramphenicol)
III. Excretion process
IV. Organ or tissues where action, metabolism, and excretion occur (*eg*, one drug exists that alters the blood flow to liver, which in turn results in altered metabolism of a second drug)

The first of the interactions at the metabolizing enzyme site involves a direct competition for binding of the drugs at the enzyme responsible for their inactivation. In this situation, the two drugs simply act as competitive inhibitors, each decreasing the extent of metabolism of the other. The degree of inhibition of each drug is influenced by its concentration at the enzyme site in relation to its respective Michaelis constant (K_m). The drug having the higher ratio between the concentration at the enzyme site and the K_m value produces the greater inhibitory effect. Inhibition of the metabolism of one or both drugs can lead to toxic manifestations, resulting in potentially serious or possibly lethal side effects of one or both drugs. (Clinical aspects of drug interactions are discussed further in Chapter 50.)

$$A \xrightarrow{\text{Enzyme}} A_{inact}$$

$$B \xrightarrow{\text{Enzyme}} B_{inact}$$

$$A \xrightarrow{\text{B present}} \text{decrease metabolism of A}$$

$$B \xrightarrow{\text{A present}} \text{decrease metabolism of B}$$

A second mechanism by which drugs can influence each other's metabolism has to do with an important property of the major enzyme system involved in the metabolism of many drugs. As discussed in greater detail in Mixed-Function Oxidase Enzyme System (Phase I Metabolism), many drugs are metabolized by the mixed-function oxidase enzyme system. This enzyme system is unique because exposure to one drug can result in an increase in the levels of the mixed-function oxidase within the liver, *ie*, *enzyme induction*; this induction results in an increase not only in that drug's metabolism but also in that of other pharmacological agents metabolized by the same enzyme system.

$$\text{Drug} \xrightarrow{\text{Enzyme}} \text{Drug}_{inact}$$

$$\text{Drug} \xRightarrow{\text{Enzyme}} \text{Drug}_{inact} \text{ (increased metabolism)}$$

For example, barbiturates have been shown experimentally to increase their own rate of metabolism and that of a variety of other drugs by a factor of two or three. The induced metabolism has been shown experimentally to be caused by an increased synthesis of the mixed-function oxidase enzyme system. This process of enzyme induction is one of the major mechanisms responsible for the metabolic tolerance that is observed with many drugs.

It is generally accepted that all agents that are metabolized by the mixed-function oxidase also are capable of inducing this enzyme. However, in some cases the toxicity of the inducing agent is greater than that for induction of the enzyme system; therefore, induction is not always observed. Induction of drug metabolism also can occur with the ingestion of certain foods or upon exposure to a variety of environmental agents that are oxidized by the mixed-function oxidase. Thus, the rate at which drugs are inactivated may be influenced and regulated by a variety of environmental factors that ultimately affect the levels of this enzyme *in vivo*.

The physiological consequence of these two types of drug interaction are of course different. Direct competitive

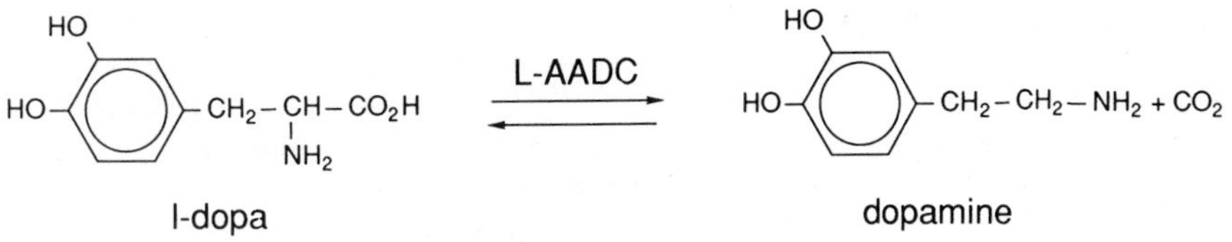

FIGURE 4–1

inhibition of drugs can result in elevated concentrations of either of the two agents, potentially leading to drug toxicity or side effects. In direct contrast, drug induction of the mixed-function oxidase enzyme system can result in the increased metabolism of drugs, thus decreasing the duration of drug action as well as the concentration of the drug required to produce a therapeutic response.

In addition, many other factors may influence drug interactions in drug metabolism; some of these factors include changes in liver blood flow and other alterations, such as inactivation, of the metabolizing enzymes.

• Drug Activation

In the preceding discussion, drug metabolism is represented as a necessary process required for the termination of the action of drugs. Although this is true for the majority of drugs used clinically, in certain instances metabolism can actually lead to a more pharmacologically active molecular species, *ie*, **drug activation**. The exploitation of drug activation is one of the newer approaches in therapeutics to maximize drug efficacy through the selective generation of pharmacologically active metabolites at specific target sites *in vivo*. A variety of methods have been employed to produce this selectivity, including the regulation of drug transport and the selective metabolism of drugs by enzymes localized in specific cells in the body.

An example of drug activation is provided by the drug levodopa for treatment of the symptoms of Parkinson's disease. This disorder is characterized biochemically by a degeneration of the dopaminergic nerve tracts that lead from the substantia nigra to the striatum, which results in an insufficient production of dopamine in the dopaminergic nerve terminals in the striatum. The neurotransmitter itself, dopamine, cannot be administered directly to these patients because of the serious side effects it would produce in the periphery and also because it cannot cross the blood-brain barrier. In addition, it would be rapidly inactivated by monoamine oxidase and catechol-*O*-methyltransferase in the periphery. Thus, the amino acid precursor of dopamine, L-dihydroxyphenylethylamine (levodopa), was developed as a treatment for Parkinson's disease. Levodopa is transported across the blood-brain barrier into the brain, where it is taken up into the dopaminergic neurons and decarboxylated by the enzyme L-aromatic amino acid decarboxylase (L-AADC) to form dopamine, as illustrated in Figure 4–1. In this instance, the agent levodopa can be referred to as a *prodrug*. (See also Chapter 21.)

• Drug Toxicity and Side Effects

As described previously, it is generally assumed that metabolism of drugs and other xenobiotics results in their detoxification. In other words, for most drugs, metabolism results in the formation of biochemically inactive products that are usually more hydrophilic and thus are more readily excreted in the urine. However, metabolism of certain drugs and xenobiotics, instead of leading to the formation of inactive compounds, in fact leads to the formation of toxic and even carcinogenic catabolites. The toxicity or carcinogenicity usually results from the formation of highly reactive intermediates that are capable of reacting with specific cellular components to produce their toxic effects. Examples of this process include halothane (Chapter 11) and 3,4-benzpyrene (Chapter 47).

For example, the widely used anesthetic agent halothane can cause hepatitis and subsequent death in appropriately sensitized individuals. It is believed that during the degradation of halothane, a reactive free radical is produced that can bind to specific sites within the liver and thereupon act as a hapten. The hapten stimulates the production of antibodies, which precipitates subsequent exposure to halothane hepatitis in susceptible individuals. The frequency of halothane hepatitis increases with an increased number of exposures to halothane (Fig. 4–2).

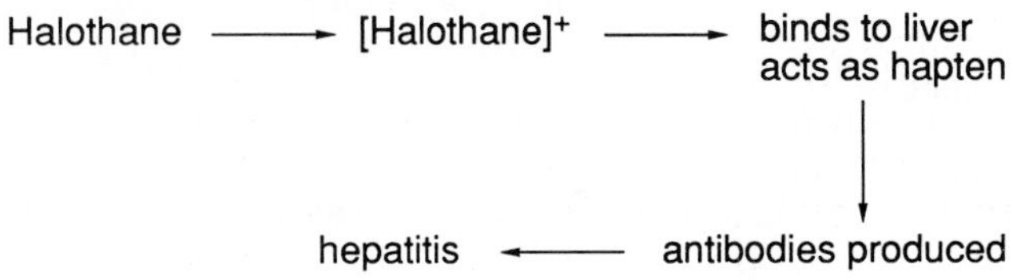

FIGURE 4–2

Another important example whereby drug metabolism leads to toxicity involves the carcinogenic polycyclic aromatic hydrocarbons, such as 3,4-benzpyrene. As illustrated in Figure 4–3, 3,4-benzpyrene is metabolized to a highly reactive epoxide intermediate that has been shown to be an active carcinogenic agent. This reactive intermediate is presumed to be capable of forming adducts with DNA within the nucleus, thus leading to the production of tumors.

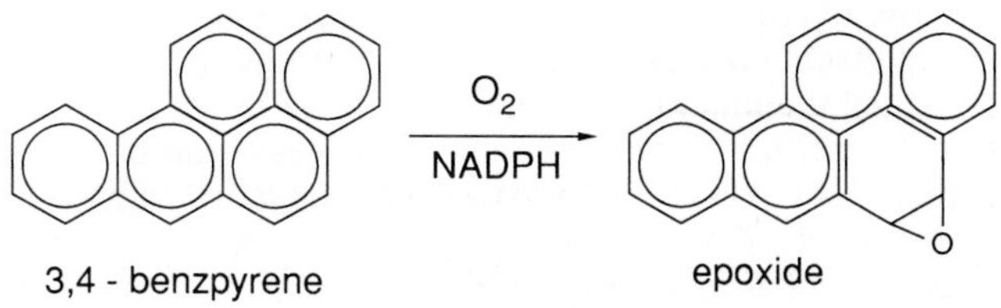

FIGURE 4–3

There are also examples in which the formation of toxic metabolites may be of practical importance and beneficial to humans. The pesticide parathion is metabolized within the liver to form the potent and toxic acetylcholinesterase inhibitor paraoxon (Fig. 4–4). Paraoxon in humans is hydro-

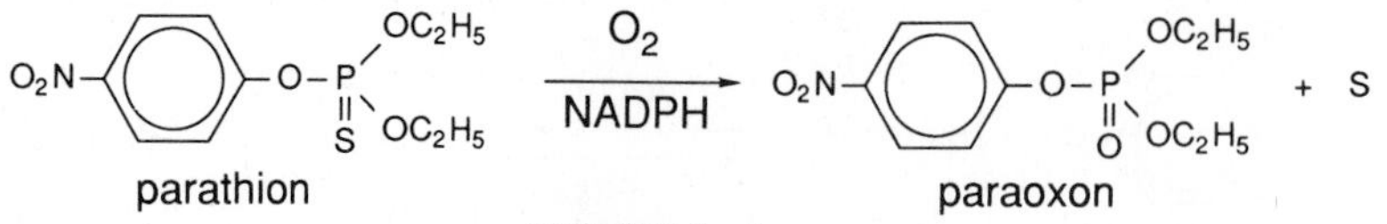

$O_2N-C_6H_4-O-P(=S)(OC_2H_5)_2 \xrightarrow[NADPH]{O_2} O_2N-C_6H_4-O-P(=O)(OC_2H_5)_2 + S$

parathion → paraoxon

FIGURE 4–4

lyzed rapidly to inactive catabolites by a variety of esterases. In general, insects lack these detoxifying esterases; therefore, toxic levels of paraoxon build up within the insects. These selective detoxifying reactions within humans permit these compounds to be effectively employed as selective toxins of insects.

PATHWAYS OF DRUG METABOLISM

> **BOX 4–2**
> **DRUG METABOLISM**
>
> 1. Major pathways and reactions involved in drug metabolism
> 2. The tissues in which these reactions take place
> 3. The enzymes catalyzing these reactions
> 4. Major factors regulating activity of drug-metabolizing enzymes

As a practical approach to studying and classifying the enzymatic pathways involved in drug metabolism, it has proved useful to divide the degradative processes into two separate stages or phases.

Drug $\xrightarrow{\text{Phase I}}$ introduction of polar group $\xrightarrow{\text{Phase II}}$ conjugation of polar group

Phase I involves the oxidation of the drug and is catalyzed by the *mixed-function oxidase enzyme system.* The mixed-function oxidase system is considered to be a principal drug-metabolizing enzyme system in the body because it has a broad substrate specificity (*ie,* it catalyzes the oxidation of a wide variety of substances) and, in addition, can catalyze a variety of reactions. As is discussed in Mixed-Function Oxidase Enzyme System (Phase I Metabolism), multiple forms of the mixed-function oxidase exist, each of which possesses unique but overlapping substrate specificity. The reactions catalyzed by this enzyme system increase the hydrophilicity (water solubility) of drugs and thus facilitate their elimination by the kidney.

Phase II of drug metabolism involves a number of enzymes that catalyze the formation of conjugates with the oxidized drug. The enzymes catalyzing these reactions are classified as *transferases,* and in all cases, the conjugates that are produced are ionized at physiological pH. A variety of transferases exist, including the *glucuronyl transferases, sulfotransferases, and glutathione transferases, as well as several specific amino acid transferases.*

The Phase II conjugation of drugs leads ultimately to the generation of highly water-soluble, ionic compounds, which are readily excreted in the urine or bile.

Therefore, the net effect of Phases I and II is the conversion of lipid-soluble drugs to ionically charged, water-soluble agents that are removed efficiently from the body.

• Mixed-Function Oxidase Enzyme System (Phase I Metabolism)

As noted in the previous section, the mixed-function oxidase system is considered the major enzyme system responsible for the metabolism of drugs and other xenobiotics. High levels of the mixed-function oxidase are present in the liver, which is quantitatively a major site of drug metabolism. However, this enzyme is present in almost all organs except muscle or fat; thus, drug metabolism can occur throughout the body. Noteworthy are the high concentrations of mixed-function oxidase in the gastrointestinal mucosa, lungs, skin, and kidneys.

In liver cells, the mixed-function oxidase is present predominantly in the smooth endoplasmic reticulum, although activity also is associated with the rough endoplasmic reticulum. The enzyme system has been purified, and three distinct components have been isolated: reduced nicotinamide-adenine dinucleotide phosphate (NADPH)–dependent cytochrome *c* reductase (cytochrome P-450 reductase), cytochrome P-450, and a phospholipid.

As illustrated in Figure 4–5, the first component, cytochrome P-450 reductase, catalyzes the initial transfer of an electron from NADPH to cytochrome P-450. The enzyme has an absolute requirement for NADPH and requires Mg^{2+} for activity. The enzyme contains one molecule each of flavin adenine dinucleotide (FAD) and flavin mononucleotide as cofactors. This reductase donates two electrons sequentially to cytochrome P-450, the first of which reduces the heme iron (Fe^{3+}) to the ferrous form (Fe^{2+}), and the second of which reduces oxygen to the superoxide anion ($Fe^{2+} \cdot O_2$ to $Fe^{2+} \cdot O_2^-$).

The second component, cytochrome P-450, is the terminal electron acceptor and the binding site of drugs. Cytochrome P-450 is actually a generic term that denotes a family of cytochromes that are immunologically and biochemically distinct, although all accept an electron from NADPH cytochrome *c* reductase. Specific antibodies have

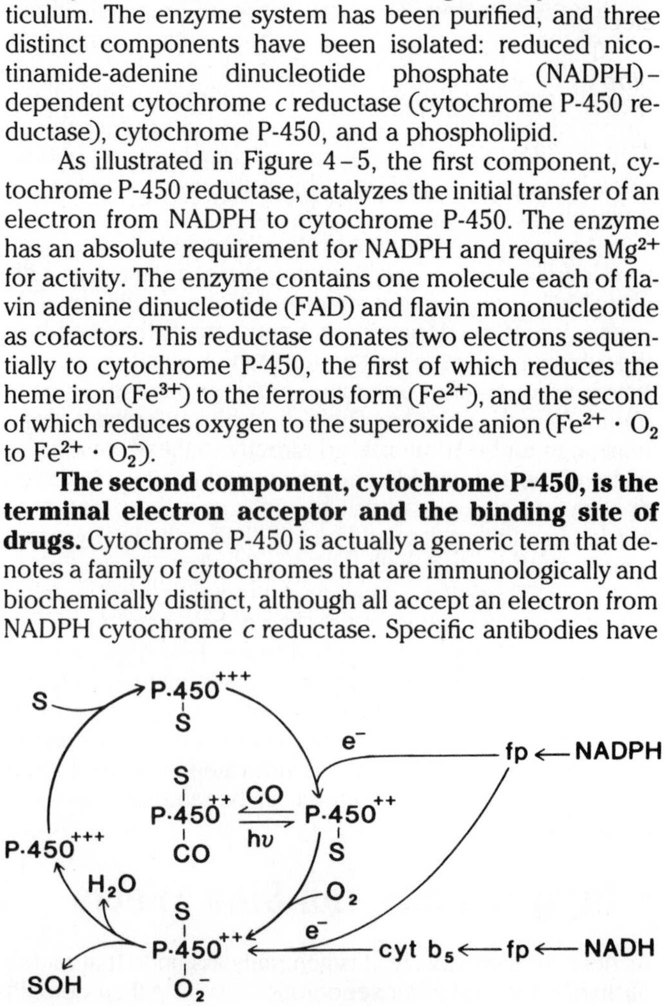

FIGURE 4–5

been raised to the different forms of cytochrome P-450, demonstrating specific structural differences between the different species of this cytochrome. Over 100 different species of the cytochrome have been identified to date, with some 20 to 30 thought to be present in the human liver. The unique substrate specificities of the different forms of cytochrome P-450 are imparted by the structure of the apoprotein. The cytochromes contain iron that is chelated to a porphyrin ring system identical to that of hemoglobin, protoporphyrin IX. Because sex steroid hormones have been shown to induce different forms of this cytochrome, males and females possess different ratios of several cytochrome P-450 species. (Selective induction of specific forms of cytochrome P-450 with various drugs and other exogenous agents has been used in the purification and characterization of the different species of this cytochrome.)

The last essential component of the mixed-function oxidase system is a phospholipid that is required to act as a membrane surface to allow for the exchange of electrons from the reductase to the iron of the cytochrome.

The second electron that oxidizes oxygen to the superoxide anion also can come from cytochrome b_5 and cytochrome b_5 reductase, a reduced nicotinamide-adenine dinucleotide (NADH)-specific reductase (Fig. 4-5). Under conditions in which NADPH is limiting, it is believed that the second electron can be donated by the cytochrome b_5 system. This latter enzyme system cannot take the place of NADPH cytochrome *c* reductase as a donor of the first electron.

The reduced cytochrome is capable of complexing *in vitro* with carbon monoxide, resulting in a complex that absorbs light at approximately 450 nm. The wavelength for the absorbance of light observed is specific for the different forms of P-450 and normally varies between 447 and 453 nm. (Because carbon monoxide is capable of binding *in vitro* to the reduced cytochrome, it can act as a potent inhibitor of the mixed-function oxidase; this interaction often is used to determine experimentally whether a drug is oxidized by this enzyme system.)

Reactions Catalyzed by the Mixed-Function Oxidase System

The mixed-function oxidase system is a relatively unique enzyme system in that it can catalyze the oxidation of a variety of types of substrates.

1. Aromatic ring hydroxylation
The example given (Fig. 4-6) is for the oxidation of benzene to phenol. Almost all drugs or xenobiotics that contain an aromatic ring system undergo ring hydroxylation. In some cases, hydroxylation can occur on a given aromatic ring at more than one site.

> **BOX 4-3**
> **REACTIONS CATALYZED BY MIXED-FUNCTION OXIDASE**
>
> 1. Aromatic ring hydroxylation
> 2. Side-chain hydroxylation
> 3. *N*-dealkylation
> 4. *O*-dealkylation
> 5. *S*-dealkylation
> 6. Sulfoxidation
> 7. Desulfuration
> 8. Deamination
> 9. Dehalogenation

Ring hydroxylation may or may not lead to the total inactivation of the drug.

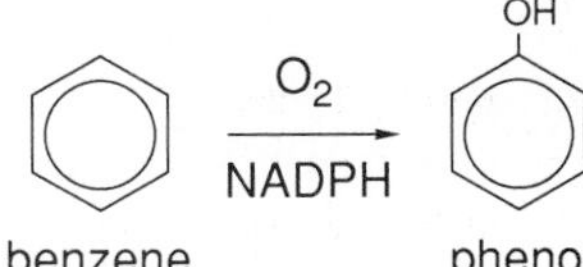

FIGURE 4-6

2. Side-chain hydroxylation
The example presented in Figure 4-7 is for the side-chain hydroxylation of pentobarbital. In general, side-chain hydroxylation occurs less frequently than ring hydroxylation, although when it does occur, it often results in the inactivation of the parent drug.

3. *N*-dealkylation
Figure 4-8 presents the *N*-demethylation of the antidepressant drug imipramine. In this case, the tertiary amine is demethylated to form the secondary amine along with production of one molecule of formaldehyde. *N*-dealkylation reactions are relatively common, in that numerous other drugs that contain a tertiary or secondary amine also undergo *N*-dealkylation reactions. Other examples of drugs undergoing *N*-dealkylation reactions include several of the phenothiazine antipsychotic and tricyclic antidepressant agents, diazepam (VALIUM), and *N*-substituted barbiturates. *N*-dealkylation does not necessarily result in the inactivation of the parent drug because the product may have either more or less pharmacological activity than the parent agent.

4. *O*-dealkylation
This reaction is similar to that for *N*-dealkylation but in this case involves the oxidation of an ether. The

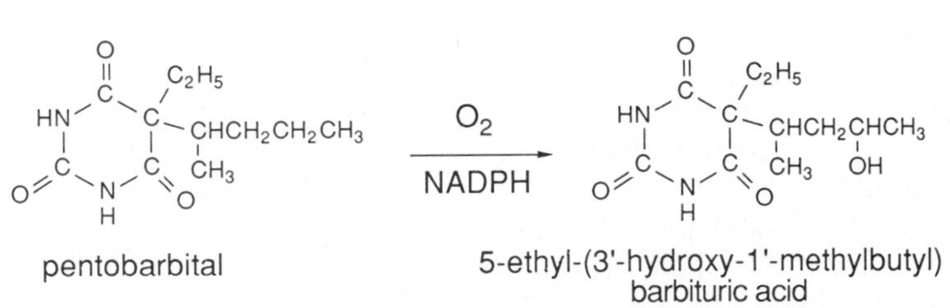

pentobarbital $\xrightarrow[\text{NADPH}]{O_2}$ 5-ethyl-(3'-hydroxy-1'-methylbutyl) barbituric acid

FIGURE 4-7

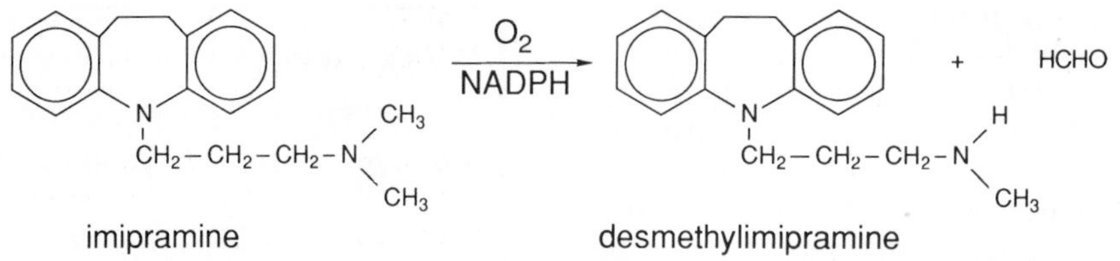

imipramine → (O_2, NADPH) → desmethylimipramine + HCHO

FIGURE 4–8

example given in Figure 4 – 9 is for the drug codeine. This example illustrates drug activation because the reaction results in a metabolite, morphine, that is ten times more potent than codeine itself (see Chapter 14).

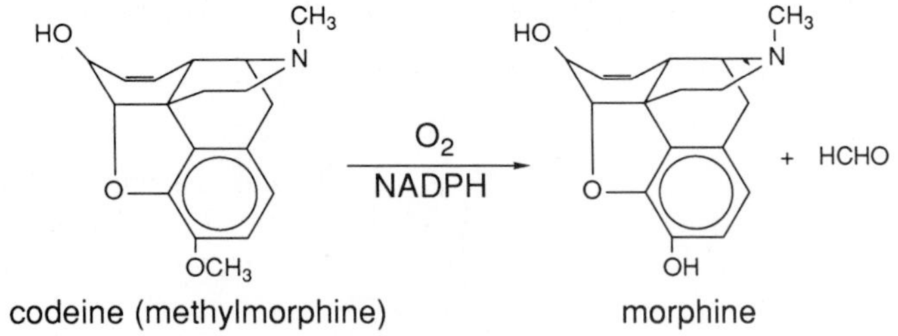

codeine (methylmorphine) → (O_2, NADPH) → morphine + HCHO

FIGURE 4–9

5. **S-dealkylation**

The reaction shown in Figure 4 – 10 is for the drug 6-methylthiopurine. This reaction results in the activation of this drug to the pharmacologically active form.

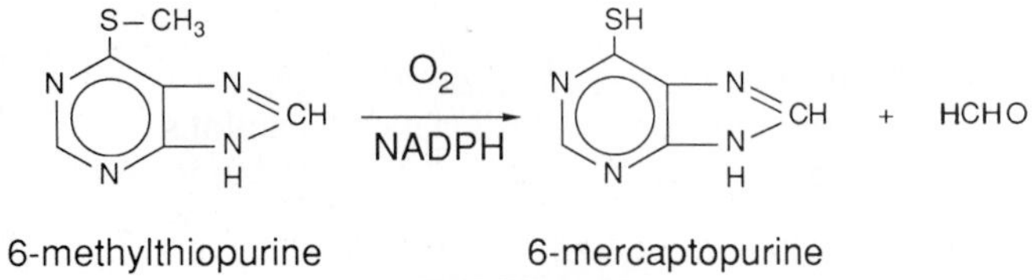

6-methylthiopurine → (O_2, NADPH) → 6-mercaptopurine + HCHO

FIGURE 4–10

6. **Sulfoxidation**

Many drugs that contain a thioether linkage can undergo oxidation to form the sulfoxide. As illustrated in Figure 4 – 11, the phenothiazines undergo sulfoxidation to form the inactive catabolite. Formation of the sulfoxide of the vitamin biotin can also be catalyzed by the mixed-function oxidase enzyme system.

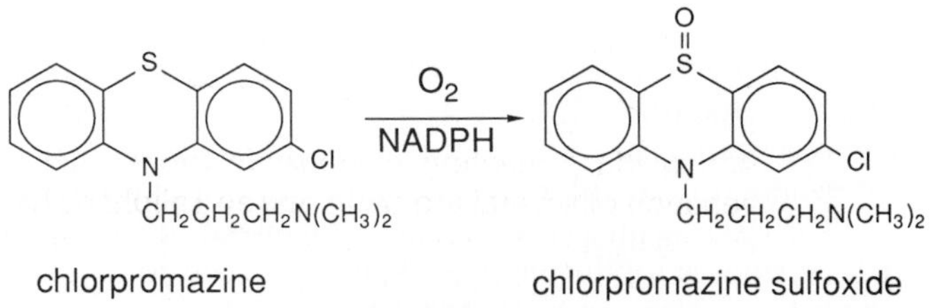

chlorpromazine → (O_2, NADPH) → chlorpromazine sulfoxide

FIGURE 4–11

7. **Desulfuration**

The example of desulfuration presented in Figure 4 – 12 is for the short-acting barbiturate thiopental. For the thiobarbiturates, desulfuration does not result in inactivation of the parent drug but leads to production of the oxy-derivative, which possesses lower pharmacological activity. As illustrated in Figure 4 – 4, parathion also undergoes a desulfuration reaction. Desulfuration of parathion leads to the formation of the acetylcholinesterase inhibitor paraoxon.

8. **Deamination**

A number of enzymes catalyze the deamination of endogenous and exogenous amines. These include monoamine oxidase (MAO), diamine oxidase (DAO), plasma amine oxidase, and the mixed-function oxidase. MAO, as well as plasma amine oxidase, catalyzes the deamination of biogenic amines and structurally related monoamine drugs, whereas DAO is specific for compounds containing diamines such as cadaverine and spermine (discussed in Deamination on p. 35). The mixed-function oxidase system is responsible primarily for the deamination of sympathomimetic amines that contain a methyl group on the carbon atom adjacent to the primary amine, as shown in Figure 4 – 13 for amphetamine.

Amphetamine is a structural analog of phenylethylamine, a compound that is readily deaminated by MAO. The presence of the methyl group on phenylethylamine causes this compound to cease to be a substrate for MAO; thus, its deamination occurs

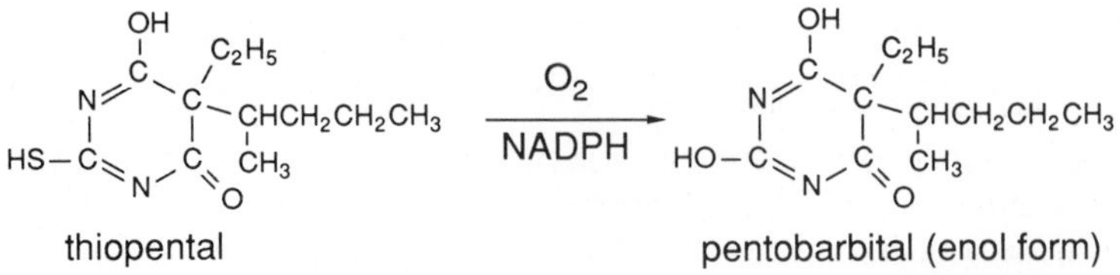

thiopental → (O_2, NADPH) → pentobarbital (enol form)

FIGURE 4–12

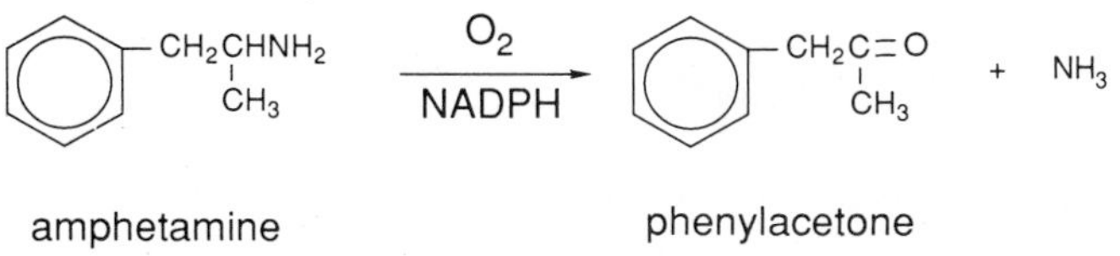

amphetamine → (O_2, NADPH) → phenylacetone + NH_3

FIGURE 4-13

exclusively through the mixed-function oxidase. This latter reaction is a slow reaction compared with the deamination of phenylethylamine by MAO.

9. **Dehalogenation**
There are a number of enzymes responsible for the dehalogenation of drugs *in vivo*. The mixed-function oxidase reaction responsible for the dehalogenation of several aromatic ring and aliphatic halogens is illustrated in Figure 4-14 for the anesthetic agent halothane (dehalogenation of aromatic hydrocarbons does occur, but is uncommon). Halothane undergoes a dehalogenation reaction that leads to the production of an unstable free radical intermediate. The majority of this intermediate is converted into trifluoroacetaldehyde and, subsequently, trifluoroacetic acid. However, a small percentage of the free radical binds to components within the liver and acts as the hapten, which ultimately can lead to hepatitis or subsequent exposure to halothane, as was mentioned in Drug Toxicity and Side Effects.

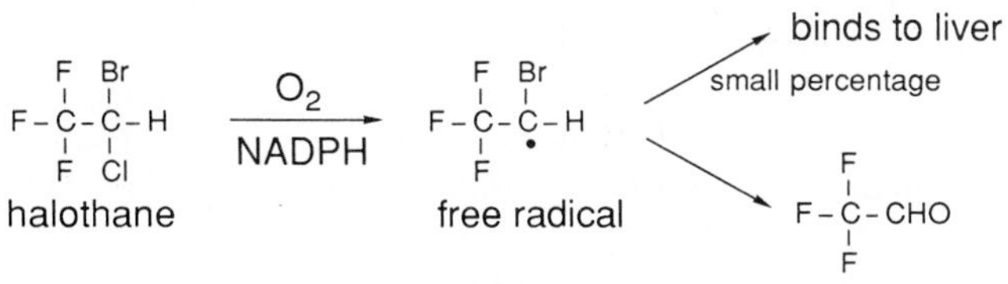

halothane → (O_2, NADPH) → free radical → binds to liver (small percentage); → F-C(F)(F)-CHO

FIGURE 4-14

Factors Regulating the Mixed-Function Oxidase System

As indicated earlier, drug metabolism may influence the pharmacological activity, toxicity, and duration of action of drugs. Therefore, it is important to understand the factors that may potentially regulate mixed-function oxidase activity *in vivo*.

• **ENZYME INDUCTION.** The mixed-function oxidase is an inducible enzyme system; exposure to a drug or a variety of other endogenous or exogenous agents (such as tobacco smoke, alcohol, and environmental toxins) has the potential to promote an increase in enzyme activity. Any one compound selectively induces the formation of specific forms of the cytochrome P-450, each of which possess unique substrate specificities. Induction of mixed-function oxidase activity involves the increased synthesis of several different forms of the cytochrome (Table 4-2).

Induction of a mixed-function oxidase activity may involve not only an increased production of the cytochrome but also an increased production of NADPH-cytochrome P-450 reductase.

TABLE 4-2. Effect of Pretreatment of Rabbits With Phenobarbital and 3-Methylcholanthrene

Substrate	Pretreatment	Enzyme Activity (μmol/mg protein/hour)
Hexobarbital	Control	0.69
	PB	1.21
	3-MC	0.27
3,4-Benzpyrene	Control	0.19
	PB	0.21
	3-MC	0.34
Aminopyrine	Control	1.07
	PB	3.40
	3-MC	1.38

From Gram TE, Rogers LA, Fouts JR: Effect of pretreatment of rabbits with phenobarbital or 3-methylcholanthrene on the distribution of drug-metabolizing enzyme activity in subfractions of hepatic microsomes. J Pharmacol Exp Ther 157:435-437, 1967,© by American Society for Pharmacology and Experimental Therapeutics.

*3-MC = 3-methylcholanthrene; PB = phenobarbital.

In addition to inhibition, the P-450 oxidase activity can be depressed by competitive inhibitors, by suicide substrates, and by any condition that impairs liver or other organ function.

• **AGE.** The specific activity of liver mixed-function oxidase normally reaches adult levels within 3-8 weeks after birth. The liver of the human fetus contains appreciable mixed-function oxidase activity and thus is capable of oxidizing a variety of drugs that cross the placental membranes.

There is also evidence suggesting that hepatic mixed-function oxidase activity is decreased in the geriatric population, thus accounting, in part, for the increased half-life of some drugs observed in older people (see Chapter 58).

• **SEX.** Differences in mixed-function oxidase activity in females and males have been observed in experimental rat studies but not in humans, illustrating one of the major problems in research in this area — the differences between human and experimental animal biochemistry.

• **GENETIC DIFFERENCES.** The most important factor regulating mixed-function oxidase activity, as well as other drug metabolism systems, is the genetic variation in the human population; these differences are one of the major factors that give rise to the wide variability among individuals in their responses to drugs and in the levels of drugs found in the body after acute, and especially chronic, dosing. The important general topic of pharmacogenetics is presented in Chapter 59.

• Conjugation Reactions (Phase II Metabolism)

Phase II of the drug-metabolizing enzyme system consists of a variety of enzymatic reactions, all of which involve conjugation of either the parent or the oxidized drug. Examples follow. For most drugs, these conjugation reactions represent important processes involved in their inactivation.

Glucuronide Conjugation

Formation of the glucuronide conjugate represents one of the major degradative processes involved in drug detoxifi-

α-D-glucose 1-phosphate + UTP → UDP-α-D-glucose (UDPG) + pyrophosphate

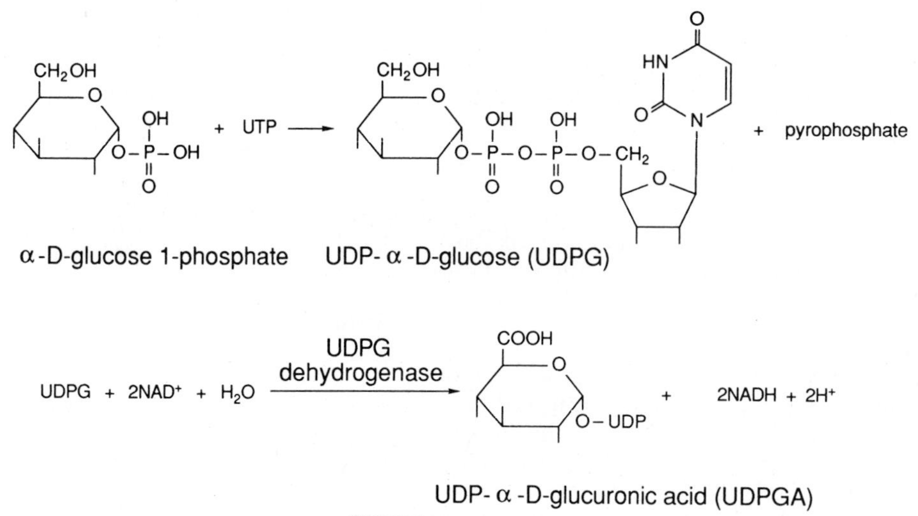

UDPG + 2NAD⁺ + H_2O —(UDPG dehydrogenase)→ UDP-α-D-glucuronic acid (UDPGA) + 2NADH + 2H⁺

FIGURE 4–15

cation and inactivation. The reactions involved in synthesis of the glucuronide donor uridine diphosphate–glucuronic acid are presented in Figure 4–15.

Uridine diphosphate–glucuronic acid transferase represents a family of enzymes that is located in the endoplasmic reticulum of the cell. Like the mixed-function oxidase, this transferase is inducible upon exposure to certain drugs. These enzymes can catalyze the conjugation of hydroxy groups, sulfhydryl groups, primary amines, and carboxylic acids. The end product of these reactions is the formation of the ionized glucuronide drug conjugate (Fig. 4–16). (Although most glucuronide conjugates are less active than the parent compound, some, such as the morphine-6-glucuronide conjugate discussed in Chapter 14, are more active than the parent drug and contribute to the pharmacological effects of the parent agent—in this example, morphine itself.)

Sulfate Conjugation

Sulfate conjugation and glucuronide conjugation are the two major Phase II conjugation reactions. The enzymatic steps involved in sulfate conjugation are presented in Figure 4–17.

The first step in the reaction catalyzed by the enzyme sulfurylase thermodynamically favors the reverse reaction. However, this reaction proceeds in the forward direction because the enzyme is coupled to adenosine-5′-phosphosulfate (APS)-kinase, which subsequently converts APS to the sulfate donor 3′-phosphoadenosine-5′-phosphosulfate (PAPS). In addition, a number of pyrophosphatases are present that rapidly break down inorganic pyrophosphate formed by the sulfurylase reaction and thus prevent the reverse reaction from occurring.

Similar to the glucuronide transferases, the sulfotransferases also represent a family of enzymes. More recent studies have identified two functionally distinct forms of phenol sulfotransferase that possess distinct but overlapping substrate specificity. These enzymes are involved in the conjugation of a wide variety of drugs and other xenobiotics. Sulfoconjugation can occur on both phenolic compounds and aromatic amines. The end product of these reactions is the ionized sulfate ester of the drug.

A variety of other sulfotransferases have been identified that appear to selectively cause the sulfate conjugation in steroids. These steroid sulfotransferases also utilize PAPS as the sulfate donor.

In general, both glucuronide and sulfate conjugation result in the formation of a biologically inert catabolite. Although this is usually the case for most drugs, in several instances conjugation has been reported to promote the biological response of drugs and other agents. For example, morphine was mentioned previously; another example involves the sulfate ester of minoxidil produced *in vivo*, which appears to be the active form of the drug, in that minoxidil sulfate is both an antihypertensive agent and a hair growth–promoting factor. Similarly, the sulfate conjugates of *N*-hydroxy-2-acetylaminofluorene and structurally related compounds have been reported to be potent carcinogens (Fig. 4–18). In the absence of formation of the sulfate ester within the cell, these unconjugated compounds have been shown to be noncarcinogenic.

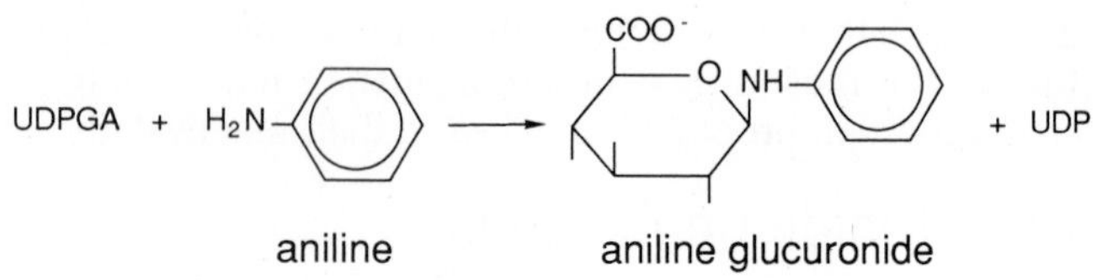

UDPGA + aniline → aniline glucuronide + UDP

FIGURE 4–16

Other Conjugation Reactions

A variety of other compounds are also capable of serving as esterifying agents for a variety of drugs. These conjugating substrates include glutathione and a variety of amino acids. In most cases, the conjugate that is formed is ionized at physiological pH, thus assuring that the esterified drug or other exogenous agent will be excreted rapidly by the kidney.

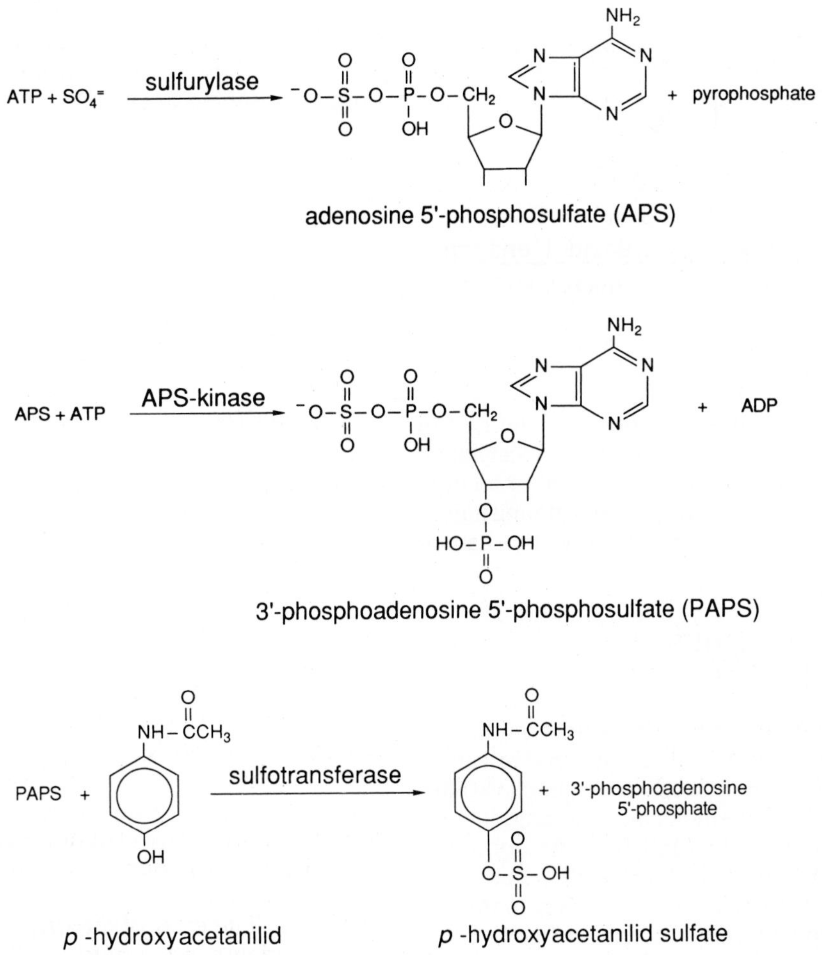

ATP + $SO_4^{=}$ —sulfurylase→ adenosine 5'-phosphosulfate (APS) + pyrophosphate

APS + ATP —APS-kinase→ 3'-phosphoadenosine 5'-phosphosulfate (PAPS) + ADP

PAPS + p-hydroxyacetanilid —sulfotransferase→ p-hydroxyacetanilid sulfate + 3'-phosphoadenosine 5'-phosphate

FIGURE 4–17

• Other Pathways Involved in Drug Metabolism

Acetylation

Aromatic amines and hydrazines undergo acetylation reactions. The reaction is catalyzed by the enzyme *N*-acetyltransferase, which proceeds by a double-displacement (ping-pong) reaction mechanism, as illustrated for isoniazid (Fig. 4–19).

In the human population, the enzyme displays genetic polymorphism and can be divided into "fast" and "slow" acetylators. The half-life of the reaction for isoniazid in fast acetylators is approximately 70 minutes, whereas in the slow acetylators, this value is longer than 3 hours (Fig. 4–19). The difference is the result of variants in the isozymes present in the liver in the different populations. From a genetic standpoint, fast acetylation is an autosomal dominant trait. In the United States, the distribution between the two groups is about 50:50. In general, Eskimos are fast acetylators, whereas Jews and white North Africans are slow acetylators.

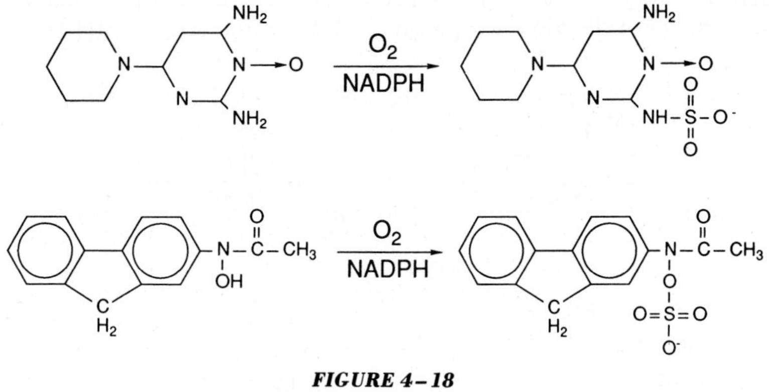

O_2, NADPH

O_2, NADPH

FIGURE 4–18

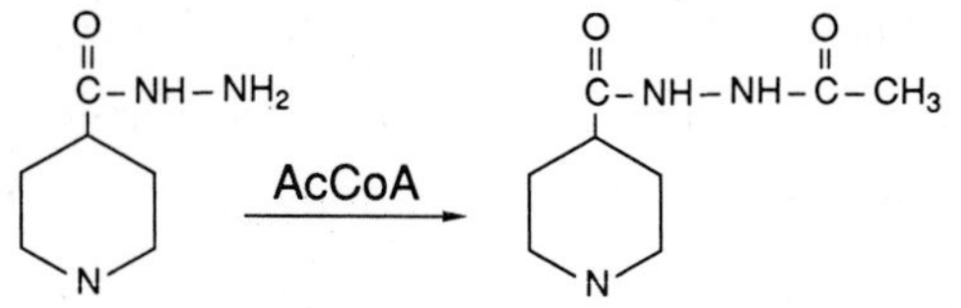

AcCoA

enzyme + AcCoA ⇌ Ac-enzyme + CoA
Ac-enzyme + isoniazid ⇌ Ac-isoniazid + enzyme
AcCoA + isoniazid $\xrightarrow{\text{enzyme}}$ Ac-isoniazid + CoA

FIGURE 4–19

Because of the rather large differences in the rate of degradation of drugs between the fast- and slow-acetylating populations, it may be important to know whether an individual patient is a fast or slow acetylator. The administration of the dose prescribed normally for fast acetylators can be toxic if given to slow acetylators.

Transulfuration Reactions (Detoxification of CN^-)

Two reactions are important in the detoxification of CN^-. The first, as illustrated in Figure 4–20, is catalyzed by a mitochondrial sulfotransferase (rhodanase; transulfuralase) that utilizes thiosulfate as the donor molecule. The second reaction utilizes *β*-mercaptopyruvic acid as the sulfur donor and is catalyzed by a cytosolic sulfotransferase. Either thiosulfate or *β*-mercaptopyruvic acid can be used clinically to treat individuals exposed to toxic levels of cyanide (Fig. 4–20).

CN^- (cyanide) + $S_2O_3^{2-}$ (thiosulfate) → CNS^- (thiocyanate) + SO_3^{2-} (sulfite)

CN^- + $HS-CH_2-C(=O)-COOH$ (β-mercaptopyruvic acid) → CNS^- + $CH_3-C(=O)-COOH$ (pyruvic acid)

FIGURE 4–20

O-, *N*-, and *S*-Methylation Reactions

A variety of methyltransferases exist that are capable of methylating hydroxyl, amine, or free sulfhydryl groups on drugs and other xenobiotics. These methyltransferases utilize *S*-adenosylmethionine as the methyl donor. An example of *O*-methylation by the enzyme catechol-*O*-methyltransferase is presented in Figure 4–21.

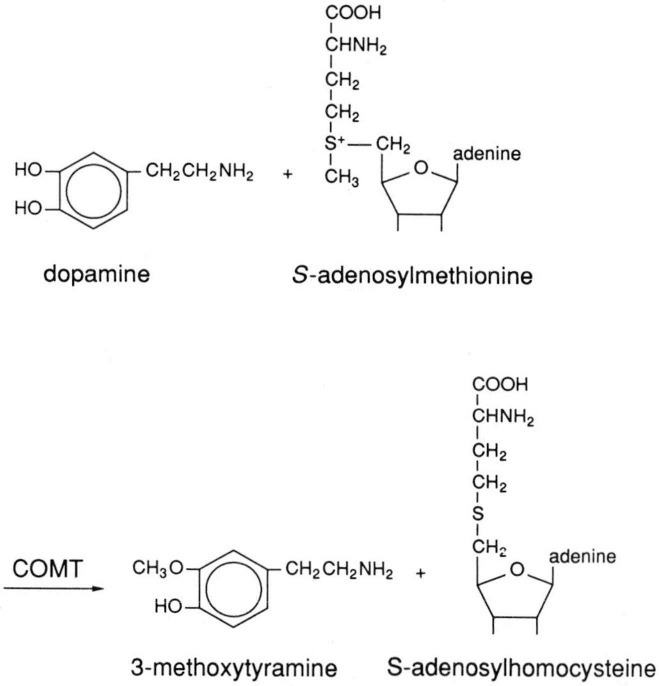

dopamine + *S*-adenosylmethionine $\xrightarrow{\text{COMT}}$ 3-methoxytyramine + S-adenosylhomocysteine

FIGURE 4–21

Alcohol and Aldehyde Oxidations

Alcohols and aldehydes are usually oxidized *in vivo* by alcohol dehydrogenase and aldehyde dehydrogenase (see Chapter 48). Both enzymes require nicotinamide-adenine dinucleotide as the cofactor and have a broad substrate specificity. The oxidation of chloral hydrate to trichloroacetic acid is illustrated in Figure 4–22.

Oxidation reactions are also important in the metabolism of aldehydes produced from the deamination of sympathomimetic amines by MAO as well as in the detoxification of ethanol.

Reduction Reactions

Aldehydes also can be reduced to the alcohol by the enzyme aldehyde reductase, which requires NADH. In general, reduction reactions are not as common as oxidation reactions,

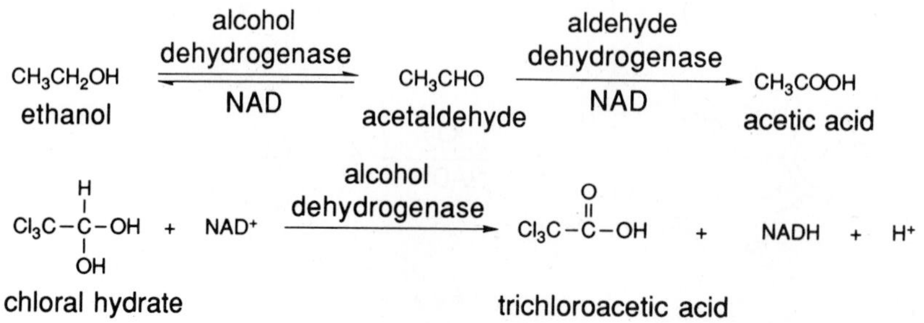

CH_3CH_2OH (ethanol) $\xrightleftharpoons[\text{NAD}]{\text{alcohol dehydrogenase}}$ CH_3CHO (acetaldehyde) $\xrightarrow[\text{NAD}]{\text{aldehyde dehydrogenase}}$ CH_3COOH (acetic acid)

$Cl_3C-CH(OH)-OH$ (chloral hydrate) + NAD^+ $\xrightarrow{\text{alcohol dehydrogenase}}$ $Cl_3C-C(=O)-OH$ (trichloroacetic acid) + NADH + H^+

FIGURE 4–22

although they do occur *in vivo*. For example, the aldehyde product of norepinephrine, 3-methoxy-4-hydroxyphenyl-β-hydroxyacetaldehyde, is preferentially reduced to form 3-methoxy-4-hydroxyphenylglycol in the brain (Fig. 4–23), whereas in the periphery, the major metabolite of this aldehyde is the oxidized acidic product.

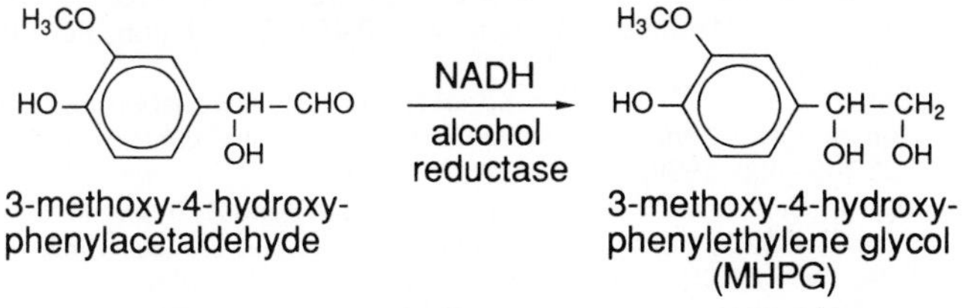

3-methoxy-4-hydroxy-phenylacetaldehyde —NADH, alcohol reductase→ 3-methoxy-4-hydroxy-phenylethylene glycol (MHPG)

FIGURE 4–23

Hydrolysis (Esterases and Amidases)

A variety of substrate-specific and -nonspecific esterases and amidases are present *in vivo* (*eg*, the ester hydrolysis of procaine [Fig. 4–24] and the hydrolysis of succinylcholine [Chapter 8]).

Deamination

As mentioned previously, several enzymes that catalyze the deamination of amines exist. These are MAO, plasma amine oxidase (benzylamine oxidase), DAO, and the mixed-function oxidase. A brief description of the properties and specificities of these enzymes follows.

• **MONOAMINE OXIDASE.** Two forms of MAO, Type A and Type B, are found on the outer mitochondrial membrane (Fig. 4–25). These enzymes have different substrate specificities and are responsible for the deamination of catechol and phenolic amines. The substrate specificities of the two enzymes follow:

Type A MAO	Type B MAO
Norepinephrine	Norepinephrine
Dopamine	Dopamine
Tyramine	Tyramine
5-Hydroxytryptamine	Phenylethylamine

The MAO enzyme is somewhat unique in that the apoenzyme is bound covalently to the 8-methyl group of FAD by a thioether linkage. In the brain, the A form is localized to neurons, whereas the B form predominates in astroglia (with the exception of B MAO in some serotonergic neurons). Studies have identified several human subjects with Norrie's disease in whom the genes for both MAO A and MAO B are deleted. These studies suggest that the genes that code for the two species of MAO are located near each other. As discussed in Chapter 24, inhibitors of MAO were the first class of drugs used clinically to treat depression. The drugs that are used clinically are irreversible nonselective inhibitors of both forms of the oxidase.

• **PLASMA AMINE OXIDASE (BENZYLAMINE OXIDASE).** The function of plasma amine oxidase is unknown, although it has a substrate specificity similar to that of the B form of MAO. It is a soluble enzyme and is found predominantly in the plasma and in the blood vessel walls. There is some debate as to whether this enzyme contains pyridoxal phosphate as a cofactor. The rate of deamination by plasma amine oxidase is extremely slow compared with that of MAO; thus, its role *in vivo* is uncertain.

• **DIAMINE OXIDASE.** As the name implies, DAO is responsible for the deamination of diamines, such as putrescine and cadaverine (Fig. 4–26). The enzyme has an absolute specificity for diamines and does not deaminate

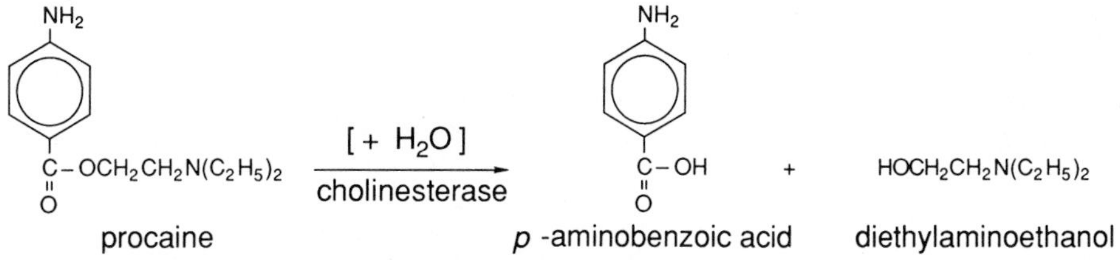

procaine —[+ H_2O], cholinesterase→ *p*-aminobenzoic acid + diethylaminoethanol ($HOCH_2CH_2N(C_2H_5)_2$)

FIGURE 4–24

Type A MAO

5-hydroxytryptamine —O_2, H_2O→ 5-hydroxyindole acetic acid + NH_3 + H_2O_2

Type B MAO

phenylethylamine —O_2, H_2O→ C_6H_5–CH_2–CHO + NH_3 + H_2O_2

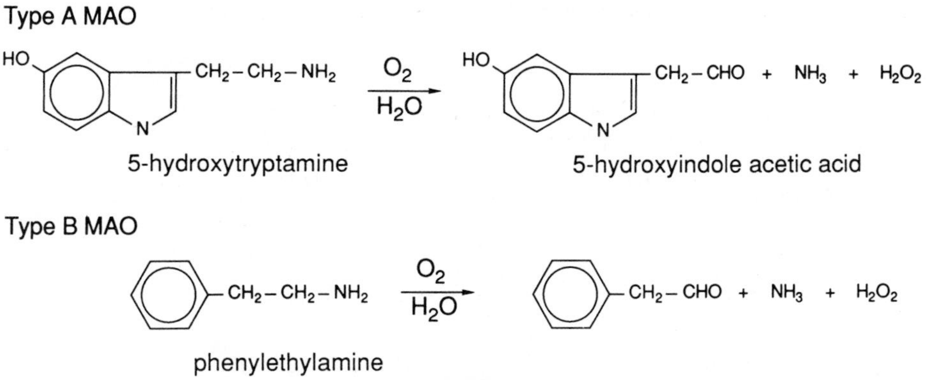

FIGURE 4–25

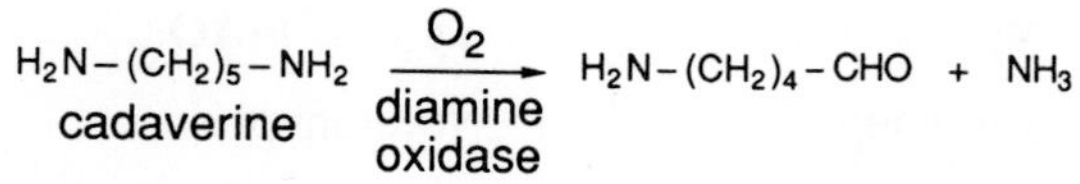

$$H_2N-(CH_2)_5-NH_2 \xrightarrow[\text{diamine oxidase}]{O_2} H_2N-(CH_2)_4-CHO + NH_3$$

cadaverine

FIGURE 4–26

monoamines. The enzyme is soluble and contains FAD as a cofactor.

REFERENCES

Alvares AP, Pratt WB: Pathways of drug metabolism. *In* Pratt WB, Taylor P (eds): Principles of Drug Action: The Basis of Pharmacology, 3rd ed, 365–422, New York: Churchill Livingstone, 1990.

Caldwell J, Davies S, Boots D, O'Gorman J: Interindividual variation in the sulfation and glucuronidation of paracetamol and salicylamide in human volunteers. *In* Mulder GJ, Caldwell J, VanKempen GMS, Vonk RJ (eds): Sulfate Metabolism and Sulfate Conjugation. London: Taylor and Francis, 1982.

Dutton G: Glucuronidation of Drugs and Other Compounds. Boca Raton, FL: CRC Press, 1980.

Guengerich FP: Characterization of human microsomal cytochrome P-450 enzymes. Annu Rev Pharmacol Toxicol 29:241–264, 1989.

Guengerich FP: Mammalian Cytochromes P-450. Boca Raton, FL: CRC Press, 1987.

Kappas A, Alvares AP, Anderson KE, et al: Effect of charcoal-broiled beef on antipyrine and theophylline metabolism. Clin Pharmacol Ther 23:445–450, 1978.

Mulder GJ, Caldwell J, Van Kempen GMJ, Vonk RJ (eds): Sulfate Metabolism and Sulfate Conjugation. London: Taylor and Francis, 1982.

Roth JA: Phenol sulfotransferase. Neuromethods 5:575, 1986

Singer TP, Von Korff RW, Murphy DL: Monoamine Oxidase: Structure, Function, and Altered Functions. New York: Academic Press, 1979.

Pharmacokinetics 5

Paul J. Kostyniak

Pharmacokinetics is a quantitative approach to the behavior of a drug or chemical in the body. (In contrast, **pharmacodynamics** is the quantitative approach to describing the **effects** over time of a drug or chemical in the body.) Mathematical models, based on certain given assumptions and data collected on the absorption, distribution, and excretion of the drug, are used to predict the quantitative pattern and time course of drug disposition in the body.

When one knows the basic mathematical model to which a specific drug conforms after being administered to a patient, the quantitative aspects of drug disposition may be followed over the time course of drug therapy by measurements of drug levels in suitable representative media, such as biological fluids (*eg*, blood, plasma, or cerebrospinal fluid), elimination products (*eg*, urine or feces), or expired air.

Two basic approaches to studying drug and chemical disposition exist: the "simplest model" approach and the "physiologically based modeling" approach. Both approaches can be useful in certain situations.

Traditionally, investigators have strived toward modeling the disposition of drugs and chemicals by applying the simplest mathematical compartmental model that would adequately fit experimentally derived data. The goal of this approach is to use samples from an easily accessible body compartment (*eg*, blood, urine, saliva) as an indicator of therapeutically relevant drug concentrations at specific drug target sites, in an effort to maintain drug levels in a therapeutically effective range without significant toxic side effects. This approach has served the needs of the clinical pharmacologist and physician for some years.

Another approach to pharmacokinetics has gained popularity lately, especially in agencies such as the Environmental Protection Agency that are responsible for the risk assessment necessary in the regulation of human chemical exposures. This approach, termed *physiologically based pharmacokinetic modeling*, strives to model exactly the disposition of chemicals in defined physiologically identifiable *compartments*. In concept it tends toward larger, more complicated mathematical models that predict tissue concentrations within specific organs, tissues, fluids, or cellular compartments. Although this is a more physiologically defined, purist approach that can in fact be of considerable use in risk assessment of chemical exposures, for the physician concerned with effective drug therapy it provides little more clinically useful information than the traditional simplest model approach. Thus, the increased complexity inherent in this more exact approach is not needed to facilitate the understanding of the kinetic behavior of a specific drug within the body. For this reason, the discussion here is limited to the simplest model approach.

FATE OF A DRUG IN THE BODY

• Absorption

The route of administration and the chemical formulation of a drug or chemical determine the amount and rate at which that agent gains access to the systemic circulation. Some drugs and drug formulations or routes of administration ensure that essentially all of the drug will be delivered to the systemic circulation, *ie*, that it has 100% *bioavailability*. Characteristically, drugs that are administered orally or that are modified before entering the circulation have a lower bioavailability, *eg*, only 5% bioavailability would mean that only 5% of the administered dose appears in the systemic circulation.

Once the drug or chemical has been absorbed, it can be modified within the organism into various states, as indicated in Figure 5-1, including:

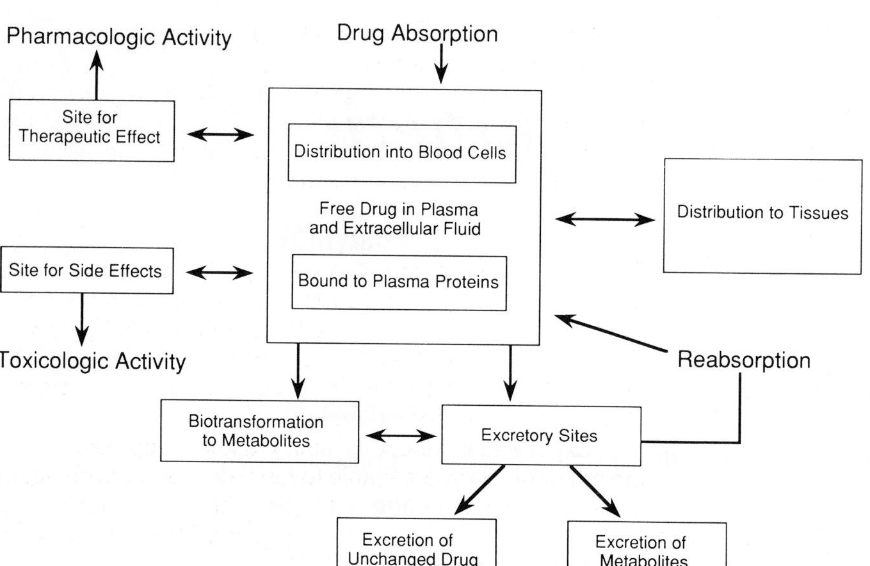

FIGURE 5–1. Possible dispositional changes that drugs and chemicals may undergo within the body.

• Compartmentalization

Compartmentalization is the distribution of a drug or chemical from the administration site into particular compartments. These may be actual physically identifiable compartments or may be mathematically defined entities. Movement of the drug among compartments is a dynamic, ongoing function whereby drug concentrations within a given compartment are constantly changing.

• Metabolism

Metabolism is the chemical or enzymatic transformation of the parent compound into chemically distinct metabolites; these transformations occur at varying rates. The resulting biotransformed metabolites may have greater or lesser activity (therapeutic or toxic) than the parent compound.

• Excretion

Excretion is the appearance of the parent compound or metabolites in elimination products, such as urine, feces, expired air, or hair.

Thus, transformations are occurring constantly from one state of a drug to another. The transformations diagrammed here are generally first-order processes, and the rate at which a particular transformation occurs can be described by a coefficient or rate constant (k). Thus, being first-order, the rate of change from one drug state (A) to another drug state (B) has a direct relation to the quantity or concentration of the substance in the first state (A), or for

$$A \longrightarrow B$$

$$dA/dt = -kA \tag{1}$$

Alternatively, stated directly, the rate of change of A with respect to time is directly proportional to the amount of A present. Similarly, the build-up of product is also a function of the amount of reactant present, or

$$dB/dt = kA \tag{2}$$

Often, the net result of these numerous first-order dispositional patterns is a kinetic profile within a central compartment (blood or plasma) that mimics a first-order process or a series of summed first-order processes. Therefore, this chapter begins by considering a simple one-compartment, first-order kinetic model and builds upon that model in an attempt to provide the tools necessary to understand the kinetic modeling of drugs and chemicals within the body. The step-by-step derivation of the various functions that are used in the modeling approach is given, because an understanding of the origin of the equations is essential in their proper application.

THE ONE-COMPARTMENT OPEN MODEL WITH RAPID INTRAVENOUS INJECTION

The simplest model of drug disposition considered here depicts the body as a single homogeneous compartment with a constant volume (V); this model is diagrammatically illustrated in Figure 5–2. Drug disposition is such a dynamic process that drug concentrations change constantly.

Just as concentration can be related to the absolute amount of solutes in a given chemical solution, the concentration of drug in the body (C) is related to the absolute amount of drug (S) by the relationship

$$C = \frac{S}{V} \tag{3}$$

Therefore, the concentration resulting from a known amount of drug (S) can be easily calculated if the volume of distribution (V) of the drug is known. This relationship is

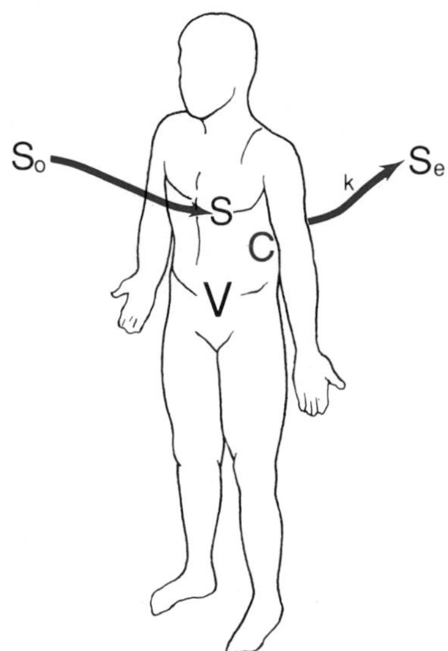

FIGURE 5–2. Diagrammatic representation of the one-compartment first-order kinetic model, where S_0 is the amount of drug injected (dose) at time = 0. It is assumed that there is *instantaneous mixing* throughout the volume of the compartment (V). S is the instantaneous amount of drug in the body at any time (t). C is the instantaneous concentration of drug in the body (*ie*, blood level of drug) at any time (t). S_e is the cumulative amount of drug excreted at any time (t). k is the first-order rate constant of elimination of drug from the body and has the units of $time^{-1}$.

used frequently in pharmacokinetic problem solving. The volume of distribution can be determined easily by measuring the extrapolated blood concentration experimentally (C_0) soon after a bolus dose of the drug (D) is given. Equation 3 then becomes

$$C_0 = \frac{D}{V}$$

where V can be calculated if the dose and concentration of drug are known.

Throughout this chapter, a one-compartment model is assumed for the sake of simplicity. In practice, however, the body consists of many compartments or volumes, some of which may behave as a single compartment; others may differ markedly in the kinetics of a drug's distribution, entry, and leaving. The overall volume of distribution can be derived from knowledge of dose, bioavailability, and concentration in the circulation. Drugs that may be sequestered or tightly bound in large amounts to tissues or to plasma proteins may exhibit a large volume of distribution that may exceed the actual physical volume manyfold.

The rate of change in the absolute amount of drug (S) in the body is described in equation 4:

$$dS/dt = -kS \quad (4)$$

which on rearrangement gives

$$dS/S = -kdt \quad (5)$$

which on integration yields

$$S = S_0e^{-kt} \quad (6)$$

This relationship in equation 6 allows the expected amount of drug (S) in the compartment at any time (t) to be calculated when the dose (S_0) and rate constant for drug elimination (k) are known.

Equation 6 also may be written in terms of concentration of drug (C) in the compartment rather than absolute amount (S). By substituting for S in equation 6 from equation 3, the following equation results:

$$C = C_0e^{-kt} \quad (7)$$

Thus, this equation indicates that a plot of drug concentration against time would produce a first-order exponential decay function with an intercept on the y axis at C_0, as indicated in Figure 5–3. Note that in first-order kinetics, the amount of drug excreted is dependent upon the plasma concentration or *body burden.*

Exponential functions and graphical representations are not particularly amenable to rapid derivation of clinically useful pharmacokinetic parameters. Therefore, a further log transformation of this function (equation 7) results in a linear function, whereby

$$\ln C = \ln C_0 - kt \quad (8)$$

As indicated in equation 8, the natural log of C declines as a linear function of time with a slope of k and an intercept of ln C_0. Thus, with first-order kinetic data, a plot of drug concentration versus time on semilog paper yields a linear function, as indicated in Figure 5–4.

By rearranging equation 8, the amount of drug in the body (S) at any time (t) can be expressed as a function of the initial dose by plotting ln S/S_0 as a function of t, where

$$\ln S/S_0 = -kt \quad (9)$$

This normalized function of the log of the percent of initial dose of drug remaining at any time (t) is depicted in Figure 5–5.

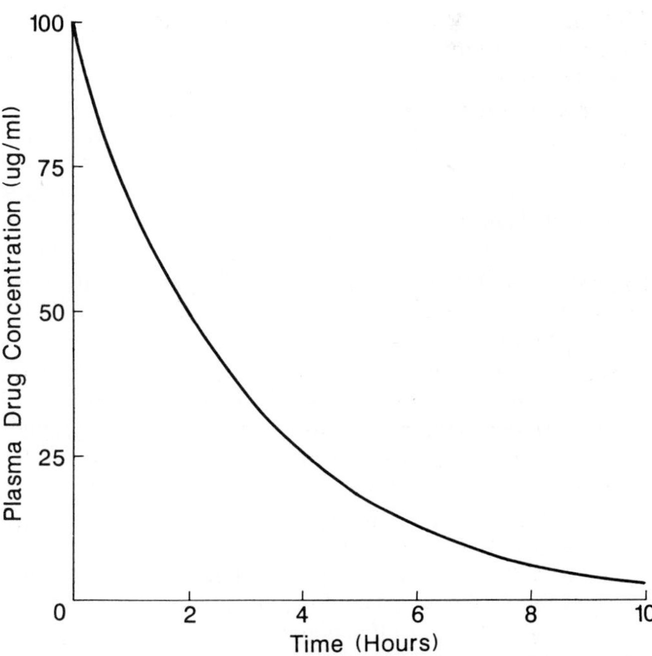

FIGURE 5–3. The concentration of drug in plasma is plotted against the time after a single bolus dose of the drug injected intravenously. The figure assumes instantaneous mixing. On linear coordinates, the blood concentration falls exponentially. The rate constant for the function plotted is 0.3465/hour.

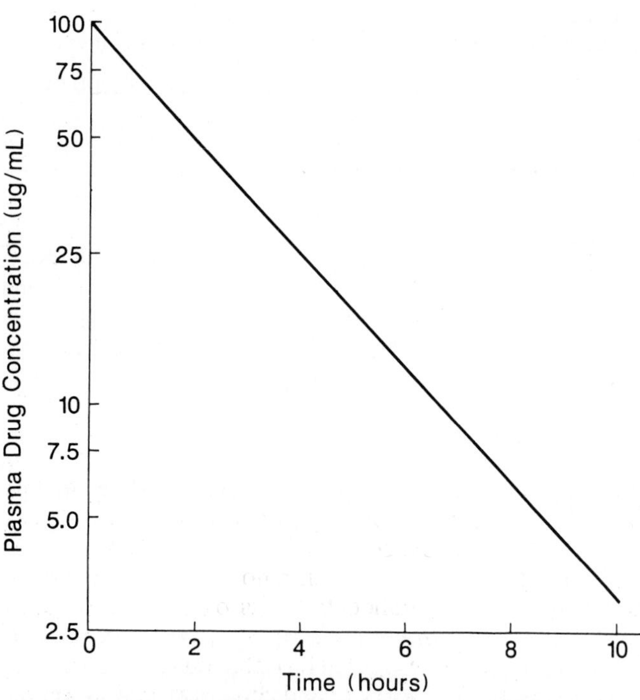

FIGURE 5-4. The concentration of drug in plasma is plotted against the time after a single bolus dose of the drug was injected intravenously. The figure assumes instantaneous mixing. On semilog paper the first-order function is a straight line. This linear plot allows for the direct graphical determination of the half-time of the function. The function plotted has a rate constant of 0.3465/hour.

Several additional clinically useful parameters may be derived from this relationship. One such parameter is the half-time for this function.

BIOLOGICAL HALF-TIME

The one-compartment open model is analogous to other first-order processes. The first-order decay of radionuclides and first-order chemical reaction kinetics may be expressed by the same equations already derived (*ie*, equation 9). The half-time is a parameter common to all of these processes, which is convenient to describe the rate at which the process proceeds. Half-time is defined as the time required for S to decline by a factor of one half. For the single-compartment open model of elimination of a drug or chemical from the body, the biological half-time of the drug or chemical is the time required to reduce the body burden of the drug or chemical by one half.

The relationship of the half-time to the rate constant k is easily demonstrated. In equation 9, one specific time can be substituted for t, namely the biological half-time ($t_{½}$) for that drug, and the equation becomes

$$\ln ½S_0/S_0 = -kt_{½} \tag{10}$$

The value of S was changed to $½S_0$, because by definition, the half-time is the time it takes for S to decrease by one half.

Rearrangement of this equation yields the relationship of the rate constant to the half-time:

$$t_{½} = \frac{\ln 2}{k} \tag{11}$$

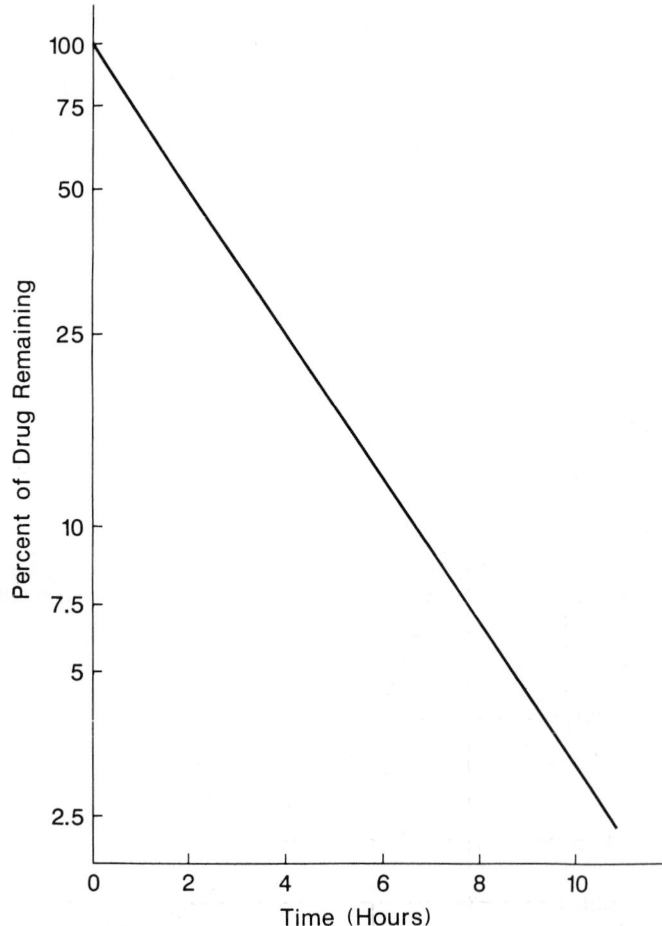

FIGURE 5-5. Normalized plot of percent of drug remaining (S/S_0 or C/C_0) against the time after a single bolus dose of the drug was injected intravenously. The figure assumes instantaneous mixing. The function plotted has a rate constant of 0.3465/hour.

or

$$t_{½} = \frac{0.693}{k} \tag{12}$$

Thus, when the rate constant for elimination of a drug or chemical is known, equation 12 allows the half-time to be easily calculated. Similarly, as indicated in Figure 5-5, graphical data on the concentration of the drug in plasma (or another suitable biofluid) allow for the graphical determination of the half-time, from which the rate constant may be easily calculated.

The amount of drug remaining in the body is depicted as a function of its half-life in Figure 5-6.

Thinking of drug kinetics in terms of the drug's half-life is an easy way to approximate drug levels in time after dosing. Because the process is first-order, with the decline in drug being proportional to the instantaneous body burden, the absolute amount of drug being excreted continues to decrease in time. As indicated in Table 5-1, nearly 94% of the initial dose of drug is eliminated in a time period equivalent to four half-times. At this point, the absolute change in body burden of drug becomes diminishingly small relative to the initial body burden.

For practical purposes, a first-order reaction is considered to have reached completion in four to five half-lives (in

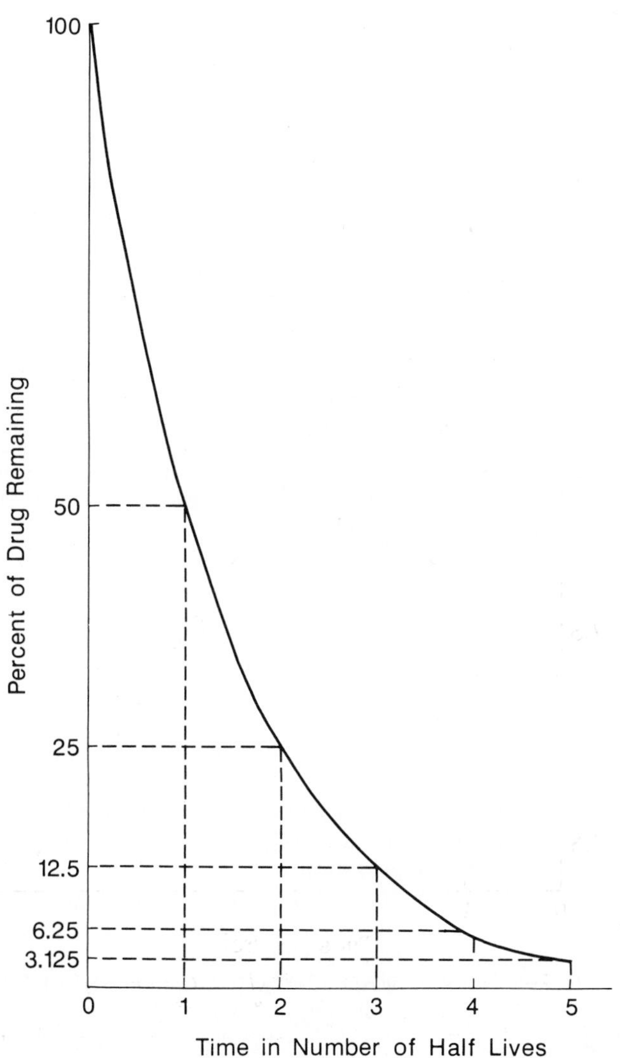

FIGURE 5–6. The percent of drug remaining (S/S_0 or C/C_0) is plotted against the number of drug half-lives after a single bolus dose of drug was injected intravenously. The drug plotted has a biological half-time ($t_{1/2}$) of 1 hour, which corresponds to a rate constant of 0.693/hour.

actuality, this is equivalent to 94–97% completion). In the case of the one-compartment open model, a single dose also can be considered to have been nearly completely excreted after four to five half-lives; one must realize, however, that as with any first-order reaction, although the drug concentration changes become negligible at infinite times (four to five half-lives), they only approach, but never become, zero.

A VARIATION OF THE SINGLE-COMPARTMENT MODEL

• A One-Compartment Open Model with Constant Dose Rate

The same single-compartment model can be altered by changing the single dose at time zero to a continuous-dosing model similar to the clinical situation in which a patient receives a continuous intravenous infusion of drug. In this case, first-order kinetics of drug elimination still prevail. Because this model has a continuous zero-order input, rather than starting off at a peak concentration as in the single-dose model, the initial drug concentration is low and then tends to increase as the infusion continues. A typical plot of drug concentration versus time for the continuous infusion model is given in Figure 5–7. Drug administration at a fixed continuous dose rate reaches a plateau, or steady-state concentration.

TABLE 5–1. The Fractional Amounts Remaining or the Percentage of Drug Remaining After a Given Number of Half-Lives

Half-Lives (n)	Drug Remaining (%)	Proportion of Drug Remaining
0	100	1
1	50	½
2	25	¼
3	12.5	⅛
4	6.25	1/16
5	3.125	1/32

In looking at the change in drug body burden over time, the following mass balance equation can be used, in which rate of drug change equals the rate of drug input minus the rate of drug output, or

$$dS/dt = I - E \tag{13}$$

where I = rate of zero-order input of drug into the patient, and E = summation of excretion of the drug by all pathways expressed as a rate.

As indicated earlier, a first-order excretion process is assumed to be in effect, as in equation 4, such that the rate of drug excretion is proportional to the instantaneous body burden (S) or

$$E = kS \tag{14}$$

where k is the same rate constant for excretion described earlier. Equation 13 then becomes

$$dS/dt = I - kS \tag{15}$$

Because the input rate is constant or zero-order, it can be described by a rate constant (m). Assume that a constant fraction (f) of a dose rate (m) is absorbed, such that I = fm; equation 15 then becomes

$$dS/dt = fm - kS \tag{16}$$

Upon integration of this function, the following exponential expression is obtained:

$$S = \frac{fm}{k}(1 - e^{-kt}) \tag{17}$$

During the period of continual dosing, the body burden approaches its steady-state value. When dosing is stopped, a simple exponential decline in body burden results, as depicted in Figure 5–8. **Steady state** may be defined as a time of no net change in S when rate of input equals rate of output

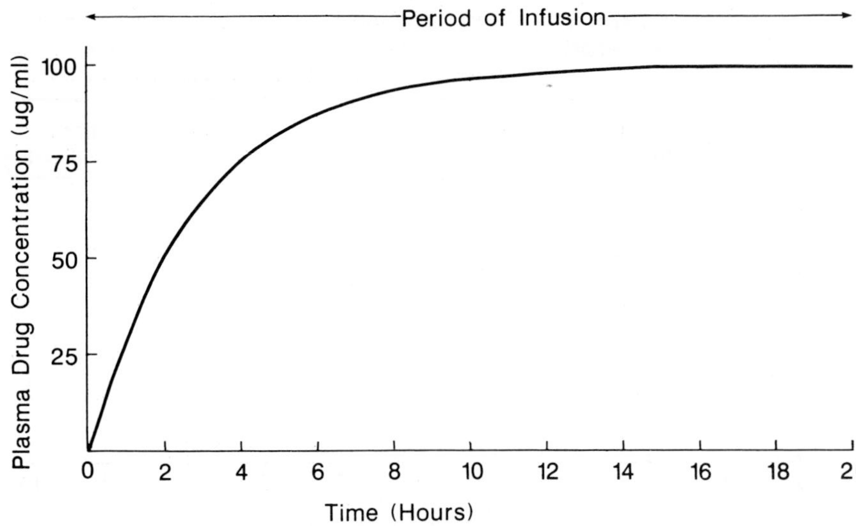

FIGURE 5–7. The plasma concentration of drug is plotted against the time from initiation of a continuous infusion of drug at a zero-order input rate (m). The drug concentration increases to a plateau, at which point the drug input and drug output are equal. The drug depicted here has a biological half-time of 2 hours.

(I = E) of the drug or chemical. This occurs when e^{-kt} is negligibly small. At $t = \infty$, $e^{-kt} \approx 0$, and

$$S_{\infty} = \frac{fm}{k} \tag{18}$$

If f and k are constant properties of the subject for a given drug, then

$$S_{\infty} \approx m \tag{19}$$

APPROACH TO STEADY STATE

How long does it take to reach steady state? The answer to this question can be put in terms of the kinetic constant already discussed for the first-order model.

In equation 17, which describes the first-order constant infusion model, S_{∞} is substituted for fm/k (from equation 18). Equation 17 then becomes

$$S = S_{\infty}(1 - e^{-kt}) \tag{20}$$

Upon rearrangement of the expression, the following is obtained:

$$S_{\infty} - S = S_{\infty}e^{-kt} \tag{21}$$

This equation states that the difference between the equilibrium body burden (S_{∞}) and any instantaneous body burden chosen for examination (S_t) declines exponentially as a function of time with the same rate constant, k, which governed the first-order excretion of that drug. Because this function is first-order, its rate is essentially identical to the first-order process for drug elimination that was already described (equation 6). Thus, as with any first-order function, the process also reaches completion in four to five half-lives; therefore, the rate of approach to steady state is easily described in terms of the half-time of the drug of interest. This is represented diagrammatically in Figure 5–9.

Because the exponent has only a rate constant and a time parameter, the rate of approach to steady state is independent of dose. Therefore, an increase in the dose rate results in a proportional change to the steady-state concentration of drug (equation 18) but does not affect the time it

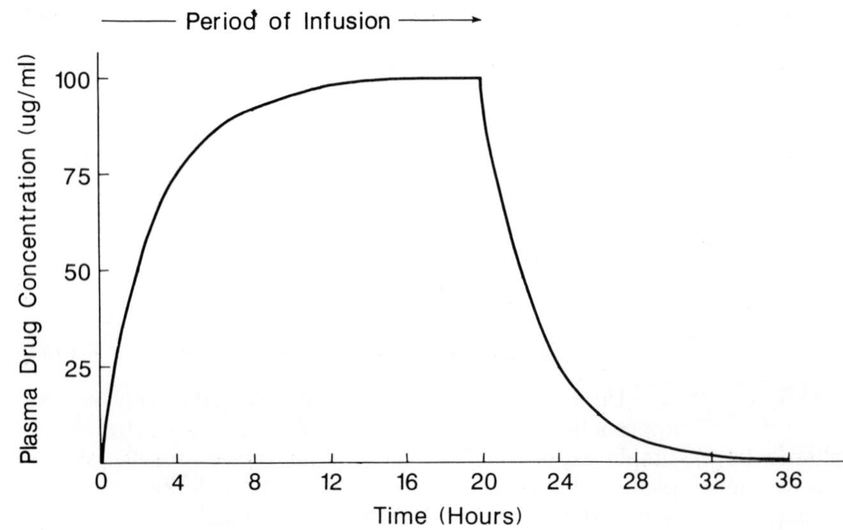

FIGURE 5–8. The plasma concentration of drug is plotted against the time from initiation of a continuous infusion of drug at a zero-order input rate (m). At 20 hours, the infusion is stopped and a first-order decline in plasma drug concentration prevails.

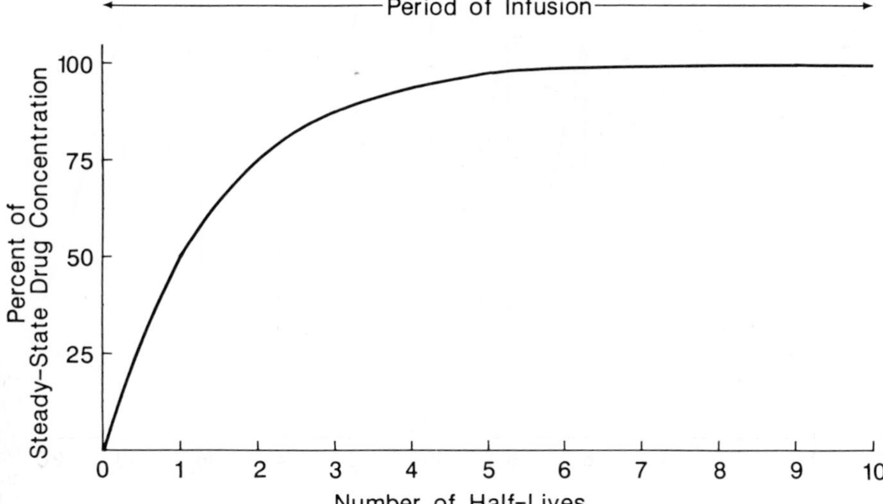

FIGURE 5-9. The plasma drug concentration expressed as the percent of steady-state drug concentration is plotted against the time measured in half-times from the time of initiation of a continuous infusion of drug at a zero-order input rate (m). Steady state or equilibrium is established within 4-5 half-lives (equivalent to approximately 94% and 97% completion, respectively).

takes to reach steady state. This is depicted graphically in Figure 5-10.

MULTIPLE-DOSE CASE

One of the most common ways to administer drugs is in divided doses separated by some time interval; for example, this is common in oral antibiotic therapy.

This case can be seen as being analogous to the constant dose rate model discussed previously. In this case, equation 20 can be applied with only a modification of the dose rate function. Instead of a continuous infusion, the input of drug has been changed into individual doses (D) separated by a dosing interval (τ), and the rate of a drug input m becomes D/τ. Substituting for $m = D/\tau$ in equation 17, the following relationship is reached:

$$\bar{S} = \frac{fD}{k\tau}(1 - e^{-kt}) \qquad (22)$$

The graphical depiction of this function is given in Figure 5-11. Rather than the smooth curve approaching equilibrium as seen in the continuous-infusion model, this intermittent-dosing model produces a saw-toothed curve that depicts a rise in drug concentration that results immediately after each dose, followed by the first-order decline that predominates until the next dose is given. At steady state, the drug concentration varies between a maximal (C_∞^{max}) and a minimal (C_∞^{min}) value. These values are also referred to as **peak** and **trough** drug concentrations.

The steady-state assumption also can be used to calculate the average steady-state value of the drug at equilibrium, just as was done for the continuous-infusion model. Because the exponential function is the same in both equations and becomes diminishingly small at large time points or as the

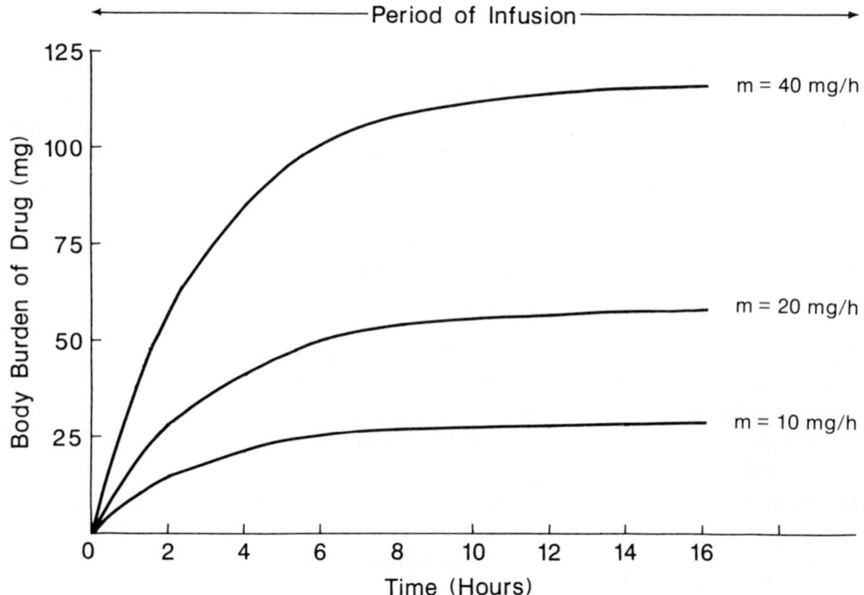

FIGURE 5-10. Body burden in milligrams is plotted against the time from initiation of a continuous infusion of drug at three different rates; m = 10 mg/hour, 2m = 20 mg/hour, and 4m = 40 mg/hour. The drug depicted here has a biological half-life of 2 hours. All three infusion rates result in similarly shaped curves, indicating that the approach to steady state is the same in each case. The drug concentrations reached at steady state are directly proportional to the rate of drug input.

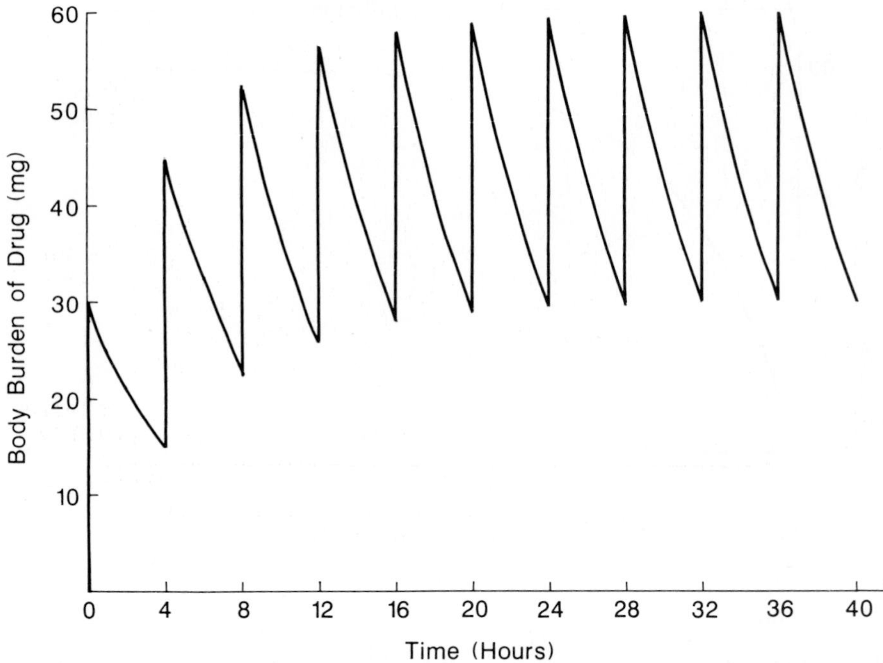

FIGURE 5–11. The body burden of drug (S) is plotted against time for a intermittent drug dosing regimen of 30 mg of drug (D) given at time 0 and at each 4-hour interval (τ) thereafter. Following each successive dose, first-order excretion kinetics prevail. As with the continuous infusion model, a steady state is reached after 4–5 biological half-lives. The difference between the peak and the trough body burden is equal to the individual drug dose (D).

process is near completion (*ie*, four to five half-times), equation 22 becomes

$$\bar{S}_\infty = fD/k\tau \qquad (23)$$

The minimal and maximal body burden for each dose also can be calculated to the nth dose using the following relationships:

$$S_n^{max} = D\,\frac{1 - e^{-nk\tau}}{1 - e^{-k\tau}} \qquad (24)$$

$$S_n^{min} = D\,\frac{1 - e^{-nk\tau}}{1 - e^{-k\tau}}\,e^{-k\tau} \qquad (25)$$

where S_n^{max} is the amount in the compartment after the nth dose, and S_n^{min} is the amount in the compartment τ hours after the nth dose.

At steady state ($t = \infty$), the values of S_∞^{max} and S_∞^{min} can be calculated as follows:

$$S_\infty^{max} = D\,\frac{1}{1 - e^{-k\tau}} \qquad (26)$$

$$S_\infty^{min} = D\,\frac{e^{-k\tau}}{1 - e^{-k\tau}} \qquad (27)$$

At steady state ($t = \infty$), the input of the drug is equal to the output of the drug over the dosing interval, and

$$S_\infty^{max} - S_\infty^{min} = D \qquad (28)$$

This occurs at approximately five half-lives after dosing is initiated (see equation 22). Thus S_∞^{max} and S_∞^{min} may be easily calculated for a drug or chemical with a known biological rate constant of excretion (k) for any dose (D) over any dosing interval (τ). At steady state, minimal sampling would be required to monitor the range of drug concentration in plasma.

As indicated in Figure 5–9, it takes a finite time to reach the steady-state drug concentration, and the length of this latent period is determined by the half-time of the drug. This has implications regarding the therapeutic effects that the drug is intended to elicit. Conceptually, there must be a threshold concentration of drug in plasma above which the expected outcome would be achieved, and below which no therapeutic effect would occur (Fig. 5–12).

Similarly, as drug concentration increases, the potential for development of adverse or toxic effects increases, and some maximal tolerated drug concentration represents a threshold for developing toxic effects. For effective therapy without serious side effects, the pharmacokinetic challenge is to maintain the drug concentration within a therapeutic range of concentration that is delineated by the threshold for effective therapy (minimal therapeutic drug concentration) and the threshold for toxic effects (maximal tolerated drug concentration).

As indicated earlier, specific steady-state concentrations can be readily achieved by selecting appropriate drug dose rates. However, the latent period for reaching steady state results in an initial period during which therapy is ineffective, despite the initiation of the drug administration as either the continuous (intravenous) or intermittent-dosing models. In order to diminish this latency period, an initial priming dose of the drug can be utilized to rapidly increase blood concentrations up to the therapeutic range. This is illustrated in Figure 5–12, in which a high primary dose (*eg*, S_∞^{max}) is given. Caution is advised in the administration of high primary doses, because it is well recognized that with drugs having a low therapeutic index, a narrow range of blood concentrations of drug exists that separates effective therapy from toxic effects.

DRUG CLEARANCE

The foregoing discussion focused on either the rate of change in total drug in the body (body burden) or the rate of

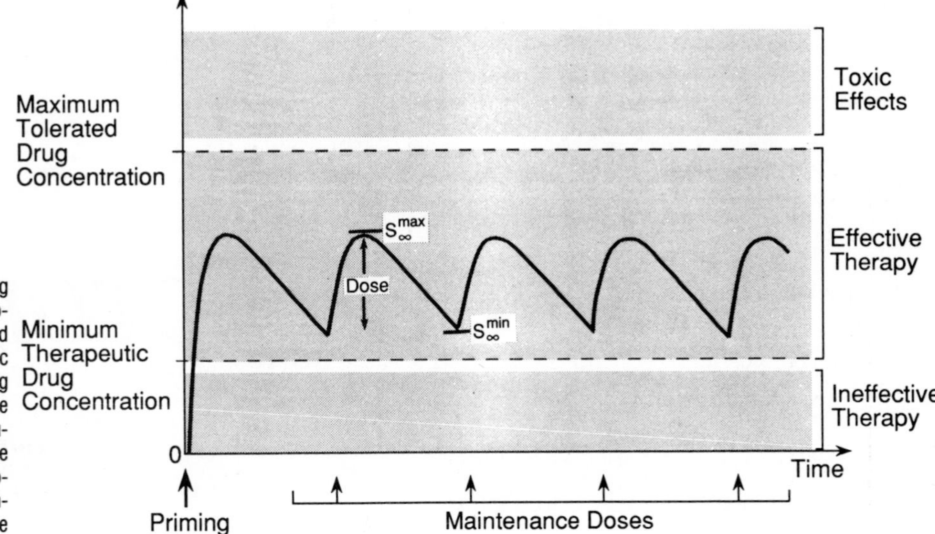

FIGURE 5–12. The blood concentration of drug is plotted in arbitrary units against time on the abscissa. The *dashed lines* are placed at the blood concentrations that bracket the minimal therapeutic drug concentration and the maximal tolerated drug concentration. After the initial *priming dose*, the peak concentration rises into the effective therapeutic, but not toxic, range of blood concentrations. The administration of *maintenance doses* with the appropriate dose frequency keeps the blood concentration out of the ineffective zone and below the level associated with toxic effects.

change in plasma concentration of a drug, both of which follow identical kinetic patterns for the ideal one-compartment model. Drug changes within the body also can be viewed in terms of *drug clearance*, a concept that mirrors certain physiological elimination processes, such as renal or biliary elimination of drugs (see Chapter 4).

Clearance in the ideal one-compartment model can be thought of as the relative volume of the total compartment cleared of the drug over a given time. A simple equation for clearance can be written as follows:

$$Cl = Vk \qquad (29)$$

where clearance (Cl) as the units of volume time^{-1}, V is the volume of distribution, and k is the first-order rate constant described earlier that has the units of time^{-1}.

To understand how the concept of clearance fits into the one-compartment pharmacokinetic model derived previously, one must start with the plasma concentration curve for a single bolus dose of drug S_0 given at zero time (see Fig. 5–3). This plasma concentration curve is described by equation 7. The area under this curve is simply the integral of that equation, or

$$AUC^{0\rightarrow\infty} = \int_0^\infty C = C_0\int_0^\infty e^{-kt}dt \qquad (30)$$

$$AUC^{0\rightarrow\infty} = -\frac{C_0}{k}(e^{-k\infty} - e^{-k0}) \qquad (31)$$

$$AUC^{0\rightarrow\infty} = -\frac{C_0}{k}(0 - 1) \qquad (32)$$

$$AUC^{0\rightarrow\infty} = \frac{C_0}{k} \qquad (33)$$

From this relationship, one can relate $AUC^{0\rightarrow\infty}$ to clearance by initially substituting for C_0

$$AUC^{0\rightarrow\infty} = S_0/Vk \qquad (34)$$

and subsequently substituting for Vk, whereby equation 34 becomes

$$AUC^{0\rightarrow\infty} = S_0/Cl \qquad (35)$$

This approach, which utilizes the concept of clearance to model drug elimination kinetics, relies on data obtained through serial monitoring of plasma drug concentrations after a single bolus dose of the drug. It is described here because many papers in the literature use this convention. This is not a different kinetic model but rather another way of looking at first-order pharmacokinetic modeling.

COMPUTER-BASED SOLUTIONS

Computer-based systems provide a variety of mathematical and graphic modeling systems. A number of the excellent and extensive software programs for pharmacokinetic modeling for both clinical applications and computer-based instruction are cited in Chapter 62.

REFERENCES

Bourne DWA, Triggs EJ, Eadie MJ: Pharmacokinetics for the Nonmathematical. Boston: MTP Press Limited, 1986.

Gladtke E, von Hattingberg HM: Pharmacokinetics. New York: Springer-Verlag, 1979.

Hug CC: Pharmacokinetics of drug administered intravenously. Anesth Analg 57:704–723, 1978.

Neubig RR: The time course of drug action. *In* Pratt WB, Taylor P (eds): Principles of Drug Action, 3rd ed, 297–364. New York: Churchill Livingstone, 1990.

Nierenberg DW, Melmon KL: Introduction to Clinical Pharmacology. *In* Melmon KL, Morrelli HF, Hoffman BB, Nierenberg DW (eds). Clinical Pharmacology: Basic Principles in Therapeutics, 3rd ed. 1–51. New York: McGraw-Hill, 1992.

Notari RE: Biopharmaceutics and Clinical Pharmacokinetics. New York: Marcel Dekker, 1987.

PART II

DRUGS AFFECTING NEUROEFFECTOR SYSTEMS

6 Autonomic Pharmacology

Oliver M. Brown

Drugs are not magic: drugs cannot make the heart secrete insulin or make the bronchioles pump blood. **Drugs can alter existing physiological functions quantitatively, not qualitatively.** The heart has the property of beating; we can make it beat faster or slower with drugs, but we cannot make it perform a different physiological function. Drug action in the autonomic nervous system results from modifying pre-existing physiological functions. Most often this modification is accomplished when drugs either mimic (as agonist) or block (as antagonist) endogenous molecules of physiological importance, usually hormones or neurotransmitters. In order to fully appreciate the pharmacology of the autonomic nervous system, one must review some aspects of autonomic anatomy and physiology.

NERVOUS SYSTEM ORGANIZATION AND FUNCTION

The nervous system is composed of the central nervous system (CNS) (brain and spinal cord) and the peripheral nervous system. It includes *peripheral afferent nerves*, which are sensory and reflex fibers carrying signals from the periphery to the CNS. With the exception of local anesthetics, relatively little drug treatment is directed toward the peripheral afferent nerves (see Chapters 12 and 13). Autonomic pharmacology primarily involves *peripheral efferent nerves*, or motor neurons. These fibers carry information from the CNS to the various organs and direct their level of activity. Modification of the interactions between motor nerves and the organs is the mode of action underlying drug therapy in the peripheral efferent system.

BOX 6–1

- CNS
- Peripheral afferent nerves (sensory and reflex fibers)—carry information to CNS
- Peripheral efferent nerves (motor neurons)—carry information from CNS

The peripheral efferent nervous system is composed of the **somatic** and the **autonomic** divisions (Fig. 6–1). The somatic, or the voluntary system, innervates skeletal muscles; whereas the autonomic, or involuntary (automatic) system, innervates most of the other organs of the body. The autonomic system is responsible for maintaining homeostasis (a constant internal environment); it controls body temperature, heart rate, blood pressure, metabolic functions, and so forth. In considering autonomic pharmacology, we also discuss the pharmacology of the somatic system because the drug principles, the mechanisms, and the neurotransmitters are the same for the two systems.

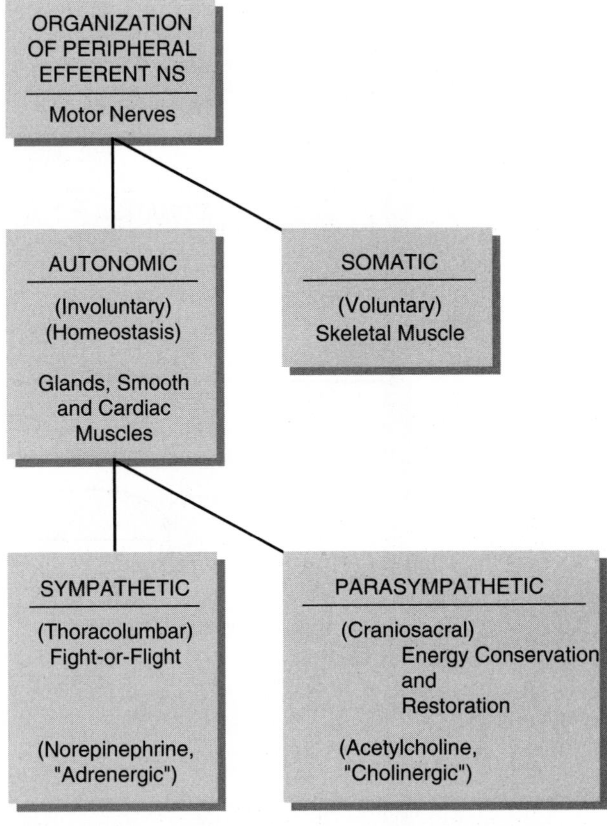

FIGURE 6–1. The peripheral efferent nervous system (NS).

BOX 6–2

CHARACTERISTICS OF NERVOUS SYSTEM COMPONENTS

CNS (Brain + spinal cord)
Peripheral Nervous System (everything else)
- *Afferent neurons* (see Chapter 13)
  - Unmyelinated fibers to CNS
  - Carry reflex and sensory signals
  - Clinical importance = relief of pain (NSAIDs, local anesthetics, surgery, transcutaneous nerve stimulation, cough suppression)
- *Efferent neurons* = motor neurons
  - Myelinated fibers to organs
  - Direct activity of organs
  - Clinical importance = control level of activity of organs

Somatic System
- Voluntary—innervates skeletal muscle
- Drugs and mechanisms = similar to ANS
- Originates in CNS (mostly spinal cord)
- Myelinated neurons travel without synapsing to skeletal muscle
- Synapse at neuromuscular junctions

Autonomic Nervous System (ANS)
- Involuntary (automatic)—innervates cardiac muscle, smooth muscle, glands
- Hypothalamus and medulla oblongata—integrate and regulate autonomic activity
- Maintains homeostasis (constant internal environment)
- Regulates: temperature, circulation, respiration, digestion, metabolism
- First neuron cell body in CNS
- Myelinated fiber to peripheral synapse in ganglion
- Second neuron (postganglionic) is unmyelinated to effector organ
- **Sympathetic** branch of ANS
- **Parasympathetic** branch of ANS

PERIPHERAL NERVOUS SYSTEM CHARACTERISTICS

Autonomic innervation can be further subdivided into the **sympathetic** and the **parasympathetic** branches. The parasympathetic system uses acetylcholine (ACh) as a neurotransmitter, and is often referred to as the cholinergic system. The end-organ neurotransmitter in sympathetic nerves is norepinephrine (NE) (with a few exceptions), and the sympathetic system is commonly called the adrenergic system (Fig. 6–2).

Somatic neurons originate in the CNS: there are no synapses in the periphery until these long myelinated neurons arrive at the junctions in skeletal muscle. The neurotransmitter at somatic neuromuscular junctions is ACh. The innervation pattern in the autonomic system is different in that there are peripheral synapses in ganglia. A myelinated preganglionic fiber arises from the CNS, it synapses in a ganglion, and a postganglionic unmyelinated fiber innervates the effector organ. In all cases the ganglia use ACh as a neurotransmitter, whereas the neuroeffector junctions use either ACh (parasympathetic) or NE (sympathetic).

The parasympathetic branch of the autonomic system is characterized by having long preganglionic neurons. Because the ganglia are usually within the organ innervated, the postganglionic fibers that innervate the cells are very short. With the exception of the gut, the parasympathetic system is characterized by having a preganglionic to postganglionic fiber ratio of 1 : 1.

The sympathetic branch is organized somewhat differently. It has short preganglionic fibers and long postganglionic fibers. Sympathetic ganglia are close to the CNS, and are primarily composed of the two chains of paravertebral ganglia. There is branching, often with a 1 : 10 or 1 : 20 preganglionic to postganglionic fiber ratio, throughout the sympathetic system. There is also considerable overlapping of postganglionic fibers to effector cells. These two features

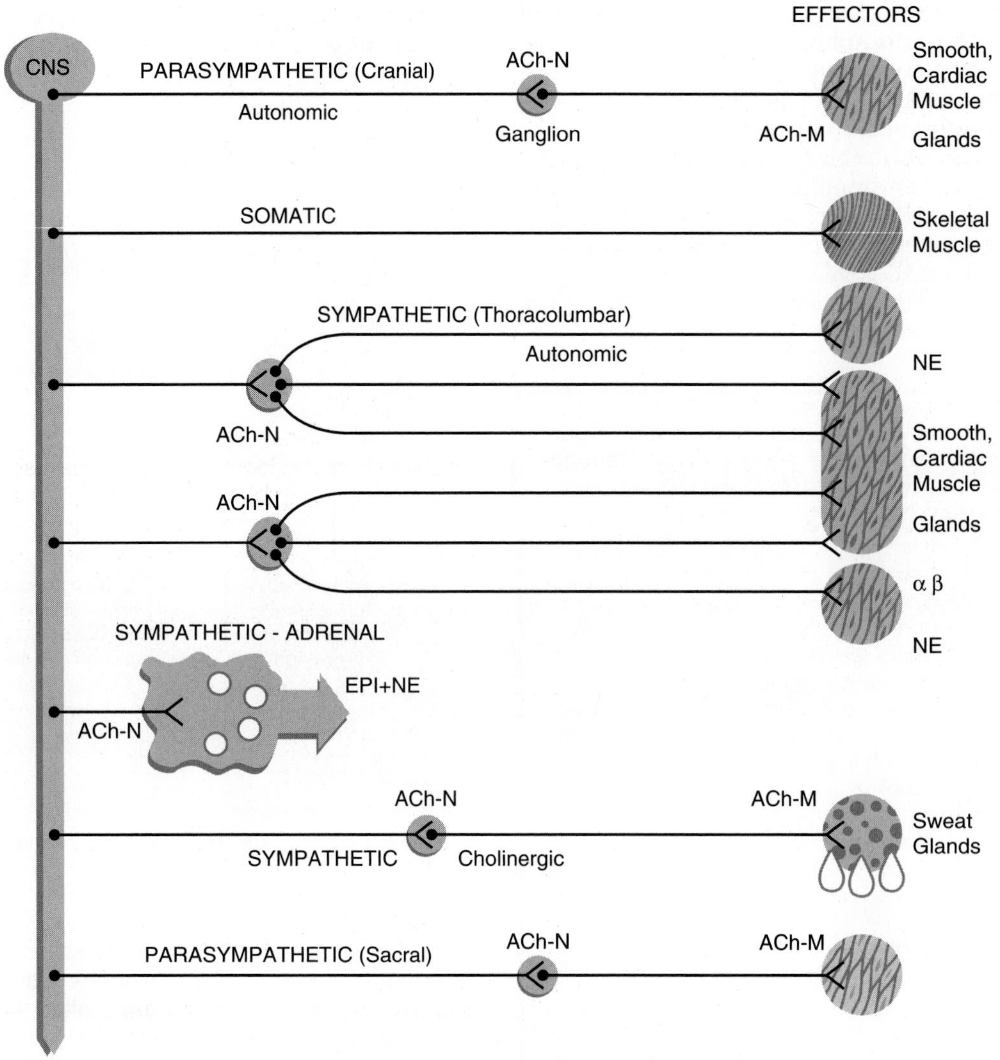

FIGURE 6–2. Peripheral efferents. (ACh = acetylcholine; ACh-M = muscarinic ACh; ACh-N = nicotinic ACh; CNS = central nervous system; EPI = epinephrine; NE = norepinephrine.)

(branching and overlap), along with the adrenal medullae, allow for a widespread sympathetic response throughout the body. For categorization, it is perhaps best to consider the adrenal medullae as being modified sympathetic ganglia: they are innervated in the same fashion as sympathetic ganglia, and ACh is the neurotransmitter. The adrenals respond to stimulation by elaborating epinephrine and norepinephrine directly into the blood stream (in humans the epinephrine-to-norepinephrine ratio is about 4 : 1).

The sympathetic system is organized so that it is capable of producing a rapid, total body response. In contrast, the parasympathetic system is more discrete: no branching, no overlapping, and no correlate to the adrenals. Most organs receive innervation from both the sympathetic and the parasympathetic branches. However, there are exceptions: most blood vessels receive only sympathetic innervation. Sweat glands and piloerector muscles also receive only sympathetic innervation. Sweat gland innervation is further unusual because sweat glands are sympathetically innervated, but the neurotransmitter is ACh; thus, a sympathetic-cholinergic system. Otherwise, the effector organ neurotransmitter in the sympathetic system is norepinephrine.

AUTONOMIC NERVOUS SYSTEM CHARACTERISTICS

Again, most organs receive innervation from both branches of the autonomic system. In those organs the two systems tend to be **physiological antagonists** of one another. That is, where stimulation of one autonomic branch may increase the activity of an organ, the other branch will inhibit it. This is similar to many public buildings wherein the air conditioning and the heat are left on all the time, opposing one another, and achieving a temperature that may be uncomfortable for everyone at all times. The sympathetic and parasympathetic branches of the autonomic nervous system counterbalance one another in an intricate fashion. In response to changes in the external and/or internal environment, the autonomic branches coordinate compensatory

BOX 6–3
PARASYMPATHETIC AND SYMPATHETIC CHARACTERISTICS

Parasympathetic
Cranial outflow
To head and neck, and to other organs via vagus
Sacral outflow
Via pelvic nerves to lower gut, kidneys, bladder, sex organs
Long preganglionic fibers
Short postganglionic neurons
Little or no branching: preganglionic to postganglionic fiber ratio = 1:1 (major exception = gut)
Characteristic transmitter = acetylcholine ("cholinergic")
Sympathetic
Thoracolumbar outflow mostly to paravertebral ganglia
Short preganglionic fibers
Long postganglionic neurons
Much branching and overlapping of fibers
Characteristic transmitter = norepinephrine ("adrenergic")
Adrenal Medullae
Secrete epinephrine and norepinephrine into blood stream

corrections to preserve homeostasis. Most organs continually receive signals from each branch in order to maintain an appropriate level of functioning. **Physiological antagonism** is the key feature of the autonomic nervous system, and it sets the stage for the *reciprocal relationships* that constitute the beauty and the nemesis of autonomic pharmacology.

BOX 6–4
AUTONOMIC ANTAGONISTS

- Most organs innervated by **both** sympathetic and parasympathetic
  One branch is usually dominant
  Some **exceptions**: sweat glands, piloerector muscles, and most blood vessels receive only sympathetic fibers
- **Sympathetic and parasympathetic are *physiological antagonists***
  Organ activity is the algebraic sum of sympathetic and parasympathetic input

Examples of this *physiological antagonism* (Table 6–1) include the eye: sympathetic nerve impulses (or drugs that stimulate the sympathetic system) stimulate the radial muscles of the iris and cause dilation of the pupil (mydriasis), whereas parasympathetic nerve impulses (or parasympathetic stimulating drugs) stimulate the pupillary sphincter,

TABLE 6–1. Physiological Antagonism Between Sympathetic and Parasympathetic Discharge—Organ Responses

Organ	Effect of Sympathetic Discharge	Effect of Parasympathetic Discharge
Eye	Mydriasis (dilate pupil)	Miosis (constrict pupil)
Heart rate	Increase	Decrease
Bronchial muscle	Relax	Contract
Stomach motility	Decrease	Increase
Intestinal motility	Decrease	Increase

causing constriction of the pupil (miosis). Heart rate will increase with sympathetic nerve impulses and decrease in response to parasympathetic (vagus nerve) activity. Bronchial muscle tone will be relaxed with sympathetic stimulation compared with bronchial constriction caused by parasympathetic influences. Stomach and intestinal motility will increase with parasympathetic activity and decrease with sympathetic.

SORTING OUT THE RELATIONSHIPS

Sympathetic stimulation changes the physiological activity of many organs in the direction appropriate for exigency: the "**fight or flight**" response. Keeping this in mind is one of the better ways to remember the essentials of autonomic pharmacology. As noted above, autonomic pharmacology is replete with potentially confusing reciprocal relationships: the sympathetic and parasympathetic branches counterbalance one another; each branch has multiple receptor types; and there are agonists and antagonists for each receptor. Recall the logical response of an organ to an emergency situation (fight or flight); this is the response one would expect from either sympathetic nerve stimulation or adrenergic agonists, and the response expected to emerge in relief if the parasympathetic effects are blocked.

BOX 6–5
DIRECTION OF SYMPATHETIC INFLUENCES

In preparation for "**fight or flight**":

- Bronchial muscles relax to open the airway
- Heart rate increases
- Blood flow is redistributed for richer perfusion of skeletal muscle
- Pupils dilate to increase light striking retina
- Gastrointestinal activity decreases
- Metabolic activity increases (elevations in blood glucose and free fatty acids)

Again, a total body discharge of the sympathetic system prepares one to respond in an emergency situation. In contrast, the parasympathetic system has a more restorative and conserving effect on bodily functions. The parasympathetic branch produces a more discrete organ to organ response, in part due to its anatomical differences from the sympathetic: the parasympathetic branch does not have an analog to the adrenals, nor does it have the branching and overlapping of neurons. Of course, most of the time we are not in emergency situations and the sympathetic system is more subtle in controlling body functions (maintaining homeostasis), as with the parasympathetic system.

An important compensating autonomic control mechanism is the baroreceptor reflex. One must recall this pressure control mechanism to understand the action of any drug with an effect on blood vessels. An increase in blood pressure is detected by stretch receptors in the aorta and carotid arteries; these receptors are the afferent input for the midbrain vasomotor center. The reflex response is a decrease in central sympathetic output and an increase in parasympathetic output. Thus, a prominent response to a sharp rise in blood pressure is a rapid, compensatory decrease in heart rate mediated over the vagus nerves. Conversely, a decrease in blood pressure causes a reflex increase in heart rate and an increase in vasoconstrictor activity to resistance and capacitance vessels.

NEUROCHEMICAL TRANSMISSION

Key concepts in any discussion of drug action in the nervous system are the *synapse* and process of *chemical transmission*. At the synapse, the nerve action potentials are converted to chemical signals; these chemical messages traverse the synaptic space and are then transduced by the effector cell. Drugs have their effects on the discrete steps involved in the process of synaptic chemical transmission (neurotransmission). This discussion will focus on chemical transmission using acetylcholine (ACh) as the neurotransmitter; however, the principles described here will apply to most chemical transmitters (norepinephrine neurotransmission will be described in detail in Chapter 9).

BOX 6–6
EVENTS INVOLVED IN NEUROCHEMICAL TRANSMISSION

- Presynaptic preparation
  - Uptake of precursor
  - Synthesis of transmitter
  - Packaging
- Arrival of action potential
  - Ca^{2+} entry
- Release of transmitter
- Receptor interaction
  - "Second messengers" (often, Ca^{2+} entry)
  - Effector cell response
- Termination of transmitter action

For neurotransmission to take place, there must first be a supply of the chemical transmitter in the presynaptic nerve varicosity (or ending), which involves uptake of precursors, enzymatic synthesis, and packaging (Fig. 6–3). In cholinergic neurons, choline is taken up into the neuron by a Na^+-dependent high-affinity transport system (in some experiments choline has been found to be synthesized *de novo* within the neuron). To synthesize ACh, choline is combined with the acetate of acetyl CoA by the cytoplasmic enzyme choline acetyltransferase (Fig. 6–4). ACh synthesized in the cytoplasm is then transported into membrane-bound synaptic

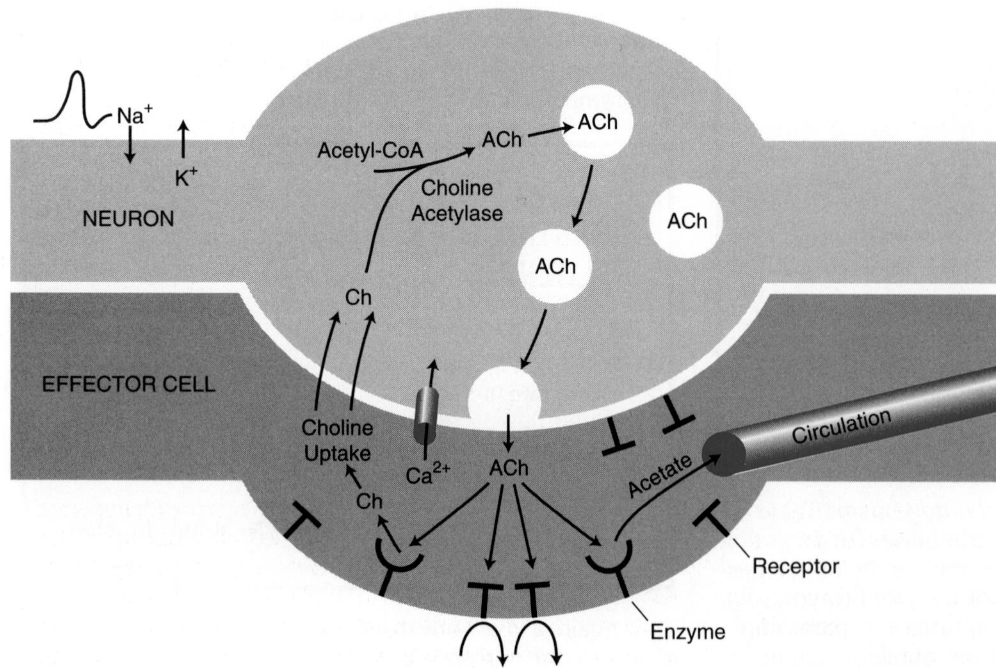

FIGURE 6–3. Cholinergic synapse. (ACh = acetylcholine; Ch = choline; CoA = coenzyme A.)

$$\underset{\text{Choline}}{CH_3\cdot\overset{+}{\underset{CH_3}{\overset{CH_3}{N}}}CH_2\text{-}CH_2\text{-}OH} + \underset{\text{Acetyl-CoA}}{CoA\text{-}O\text{-}\overset{O}{\overset{\|}{C}}\text{-}CH_3} \xrightarrow[CAT]{} \underset{\text{Acetylcholine}}{CH_3\cdot\overset{+}{\underset{CH_3}{\overset{CH_3}{N}}}CH_2\text{-}CH_2\text{-}O\text{-}\overset{O}{\overset{\|}{C}}\text{-}CH_3}$$

FIGURE 6–4. Synthesis of acetylcholine. (CAT = cholineacetyltransferase; CoA = coenzyme A.)

vesicles, the storage site for ACh. The signal for ACh release is the arrival of a nerve action potential. Among other events that accompany the action potential arrival and the localized membrane depolarization is the entry of calcium ions through calcium channels in the presynaptic membrane. Although the entry of calcium is essential for evoked neurotransmitter release, its exact role in the process is not certain (calcium may play a part in the fusion of the synaptic vesicle membrane with the plasma membrane). Calcium-dependent ACh release takes place, presumably by vesicular fusion and exocytosis (there are other theories that propose the release of cytoplasmic ACh). The released transmitter then diffuses across the synaptic cleft to interact with its receptor sites on the effector cell, and thus complete the chemical signal. There are, however, actually several possible fates for the ACh that has been released:

- Interaction with postsynaptic receptors
- Interaction with presynaptic receptors
- Diffusion out of the cleft
- Hydrolysis by acetylcholinesterase

The primary purpose for the transmitter release is to complete the chemical signal by interacting with postsynaptic receptors. However, in addition the transmitter may also interact with presynaptic receptors, initiating an auto-inhibitory feedback control mechanism, which decreases further release of neurotransmitter. Two other possible fates will stop the action of the transmitter: simple diffusion out of the cleft and into the circulation; and hydrolysis by the enzyme acetylcholinesterase, which is located on the postsynaptic membrane or on the basal lamina.

Autonomic Receptors

Enough interactions between ACh or an agonist and the postsynaptic receptors will create sufficient localized depolarization to trigger the effector cell. If the effector cell is another nerve cell, it will initiate an action potential; if a muscle cell, it will contract; and if a glandular cell, it will secrete. Two major kinds of receptors are important to autonomic pharmacology. One type of receptor has an *ion channel* as an integral part of the receptor complex itself (Fig. 6–5). When a ligand (neurotransmitter or drug) binds to the receptor, there is an immediate opening of the ion channel. The nicotinic acetylcholine receptor (see Chapter 7) is an example of this type of receptor.

Most of the other receptors in the autonomic system (α and β norepinephrine, and muscarinic acetylcholine receptors, see following chapters) are of the so-called *G-protein–linked* type (guanine nucleotide-binding regulatory protein). The G-protein–linked receptors are coupled to various *second messenger* systems: cyclic AMP, cyclic GMP, and phosphatidylinositol hydrolysis (Fig. 6–5).

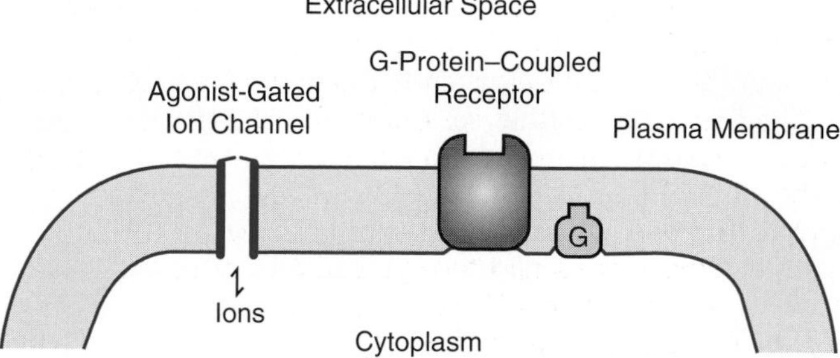

FIGURE 6–5. Agonist-gated ion channel receptors and G-protein–linked receptors.

Effector Cell Response

The interaction between the neurotransmitter (or agonist) and the effector cell receptor is transduced, and then amplified by a second messenger system. Several such second messenger mechanisms are outlined in Figure 6–6. Stimulation of the messenger systems is amplified by the activation of protein kinases and/or the modification of internal calcium levels. Generally, raising intracellular free calcium concentration affects a contraction of the effector cell, whereas lowering or sequestering free calcium concentration inhibits or relaxes the cell. Thus, the initial chemical signal has been transduced to a biological response in the effector organ.

Receptors are themselves subject to regulatory control; superstimulation or subnormal response may occur if the receptor activity or receptor numbers have been modified by up- or down-regulation. Such regulatory mechanisms are usually evident with chronic use of an agonist or an antagonist. (Note: some dangerous situations can result from these phenomena, and will be discussed in later chapters.)

- Receptor down-regulation (desensitization)

  May follow continued stimulation of cells with agonists

  Several mechanisms possible

  - Phosphorylation, relocalization, sequestration (time course = seconds)
  - Decreased synthesis (time course = hours to days)

- Receptor up-regulation (supersensitivity)

  May follow continued use of antagonists (or denervation)

  Usually synthesis of additional receptors (time course = hours to days)

Termination of Neurotransmission

Once the chemical transmitter has interacted with the effector cell receptors and initiated a biological response, it has served its function. Neurotransmitters must be rapidly removed from the synapse to prevent exaggerated or extended stimulation of effector organs. Thus, mechanisms responsible for terminating transmitter action are a critical

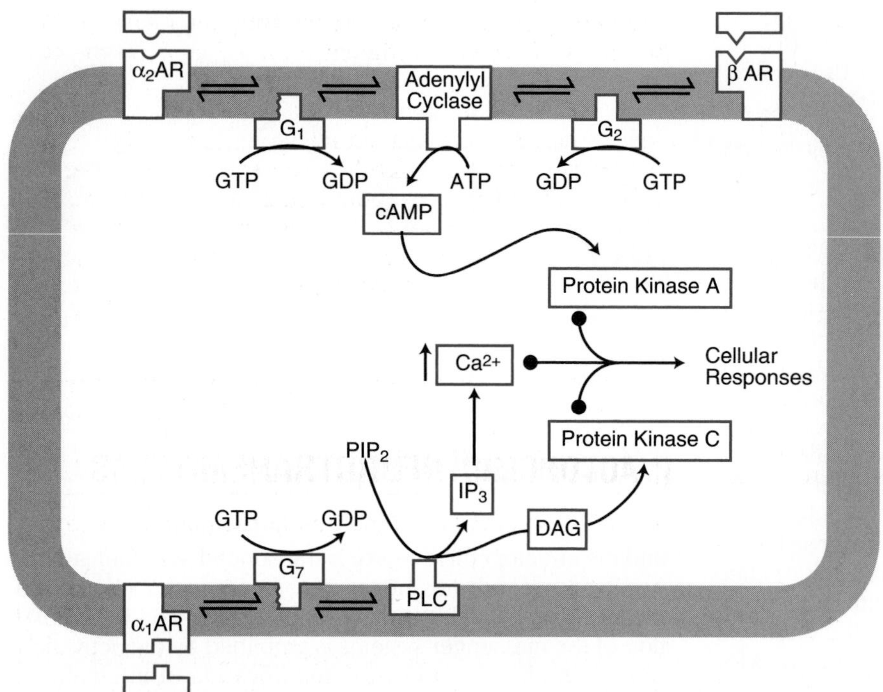

FIGURE 6–6. Second messenger cellular amplification systems. (AR = adrenergic receptors; ATP = adenosine triphosphate; cAMP = cyclic AMP; DAG = diacylglycerol; GDP = guanosine diphosphate; Gi = inhibitory G-protein; Gs = stimulatory G-protein; GTP = guanosine triphosphate; IP_3 = inositol 1,4,5-triphosphate; PIP_2 = phosphatidylinositol 4,5-biphosphate.)

step in the neurotransmission process. There are three primary mechanisms for terminating the action of a neurotransmitter (Fig. 6–7):

- Diffusion out of the cleft — ACh and NE
- Enzymatic conversion — ACh, not NE
- Uptake (uptake$_1$ and uptake$_2$) — NE, not ACh

Diffusion is nonspecific and contributes to the termination of transmitter action at all synapses. The major terminating step for ACh is hydrolysis by the extremely rapid-acting enzyme acetylcholinesterase. This very specific enzyme is membrane-bound and is located on the postsynaptic membrane or the basal lamina. Acetylcholine is enzymatically hydrolyzed into its component parts: acetate (inactive), and choline (about 1/600th the potency of ACh at receptors). A

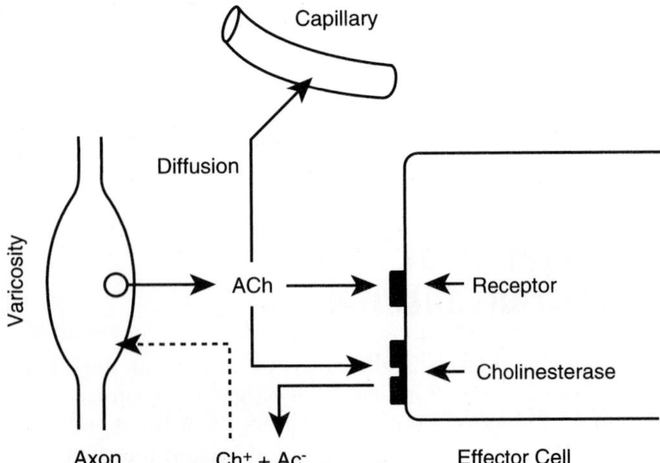

FIGURE 6–7. Termination of neurotransmission. (Ac = acetate; ACh = acetylcholine; Ch = choline.)

less specific family of enzymes, the pseudocholinesterases (or plasma cholinesterase), also circulates in the blood stream. These enzymes are capable of hydrolyzing not only ACh, but ester groups in other compounds as well (*eg*, succinylcholine and cocaine). Much of the choline that results from hydrolysis of ACh in the synapse is taken up into the neuron and recycled into ACh.

Diffusion also contributes to terminating the effects of norepinephrine (NE) as a chemical transmitter. However, the primary step for terminating NE transmission is a very specialized re-uptake system (uptake$_1$) that transports NE back into the nerve varicosity. Inside the neuron it is repackaged, to be used in transmission again. There is no correlate to acetylcholinesterase at NE synapses. There are, of course, enzymes that metabolize NE, but they are not strategically located at the postsynaptic membrane, and they do not play a role in the rapid termination of NE transmission. (NE is further discussed in Chapter 9.)

Altering Neurotransmission with Drugs

The processes involved in chemical transmission are the sites of drug action in autonomic pharmacology (Table 6–2). Each step is subject to modification by clinically useful or investigational compounds. The specifics of cholinergic transmission will be discussed here; although listed here for comparison, the adrenergic system will be detailed in Chapter 9. The synthesis of ACh can be disrupted by blocking the high-affinity choline uptake with the experimental drug hemicholinium-3 (HC-3). Application of this agent to a cholinergic system will decrease the net synaptic transmission (thus, the downward arrow in Table 6–2).

Botulinum food poisoning results from neurotoxic polypeptides made by the bacterium *Clostridium botu-*

Table 6–2. Modification of Chemical Transmission by Drugs

Step	Cholinergic (Parasympathetic)	Adrenergic (Sympathetic)
Synthesis of transmitter (Presynaptic Ca^{2+} influx)	HC-3(↓)	α-m-Tyrosine (↓)
Release of transmitter	Botulinum toxin (↓)	Bretylium (↓) Amphetamine (↑)
Combination with receptor	Methacholine (↑) Atropine (↓)	Isoproterenol (↑) Propranolol (↓)
(Postsynaptic Ca^{2+} influx and second messenger systems)		
Termination step	Neostigmine (↑)	Cocaine (↑)

HC-3 = hemicholinium-3.

linum. Type A toxin, a 150-kD protein, specifically blocks the release of ACh wherever ACh is a neurotransmitter. Thus, individuals who succumb to botulism food poisoning die of respiratory paralysis. This polypeptide has been approved for treating several conditions characterized by facial muscle or ocular muscle spasms. Botulinum toxin injected locally into the offending muscle will stop muscle contractions by preventing the release of ACh.

The entry of calcium is required for release of the neurotransmitter. Postsynaptic calcium entry and second messenger mechanisms are also components of effector cell response. Calcium channel blockers, acting at either presynaptic or postsynaptic channels, will be discussed in Chapter 32.

Most of the clinically useful autonomic drugs act on the postsynaptic receptor. They are either agonists (*eg*, methacholine) and mimic the endogenous transmitter, or they are antagonists (*eg*, atropine) and block the endogenous transmitter. The postsynaptic receptor is a logical site for optimizing the specificity of drug action because receptors are inherently very specific macromolecules that recognize unique neurotransmitters.

Drugs can also interfere with the termination step. If the enzyme acetylcholinesterase is blocked by neostigmine, high levels of ACh will accumulate in the synapse, resulting in a more dramatic and more persistent effector cell response.

Receptor Location and Selective Drug Action

It is clear that autonomic activity can be modified by blocking or stimulating the various steps in neurotransmission with drugs. However, there is no therapeutic benefit in inhibiting or activating the whole autonomic nervous system (a minor, limited exception is ganglionic blockers, discussed in Chapter 8). A finer degree of control is required for drug treatment to be clinically helpful. **Neurotransmitter receptor specificity is the key to controlling drug effects.** The first level of receptor differentiation is based on the two major autonomic neurotransmitters, ACh and NE; thus, there are receptors that specifically recognize ACh, and compounds with a similar structure, and those that recognize NE and analogs. It should be noted that there are other neurotransmitters in the autonomic nervous system, the prominent example being the *enteric system of the gut*, which functions as an independent nervous system and utilizes several chemical transmitters.

BOX 6–7
AUTONOMIC NEUROTRANSMITTERS

- Major transmitters (throughout the peripheral nervous system):
  - Acetylcholine (ACh)
  - Norepinephrine (NE)
- Other transmitters:
  - Dopamine (DA)—vascular beds in the kidney
  - Serotonin, adenosine triphosphate (ATP), substance P, endorphins, vasoactive intestinal polypeptide (VIP)—enteric system
- Characteristics of the *enteric nervous system of the gut*: much branching in intrinsic submucosal and myenteric neural plexuses, functional reflex loops, several neurotransmitters

As can be seen by examining Figure 6–2, ACh is the transmitter at all junctions shown except for the postganglionic neuroeffector junctions in the sympathetic system, which use NE as a transmitter. That is, ACh is the neurotransmitter in all autonomic ganglia (both parasympathetic and sympathetic) and in the adrenals. ACh is also the characteristic transmitter at the effector organ junctions in the parasympathetic system, and at the neuromuscular junctions in the somatic system. An exception to the rule of NE being the sympathetic end-organ transmitter is that in the sympathetic innervation of the sweat glands, ACh is the end-terminal transmitter. This is an unusual case of sympathetic-cholinergic innervation.

BOX 6–8

- **Acetylcholine ("cholinergic") receptor** locations
  - Parasympathetic postganglion neuroeffector junctions
  - Somatic (neuromuscular junction)
  - Autonomic ganglia
  - Sympathetic adrenals
  - (Sympathetic sweat glands)
- **Norepinephrine ("adrenergic") receptor** locations
  - Sympathetic postganglionic neuroeffector junctions

SELECTIVE DRUG ACTION: NICOTINIC AND MUSCARINIC RECEPTORS

Administration of a drug that blocks all ACh receptors is not very selective; it blocks transmission in the entire peripheral system. Even in the sympathetic system, where NE is the end-effector transmitter, ACh is the transmitter upstream at the sympathetic ganglia. Another degree of selectivity is required for useful drug action at ACh receptors. A further level of discrimination was provided by Sir Henry Dale in 1914. He characterized the actions of ACh in experiments with two plant alkaloids, muscarine and nicotine, that mimic various effects of injected ACh.

> **BOX 6–9**
>
> - Muscarine (mushroom alkaloid)—"**Muscarinic**" effects of ACh = lowering of blood pressure and heart rate, and increase in gut activity
> - Nicotine (tobacco alkaloid)—"**Nicotinic**" effects of high doses of ACh = increase in blood pressure

The concept of neurotransmitter receptors was introduced long after Dale's experiments; however, his terminology is still used: currently, ACh receptors are described as being either "nicotinic receptors" or "muscarinic receptors." These two very distinct families of receptors have different functions and distributions, and allow for drug discrimination within the peripheral efferent nervous system.

> **BOX 6–10**
>
> - **Muscarinic (ACh) receptor** locations
>   - Parasympathetic postganglion neuroeffector junctions
>   - (Sympathetic sweat glands)
> - **Nicotinic (ACh) receptor** locations
>   - Somatic (neuromuscular junction)
>   - Autonomic ganglia (parasympathetic and sympathetic)
>   - Sympathetic to adrenal medullae

Fortunately, for practical application, the nicotinic ACh receptors in the skeletal muscle junctions bind to different types of chemicals than the ones in the ganglia; such differences are exploited with different drugs. However, there apparently is little or no difference between the *ganglionic* receptors in the sympathetic branch and those in the parasympathetic. A drug that has actions on autonomic ganglia stimulates or blocks both branches of the autonomic system. In a similar fashion to this characterization of ACh receptors as being either muscarinic or nicotinic, a characterization of NE receptors in the sympathetic system as being either alpha or beta will be described in Chapter 9.

Biological Model Systems and Receptor Characterization

Understanding receptor characteristics is essential in designing drugs that are selective for specific pharmacological therapeutics. The pharmaceutical industry has expended a tremendous amount of energy to characterize various receptors throughout the body. Their organic chemists hope to synthesize drug molecules that fit very precisely into the topography of certain receptors and achieve more drug specificity, and perhaps greater potency.

Several biological model systems have served an invaluable role in characterizing receptors and the etiology of various diseases. Some of these systems might seem a bit obscure at a distance—for example, the venom of the Korean krait snake. This venom contains a toxic polypeptide, α-bungarotoxin, that binds very specifically to nicotinic ACh receptors. Studies with radiolabeled α-bungarotoxin were pivotal in elucidating the pathophysiology of myasthenia gravis (see Chapter 7).

Another unique model system is the electric organ of several fishes. Most of these electric tissues are modified neuromuscular end-plates and thus are pure cholinergic organs. They are a simple and powerful system in which to study all aspects of cholinergic chemistry. It was from the Torpedo ray electric organ that the first neurotransmitter receptor was isolated, identified, and synthesized—the nicotinic ACh receptor.

ACh receptor characteristics were also defined, in part, by studies with the clam heart. The heart of a clam removed and placed into a beaker of sea water will beat for hours. The beating rate and amplitude of the heart can easily be monitored by tying it to a kymograph pen, producing a record like that shown in Figure 6–8. If ACh is added to the bathing solution, the force of contraction decreases dramatically (and the rate slows). When the ACh is washed out with fresh sea

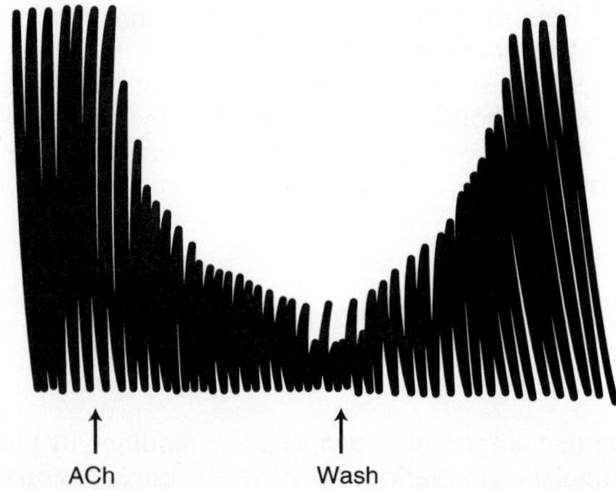

FIGURE 6–8. Characteristic effect of acetylcholine (ACh) on a spontaneously beating clam heart. The record on a kymograph drum is shown. Contractions cause upward deflection. Addition of acetylcholine (ACh) and removal by washing are shown by arrows. (From Goldstein A, Aronow L, Kalman SM: Principles of Drug Action: The Basis of Pharmacology, 2nd ed. New York: Churchill Livingstone, 1986, p 24.)

Compound	Relative Potency
$CH_3-{}^{+}N(CH_3)_2-CH_2-CH_2-O-C(=O)-CH_3$ (ACh)	100
$-CH_2-CH_2-CH_2-C(=O)-CH_3$	8
$-CH_2-CH_2-O-CH_2-CH_3$	1
$-CH_2-CH_3$	0.007
$-CH_2-CH_2-CH_2-CH_3$	0.4
$-CH_2-CH_2-CH_2-CH_2-CH_3$	1
$-CH_2-CH_2-CH_2-CH_2-CH_2-CH_3$	0.2

FIGURE 6–9. Relative potency of ACh analogs on clam heart contractions. (Modified from Goldstein A, Aronow L, Kalman SM: Principles of Drug Action. The Basis of Pharmacology, 2nd ed. New York: Churchill Livingstone, 1986, p 25.)

water, the contractions return to normal. A series of chemical analogs to ACh were also tested on this preparation, and the resulting amplitudes of contraction were compared with that from ACh to determine a relative potency for each compound. Altering the molecular carbon chain length reveals that a length of five atoms from the quaternary nitrogen is optimal for muscarinic activity. The relative importance of the esteratic and the ether oxygen of ACh was also indicated by the data given in Figure 6–9. These results suggest that the receptor recognition site might contain an anionic group that interacts electrostatically with the quaternary nitrogen of ACh (Fig. 6–10). As suggested by varying the analog chain length, we expect to find a group that will hydrogen bond to that esteratic oxygen about 5 Å from the anionic site.

Thus, such studies have helped determine what structural features of the ACh molecule are likely to have important complementary structural features at the receptor recognition site. Other similar experimentation has shown that the nicotinic and the muscarinic ACh receptors have very different sensitivities to a group of test drugs, indicating that the two receptor types have very different molecular topographies at their recognition sites. The characteristic classification that has emerged from these studies is that atropine is a very specific antagonist at muscarinic ACh receptors, whereas d-tubocurarine (curare) is a specific antagonist for nicotinic ACh receptors (especially in the skeletal muscle synapses).

> **BOX 6–11**
> **CLASSIC ACh RECEPTOR ANTAGONISTS**
>
> - **Muscarinic—Atropine**
> - **Nicotinic—d-Tubocurarine (curare)**

ACh is a small and very simple molecule; how does it have activity at two different receptor sites with very different molecular requirements (the muscarinic and nicotinic receptors)? This question has been addressed in several ways, including the following two simple and revealing approaches. The structural characteristics of numerous drugs with well-defined nicotinic or muscarinic activities have been compared on the basis of three-dimensional models and of x-ray crystallography data. All of the compounds examined had two active groups: a quaternary nitrogen and another hydrogen-bonding site (*eg*, an esteratic oxygen). One observation was that the distances between the two critical functional sites were found to be 5.9 Å in the nicotinic compounds, and 4.4 Å for the muscarinics (Fig. 6–11). It was also noted that the methyl side of the ACh molecule was unobstructed in all muscarinic compounds, whereas the carbonyl side was open in all nicotinic compounds. Both of these views suggest that the methyl side of ACh, which also has the ether oxygen 4.4 Å from the quaternary nitrogen, fits the recognition site of muscarinic receptors (thus, the "muscarinic side" of ACh). The corollary is that the carbonyl side, with the esteratic oxygen 5.9 Å from the nitrogen, is the "nicotinic side" of ACh. This model, which can explain how such a simple molecule can be fully active at two very different receptor sites, is shown in Figure 6–11.

RECEPTOR STRUCTURE

Much is now known about the molecular structure of receptors. As noted above, the nicotinic ACh receptor, first iso-

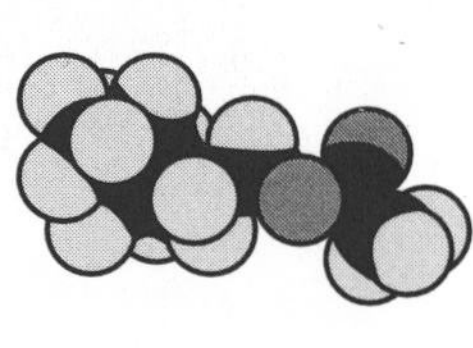

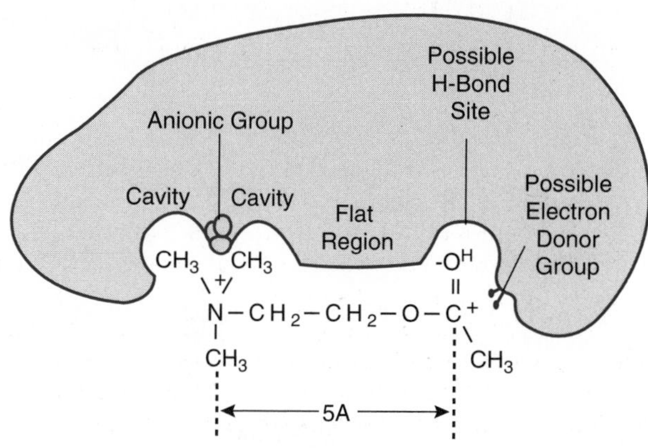

FIGURE 6–10. Possible topography of acetylcholine (ACh) receptor recognition sites.

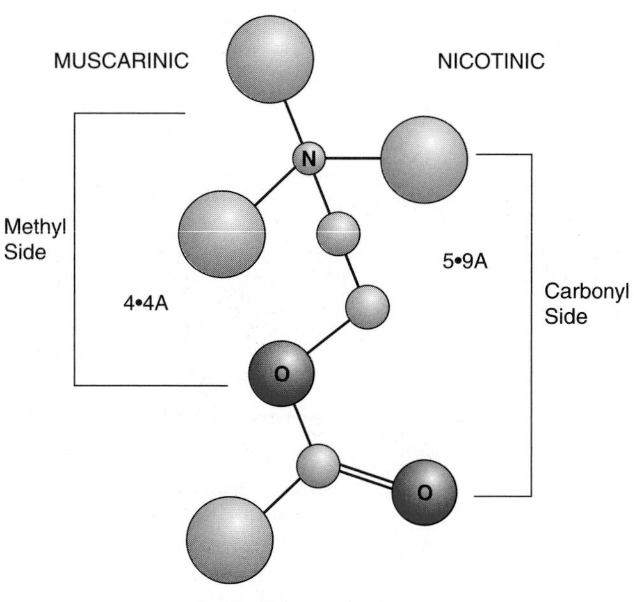

FIGURE 6–11. Muscarinic and nicotinic sites of ACh. (Reprinted with permission from *Nature*. Chothia C: Interaction of acetylcholine with different cholinergic nerve receptors. Nature 225:36–38, 1970. Copyright 1970 Macmillan Magazines Limited.)

lated from the electric organ of the Torpedo ray, has an ion channel as an integral part of its structure. The binding of the ligand (ACh) to its receptor results in opening of the ion channel. Such ligand-gated ion channels mediate very rapid onset and rapidly reversible transmission. The receptor is composed of four different membrane-spanning glycoprotein subunits. Five subunits (two copies of the alpha subunit) are arranged to form a channel (Figs. 6–5 and 6–12). Two molecules of ACh are necessary to interact with the two ACh binding sites on the alpha subunits to open the ion channel. Molecular cloning approaches have been used to determine the amino acid sequences of the receptor subunits. Each subunit has four membrane-spanning hydrophobic domains. Functional nicotinic receptors have now been synthesized and inserted into artificial membranes; the permeability of such membranes to ions is tremendously increased upon exposure to ACh.

Muscarinic ACh receptors are of the G-protein–linked receptor type, wherein receptor and channel proteins interact with each other through information transduced by a guanyl nucleotide-binding protein. As noted above, activation of these receptors is amplified by one or more of the second messenger mechanisms. Cloning techniques have also been applied to the study of these macromolecules, and the amino acid sequences for several muscarinic receptors

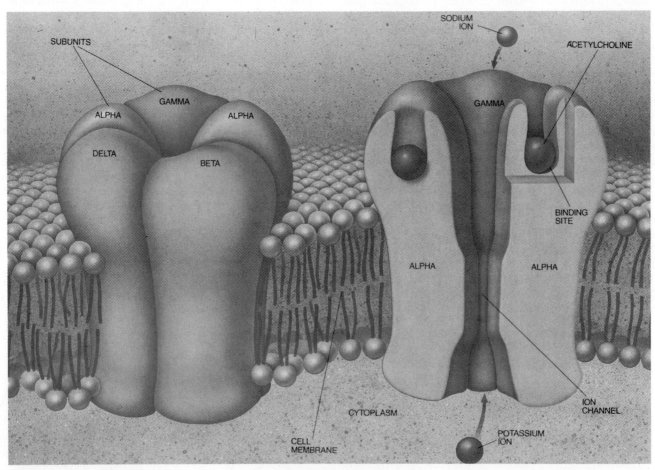

FIGURE 6–12. Acetylcholine (ACh) receptor, which consists of five subunits (left), was the first neurotransmitter receptor to be isolated. Later work showed it to include not only neurotransmitter binding sites but also an ion-transporting channel (right). (The beta and delta subunits and part of one alpha subunit have been cut away for clarity.) The channel is closed when the receptor is at rest, but it opens rapidly when the two alpha subunits both combine with ACh. (Appears in Changeaux J: Chemical signaling in the brain. Sci Am Nov:59, 1993. Reprinted with permission from Kistler J, Stroud R, Klymrowsky M, et al: Structure and function of an acetylcholine receptor. Biophys J 37:371–373, 1982; and Changeaux J, Devillers-Thiery A, Chemouilli P: Acetylcholine receptor: An allosteric protein. Science 225:1335–1345, 1984. Copyright 1993 American Association for the Advancement of Science.)

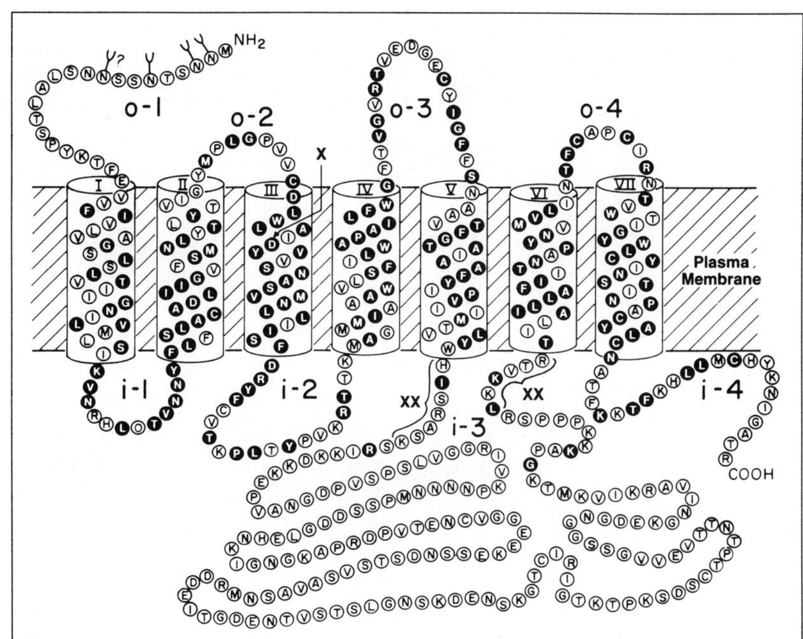

FIGURE 6–13. Structure of muscarinic acetylcholine (ACh) receptor. (Reprinted by permission of *The New England Journal of Medicine*. Modified from Goyal RK: Muscarinic receptor subtypes. Physiology and clinical implications. N Engl J Med 321:1022–1029, 1989. ©1989 Massachusetts Medical Society.)

have been determined. As with the other members of this family of receptors, the muscarinic ACh receptors have seven membrane-spanning alpha helices (Figs. 6–5 and 6–13). Several phosphorylation sites that control the activity of the receptor are within the cytoplasmic domain. Muscarinic receptor–mediated responses have a slower onset and last much longer than nicotinic responses.

TWO OTHER AUTONOMIC CONTROL MECHANISMS

Two other synaptic control mechanisms bear mentioning before closing this introduction to autonomic pharmacology: presynaptic heteroreceptors and endothelium-derived relaxing factors (EDRFs). Mentioned above was the concept of presynaptic autoreceptors that mediate inhibitory control mechanisms. A similar, more recently recognized concept, presynaptic heteroreceptors, allows a fine degree of autonomic control between NE and ACh nerve endings innervating the same organ. This dual innervation provides for potential cross-talk of feedback receptors, wherein parasympathetic neurons may control the release of NE from proximate sympathetic nerve varicosities. Likewise, sympathetic neurons may exert a control over the release of ACh from nearby parasympathetic fibers. Clear examples of such heteroreceptor control mechanisms have been demonstrated in the gut and in the heart (see Fig. 9–3).

Many blood vessels have ACh receptors that do not receive nerve input; further, these muscarinic receptors are located on endothelial cells rather than on the smooth muscle cells themselves. Stimulation of the endothelial muscarinic receptors with agonists results in the secretion of one or more EDRFs. In several systems, the EDRF has been identified as the simple inorganic molecule nitric oxide (NO). The EDRF (NO) activates second messenger systems in the smooth muscle cells, causing them to relax (the clinical relevance of this system is made obvious in the treatment of angina [see Chapter 30]).

REFERENCES

Axelsson J, Thesleff S: A study of supersensitivity in denervated mammalian skeletal muscle. J Physiol (Lond) 147:178–193, 1959.

Bannnister R (ed): Autonomic Failure: A Textbook of Clinical Disorders of the Autonomic Nervous System. Oxford: Oxford University Press, 1983.

Bartfai T: Presynaptic aspects of the coexistence of classical neurotransmitters and peptides. Trends Pharmacol 6:331–334, 1985.

Changeaux J-P: Chemical signaling in the brain. Scientific American November, 1993, pages 58–62.

Chothia C: Interaction of acetylcholine with different cholinergic nerve receptors. Nature 225:36–38, 1970.

Cooper JR, Bloom FE, Roth RH: The Biochemical Basis of Neuropharmacology, 6th ed. New York: Oxford University Press, 1991.

Day MD: Autonomic Pharmacology: Experimental and Clinical Aspects. New York: Churchill Livingstone, 1979.

Dunant Y: On the mechanism of acetylcholine release. Prog Neurobiol 26:55–92, 1986.

Furchgott RF: Role of endothelium in response of vascular smooth muscle. Circ Res 53:557–573, 1983.

Gilman AG, Rall TW, Nies AS, Taylor P (eds): Goodman and Gilman's The Pharmacological Basis of Therapeutics, 8th ed. New York: Pergamon, 1990.

Goldstein A, Aronow L, Kalman SM: Principles of Drug Action: The Basis of Pharmacology, New York: Churchill Livingstone, 1986.

Goyal RK: Muscarinic receptor subtypes. Physiology and clinical implications. N Engl J Med 321:1022–1029, 1989.

Howard BD, Gunderson CB Jr: Effects and mechanisms of polypeptide neurotoxins that act presynaptically. Annu Rev Pharmacol Toxicol 20:307–336, 1980.

Jope RS: High-affinity choline transport and acetyl CoA production in brain and their roles in regulation of acetylcholine synthesis. Brain Res Rev 1:313–344, 1979.

Laduron PM: Presynaptic heteroreceptors in regulation of neuronal transmission. Biochem Pharmacol 34:467–470, 1985.

McCarthy MP, Earnest JP, Young EF, et al: The molecular neurobiology of the acetylcholine receptor. Annu Rev Neurosci 9:383–413, 1986.

North RA: Electrophysiology of the enteric nervous system. Neuroscience 7:315–325, 1982.

Pratt WB, Tayor P (eds): Principles of Drug Action: The Basis of Pharmacology. 3rd ed. New York: Churchill Livingstone, 1990.

Rahamimioff R: The role of calcium in transmitter release at the neuromuscular junction. *In* Thesleff S (ed): Motor Innervation of Muscle, 117–149. London: Academic Press, 1976.

Reichardt LF, Kelly RB: A molecular description of nerve terminal function. Annu Rev Biochem 52:871–926, 1983.

Simpson LL: The origin, structure, and pharmacological activity of botulinum toxin. Pharmacol Rev 33:115–188, 1981.

Vanhoutte PM, Barnard EA, Cosmides GJ, et al: I. International Union of Pharmacology Committee on Receptor Nomenclature and Drug Classification. Pharm Rev 46:111–116, 1994.

Cholinergic Agonists

7

Oliver M. Brown

The pharmacology of the peripheral efferent nervous system is primarily based on the use of agonists and antagonists at cholinergic or adrenergic synapses; we will examine these four areas in four separate chapters. We first focus on a group of drugs that has its effect by stimulating acetylcholine (ACh) receptors, starting with muscarinic receptors. Drugs that mimic ACh at muscarinic receptors at the postganglionic neuroeffector junctions of the parasympathetic system are, thus, parasympathomimetics. The effects of administering a parasympathomimetic drug are easily predicted; they are nearly the same as the expected physiological responses of stimulating the parasympathetic system.

Muscarinic stimulation (with a drug like bethanechol) will result in the responses anticipated from autonomic (parasympathetic) physiology: miosis (constriction of the pupils), possibly spasm of accommodation, increased salivation, increased gastrointestinal activity, and bradycardia (Table 7 - 1). A couple of responses — excessive sweating and flushing — might not be obvious. Sweating is a sympathetic function, so sweating will not occur as a result of stimulating the parasympathetic nervous system. However, recall that the sweat glands receive anomalous sympathetic-cholinergic innervation. Thus, giving drugs that are active at muscarinic receptors will chemically induce sweating. Flushing (dilation of blood vessels in the skin) might also not be an expected muscarinic response, and probably occurs for two reasons. There are numerous muscarinic receptors in most vascular beds, and because these receptors do not receive nerve input, vasodilation does not occur as a physiological response; however, dilation will result from activating these receptors with muscarinic agonists. Also, bradykinin, produced in conjunction with sweating, is a powerful vasodilator and could contribute to parasympathomimetic flushing.

Blocking muscarinic receptors (with a drug like atropine) will produce essentially the opposite effects: we will see the sympathetic influence over these functions come out in relief. Muscarinic blockade results in mydriasis (dilation of the pupils), cycloplegia (paralysis of accommodation), drying of secretions, decrease in gut motility, and tachycardia (from suppressing the influence of the cardiac vagus). (Flushing, peripheral vasodilation, also occurs with large doses of atropine, in part in response to hyperthermia produced by absence of sweating.)

Unfortunately for therapeutics, the clinician has to choose either "Column A" or "Column B" from Table 7 - 1; that is, parasympathomimetics will produce essentially all of the effects listed in the left-hand column. Likewise, antimuscarinic drugs will produce the effects listed in the right-hand column. Depending on what problem a patient is being treated for, one must choose the effect that is therapeutically beneficial — the remaining effects in the column will be the side effects. For example, in treating a patient for hyperactive bowel, one may choose atropine for its constipating effect — one of the side effects will be dry mouth.

CLASSES OF CHOLINERGIC AGONISTS

- Choline esters
- Cholinergic alkaloids
- Cholinesterase inhibitors

Drugs from these three classes stimulate muscarinic sites by mimicking the actions of ACh; accordingly, these drugs are referred to as muscarinics, cholinergics, cholinomimetics, or parasympathomimetics. The esters and alkaloids that are used therapeutically have agonist activity at muscarinic receptors. For the most part, these drugs are used to stimulate smooth muscle activity in several clinical situations. The cholinesterase inhibitors are not primarily receptor agonists; they block the enzyme acetylcholinesterase (the termination step). This allows the concentration of ACh to build up in synapses, and results in increased activity at those synapses. Thus, these agents (cholinesterase inhibitors) are not specific for muscarinic sites, they also have significant activity at some nicotinic sites (see below). This latter group of drugs is also useful in augmenting skeletal neuromuscular transmission.

TABLE 7-1. Typical Effects of Drugs That Stimulate (or Block)* Muscarinic ACh Receptors

Muscarinic Stimulation (*eg*, bethanechol)	Muscarinic Blockade (*eg*, atropine)
Miosis	Mydriasis and cycloplegia
Excessive sweating	Dry skin
Flushing	[Flush, as reflex to hyperthermia]
Salivation	Dry mouth
Increased GI motility	Constipation
	Urinary retention
Bradycardia	Tachycardia

**Stimulants* = muscarinics, cholinergics, cholinomimetics, parasympathomimetics; *blockers* = antimuscarinics, anticholinergics, parasympatholytics.

CHOLINE ESTERS

As might expect be expected from the name, choline esters are close structural analogs of ACh. Obviously, ACh itself is a choline ester. Why consider other choline esters if we have ACh and we know that it works? Actually, there are two good reasons why ACh is not a useful therapeutic drug:

1. ACh is not specific for muscarinic receptors.
2. ACh is rapidly hydrolyzed.

Structure and Activity of Choline Esters

ACh is not selective for muscarinic receptors; it also has activity at all nicotinic receptors because it is the neurotransmitter at both sites. Nicotinic activity is generally an undesirable characteristic for drugs in this group because it imparts ganglion-stimulating properties. Such stimulation of ganglia would lead to widespread effects throughout the autonomic nervous system: nicotinic side effects.

Another reason that ACh is not a useful drug is that it is rapidly hydrolyzed by plasma cholinesterase. Even doses of ACh large enough to produce some effect would be extremely short-lasting.

These two problems, specificity and hydrolysis, were addressed by chemists, who modified the ACh molecule. Figure 7-1 shows the structures of choline and several choline esters. If a methyl group is added to the ACh molecule, adjacent to the ether oxygen, methacholine results. Compare the structures of ACh and methacholine in Figure 7-1 and in the projection structures of the same two molecules in Figure 7-2. From the previous chapter (Fig. 6-11) it is clear that this additional methyl group is jutting out into the nicotinic side of the ACh molecule. Thus, this methyl group confers selective muscarinic receptor-binding properties to methacholine by obstructing the nicotinic-binding face. However, as with ACh, methacholine is rapidly hydrolyzed by cholinesterase enzymes.

Another pharmacologically active analog of ACh, carbachol, terminates in a carbamate group rather than an ester group (Fig. 7-1). This carbamate structure is resistant to hydrolysis by the enzymes, but carbachol is not selective for muscarinic receptors.

Choline $(CH_3)_3\overset{+}{N}CH_2CH_2OH$

Acetylcholine $(CH_3)_3\overset{+}{N}CH_2CH_2O\overset{\overset{O}{\|}}{C}CH_3$

Methacholine $(CH_3)_3\overset{+}{N}CH_2\underset{\underset{CH_3}{|}}{C}HO\overset{\overset{O}{\|}}{C}CH_3$

Carbachol $(CH_3)_3\overset{+}{N}CH_2CH_2O\overset{\overset{O}{\|}}{C}NH_2$

Bethanechol $(CH_3)_3\overset{+}{N}CH_2\underset{\underset{CH_3}{|}}{C}HO\overset{\overset{O}{\|}}{C}NH_2$

FIGURE 7-1. Choline esters.

Based on these observations, an obvious solution to the problems of specificity and hydrolysis is to incorporate *both* structural analogs into one molecule. That molecule is bethanechol, which embodies both the muscarinic-directing methyl group and the hydrolysis-resisting carbamate moiety (Fig. 7-1). Thus, in bethanechol we have a choline ester drug that is useful because it is muscarinic-selective and it is not hydrolyzed (therefore it has a serviceable half-life of several hours).

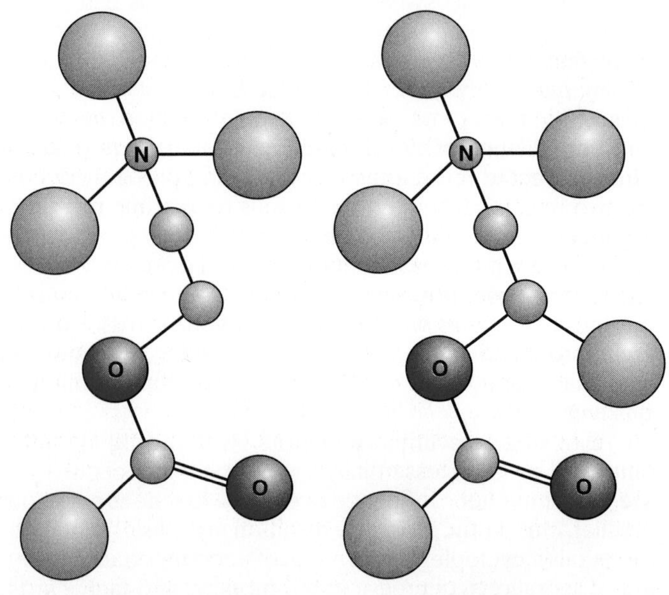

FIGURE 7-2. Structures of ACh and methacholine.

BOX 7-1

THERAPEUTIC USES OF CHOLINE ESTERS

• Acetylcholine	nonselective	rapidly hydrolyzed
• Methacholine	muscarinic-selective	rapidly hydrolyzed
• Carbachol	nonselective	not hydrolyzed
• Bethanechol	muscarinic-selective	not hydrolyzed

BOX 7-2

THERAPEUTIC USES OF CHOLINE ESTERS

Problems that require smooth muscle stimulation include:

- Atonic intestine (postoperative and neurogenic)
- Urinary retention (postoperative and postpartum, nonobstructive [functional])
- Reflux esophagitis

In some patients these are chronic problems, in other cases adynamic intestine and abdominal distention follow surgical procedures.

Each of the other esters—ACh, methacholine, and carbachol—has some very specialized applications, such as during ocular surgery. In this instance, the surgeon may require the brief contraction of a muscle; nonselective systemic effects are not problematic with such a localized application.

CHOLINERGIC ALKALOIDS

The concept of muscarinic receptors originated from Sir Henry Dale's experiments (in 1914) with the mushroom (*Amanita muscaria*) alkaloid muscarine. Currently, the only cholinergic plant alkaloid used clinically is **pilocarpine** (from the South American shrub *Pilocarpus*). Furthermore, pilocarpine has only one major clinical application: to treat open angle **glaucoma**.

The elevated intraocular pressure characteristic of glaucoma usually causes pain and blurred vision, and can progress to blindness. One approach to lowering the intraocular pressure is to facilitate the drainage of aqueous humor from the anterior chamber through the normal passageway, the canal of Schlemm. Application of pilocarpine to the eye contracts the ciliary muscle and the iris sphincter muscle. This contraction mechanically relieves the constriction in the region of the canal of Schlemm and allows for better outflow of aqueous humor from the anterior chamber (Fig. 7-3).

Dropping pilocarpine into the eye several times a day usually causes pupillary constriction, strong accommodation for near vision, and some burning and tearing. One solution to relieving these uncomfortable effects is by using a drug-delivery system called Ocusert. A permeable membrane containing pilocarpine that is inserted under the lower eyelid, Ocusert releases small amounts of pilocarpine constantly throughout the day.

A number of other approaches to treating glaucoma are available. Beta blockers, epinephrine, carbonic anhydrase inhibitors, and tetrahydrocannabinol all decrease the synthesis of aqueous fluid. The ciliary process produces aqueous humor as an ultrafiltrate, the vascularity of that organ is critical to the production of this ultrafiltrate, and these drugs all have an effect on that process. Physostigmine, a cholinesterase inhibitor, lowers intraocular pressure by facilitating outflow of aqueous humor by the same mechanism as pilocarpine (see next section). In some severe cases of glaucoma that do not respond to drug approaches, a drainage pathway larger than the canal of Schlemm can be created with laser surgery.

BOX 7-3

TREATMENTS FOR (OPEN ANGLE) GLAUCOMA

1. Pilocarpine (drops or Ocusert)
2. Physostigmine (cholinesterase inhibitor) (drops)
3. Timolol (β blocker) (drops)
4. Epinephrine (drops)
5. Acetazolamide (carbonic anhydrase inhibitor) (oral)
6. Δ^9-Tetrahydrocannabinol (marijuana) (oral or smoked)
7. Surgery (including laser)

CHOLINESTERASE INHIBITORS

We can also stimulate muscarinic sites, indirectly, by blocking the terminating step for ACh as a neurotransmitter. These cholinesterase inhibitors are not specific for muscarinic sites; they also have significant activity at some nicotinic sites. The cholinesterase inhibitors (anticholinesterase agents) are not primarily receptor agonists, they block the enzyme acetylcholinesterase (plasma cholinesterases are also inhibited). This inhibition of cholinesterase allows the concentration of ACh to build up in synapses, and more effector cell activity will result. The problem with this approach is that we have the potential of increasing activity wherever ACh is the neurotransmitter: at muscarinic sites, somatic sites, all autonomic ganglia, and in the central nervous system (CNS). This profile implies a potential for a wide variety of side effects, some extremely toxic, from such agents. However, with appropriate administration, some therapeutic gains can be obtained with this group of drugs without prohibitive side effects. The side effects can be minimized by using small doses of the drugs, and by selecting agents that contain quaternary nitrogen groups, so that they are very poorly translocated across membranes (thus, no CNS effects). Furthermore, the various organs have differences in sensitivity to these drugs, and some of the cholinesterase inhibitors have direct activity on the nicotinic ACh re-

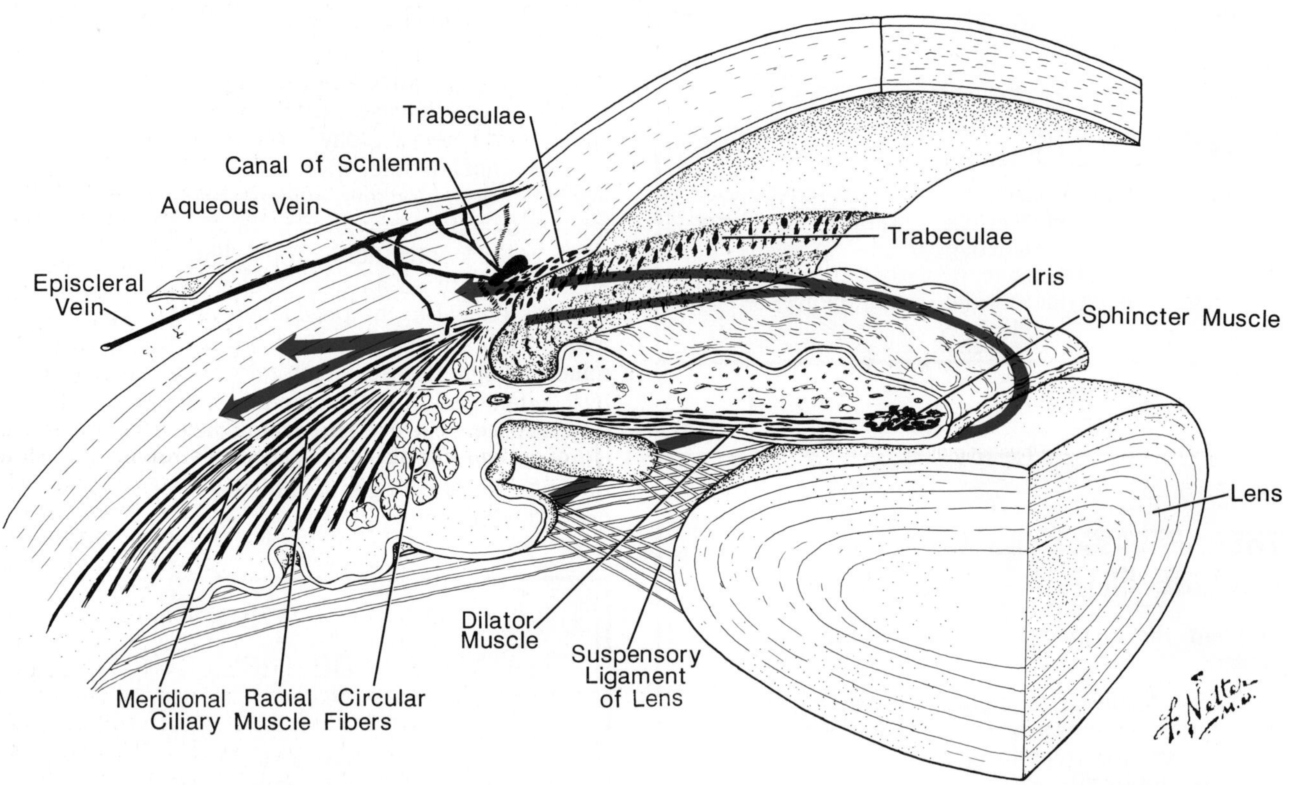

FIGURE 7–3. The eye. The lens is shown in relation to the ciliary muscles and the muscles of the pupil. The *colored arrows* indicate the flow of the aqueous humor—originating from the ciliary processes into the posterior chamber; through the pupil into the anterior chamber, leaving at the angle through the trabeculae and through uveoscleral routes. (Modified; copyright 1989 CIBA-GEIGY Corporation. Reproduced with permission from Atlas of Human Anatomy by Frank H. Netter, M.D. All rights reserved.)

ceptors in the somatic system. With all of these factors considered, cholinesterase inhibitors are used therapeutically to treat conditions of the eye, the intestine, and the skeletal muscular system.

BOX 7–4
CHARACTERISTICS OF CHOLINESTERASE INHIBITORS

- *Reversible*—therapeutic agents

  Quaternary—carbamates
  Poorly absorbed
  Some have direct activity (at nicotinic receptors)

- *Irreversible*—toxic agents

  Organophosphates
  Very lipid soluble
  Easily enter CNS

There are two major classes of cholinesterase inhibitors: the *reversible* drugs are used therapeutically, and most of them are carbamates; the *irreversible* agents are primarily used as insecticides and chemical warfare agents, and most of them are organophosphates.

The **model drug** for the reversible/therapeutic group is the quaternary carbamate **neostigmine**. Two other reversible drugs with slightly different structural characteristics and uses are physostigmine (ESERINE; ANTILIRIUM) and edrophonium (TENSILON) (Fig. 7–4). Physostigmine is not a quaternary compound and thus gains access to the CNS; it is useful in reversing the central effects of antimuscarinic drugs (*eg*, atropine). Edrophonium does not contain a carbamate group, and is very short acting in low doses; it is useful in diagnosing both the disease of, and the cholinergic crisis in, myasthenia gravis.

There are over 50,000 irreversible acetylcholinesterase inhibitors; these organophosphate compounds are notable for being important pesticides (*eg*, parathion, malathion) and nerve gases used in chemical warfare (*eg*, soman and sarin) (Fig. 7–4).

Acetylcholinesterase: Mechanism of Inhibition

The scheme for the hydrolysis of ACh by acetylcholinesterase is shown in Figure 7–5. Also seen in Figure 7–5 is the interaction of the enzyme with several other agents. Analogous to the characteristics discussed earlier for receptor selectivity, the enzyme has somewhat similar anionic and esteratic recognition sites.

Some agents interact with the esteratic site of acetylcholinesterase, some with the anionic site, and some bind to both (as does ACh). In the association of ACh with the active site of the enzyme, there is an ionic interaction with its quaternary nitrogen and a covalent bond with the esteratic carbon (Fig. 7–5*A*). The actual hydrolysis of the ACh molecule

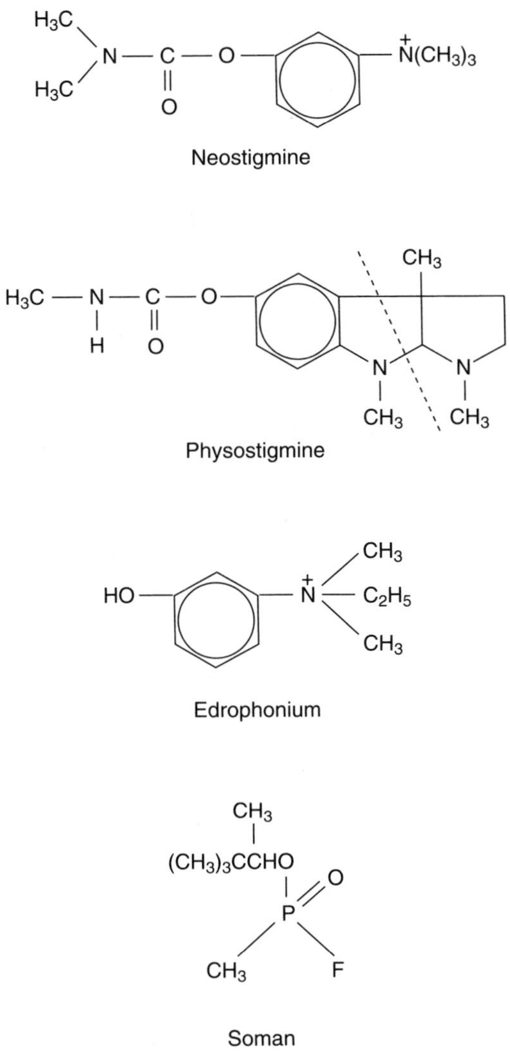

Neostigmine

Physostigmine

Edrophonium

Soman

FIGURE 7-4. Cholinesterase inhibitors.

is extremely fast and rapidly releases free choline. The subsequent hydrolysis of the remaining acetylated enzyme intermediate is the slow step in the process, with a half-time of about 100 microseconds.

Neostigmine (Fig. 7-5*B*) interacts with acetylcholinesterase in a similar fashion as does ACh, resulting in a carbamylated enzyme intermediate. The half-time for the hydrolysis of the carbamylated intermediate is 30 minutes—several million times slower than for ACh. Thus, the carbamate ties up the enzyme for long enough to prevent the hydrolysis of many million molecules of ACh.

Edrophonium (Fig. 7-5*C*) is not a carbamate; it associates ionically as does ACh, but it forms only a hydrogen bond with the esteratic binding site on the enzyme. Because edrophonium does not form a covalent-bonded enzyme intermediate, it is short-acting compared with neostigmine.

The irreversible organophosphate agents (*eg*, soman, Fig. 7-5*D*) form covalent bonds with the esteratic binding site of the enzyme. However, hydrolysis of the phosphorylated complex does not occur; this is a permanent covalent bond. Thus, recovery occurs only after the synthesis of new enzyme.

BOX 7-5
THERAPEUTIC USES OF CHOLINESTERASE INHIBITORS

Reversible cholinesterase inhibitors are used to stimulate smooth muscle activity (muscarinic sites) and skeletal muscle activity (nicotinic sites) in several clinical situations. Neostigmine and other similar agents can be used in conditions analogous to those described above for other muscarinic-stimulating drugs (*eg*, pilocarpine or bethanechol); namely, cholinesterase inhibitors are occasionally used to treat glaucoma and to increase intestinal activity. Neostigmine is used to reverse the peripheral effects of antimuscarinic agents, such as atropine, that slow intestinal activity. Atropine poisoning, particularly in children (see Chapter 8), is specifically treated with physostigmine, which crosses the blood-brain barrier and reverses both the central and peripheral effects of atropine.

These agents are uniquely used to increase activity at skeletal muscle junctions (nicotinic sites). Some cholinesterase inhibitors, notably neostigmine and edrophonium, have a dual effect; they not only increase the concentration of ACh but also directly act on the somatic nicotinic ACh receptor. These properties are taken advantage of in reversing the action of muscle relaxers (*eg*, curare) and in treating myasthenia gravis.

Thus, the effects of neostigmine (and other cholinesterase inhibitors) are reciprocal to some actions of both atropine (at muscarinic sites) and curare (at nicotinic sites).

BOX 7-6
USES OF CHOLINESTERASE INHIBITORS

- Treat glaucoma
- Reverse atropine
- Reverse curare and related neuromuscular blocking agents
- Treat myasthenia gravis

Myasthenia Gravis

Myasthenia gravis is a disease of progressive skeletal fatigue and muscle weakness. Facial and eye muscles are usually the first to be affected (drooping eyelids and facial flaccidness), with progression that includes all skeletal muscle, and ultimately those of respiration.

As noted in Chapter 6, characterization of the pathophysiology of myasthenia gravis was made possible by using elements from two unusual biological systems. Radiolabeled alpha-bungarotoxin, from the venom of the Korean krait snake, specifically binds to nicotinic ACh receptors and was used to demonstrate that muscle biopsy specimens of myasthenia gravis patients have fewer ACh receptors than

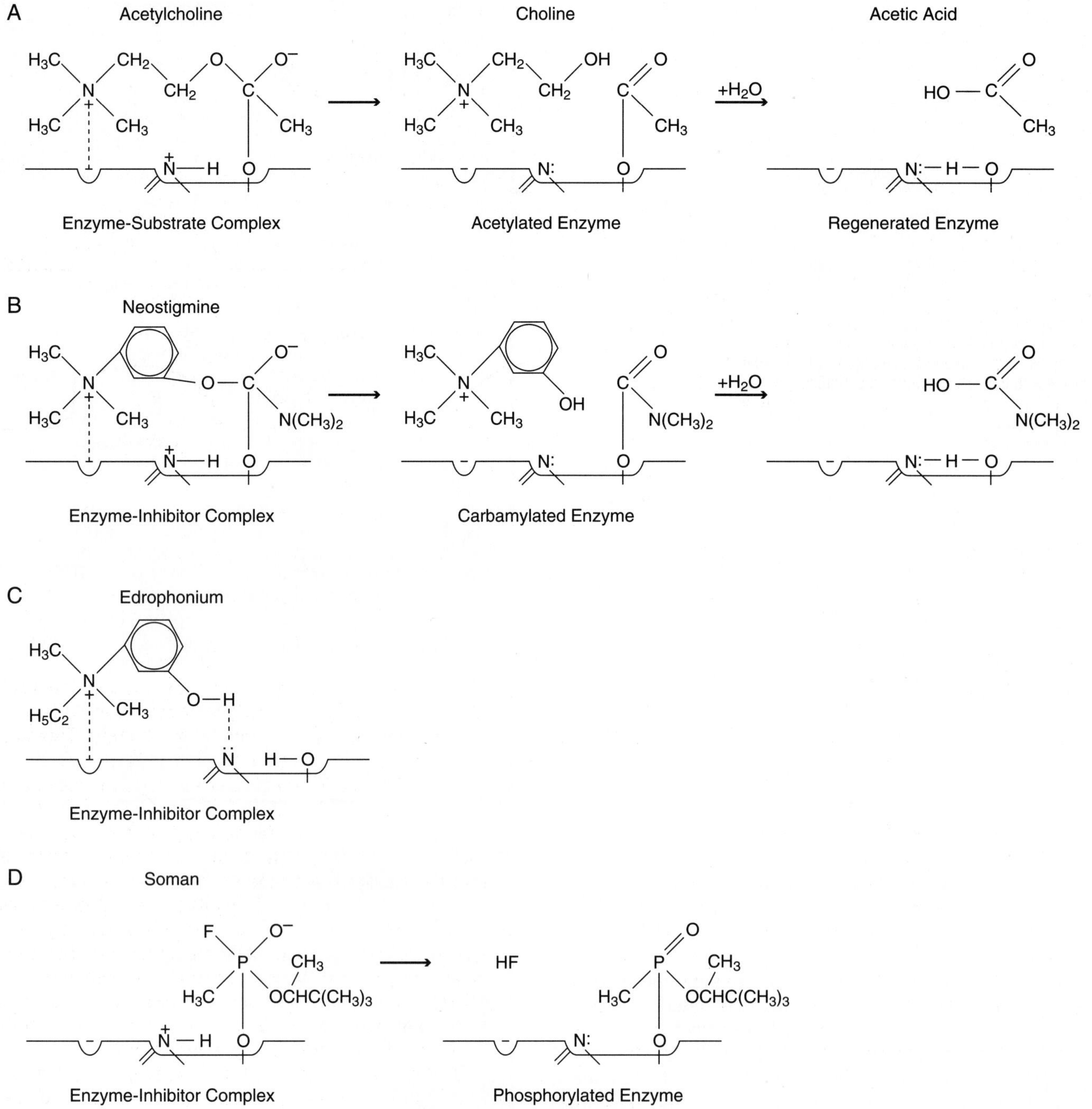

A Acetylcholine — Choline — Acetic Acid

Enzyme-Substrate Complex — Acetylated Enzyme — Regenerated Enzyme

B Neostigmine

Enzyme-Inhibitor Complex — Carbamylated Enzyme

C Edrophonium

Enzyme-Inhibitor Complex

D Soman

Enzyme-Inhibitor Complex — Phosphorylated Enzyme

FIGURE 7–5. Acetylcholinesterase reactions.

controls. In other experiments, rabbits were injected with nicotinic ACh receptor proteins purified from the electric organ of the electric eel. The rabbits made antibodies to the eel receptors, and the antibodies attacked their own skeletal muscle nicotinic ACh receptors, producing a condition nearly identical to the myasthenia gravis disease. The conclusion of these and other studies is that *myasthenia gravis is an antibody-mediated autoimmune disease*—an antibody attack on the patient's own somatic nicotinic ACh receptors, resulting in far fewer functional receptors. The application of cholinesterase inhibitors decreases the destruction of released ACh, increasing its concentration and prolonging its action, thus improving skeletal muscle strength and reducing fatigability (Fig. 7–6).

Treatment with neostigmine or other such drugs may also produce muscarinic side effects, including increased salivation and gastrointestinal (GI) activity, bradycardia, constriction of pupils, and possibly some bronchconstriction. In some patients these side effects are counteracted by concomitant administration of an antimuscarinic drug such as atropine. (If both drugs are used in appropriate doses, a net cancellation of the muscarinic effects and an increase in skeletal muscle nicotinic activity can be produced.)

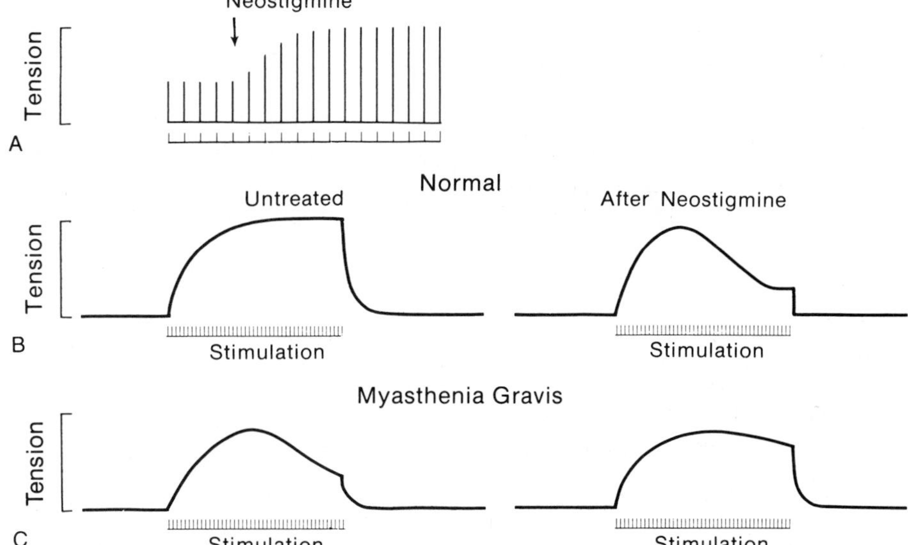

FIGURE 7–6. Effects of neostigmine on muscle contractions produced by supramaximal nerve stimulation in three different conditions: (*A*) Normal muscle with the nerve stimulated periodically at 10-second intervals. (*B*) Normal muscle with the nerve stimulated repetitively, 25 times per second. (*C*) Myasthenic muscle with the nerve stimulated repetitively, 25 times per second.

BOX 7–7

CHOLINESTERASE INHIBITOR + ATROPINE: ALGEBRAIC SUM OF ACTIVITIES

	Neostigmine	*Atropine*	*Net*
Muscarinic	↑	↓	0
Nicotinic	↑	0	↑

Because myasthenia gravis is an autoimmune condition, suppressing the immune response with corticosteroids (or azathioprine) is another successful approach to treatment in some patients. Also, because many of the antibodies to the nicotinic receptors appear to arise from the thymus, a surgical thymectomy is sometimes curative, especially in younger patients.

BOX 7–8

MYASTHENIA GRAVIS

- Is progressive skeletal muscle weakness
- Is an antibody-mediated autoimmune disease
- Cholinesterase inhibitors improve muscle strength
  Atropine prevents muscarinic side effects
- Other treatments
  Immune suppression
  Thymectomy
- Cholinergic crisis: overdose or underdose
  Mechanical respiration
  Edrophonium test

Cholinesterase Inhibitor Overdose and the Cholinergic Crisis

Another aspect of treating myasthenia gravis patients is the *cholinergic crisis.* Occasionally, a myasthenic patient may experience a paroxysm of breathing difficulty. This emergency situation may result from *either underdosing or overdosing* with cholinesterase inhibitors. Because neostigmine and similar drugs are quaternary compounds, they move across membranes with great difficulty, if at all. Thus the absorption of these drugs may be affected fairly dramatically by the timing and the nature of meals. Consequently, myasthenic patients may end up either underdosed or overdosed by changing their daily habits, or by forgetting to take a tablet or by taking an extra tablet. It should be obvious that a myasthenic patient who is undertreated would experience the characteristic weakness of the disease and have trouble breathing. Not so obvious is the muscle paralysis resulting from overdoses of cholinesterase inhibitors.

As noted in Chapter 1, log dose-response curves for most drugs form an S-shaped curve (note the dashed line in Fig. 7–7). However, log dose-response curves for cholinesterase inhibitors follow a bell-shaped curve (the solid line in Fig. 7–7). Once a maximum skeletal muscle response has been achieved, greater amounts of drug can actually cause blockade. As more drug is added, more and more depolarization at the neuromuscular end-plate (nicotinic receptors) results. At a certain point, the muscle membrane cannot recover its normal membrane polarity in order to be discharged again, and the membrane is persistently depolarized—a depolarization block. Figure 7–7*A* shows a hypothetical log dose-response curve for muscle strength in a myasthenic patient treated with a cholinesterase inhibitor; Figure 7–7*B* is a similar hypothetical curve for a normal individual.

Thus, in myasthenia gravis, muscle weakness can occur at either of two ends of the dose-response curve (Fig. 7–

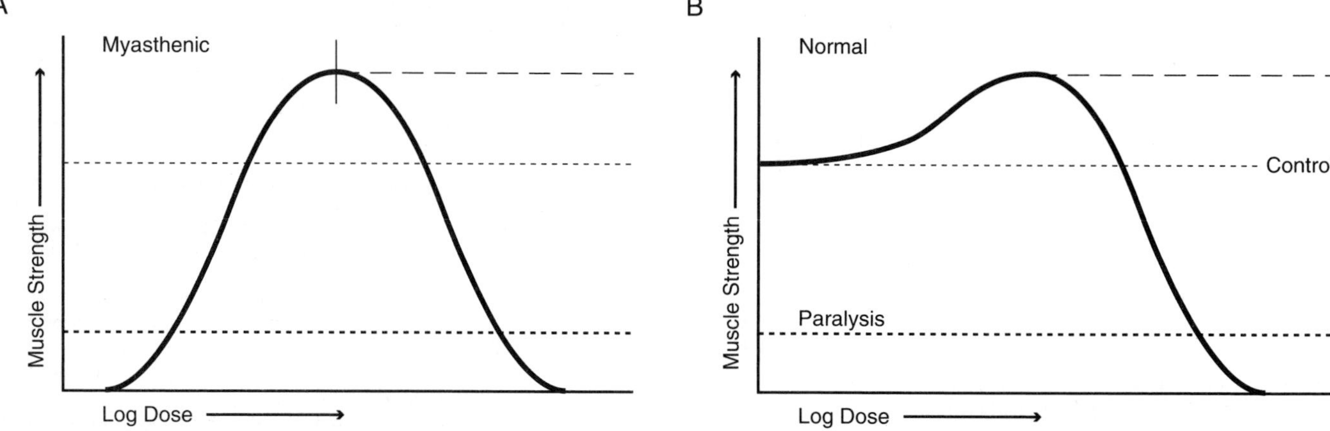

FIGURE 7–7. Hypothetical log dose-response curves for cholinsterase inhibitor: effects on skeletal muscle strength.

7*A*)—at one end, insufficient transmitter ACh; at the other end, an excess of cholinergic-induced depolarization, the cholinergic crisis. The physician's dilemma is that he or she must treat the crisis patient who is either underdosed or overdosed with a cholinesterase inhibitor. Of course, patients must be artificially respired in either case. The best test to determine if the patient is underdosed or overdosed is the "edrophonium test." Edrophonium is uniquely valuable in this situation (and diagnostic for myasthenia itself) because low doses of it are very short-acting. Thus, an injection of edrophonium will result in either a brief remission (in an underdosed patient) or a brief exacerbation (in an overdosed patient) of the patient's weakness and breathing difficulties. Following the test results, underdosed patients are given more of their usual anticholinesterase drug, whereas overdosed patients may require breathing support until they clear the drug (there is no antidote).

Organophosphate Cholinesterase Inhibitors

Although their clinical application is only extremely rare ("last resort" for severe glaucoma), the organophosphate compounds are clinically very important because of their toxicity. Inasmuch as hundreds of tons of these chemicals are manufactured and used in this country every year, there is a continuing problem of individuals who are exposed to pesticides in agriculture fields and nerve gas compounds at chemical plants. Public awareness of these compounds was heightened with the advent of the war in the Persian Gulf. The toxic effects of these agents are essentially an exaggeration of the expected muscarinic symptoms—tremendous salivation and respiratory secretions, tearing, blurring and burning of the eyes, and the like. Furthermore, the nicotinic signs can include profound muscle twitching, fasciculations, and cramps, followed by flaccid paralysis (again, "depolarization block"). Death is from both peripheral and centrally mediated respiratory paralysis. The organophosphates are very lipid soluble, are readily absorbed through the skin, and easily enter the CNS.

Treatment of organophosphate toxicity includes assisting respiration and administering large amounts of atropine to reverse the muscarinic effects. Atropine will also improve the CNS toxicity because most of the receptors for acetylcholine in the brain are muscarinic in nature. There is only a limited capability to reverse the peripheral nicotinic poisoning, namely, skeletal muscle paralysis. A class of drugs, the oxime reactivators, is used to reactivate the phosphorylated cholinesterase enzyme (Fig. 7–5*D*). The oxime reactivators (e.g., pralidoxime [2-PAM]) bind electrostatically to the anionic site of the phosphorylated cholinesterase molecule and perform a nucleophilic attack on the phosphorus, breaking the covalent bond between the phosphate and the enzyme, regenerating the enzyme.

Unfortunately, with the passage of time the phosphorylated form of the enzyme undergoes unexplained changes referred to as "aging." Once the phosphorylated enzyme "ages," it can no longer be recovered with the oxime compounds. The time period for the aging reaction is different for differing organophosphate compounds: the aging half-time for many of these compounds ranges between 24 and 48 hours; however, the half-life for aging of the soman-bound enzyme is only 2 minutes! Note also that the oxime reactivators are not effective in recovering enzyme activity from the effects of the carbamate agents (*eg*, neostigmine). For example, in the case of an overdosed myasthenic patient, the use of an oxime compound will only make the patient weaker.

BOX 7–9

TREATMENT OF ORGANOPHOSPHATE ANTICHOLINESTERASE TOXICITY

- Assist respiration
- Atropine in adequate doses
- Cholinesterase reactivator (oxime)

SIDE EFFECTS OF PARASYMPATHOMIMETICS

The side effects of drugs that stimulate the parasympathetic system (*eg*, bethanechol, pilocarpine, and the cholinesterase inhibitors) should be apparent from autonomic physiology. From Table 7 – 1, we would expect the following *possible side effects*:

- Miosis, spasm of accommodation
- Excessive sweating
- Marked salivation
- Increased GI motility, diarrhea
- Bradycardia
- Urinary urgency

CONTRAINDICATIONS FOR PARASYMPATHOMIMETICS

An obvious extension of the possible side effects of cholinergic agents suggests the major contraindications of parasympathomimetics. A patient who has a compromised cardiovascular system (bradycardic or hypotensive) would not be improved by further slowing of the heart caused by parasympathetic stimulation. The bronchoconstriction resulting from parasympathetic stimulation might precipitate an asthmatic attack in an asthmatic patient. Hyperthyroid patients are notably prone to atrial arrhythmias; cholinergic stimulation shortens atrial muscle refractory period, and can cause atrial flutter or fibrillation in hyperthyroid patients. Drugs that increase GI activity and gastric acid secretion will certainly only aggravate peptic ulcer. Thus, the *contraindications for parasympathomimetic drug use* are:

- Bradycardia or hypotension
- Asthma
- Hyperthyroidism
- Peptic ulcer

REFERENCES

Also see references for Chapter 6.

Adou-Donia MB: Organophosphorus ester-induced delayed neurotoxicity. Annu Rev Pharmacol Toxicol 21:511 – 548, 1981.

Brimijoin S: Molecular forms of acetylcholinesterase in brain, nerve and muscle: Nature, localization and dynamics. Prog Neurobiol 21:298 – 322, 1983.

Drachman DB: Myasthenia gravis. New Engl J Med 330: 1797 – 1810, 1994.

Dunant Y: On the mechanism of acetylcholine release. Prog Neurobiol 26:55 – 92, 1986.

Ellin RI: Anomalies in theories and therapy of intoxication by potent organophosphorus anticholinesterase compounds. Gen Pharmacol 13:457 – 466, 1982.

Goyal RK: Muscarinic receptor subtypes. Physiology and clinical implications. N Engl J Med 321:1022 – 1029, 1989.

Hobbiger F: Pharmacology of anticholinesterase drugs. *In* Zaimis E (ed): Neuromuscular Junction, 487 – 581. Vol 42 of Handbook of Experimental Pharmacology. Berlin: Springer-Verlag, 1976.

Johnson MK: The target for initiation of delayed neurotoxicity by organophosphorus esters: Biochemical studies and toxicological applications. Rev Biochem Toxic 4:141 – 212, 1982.

Karlin A: Explorations of the nicotinic acetylcholine receptor. Harvey Lectures 85:71 – 107, 1991.

Kaufman PL, Wiedman T, Robinson JR: Cholinergics. *In* Sears ML (ed): Pharmacology of the Eye, 149 – 192. Vol 69 of Handbook of Experimental Pharmacology. Berlin: Springer-Verlag, 1984.

Kerkut GA: Acetylcholinesterase (ACHE) (EC.3.1.1.7). Gen Pharmacol 15:375 – 378, 1984.

Marquis JK: Non-cholinergic mechanisms in insecticide toxicity. Trends Pharmacol Sci 6:59 – 60, 1985.

Tautant J-P, Massoulie J: Cholinesterases: Tissue and cellular distribution of molecular forms and their physiological regulation. *In* Whittaker VP (ed): The Cholinergic Synapse, 255 – 265. Vol 86 of Handbook of Experimental Pharmacology. Berlin: Springer-Verlag, 1988.

Unwin N: Nicotinic acetylcholine receptor at 9 Å resolution. J Mol Biol 229:1101 – 1124, 1993.

8 Cholinergic Antagonists: Antimuscarinic and Antinicotinic Drugs

Oliver M. Brown

The previous chapter concerned itself with cholinergic agonists—drugs that stimulate acetylcholine (ACh) receptors. We now turn our attention to cholinergic antagonists—drugs that block ACh receptors. Both muscarinic and nicotinic blockers will be considered, as well as two *different mechanisms of blockade.*

The *competitive* (nondepolarizing) antagonists have no intrinsic activity of their own; they simply occupy the receptor site and prevent access by ACh. This type of blockade is possible at both muscarinic and nicotinic ACh receptors.

Classic **competitive antagonists** (nondepolarizing) include:

- *Atropine* (at muscarinic sites)
- *Curare* (at nicotinic sites)

At nicotinic receptors in the ganglia and the somatic neuromuscular junction, there is another possible blocking mechanism. There are *depolarizing* antagonists that have biphasic action at these nicotinic sites: they produce an initial stimulation of activity, followed by a more persistent block of activity. (This mechanism does not occur at muscarinic sites.) As noted previously (see Fig. 7-7 and related discussion, Chapter 7), the simplest explanation for this type of block is a persistent depolarization (overstimulation) of the effector cell membrane.

Classic **depolarizing antagonists** include:

- *Nicotine* (at ganglia)
- *Succinylcholine* (at somatic junctions)

ANTIMUSCARINIC AGENTS

Drugs that block muscarinic ACh receptors can be regarded as parasympatholytic; thus, in the presence of antimuscarinic agents, the sympathetic influence on organs is brought out in relief. Antimuscarinics generally cause drying of secretions, dilation of the pupils, tachycardia, and decrease in gut motility. Muscarinic antagonists are all of the competitive type (block can be overcome by increasing the concentration of ACh; there are no depolarizing muscarinic blockers). The classic antimuscarinic drug is **atropine**. Atropine and the similar compound scopolamine are belladonna alkaloids. These agents occur naturally in several plants, including *Atropa belladonna*, the deadly nightshade (also in Jimson weed, henbane, and others). The belladonna alkaloids are tertiary amines, and readily cross the blood-brain barrier. There are also many synthetic antimuscarinic compounds, a number of which are quaternary amines that do not gain access to the CNS. The following is a partial listing of several characteristic antimuscarinic drugs; the structures of atropine, cyclopentolate, ipratropium, and pirenzepine are shown in Figure 8-1.

Belladonna alkaloids (naturally occurring antimuscarinic alkaloids) include:

- **Atropine**
- Scopolamine

Synthetic antimuscarinics (there are many more) include:

- Cyclopentolate
- Tropicamide
- Pirenzepine
- Ipratropium

Activity of Antimuscarinic Agents

Most of the drugs in this group, synthetic and naturally occurring, have a pharmacological profile similar to that of atropine—the major exception being that quaternary synthetic agents are poorly absorbed and have no CNS activity. Antimuscarinic drug effects depend on the differing sensitivities of the various organs to parasympathetic stimulation. Because the most sensitive system is the organs of secretion, very low doses of atropine produce dry mouth, dry eyes, and

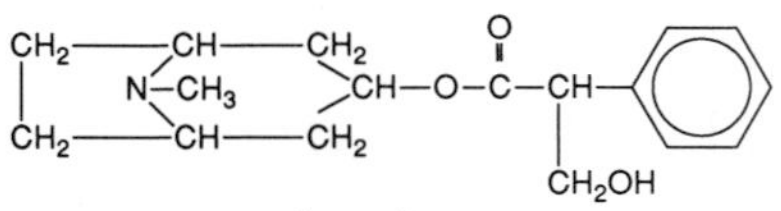

FIGURE 8–1. Structures of antimuscarinics: atropine, cyclopentolate hydrochloride, ipratropium bromide, and pirenzepine.

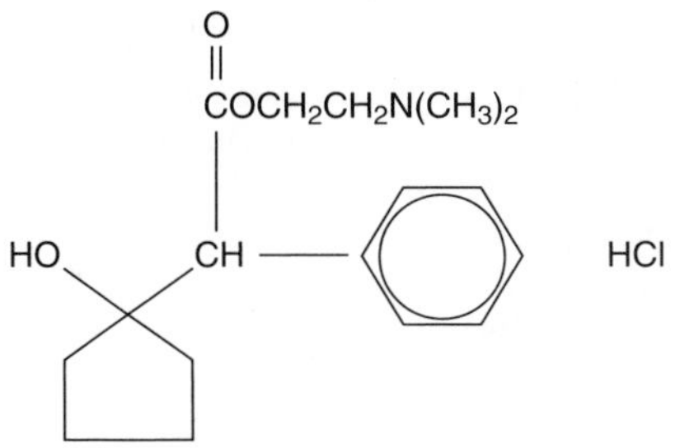

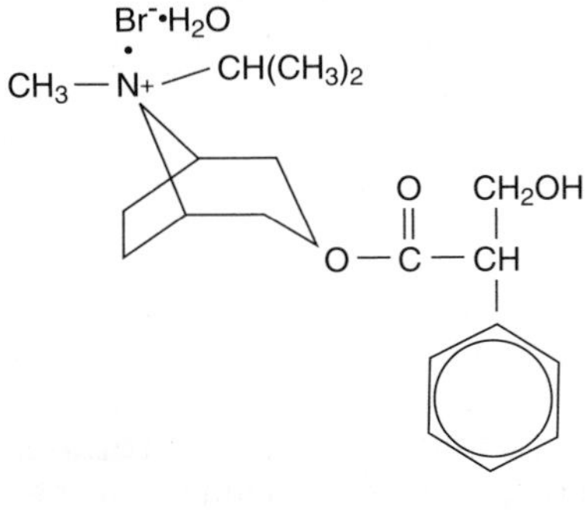

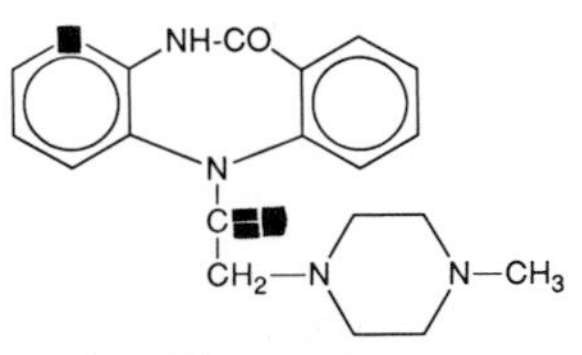

a dry respiratory tract. Next in sensitivity are the eyes, then heart, gut, and finally CNS (Table 8–1).

Antimuscarinics and the Gut

That there are so many synthetic antimuscarinics is a tribute to one of our national diseases, peptic ulcer. Logically, if the parasympathetic influences to the gut are blocked, there would be a decrease in motility and a decrease in acid secretion. Unfortunately, the synthetic antimuscarinic agents have pharmacological profiles virtually identical to that of atropine. As seen in Table 8–1, one of the more resistant functions is gastric acid secretion. Thus, patients treated with an antimuscarinic dose large enough for an effective decrease in gastric acid secretions are made very uncomfortable by difficulties with vision, urination, and the like. Thus, this theoretically valuable application for antimuscarinics is of limited usefulness due to significant side effects.

Fortunately, there is now an exception to this situation: research on muscarinic receptor subtypes has identified at least five types of muscarinic receptors. Atropine blocks the traditional parasympathetic muscarinic receptors, now referred to as M2-muscarinic receptors. Of special interest here are the newly described M1-muscarinic receptors, which are localized in the brain and in the ganglia of the enteric nervous system of the gut. Further, a new agent, **pirenzepine**, binds with very high affinity to M1 receptors, where it is an antagonist. Clinical experience has shown that pirenzepine is a far more effective and specific blocker of gastric acid secretion and has far fewer side effects than atropine itself. Upon food stimulation, pirenzepine (blocking M1 receptors) decreased gastric acid secretions from parietal cells by 50–60% in experimental subjects. This effect is compared with atropine administration (blocking M2 receptors), which caused a 30% decrease. At this writing, pirenzepine is not yet in clinical use in the United States; it is being used successfully in Europe. Currently, a very effective approach to treating ulcer in the United States is to block histamine-2 receptors with H2 antagonists such as cimetidine. The relationship between these three receptor types and the enteric innervation of the parietal cells is shown in Figure 33–1.

TABLE 8–1. Dose-Related Effects of Atropine in an Adult

Dose	Effect
0.5–1 mg	Dry mouth, dry skin
2 mg	Dilated pupils, accommodation paralyzed, tachycardia
5 mg	Very dry, ↓ GI and bladder tone, ↓ gastric acid secretion, CNS effects
10 mg	CNS toxicity
100–200 mg	Coma

BOX 8–1
MUSCARINIC RECEPTOR SUBTYPES (there are at least 5)

M1 High-affinity binding to the antagonist drug **pirenzepine**
In brain and enteric ganglia

M2 "Traditional" muscarinic receptors
High-affinity binding to antagonist **atropine**
In heart, eyes, GI smooth muscle, etc . . .

BOX 8–2
THERAPEUTIC USES OF ANTIMUSCARINIC AGENTS

There are many clinical applications for drugs which block muscarinic ACh receptors, including:

- Reverse bradycardia—atropine
- Produce mydriasis and cycloplegia—tropicamide
- Adjunct to anesthesia—atropine
- Parkinson's disease—trihexyphenidyl

Continued

BOX 8-2

THERAPEUTIC USES OF ANTIMUSCARINIC AGENTS (*Continued*)

- GI disorders—pirenzepine
- Chronic obstructive pulmonary disease (COPD)—ipratropium
- Treat anticholinesterase poisoning—atropine
- Motion sickness—scopolamine

Atropine is often used to *reverse the bradycardia* that frequently follows a myocardial infarction and results from excessive vagal tone.

Atropine and atropine-like compounds are useful in ophthalmology in some therapeutic situations and to facilitate examinations, by causing *dilation of the pupil*, and *paralysis of accommodation* (cycloplegia). One problem with applying atropine itself is that the effect will last for up to fourteen days. Short-acting synthetic antimuscarinics include cyclopentolate, which lasts about a day, or tropicamide, which is effective for only 3 or 4 hours (Fig. 8–1).

Antimuscarinics are commonly used *before, during, and after surgery*. Preanesthetic atropine antagonized, copious secretions produced by now obsolete anesthetics; the newer halogenated hydrocarbon anesthetics are far less aggravating. Atropine is still useful to protect against bradycardia during anesthesia. It is also used following surgery to prevent the muscarinic side effects during reversal of neuromuscular blockade with neostigmine.

Centrally acting antimuscarinic agents (such as trihexyphenidyl) are used to treat *Parkinson's* disease, usually in conjunction with L-dopa (see Chapter 21).

Some *GI disorders* do find an application for atropine: spastic colon and the like. Pirenzepine (Fig. 8–1) is a special M_1 muscarinic receptor antagonist that is effective in treating ulcers, while producing far fewer side effects than atropine.

The bronchioles constrict in response to parasympathetic stimulation; thus antimuscarinics produce relaxation. However, in *asthma* and *COPD* most antimuscarinic drugs not only produce *bronchial dilation* but also reduce the volume of and increase the viscosity of bronchial secretions. The quaternary compound ipratropium bromide (Fig. 8–1), a drug that dilates the bronchioles without significantly affecting respiratory secretions, is a useful agent in treating some COPD and asthma patients (other approaches to treating asthma and COPD are given in Chapter 17).

As discussed in Chapter 7, atropine is an essential *antidote* in treating poisoning with *anticholinesterase* agents.

There are several other miscellaneous uses of antimuscarinics. For example, scopolamine (often as dermal patches) is effective for many in preventing motion sickness.

Side Effects of Antimuscarinic Drugs

The side effects of these agents are obvious from Table 8–1. Dry mouth, dilated pupils (thus, photophobia), tachycardia, and decreased gut and bladder activity are often experienced when antimuscarinics are used. Higher doses of agents that cross the blood-brain barrier also cause CNS effects: initially sedation with scopolamine. Still higher doses of scopolamine and atropine cause CNS excitation, delirium, and hallucinations. Coma and death are possible; they are very rare in adults but a real possibility with children. It is unfortunately fairly common for young children to ingest large quantities of antimuscarinic-containing medications, or belladonna-containing plants. Atropine-poisoned children experience dramatic elevations in body temperature—they stop sweating, and central temperature regulation is also lost. Intoxicated children become red, hot, and delirious; they may die without prompt treatment with the specific antidote, physostigmine (see Chapter 7).

It is worth keeping in mind that a number of other (especially centrally acting) agents such as antihistamines, phenothiazines, and tricyclic antidepressants (see Chapters 16 and 24), have significant antimuscarinic side effects. Some of these agents may contribute to memory loss and confusion, especially in the elderly.

BOX 8-3

ANTIMUSCARINIC SIDE EFFECTS

- Dry mouth, dry skin
- Dilated pupils (photophobia)
- Tachycardia
- Decreased gut and bladder activity
- *CNS effects*: sedation, excitation, confusion

Especially children: coma and death (first: red, hot, and delirious)

Especially elderly: memory loss and confusion

NICOTINIC BLOCKING AGENTS

There are two major types of nicotinic receptors, those at the **neuromuscular junction** of the somatic system and those at the autonomic **ganglia** (both sympathetic and parasympathetic). Fortunately, for therapeutic usefulness, we have drugs that distinguish between these two receptor types. Also recall that, at nicotinic receptors, there are two different antagonist mechanisms: *competitive* (nondepolarizing) antagonists, which have no intrinsic activity of their own (*eg*, curare and trimethaphan); and *depolarizing* antagonists that produce an initial stimulation, followed by a more persistent block (*eg*, succinylcholine and nicotine) (see structures of these drugs in Fig. 8–2).

Ganglionic blockers:

- Nondepolarizing = **trimethaphan**
- Depolarizing = **nicotine**

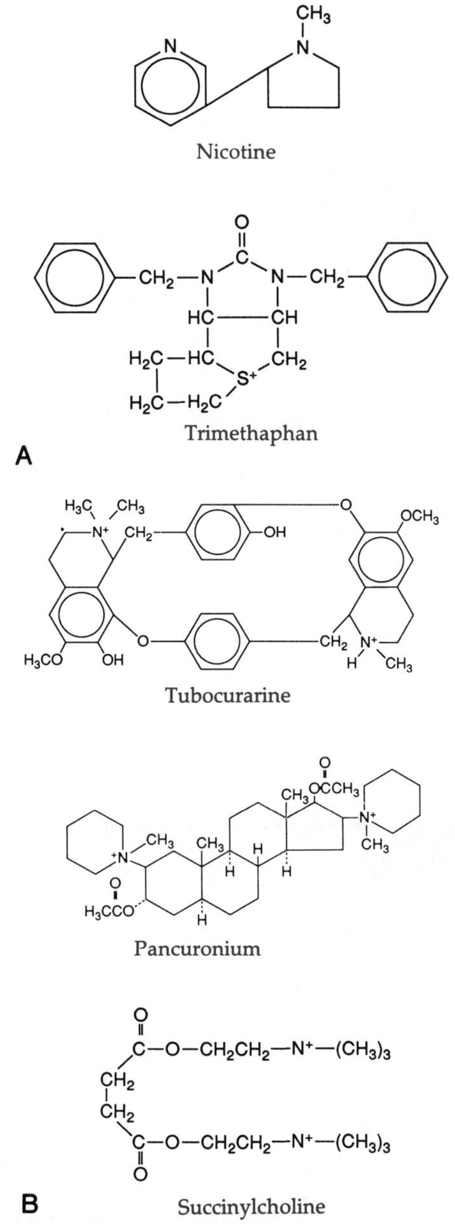

Nicotine

Trimethaphan

A

Tubocurarine

Pancuronium

B Succinylcholine

FIGURE 8–2. Structures of nicotinic receptor–blocking drugs. (*A*) Blockers at autonomic ganglia (nicotine and trimethaphan).

(*B*) Blockers at somatic neuromuscular junction (tubocurarine chloride [curare], pancuronium, and succinylcholine).

Neuromuscular blockers:

- Nondepolarizing = **curare**
- Depolarizing = **succinylcholine**

Ganglionic Blockers

Application of a drug that blocks all ganglionic nicotinic ACh receptors has the potential to shut down the entire autonomic nervous system, both sympathetic and parasympathetic branches. Obviously, such a drug application causes widespread effects, many of them undesirable. Thus, ganglionic blockers have only very limited clinical uses, namely to acutely reduce blood pressure in certain situations.

The outcome of ganglionic blocker application can be predicted by recalling which autonomic tone (sympathetic or parasympathetic) is dominant in each organ system. For instance, we know that vagal (parasympathetic) tone is the dominant tone in controlling heart rate. When all autonomic input is blocked, the heart rate will increase as it is released from its dominant tone. The dominant tone in the vasculature is sympathetic; administration of a ganglionic blocker will cause a rapid fall in blood pressure as the vasculature is released from the constricting influence of the sympathetic system—herein lies the potential therapeutic application for these drugs.

BOX 8–4
CHARACTERISTICS OF GANGLIONIC BLOCKERS

- Depolarizing and nondepolarizing mechanisms
- Block all autonomic ganglia: sympathetic and parasympathetic
- Produce widespread dysautonomia
- Notable (useful) effect = lower blood pressure

BOX 8–5
THERAPEUTIC USES OF GANGLIONIC BLOCKERS

The ability to cause a rapid and reversible **fall in blood pressure** has made ganglionic blockers valuable in their ability to immediately reverse an emergency hypertensive crisis. Clearly, one would choose a **nondepolarizing** agent (*eg*, trimethaphan) for this use because a depolarizing agent would first cause additional vasoconstriction before producing the desired relaxation. Ganglionic blockers have found some application in other clinical situations requiring the acute lowering of blood pressure: acute dissecting aortic aneurysm, and "bloodless field" surgery (*eg*, some orthopedic and vascular surgeries and neurosurgery). Of late, much of the use of ganglionic blockers has been replaced by using direct-acting vasodilators such as sodium nitroprusside (see Chapter 29).

Ganglionic blockers acutely lower blood pressure for:

- Emergency hypertensive crisis
- Acute dissecting aortic aneurysm
- "Bloodless field" surgery
- **Use nondepolarizing agents only** (*eg*, trimethaphan)

Depolarizing Ganglionic Blockers—Nicotine

The classic depolarizing ganglionic blocker is **nicotine**. Again, depolarizing agents first produce **stimulation followed by a block** at ganglionic nicotinic receptors. Nicotine is important as an experimental tool, but it is not used therapeutically. It is, however, clinically important because of its **toxicology**: nicotine is used in a number of pesticide preparations to poison insects, and in many tobacco preparations to poison human beings. Because nicotine is biphasic, its pharmacology is very complicated. It is highly lipid soluble, and is readily absorbed across all membranes. There is often simultaneous stimulation and blocking of various autonomic ganglia throughout the body. The nicotine in tobacco smoke usually produces a net stimulation of the CNS and cardiovascular systems.

The real health concern with tobacco smoke is not so much the nicotine itself (although it may constitute the major habit-forming component), but the several thousand other compounds in tobacco smoke. It has been known and widely accepted for 30 years that **cigarette smoking is the single most important preventable cause of death** in this country. More than 1000 people a day die in this country from the numerous diseases resulting from tobacco smoking; furthermore, the Environmental Protection Agency has acknowledged that second-hand smoke is also dangerous. Fortunately, more smokers are trying to quit, and more public spaces are becoming smoke-free. Unfortunately, the tobacco industry response to this is to push hard for new customers in Asia, creating health problems there. And unfortunately, cigarette ads, promotions, and vending machines appeal to youngsters; cigarette smoking usually starts at a young age (see Chapter 49).

Neuromuscular Blockers

Let us consider drugs that block the other family of nicotinic ACh receptors, antagonists at the somatic neuromuscular junction. Again, there are both nondepolarizing and depolarizing blockers (model compounds = curare and succinylcholine, respectively) (structures shown in Fig. 8-2). The primary use of these compounds is to produce profound **skeletal muscle relaxation**, especially for major **surgery**.

Many anesthetists have replaced curare with several newer steroid-based drugs, primarily pancuronium. Pancuronium has about the same duration of action as curare, but causes less hypotension as a side effect. Curare has some ganglionic blocking properties and causes some histamine release, both of which produce hypotension. However, in some clinical situations, such as hypertensive patients, this property of curare is useful. Because pancuronium has a bit of muscarinic blocking property, an elevated heart rate (block of cardiac vagus) is an expected side effect; this often helps offset the decrease in heart rate caused by many anesthetic agents.

Succinylcholine is a depolarizing blocker that has a biphasic mode of action. In patients who are not otherwise heavily drugged, one will often see fasciculations briefly before flaccid relaxation is achieved. Succinylcholine is very rapidly hydrolyzed by plasma cholinesterase enzymes, such that the duration of action is only approximately 5 minutes (Table 8-2, Fig. 8-3).

BOX 8-6
CHARACTERISTICS OF NEUROMUSCULAR BLOCKERS

Nondepolarizing Agents

- **d-Tubocurarine (curare)**—long-acting ($t_{1/2}$ approx. 1 hr)
  Some hypotension (from ganglionic blockade and histamine release)
- **Pancuronium** (PAVULON)—similar to curare, but less hypotension as a side effect
  Some heart rate increase (from block of cardiac vagus), weak anticholinesterase activity
- Several intermediate agents ($t_{1/2}$ approx. ½ hr)
  Including: atracurium (TRACRIUM) and vecuronium (NORCURON)

Depolarizing Agent

Succinylcholine (ANECTINE)—short-acting ($t_{1/2}$ approx. 5 min)

- Brief initial fasciculations
- Hydrolyzed by serum cholinesterase

BOX 8-7
CLINICAL USES OF NEUROMUSCULAR BLOCKERS

Muscle Relaxation for:

- Surgery
- Orthopedic maneuvers
- Intubations

TABLE 8-2. Comparison of the Major Properties of Competitive and Depolarizing Neuromuscular Blocking Drugs

Response	Competitive Drugs (Tubocurarine or Pancuronium)	Depolarizing Drugs (Succinylcholine)
Effect on resting potential at end-plate	None	Depolarized
Effect on end-plate potential	Reduction	End-plate is depolarized
Effect on tetanic volley to motor nerve	Fatigue during tetanus; posttetanic antagonism	No change during tetanus; no posttetanic antagonism
Inhibition of AChE	Antagonism of block	Enhanced block
Duration of block	Moderate to long depending on dose	Very short
Effect on muscle membrane away from synaptic region	None	None

AChE = acetylcholinesterase.

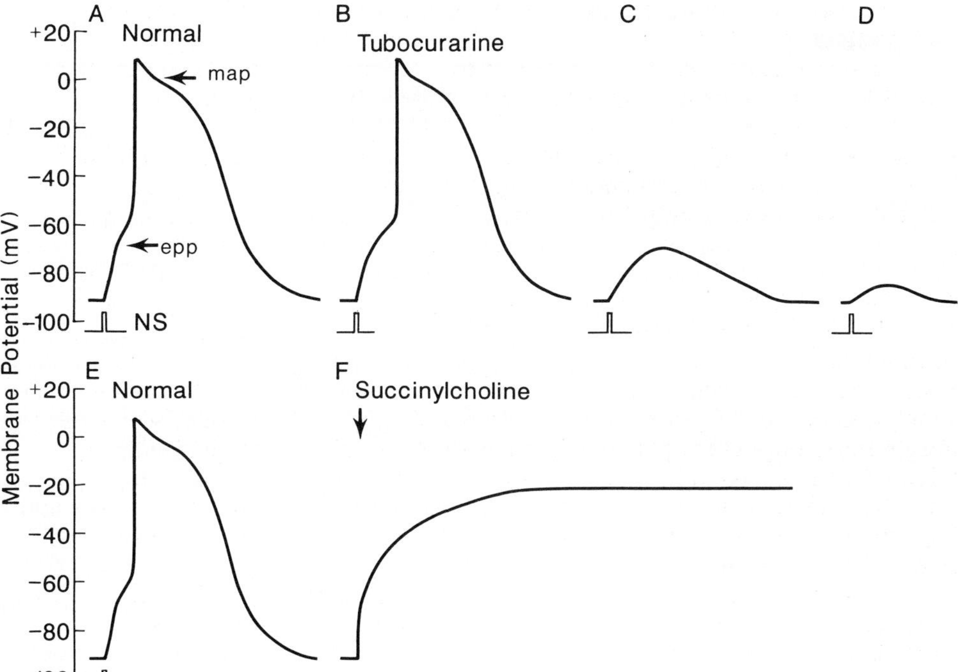

FIGURE 8–3. Comparison of the effects of tubocurarine and succinylcholine on the intracellular potential recorded from an end-plate of an isolated muscle preparation. In normal muscle (*panels A* and *E*) the end-plate potential (epp) gives rise to a muscle action potential (map). The initial effect of tubocurarine (*panel B*) is to slow the rate of rise of the epp; the amplitude of the epp is progressively reduced and eventually fails to reach threshold for the initiation of an action potential (*panels C* and *D*). Note that the resting potential does not change after tubocurarine.

In contrast, the addition of succinylcholine (*panel F*) results in a prolonged depolarization of the end-plate, even in the absence of any nerve stimulation. (NS and square wave symbols indicate nerve stimulation with single shocks.)

With all uses of neuromuscular blocking drugs, one should always secure an airway, or be prepared to do so immediately. After all, one is about to paralyze the patient. The longer acting (nondepolarizing: *eg,* curare and pancuronium) agents are used to produce muscle relaxation during surgery. Succinylcholine is used to produce muscle relaxation for shorter procedures such as intubations and orthopedic maneuvers, and to prevent dislocations and fractures during electroconvulsive shock therapy.

On occasion, an **anomalous response to succinylcholine** occurs; namely, the patient responds to succinylcholine as if he or she had been given curare. Some individuals have a genetically determined **low activity of blood cholinesterase** enzymes, effectively prolonging the effect of succinylcholine. Also, some chemical plant and agricultural workers are chronically exposed to low levels of (organophosphate) cholinesterase inhibitors and may have depressed plasma cholinesterase enzyme activity. Such patients may respond with a long-duration paralysis from succinylcholine.

Some other **drugs** will **potentiate** the action of the **neuromuscular blockers**. Most of the general anesthetic agents (*eg,* halothane, enflurane) will themselves cause some degree of muscle relaxation. Some antibiotics, notably tetracycline and streptomycin, may interfere with the calcium movement that is critical for neuromuscular contraction. A number of other miscellaneous drugs cause some degree of interference with membrane ion movement and will potentiate the effects of the neuromuscular blockers, for example, digitalis, quinidine, and opioids.

BOX 8–8

OTHER DRUGS MAY POTENTIATE NEUROMUSCULAR BLOCKERS

- General anesthetic agents: *eg,* halothane, enflurane
- Antibiotics: *eg,* tetracycline, streptomycin
- Miscellaneous: *eg,* digitalis, quinidine, opioids

Side Effects of Neuromuscular Blockers

As you would expect, the major danger of these drugs is too much, or too persistent a **paralysis**; the patient cannot breathe. Always be prepared to breathe (with **oxygen**) for someone when these agents (including succinylcholine) are applied. Administration of a cholinesterase inhibitor, such as neostigmine, will reverse the effects of a nondepolarizing blocker. **Neostigmine** will inhibit the enzyme and increase the local concentration of ACh; this can overcome the block of a competitive antagonist such as curare. Note this caveat: neostigmine will likely exacerbate, not reverse, the paralysis from succinylcholine. First, neostigmine may add to the depolarization of the depolarizing block; second, it will prevent the hydrolysis of succinylcholine by inhibiting cholinesterase activity.

TABLE 8–3. Cholinergic Drugs

Agents	Receptor	Therapeutically Useful Property
Cholinergic Agonists		
Acetylcholine	Nonselective	Increase smooth muscle tone during ocular surgery
Methacholine	Muscarinic	Increase smooth muscle tone during ocular surgery
Carbachol	Nonselective	Increase smooth muscle tone during ocular surgery
Bethanechol	Muscarinic	Increase smooth muscle tone—treat atonic gut, urinary retention, and reflux esophagitis
Pilocarpine	Muscarinic	Increase smooth muscle tone—treat open angle glaucoma
Nicotine	Nicotinic	Addictive toxin
Cholinesterase Inhibitors—Indirect Cholinergic Agonists		
Neostigmine	Nonselective	Reverse atropine and curare; increase skeletal muscle strength—treat myasthenia gravis
Physostigmine	Nonselective	Reverse atropine poisoning; alter muscle tone—treat open angle glaucoma
Pyridostigmine	Nonselective	Increase skeletal muscle strength—treat myasthenia gravis
Ambenonium	Nonselective	Increase skeletal muscle strength—treat myasthenia gravis
Edrophonium	Nonselective	Increase skeletal muscle strength (briefly)—diagnostic for myasthenia gravis
Cholinergic Antagonists		
Atropine	Muscarinic (M2)	Reverse bradycardia, treat anticholinesterase poisoning; decrease smooth muscle tone—treat some GI disorders (*eg*, irritable bowel syndrome); dries secretions—preanesthetic medication
Scopolamine	Muscarinic (M2)	Dries secretions—treat motion sickness, produce amnesia
Cyclopentolate	Muscarinic	Produce mydriasis for ophthalmology treatment and examinations
Tropicamide	Muscarinic	Produce mydriasis for ophthalmology treatment and examinations
Ipratropium	Muscarinic (M2)	Relax bronchial smooth muscle—treat chronic obstructive pulmonary disease
Pirenzepine	Muscarinic (M1)	Decrease gastric acid secretions and smooth muscle tone—treat peptic ulcer
Homatropine	Muscarinic	Decrease smooth muscle tone—treat GI spastic disorders (*eg*, irritable bowel syndrome)
Methantheline	Muscarinic	Decrease smooth muscle tone—treat GI spastic disorders (*eg*, irritable bowel syndrome)
Propantheline	Muscarinic	Decrease smooth muscle tone—treat GI spastic disorders (*eg*, irritable bowel syndrome)
Glycopyrrolate	Muscarinic	Decrease smooth muscle tone—treat GI spastic disorders (*eg*, irritable bowel syndrome)
Dicyclomine	Muscarinic	Decrease smooth muscle tone—treat GI spastic disorders (*eg*, irritable bowel syndrome)
Benztropine	Muscarinic	Treat parkinsonism
Trihexyphenidyl	Muscarinic	Treat parkinsonism
Trimethaphan	Nicotinic	Decrease blood pressure—control of dissecting aortic aneurysm, and for "bloodless" surgery
Mecamylamine	Nicotinic	Decrease blood pressure—control of dissecting aortic aneurysm, and for "bloodless" surgery
Nicotine	Nicotinic	Addictive toxin
d-Tubocurarine	Nicotinic	Decrease skeletal muscle tone for surgery
Pancuronium	Nicotinic	Decrease skeletal muscle tone for surgery
Atracurium	Nicotinic	Decrease skeletal muscle tone for surgery
Gallamine	Nicotinic	Decrease skeletal muscle tone for surgery
Vecuronium	Nicotinic	Decrease skeletal muscle tone for surgery
Succinylcholine	Nicotinic	Decrease skeletal muscle tone for brief procedures (*eg*, intubations, resetting dislocations)
Nerve Ending Blocker		
Botulinum toxin	ACh release	Skeletal muscle relaxation—treat facial muscle spasms

Malignant hyperthermia is a life-threatening condition with a genetic predisposition, which is manifest occasionally in patients simultaneously treated with a halogenated anesthetic agent plus succinylcholine. Patients so affected may end up with precipitous muscle rigidity, hypermetabolism, and extreme high temperature, which can cause tissue damage and death unless treated immediately (see Chapter 22).

REFERENCES

See also references in Chapters 6 and 7.

Adams PR: Transmitter action at endplate membrane. *In* Salpeter MM (ed): The Vertebrate Neuromuscular Junction, 317–359. Vol 23 of Neurology and Neurobiology. New York: AR Liss, 1987.

Ali HH: Monitoring of neuromuscular function. Semin Anesthes 3:284–292, 1984.

Azar I (ed): Muscle Relaxants: Side Effects and a Rational Approach to Selection. Vol 7 of Clinical Pharmacology. New York: Marcel Dekker, 1987.

Denborough M: The pathopharmacology of malignant hyperpyrexia. Pharmacol Ther 9:357–365, 1980.

Gil DW, Wolfe BB: Pirenzepine distinguishes between muscarinic receptor-mediated phosphoinositide breakdown and inhibition of adenylate cyclase. J Pharmacol Exp Ther 232:608–616, 1985.

Gross NJ, Skorodin MS: Anticholinergic, antimuscarinic bronchodilators. Am Rev Respir Dis 129:856–870, 1984.

Kharkevich DA (ed): Neuromuscular blocking agents. Vol 79. Handbook of Experimental Pharmacology. Berlin: Springer-Verlag, 1986.

Kohl RL, Homick JL: Motion sickness: A modulatory role for the central cholinergic nervous system. Neurosci Biobehav Rev 7:73–85, 1983.

Vakil DV, Ayiomamitis A, Nizam RM: Use of ipratropium aerosol in long-term management of asthma. J Asthma 22:165–170, 1985.

9 Adrenergic Drugs

Oliver M. Brown

The pharmacology of cholinergic neuroeffector junctions was discussed in preceding chapters. This chapter describes drugs that have their primary actions at neuroeffector junctions that utilize the other major autonomic neurotransmitter, **norepinephrine (NE)**. Because NE is the transmitter at most postganglionic neuroeffector junctions in the **sympathetic** branch of the autonomic nervous system, the agonists at these sites are commonly referred to as sympathetic, sympathomimetic, or adrenergic drugs.

As was the case for drugs affecting acetylcholine (ACh) synapses, drugs are available that affect selectively the synthesis, packaging, release, receptor interaction, and termination of NE as a neurotransmitter. As with cholinergic agents, most of the adrenergic drugs in clinical use have their **main site of action at the neurotransmitter receptor** either to mimic the action of NE at such receptors (**agonists**, sympathomimetics) or to block access to the receptor binding sites (**antagonists**, sympatholytics).

Inasmuch as the sympathetic nervous system has important influences over cardiovascular and respiratory functions, it is obvious that drugs that stimulate or block NE receptors may have profound effects on these functions (sympathetic nerves also innervate many other organs). Thus, adrenergic drugs are **primarily used to treat several cardiac conditions**, **blood pressure problems**, **and asthma**. Those drugs that cross the blood-brain barrier also have effects on the central nervous system (CNS).

> **BOX 9–1**
> **CHARACTERIZATION OF ADRENERGIC DRUGS**
>
> - Affect NE transmission at synapse
> - Most act on NE receptors
> - Primary system: sympathetic branch of autonomic and CNS
> - Primary organs: blood vessels, heart, bronchial muscle, eye, CNS

CHEMICAL TRANSMISSION INVOLVING NOREPINEPHRINE

A schematic of NE chemical transmission at an autonomic nerve varicosity is shown in Figure 9–1. The events involved in NE transmission can be summarized as:

- Uptake of precursor (circulating tyrosine)
- Synthesis of NE (several enzyme steps)
- Packing of NE (into synaptic vesicles)
- Release of NE (upon action potential arrival and Ca^{2+} entry)

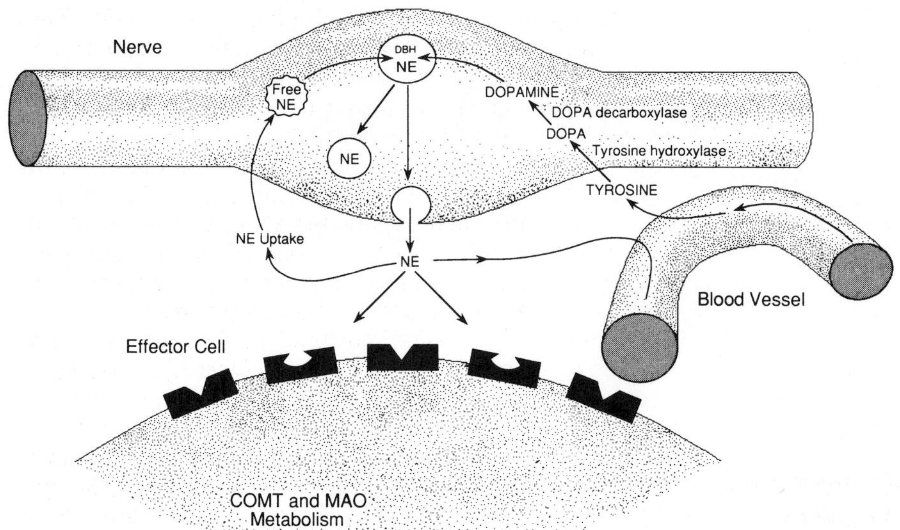

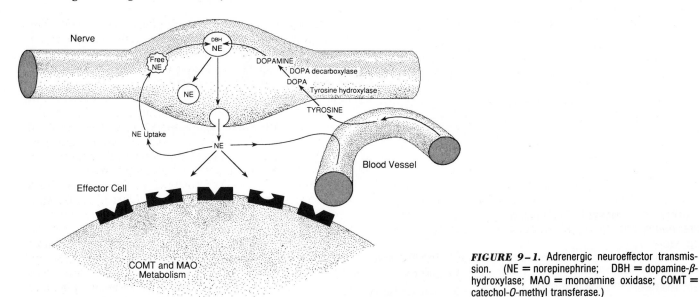

FIGURE 9-1. Adrenergic neuroeffector transmission. (NE = norepinephrine; DBH = dopamine-β-hydroxylase; MAO = monoamine oxidase; COMT = catechol-*O*-methyl transferase.)

- Receptor interaction (second messengers engaged)
- Effector cell response — effect
- Termination (NE uptake and diffusion)

Synthesis of Norepinephrine

Norepinephrine is synthesized from tyrosine by a series of steps that are shown in Figure 9-2. Tyrosine is taken up (by active transport) from the circulation into the nerve varicosity, and the following conversions take place:

- Tyrosine to dihydroxyphenylalanine (DOPA)

  Enzyme: tyrosine hydroxylase, cytoplasmic

  Rate-limiting step in pathway

- DOPA to dopamine

  Enzyme: 1-aromatic amino acid decarboxylase, cytoplasmic

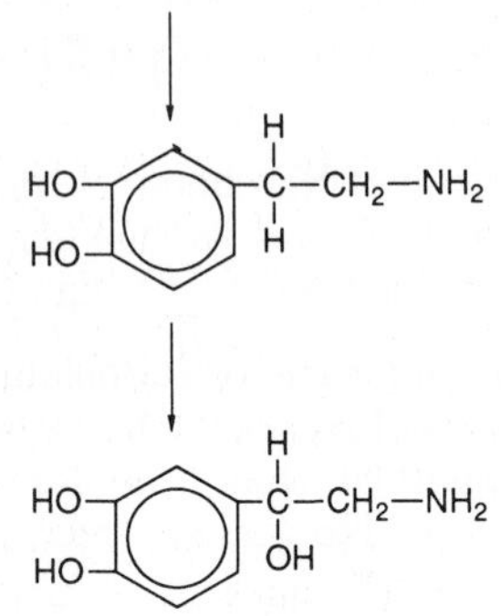

tyrosine: HO–C_6H_4–CH(H)–CH(NH$_2$)–COOH

↓

DOPA: (HO)$_2$–C_6H_3–CH(H)–CH(NH$_2$)–COOH

↓

dopamine: (HO)$_2$–C_6H_3–CH$_2$–CH$_2$–NH$_2$

↓

norepinephrine: (HO)$_2$–C_6H_3–CH(OH)–CH$_2$–NH$_2$

FIGURE 9-2. Biosynthetic steps leading to the synthesis of norepinephrine.

  Dopamine is transported into the vesicles
  (Dopamine is also a neurotransmitter in some areas)

- Dopamine to NE

  Enzyme: dopamine-β-hydroxylase, in synaptic vesicles

The final step in NE synthesis takes place in the synaptic vesicles (or "granules"). Dopamine is transported into the vesicles, where it is hydroxylated to NE by dopamine-β-hydroxylase; thus, there is **no synthesis of NE in the cytoplasm**. The **vesicles** not only **take up dopamine** but will **also package soluble NE** that has been **taken up by the neuron** (see below). The NE packaged in these vesicles (granules) is complexed with adenosine triphosphate (ATP), calcium, and chromogranin A (a protein).

In the adrenal medulla and in other chromaffin cells, there is a further conversion of much of the NE to epinephrine (adrenaline) (EPI) by the enzyme phenylethanolamine-*N*-methyltransferase (PNMT). Newly synthesized NE leaves the vesicles and is methylated to EPI in the cytoplasm by PNMT. The EPI is taken up by a different set of vesicles (chromaffin granules), where it is stored for release. Chromaffin granules contain EPI and NE in a 4 : 1 ratio, complexed with ATP, calcium, and chromogranin A.

Note the distinction that NE is primarily a **neurotransmitter**; that is, it is released into a synaptic cleft for interaction at the immediately adjacent postjunctional effector cell. In contrast, **EPI** is primarily a **neurohormone**; that is, it is secreted into the blood stream by the adrenal medulla and interacts with effector sites throughout the body.

Release of Norepinephrine

With the arrival of an action potential at an adrenergic varicosity, there is an influx of calcium ions that triggers the fusion of synaptic vesicles with the presynaptic plasma membrane. This is followed by an exocytosis of the vesicle contents (NE, ATP, and dopamine-β-hydroxylase are released) into the synaptic cleft. The **released NE** is then free to **diffuse** and encounter several fates (Fig. 9-1).

Possible fates of released NE:

1. Interact with receptors on the postjunctional membrane.
2. Interact with receptors on the prejunctional membrane (*autoreceptors*).
3. Diffuse out of the cleft and be lost to the circulation.
4. Be taken back up through the prejunctional membrane ($uptake_1$).
5. Be taken up through the postjunctional membrane ($uptake_2$).

Of the above possibilities, number 1 fulfills the **neurotransmitter function** of the released NE; NE interacts with **postsynaptic receptors** and depolarizes the effector cell membrane, completing **transmission of the signal** from the nerve.

Possibility number 2 represents an **autoinhibitory** control mechanism: stimulation of presynaptic receptors (autoreceptors) by NE inhibits further release of NE. The remaining three (nos. 3–5) of the possible fates for released NE represent mechanisms for **terminating** neurotransmission.

Norepinephrine-Receptor Interaction

Activation of specific postjunctional adrenergic receptors by NE or other adrenergic agonists causes biochemical and physiological responses that involve "**second-messenger**" transduction mechanisms. These mechanisms generally either:

- **Increase** available cytosolic calcium **concentration**, which results in smooth muscle **contraction**, or
- **Decrease** available **calcium**, which results in **relaxation** of smooth muscle.

Both subtypes of **β-adrenergic** receptors (β_1 and β_2) are coupled through a **stimulatory G-protein** (guanine nucleotide-binding regulatory protein) to adenylate cyclase. Thus, activation of these receptors by agonists increases cellular concentrations of the second messenger, cyclic adenosine monophosphate (cAMP). The **increase in cAMP** amplifies the receptor signal by activating a protein kinase, which in turn phosphorylates a variety of intracellular enzymes. The activity of the phosphorylated enzymes is thought to be responsible for all the responses to β-adrenergic receptor activation, including excitatory effects on the heart, increased metabolic activity, and relaxation of smooth muscle in bronchi and some blood vessels.

In contrast **$alpha_2$ receptors** are coupled to adenylate cyclase through an **inhibitory G-protein**. Thus, activation of α_2 receptors results in a **decrease** in the second messenger, **cAMP**.

A different second messenger is involved in the activation of the **α_1-adrenergic** receptor. They are coupled (through another G-protein) to a system that hydrolyzes phosphatidylinositol. The products of phosphatidylinositol breakdown serve as second messengers by releasing intracellular calcium stores. This initiates the phosphorylation of a number of regulatory enzymes that are responsible for the cell response to α_1 activation.

As described in Chapter 8, chronic treatment with adrenergic agonists can result in a decrease in the number of neurotransmitter receptors (**down-regulation**). Conversely, the adaptive response to chronic treatment with antagonists is an increase in the number of receptors (**up-regulation**). For example, treatment with an antagonist may result in an adaptive increase in adrenergic receptors in a fashion analogous to the phenomenon of denervation supersensitivity. If chronic treatment with such an antagonist is terminated (especially if the antagonist is rapidly eliminated), activation of the now-increased number of receptors will result in an exaggerated effector cell stimulation. In the case of the β blocker propranolol (discussed in Chapter 10), rapid withdrawal could cause life-threatening cardiac arrhythmias. As a general principle, agents that stimulate or inhibit the autonomic or central nervous system should be withdrawn from chronic use gradually in a stepwise fashion. (The up- and down-regulation is accomplished by at least two mechanisms—sequestration of the receptor complex and decreasing or increasing synthesis.)

Termination of Norepinephrine Transmission

Several mechanisms contribute to the termination of NE synaptic transmission (Fig. 9–2) As with all neurotransmitters, diffusion out of the cleft contributes to terminating the effects of NE. However, the main mechanism by which the effect of **NE is rapidly terminated** is the specific **uptake of NE** into the presynaptic varicosity (often referred to as reuptake, or **$uptake_1$**). The NE that has been taken back up by the nerve forms the cytoplasmic pool of NE; much of this soluble NE is recycled by packaging into synaptic vesicles. Other tissues also take up NE and related compounds by a less specific, higher-capacity uptake mechanism, $uptake_2$. Most **metabolism** of NE and other catecholamines takes place in nonneural cells following uptake by **$uptake_2$**.

Metabolism of Norepinephrine

The catecholamines (NE, EPI, dopamine, and some synthetic analogs) are taken up (**$uptake_2$**) by many tissues of the body, metabolized, and excreted primarily as sulfated conjugates. The **mitochondria** of most cells, including nerve cells, contain **monoamine oxidase (MAO)**. The other major catecholamine-metabolizing enzyme, **catechol-*O*-methyl transferase (COMT)**, is found primarily in the **cytoplasm** of **nonneural** cells (especially in the liver). Other enzymes (aldehyde dehydrogenases and aldehyde reductases) contribute to the formation of the final metabolic products of catecholamines. The major metabolites of NE found in human plasma and urine are 3-methoxy-4-hydroxyphenylethylene glycol (MHPG), free and conjugated, vanillylmandelic acid (VMA), and normetanephrine (NMN), free and conjugated. The same, or analogous, deaminated and methoxylated metabolites are formed from other catecholamines. Unlike acetylcholine neurotransmission, wherein enzymatic action (by acetylcholinesterase) plays the major role in ending transmission, enzymatic metabolism of NE plays no role in terminating neurotransmission.

Modification of Norepinephrine Neurotransmission by Drugs

Each of the steps in the process of NE chemical transmission can be modified by drugs, resulting in either a potentiation or an inhibition of activity at NE synapses. Some examples of drug modification are:

- **Synthesis of NE** is blocked by inhibiting tyrosine hydroxylase with methyltyrosine, thus inhibiting NE synaptic transmission.
- **Vesicle uptake** of dopamine and NE is prevented by reserpine, depleting the nerve of transmitter and inhibiting transmission.
- **Release of NE** from the nerve varicosity is enhanced by amphetamine (potentiating) and prevented by bretylium (inhibiting).
- **Receptor interaction** with NE is blocked by antagonists such as propranolol (inhibiting) and mimicked by agonists such as isoproterenol (potentiating).
- **Termination of NE** as a transmitter by uptake$_1$ is blocked by cocaine, thus potentiating neurotransmission.

Most adrenergic agonists and antagonists in clinical use exert their effects by interacting directly with adrenergic receptors, as either agonists or antagonists.

TABLE 9–1. Receptor Types in the Sympathetic (Adrenergic) System

Receptor Type	Prominent Effector Organs	Response to Receptor Activation
α_1	Arterioles in skin, mucosa, viscera, and kidney (resistance vessels)	Constriction
	Veins	Constriction
	Uterus	Contraction
α_2	Presynaptic nerve endings	Inhibit NE release
	Postsynaptic in CNS	Decreased sympathetic tone
β_1	Heart	Increased heart rate Increased force of contraction
β_2	Arterioles (and arteries in skeletal muscle)	Dilation
	Bronchial and uterine smooth muscle	Relaxation
	Several sites	Metabolic effects
Dopamine	Arterioles in kidney, brain, and mesentery	Dilation

CNS = central nervous system; NE = norepinephrine.

RECEPTOR TYPES IN THE SYMPATHETIC SYSTEM

Administration of EPI (adrenaline) produces effects similar to those achieved by stimulating the sympathetic nerves. Both perturbations cause the contraction of some smooth muscles and the relaxation of others. This can be best explained by the fact that there are two major types of adrenergic receptors; as originally characterized:

- **Alpha (α) receptors** — responsible for most of the **excitatory** effects such as vasoconstriction and contraction of the uterus and spleen.
- **Beta (β) receptors** — responsible for most of the **inhibitory** effects such as vasodilation and relaxation of respiratory smooth muscle.
- **Two important exceptions** to this characterization: some α receptors mediate relaxation of gastrointestinal (GI) smooth muscle, and some β receptors mediate increases in the force and rate of contractions of the heart.

Adrenergic receptor subtypes are currently defined in much greater detail. A knowledge of the locations and characteristic responses of the various adrenergic receptor subtypes allows one to predict the effects of specific adrenergic drugs. A classification of adrenergic receptors and their responses to activation is outlined in Table 9–1.

Alpha Receptors

Alpha$_1$ receptors are the originally defined excitatory receptors that mediate constriction or **contraction** of smooth muscle in a number of locations, including:

- Arterioles in skin, mucosa, viscera, and kidneys. These arterioles are numerous and small, and account for a large proportion of peripheral resistance.
- Veins throughout the body.
- Uterus, spleen, male sex organ, and radial muscle of the iris.

Alpha$_2$ receptors are a more recently described subtype that are located primarily on prejunctional membranes (Fig. 9–3), where they serve to **regulate the release of NE**. Activation of these prejunctional receptors inhibits further release of the transmitter. Alpha$_2$ receptors can also be found postsynaptically in the **CNS** (see discussion later in this chapter) and in some peripheral sites. Alpha$_2$ receptors are responsible for **relaxation of GI** smooth muscle.

Beta Receptors

Beta$_2$ receptors mediate relaxation of smooth muscle in various locations:

- Arterioles in skeletal muscle and liver (and to some degree, other locations).
- Many veins throughout the body.
- Bronchial and uterine smooth muscle.

Beta$_1$ receptors are a very important exception to the generalization that β receptor activation is inhibitory to the end-organ; β_1 receptor activation results in an increase in heart rate (positive chronotropic effect) and an increase in the force of contraction (positive inotropic effect).

In addition to smooth and cardiac muscle activity, β receptors also subserve several **metabolic functions** by in-

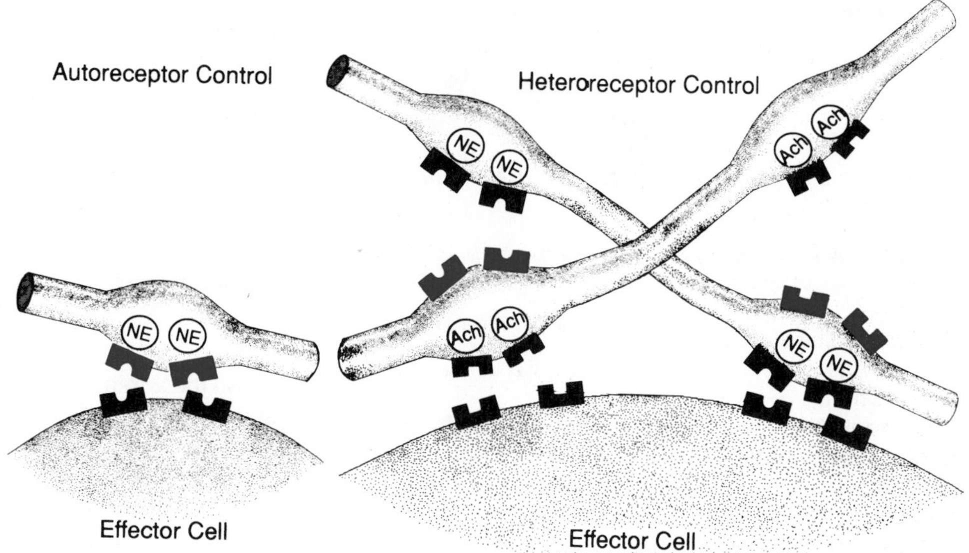

FIGURE 9–3. Autoreceptor and heteroreceptor regulation. (ACh = acetylcholine; NE = norepinephrine.)

creasing cellular cAMP levels. For example, EPI stimulates the conversion of liver glycogen to glucose, glycogenolysis (thus elevating blood sugar, hyperglycemia), by interacting with β_2 receptors. Similarly, EPI activates β_1 receptors in adipose tissue to stimulate the breakdown of triglycerides to free fatty acids, lipolysis (elevating blood fatty acids, hyperlipidemia).

Although not truly an adrenergic receptor, a receptor for another catecholamine, **dopamine**, is included in Table 9–1. There is evidence that dopamine may serve as a neurotransmitter in certain arterioles of the brain, kidney, and mesentery. Activation of dopamine receptors found in these areas results in **dilation of these vessels**.

Presynaptic Control Mechanisms

As described above and in Chapter 8, activation of prejunctional α_2 receptors results in a **feedback inhibition** of further NE release, a presynaptic **autoreceptor** control mechanism. Evidence has also accumulated to support an additional autonomic checks-and-balances control system: presynaptic **heteroreceptor** regulation, shown in Figure 9–3. This scheme allows a fine degree of autonomic control between NE and ACh nerve endings innervating the same organ: prejunctional muscarinic acetylcholine receptors serve to inhibit release of NE from sympathetic varicosities, and prejunctional α-adrenergic receptors inhibit release of acetylcholine from parasympathetic varicosities. These mechanisms contribute to the balance of most organ functions that results from concurrent activity of both the sympathetic and parasympathetic systems. It is proposed, for example, that adrenergic drugs (or sympathetic stimulation) decrease GI activity by activating prejunctional α heteroreceptors that inhibit acetylcholine release from parasympathetic nerves. (Note: the functionally dominant innervation of the gut is parasympathetic.)

Receptor Distribution and Sensitivity

Important factors that help determine the response of an organ to adrenergic drugs are the relative **proportion and density** of α and β receptors in the tissue. Furthermore, receptors have different sensitivities to NE and EPI and other adrenergic drugs: NE and EPI have similar potencies at α_1, α_2, and β_1 receptors, but EPI is much more potent than NE at β_2 receptors. The **heart** is generally considered to have **predominantly β_1 receptors**, and most **blood vessels** to have **predominantly** α_1 receptors; thus, drug effects at these sites should be quite predictable.

The **vascular beds in skeletal muscle**, on the other hand, are plentiful in **both β_2 and α_1 receptors; accordingly, an agent such as EPI with activity at both receptor types has the potential to produce both dilation and constriction** of these vessels. An important consideration in this case is that the threshold of sensitivity to EPI is lower for the β_2 receptors than for the α_1 receptors. As illustrated in Figure 9–4, lower (physiological) concentrations of EPI cause (β_2-mediated) vasodilation (which facilitates increased skeletal muscle perfusion during the *fight or flight* response). Only at very high concentrations of EPI (above those found *in vivo*) do the constricting effects of α_1 receptor activation become evident. This constricting effect will predominate at high levels of EPI, levels that are usually obtained only under experimental conditions.

The differences in receptor **specificity** and sensitivity to various adrenergic drugs can be explored by examining the **chemical structures** of the drugs in a systematic way (a structure-activity relationship study). A number of such studies have concluded that the addition of alkyl groups to the amine substituent of catecholamines increases β activity and decreases α activity. This effect is shown for the three compounds with identical catecholamine backbones listed in Table 9–2: NE, EPI, and isoproterenol (ISO).

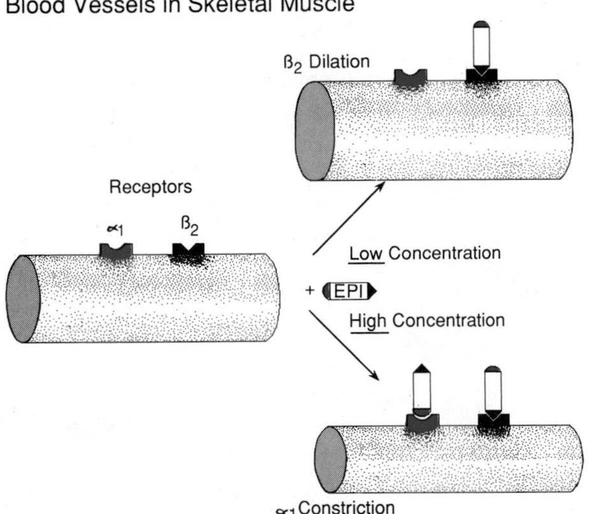

FIGURE 9–4. Differential receptor-related effects of low and high concentrations of epinephrine (EPI) on blood vessels in skeletal muscle.

Not only does the **chemical structure** of adrenergic drugs correlate with their specificity at receptor sites; the structure is also correlated with their **potency** at those receptors. Table 9–3 indicates the relative potencies for several characteristic adrenergic agonists at the α and β receptor types described earlier. For example, at β_1 receptors, ISO is more potent than EPI, which is equal to or more potent than NE, which is more potent than dopamine.

Direct Versus Indirect Agonists

Some drugs that stimulate sympathetic functions do so at least in part by causing the **release of NE** from the prejunctional membrane. Such drugs are referred to as having **indirect** activity, as contrasted with those that have direct activity on the adrenergic receptor itself. Obviously, the receptor specificity profile of indirect-acting drugs is similar to that of NE because it is NE that is actually stimulating the receptors. The structural features that determine the direct-acting or indirect-acting properties are the **alkyl hydroxyl group** and the **phenyl hydroxyl group meta** to the alkyl side chain (the hydroxyls shown in color on the structure of NE, Table 9–4). Tyramine, which has neither of the two critical hydroxyl groups, is a weak agonist that owes all its activity to the release of NE. The addition of **one hydroxyl** group (to the tyramine structure) imparts **partial direct-acting** properties to phenylpropanolamine and dopamine, and the addition of both hydroxyl groups results in the purely direct-acting NE.

The **indirect-acting** drugs, such as **tyramine** (and amphetamine and ephedrine), release NE through a calcium-independent mechanism that does not involve exocytosis. It is thought that they displace and cause the **release of NE from the soluble cytoplasmic pool**. This cytoplasmic pool of NE is quite small and can be rapidly depleted; thus **tachyphylaxis** is observed with repeated administrations of tyramine. That is, the increase in blood pressure that results from an injection of tyramine fails to occur after the injection is repeated several times every 10 to 30 minutes. (**Tachyphylaxis** is defined as **tolerance with a very**

TABLE 9–3. Agonist Potencies at Adrenergic Receptors

Receptor	Potency
β_1	ISO > EPI ≥ NE > DA
β_2	ISO > EPI ≫ NE ≫ DA
α_1	EPI ≥ NE > DA ≫ ISO
α_2	CLO > EPI ≥ NE ≫ ISO

CLO = clonidine; DA = dopamine; EPI = epinephrine; ISO = isoproterenol; NE = norepinephrine.

TABLE 9–2. Structure-Activity Relationship of Norepinephrine, Epinephrine, and Isoproterenol

Adrenergic Agent	Structure	Receptor Selectivity	Activity at Receptor
Norepinephrine	(3,4-di-HO-phenyl)–CH(OH)–CH_2–NH_2	α	Norepinephrine (with no alkyl groups on the amine) is the most α-specific of the three compounds, with activity at α_1, α_2, and β_1 receptors; it has almost no activity at β_2 sites.
Epinephrine	(3,4-di-HO-phenyl)–CH(OH)–CH_2–NH–CH_3	$\alpha + \beta$	Epinephrine (with the addition of one methyl group on the amine) is active at all α and β receptors; the addition of the methyl group has imparted β_2 activity to this compound.
Isoproterenol	(3,4-di-HO-phenyl)–CH(OH)–CH_2–NH–$CH(CH_3)_2$	β	Isoproterenol (with the addition of an isopropyl group on the amine) is active at β_1 and β_2 receptors, with almost no activity at α sites. This most "alkyl" of the three drugs has lost all its ability to bind to α receptors.

Modified from Day M: Autonomic Pharmacology, 130. New York: Churchill Livingstone, 1979.

TABLE 9–4. Indirect Versus Direct Structures

Adrenergic Agonist	Structure	Type of Activity
Tyramine	HO–C_6H_4–$CH_2-CH_2-NH_2$	Indirect
Phenylpropanolamine (PPA)	C_6H_5–CH(OH)–CH(CH_3)–NH_2	Mixed, indirect, and direct
Dopamine	(HO)$_2$$C_6H_3$–$CH_2-CH_2-NH_2$	Mixed, indirect, and direct
Norepinephrine	(HO)$_2$$C_6H_3$–CH(OH)–$CH_2-NH_2$	Direct

Modified from Day M: Autonomic Pharmacology, 129. New York: Churchill Livingstone, 1979.

short onset—a decrease in the response to a given dose of drug with its repeated administration.)

Cardiovascular Effects of Adrenergic Receptor Activation

Drugs that activate adrenergic receptors have important effects on the cardiovascular system. The cardiovascular changes that result are complicated because they consist of the direct effects plus the consequence of the **compensatory baroreceptor reflexes**. These reflex responses may, in fact, be used to therapeutic advantage. For example, cases of paroxysmal atrial tachycardia may be converted to a sinus rhythm with the α agonist phenylephrine. Phenylephrine stimulates vascular α_1 receptors, causing an increase in arterial blood pressure. This pressure increase elicits a baroreceptor-mediated reflex increase in vagal tone, which results in a slowing of the heart rate.

Thus, just knowing the α and β receptor activities of a given drug is not sufficient to completely predict the outcome of administering the drug; baroreceptor reflexes must always be considered. The cardiovascular profiles of α and β receptor activation without complication by the reflexes have been determined using experimental preparations. Figure 9–5 presents experimental results from an anesthetized dog with the cervical vagus nerves cut (afferent and efferent) to eliminate baroreceptor reflex activity. Heart rate (HR) and mean arterial pressure (MAP) were monitored, and the dog was given intravenous (IV) injections of NE, EPI, and ISO.

In contrast, when the same drugs are given in the presence of intact baroreceptor reflexes, the resultant actions are somewhat different. Figure 9–6 shows the heart rate (HR), blood pressure (BP), and total peripheral resistance (TPR) for a human who received IV infusions of NE, EPI, and ISO.

BOX 9–2

SUMMARY OF CARDIOVASCULAR EFFECTS (Figs. 9–5 and 9–6)

EPI (epinephrine) (α_1, β_2, β_2 activity)

- **Heart rate—increases**, β_1 effect
- **Blood pressure—usually increases**, result of competing influences:

  α_1 vasoconstriction + β_2 vasodilation + β_1 effects on heart

ISO (isoproterenol) (β_1, β_2 activity)

- **Heart rate—increases**, β_1 effect
- **Blood pressure—decreases**, β_2 vasodilation

NE (norepinephrine) (α_1, β_1 activity)

- **Heart rate—decreases**, result of competing influences:

  β_1 primary effect on heart overwhelmed by **vagus discharge** resulting from baroreceptor response to increase in blood pressure

- **Blood pressure—increases**, α_1 vasoconstriction

ADRENERGIC AGONISTS AND THEIR THERAPEUTIC USES

The three endogenous catecholamines, NE, EPI, and dopamine, activate adrenergic receptors to varying degrees (Table 9–3). In addition to these agents, there are numerous synthetic drugs that also have adrenergic agonist properties.

Many adrenergic drugs have similar properties to one another, and clinicians may vary in their choice of drug in a

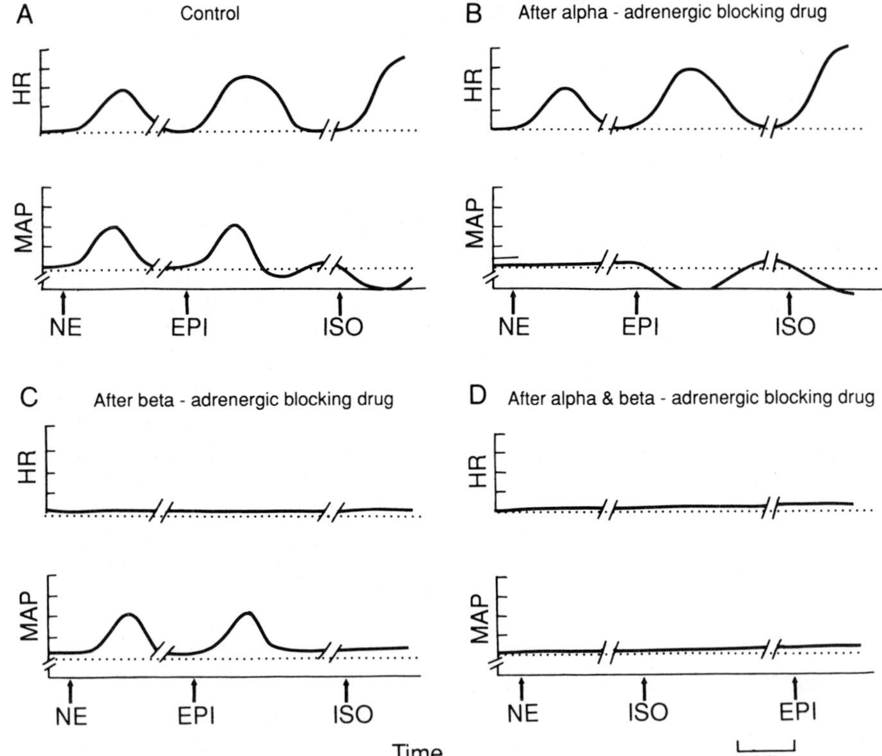

FIGURE 9–5. Results from an experimental study on the dog. (*A*) The potent α_1 agonist activity of norepinephrine (NE) constricts most blood vessels, increasing peripheral resistance, which results in an increase in mean arterial pressure (MAP). Beta$_1$ receptor activation by NE causes positive chronotropy (increased heart rate [HR]) and positive inotropy (not shown). Epinephrine (EPI) activates β_1 receptors, increasing HR. EPI also is a potent α_1 agonist and raises MAP when given in a large dose, but note that the effect is biphasic —as the blood level of EPI declines, EPI stimulation of β_2 receptors to dilate skeletal muscle vascular beds can be seen (this effect was present throughout but was masked by α_1 vasoconstriction; see *panel B*). ISO has β_1 and β_2 activity: HR is elevated from β_1 activation; MAP is decreased from β_2-mediated dilation of vascular beds in skeletal muscle.

(*B*) After pretreatment with an α antagonist, the responses to the same drugs were determined. All α_1-mediated vasoconstriction (increased MAP) has been prevented. The β_1 dilation of skeletal muscle vessels by EPI is now clearly revealed. Beta$_1$ effects on HR are not changed by α blockade.

(*C*) After pretreatment with a β antagonist only the α-mediated vasoconstriction (increased MAP) of NE and EPI is seen.

(*D*) Pretreatment with a combination of an α antagonist and a β antagonist blocks the actions of all three drugs. (ISO = isoproterenol.)

(*Panels A–D* from Carrier O Jr: Pharmacology of the Peripheral Autonomic Nervous System, 97. Chicago: Year Book Medical, 1972.)

given situation. For these reasons, only the model drugs used for a given therapeutic application are discussed here. A more comprehensive listing of adrenergic drugs and their receptor specificities appears in Table 10–1.

Adrenergic agonists that mimic NE at α_1 receptors cause **vasoconstriction**. This property is useful in many situations in which control of blood flow is required. Agents with β_1 activity have some application in **stimulating the heart**. Bronchial **smooth muscle is relaxed** with β_2 stimulation, making drugs with this property valuable in treating asthma.

Alpha Agonists

Alpha$_1$ Agents—Vasoconstriction

CONTROL HEMORRHAGE. An agent with α_1 agonist properties, often epinephrine (adrenaline), is used to constrict vessels in the area of superficial surgery. This application controls capillary bleeding and is especially useful in tooth extractions. (Caution: Alpha agonists should not be used to control bleeding in anything other

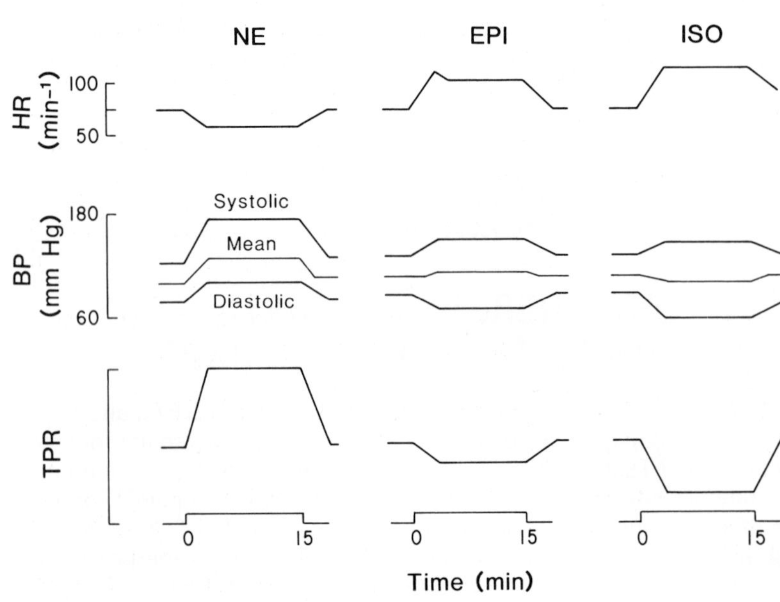

FIGURE 9–6. Norepinephrine (NE) causes a dramatic α-mediated increase in total peripheral resistance (TPR) and blood pressure (BP). The β_1 effect of NE would be expected to produce an increase in heart rate (HR), yet a decrease in HR is seen here. This results from baroreceptors responding to the increased BP and reflexively increasing the discharge of vagal nerves to the heart. The baroreceptor reflex effect (mediated through the vagus nerves) to lower HR overrides the direct β_1 receptor effect to raise the HR.

Epinephrine (EPI) causes a redistribution of blood flow (an effect consistent with the fight-or-flight generalization); α_1 activation results in vasoconstriction in many areas, and concurrent β_2 activation dilates vessels in the skeletal muscles. The algebraic sum of these simultaneous effects in the individual studied is a net lowering of TPR (this will vary among individuals depending on relative muscle mass and other factors). Although TPR dropped in this case, there was no decrease in BP; BP was maintained by the increase in HR and in pulse pressure (positive inotropy), both resulting from β_1 activation by EPI.

Isoproterenol (ISO) increases HR by β_1 activation and lowers TPR by β_2 activation; net decreases in BP are small, as these two effects tend to oppose one another. (Modified from Allwood MJ, Cobbold AF, Ginsburg J: Peripheral vascular effects of noradrenaline, isopropylnoradrenaline, and dopamine. Br Med Bull 19:132–136, 1963.)

than superficial surgery; deep bleeding would recur after surgical closure and drug absorption.)

CONTAIN LOCAL ANESTHETIC. Alpha$_1$ agonists (again, usually epinephrine) are sometimes injected along with local anesthetics to cause localized vasoconstriction. The decreased blood flow in the area slows the absorption of the anesthetic and localizes the effect of the anesthetic. This gives more effective anesthesia in the area of surgery, and it minimizes systemic toxicity from the anesthetic. (Caution: Special care must be taken to avoid injection into a vessel; a bolus of epinephrine could be life-threatening.)

NASAL DECONGESTANT. Alpha agonists are applied locally or taken orally to constrict the swollen vessels in edematous tissue in order to relieve the symptoms of mucosal congestion in the common cold, hay fever, and other allergic rhinitis. Both indirect-acting agents (which act by causing NE release), such as phenylpropanolamine, and direct-acting agents, such as phenylephrine (NEO-SYNEPHRINE), are used in many over-the-counter nasal decongestant products. (Caution: Repeated application of these agents often results in a "rebound" after-congestion that is possibly more severe than the original rhinitis.)

ALLERGIC SHOCK (ANAPHYLAXIS). Epinephrine is the drug of choice in treating the medical emergency of anaphylactic shock. The α_1 properties of epinephrine will relieve the swelling of edematous mucosa, glottis, and facial tissue. In addition, the β_2 activity of epinephrine relaxes the contracted bronchial smooth muscles. Both receptor-activating properties of epinephrine contribute to reversing the life-threatening respiratory crisis of allergic shock. (Caution: Epinephrine is also a potent β_1 agonist; care must be used to avoid excessive cardiac stimulation or arrhythmia.)

HYPOTENSION. In some hypotensive situations (*eg*, during spinal anesthesia, following pheochromocytoma surgery, and in certain cases of shock), α_1 agonists (or dopamine [INTROPIN]) are used for their pressor action. They are administered by IV infusion to raise blood pressure until the hypotensive crisis has passed or until other long-term measures are taken. (Cautions: Care should be taken to frequently change the site of administration of the IV drip; localized ischemia may cause tissue necrosis. Ischemia may occur in the extremities or in some organs with prolonged administration of a pressor agent. When blood pressure is supported by administration of a pressor agent, withdrawal of the agent should be done cautiously and slowly to avoid a precipitous drop in blood pressure.)

SHOCK. Shock is a cardiovascular syndrome distinguished by inadequate perfusion of tissue. Several insults to the body can bring about shock: hypovolemia (usually due to hemorrhage), cardiac insufficiency, or venous pooling (*eg*, that which can occur with septicemia or some drug overdoses). Usually characterized by hypotension, clouding and loss of consciousness, and metabolic acidosis, the ischemia of shock may progress to cause extensive organ damage and death.

Because of the obvious hypotension, sympathomimetic vasopressor drugs have often been employed in the past in the treatment of various types of shock. However, the wisdom of this approach has been effectively challenged. The response of the autonomic nervous system to the stressful condition of shock is a compensatory sympathetic discharge, resulting in high circulating levels of the adrenal catecholamines, NE and EPI. Thus, the addition of more vasoconstrictors is of little benefit. Rather, much evidence indicates that in many situations treatment with a vasodilator (including α blockers; see Chapter 10) may be more rational.

Any pharmacological intervention in shock should be considered only after intravascular fluid volume has been replaced and the causative problem has been addressed. One catecholamine that currently is widely used to treat various forms of shock is dopamine. Dopamine does have some α_1 vasoconstricting and β_1 cardiac-stimulating properties, but its value in shock stems from its ability to improve the perfusion of the kidneys, brain, and intestines. Renal, cerebral, and mesenteric vascular beds are rich in dopamine receptors, and these vessels respond to dopamine by dilating (even in the presence of high circulating levels of NE).

Ergot Alkaloids

Ergot alkaloids are naturally occurring or semisynthetic derivatives of lysergic acid. The source for these powerful and unusual compounds is the ergot fungus that can infect rye and other grain grasses. The fungus contains 30 to 40 lysergic acid derivatives, many of them pharmacologically active. The classification of these agents is complex because some of them are either agonists or antagonists (or have mixed actions) at adrenergic, dopaminergic, or serotonergic receptors. However, since most of the clinically important actions of the ergot alkaloids are blocked by the α-antagonist phentolamine, these agents can be classed as α-agonists.

The ergot alkaloids, primarily by α receptor activation, cause very strong contraction of smooth muscles, including vascular smooth muscle, resulting in **dramatic vasoconstriction**. Throughout history, there have been a number of mass poisonings resulting from the consumption of bread baked from ergot-infected rye. The resulting condition is characterized by a profound vasoconstriction in the extremities, which can result in necrosis. This **ergotism** is also distinguished by significant CNS effects: confusion, depression, delirium, and hallucinations (note that lysergic acid diethylamide [LSD] is an ergot derivative).

The ergot alkaloids have limited clinical application, being used primarily for their ability to cause contraction of vascular and uterine smooth muscles (see Chapter 18).

HYPERPROLACTINEMIA. High serum levels of prolactin are effectively reduced in most patients by treatment with another ergot derivative, bromocriptine (PARLODEL). Bromocriptine is a dopamine (D2) receptor agonist, and as such it inhibits the release of prolactin from the pituitary.

Alpha$_2$ Agents — Central Control of Blood Pressure

Studies on central blood pressure control mechanisms suggest that the nucleus tractus solitarius exerts an inhibitory effect on sympathetic outflow from the medulla. The receptors on the solitary tract nuclei are of the α_2-adrenergic subtype.

Thus, activation of these postsynaptic receptors with selective α_2 agonists results in a reduced sympathetic outflow from the CNS and a lowering of blood pressure. Two centrally acting α_2-adrenergic agonists that are effective in lowering the blood pressure of hypertensive patients are clonidone (CATAPRES) and α-methyldopa (ALDOMET); the activity of α-methyldopa is due to its enzymatic conversion to α-methylnorepinephrine.

Alpha-methyldopa was originally thought to inhibit the enzyme DOPA-decarboxylase in the biosynthetic pathway for NE (Fig. 9-2). However, it was later learned that α-methyldopa is actually a substrate for DOPA-decarboxylase, and it is modified in a fashion parallel to that of endogenous DOPA. Enzymatic transformation of α-methyldopa results in the production of the NE analog α-methylnorepinephrine. It is now recognized that α-methylnorepinephrine is a unique agonist for the α_2 subclass of adrenergic receptors found in the midbrain neural systems involved in the control of blood pressure. Thus, α-methyldopa is actually a "prodrug." Clonidine (CATAPRES) is also a potent α_2 agonist that lowers blood pressure through this central mechanism (clonidine does not require prior enzyme modification to be effective).

Both α-methyldopa and clonidine are widely used and well tolerated in the treatment of hypertension. Because peripheral sympathetic reflexes are little affected by these drugs, orthostatic hypotension is not pronounced. The most common side effects of both drugs are sedation, dizziness, and dry mouth (see Chapter 29).

Clonidine also prevents many of the symptoms of withdrawal from chronic opioid and alcohol use. Withdrawal from chronic opioid use increases adrenergic activity in the locus ceruleus and in the peripheral sympathetic system. This "hypersympathetic state" can be ameliorated by treating with either an opioid or clonidone. Clonidine is currently a part of the pharmacological regimen used in some narcotic and alcoholism treatment programs. (Caution: The sudden withdrawal from chronic treatment with clonidine has been reported to result in a life-threatening hypertensive crisis due, presumably, to a sudden increase in sympathetic activity in an up-regulated receptor system.)

Beta Agonists

Beta$_1$ Agents — Cardiac Stimulation

Stimulation of β_1-adrenergic receptors increases both heart rate and force of contraction. In cases of bradycardia, heart block, congestive heart failure, or cardiac arrest, isoproterenol (ISUPREL) or the β_1-selective agent dobutamine (DOBUTREX) can be used as cardiac stimulants.

Beta$_2$ Agents — Bronchial Relaxation

Stimulation of β_2 receptors causes relaxation of bronchial smooth muscle, thus decreasing airway resistance. This effect is taken advantage of in treating bronchial asthma. Both epinephrine (adrenaline) and isoproterenol (ISUPREL) are used in personal metered-dose inhalers to relieve an asthmatic attack. A severe asthmatic attack or the medical emergency status asthmaticus usually requires subcutaneous injections of epinephrine or isoproterenol.

Epinephrine and isoproterenol are rapid-acting and effective, but they have several disadvantages. Owing to rapid tissue uptake and metabolism, their duration of action is very short and they are not effective when administered orally. Most importantly, both agents are active at β_1 as well as β_2 receptors; thus they have significant cardiac stimulation side effects.

Fortunately, there are now available several orally active, **β_2-selective** agents: for example, terbutaline (BRETHINE) and albuterol (VENTOLIN), which are effective and widely used, both in oral preparations and in metered-dose inhalers (see Chapter 17).

Miscellaneous Uses of Adrenergic Agonists

Ophthalmic

Epinephrine is used to lower intraocular pressure in some patients with wide angle glaucoma. The vasoconstricting (α_1) effect of topically applied epinephrine decreases the production of aqueous humor by the ciliary processes. The α_1 activity of epinephrine also causes dilation of the pupil. This mydriatic property facilitates eye examination and is useful in ophthalmic surgery (see Chapter 7).

Central Nervous System

A number of adrenergic agents cross the blood-brain barrier and cause CNS stimulation, which includes increased wakefulness, nervousness, irritability, excitation, appetite suppression, and often, euphoria. These effects are usually not seen with clinically useful doses of EPI, NE, or ISO. However, CNS stimulation is a prominent feature of the amphetamines (indirect-acting adrenergic agonists). Tolerance develops to the stimulant properties of such drugs, and drug habituation or dependence can occur, notably with the amphetamines.

NARCOLEPSY. Dextroamphetamine (DEXEDRINE) and other stimulants are used to prevent daytime sleepiness in patients with narcolepsy. A careful schedule of timing and dose must be adjusted for each patient to allow effective nighttime sleep (see Chapter 25).

ATTENTION-DEFICIT HYPERACTIVITY DISORDER. Hyperkinesis — a syndrome consisting of inattentiveness, easy distractibility, impulsive behavior, and often hyperactivity — is seen most often as a developmental disorder of children. The amphetamines have an apparently paradoxical, calming effect on this condition; the mechanisms are unknown. Dextroamphetamine and other stimulants (notably, methylphenidate [RITALIN]) appear to be quite effective in many of these children: attention span is increased, impulsiveness is decreased, and classroom behavior is improved. However, this is an area of much controversy in terms of when medication is warranted, and the consequences of years of chronic administration (see Chapter 26).

BOX 9-3

SUMMARY: THERAPEUTIC USES OF ADRENERGIC AGONISTS

- **Control superficial hemorrhage**—α_1—vasoconstrictor—epinephrine
- **Contain local anesthetic**—α_1—vasoconstrictor—epinephrine
- **Nasal decongestant**—α_1—vasoconstrictor—phenylephrine
- **Allergic shock (Anaphylaxis)**—α_1—vasoconstrictor—epinephrine and β_2 relaxation of bronchial smooth muscle—epinephrine
- **Hypotension**—α_1—vasoconstrictor—often dopamine
- **Shock**—α_1—dopaminergic vasodilator—dopamine
- **Postpartum bleeding**—ergot (α_1) vasoconstrictor—ergonovine
- **Migraine headaches**—ergot (α_1) vasoconstrictor—ergotamine
- **Hyperprolactinemia**—dopaminergic prolactin release inhibitor—bromocriptine
- **Hypertension**—CNS α_2 agonists—clonidine and α-methyldopa
- **Cardiac stimulation**—β_1 agonists—isoproterenol and dobutamine
- **Bronchial relaxation (asthma)**—β_2-agonists—terbutaline and albuterol
- **Wide angle glaucoma**—α_1—vasoconstrictor—epinephrine
- **Narcolepsy**—CNS stimulant—dextroamphetamine
- **Hyperkinesis**—CNS stimulant—methylphenidate
- **Weight loss**—CNS stimulant—phenteramine

WEIGHT LOSS. The anorexic central action of many adrenergic agonists has become an enormous commercial, if not medical, success. Drugs such as phenteramine and fenfluramine can be used as adjuncts to a weight loss program for some patients. This topic is examined in more detail in Chapter 26.

ADVERSE EFFECTS OF ADRENERGIC AGONISTS

- **Tachyarrhythmias**, palpitations, and even ventricular fibrillation are possible adverse effects of agents with **β_1 activity**.
- **Hypertension** is a potential side effect of any agent with **α_1 activity.**
- **Localized ischemia** can occur at the infusion of **α_1 agonists**. If the site of an IV infusion is not changed periodically, localized vasoconstriction can result in necrosis. As a related caution, great care must be taken to avoid extravasation of these drugs.
- **Precipitous hypotension on withdrawal** can occur from an infusion of an **α_1 agonist**. Such infusions must be discontinued gradually to allow receptor and reflex regulation mechanisms to readjust.
- **CNS stimulation** in the form of nervousness, anxiety, insomnia, and drug dependence can result from the use of adrenergic agonists that cross the **blood-brain barrier** (the amphetamines are notable in this respect).

REFERENCES

See also references for Chapter 6.

Ornato JP: Use of adrenergic agonists during CPR in adults. Ann Emerg Med 22:411–416, 1993.

10 Adrenergic Antagonists

Oliver M. Brown

The major clinical application for adrenergic antagonists is to **lower blood pressure** in hypertensive patients by decreasing the sympathetic influence on the vasculature. This result can be accomplished by blocking the α_1-adrenergic receptors that mediate vasoconstriction, by blocking β_1-mediated renin release, by blocking peripheral sympathetic neuron activity, or by altering central nervous system (CNS) mechanisms and decreasing centrally mediated sympathetic outflow (see Chapter 9). Other important applications for adrenergic blocking drugs include **decreasing sympathetic stimulation of the heart** in patients with certain cardiac diseases. As in Chapter 9, the following discussion focuses on several model drugs.

BETA (β) BLOCKERS

The β blockers are competitive antagonists for norepinephrine (NE) and epinephrine (EPI) receptor sites in the heart (β_1 receptors), the bronchioles (β_2), and the blood vessels in skeletal muscle (β_2). Four widely used β blockers are propranolol (see structure), metoprolol, atenolol, and timolol. Propranolol (INDERAL) and timolol (TIMOPTIC, BLOCADREN) are **nonselective antagonists**, with β_1 and β_2 antagonist properties. Agents with β_2-blocking activity increase airway resistance by antagonizing β receptor–mediated relaxation of bronchial smooth muscle. Thus, the use of these agents to treat cardiovascular problems runs the risk of precipitating an asthmatic attack in patients with a history of asthma or bronchitis. This consideration has encouraged the search for β blockers that are selective for β_1-adrenergic receptors. Two agents that are relatively more β_1-selective are metoprolol (LOPRESSOR) and atenolol (TENORMIN).

OH, CH3, OCH2—C—CH2NHCH, H, CH3

Propranolol

> **BOX 10-1**
> **BETA BLOCKERS**
>
> - Propranolol—nonselective β_1 and β_2
> - Timolol—nonselective β_1 and β_2
> - Metoprolol—β_1-selective (less bronchoconstriction)
> - Atenolol—β_1-selective (less bronchoconstriction)

CLINICAL APPLICATIONS OF BETA BLOCKERS

Hypertension

Beta blockers are very effective in lowering the blood pressure in individuals with hypertension. The **mechanism** for this effect is unknown; however, several have been suggested:

- *Decreased cardiac output*—this effect is seen soon after administration of a β blocker, but the decrease in blood pressure develops only slowly thereafter.
- *CNS effect*—that decreases central sympathetic output.
- *Presynaptic β receptor inhibition*—analogous to the previously described presynaptic autoinhibitory α receptors. Presynaptic β receptor activation may enhance NE release; β antagonists would block these receptors, decreasing NE release.
- *Inhibition of renin release*—renin is released by activating β_1 receptors on the juxtaglomerular apparatus; this release can be blocked by a β_1 antagonist. (Note that β blockers are nearly always effective in reducing high-renin hypertension.)

Propranolol is both nonselective for β_1 and β_2 receptors and displays a remarkable degree of **variation in bioavailability**, both among individuals and within the same individual (possibly owing to wide differences in plasma protein binding and metabolism). Metoprolol and atenolol are longer-acting and more predictable than propranolol in producing therapeutic plasma levels. They also have the advantage of being **more β_1-selective**, making them safer to use in patients with a history of asthma or bronchitis. Atenolol is the least lipid-soluble of the β blockers; consequently it does not readily cross the blood-brain barrier and has fewer CNS side effects than the other agents. The clinical application of β blockers in the management of hypertension is covered in Chapter 29.

Cardiac Arrhythmias and Angina Pectoris

Beta antagonists attenuate the cardiac responses to sympathetic stimulation: they decrease heart rate and contractility, cardiac output, and myocardial oxygen demand (see Fig. 9-5). These effects are valuable in treating angina pectoris and supraventricular and ventricular tachyarrhythmias. The resulting decrease in cardiac work and oxygen demand makes β blocker therapy effective in reducing the incidence of reinfarction and death after myocardial infarction. For the clinical application of β blockers in managing these cardiac diseases, see Chapters 28 and 30.

Glaucoma

Topical application of a β blocker such as timolol decreases the production of aqueous humor by the ciliary body. The resulting lowering of intraocular pressure brings relief in most types of glaucoma. Unlike pilocarpine, β blockers do not cause miosis or spasm of accommodation; thus they are especially valuable in treating younger patients who possess active accommodation.

Migraine Headaches

When used chronically, propranolol produces a marked reduction in the number of attacks in approximately one third to one half of individuals with migraine. Such β blocker therapy is useful for prophylaxis of migraine attacks, but it is not usually effective in the acute treatment of headache, although it can be in some patients. The mechanism for the prophylactic effect is not known, but the β_2 activity of propranolol may block dilation of extracranial arteries and thus prevent the pain associated with the expansion of these vessels (see Chapter 18).

Stage Fright

Beta blockers appear to relieve the anxiety of "anticipational anxiety" of performing artists and public speakers by preventing the palpitations associated with stage fright.

Caution: β blockers can cause dramatic bradycardia, hypotension, and bronchial constriction. Moreover, the sudden cessation of β blocker treatment can precipitate ventricular tachycardia, myocardial infarction, unstable angina, and even sudden death.

> BOX 10-2
>
> **BETA BLOCKERS**
>
> **Effects:**
> - **Bradycardia**
> - **Hypotension**
> - **Bronchial constriction**
>
> **Applications:**
> - **Hypertension**—decrease blood pressure
> - **Cardiac arrhythmias**—decrease heart rate
> - **Angina pectoris**—decrease myocardial oxygen demand
> - **Glaucoma**—decrease aqueous formation
> - **Migraine headaches**—primarily prophylaxis
> - **Stage fright**—decrease palpitations

ALPHA (α) BLOCKERS

The α blockers are reversible, competitive antagonists for NE receptor sites, primarily in vascular smooth muscle. However, phenoxybenzamine is unusual in that it forms a covalent bond with the α receptor (thus producing long-lasting effects); it is an alkylating agent with a nitrogen mustard-like structure. The older α antagonists phentolamine (REGITINE) and phenoxybenzamine (DIBENZYLINE) are nonselective, with affinity for both α_1 and α_2 receptors. Several newer agents, such as prazosin (MINIPRESS), are selective for α_1 receptors. (Structures of these three agents are shown.) Alpha blockers **decrease sympathetically mediated vasoconstriction** (see Fig. 9-5). Because these drugs are antagonists, they owe their pharmacological activity to blocking the action of the agonists NE and EPI. Thus, the **degree of vasodilation produced by α blockers is dependent on the level of adrenergic tone of the vascular beds**. The level of **sympathetic activity will vary** among and within vascular beds and will also vary with physiological state (*eg*, exercise, stress).

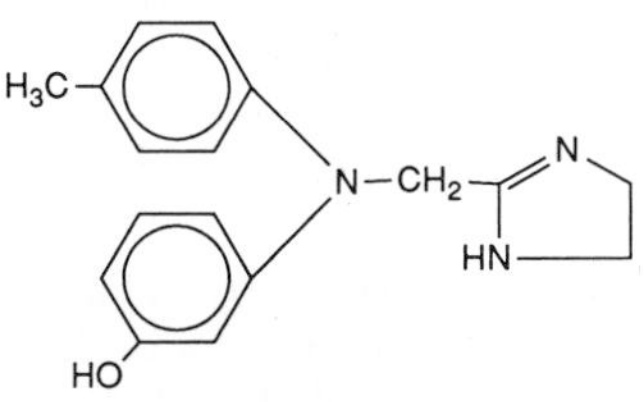

H_3C · N–CH_2 · N · HN · HO

Phentolamine

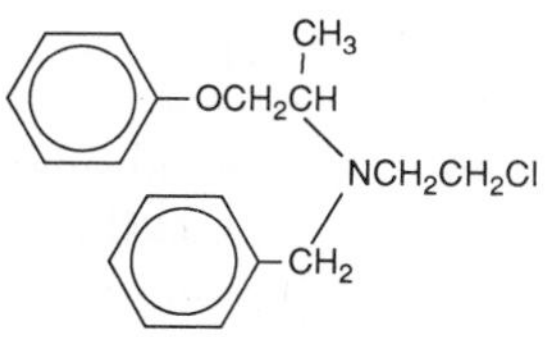

CH_3 · OCH_2CH · NCH_2CH_2Cl · CH_2

Phenoxybenzamine

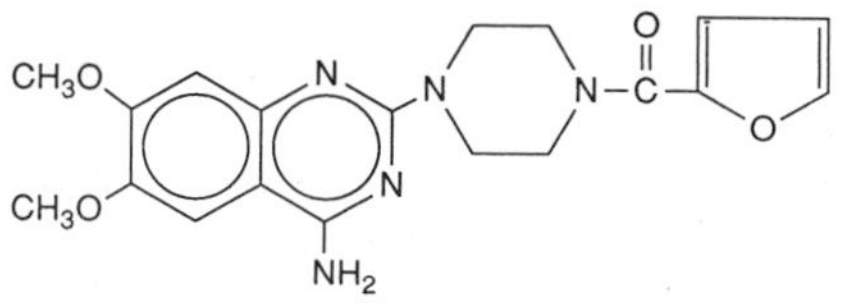

CH_3O · CH_3O · N · N · N · N–C · O · O · NH_2

Prazosin

BOX 10–3
ALPHA BLOCKERS

- Phentolamine—nonselective α_1 and α_2 (competitive)
- Phenoxybenzamine—nonselective α_1 and α_2 (noncompetitive)
- Prazosin—α_1 (less tachycardia)

CLINICAL APPLICATIONS OF ALPHA BLOCKERS

Hypertension

Because α blockers can produce a marked degree of vasodilation, they would seem a logical choice of drug to lower blood pressure in the treatment of hypertension and other hemodynamic problems. Unfortunately, the nonspecific α antagonists also produce a profound orthostatic (postural) hypotension and reflex tachycardia. These adverse effects are severe enough to limit the clinical utility of such α blockers. A major exception to this limitation is the newer α_1-selective agent prazosin. Some degree of orthostatic hypotension occurs with prazosin use, but this effect decreases with repeated administration. Prazosin produces considerably less tachycardia than the nonselective agents; it has thus become a useful antihypertensive medication. The clinical application of prazosin and other drugs used to treat hypertension is covered in Chapter 29.

It is unclear why **prazosin produces milder side effects** than the nonselective α blockers. One suggested mechanism is that the nonselective α antagonists (phentolamine and phenoxybenzamine) not only block the (desired) postjunctional α_1 receptors; they also block the prejunctional α_2 receptors. This would reduce the negative feedback inhibition of NE release, resulting in increased NE release, which produces tachycardia. Because prazosin has negligible activity at α_2 receptors, it will have only the intended postjunctional α_1 blockade, and not enhance NE release. An additional contribution to the lack of significant tachycardia after prazosin administration may involve heteroreceptor regulatory mechanisms (see Fig. 9–3). There is evidence that presynaptic α_1 receptors exert control on the release of acetylcholine nerve endings in the heart. Prazosin would block this α_1-adrenoceptor inhibition of acetylcholine release. The combination of increased acetylcholine release and decreased NE release may explain the low incidence of tachycardia with prazosin therapy (Fig. 10–1).

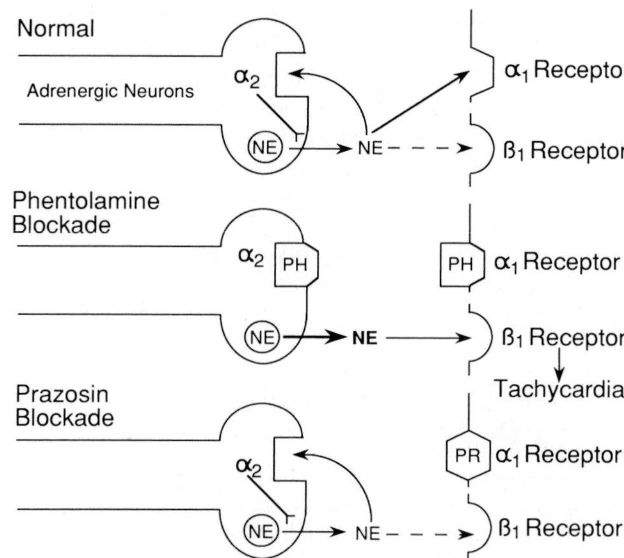

FIGURE 10–1. Action of prazosin.

Peripheral Vascular Disease

Most cases of vascular disease, including multi-infarct dementia, involve chronic occlusive atherosclerosis. The vessels in the ischemic areas of these patients are coated with plaque, damaged, and no longer resilient. Such vessels do not respond to vasodilator therapy. Introduction of an α blocker will cause a "stealing" of blood from already poorly perfused areas to other parts of the body with healthy, compliant vessels, which do respond to vasodilators. Thus, although the use of α blockers and other vasodilators to treat peripheral vascular disease is widely promoted, the wisdom of such therapy is questionable.

There are some instances of peripheral ischemia that result from **vasospasm**; such conditions can often be improved with α blockers. The vigorous vasoconstriction of the extremities resulting from exposure to the cold in **Raynaud's disease** is relieved by phenoxybenzamine or prazosin. Likewise, the sequelae of **frostbite** and **intermittent claudication** are effectively treated with α blockers.

Pheochromocytoma

A pheochromocytoma may release large amounts of EPI and NE into the blood stream, especially when it is manipulated during surgery. This can, of course, result in dramatic changes in heart rate and blood pressure. Thus, before and during surgery to remove such an adrenal tumor, patients are protected from the cardiovascular effects of catecholamines by treatment with a combination of α and β blockers.

Shock

Compensatory mechanisms during shock usually release large quantities of adrenal catecholamines into the blood stream, producing a profound vasoconstriction. Such constriction in postcapillary resistance vessels results in the concentration of blood. Concentrated, viscous blood exacerbates the already inadequate perfusion characteristic of shock. In some cases, α blockers and other vasodilators have been shown to reverse this vasoconstriction and improve the survival rate from shock.

Caution: α blockers can produce a number of side effects, including postural hypotension, reflex tachycardia, nasal stuffiness, and inhibition of ejaculation.

BOX 10-4
ALPHA BLOCKERS

Effects:
- **Vasodilation**
- **Lower blood pressure**
- **Orthostatic hypotension** (less with α_1-selective agents)
- **Tachycardia** (less with α_1-selective agents)

Applications:
- **Hypertension**—decrease blood pressure
- **Raynaud's disease**—decrease vasospasm
- **Sequelae of frostbite**—decrease vasospasm
- **Pheochromocytoma surgery**—protect against catecholamines
- **Shock**—protect against catecholamines

AGENTS WITH BOTH ALPHA AND BETA BLOCKING ACTIONS

Labetalol (NORMODYNE) is unique in having both α (α_1-selective) and β (nonselective β_1 and β_2) blocking activity. Labetalol is actually a mixture of drugs: it is given as a racemic mixture of four optical isomers. Two of the isomers are inactive, one is a potent α blocker, and one is a potent β blocker.

Labetalol lowers total peripheral resistance without producing tachycardia and has thus proved useful in treating hypertension. An oral preparation is given to treat essential hypertension, and labetalol is administered intravenously to treat hypertensive emergencies.

NEURON-BLOCKING DRUGS

In addition to the actions of α- and β-adrenergic receptor antagonists considered earlier, drugs may decrease the effects of sympathetic activity by several other mechanisms. Included among these mechanisms is the depression of the output of NE from peripheral sympathetic neurons; drugs with this action are referred to as neuron-blocking drugs. As with the receptor antagonists, the primary clinical interest in these drugs is in **treating essential hypertension**.

Neuron-blocking drugs interfere with:

- **Synthesis of NE** (α-methyl tyrosine)
- **Packaging of NE** (reserpine)
- **Release of NE** (bretylium and guanethidine)

Several steps in the process of neurotransmission by norepinephrine are susceptible to interference by drugs, as described in the following paragraphs.

Synthesis of Norepinephrine

The rate-limiting step in the synthesis of NE is the conversion of tyrosine to L-DOPA by tyrosine hydroxylase (see Fig. 9-2). Thus, an inhibitor of this enzyme should markedly decrease the synthesis of neuronal NE and lower adrenergic nerve activity. The tyrosine analog α-methyl tyrosine (DEMSER) effectively inhibits tyrosine hydroxylase. However, this drug produces such severe side effects (pronounced sedation, diarrhea, anxiety, and tremors) that it is not useful in the management of essential hypertension. **Alpha-methyl tyrosine** is occasionally used in the **management of pheochromocytoma** in those patients who are hypersensitive to or unresponsive to combined α and β blockers (see earlier discussion).

Packaging of Norepinephrine

The alkaloid **reserpine** is transported into adrenergic neurons, where it associates with the synaptic vesicle membrane and prevents the packaging of both dopamine (for conversion to NE) and cytoplasmic NE into synaptic vesicles. This leads to a long-lasting and nearly complete depletion of neuronal NE and dopamine, both in the peripheral sympathetic system and in the CNS. With reserpine treatment, a lowering of blood pressure does ensue, and it has been used to treat hypertension. However, as with many sympatholytic agents, reserpine produces orthostatic hypotension. The peripheral NE depletion caused by reserpine also results in an up-regulation of postjunctional adrenergic receptors, producing a supersensitivity to sympathetic agonists that is similar to denervation supersensitivity. Extreme GI discomfort (diarrhea and abdominal cramps) also occurs as parasympathetic tone is unopposed by sympathetic activity following the "chemical sympathectomy" produced by reserpine. The depletion of NE in the CNS can lead to severe depression.

Release of Norepinephrine

Bretylium (BRETYLOL) and **guanethidine** (ISMELIN) decrease adrenergic nerve activity by blocking neuronal NE release. In the same fashion as for reserpine, bretylium and guanethidine are taken into the adrenergic neuron by the specific amine uptake pump used for NE re-uptake (uptake$_1$). As these drugs are transported into the neuron they displace cytoplasmic NE and cause its release, producing a transient sympathomimetic effect. Following the brief period of increased adrenergic activity, all three drugs produce a prolonged decrease in adrenergic activity. Bretylium and guanethidine, like reserpine, produce the side effects of severe orthostatic hypotension and supersensitivity to sympathomimetic drugs.

Despite the similarities between guanethidine and bretylium, there are some differences in their mechanisms and their applications. They both appear to block the process of release of NE from the neuronal membrane. However, guanethidine causes depletion of neuronal NE, whereas bretylium does not. Guanethidine is considered to be a "false transmitter," because it is packaged in synaptic vesicles and can be released by nerve stimulation. The use of **guanethidine** is reserved for patients with **severe hypertension**.

Bretylium is currently used as an **antiarrhythmic** agent, with extremely limited use in emergency situations.

TABLE 10–1. Adrenergic Drugs

Agents	Receptor	Therapeutically Useful Property
Alpha Agonists		
Epinephrine	Nonselective	Vasoconstriction (α_1)—prevent bleeding or hypotension, in CPR
Norepinephrine	Nonselective	Vasoconstriction (α_1)—control hypotension
Dopamine	Indirect	Vasoconstriction (α_1)—control hypotension
	Dopamine	Vasodilatation—of certain areas (*eg*, kidneys) during shock
Phenteramine		Anorexia (CNS)—component of weight-loss program
Phenylpropanolamine	Indirect	Vasoconstriction (α_1)—nasal decongestant
Pseudoephedrine	Nonselective	Vasoconstriction—nasal decongestant
Phenylephrine	α_1-Selective	Vasoconstriction—treat hypotension, nasal decongestant
Methoxamine	α_1-Selective	Vasoconstriction—treat hypotension
Metaraminol	α_1-Selective	Vasoconstriction—treat hypotension
Mephentermine	α_1-Selective	Vasoconstriction—treat hypotension
Ergotamine	α_1-Selective	Vasoconstriction—treat migraine headache
Ergonovine	α_1-Selective	Vasoconstriction—treat postpartum bleeding
Methyldopa	α_2-Selective	Decrease sympathetic output (CNS)—treat hypertension
Clonidine	α_2-Selective	Decrease sympathetic output (CNS)—treat hypertension
Guanfacine	α_2-Selective	Decrease sympathetic output (CNS)—treat hypertension
Guanabenz	α_2-Selective	Decrease sympathetic output (CNS)—treat hypertension
Beta Agonists		
Epinephrine	Nonselective	Bronchial relaxation (β_2)—treat asthma and anaphylactic shock
		Cardiac stimulation(β_1)—treat depressed contractility
Isoproterenol	Nonselective	Bronchial relaxation (β_2)—treat asthma
		Cardiac stimulation (β_1)—treat depressed contractility
Ethylnorepinephrine	Nonselective	Bronchial relaxation (β_2)—treat asthma
		Local vasoconstriction (α_1)—treat asthma
Dobutamine	β_1-Selective	Cardiac stimulation—treat depressed contractility
Terbutaline	β_2-Selective	Bronchial relaxation—treat asthma
Albuterol	β_2-Selective	Bronchial relaxation—treat asthma
Pirbuterol	β_2-Selective	Bronchial relaxation—treat asthma
Bitolterol	β_2-Selective	Bronchial relaxation—treat asthma
Ritodrine	β_2-Selective	Uterine relaxation—treat premature labor
Miscellaneous Agonists		
Dopamine	Dopamine	Vasodilatation—of certain areas (*eg*, kidneys) during shock
Bromocriptine	Dopamine	Inhibit prolactin release—treat hyperprolactinemia
Phenylpropanolamine	Indirect	Anorexia (CNS)—component of weight-loss program
Pemoline	Indirect	CNS stimulation—treat attention-deficit hyperactivity
Amphetamine	Indirect	CNS stimulation—treat narcolepsy and hyperactivity
Methylphenidate	Indirect	CNS stimulation—treat narcolepsy and hyperactivity
Fenfluramine	Indirect	Anorexia (CNS)—component of weight-loss program
Alpha Antagonists		
Phenoxybenzamine	Nonselective	Vasodilatation—treat vasospasm of Raynaud's disease and frostbite; protect against pheochromocytoma
Phentolamine	Nonselective	Vasodilatation—treat vasospasm of Raynaud's disease and frostbite; protect against pheochromyocytoma
Prazosin	α_1-Selective	Vasodilatation—treat hypertension
Terazosin	α_1-Selective	Vasodilatation—treat hypertension
Beta Antagonists		
Propranolol	Nonselective	Inhibit renin release(?)—treat hypertension
		Decrease cardiac output—treat angina, arrhythmia, migraine headache, essential tremor
Timolol	Nonselective	Decrease cardiac output—prophylaxis of myocardial infarction
		Decrease aqueous humor production—treat glaucoma
Nadolol	Nonselective	Inhibit renin release(?)—treat hypertension
		Decrease cardiac output—treat angina
Pindolol	Nonselective	(?)—treat hypertension
Metoprolol	β_1-Selective	Inhibit renin release(?)—treat hypertension
		Decrease cardiac output—treat angina and arrhythmia
Acebutolol	β_1-Selective	Inhibit renin release(?)—treat hypertension
		Decrease cardiac rate—tachyarrhythmia
Atenolol	β_1-Selective	Inhibit renin release(?)—treat hypertension
Esmolol	β_1-Selective	Decrease cardiac rate—treat tachyarrhythmia
Labetalol	β_1, β_2, and α_1	Lower peripheral resistance—treat hypertension
Neuron-Blocking Drugs		
Alpha-methyl tyrosine	NE synthesis	Decrease NE—protect against pheochromocytoma
Reserpine	NE packaging	Deplete NE—treat hypertension
Guanethidine	NE release	Prevent NE release—treat hypertension/antiarrhythmic
Bretylium	NE release	Block NE release—antiarrhythmic

CNS = central nervous system; CPR = cardiopulmonary resuscitation; NE = norepinephrine.

The antiarrhythmic action of bretylium appears to be unrelated to its adrenergic neuron-blocking property. Through unknown mechanisms bretylium increases cardiac action potential duration and effective refractory period (see Chapter 28).

Caution: Note the severe side effects of these drugs. Reserpine, guanethidine, and bretylium can produce severe orthostatic hypotension and a potentially dangerous supersensitivity to sympathomimetics (the use of even some over-the-counter cold preparations may precipitate a life-threatening hypertensive or cardiac crisis). Use of reserpine must be avoided by all who have a history of depression. Unlike reserpine, guanethidine and bretylium do not cause CNS side effects because they fail to cross the blood-brain barrier.

BOX 10–5

NEURON-BLOCKING DRUGS

Effects:
- Hypotension
- Orthostatic hypotension
- Increased gastrointestinal (GI) activity
- Supersensitivity to sympathomimetics

Applications:
- **Hypertension**—decrease blood pressure
- **Management of pheochromocytoma**—protect against catecholamines
- **Cardiac arrhythmia**—emergency antiarrhythmic

ADVERSE EFFECTS OF ADRENERGIC ANTAGONISTS

- **Hypotension**, in particular orthostatic (postural) hypotension, is a potential side effect of any agent with α antagonist or neuron-blocking activity.
- **Nasal congestion** is a complication of α antagonist use.
- **Inhibition of ejaculation** can also result from the use of agents with α antagonist or neuron-blocking activity.
- **Bradycardia** is a likely side effect when using agents with β blocking properties.
- **Bronchoconstriction** (precipitation of an asthmatic attack) can result from using agents with β antagonist properties.
- **Sedation** is a possible consequence of administration of any of these agents (*eg*, propranolol) that cross the blood-brain barrier.
- **Severe CNS depression** is uniquely associated with the use of reserpine.

A comprehensive list of adrenergic antagonists appears in Table 10–1.

REFERENCES

See also references for Chapter 6.

Day MD: Autonomic Pharmacology: Experimental and Clinical Aspects. New York: Churchill Livingstone, 1979.

DiStefano PS, Brown OM: Biochemical correlates of morphine withdrawal. 2. Effects of Clonidine. J Pharmacol Exp Ther 233:339–344, 1985.

PART III

DRUGS FOR THE PREVENTION AND TREATMENT OF PAIN, PAIN SYNDROMES, AND INFLAMMATION

11 General Anesthesia and General Anesthetics

Paul R. Knight III and Cedric M. Smith

THE SYNDROME OF ANESTHESIA

The first studies into what we today can recognize as anesthesia occurred in the 1800s as casual social experimentation with a variety of intoxicants, including nitrous oxide and diethyl ether. The first known successful use in a patients was in 1842 when Crawford W. Long, a rural practitioner in Georgia who had witnessed "ether frolics," administered diethyl either for surgery to incise a boil. Unfortunately, at this time most attempts to reduce the pain and suffering of surgery went unpublicized. It was not until October 1846, 4 years later, that a medical student, William T. G. Morton, convincingly demonstrated to a small skeptical medical audience that inhalation of the pungent vapors from a secret substance, later revealed to be diethyl ether, could produce such a profound sleep that the surgical removal of a tumor of the jaw was accomplished without pain or struggling.

Although perhaps the most celebrated event in American medical history, the magic of anesthesia was born amid controversy, not only over who should receive the credit and potential financial rewards, but whether relief of the pain, such as was associated with childbirth, was contrary to religious scripture.

In the following years a large variety of agents were tested, and within a few years both chloroform and nitrous oxide were added to the list of practical agents. During the middle of this century with the development of accurate and reliable vaporizers and anesthetic gas machines, a number of agents (notably cyclopropane and ethylene) were introduced. Explosions and fires, particularly with the use of cyclopropane, plagued the operating rooms during this era.

It was not until nearly 100 years after the demonstration of the effects of diethyl ether that the nonflammable halogenated alkane (halothane) and halogenated methylethyl ethers (enflurane, isoflurane) had been studied sufficiently for their introduction into clinical medicine. In spite of the passage of many years and extensive investigations, the two agents first discovered, diethyl ether and nitrous oxide, remain in some use. Nitrous oxide continues to be extensively employed in combination with other anesthetic agents because its effects are additive and will permit decreasing the concentrations required of the more potent agents. Nitrous oxide also decreases the oxygen concentration in the inspired gas mixtures, reducing the risk of pulmonary oxygen toxicity. (Although slow in onset and recovery, and relatively unpleasant to receive or administer, diethyl ether is very inexpensive and is still probably the safest general anesthetic agent to be administered by inexperienced medical personnel. These qualities cause it to still enjoy some usage in developing countries.)

For the modern use of the words anesthesia and anesthetics we are indebted to Oliver Wendell Holmes.

Definition

Anesthesia is a reversible state in which there is a loss of awareness without conscious recall, a lack of overt muscular movement (possibly with some muscle relaxation), and an attenuation of the autonomic responses to surgical stimulation. Essential to understanding anesthesia is the recognition of its reversibility. It is critical that there should be no sustained impairment of cardiovascular or respiratory functions. Substances that produce this altered state are called anesthetics. Anesthesiology is a recognized medical specialty practiced by trained physicians.

The term *anesthesia* comes from the Greek *anaisthēsis*, meaning insensible and is defined in the 1771 copy of the Encyclopedia Britannica as "a privation of the senses." At one extreme, it can be viewed as a neural phenomenon reflecting specific changes in the neuronal systems of the brain and peripheral nervous system; at the other extreme, it is a unique behavioral state of nonresponsiveness to noxious stimuli that would otherwise produce an excitatory condition similar to the "fight or flight" state of arousal.

Basic Risk-Benefit Analysis

Because anesthesia decreases the ability of patients to maintain normal physiological homeostasis in response to changes in their environments, it intrinsically places the patient at risk for untoward cardiopulmonary sequelae; thus, all anesthesias require continuous, vigilant monitoring by specially trained individuals.

The minimal requisite that anesthesia must provide in order to carry out surgery is to keep the patient from moving in response to surgical cutting or other traumatizing of tissues. Important additional objectives are the provision of amnesia for the procedures, the maintenance of physiological homeostasis, and the avoidance of untoward reflex responses.

Most of the current major anesthetic agents (Table 11–1) have been recently introduced. The use of the potent inhalational anesthetics became feasible only with the development of sophisticated techniques and the equipment for their delivery to the patient. Among the techniques essential to the development of modern anesthesia and surgery were precise and reliable machines for delivery of gases, instruments for measuring the physiologic effects of anesthetics, knowledge obtained from scientific investigation into the effects of anesthetic agents on the pathophysiological processes of the patient, and the availability of adjunct medications that permit tailoring the anesthetic procedure to the patient's condition and surgical intervention. The advances in anesthesia and anesthetic techniques have paralleled the

TABLE 11–1. General Anesthetics Currently in Use

Administered by Inhalation	Boiling Point (°C)	MAC	Blood/Gas Partition Coefficient	Oil/Gas Partition Coefficient
Nitrous oxide—N_2O	Gas	101%*	0.47	37.3
Halothane (FLUOTHANE) ($CF_3CHBrCl$)	50	0.77%	2.4	310
Enflurane (ETHRANE) (CHF_2-0-CF_2-CHFCl)	57	1.68	1.8	128
Isoflurane (FORANE) (CHF_2-0-$CHClCF_3$)	48	1.15	1.4	170
Desflurane (SUPRANE) (CHF_2-0-CHF-CF_3)	23	7.3	0.42	18.7
Sevoflurane (SEVOFRANE) ($[CF_3]_2$-CH-0-CH_2F)	59	1.71–2.05	0.69	55
Administered Intravenously				
Barbituates				
Thiopental (PENTOTHAL)				
Methohexital (BREVITAL)				
Thiamytal (SURITAL)				
Benzodiazepines				
Diazepam (VALIUM)				
Midazolam (VERSED)				
Lorazepam (ATIVAN)				
Profolol (DIPRIVAN)				
Ketamine (KETALAR)				
Etomidate (AMIDATE)				
Droperidol (INAPSINE)				

Data from Firestone LL, Miller JC, Miller KW: Tables of physical and pharmacological properties of anesthetics appendix. *In* Roth SH, Miller KW (eds): Molecular and Cellular Mechanisms of Anesthetics. New York and London: Plenum Medical Book Company, 1986; and Wrigley SR, Jones RM: Inhalational agents: An update. Eur J Anesthesiol 9:185–201, 1992.

*MAC (minimal alveolar [anesthetic] concentration) not reached alone with concentrations that cannot safely exeed 70% with the remaining 30% devoted to oxygen. However, larger amounts can be achieved using hyperbaric chambers, and under hyperbaric conditions nitrous oxide can produce the defined minimal anesthesia required for the MAC.

remarkable progress in surgical techniques and improvements in pre- and postoperative care.

ASSESSING POTENCY AND DEPTH

Minimal Alveolar (Anesthetic) Concentration

The depth of anesthesia can be defined in terms of the relationship between the concentration of an inhalational anesthetic being administered and the responsiveness of the patient to noxious stimulation—an applied example of the dose (concentration)-response relationship. To standardize a measure of potency of the different anesthetic agents, the concept of MAC (the *m*inimum *a*lveolar *c*oncentration of a volatile anesthetic at one atmosphere in which 50% of the subjects will move to a standardized noxious stimulus) was developed. This was possible because the concentration in the brain of an inhaled anesthetic gas and the alveolar anesthetic concentration are at relatively steady states.

Stages of Anesthesia

The stages of anesthesia associated with the use of diethyl ether were introduced by Guedel largely as a teaching tool for training anesthesiologists and technicians at the time of World War I. Although attempts to use specific criteria (signs) to describe the levels and progression of diethyl ether anesthesia is outmoded, the general concepts may be adapted to provide conceptual and practical help in learning clinical anesthesia. The signs of anesthetic depth vary considerably among anesthetic agents as a consequence of the variations of "side" effects among agents; knowing these unique "side" effects, one can ascertain the depth of anesthesia. Although somewhat artificial with blurry lines of demarcation, the stages of anesthesia can be adapted for general use to help describe the clinical picture seen when patients receive an inhalational anesthetic.

- **Stage I**—the time the patient first receives the anesthetic to the time he or she becomes unconscious. Patients may demonstrate analgesia, if it is a side effect of the agent being used (*ie*, nitrous oxide, diethyl ether) and may also develop amnesia, while responding appropriately to verbal commands.
- **Stage II** (The stage of delirium)—begins when the patient becomes unconscious and stops obeying verbal commands. The patient may be agitated an/or combative. A period of heightened reflex responses and involuntary movements and actions that may include thrashing about, fluctuating respiration and blood pressure, fighting, and struggling occurs. Nonpurposeful rapid eye movements, swallowing, breath-holding, vomiting, and larnygospasm are also hallmarks of this stage. Upon recovery the individual is amnesic for this entire period. One of the major ad-

vantages of the use of intravenous agents is to induce anesthesia and rapidly move the patient out of this stage.

- **Stage III** — the stage of surgical anesthesia; it may be divided into light and deep anesthesia based on the responses of the patient to surgical stimuli and the requirement of adjuncts to render the patient suitable for performing the surgery (*ie*, muscle relaxants). This stage is marked by the onset of more regular respiration in which the tidal volume tends to decrease as the depth of anesthesia deepens. During surgical anesthesia, with the increasing concentrations of the anesthetic in the blood and brain, there occurs a progressive depression of a variety of autonomic reflex responses, as well as muscle tone (variable depending on the agent used) of the extremities and of the abdomen; and changes in the cardiovascular reflex responses to skin stimulation, traction on the mesentery, and to stimulation of the bronchi. Within the stage of surgical anesthesia, levels of anesthesia can also be used to describe qualitatively the response in relation to the intensity of the surgical stimulation.
- **Stage IV** — the stage of relative overdose, associated with pending cardiovascular collapse and severe respiratory depression. The patient's pathology may result in stage IV becoming manifest prior to stage III, which necessitates the use of other adjuncts to provide for the proper conditions to allow the surgeon to operate.

SITES AND MECHANISMS OF ACTION OF GENERAL ANESTHETICS (TABLE 11-1)

Variety of Anesthetics

General anesthesia involves depressive effects on the entire body, in contrast with local or regional anesthesia in which only a portion of the patient is made unresponsive to the surgical trauma. General anesthetics can be classified into intravenous agents and inhalational agents. Intravenous agents are, for the most part, opioids, sedatives, or derivatives of these agents designed structurally to have properties suited for anesthetic states, for example, a short duration of action. These parenterally administered drugs are used for anesthetic purposes in concentrations that would be toxic outside the protected operative setting. Because their sites and mechanisms of action are the same as when they are used for other therapeutic conditions, they are presented in other chapters (14 and 25).

Spectrum of Effects of Anesthetics

Although general anesthetics appear to act selectively or specifically on nervous tissue, they potentially affect all body functions; nevertheless, they exhibit relative selectivity regarding variations in the potency of their actions on different tissues and organ systems. Exposure of tissues to concentrations of the agents required for anesthesia results in graded effects on specific neuronal networks and organ functions. For example, the auditory centers of the brain stem can remain active even during deep anesthesia. Without concurrent pathology, the respiratory and cardiovascular systems remain functionally adequate while the systems of memory, sensation, autonomic response, and volitional movement are depressed.

Thus, explanations of the mechanisms of general anesthesia necessarily entail a description of the selectivity and the spectrum of actions of each of the anesthetic agents. Understanding the mechanisms underlying these actions will ultimately provide a picture of the relationships among their molecular actions on single cells, their actions on the activity of neural networks and functional components of other organ systems, and the resultant changes in functions and behavior of the whole individual. The functional interactions among the various intervening levels of neural organizations constitute the basis for theories of anesthesia. (As will be seen below, it is probable that different general anesthetics act by more than one ultimate molecular mechanism.)

Although the central nervous system is considered the target organ for these agents, inhalational anesthetics are also general body depressants in the sense that direct depression of the heart may be produced by molecular mechanisms similar to that which occur in the brain. Such side effects are integral components of the overall state of general anesthesia inasmuch as they may include the depression of untoward responses associated with the surgical insult. Finally, any theory of anesthetic action must account for the ability of high levels of hyperbaric pressure to antagonize the anesthetic state, as observed experimentally in intact animals and isolated tissues.

- **Reversible interaction with tissue components — not covalent or ionic binding.** How is it that simple chemical substances can be inhaled, not be metabolized, not be tightly bound to tissues, and rapidly reversed by exhalation through pulmonary expiration, yet can affect the brain and other organ systems in such a profound and selective fashion? It has been believed that the inhalational anesthetic agents act "nonspecifically" to produce changes through alterations of physicochemical processes such as weak Van Der Waals types of interactions between the site of action and the anesthetic molecule, rather than covalent or ionic bonds.
- **Hydrophobic lipid and protein domains of the cell membranes** are sites where general anesthetics are distributed preferentially because of their high lipid solubilities. Anesthetic potency is known to correlate almost directly with lipid solubility (Fig. 11-1).

  Anesthetics applied *in vitro* to membrane preparations produce an **increase in membrane thickness or volume, associated with an increased fluidity of membranes**. It is postulated that the critical site of the anesthetic-cell interaction involves regions of the cell membrane containing intercalated proteins, possibly receptors or ion channels, which are altered secondary to physical changes in the lipid matrix.

  Nevertheless, the fact that the anesthetic is present in a high concentration in lipid or hydrophobic regions of cell membranes describes the cellular and subcellular distribution of the anesthetic molecules; it does not provide any direct information about the functional significance of any selective distribution. Moreover, such theories alone are limited inasmuch as they fail to provide insight regard-

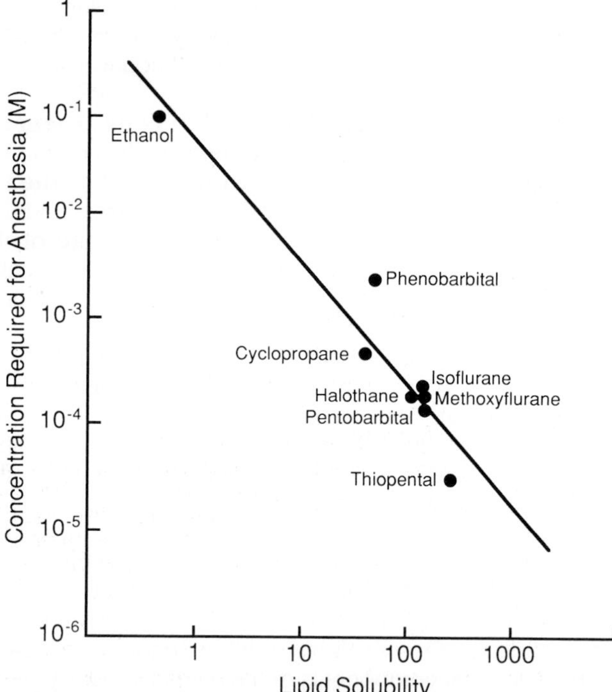

FIGURE 11–1. Concentrations of inhalation anesthetics required to produce anesthesia are inversely correlated with their solubilities in lipids. The lower the concentration required, the more potent the agent; thus, the potency of anesthetics is directly correlated with their solubilities in lipids. (Adapted from Strichartz G, Krieger N: Neurobiology of Anesthesia—Supplement to the Grass Calendar for 1988. Quincy, MA: Grass Instrument Co, 1988; and Miller KW: The nature of the site of general anesthesia. Int Rev Neurobiol 27:1–61, 1985, based on data summarized by Janoff and colleagues on the aqueous concentrations required to abolish the righting reflex in tadpoles plotted against the lipid/aqueous partition coefficient [Janoff AS, Pringle MJ, Miller KW: Correlation of general anesthetic potency with solubility in membranes. Biochim Biophys Acta 649:125–128, 1981].)

ing the origin of the selectivity of action among the various specific neuronal systems that is a hallmark of a practically useful anesthetic.

- **The "Protein Theory of Anesthesia"** hypothesizes that anesthetics directly bind to hydrophobic domains of the secondary structure of a critical protein(s) in the cell, thereby altering those proteins' functions. Interestingly, the lipid and protein theories of anesthetic action are both in agreement that the target molecule is probably a functional membrane protein. Where they differ is that in the one theory the anesthetic agent acts directly, whereas it acts indirectly in the lipid theory in the cell. A protein site of action is supported by evidence of differential effects of optically active isomers on neurons and myocardium (Moody et al, 1994).

Actions of Anesthetics on Neuronal Systems

The exact neuronal targets of anesthetic action—groups of specific neurons or the components of such neurons—have not as yet been unambiguously identified. This is not surprising inasmuch as the specific groups of neurons responsible, for example, for the altered functions such as consciousness have yet to be fully identified or understood. Nevertheless, the levels of neural integration can be identified (Table 11–2).

NEURONAL MEMBRANES. Exposure of nerves to an inhalational anesthetic increases the likelihood that the sodium ion channels responsible for the excitatory depolarization of the conducted action potential remain in the closed state. Although the concentrations of anesthetics necessary to interfere with conduction in single neurons are higher than are required in clinical anesthesia, this mechanism is attractive because this is an effect of anesthetics that can be antagonized by hyperbaric pressure. Nevertheless, it may be hypothesized that very small changes in action potential conduction in single cells brought about by clinical concen-

TABLE 11–2. Sites and Mechanisms of Action of General Anesthetics (A partial integration of actions across systems)

I. *Direct effects on neurons:*
   - General anesthetics are selectively localized to lipids and hydrophobic regions of proteins; anesthetic potencies are correlated with lipid solubility as well as with hyperpolarization of small nerve fibers
   - Depression of membrane excitability, decrease in sodium conductance, possibly the consequence of increased membrane thickness/volume and increased fluidity of membranes
   - Intracellular components: mitochondria oxidative systems depressed (hypoxia produces unconsciousness, hypoxia and anesthetics are additive or synergistic in actions); calcium-mediated mitochondrial functions are depressed by anesthetics

II. *Synaptic processes potentially affected by general anesthetics:*
   - Transmitter synthesis
   - Transmitter release—halothane in cerebral cortex
   - Transmitter metabolism
   - Postsynaptic effects:
     - Augmentation of inhibition
       - Augmented and/or prolonged presynaptic inhibition (benzodiazepines, barbiturates, ethanol, ether)
       - Augmented endorphin release (nitrous oxide and possibly ether, but not halothane)
       - Augmented GABA-induced inhibition
     - Depression of transmitter-induced postsynaptic excitation
       - (All inhalation anesthetics in high concentrations as well as barbiturates, ethanol)
     - Alteration of neurotransmitter receptor proteins
     - Anesthetics cause desensitization of the receptor and accelerated closing of the ion channels associated with the receptor (demonstrated to date with an acetylcholine receptor)

III. *Neuronal systems selectively influenced by general anesthetics (by function):*
   - Consciousness
     - Cerebral cortex
     - Reticular and other ascending activating systems
     - Electroencephalograms reveal at least two classes of anesthetics: one exemplified by halothane (chloroform and trichloroethylene), and another that includes nitrous oxide, diethyl ether, and cyclopropane
   - Memory/amnesia—cerebral cortex, hippocampus, amygdala
   - Analgesia/pain perception—descending pain modulating systems, mid-brain periaqueductal gray matter, spinal cord dorsal horn gray matter (endorphin release after nitrous oxide, ethanol)

TABLE 11–2. Sites and Mechanisms of Action of General Anesthetics (A partial integration of actions across systems) *Continued*

IV. *Neuronal systems functionally impaired by higher concentrations of most general anesthetics:*

- Respiration—respiratory centers; carotid chemoreceptors by halothane, enflurane
- Blood pressure—hypothalamic center control of cardiovascular system via autonomic outflow
- Skeletal muscle movement and tone—cerebellum, mid-brain, basal ganglia, cerebral cortical systems involved in initiation of movement, spinal cord

V. *Outline of differential actions of various "general" anesthetics:*

- Markedly different chemical structures and physical properties; some actions appear to be "receptor mediated" whereas for others the "receptors" not readily identified
- Different electroencephalograms with different agents
- Different margins of safety and spectra of neural actions
- Differential sensitivities of various synaptic and neural systems to different agents
- Differential genetically determined sensitivities among agents
- Genetic influences occur as demonstrated in mice, Drosophila, and nematodes

GABA = gamma-aminobutyric acid.

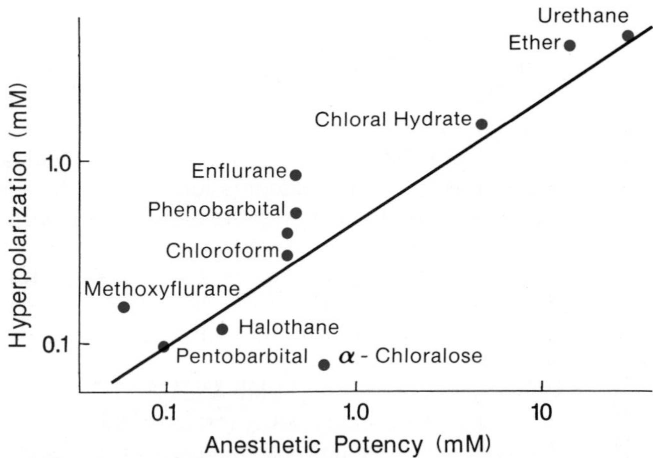

FIGURE 11–2. Hyperpolarization of spinal motor neurons by general anesthetics. Minimal effective hyperpolarizing concentration (mM) of the anesthetic (ordinate) plotted against the anesthetic potency of the agent (expressed as mM). (Redrawn from Nicoll RA, Madison DV: General anesthetics hyperpolarize neurons in the vertebrate central nervous system. Science 217:1055–1057, 1982. Copyright 1982 by the AAAS.)

trations of the anesthetics may be amplified in large networks of neurons.

NEURONAL MEMBRANE HYPERPOLARIZATION. An important effect of general anesthetics is increased membrane potential in some small fibers, *ie*, hyperpolarization (Fig. 11–2). Although cortical neuronal systems have received little research attention because of the technical difficulties of such experiments, such an increase in membrane potential would have profound effects if it occurred in the cells and neuropile of the cerebral cortex.

INTERFERENCE WITH SYNAPTIC TRANSMISSION. Anesthetic agents selectively disrupt synaptic transmission; both neuron cell bodies and axons tend to be less influenced by the anesthetics than are synapses. Moreover, as a general rule the more complex the synaptic and neuronal arrangement, the more susceptible the system is to disruption by anesthesics. For example, thought processes, muscular coordination, and alertness appear to be more sensitive to anesthetics than are simple reflexes or respiration.

Among the possible mechanisms of depression of synaptic transmission is the inhibition of the release of neurotransmitters from presynaptic terminals. Although it is feasible, the inhalation anesthetics have not been extensively investigated for their effects on neurotransmission in the central nervous system. It is probable that anesthetics do depress the neurotransmitter release that involves calcium signal transduction.

In high concentrations all anesthetics depress postsynaptic excitatory transmission and the binding of neurotransmitters to postsynaptic receptors. The postsynaptic binding of certain ligands, namely acetylcholine, to nicotinic receptors at clinical concentrations of the anesthetic agents, provides one of the most studied models for the synaptic effects of anesthetics. However, it cannot serve as a general model because anesthetics do not inhibit the binding of all neurotransmitters to postsynaptic receptors. Furthermore, although hyperbaric conditions can antagonize anesthetic-induced inhibition of some ligand-binding parameters, other parameters involved in anesthetic-induced inhibition of neurotransmitter binding are not affected.

STIMULATION OF INHIBITORY PATHWAYS. Anesthetics may also act by stimulating inhibitory pathways in the brain and spinal cord. Both benzodiazepines and barbiturates have binding sites on the chloride ion channel, which is modulated by gamma-aminobutyric acid (GABA). Although the GABA-mediated inhibitory pathway may represent one of many sites of action of the volatile anesthetics, this pathway is not antagonized by hyperbaric conditions. Stimulation of other inhibitory neuronal pathways, such as those activated by α_2 agonists, *eg*, clonidine, are also possibly involved in the anesthetic state.

Thus, the mechanisms of anesthesia may be a culmination of all these actions in specific neuronal circuits—neuronal circuits that are difficult to study and whose altered functions may not be readily apparent in isolated nerve cell preparations.

SYSTEMS AND NETWORKS OF NEURONS. A comprehensive account of anesthesia will be possible when the sensitivities of the various neuroreceptor and neuronal systems to anesthetics have been elucidated. Although the anesthetics have effects on synaptic systems in concentrations used clinically, it is not yet possible to correlate the effects of the anesthetics on these systems with the selective alterations of specific neurons.

A useful approach to examining the effects of the anesthetics is to ask, "What are the major effects observed and what are the neuronal sites and systems that are associated with the functional deficit or change in function induced by the anesthetic agent?" For example, with respect to **consciousness**, the loss of awareness is obviously an interference with a cerebral cortical function, functions that are under the influence of a variety of neuronal activating systems. Of these, the most extensively studied is the reticular activating system originating in the midbrain whose anterior elaboration innervates the entire cerebral cortex. Activation of this reticular system is associated with awakening and a shift toward low-voltage, high-frequency activity in the electroencephalogram (EEG). Anesthetic agents selectively depress the activation of the cerebral cortex induced by sensory stimulation or by stimulation of the reticular activating system. This anesthetic-induced depression of the recticular system is correlated temporally with the depression of consciousness and the induction of sleep.

The anesthetic-induced impairment of memory, **amnesia**, probably results from effects on the cerebral cortex, on the hippocampus, and on the amygdala—systems known to be involved in memory.

ANALGESIA PRODUCED BY SOME ANESTHETICS. Another cardinal sign of anesthesia is depression of the reflexes induced by otherwise nociceptive stimulation. Certain anesthetic agents, namely nitrous oxide, methoxyflurane, and diethyl ether, produce analgesia, that is, reduction of pain (in the absence of any loss of consciousness, inasmuch as one cannot talk of analgesia in the absence of conscious perception). The analgesia produced by these agents may result from the release of endorphins and enkephalins in the midbrain periaqueductal gray matter. The analgesia seen with these agents may also be the consequence of direct effects of the anesthetic on the midbrain and hypothalamus as well as the cerebral cortex.

Other anesthetics, such as halothane, do not produce analgesia, although in the unconscious, anesthetic state they do depress reflex responses to stimulation of nociceptive systems by virtue of their effects on neurons in the spinal cord and those involved in transmission to higher centers.

ANESTHETIC EFFECTS AND THE EEG. The electrical activity of the cerebral cortex, as recorded with an EEG, provides direct information about the effects of anesthetic agents. Not only does the qualitative and quantitative nature of the electrocortical effects reflect different levels of anesthesia, they vary with the anesthetic agent and with the individual's unique encephalographic pattern. The electroencephalographic changes during anesthesia allow the categorization of the anesthetics into two major classes. The group exemplified by halothane anesthesia is associated with a depressed EEG pattern with an absence of high-voltage fast activity, leaving only rather low voltage slow waves.

Early comparisons of diethyl ether, cyclopropane, and nitrous oxide revealed that during ether anesthesia the fast (higher frequency) EEG activity decreased and was replaced by relatively high-voltage slow waves. In contrast, other anesthetics produce a different EEG pattern. For example, enflurane, a halogenated methylethyl ether, produces "spike-dome" epileptic seizure activity in clinically used concentrations. Such differences in the EEG among anesthetic agents may not be clinically of much import, but the fact that they vary with level of anesthesia and are unique for different agents clearly demonstrates that different general anesthetics have distinguishing neuronal actions. The different EEGs reflect differential effects of the anesthetic on the electrical activity in the neurons in the cortex and in the neuronal input to the cortex.

Thus, general anesthetics may act at many sites and influence many functions within the central nervous system—from inhibiting excitatory pathways to exciting inhibitory pathways. Establishment of the specific mechanisms listed in Table 11-2 or a combination thereof may ultimately provide the explanation of anesthesia. Already it is evident that the mechanism of the effects of low concentrations of barbiturates—that is, to augment GABA-induced inhibition—is distinctly different from the generalized depression of the neuronal excitability observed with lethal levels.

MULTIPLE MECHANISMS AND OVERLAPPING IN THE DESCRIPTIONS OF THE ACTIONS OF ANESTHETICS. Note that many of different categories of action listed in Table 11-2 are not necessarily mutually exclusive; for example, an anesthetic could both produce changes on nerve membranes and have selective effects on the cerebral cortex. Although the table is extensive, it is not exhaustive; many of the potential sites for anesthesia have yet to be examined experimentally, and even for those potential mechanisms listed, many have yet to be investigated for each of the various neuronal sites.

ORGAN SYSTEM EFFECTS OF ANESTHETICS

Action of Anesthetics on the Cardiovascular and Skeletal Muscle Systems

The side effects of anesthetics on the function of the heart and the peripheral circulatory system as well as the skeletal muscle system must also be taken into account when describing the condition of general anesthesia. The depth of anesthesia is monitored primarily on the basis of:

- Responses to the stimuli of surgery
- Skeletal muscle relaxation
- Control of blood pressure and heart rate
- Autonomic activation of the cardiovascular system

Volatile anesthetics are potent direct myocardial depressants and produce variable degrees of vascular vasodilation and skeletal muscular relaxation. Anesthetics directly interfere with the cardiac calcium-activated excitation-contraction cycle, and the extent to which they do interfere correlates with the amount of myocardial depression or skeletal muscle relaxation seen with each agent. The regulation of the intracellular pool of calcium, which is necessary for the correct functioning of muscle tissue, is also important in the release of neurotransmitters from presynaptic nerve terminals. Anesthetic-induced perturbations of these calcium-regulating mechanisms may reflect common sites of action in all the tissues affected by inhalational anesthetics, an idea consistent with a unitary hypothesis of anesthetic action.

Recent studies have established that the risk of adverse cardiovascular events during and following anesthesia can be ". . . reasonably predicted from preoperative findings that include general physical state and cardiovascular status, including evidence or suspicion of coronary artery disease, hypertension and left ventricular hypertrophy" (Killip, 1993).

Depression by anesthetics of voluntary muscle control, spinal reflexes, and baroreceptor responses would be expected to be additive with the direct depression of muscle contraction produced by the anesthetic.

Skeletal muscle movement and tone are decreased during anesthesia. Movement is limited generally to small movements or none at all, although reflex muscle contractions can occur, for example, to sudden noxious stimuli. Thus, the initiation of muscle movement is depressed, although not necessarily completely abolished. The control of muscle movement is more markedly depressed than is movement itself, and the cerebellar and spinal cord regulation is reduced significantly. Of particular interest in anesthesia is the degree to which the responses to muscle stretch and the sustained muscle tone are retained. The various anesthetic agents differ in the degree to which they produce muscle relaxation relative to depression of the central nervous system.

Muscle relaxation is essential for certain surgical procedures, such as an exploratory laparotomy. In such patients, further supplementation of anesthesia with neuromuscular blocking agents is necessary because relaxation of skeletal muscles is usually incomplete except at high concentrations with certain agents (for example, enflurane or diethyl ether).

Action of Anesthetics on the Respiratory System

A number of neuronal systems including the respiratory system are impaired functionally by higher concentrations of most of the general anesthetics. Depth of respiration is depressed whereas rate tends to be increased with most agents, although overall minute ventilation is decreased. A reduction in the reflex responsiveness of the respiratory center to increases in carbon dioxide level and decreases in oxygen tension also occurs. Halothane is unique among the anesthetics in that its respiratory depressant effects are due not only to depression of central respiratory centers but also to its effects on the carotid body chemoreceptors. (It and other drugs with effects on sensory receptor systems are discussed in Chapter 13.)

All inhalation anesthetics have a small safety margin. A major hazard in any anesthesia (with the possible exception of nitrous oxide given alone with ample oxygen) is respiratory and cardiovascular depression that, if not alleviated and reversed quickly, can be fatal. Such ultimately fatal effects may well be due in the end to a generalized effect on many different neuronal elements and many different tissue elements that have in common excitable membranes or involve calcium translocation (*eg*, the depression of the rhythmic neuronal activity associated with respiration or depression of the responses of skeletal muscle and autonomic nerves as well as depression of cardiac function). Widespread central nervous system (CNS) depression by general anesthetics of any one of the systems just mentioned is life-threatening.

FACTORS THAT INFLUENCE DEPTH OF ANESTHESIA

Genetic

The susceptibility to, and character of, anesthesia are under a variety of genetic influences. These influences are currently being explored in various model systems; *Drosophila* mutants and mutants of a species of *Nematoda* exhibit differential sensitivities to anesthetics. Such observations clearly conflict with the concept of a singular uniform molecular mechanism responsible for anesthesia. Rather, **it suggests that more than one molecular mechanism or site of action underlies anesthesia, which is consistent with the striking differences of the spectrum of the actions of inhalational anesthetics. More than one mechanism is also consistent with the fact that an anesthetic state can be produced by a variety of diverse molecules ranging from nitrogen under pressure to nitrous oxide, diethyl ether, carbon dioxide, and the inert gas Xenon, as well as a variety of halogenated hydrocarbons.**

Pregnancy

Anesthetic actions are also under a wide variety of other influences, among these is pregnancy. Pregnant women are more susceptible not only to general anesthetics but to local anesthetics than are nonpregnant individuals.

Stress and Anxiety

Conditions of stress and anxiety have complex interactions with anesthesia. Undoubtedly, anxiety not only alters the susceptibility to agents that produce unconsciousness but clearly modifies pain reflexes and the responses of pain systems. Certain kinds of stress can decrease the perception of pain. On the other hand, anxiety by itself tends to decrease the pain threshold and thus increase the amount of an analgesic drug required to alleviate a given level of pain. Usually, anxious patients have higher anesthetic requirements than relaxed patients. This is an important reason for an effective preoperative visit by the anesthesiologist and the judicious use of anxiolytic agents preoperatively.

Metabolic Rate and Age

Other influences on anesthetic needs include increased requirements in the presence of elevated body temperature or a high basal metabolic rate. On the other hand, patients at the extremes of age usually require less anesthetic for a given operative procedure.

Drug Interactions

Essentially all of the drugs that produce CNS depression, including anesthetics, are at least additive in their effects with other CNS depressants such as opioids, barbiturates, and benzodiazepines. Amphetamines and related compounds, conversely, tend to increase the anesthetic requirements. When certain substances are taken chronically, such as alcohol, the anesthetic requirements depend on the level of tolerance and on the time and amount of the last "dose." If the last dose was relatively recent there will be an additive effect with the anesthetic; if a somewhat longer time has elapsed there may be either tolerance to the anesthetic or even antagonism due to increased neuronal excitability resulting from a withdrawal syndrome.

Analogous, but of opposite sign, changes appear with chronic administration of amphetamines or cocaine. Administered together with an anesthetic, amphetamines increase the anesthetic requirement, whereas during withdrawal from chronic amphetamine use the individual may be more sensitive to anesthetics. More importantly, the interaction of the potent inhalational anesthetics, especially halothane, with these sympathomimetic agents may increase the risk of cardiac arrhythmias during surgical procedures.

UPTAKE AND DISTRIBUTION OF INHALATIONAL ANESTHETICS

A diagram of a closed system for administration of inhalational anesthetics is presented in Figure 11-3. Components include a source of the gas and a method of vaporization. The agents are inhaled in the form of gases, not aerosols. Accurate and reliable flow meters for control of inhaled gases are important to ensure adequate oxygen concentrations in the inspired mixture. Upon initiation of the flow of gases, oxygen and the anesthetic(s) fill the bag; one-way valves and electrically conductive rubber tubing and noncorrosive connectors complete the system. In the closed system shown in Figure 11-3, the patient inhales from the bag and exhales through a carbon dioxide absorber back into the bag. Due to changes in gas exchange that occur as a result of the anesthetic state, the inhaled mixture has to include at least 30% oxygen. Therefore, the maximal anesthetic gas concentration, such as nitrous oxide plus possibly a more potent agent, can constitute no more than 70% of the total mixture.

Upon inhalation by the patient the gas mixture fills the lungs; the gases—anesthetic and oxygen—diffuse into blood across the alveolar-capillary boundary. Because only a finite amount can be taken up by blood within a given respiratory cycle, each breath results in the incorporation of a certain limited amount of anesthetic into the blood stream. This blood is then distributed to the various tissues via the circulation, and gases diffuse into tissues across the capillary membranes. In each respiratory cycle, the gas that diffuses into the blood stream is constantly restored with each breath so that the alveolar concentration to which the blood is exposed remains relatively constant. Therefore, there is net movement of anesthetic molecules from the respiratory tract to the tissues until such time as the partial pressure of the agent in the tissues approaches that in blood, and that, in turn, approaches that in the alveoli.

Kinetics of Anesthetics

The rates at which the concentration of anesthetic in the organs and tissues increases vary directly with the concentration in the blood, which in turn is directly correlated with the concentration in the inhaled mixture, the physical properties of the agent, and the blood flow through the lungs and other organs. Because the brain is among the organs that have relatively high blood flows, equilibrium occurs between this organ and the blood and the alveoli more rapidly than those other tissues that are more poorly perfused.

Eventually, all the high and moderately perfused tissues of the body reach a relatively steady state and only the vascular-poor tissues continue to slowly draw off anesthetic from the vascular and alveolar pools. This relatively steady state is characterized by near equal partial pressures in the majority of tissue compartments of the body with that in the alveolar gas. Therefore, knowing the **end-expired anesthetic concentration** at a relatively steady state gives the anesthesiologist a direct guide as to the amount of anesthetic in the brain and other blood rich organs. (Such an indirect determination of the anesthetic concentration in the brain is analogous to the concentration at the target tissue of a parenterally administered drug that is constantly being infused to replace any drug that is lost through metabolism or redistribution.)

In studies of the time course, that is, the kinetics, of anesthesia, the concept of equilibrium is important (see Figs. 11-4 and 11-5). Equilibrium is the condition in which there is no net movement of a gas such as an anesthetic in or out of tissues, blood, or the inhaled mixture in the alveoli. The kinetics of onset and recovery from anesthetics have been studied extensively and mathematically modeled usually using artificially fixed conditions. The anesthetic concentration in the inhaled gases is kept constant and the anesthetic concentrations in the alveoli estimated; the anesthetic con-

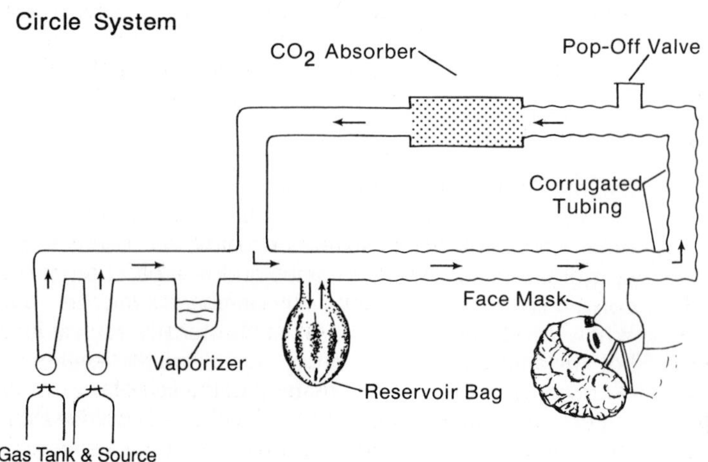

FIGURE 11-3. A simplified sketch of a closed "circle" anesthetic system showing the essential components and direction of flow of gases: source, vaporizer for volatile agents, reservoir or rebreathing bag, face mask (or endotracheal tube), and carbon dioxide (CO_2) absorber. Anesthetics and other agents are supplied as gases, and the flow rate of supply equals that stored or metabolized in the body plus that exhaled. The excess, if any, escapes from the pop-off valve or from any loose hosing connections. As the anesthetic and oxygen are administered, they displace the gases present in the body and nitrogen accumulates in the reservoir bag.

TABLE 11 – 3. Factors Regulating Rates of Onset on Anesthesia and Differences Among Agents

I. *Respiration* rate, depth, respiratory minute volume probably most important quantitatively
II. *Concentration (ie, partial pressure) of anesthetic* in the inspired mixture
III. *Cardiac output*—and functional perfusion of brain and tissue
IV *Alveolar membrane—blood translocation*—very rapid relative to other processes, in absence of lung pathology
V. *Solubility in blood and tissues*—(*ie*, solubility in water as measured as blood : gas partition coefficient) the more soluble in tissues, the slower the rate of rise of alveolar blood concentration at a given inhaled concentration (Fig. 11 – 5)

centration at the time of maximal exhalation (end tidal) is used for these determinations because it directly approximates the anesthetic concentration in the alveoli. The gas concentrations in the capillary blood come into temporary equilibrium with the alveolar gas concentrations, that is, the partial pressures of the gases in the pulmonary capillaries and within the alveoli are approximately equal. These end-tidal concentrations are analyzed relative to time after the introduction of the specific inhaled mixture.

Thus, at any given time following the beginning of such inhalation, the condition of the individual can be assessed and correlated with the level of the anesthetic in the blood and, more importantly, correlated with the concentration of the anesthetic in the different organs. For many of the general anesthetics this is a relatively simple relationship, because the anesthetic agent does not bind strongly to any of the tissues and is distributed predictably according to the physical properties of the agent (largely its solubilities in various tissues) and the biological systems with which it interacts. Thus, the anesthetic effects can be described in relation to the concentration of the anesthetic in a tissue, that is, a dose or concentration-response relationship.

The factors that regulate the rates of onset and recovery of anesthesia are presented in Table 11 – 3. Note that only two of these important factors are under the direct control of the anesthetist:

- The composition of the inhaled gas mixture, especially the concentration of the anesthetic
- The respiration rate and depth

Practical matters include ensuring that the anesthetic mixture does not interact with the soda lime in the carbon dioxide absorber or with the material in the hoses and mask. For example, some anesthetics such as halothane are absorbed extensively by rubber tubing.

Solubility of the Anesthetic Gas in Tissues

After the introduction of an inhalational anesthetic agent, the alveolar capillary concentration rises rapidly as the individual inspires the gas mixture containing the anesthetic (Fig. 11 – 4). After a few minutes of active respiration and normal cardiovascular function, significant differences among various agents appear with respect to the rate at which the alveolar capillary concentration approaches the concentration that it will reach at equilibrium. This final rate at which the alveolar air, in equilibrium with pulmonary capillary blood, reaches equilibrium with the inspired mixture is correlated inversely with the solubility of the gas in tissues. For example, equilibrium with nitrous oxide with a low solubility in blood and tissues (Table 11 – 1) is approached quite rapidly, whereas with the more soluble agents the rate at which equilibrium is established is slower.

The differences in the times required to establish equilibrium of tissue and blood levels with the inspired concentration are primarily due to the tremendous tissue reservoir for soluble agents; a high solubility in tissues in effect results in a large volume of distribution. In this situation the capacity of the respiratory and cardiovascular systems to fill this large volume with anesthetic molecules constitutes the major rate-limiting step. Fortunately, the brain and selected other organs (*ie*, the heart, liver, and kidney) are well perfused by arterial blood and the anesthetics readily diffuse into brain tissue and rapidly approximate the arterial concentration.

Clinically, knowledge of the speed of anesthetic uptake is useful in performing closed-circuit anesthesia. Because the concentration of an anesthetic agent at its neural sites of action is the critical factor in establishing the state of anesthesia, the administration initially of anesthetic concentrations higher than those required for maintenance can accelerate the induction of anesthesia. This technique is especially useful with agents with high solubility in tissues that have a slow rate of establishment of equilibrium between inhaled gas and tissues if given as a fixed concentration. Unfortunately, other factors, such as diffusion across the alveolar-capillary border and pulmonary blood flow, do not permit overcoming completely the slowness of induction with soluble agents. The newer potent inhalational agents, sevoflurane and desflurane, have low blood and tissue solubilities and a very fast onset and recovery. The cost of the use of these two new, expensive agents may well be compensated for by a decrease in the time spent in the recovery room.

ROLE OF NITROGEN

Note that the anesthetic mixture (oxygen and anesthetic) displaces the gases, primarily nitrogen, normally present in air and dissolved in body tissues. With continued respiration of the anesthetic mixture, the nitrogen concentration in the rebreathing bag rises, diluting the anesthetic mixture. Thus, the anesthetic mixture must be replaced and refreshed periodically, especially during the first few minutes after the initiation of the anesthetic gas mixture.

Second Gas Effect

The uptake of anesthetics and other gases is influenced not only by respiratory exchange, relative solubilities, and related partial pressures but by other factors such as differences in diffusibility between nitrogen and nitrous oxide. Because nitrous oxide diffuses into the blood stream faster than nitrogen diffuses out, the remaining alveolar gases and vapors are concentrated in the alveoli. This concentrating effect increases the concentration of second anesthetic that

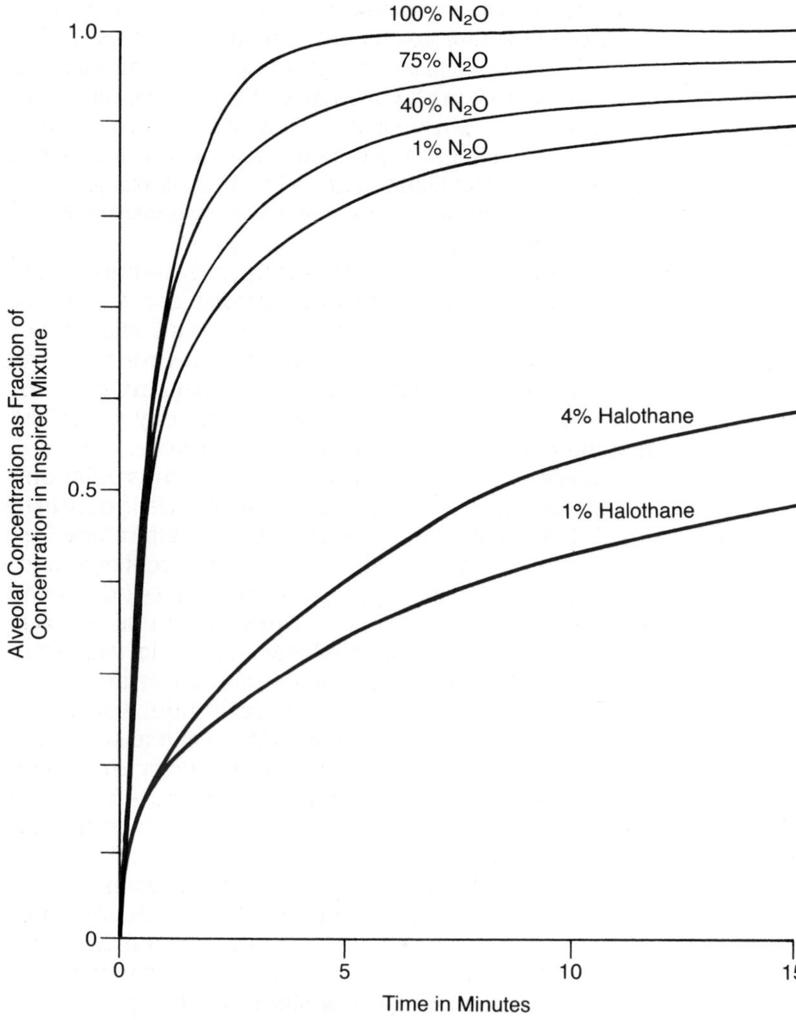

FIGURE 11–4. The effect of increasing the concentration of an anesthetic in the inspired mixtures (theoretical simulation). Y axis: Alveolar concentration as a *fraction of the concentration in the inspired mixture*. For example, a value of 1.0 is obtained when the partial pressure of anesthetic in blood returning to the alveolus is equal to that in the anesthetic being inspired. For the initial few minutes, the *rate* of rise of anesthetic concentration in the alveolus is similar for both agents and for different concentrations; this fast increase in concentration reflects primarily the rate at which the anesthetic reaches all the alveolar space. Over time, the differences relating to absolute concentration become apparent.

After 15 minutes of inhalation, the alveolar concentration of halothane, as a correlate of its great solubility in tissues, reaches a level less than half its concentration in the inspired mixture; so long as anesthetic is supplied and adequate respiratory and cardiac functions are maintained, its alveolar concentration continues to increase gradually over hours until if finally reaches equilibrium with the inspired mixture. (Data from Eger EI: Anesthetic Uptake and Action. Baltimore: Williams & Wilkins, 1974.)

the pulmonary blood is exposed to and increases the uptake of the anesthetic into the circulatory system, thereby increasing the speed of induction. This phenomenon is termed the "second gas effect" of nitrous oxide. This effect is important during the first couple minutes of induction. The reverse of this phenomenon occurs when the nitrous oxide is discontinued at the end of the case. Nitrous oxide rushes out of the blood into the alveoli much faster than nitrogen diffuses from the alveoli into the blood, resulting in a decrease in the concentrations of gases in the alveoli. If supplemental oxygen is not given during this period of time, which lasts for some 5 to 10 minutes after stopping nitrous oxide, diffusion hypoxia may result.

During Maintenance Anesthesia

As anesthesia proceeds, the concentrations of anesthetics in tissues with lower blood flow tend to rise slowly. Hydrophobic tissues, which can constitute up to 20–60% of body weight, generally have less blood flow per gram of tissue, and equilibrium between the concentrations in these tissues with those in the inspired gas mixture occurs only after many hours of anesthesia. The longer the anesthetic is administered, the greater is the concentration in the poorly perfused organs and body lipids. Moreover, the more that is dissolved

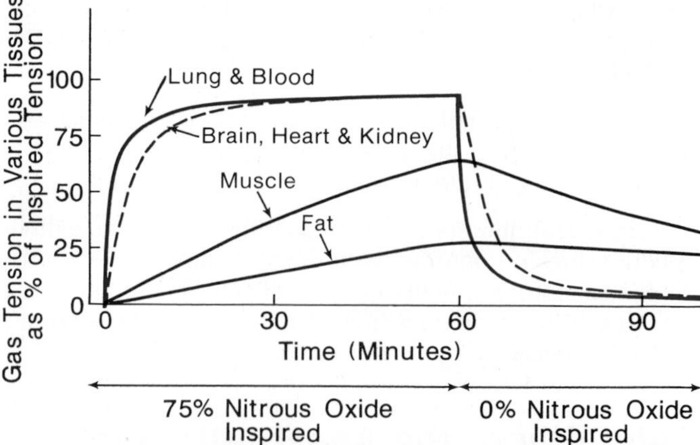

FIGURE 11–5. Time course of changes in gas tension in various tissues with the inspiration of nitrous oxide. The gas tension is expressed as a percentage of that in the inspired mixture; 100% would signify equal gas tensions in the tissues and in the inspired mixture, *ie*, equilibrium. Note that the concentrations in tissues that have ample blood supply (exemplified by brain, heart, and kidney) are almost the same as those in the lung and blood. On the other hand, the tensions in muscle and fat, tissues with much more limited blood flow, lag behind the changes in tensions in blood by minutes to hours. (Modified from Cowles AL, Borgstedt HH, Gillies AJ: Uptake and distribution of inhalation anesthetic agents in clinical practice. Anesth Analg 47:404–414, 1968.)

TABLE 11-4. Factors Regulating Rate of Recovery from Anesthesia

I. All of factors involved in *rate of onset* (Table 11-3) plus the following:
II. Solubility in adipose tissues
III. Circulatory perfusion of tissues, especially adipose, for potent, highly lipid soluble agents

in lipids and poorly perfused tissues, the slower is the overall recovery from the anesthetic (Fig. 11-5). **Thus, the more lipophilic the anesthetic, the fatter the patient, and the longer the anesthesia, the more prolonged is the elimination of the anesthetic and subsequent recovery** (Table 11-4). For example, halothane's solubility in oil is 200 times greater than its solubility in water, and the proportion present in the lipid compartment (at equilibrium) would be more than 95% of the total anesthetic present in the entire body.

PRESENT AND FUTURE PRACTICE OF ANESTHESIA AND SURGERY

Because of the significant risk, historically, of general anesthesia, it was primarily given in the hospital setting, where the individual was interned for one or more days prior to and for many days following surgery. Anesthesiology has made great strides in the area of patient safety. Indeed, the virtual explosion of surgical intervention that has occurred over the last 50 years is a direct result of improved care of the patient in the perioperative period, of which anesthesiology is the major component. Now patients can enjoy the benefits of receiving anesthesia and surgery as outpatients—procedures that in the past would have required 2 or more weeks of hospitalization. Not only has this approach decreased the cost of medical care, many minor types of invasive procedures, which formerly required general anesthesia, are now performed using local or regional anesthesia and conscious sedation; usually there is added benefit of receiving lower doses of the anesthetics. Thus, drug-induced facilitation of surgical procedures now ranges from no anesthesia to mild analgesia, antianxiety medication, opioid analgesia, opioid/local anesthesia, amnestic/sedation medication, to small or large amounts of a general anesthetic.

The agents currently in use that are discussed in this section start with those that are gases at standard temperature and atmospheric pressure, followed by the volatile liquids.

Gas Inhalational Anesthetics

Nitrous Oxide

ACTIONS. Nitrous oxide is available as a medical gas in blue tanks under pressure. It is nonflammable (but supports combustion in the same way as oxygen) and odorless; it lacks any irritating qualities. This agent is administered using a gas machine with the concentration monitored by the use of accurately calibrated flow meters. The major drawback of nitrous oxide is its lack of potency. Maximal safe concentrations of nitrous oxide (70% in 30% oxygen) produce intoxication, analgesia, amnesia, and stage II anesthesia in some patients, but by itself nitrous oxide lacks sufficient potency to produce surgical anesthesia (Table 11-1).

The subjective effects of nitrous oxide alone are usually reported as pleasant, with euphoria and a sense of well-being frequently accompanied by fantasies. Emotional lability is present and may be manifested, for example, by uncontrollable laughing ("laughing gas") or crying. The subjective effects are commonly described as similar to intoxication with ethyl alcohol

Analgesia is a useful side effect of nitrous oxide. Inhaled concentrations of 25% are equivalent in intensity to that obtainable with therapeutic doses of morphine (*eg*, 10 mg in a 70-kg adult) and may be due to endorphin release. This analgesic property has been exploited outside the operating room setting, and special containers that deliver nitrous oxide in fixed nonanesthetic, analgesic concentrations have been marketed.

In addition to analgesia, nitrous oxide produces a marked amnesia for the events taking place while exposed to the agent. This amnesia is frequently not explicitly recognized by the patient, but may be a desirable aspect of nitrous oxide when it is used for either its analgesic or anesthetic effects.

Because of the limited potency of nitrous oxide, it is usually combined with other CNS depressants: other potent inhalational anesthetics, sedatives, opioids, or antianxiety agents such as thiopental, morphine, or a benzodiazepine. Nitrous oxide is still in wide use due to its low cost, long record of safety, and the ability of the anesthetist to decrease the oxygen concentration of the inspired mixture to prevent untoward sequelae of oxygen toxicity.

KINETICS AND TIME COURSE OF ACTION. The effects of nitrous oxide are extremely rapid in onset, within a few circulation times, and there is an equally rapid rate of recovery. In correlation with its low solubility in blood and tissues, equilibrium between the concentration in the inhaled mixture and the concentration in body tissue can be established within a few minutes (Fig. 11-4).

ORGAN SYSTEM EFFECTS. By itself in concentrations up to 70% in the inhaled mixture, nitrous oxide has only negligible effects on the cardiovascular system, respiration, or skeletal muscle tone. Mild activation of the sympathetic system has been reported. When combined with other potent inhalational or intravenous agents, nitrous oxide can contribute significantly to cardiovascular and respiratory depression.

TOXICITIES AND SIDE EFFECTS OF NITROUS OXIDE. Acute toxicity of nitrous oxide is of relevance almost exclusively as a hazard of inadvertent exposure or of nonmedical self-administration. The subjective effects, as noted earlier, may be quite enjoyable or reinforcing to repeated use. The major *acute* hazards of such exposure as an anesthetic or in its nonmedical use consist of altered judgment, confusion or loss of consciousness, decrease of pain perception, and minor to profound amnesia. When self-administered, the confusion, impaired judgment, plus possible concomitant hypoxia, have resulted in tragic accidental deaths; such deaths are frequently the result of suffocation associated with rebreathing from a plastic or paper bag to the point of unconsciousness (see Chapter 49). Homemade nitrous oxide presents the additional hazard owing to the probable presence of the highly toxic contaminants nitrogen dioxide and nitrogen oxide.

CHRONIC TOXICITY. Scavenging any nitrous oxide released into the operating room atmosphere is critical because of toxic effects to operating room personnel exposed chronically to low levels of the agent. Chronic toxicity associated with repeated exposure in the operating room setting or repeated nonmedical use consists of bone marrow suppression, blood dyscrasias, peripheral neuropathy, increased rate of spontaneous abortion, and deficits in cell-mediated immunity. Chronic exposure to nitrous oxide results in inactivation of vitamin B_{12} and clinical signs of cobalamin deficiency. Inactivation of methionine synthetase by this mechanism mimics folate deficiency, with secondary depression of the hemopoietic system. These hemopoetic sequelae of nitrous oxide exposure can be reversed by folinic acid (leucovorin).

Volatile Inhalational Anesthetics

Halothane

ACTIONS. In the 1960s and 1970s halothane (FLUOTHANE) was the most widely used general inhalation anesthetic and it still enjoys some advantages over the newer agents. Halothane is considered in detail because our extensive knowledge about its effects allows it to serve as the prototype. The other halogenated inhalational agents will be compared with halothane.

Halothane is liquid, nonflammable, nonirritating, with a distinct odor usually described as pleasant. It is a potent anesthetic agent with an MAC of less than 1% (0.77%). In contrast to diethyl ether and cyclopropane, the signs of the depth of halothane anesthesia are different. There is a time- and concentration-dependent depression of reflex responses, depression of respiration, and depression of blood pressure and heart rate. In distinction to nitrous oxide and diethyl ether, it produces no analgesia.

KINETICS. As with all potent anesthetics, halothane can be administered initially in relatively high concentrations in order to decrease the time taken to induce surgical anesthesia. (After induction the concentration is decreased to that desired for the maintenance period of anesthesia.) Inhalational induction of anesthesia with halothane is usually smooth and uneventful, although stage II delirium occurs in some patients. Induction is faster than possible with diethyl ether, but slower than with the newer halogenated agents.

Recovery is the result largely of exhalation of the anesthetic gas; 80% or more is excreted through the lungs. The remainder, some 15% or more, is destroyed by metabolism by the liver microsomal mixed-function oxidase system. Chloride and bromide ions are removed from the halothane molecule, with the ultimate excretion by way of the urine of fluorine-containing compounds, mostly trifluoroacetic acid and trifluoroethanol.

ORGAN SYSTEM EFFECTS

Respiration. Because halothane has a pleasant odor, it is particularly well suited for an inhalational induction. As the depth of anesthesia increases, respiration with halothane becomes more shallow and rapid. The degree of respiratory depression is concentration-related; however, the stimulation from the surgery tends to oppose this respiratory depression with the result that the patient tends to take deeper, slower breaths. As with diethyl ether, the respiratory pattern may be used as a guide to titrate the depth of anesthesia; however, halothane-induced decreases in blood pressure may limit the use of this parameter in many patients. The respiratory and chemoreceptor reflexes are also markedly obtunded by halothane due to both the peripheral and central actions of the agent.

Circulation. With halothane anesthesia there is a progressive, dose-related, decrease in blood pressure due primarily to a depression of cardiac contractility. The faster the induction, the more profound and the more rapid is the drop in blood pressure. In addition to the direct effects on cardiac output, halothane also alters the cardiac rhythm. Halothane directly slows heart rate due to both its actions on autonomic function and directly on the heart. This may be an advantage in the care of certain surgical patients. The appearance of nodal rhythm is common and usually of no clinical consequence except in patients who are dependent on atrial contraction to support cardiac output. Of some concern is the sensitization of the myocardium to the arrhythmic effects of catecholamines, and care must be taken when the use of epinephrine is required. In addition, excessive autonomic stimulation such as that associated with the lighter planes of anesthesia or hypercarbia should be avoided.

Muscular System. Halothane depresses uterine tone. Although this property can be viewed as a disadvantage because uterine contraction is necessary to control bleeding immediately after delivery, it may be useful in facilitating certain obstetrical manipulations.

Skeletal muscle relaxation is minimal and insufficient for major abdominal surgery and requires supplementation with skeletal muscle relaxants. The small amount of muscle relaxation produced by halothane is, however, additive with nondepolarizing neuromuscular blocking agents.

A rare but serious abnormality of skeletal muscle function, *malignant hyperpyrexia* has been associated with exposure to halogenated anesthetics, as well as other drugs, especially succinylcholine. This syndrome is characterized by a rapid rise in body temperature, muscle rigidity, and an increase in oxygen consumption and carbon dioxide production. However, not all of these symptoms become manifest in a given occurrence. Malignant hyperpyrexia appears to be due to abnormalities in the calcium homeostasis of skeletal muscle, particularly sarcoplasmic reticular release and re-uptake in genetically susceptible individuals (also see Chapter 22).

Liver. There is little evidence that halothane directly produces liver damage. However, *hepatitis* has been reported in approximately 1 in 3000 to 7000 halothane anesthesias. The liver damage is not explainable on the basis of viral infections or known hepatotoxic drugs. In certain cases, repeated exposures to halothane are associated with an increased likelihood of the occurrence of hepatitis, and it is generally concluded that it is either a hypersensitivity reaction or toxic metabolic product injury. (Nevertheless, the most common causes of hepatitis in the postoperative period are viral infections and exposure to known hepatotoxic agents.) Furthermore, careful selection of patients who are at risk for this problem can all but eliminate this possible cause of serious intraoperative liver injury.

Enflurane

ACTIONS. Enflurane (ETHRANE) is 2-chloro-1,1,2-trifluoroethyl difluoromethyl ether, a colorless, nonflammable liquid with a sweet, pungent odor. The anesthesia produced by enflurane is similar to that of halothane; however, at higher concentrations (>2.5%), seizure activity can occur, especially in patients who are hyperventilated (low CO_2). The seizure activity is usually only seen on the EEG and consists of a "spike and dome" (petit mal) pattern. Actual muscle clonus occurs only rarely and is usually without any long-term consequences; however, because of this property, patients with epileptic foci or history should probably not receive this anesthetic agent.

Enflurane is relatively potent, with an MAC of 1.68%, and modest increases above this amount permit a fairly smooth and rapid induction of anesthesia. However, because of its pungent odor, inhaled induction is difficult due to breath holding. It is therefore recommended that a barbiturate be used to produce unconsciousness, after which the anesthetic gas mixture can be slowly introduced.

ORGAN SYSTEM EFFECTS. As with halothane, enflurane anesthesia is accompanied by a gradual decrease in both respiratory minute ventilation and blood pressure. The depression of blood pressure is due primarily to a decrease of myocardial contractility and vascular smooth muscle relaxation. Some tachycardia may occur although not to the same extent as with isoflurane. Clinically, enflurane produces the greatest amount of myocardial depression, and patients on calcium channel antagonists may be the most affected.

Overall, there is a smaller likelihood of arrhythmias with enflurane than with halothane. As with halothane, the respiratory depth decreases and the rate increases as the concentration of enflurane is increased. The depression in reflex respiratory responses to both hypoxia and hypercarbia is approximately equal to halothane.

The skeletal muscle relaxation seen with enflurane is greater than with either halothane or isoflurane and may be sufficient to permit abdominal surgery without the use of additional agents in selected patients. As with isoflurane and halothane, the muscle relaxation secondary to enflurane is additive to that produced by nondepolarizing muscle relaxants. Relaxation of uterine muscle is also apparent with use of this agent.

Liver damage has occurred during and after anesthesia with enflurane, but its mechanism remains obscure. Obviously, it should be avoided if the individual patient had exhibited liver damage following a previous exposure.

• KINETICS AND TIME COURSE. The onset and recovery from enflurane is satisfactorily rapid. The bulk of the anesthetic is excreted unchanged in the expired gas. Only some 2–5% is metabolized by the liver. Fluoride ions are produced as metabolites of this agent and represent a theoretical concern for nephrotoxicity. However, blood levels of fluoride ion do not usually reach toxic (>50 μM) levels even with prolonged use at high concentrations. Therefore, the presence of renal disease in the surgical patient represents only a relative contraindication to the use of this agent.

Isoflurane

ACTIONS. Isoflurane (FORANE), 1-chloro-2,2,2-trifluoroethyl difluoromethyl ether, is an isomer of enflurane and clinically the most commonly used inhalation anesthetic in clinical practice. Isoflurane is a potent agent with a pungent smell. This pungent quality may result in breath-holding, retching, and bucking when attempting an inhalational induction; therefore, as with enflurane, an intravenous barbiturate is usually used to facilitate induction of anesthesia. The optically active isomers of isoflurane differ in anesthetic potency (see page 96), an observation supporting a protein site of action.

This agent is very inert, with less than 2% of the inspired amount undergoing metabolism.

ORGAN SYSTEM EFFECTS. Isoflurane depresses respiration progressively as the concentration in the inhaled mixture is increased. The effects of this agent on the respiratory pattern are similar those of halothane and enflurane.

The myocardial depression produced by isoflurane is similar qualitatively to halothane and enflurane; however, at higher anesthetic concentrations (above 1 MAC) the depression does not appear to be as great. Isoflurane also produces a dose-related vasodilation with a reflex tachycardia at higher anesthetic concentrations. As a consequence of these properties, isoflurane must be used with caution in cardiac patients with ischemic heart disease. Furthermore, with prolonged use at higher concentrations, vascular volume is expanded, which can result in a relative intravascular volume overload when the anesthetic is terminated. Patients with impaired ventricular function may demonstrate signs and symptoms of myocardial failure as a result. Finally, because of significant tachycardia and the secondary activation of the autonomic system that accompanies the use of this agent, healthy patients may be difficult to maintain on just isoflurane. For all these reasons isoflurane is usually used in concentrations of 1.5% or less and is supplemented with an intravenous agent or is used to "top off," an anesthetic technique that utilizes primarily an intravenous agent.

Isoflurane can provide greater skeletal muscle relaxation than halothane; however, it is not as effective in this regard as enflurane. The muscle relaxant activities are the result of central actions as well as effects on the neuromuscular junction. Like enflurane and halothane, isoflurane potentiates the neuromuscular blocking effects of nondepolarizing muscle relaxants. Uterine muscle is also relaxed by isoflurane.

Sevoflurane and Desflurane

(The desflurane molecule is a methyl ethyl ether identical to isoflurane except for the substitution of a fluorine for a chlorine. Sevoflurane (SEVOFRANE) is a fluorinated methyl isopropyl ether.) Desflurane (SUPRANE) is a new agent just released for clinical use and sevoflurane is in the last stages of clinical trials prior to its release for clinical usage. Sevoflurane has had extensive clinical use in Japan. Both agents have very rapid induction and recovery times, consistent with their low blood/gas partition coefficients, making them ideal for outpatient anesthesia.

Both of these agents affect the respiratory and cardiovascular systems similarly to isoflurane, although sevoflurane slows the heart rate. Desflurane and sevoflurane relax the skeletal musculature similarly to isoflurane and enflurane, and potentiate the neuromuscular blocking effects of nondepolarizing muscle relaxants like the other halogenated inhalational agents.

In comparing these two agents, onset of anesthesia and recovery is faster with desflurane, whereas sevoflurane has a less irritating odor, making it better suited for an inhalational induction. The major disadvantage to the use of desflurane is that this anesthetic must be given in a special vaporizer.

Sevoflurane is metabolized similarly to enflurane, resulting in free fluoride ions in the blood; nevertheless, there have been over 350,000 anesthetic inductions with this agent without renal or hepatic toxicity. Sevoflurane interacts with soda lime and therefore theoretically should not be used with "low-flow" anesthesia. Because both agents are patented and expensive, cost-benefit analyses need to be carried out in order to establish the appropriate justifications for their selection.

Volatile Anesthetics of Historical Interest

Diethyl Ether

Diethyl ether, the first and arguably the safest anesthetic, has a pungent odor that is irritating to the respiratory tract. It is flammable and explosive. The induction is slow owing to the combination of its relatively high lipid solubility and marked irritation of the respiratory tract; this irritation may lead to voluntary and involuntary breath-holding, retching, vomiting, and copious production of mucous secretions.

A variety of other anesthetic agents have been introduced and used for a while, only to be replaced by newer and better ones, *eg*, cyclopropane, ethylene, chloroform, vinyl ether, and methoxyflurane.

Intravenous Anesthesia

Thiobarbiturates (Thiopental, Thiamylal, Methohexital)

A few barbiturates that have the desirable properties of rapid action and short duration of action (**thiopental, thiamylal, methohexital**) are used extensively for induction of anesthesia because of their ease of delivery and patient acceptance. More importantly, these drugs allow the anesthetist to avoid the "stormy" stage II phase seen with the slower inhalational inductions such as ether. Intravenous administration results in sleep, as well as subsequent amnesia, and is usually followed by maintenance with other anesthetic agents. The fast onset of sedation and sleep is the direct result of the rapid translocation of the agent from the vascular compartment to the brain due to its high blood flow. The short duration of action of a single bolus dose is due to the subsequent redistribution of the agent from the well-perfused brain to tissues that are less well perfused. The overall amount of the thiobarbiturates in the body is determined by their distribution to the hydrophobic (fat) compartment and their eventual metabolism in the liver.

The barbiturates have all the expected effects of a general anesthetic agent—including respiratory depression, cardiovascular depression after large doses, and ultimately death if given in excess. Their effects are at least additive and may be synergistic with other CNS depressants.

Benzodiazepines (Diazepam, Lorazepam, Midazolam)

The benzodiazepines (especially **diazepam, lorazepam and midazolam**) are important adjuncts in the practice of anesthesiology. They may be used as preoperative sedatives and induction agents, as well as supplemental agents for the maintenance of anesthesia. They are also useful in producing conscious sedation (see Chapter 25 and below).

Each of these three agents, diazepam, lorazepam, and midazolam, has found a role in the practice of anesthesiology. Midazolam and diazepam offer major advantages over the short-acting barbiturates in that they produce relatively less depression of the cardiovascular and respiratory functions and are therefore better suited for induction and maintenance in patients with significant pathology of these organ systems. Benzodiazepines have a longer duration of action than the short-acting barbiturates but resemble them in other respects.

Midazolam has largely replaced diazepam as the most commonly used benzodiazepine for induction. In addition, it has gained popularity as a component (with a short-acting narcotic and muscle relaxant) of a total intravenous anesthetic mixture given by continuous infusion. Although it has many of the same properties as diazepam, it is less irritating on intravenous administration because of greater water solubility. Midazolam has a shorter half-life than diazepam and is not metabolized to any active metabolites; these properties allow the patient to recover faster. Respiratory complications with midazolam were encountered more frequently than with the other benzodiazepines when it was first introduced clinically. These complications have mostly been corrected by proper attention to dose and to the fact that the onset of action is slower than with diazepam. Nevertheless, caution in avoiding overdosing must still be practiced when using this drug for conscious sedation.

Lorazepam is the agent of choice when loss of recall is required. Because of its profound amnesia this agent is particularly useful in procedures such as cardiopulmonary bypass where major changes in intravascular volume coupled with predominantly opioid (narcotic) anesthetic techniques make recall more likely. Midazolam is also a good amnestic agent, although not as profound as lorazepam; in this regard midazolam may be useful in cases of shorter duration.

FACTORS INFLUENCING ACTION AND DOSAGE. The dose for intravenous administration should be decreased for elderly and debilitated patients. In addition, the sedative effects of these agents are magnified by opioid analgesics, by secobarbital, and by alcohol. These agents also, expectedly, decrease the minimal anesthetic concentration required for general anesthesia by inhalation anesthetics.

ANTAGONISM. **Flumazenil**, a benzodiazepine antagonist, may be used to reverse the residual effects of benzodiazepines in the event of an overdose (see Chapter 25).

Propofol

Propofol (DIPRIVAN Injection) is a relatively new agent of unique chemical structure (2,6-diisopropylphenol). It is marketed as an emulsion for intravenous administration for induction and maintenance of anesthesia. It has the advantages of a very rapid onset after infusion or bolus injections (similar to thiobarbiturates) plus a very short recovery period of some 8 minutes or less. A subjective feeling of well-being and a low incidence of postoperative nausea following use of this agent make it ideally suited for outpatient anesthesia.

The plasma levels after a bolus injection reveal two phases: a rapid phase with a half-life of 1.8 to 8.3 minutes and a slower phase with a half-life of 34 to 64 minutes. These two phases are analogous to similar changes by the thiobarbiturates and reflect a similar initial movement of the agent into highly perfused tissue, followed by its redistribution to less well perfused tissue.

Its disadvantages are similar to those reported for the short-acting barbiturates and include respiratory and myocardial depression. The lipid emulsion may also increase bleeding due to its effects on platelets. Moreover, there is a slightly greater risk for anaphylactoid reactions with the use of this agent, probably as a result of the hydrophobic emulsion, although these reactions have been decreased by a change in the lipid carrier.

Etomidate

Etomidate (AMIDATE) is a short-acting induction agent that is chemically distinct but pharmacologically similar to the short-acting barbiturates discussed above. This agent produces less respiratory and cardiovascular depression when compared with other commonly used induction agents. Mild coronary vasodilation has also been reported with the use of this drug. For these reasons etomidate has been highly touted for induction of anesthesia in patients whose cardiac disease renders them hemodynamically unstable. Etomidate is suspended in propylene glycol for intravenous administration and, therefore, must be given slowly to avoid venous irritation. Other disadvantages of this agent are the appearance of myoclonic muscle contractions in some patients, and adrenocortical suppression, which can last for up to 12 hours following its usage. This drug is metabolized primarily in the liver.

Droperidol

Droperidol (INAPSINE) is an antidopaminergic anesthetic adjuvant that produces a neuroleptic state of detachment. When used with an opioid to produce conscious sedation, the term *neuroleptoanalgesia* has been used, and when it is given in anesthetic concentrations, the state is referred to as *neuroleptoanesthesia*. This agent produces some peripheral vasodilation. Droperidol decreases nausea and vomiting and has been used in small doses for this purpose as well as to decrease the levels required of other anesthetic agents in the outpatient setting.

Disadvantages include unpleasant extrapyramidal side effects and dysphoria in some patients, particularly the aged. Because of the heightened sensitivity and increased frequency of side effects, this compound must be carefully titrated in the aged patient.

Opioids

Morphine and meperidine have been long used for preoperative medication, as an adjuvant for the maintenance of anesthesia, and postoperatively to provide analgesia. With the introduction of the shorter acting anesthetic agents, opioids have recently found much wider and more varied use. With such agents, patients can be rapidly obtunded and are markedly analgesic without appreciable cardiovascular risk. Opioids are a major component of the *balanced anesthetic technique*. This technique uses multiple agents, each chosen for its selective, and additive or synergistic effects; one of the prime objectives of such techniques is the reduction of undesirable side effects associated with large doses of any one agent. For example, in the surgical patient, opioids may be combined with nitrous oxide, a sedative such as diazepam, a muscle relaxant, and a potent volatile anesthetic — this combination permits excellent control of hemodynamic functions.

Patients who receive opioids as part of their anesthetic procedure must be closely monitored for adequacy of ventilation in view of the depression of the response of respiratory drive to carbon dioxide and oxygen. When high doses are used, the patient must be artificially ventilated.

FENTANYL, ALFENTANIL, AND SUFENTANIL. Anesthesia with fentanyl (SUBLIMAZE), and related drugs, alfentanil (ALFENTA), and sufentanil (SUFENTA), occurs very shortly after intravenous injections. These agents differ from each other somewhat in terms of potency and duration of action (see also Chapter 14). The degree of analgesia or anesthesia is dose-related. These agents can be used for conscious sedation techniques, for induction, as the primary anesthetic, as an adjunct with other anesthetics, and as part of a continuous infusion with other intravenous anesthetics for maintenance of anesthesia.

Because these agents are opioid agonists, respiratory depression and muscle rigidity of the chest can occur during induction. Histamine release is not marked, although itching can sometimes be a troublesome side effect. These agents can be antagonized by the competitive opioid antagonist naloxone. Nevertheless, naloxone should *not* be necessary in an appropriately managed patient. Moreover, by antagonizing all opioids possibly present in a patient, its administration may result in the sudden onset of severe pain as well as marked sympathetic activation. Pulmonary edema and other untoward adverse reactions have also been observed after naloxone administration following anesthesia.

Ketamine

Ketamine (KETALAR) administration produces a catatonic state in which the patient does not respond to noxious stimuli. In this state of catalepsy, muscle tone is sustained and posture or position is maintained, although movement is nonpurposeful. Phonation may also occur. The eyes frequently remain open and appear to stare or to move with slow nystagmoid movements but without significant awareness. The term *dissociative* has been used to describe the disassociation between the individuals's response and the environment—a functional disassociation of the thalamocortical and limbic systems, probably the result of noncompetitive blockade of *N*-methyl-D-asparate receptors.

Ketamine directly depresses myocardial function although this effect is masked due to a concomitant activation of the sympathetic nervous system. This activation results in small increases in heart rate and blood pressure. The airway and respiration are usually adequate; however, vigilance must be maintained because aspiration and laryngospasm may also occur.

In light stages of this anesthetic state, or during emergence from deeper levels, bizarre dreams and hallucinations may occur, and these may be remembered by the patient as unpleasant. These unpleasant side effects can be drastically decreased by the concomitant use of sedative adjuvants such as droperidol or a benzodiazepine.

The state produced by ketamine is quite similar to that produced by a chemically close relative, phencyclidine (PCP), a drug used in veterinary medicine to produce anesthesia. PCP has also been widely used nonmedically and is discussed further in the chapter on substance abuse (Chapter 49) and that in relation to drug-induced psychiatric symptoms (Chapter 50).

Because during ketamine anesthesia the cardiovascular system is under sympathetic activation, it is used in patients who are unstable (*eg*, those who have bled excessively following trauma). In addition, because of ketamine's apparent lack of toxicity with repeated use, it is frequently used in burn patients who must have repeated harvesting and grafting of skin. Ketamine also has analgesic properties and can be used in low doses in obstetrics to ease the pain of labor. Care must be taken to keep the doses low in order to reduce the incidence of a hypertonic uterus and untoward fetal depression.

When it is given intravenously, the onset is within 1 minute with a duration of 5 to 10 minutes, although the half-life of ketamine is 3 hours. Anesthesia can be maintained by repeated injections. There are no known antagonists.

Conscious Sedation

The term conscious sedation has become widely used to describe a drug-induced state that facilitates surgical interventions or endoscopic procedures, and that provides improved patient comfort. The essential features of this state are a sedated, calm patient, who may or may not require analgesia and/or amnesia. Patients receiving a conscious sedation technique should retain the ability to respond to simple questions and commands, although they may sleep when not stimulated. Respiratory depression, agitation, delirium, and combativeness are potential complications of this state, particularly in the aged patient.

An opioid, such as meperidine or morphine, given in combination with a sedative such as a benzodiazepine (*eg*, diazepam or midazolam), propofol, droperidol, or a barbiturate can result in a patient who is calm, analgesic, with amnesia for most of the events taking place. Blood pressure and respiration are well maintained and the patient is usually oriented to person, place, and time. Typically, the sedative is given slowly over minutes starting with a small dose with increments given to achieve the desired end-point of a patient who is comfortable but also has the ability to respond to simple direct commands and questions, such as "open your eyes, lift your arm," or questions of person and place. Most important is a decrease in anxiety level so that patients are cooperative and unperturbed by the events around them. If left alone, patients usually tend to go to sleep, a sleep from which they usually can be aroused. Speech tends to be slurred and nystagmus is usually prominent at least during the initial phases.

Amnesia is present in many of these patients, especially if a benzodiazepine is used. This amnesia may only be partially appreciated by the patient and is characterized by a patchy recollection of a small portion of the events that transpired during the drug action. Bizarre dreams or sexual fantasies have also been reported. To such a baseline state produced by a sedative other agents may be added, primarily narcotics but occasionally other hypnotic agents depending on the nature of the procedure being performed. In addition to the antianxiety and analgesic medications, local anesthetics are used for procedures in which appreciable pain is anticipated, such as tooth extractions or dental restorations.

As in all cases requiring anesthetic care, the drugs employed and the doses are largely adjusted on the basis of the patient's responses to the procedures undertaken. Although they do not require the intensity of monitoring as in general anesthesia, continuous monitoring of respiration, electrocardiogram, and blood pressure is necessary. Such combinations enjoy a relatively large safety margin and at the same time are adequate for a variety of painful or discomforting procedures. There remain significant potential risks of excessive respiratory depression or behavior agitation. Because patients may not be receiving oxygen inhalation, covert unrecognized levels of hypoxia may result. Monitoring of oxygenation by pulse oximetry is standard practice.

Appropriately managed, recovery from conscious sedation is rapid and smooth. Amnesia may be present for most of the events that transpire. Nausea, vomiting, and other postoperative events common with general anesthetics are rare. In fact, in skillful hands the recovery is so uneventful as to be deceptive. It is absolutely necessary that outpatients have somebody else present to take them home for eventual recovery. All patients postoperatively are at serious risk for a wide variety of accidents. It is essential that there is appropriate postoperative monitoring. Although patients may appear to be conscious, awake, and hearing what is being told, many are actually unable to recall the events subsequently. Thus, any kind of direction must be given to the patient days in advance of the drug administration. Directions need to be written down and also provided to a responsible third party.

Clinical tests of recovery from conscious sedation do

not provide a valid prediction of a patient's ability to operate machinery or an automobile. At least a day or so should elapse before driving is permitted. As with all anesthetic agents and all kinds of anesthesia, including local anesthesia, the provision of devices and staff for immediate monitoring, detection, and correction of any cardiorespiratory adverse events, including oxygen levels, should be routine. Equipment and personnel prepared for resuscitation should be available with no more than 2- to 5-second delay. *The patient must be monitored at all times directly by trained personnel. This should include regular routine measurements of respiration, oxygen level, and cardiovascular function including adequacy of organ perfusion as well as determinations of the depth of sedation and patient comfort. Protocols need to be established regarding the level of care required (eg, skilled nursing care vs anesthesia care) based on the patient's health status and complexity of the procedure. Regardless of the level of care, arrangements for emergency back-up by anesthesia services must be established prior to implementation of any procedures involving conscious sedation.*

ANESTHETIC ACCIDENTS

Fortunately, serious life-threatening reactions to anesthetics and anesthesia are rare. Furthermore, over the past two decades the standards of care have improved and anesthesiologists have received improved training. As a consequence, the frequency of untoward adverse events has decreased to less than one sixth the previous occurrence rate. Despite this rate reduction, when anesthetic complications do occur they can be truly tragic because of the extremely altered state that patients are placed in by being exposed to these potent agents with low therapeutic indices.

Anesthetic accidents can lead to consequences that affect not only the patient but also the family, physician, and institution. Retrospective studies of accidents that have occurred around anesthetics, and that have been attributed in some way or another to the anesthesia, reveal that most involve the airway and respiratory tract and *that more than 70% of all anesthetic "accidents" are preventable.* Tragedies based on ignorance of facts, lack of technical skills, or errors in judgment that the well-trained anesthesiologist or nurse anesthetist should have, must be avoided. The conclusions of these studies are heartening in the sense that they identify the sources of the already infrequent problems and the means for their solutions. It is also apparent from such studies that the information needed for the safe use of anesthetic agents has been, or at least can be, obtained by research and using the methods of Total Quality Improvement (TQI). The agents and their effects are sufficiently predictable and safe for the benefit-risk evaluations of most individuals. Moreover, well-designed studies can establish the potential for untoward effects.

DRUG COMBINATIONS AND INTERACTIONS IN ANESTHESIA

Because of the nature of modern anesthesia and surgery, surgical procedures involve the administration of numerous drugs before the procedure, during anesthesia and surgery, and in the recovery period. Awareness of all the agents involved, as well as the disease state and operative procedure, is important inasmuch as there are interactions, in terms of effects as well as pharmacokinetics. For example, midazolam and alfentanil potentiate each other and are synergistic with propolol (Vinik et al., 1994). The following provides a scheme and *minimal examples* of the agents that could be used in a patient, arranged according to the time course:

BOX 11–1
EXAMPLES OF DRUGS IN AN ANESTHESIA

The night before:

- Assessment of patient by anesthesiologist as well as surgeon
- Hypnotic—a benzodiazepine to reduce anxiety and promote sleep
- Nothing to eat or drink after a given time, *eg*, midnight

The day of surgery:

- Preanesthetic medications

  Analgesic—opioid

  Antianxiety—a benzodiazepine

  Anticholinergic—atropine or scopolamine

- Establish intravenous (IV) lines and start IV fluids
- Induction of anesthesia

  Intravenous induction—thiopental, benzodiazepine (*eg*, midazolam), propofol, etomidate, or ketamine

  Opioids (*eg*, fentanyl)

  Inhalation induction, *eg*, halothane

  Neuromuscular blockade (*eg*, succinylcholine) to facilitate endotracheal intubation if necessary

- Maintenance of anesthesia (during anesthesia and surgery)

  Inhalation agents—nitrous oxide, halothane, enflurane, isoflurane, desflurane, or sevoflurane

  Opioids—morphine, fentanyl

  Spinal or epidural anesthetic in conjunction with a light plane of general anesthesia

  Sedatives and hypnotics (from the list of intravenous induction agents)

Anesthetic adjuncts and procedures (during and after anesthesia and surgery):

- Neuromuscular blocking agent(s)—succinylcholine, pancuronium, dimethylcurare, atracurium, and/or vecuronium
- Cardiovascular drugs—hypotensive agents (nitroglycerin), vasopressors (metaraminol), or antiarrhythmic agents (lidocaine, atropine)
- Fluid and blood replacement

Continued

BOX 11–1
EXAMPLES OF DRUGS IN AN ANESTHESIA *Continued*

Termination of anesthesia and recovery:

- Turn off the inhalational anesthetic agents, such as halothane
- Assess and provide analgesia for the awakening patient
- Reverse nondepolarizing muscle relaxants if used (neostigmine, usually with an anticholinergic agent such as atropine)
- Support respiratory and cardiovascular systems as needed

Postoperative period:

- Reverse narcotic or benzodiazepine, but caution is in order and only when absolutely necessary
- Antinausea and vomiting medication—droperidol, ondansetron
- Pain management—morphine, patient-controlled analgesia, or continuous epidural analgesia
- Cough induction or antitussive
- Antianxiety agent or hypnotic
- IV fluids

REFERENCES

Barash PG, Cullen BF, Stoelting RK (eds): Clinical Anesthesia, 2nd ed. Philadelphia: JB Lippincott, 1992.

Biebuyck JF: The role of the $GABA_A$ receptor/chloride channel complex in anesthesia. Anesthesiology 78:757–776, 1993.

Bowdle TA, Horita A, Kharasch ED (eds): The Pharmacologic Basis of Anesthesiology. New York: Churchill Livingstone, 1994.

Eger EI II: Nitrous Oxide/N_2O. New York: Elsevier, 1985.

Feldman S (ed): Anesthetic Pharmacology Review [Quarterly]. London: Castle House Publications.

Feldman S, Scurr CF, Paton W (eds): Mechanisms of Drugs in Anesthesia. London: Edward Arnold, 1993.

Firestone LL, Miller JC, Miller KW: Tables of physical and pharmacological properties of anesthetics appendix. *In* Roth SH, Miller KW (eds): Molecular and Cellular Mechanisms of Anesthetics. New York and London: Plenum Medical Book Company, 1986.

Franks NP, Lieb WR: Molecular and cellular mechanisms of general anesthesia. Nature 367:607–614, 1994.

Franks NP, Lieb WR: Stereospecific effects of inhalational general anesthetic optical isomers on nerve ion channels. Science 254:427–430, 1991.

Killip T: Anesthesia and major noncardiac surgery. JAMA 268:252–253, 1992.

Knight PR, Tait AR: Immunological aspects of anesthesia. *In* Nunn J, Utting J, Brown BR (eds): General Anesthesia, 5th ed, 283–293. Boston: Butterworths, 1988.

Krystal JH, Karper LP, Seibyl JP, et al: Subanesthetic effects of the noncompetitive NMDA antagonist, ketamine, in humans. Arch Gen Psychiatry 51:199–214, 1994.

Miller RD (ed): Anesthesia, 4th ed. New York: Churchill Livingstone, 1994.

Moody EJ, Harris BD, Skolnick P: The potential for safer anesthesia using stereoselective anaesthetics. Trends Pharmacol Sci 15:387–391, 1994.

Nakahiro M, Yeh JZ, Brunner E, Narahashi T: General anesthetics modulate GABA receptor channel complex in rat dorsal root ganglion neurons. FASEB J 3:1850–1854, 1989.

Nicoll RA, Madison DV: General anesthetics hyperpolarize neurons in the vertebrate nervous system. Science 717:1055–1057, 1982.

Nunn J, Utting J, Brown BR: General Anesthesia, 5th ed. Boston: Butterworths, 1989.

Papper EM, Kitz RJ: Uptake and Distribution of Anesthetic Agents. New York: McGraw-Hill Book Co, 1963.

Prys-Roberts C, Hug CC Jr: Pharmacokinetics of Anaesthesia. Boston: Blackwell Scientific Publications, 1984.

Vinik HR, Bradley EL Jr, Kissin I: Triple anesthetic combination: Profololmidazolam-alfentanil. Anesth Analg 78:354–358, 1994.

Wrigley SR, Jones RM: Inhalational Agents: An update. Eur J Anesthesiol 9:185–201, 1992.

Local Anesthetic Agents 12

Mark J. Lema

The coca leaf was first brought back to Europe by Pizarro's conquistadors in the 1500s after witnessing its euphoric and anesthetic effects on the Incas. Its extract, cocaine, was first used medically as a local anesthetic in 1884 when Dr. Carl Koller, a Viennese surgeon, irrigated a patient's eye with a 2% cocaine solution to anesthetize the cornea. Since that time a number of local anesthetic congeners have been developed, providing both superior and safer anesthesia when compared with cocaine. The main advantage to using local anesthetics in the nineteenth century was to eliminate the need for general anesthesia, which carried with it a high mortality risk of about 1 : 500. Today, regional anesthesia is still used to provide an added measure of patient safety during surgery.

CHEMISTRY

Prototype Agents—Procaine and Lidocaine

All local anesthetic agents consist of four basic components: an aromatic lipophilic ring, the ester or amide linkage, an intermediate hydrocarbon chain, and a hydrophilic tertiary amine terminus (Fig. 12-1). The aromatic ring is usually a benzene ring with methyl amide substitutions. The linking arrangement divides all of the local anesthetics into either an ester (-COO-) or an amide (-NH-) compound (Fig. 12-2). The currently used ester compounds are cocaine, procaine, tetracaine, and chloroprocaine. Contemporary amide compounds include lidocaine, mepivacaine, etidocaine, prilocaine, bupivacaine, and ropivacaine. Both lidocaine (XYLOCAINE) and procaine (NOVOCAIN) are considered the prototypic agents of the amide and ester classes, respectively. Clinically, the distinction between these two compounds lies with their different metabolic pathways and their propensity toward hypersensitivity reactions. The ester compounds are hydrolyzed by plasma esterases to a para-amino benzoic acid (PABA), which is cross-reactive with a known allergen, methylparaben. Amide compounds are metabolized by the hepatic microsomal oxygenases and are rarely associated with allergic reactions; the preservative in some local anesthetic solutions (benzoic acid; parabens) can also induce a hypersensitivity response.

NEUROPHYSIOLOGY

Site of Action

Local anesthetics are one of the most commonly used drugs in clinical practice today. Although their principal purpose is to provide insensitivity to pain and sensation for surgery, these agents produce clinically significant depression of all excitable membranes including heart, brain, vascular, muscle, and autonomic tissues. Interestingly, lidocaine was used as an antiarrhythmic agent for almost a decade until the Food and Drug Administration approval for that use was granted.

Both ester and amide local anesthetics reduce the discharge frequency of nerve conduction and decrease the total number of nerve fibers activated by a given stimulus. The primary action for accomplishing this reduction is alteration of inward ionic fluxes Na^+, Ca^{++}, which elevates the action potential threshold (Fig. 12-3). This action prevents certain nerve fibers from firing, depending on their diameter size. Consequently, in a mixed nerve bundle, as a decrease in the discharge frequency is recorded, pain and sensation responses are attenuated (Fig. 12-4).

Effect of Nerve Diameter

Fiber size affects the onset of nerve blockage. Pain and temperature sensation are carried by their unmyelinated C fibers and poorly myelinated A-delta fibers. Preganglionic autonomic fibers control vascular smooth muscle tone. Finally,

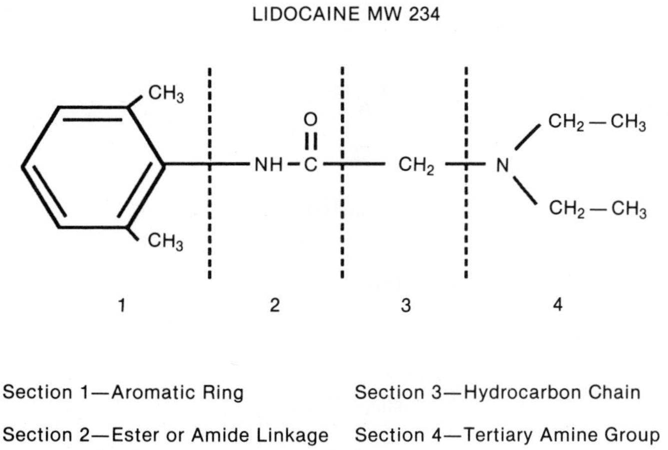

LIDOCAINE MW 234

Section 1—Aromatic Ring | Section 3—Hydrocarbon Chain

Section 2—Ester or Amide Linkage | Section 4—Tertiary Amine Group

FIGURE 12–1. Component structures of local anesthetics that form four distinct chemical subunits.

A-gamma, A-beta, and A-alpha nerve axons are responsible for sending muscle spindle tone; pressure, touch and muscle tone; and muscle movement, reflex activity, and proprioception, respectively. When one instills local anesthetic near a nerve bundle, the different fibers are blocked as the concentration at the axon site increases, known as Cm (minimum blocking concentration). Hence, a differential nerve blockage occurs in the following order: C < B < A-delta < A-gamma < A-beta < A-alpha fibers last. Clinically, the loss of sensation to needle prick, coldness, and vasodilation herald the early onset of an anesthetic block. As full neural blockade develops, position sense (proprioception), skin sensation and voluntary muscle movement, and involuntary muscle motion (paralysis) sequentially occur.

Effect on Ionic Channels

Local anesthetics act by blocking primarily open and inactive sodium channels, preventing the influx of Na^+ during the depolarization phase of the action potential. When the channels are in the resting or closed state, local anesthetic will dissociate from the binding site and the channels will recover from the block. On unmyelinated C fibers, sodium channels reside along the entire axon, whereas in myelinated nerves, high concentrations of channels exist in the open gaps between myelin segments (nodes of Ranvier).

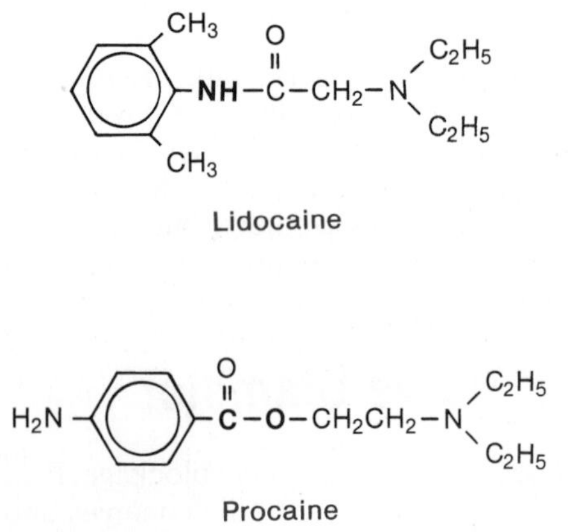

Lidocaine

Procaine

FIGURE 12–2. Differences in structure between amide and ester local anesthetics lie in section 2, as shown in bold face type.

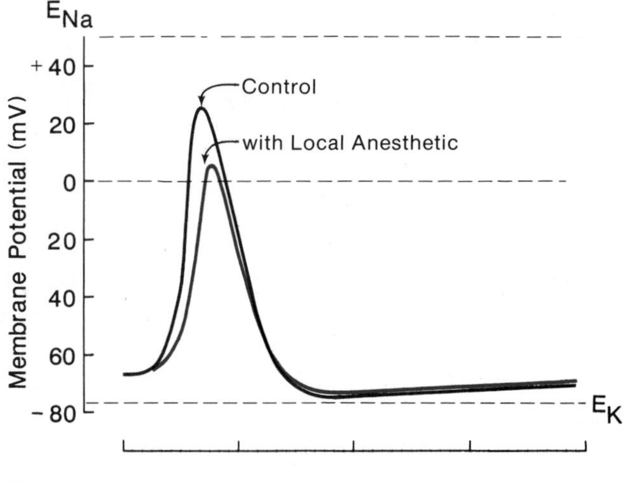

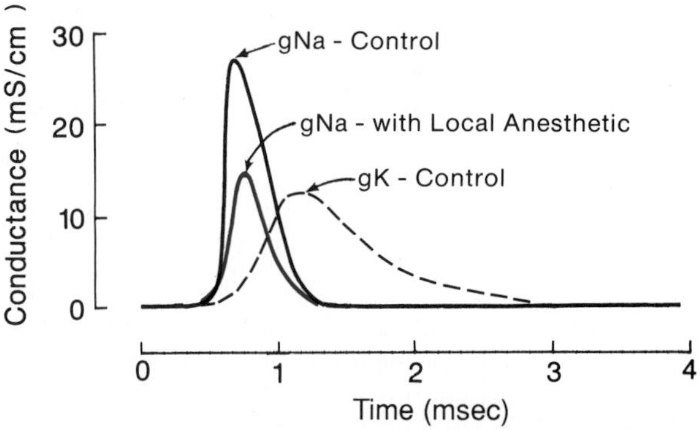

FIGURE 12–3. Action potential and associated changes in permeability of the nerve membrane to sodium and potassium ions. The ordinate of the top recording shows the nerve membrane potential recorded intracellularly, and the ordinate of the bottom recording gives the associated ion conductances. The effects of a local anesthetic are shown in color—a decrease in the rate of rise and in the size of the action potential in association with a corresponding decrease in sodium permeability. (Local anesthetics have only small effects directly on potassium conductances.) (This figure is a general illustration based ultimately on the pioneering work of Hodgkin and Huxley [1952] relating the membrane electrical properties and ionic permeabilities.) Membrane potential is recorded as the difference in potential between the intracellular electrode and the external service expressed in millivolts (mV). (E_{Na} = sodium equilibrium potential—the membrane potential at which there would be no net influx or efflux of sodium ions; F_K = potassium equilibrium potential.) Conductance is expressed as gNa = sodium conductance; gK = potassium conductance.

Frequency-Dependent Blockade

The effectiveness of local anesthetic binding is a property of both the molecular shape and the conformational state of the channel. Moreover, nerve axons become more sensitive to local anesthetic action as nerve activity increases because more channels reside in the open and inactive states. Lidocaine, a smaller, less lipophilic compound, can rapidly bind and dissociate and thus would seem to act best when there is a high frequency of activity. Conversely, bupivacaine, a larger, more lipophilic agent, acts more slowly and would favor a lower frequency of activity. Thus, one can understand how lidocaine functions more effectively as an antiarrhythmic whereas bupivacaine promotes myocardial depression. Moreover, evidence suggests that bupivacaine also

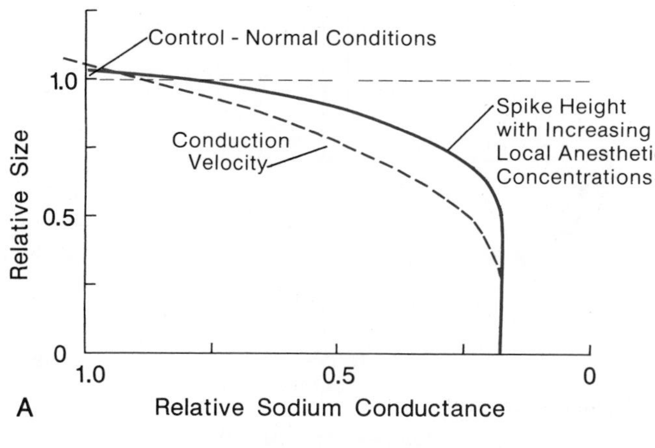

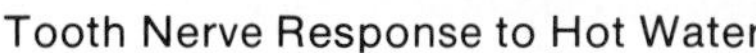

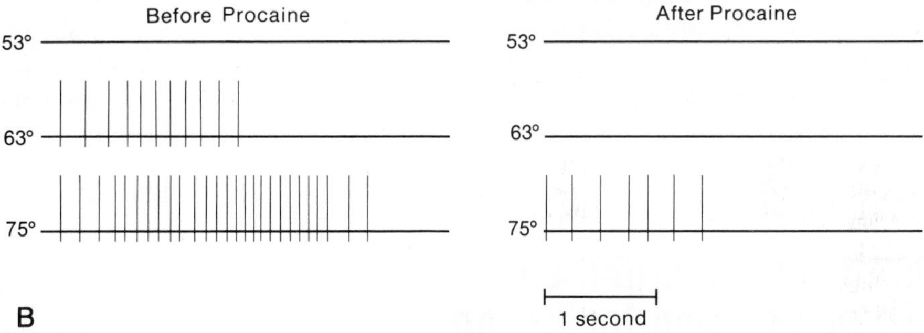

FIGURE 12–4. (*A*) Relation of nerve conductance velocity and action potential spike height to maximal sodium conductance. With a decrease in sodium conductance, as might be produced by a local anesthetic, both the spike height and the conduction velocity fall. Finally, as the conductance decreases to about one sixth of the normal sodium conductance (the normal is shown as 1.0 at the origin on this graph), impulse conduction fails; i.e., there is a safety factor of 6. (This example is plotted from a computer simulation of data pertaining to frog nerve of 20 μm diameter at 20° C. Replotted from Ritchie JM: An overview of the mechanisms of local anesthetic action past, present, future. *In* Roth SH, Miller KW [eds]: Molecular and Cellular Mechanisms of Anesthetics, 196. New York: Plenum, 1984.)

(*B*) Electrical responses of a single afferent nociceptive ("pain") fiber from the tooth pulp induced by application of hot water to the crown of the tooth. The greater the temperature, the greater the frequency and the longer the repetitive discharge of action potentials. Each upward spike is a propagated action potential. Note that at rest at temperatures of 53° C (and below), there are no action potentials. After the application of procaine to the pulp (in this preparation through the circulation), the threshold for activation is increased and the discharge frequency decreased or abolished. (The rationale for studying the tooth pulp is that stimulation of the afferent nerves from tooth pulp gives rise almost exclusively to sensations of pain.) (Adapted from Wagers PW, Smith CM: Responses in dental nerves of dogs to tooth stimulation and the effects of systematically administered procaine, lidocaine and morphine. J Pharmacol Exp Ther 130:89–105, 1960.)

blocks calcium channels more specifically than lidocaine, increasing the cell's resting membrane potential.

The result of this action is a decrease in both myofibril contraction and myocardial nerve conduction. Toxic concentrations of bupivacaine can produce cardiovascular collapse and bradyarrhythmias, resulting in asystole. The concept of **frequency-dependent blockade** is also called **use-dependent blockade**.

PHARMACOKINETICS

Drug Delivery

Clinically, local anesthetics are injected as close to the targeted nerves as possible. Administration is peripheral rather than systemic because of the number of physicochemical barriers that the local anesthetic must traverse. The agent can be diluted by body fluids, confronted with fibrous tissue, absorbed into adipose tissue, be systemically absorbed, or be affected by tissue pH.

When a drug is injected into peripheral tissue, the following sequence occurs before an anesthetic effect is noticed:

1. Local anesthetic moves away from injection site in all directions.
2. Local anesthetic reaches the neural membrane by mass action, which requires both drug concentration and an adequate volume.
3. Diffusion across membrane barriers is dependent on the magnitude of the concentration gradient.
4. Because diffusion is slow, drug dilution, systemic absorption, and nonspecific binding occur.
5. Once in the nerve bundle, drug action occurs in the outer fibers first and the core last. Thus, fibers more proximal to the block site are anesthetized first and distally served structures last.
6. After equilibrium is reached between the nerve membrane and surrounding medium, the block begins to regress.
7. The core retains drug the longest and therefore outer fibers recover before central fibers.
8. Rate of diffusion is more dependent on lipid solubility than concentration. Highly lipophilic agents (bupivacaine, etidocaine) form tissue depots and diffuse very slowly, resulting in prolonged neural blockade.

Factors Affecting Drug Action

Virtually all drugs enter tissue in an un-ionized form but must become cationically (+) charged to bind to the active site. Thus, body fluids play a key role in modifying the degree of ionization, in relation to each agent's pK_a. However, the onset of action is dependent on how quickly the drug penetrates biological tissue to undergo receptor binding. Only un-ionized, free (unbound to protein) drug is capable of passing through neural membranes (Fig. 12–5).

The following factors are important in determining both the rate and extent (onset) of local anesthetic diffusion.

1. Molecular weight
2. Lipid solubility

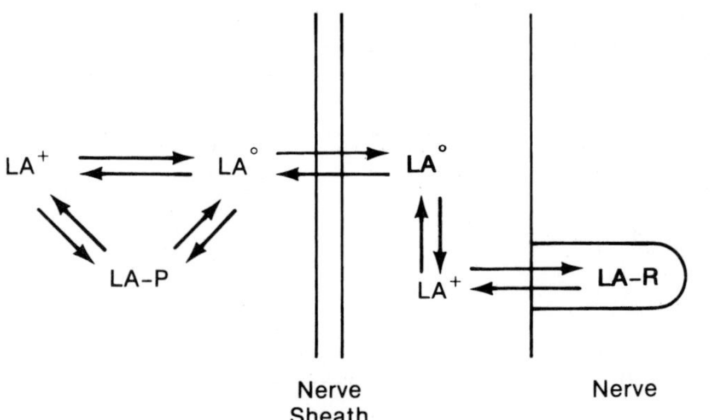

FIGURE 12–5. Diffusion and binding of local anesthetics to receptor site.

3. Degree of ionization
4. Drug concentration
5. Drug volume
6. Protein binding
7. Site of drug introduction

Molecular Weight, Lipid Solubility, and Ionization

For currently used local anesthetics, the molecular weights range from 220 to 288 daltons. Even though diffusion is proportional to the square root of the molecular weight ($\delta = \sqrt{mw}$), this factor is not clinically significant.

Lipid solubility is a more critical factor for two reasons: it promotes drug entry into biological membranes and it encourages protein binding. Rapid entry into tissue hastens onset, whereas enhanced protein binding delays onset. Therefore, it is difficult to determine if lipid solubility actually hastens or delays the clinical onset of action. Lipid solubility is independent of side chain grouping; both bupivacaine (amide) and tetracaine (ester) are highly lipid soluble.

Some local anesthetics exist as weak bases ($pK_a > 7.4$) and are poorly water soluble. They are packaged as highly ionized hydrochloric acid (HCl) salts (pH 4–7). When injected, body buffers raise pH (alkalinize), which increases the free base, producing a more lipid soluble moiety, promoting membrane transfer. Thus, ionization is related to local anesthetic action, solubility, and the distribution throughout the body.

Protein Binding

Local anesthetics predominantly bind with albumin but also with α_1-acid glycoprotein (α_1GP). Although α_1GP has a much higher binding affinity for local anesthetics, albumin has a higher capacity for binding them. Changes in protein concentration can affect the availability of free drug. When local anesthetic plasma concentrations are less than 10 μg/ml, which is the case for all therapeutically used agents, α_1GP binding predominates. Thus, during acute phase reactions (infection, cancer, autoimmune diseases), increased levels of α_1GP are detected, which will bind free local anesthetic and reduce its activity.

In neonates, α_1GP levels are about 60% of that detected in adults. Thus, less protein binding will occur for such amide agents as bupivacaine and etidocaine, making more drug available in the free form. The likelihood of toxic levels developing is also increased. Agents such as lidocaine and mepivacaine, which have lower protein binding capabilities, would be safer choices in these young patients.

Effects of Tissue Binding

The major portion of local anesthetics remains in or on cell structures (tissue). The presence of many nonspecific binding sites around excitable tissue will delay equilibrium in that tissue by acting as a "sink."

The size and impact of this local anesthetic sink depends on:

- Size of the tissue (volume)
- Blood flow through tissue (rate)
- Lipid content of tissue
- Membrane permeability of tissue
- pH gradient
- Binding to tissue and plasma proteins

Inasmuch as most local anesthetics have volumes of distribution (V_d) much larger than tissue body water, extensive tissue uptake and sequestration occur after injection. In fact, animal studies using radiolabeled local anesthetics show that most of the drug is sequestered into highly perfused organs and not the fat. Lung tissue will take up 95% of all first-pass drug, only to release it after about 15 seconds. Its purported role is the buffering of the body against rapid rises in serum levels.

Local Anesthetic Absorption

Absorption from tissue and bioavailability of injected (nonintravenously) drug is virtually 100%. Local anesthetics rapidly diffuse through tissue and eventually become absorbed into the systemic circulation. As an example, a brachial plexus local anesthetic injection of 40 ml produces **peak** plasma concentrations in only 15 minutes. Systemic absorption is thought to proceed by a biphasic, first-order mechanism of an initial rapid phase and a slow second phase.

Rates of absorption from various body locations commonly injected with local anesthetic relate to the proximity and distribution of vascular structures (both arterial and venous systems). The following figure lists the anatomical locations in descending order from the fastest rate to the slowest rate of systemic drug absorption:

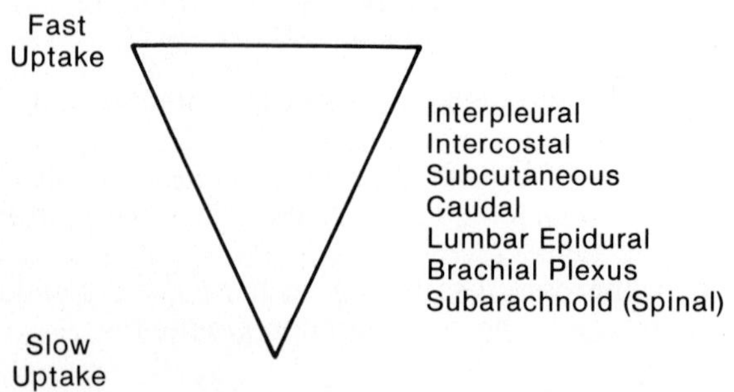

If one adds a vasoconstrictor such as epinephrine or phenylephrine to the local anesthetic solution, systemic absorption can be slowed and anesthetic action clinically prolonged by about 50%.

Drug Distribution

Once absorbed, local anesthetic is distributed primarily to such vessel-rich organs as the brain, heart, lungs, liver, and kidneys (central compartment). Factors influencing rate (onset) and extent (duration) of local anesthetic action are:

- Amount of blood flowing to organ
- Rate of organ blood flow
- Tissue pH
- Protein binding of local anesthetic
- Tissue : blood partition coefficient

At the same time, local anesthetics in the blood are being distributed to less well perfused organs at a much slower rate. Muscle, fat, bone, and connective tissue comprise the peripheral compartment, and its total volume can have an impact on both drug accumulation and eventual elimination. Obese patients can have as much as 30% of total cardiac output going to fat. Consequently, they are slow to recover from the effects of most drugs, which must be given in larger amounts to compensate for this increased fatty distribution. The volume of distribution for most local anesthetics is between 72 and 133 liters, much larger than the V_d for free water.

Drug Elimination

Amide local anesthetics undergo hepatic metabolism as their sole mechanism of irreversible elimination. About 5% of all drug is eliminated unchanged by the kidney. Hepatic clearance depends on:

- Liver blood flow
- Efficiency of drug extraction (extraction ratio)

Local anesthetics with high extraction ratios (lidocaine and etidocaine) are completely metabolized on first pass and are designated as "flow-limited" agents. Conditions that change liver blood flow will alter the local anesthetic clearance. Conversely, such drugs as bupivacaine and mepivacaine, with low extraction ratios, must rely on the intrinsic clearance of free drug concentration, and are known as "rate-limited" agents. Changes in enzyme activity and plasma protein binding have a more profound impact on their clearance.

Ester drugs are cleared predominantly by plasma esterases, with only 5% being excreted unchanged in the urine.

Total clearance (Cl) of all compounds is the sum of all clearing mechanisms. All amide agents have active metabolites that have been implicated in slowing down clearance rates if doses are high or continuous infusions are used. Lidocaine is converted to monoethylglycinexylidine (MEGX) by hepatic N-dealkylation. This compound is only slightly less potent and toxic when compared with lidocaine. Thus, those patients with impaired renal clearance may experience prolonged effects from repeated amide local anesthetic usage.

TABLE 12–1. Pharmacokinetics of Commonly Used Local Anesthetics

	V_d (L/kg)	Cl (L/kg/hr)	$t_{1/2}$ (hrs)
Amides			
Lidocaine	1.30	0.85	1.6
Mepivacaine	1.20	0.67	1.9
Prilocaine	2.73	2.03	1.6
Etidocaine	1.90	1.05	2.6
Bupivacaine	1.02	0.41	3.5
Ropivacaine	0.84	0.63	1.9
Esters			
Cocaine	2.06	2.01	0.71
Procaine	0.93	5.62	0.14
Chloroprocaine	0.50	2.96	0.11
Tetracaine*			

*Restricted to topical and occasional spinal usage.
Cl = total clearance; $t_{1/2}$ = elimination half-life in plasma; V_d = volume of distribution at steady state.

A useful parameter to gauge local anesthetic duration is the **elimination half-life**—the time required for the body to eliminate 50% of the remaining drug. Both Cl and V_d affect the half-life of a drug as follows:

$$\begin{aligned} \text{elimination constant (k)} &= \text{Cl}/V_d \\ \text{and } t_{1/2} &= 0.693/\text{k} \\ \text{thus substituting } t_{1/2} &= 0.693V_d/\text{Cl} \end{aligned}$$

Thus, the half-life is directly proportional to the volume of distribution and inversely proportional to the clearance. So low V_d and high Cl produce short half-lives, while high V_d and low Cl cause long half-lives. However, if both V_d and Cl are increased or decreased proportionately, $t_{1/2}$ remains unchanged. Table 12–1 lists the pharmacokinetic values for the currently used amide and ester local anesthetics.

SYSTEMIC ACTIONS

As previously stated, local anesthetic action can occur on any electrically excitable cell—central or peripheral nervous tissue and smooth, striated, or cardiac muscle. All systemic actions are based on:

- Dose (volume and amount)
- Site of injection
- Method of metabolism

The three major systems to be discussed regarding local anesthetic action are the central nervous system, the peripheral nervous system, and the cardiovascular system.

Central Nervous System

The central nervous system (CNS) is particularly sensitive to the action of local anesthetics; yet opposite effects can be manifested at different concentrations. All agents are capable of crossing the blood-brain barrier because of high lipophilicity and low molecular weight. At lower concentrations, local anesthetics raise seizure thresholds and act as anticonvulsants, but at higher concentrations they are proconvulsants. At the highest levels, they produce profound CNS depression resulting in coma. In Table 12–2, maximum single

TABLE 12–2. Maximum Single-Dose Levels and CNS Toxic Plasma Threshold Levels for Clinically Used Local Anesthetics

	Maximum Single Dose (mg) ( ) = with epinephrine	Maximum Dose (mg/kg)	Threshold Toxic Plasma Concentration (μg/ml)
Amides			
Lidocaine	300 (500)	6.4	5–6
Mepivacaine	300 (500)	9.8	5–6
Prilocaine	400 (600)	6.0	5–6
Etidocaine	300 (400)	3.4	2
Bupivacaine	175 (250)	1.6	1.6
Ropivacaine*	250 (350)	3.0	—
Esters			
Cocaine†	150 (—)	(topical)	—
Procaine†	500 (600)	19.2	—
Chloroprocaine†	600 (650)	22.8	—
Tetracaine	100 (—)	2.5	—

*Drug not released for clinical use in United States. Numbers are estimated based on ¾ potency compared with bupivacaine.

†Rapidly cleared by plasma esterases.

CNS = central nervous system.

dosage and plasma toxicity threshold levels are listed for commonly used agents.

Initially, local anesthetics block inhibitory pathways in the brain to produce excitation such as shivering, muscle twitching, and tonic-clonic seizures. Higher doses cause blockade of both inhibitory and facilitory pathways to produce CNS depression, manifested as coma and respiratory arrest.

Peripheral Nervous System

Intravenous injection of local anesthetics can depress peripheral nerve activity (for discussion of local anesthetic action of nerve blocks, see the earlier discussion under Neurophysiology). Most notably, lidocaine given in 30- to 40-mg doses is capable of suppressing the cough reflex. Neuromuscular blockade is seen when toxic levels produce respiratory depression. However, central mechanisms also contribute to this response. Loss of autonomic and smooth muscle reflexes is manifested as hypotensive episodes, increased gastrointestinal activity, or decreased uterine contractions.

Cardiovascular System

Although somewhat more resistant than the CNS, profound cardiovascular system (CVS) changes can occur as local anesthetic levels increase. Both cardiac and smooth muscle fibers are directly affected. It appears that CVS effects require about three times higher levels than CNS toxic effects. Serum ratios of CVS : CNS toxicity are about 3.5 to 6.7 : 1 for bupivacaine > tetracaine > etidocaine > lidocaine, respectively. Lidocaine is the *least* cardiotoxic because it has the *highest* CVS : CNS ratio, whereas bupivacaine is the *most* cardiotoxic because it has the lowest CVS : CNS ratio. The first sign of CVS toxicity is hypotension due to negative inotropy, **not** vasodilation. As serum levels rise, profound hypotension and cardiovascular collapse are due to negative inotropic, chronotropic, and vasodilatory effects. Sinoatrial conduction blockade is seen at very high levels.

Bupivacaine appears to be more cardiotoxic than other agents, owing to its more potent, highly lipid soluble, high protein bound state. It can produce sinoatrial suppression resulting in nodal and ventricular arrhythmias at levels far below those detected for CNS toxicity. Even though bupivacaine is 4 times more potent than lidocaine as a local anesthetic, it is 16 times more cardiotoxic. The cardiotoxicity is due primarily to its blockage of cardiac muscle sodium channels five times longer than lidocaine. However, the impact of early hypoxemia, hypercapnia, and acidosis on both bupivacaine's and lidocaine's cardiodepressant effects is significant. In particular, the combination of hypoxemia, acidosis, and local anesthesia potentiates negative chronotropic and inotropic agents when compared with similar local anesthetics alone.

TOXICITY

Allergic Reactions

Allergic (hypersensitivity) reactions can occur and are almost always associated with the para-aminobenzoic acid (PABA) metabolite of ester local anesthetics. Its apparent cross-reactivity with a known common allergen, methylparaben (a preservative) produces dermatitis, urticaria, bronchospasm, angioedema, pruritus, and anaphylaxis. All reported cases of amide local anesthetic hypersensitivity have proved to be related to preservatives. Skin wheal tests using various local anesthetic agents, metabolites, and preservatives can be performed to identify the active compound.

Systemic Toxicity

There is a fine distinction between therapeutic inhibition of the excitation-conduction mechanism of nervous and muscle tissues and the toxic effects. While nerve blocks and antiarrhythmic therapies are dosed to prevent untoward effects, unintentional vascular injections of large amounts of drug affect CNS before CVS tissue. Figure 12–6 shows the order in which the various tissues are affected as toxic serum levels rise.

Rising blood concentration clearly promotes local anesthetic toxicity. The factors that can affect the rate of rise and magnitude of these blood levels are:

1. Site of drug injection—blood-rich areas favor rapid absorption.
2. Drug used—bupivacaine and etidocaine are more cardiotoxic even at lower doses.
3. Dosage administered—maximum single dose injection levels must be followed. Mixing two agents results in their maximum doses to be additive.
4. Use of vasoconstrictors—epinephrine can delay systemic absorption with most agents. Its cardiac actions must also be considered in cardiac patients.
5. Speed and volume of injectate—rapid injection of 5 to 10 ml will increase plasma levels more quickly than three slowly injected 3-ml bolus doses.

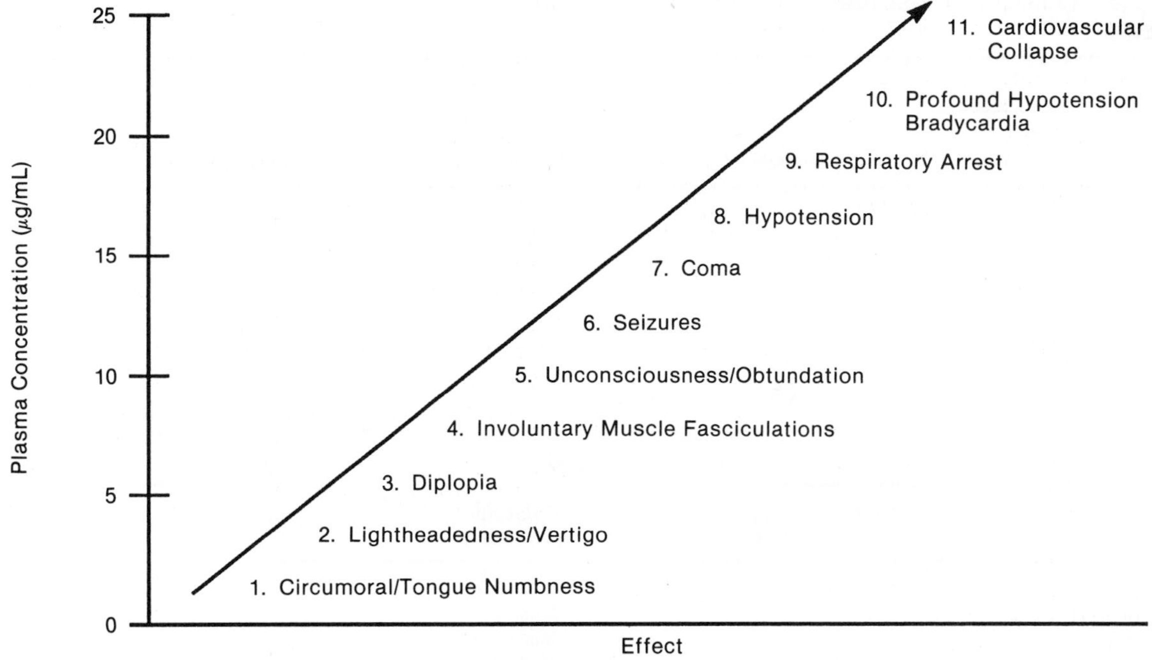

FIGURE 12–6. **Relationship between rising plasma concentrations and toxic effects.**

6. Patient's medical condition — cardiac and hypovolemic patients have reduced compensatory mechanisms against high local anesthetic levels.

CLINICAL APPLICATIONS

Clinical uses fall into three basic categories:

- Anesthetic actions
- Antiarrhythmic actions
- Analgesic/antineuropathic actions

Anesthetic Actions

Local anesthetics are employed ubiquitously to render peripheral or central nervous tissue insensitive to stimuli. One can apply these agents cutaneously (topical), subcutaneously (infiltrative), via peripheral nerve blocks, interpleurally, spinally, and epidurally in order to produce surgical anesthesia. A wide variety of agents are employed to accomplish these procedures. Table 12–3 explains the clinical characteristics of selected local anesthetics. The major distinctions elucidated by this table are that local anesthetics differ in onset, penetration, and duration. Chloroprocaine and procaine have the shortest durations, whereas tetracaine, bupivacaine, and etidocaine have the longest durations.

Topical to Skin or Mucous Membranes

Most of the local anesthetics on the market are water soluble and poorly soluble in oil; most are also poorly absorbed through the skin. An exception to this general rule are agents used for topical anesthesia. One of the most widely used drugs for topical anesthesia is benzocaine, which both is oil soluble and permeates the skin. Hence, benzocaine is available in ointments and creams for topical application on intact skin to relieve pain or itch associated with such conditions as skin rashes and sunburn.

For application to mucous membranes, cocaine, lidocaine, and a number of other agents (such as tetracaine [CETACAINE] and proparacaine [ALCAINE, OPHTHAINE] have been found to be effective. For both skin and mucous membranes, only the most superficial layers are exposed to effective concentrations of the anesthetic agent.

Antiarrhythmic Actions

Lidocaine is a class IB antiarrhythmic agent that blocks fast sodium channels to produce:

- Shortened AP duration and repolarization
- Unchanged QRS duration and conduction
- Increased fibrillation threshold

It is considered the drug of choice for ventricular ectopy such as fibrillation or tachycardia. No other parenteral local anesthetics are currently used as antiarrhythmics.

Analgesic/Antineuropathic Actions

Local anesthetics given intraspinally in low doses or in combination with opioid analgesics can selectively block pain while sparing sensory and motor nerve function. In fact, epidural local anesthetic agents are the drugs of choice for labor analgesia and postcesarean analgesia, and are commonly used for postoperative analgesia. The synergy found between simultaneous blockade of nerve conduction by local anesthetics and substance P release (pain neurotransmitter) by opioids in low doses has greatly enhanced the use of this technique while dramatically reducing the side effects of each agent.

Investigative studies have shown that delivery of local anesthetic to thalamic pain centers by intravenous or in-

TABLE 12–3. Clinical Characteristics and Concentrations of Selected Local Anesthetics

Low Potency, Short Duration

	Procaine (NOVOCAINE)	*2-Chloroprocaine (NESACAINE)*	*Lidocaine (XYLOCAINE)*
CHARACTERISTIC			
Latency (speed of onset)	Moderate	Fast	Fast
Penetration (diffusibility)	Moderate	Marked	Marked
Duration	Short	Very short	Moderate
CONCENTRATION			
Optimal concentrations (%)			
Infiltration	0.5	0.5	0.25
Spinal nerve and plexus block	1.5–2	1.0–2	0.5–1.0
Maximal amount (mg/kg)	12	15	6

Intermediate

	Mepivacaine (CARBOCAINE)	*Prilocaine (CITANEST)*
CHARACTERISTIC		
Latency (speed of onset)	Moderate	Moderate
Penetration (diffusibility)	Moderate	Moderate
Duration	Moderate	Moderate
CONCENTRATION		
Optimal concentrations (%)		
Infiltration	0.25	0.25
Spinal nerve and plexus block	0.5–1.0	0.5–1.0
Maximal amount (mg/kg)	6	6

Potent, Long Duration

	Tetracaine (PONTOCAINE)	*Bupivacaine (MARCAINE, SENSORCAINE)*	*Etidocaine (DURANEST)*	*Ropivacaine*
CHARACTERISTIC				
Latency (speed of onset)	Very slow	Fast	Very fast	Fast
Penetration (diffusibility)	Poor	Moderate	Moderate	Moderate
Duration	Long	Long	Long	Long
CONCENTRATION				
Optimal concentrations (%)				
Infiltration	0.05	0.05	0.1	—
Spinal nerve and plexus block	0.1–0.2	0.25–0.5	0.5–1.0	0.5–1.0
Maximal amount (mg/kg)	2	2	2	3

trathalamic injection can markedly reduce intractable pain associated with phantom limb phenomena, postherpetic neuralgia, thalamic pain syndromes, and peripheral neuropathic (deafferentation) pain. An oral lidocaine-like compound, mexiletine, has been successfully used to treat some of these aforementioned conditions. In addition, mexiletine has become useful in treating the neuropathic aspects of cancer pain produced by tumor invasion, chemotherapy, surgery, or radiation damage.

REFERENCES

Arthur GR: Pharmacokinetics of local anesthetics. *In* Strichartz GR (ed): Local Anesthetics, 165–186. Berlin: Springer-Verlag, 1987.

Covino BG: Clinical pharmacology of local anesthetic agents. *In* Cousins MJ, Bridenbaugh PO (eds): Neural Blockade in Clinical Anesthesia and Management of Pain, 2nd ed, 111–144. Philadelphia: JB Lippincott Co, 1988.

Covino BG, Vassallo HG (eds): Local Anesthetics: Mechanisms of Action and Clinical Use. New York: Grune & Stratton, 1976.

Denson DD, Mazoit JX: Physiology and pharmacology of local anesthetics. *In* Sinatra RS, Hord AH, Ginsberg B, Preble LM (eds): Acute Pain: Mechanisms and Management, 124–139. St Louis: Mosby Year Book, 1992.

DiFazio CA, Woods AM: Pharmacology of local anesthetics. *In* Raj DP (ed): Practical Management of Pain, 2nd ed, 685–700. St Louis: Mosby Year Book, 1992.

Smith CM: Local anesthesia and local anesthetics. *In* Smith CM, Reynard AM (eds): Textbook of Pharmacology, 213–225. Philadelphia: WB Saunders Co, 1992.

Strichartz GR: Neural physiology and local anesthetic action. *In* Cousins MJ, Bridenbaugh PO (eds): Neural Blockade in Clinical Anesthesia and Management of Pain, 2nd ed, 25–46. Philadelphia: JB Lippincott Co, 1988.

Tucker GT, Mather LE: Properties, absorption, and disposition of local anesthetics. *In* Cousins MJ, Bridgenbaugh PO (eds): Neural blockade in clinical anesthesia and management of pain, 2nd ed, 47–110. Philadelphia: JB Lippincott Co, 1988.

Wagers PW, Smith CM: Responses in dental nerves of dogs to tooth stimulation and the effects of systemically administered procaine, lidocaine and morphine. J Pharmacol Exp Ther 130:89–105, 1960.

Sensory Pharmacology 13

Cedric M. Smith

Sensory pharmacology is the study of actions of drugs on neuronal sensory receptors, resulting in an increase, decrease, or modification of afferent nerve activity. Sensory refers to both (1) afferent to the central nervous system (CNS) and (2) afferent to local nervous reflexes such as in the axon reflex and intrinsic nerve circuits of the gastrointestinal (GI) tract. Thus, in analogy with other drug classifications, drugs that have effects on sensory and afferent system are described as sensory or afferent drugs.

An important reason for examining the drugs that alter sensory afferent systems is the fact that most drugs alter sensory systems either directly or indirectly. In so doing, they have the potential to affect many organ systems, inasmuch as most body functions are under nervous control and are thus potentially affected by drugs that alter the afferent limb of nervous reflexes.

Knowledge of drug effects on sensory systems makes possible three classes of applications: *therapeutic use*; *detection of side effects*; and *tools for research.*

THERAPEUTIC USES OF DRUGS ACTING ON SENSORY RECEPTORS

A compilation of the therapeutic uses of drugs acting on sensory receptors is presented in Table 13-1. Those that illustrate the therapeutic applications best are listed first. This chapter will refer the reader to other chapters for agents described in detail elsewhere.

• Depression of Sensation, Analgesia, and Local Anesthesia

The local anesthetics (or cold), by their very nature, act to modify sensory input. Usually they are given locally so that they act directly on the endings or the nerve axon, but systemic administration also has had limited use (see Chapter 12).

• Nonsteroidal Anti-inflammatory Drugs

Nonsteroidal anti-inflammatory drugs (NSAIDs) (as well as capsaicin, discussed later in this section) act specifically on peripheral afferent receptor systems to decrease nociceptive receptor sensitivity and nerve activity, as well as to antagonize the process of inflammation (see Chapter 15). This class of agents illustrates, perhaps better than any other, the potential for drug actions at specific sensory targets. Although all agents of this class have similar pharmacological effects, there are differences in their relative potency for analgesia and for the reduction of inflammation, as well as for a variety of side effects.

• Opioids

Morphine and related analgesics have now been found to act, in addition to their multiple sites of action in the central nervous system, on opioid receptors in peripheral nociceptive systems. Thus, the analgesic actions of opioids are the result of both peripheral and central actions on sensory systems (see Chapter 14).

• Capsaicin and Methyl Salicylate—So-Called Counterirritants

Counterirritant is an ill-defined classification that is used for the lack of any other; unfortunately, it implies a probably incorrect mechanism of action. Capsaicin and methyl salicylate do produce some of the signs of inflammation and irritation, but the "irritating" properties of these agents are an insufficient and incomplete characterization. This group in-

TABLE 13–1. Therapeutic and Potential Uses of Drugs Affecting Afferent Input

Therapeutic Action	Some Examples
Depression of sensation, analgesia	Local anesthetics, ethylchloride spray
Analgesia	Salicylates, NSAIDs, caffeine antagonism of adenosine, bradykinin and substance P antagonists, counterirritants, capsaicin, methyl salicylate (amitriptyline, mexiletine)
Anti-inflammatory	NSAIDs, capsaicin, substance P antagonists, heat, cold
Local vasodilation, counterirritation	Capsaicin, methyl salicylate
Relief of cluster headache	Capsaicin intranasal
Abolition of triggers of neuralgic attacks	Carbamazepine, phenytoin, capsaicin, amitriptyline, desipramine, mexiletine
Muscle relaxation	Phenytoin, mephenesin, carbamazepine
Decreased muscle tremor	(*eg*, a sensory site of action of propranolol in reducing essential tremor is conceivable)
Antitussive	Benzoantate (TESSALON), menthol, camphor (?peripheral effects of diphenhydramine)
Relief of dyspnea	Morphine insuffiation
Nausea, vomiting	Apomorphine, ipecac, lithium (many drugs as side effect)
Modification of intestinal motility	Irritant laxatives, alcohol
Decreased blood pressure	Veratrum alkaloids, calcium channel blockers
Sensitization of warm receptor	Capsaicin, methyl salicylate
Sensitization/stimulation of cold receptors	Menthol, eugenol
Prevention of loss of smell—postmenopausal	Estrogens
Respiratory stimulation	Nicotine, choline esters, carbon dioxide, cyanide, doxapram
Antiemetic, antivertigo	(Possible sensory effects of phenothiazines, nabilone, diphenidol, scopolamine, cinnarizine)
Relief of tinnitus	Alprazolam, terfenadine, lidocaine, carbamazepine, phenytoin, trazadone
For diagnosis of:	
Panic disorder—caffeine taste test (DeMet et al, 1989)	
Digoxin toxicity—color vision test	

NSAIDs = nonsteroidal anti-inflammatory drugs.

cludes a rather wide variety of substances that have in common only the fact that they produce some of the signs of inflammation and irritation. They are used therapeutically by topical applications to the skin as creams or ointments for the symptomatic relief of muscle stiffness and soreness following

1. Bruises, extensive muscle use, or exposure to cold;
2. Tendinitis or bursitis associated with specific repeated movements; and
3. The pain and muscle stiffness frequently accompanying rheumatoid arthritis and osteoarthritis.

Capsaicin is also used for neuralgias. A Food and Drug Administration (FDA) advisory review panel has recognized the agents and classes shown in Table 13–2 as being "safe and effective."

In sufficient concentrations the compounds in Groups A and D (Table 13–2) produce reddening and erythema of the skin. The most widely used of all of these agents is methyl salicylate (oil of wintergreen; note the marked differences in action between methyl salicylate and aspirin, acetyl salicylate, and salicylic acid). When applied to intact skin, methyl salicylate, like most of the agents in this class, produces a sense of warmth and skin reddening. It is widely available in numerous creams by itself or in a variety of combination with other agents; for example, BEN-GAY preparations consist of methyl salicylate (15–29%) and menthol (7–16%) in a variety of bases. It is used for the topical treatment of muscle and joint pain. (Oil of wintergreen is also used in low concentrations for its pleasant taste and aroma. However, it is extremely toxic; as little as 4 ml of methyl salicylate has been fatal in children. However, as a topical ointment it has had a long and safe marketing history.)

• Mustard Oil (Allyl Isothiocyanate) and Turpentine

These agents not only cause irritation and erythema but also have the potential to produce blisters, vesication, urticaria, and tissue damage.

• Capsaicin

Capsaicin is the active ingredient in hot pepper of the genus *Capsicum*; as most people who have had direct experience with hot pepper know, capsaicin is not only hot to the taste, it produces the sensation of heat when applied to the skin and augments the intensity of any warm stimulus (temperature or infrared radiation). It has a remarkable specificity and potency. The threshold concentration for its perception in the taste of foods is of the order of 0.07 micromolar! Beyond its fascinating history and variety of its uses as a food flavoring, it has found widespread therapeutic use, and it has taken on major importance as a tool for unraveling the neurophysiology of a variety of neural and sensory systems.

Functional tolerance, "desensitization," develops to the taste, heat, and pain induced by oral or topical capsaicin when applied in low concentrations over a period of hours to days. In very high concentrations, or in neonatal animal experiments, capsaicin administration can result in death and degeneration of C fibers of the nerves on which it is applied.

TABLE 13–2. Counterirritants

Group	Characteristic Actions	Active Ingredients
A	Erythema, irritation	Mustard (allyl isothiocyanate), methy salicylate, turpentine oil
B	Cooling followed by warmth	Menthol, camphor
C	Warmth	Eucalyptus oil
D	Erythema, vasodilation	Histamine, methyl nicotinate
E	Irritation, sensation of warmth, erythema, and pain with large concentrations	Capsaicin, capsicum, capsicum oleoresin

ACUTE TOPICAL EFFECTS. Capsaicin selectively stimulates certain primary afferent neurons at their sensory endings, sometimes along their axons as well as at their terminations. When applied to the intact skin or mucous membranes in low concentrations, it may not have any directly detectable effects; however, it sensitizes warm receptors such that upon exposing the skin to a mild heat source, a sense of warmth localized to the area of the capsaicin application results. After application of higher concentrations, the agent alone produces the characteristic sensation of warmth and heat; in large concentrations it causes both pain and heat. Thus, capsaicin results in a local warming effect coupled with a decrease in the pain threshold to heat sufficient to produce spontaneous burning pain. These sensations can be reduced rapidly by cooling the skin surface (Fig. 13-1).

The symptomatic relief of pain following application of capsaicin is commonly accompanied by a feeling of warmth and erythema at the site of application. Although capsaicin can produce profound stimulation of warm receptors of skin or of mucous membranes, it produces almost no evidence of tissue damage or destruction. Thus, although it activates one of the systems critically involved in inflammation, it cannot be considered as an inflammatory substance.

MECHANISMS OF ACTION. The effects of capsaicin are, in the lowest concentrations, due to selective actions on afferent nerves mediating heat. Although capsaicin appears to be without appreciable effects on cold receptors, its application results in increased responses to stimulation by other modalities such as mechanoreception; that is, it produces hyperalgesia of mechanoreceptors.

Capsaicin selectively excites certain afferents responding to nociceptive chemical stimuli, including some of the so-called polymodal C fiber nociceptors. These endings are assumed to possess at least two membrane conductance systems, one of which is a transducer to heat while others transduce mechanical and other chemical stimuli. This concept implies that chemicals such as capsaicin act proximally to the sensory receptor-nerve activity transducer mechanisms. (Alternatively, the cross-modality perceptual responses that have been observed could take origin from two different afferent receptors and nerves that converge on a second-order sensory neuron.)

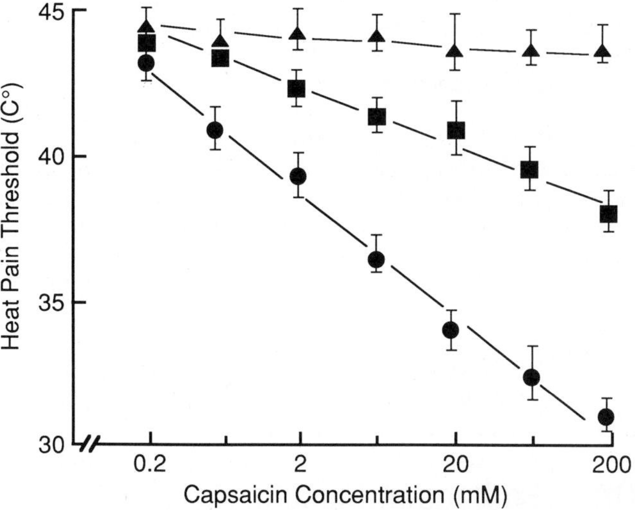

FIGURE 13-1. The dependence of threshold for heat pain (ordinate) on capsaicin concentration and time. Capsaicin was applied at the indicated concentrations (abscissa) to a linear array of skin patches on the anterior aspect of the forearm. The heat threshold was determined at 4 hours (*circles*), 11 hours (*squares*), and 21 hours (*triangles*) following application. (From Culp WJ, Ochoa J, Cline M, Dotson R: Heat and mechanical analgesia induced by capsaicin—Cross modality threshold in human C-nociceptors. Brain 112:1317-1331, 1989. By permission of Oxford University Press.)

Among the prime possible actions of capsaicin underlying the pharmacological effects observed after systemic as well as local administration are (1) **depletion of the peptide, substance P, from certain sensory neurons**; and (2) **blockade of the intraneural transport of nerve growth factor (NGF) and probably a variety of other peptides**. Substance P, an undecapeptide, is thought be a neurotransmitter or neuromodulator involved in certain afferent C fibers. Capsaicin-sensitive neurons possess specific *capsaicin receptors*. However, the mechanisms of action and origins of specificity are complex because not all neurons and sensory endings of certain modalities or size possess capsaicin receptors. It is probable that some sensory neurons containing substance P are not sensitive to capsaicin; and there may be primary afferents altered by capsaicin that do not contain substance P.

Not only is substance P important—a number of other neuropeptides including NGF are affected by capsaicin. Interestingly, the possible endogenous ligand(s) for capsaicin remain to be discovered. Although highly specific, the neurons sensitive to capsaicin do not correspond to any particular classification of afferent neurons; the degree of specificity varies for the acute and long-term effects, as well the dose/concentration, organ examined, age, strain, species, and route of administration (see comprehensive review of Holzer, 1991).

These hypotheses address the acute effects of capsaicin on the more sensitive of sensory systems. In addition, capsaicin has chronic effects that may oppose the acute actions, and higher concentrations of capsaicin affect a number of neuronal systems—the so-called cell-nonselective effects of capsaicin.

Note that capsaicin can be antagonized by the competitive antagonist capsazepine, a compound of immense value in the exploration of capsaicin's actions; ruthenium red has also been extensively studied as a selective antagonist. From a practical point of view, relief of intense oral burning from eating a high concentration of red peppers can be achieved, at least to a limited degree, by casein—most readily available in milk (Henkin, 1991).

BOX 13-1
THERAPEUTIC USES

The major therapeutic use of capsaicin is in over-the-counter topical ointments and creams used to facilitate relief of pain and muscle spasm in conditions of skeletal muscle aches, strains, sprains, or inflammatory states such as rheumatoid arthritis. In addition, it sometimes relieves postherpetic neuralgia, local stump pain, and some otherwise refractory painful diabetic neuropathy. (Examples of many preparations available are ZOSTRIX, with 0.025% capsaicin in a cream base; ZOSTRIX-HP, 0.075% capsaicin; and HEET, which contains oleoresin capsicum, 0.4%, camphor, 3.6%, methyl salicylate, 15%, and alcohol, 70%.)

SYSTEMIC AND CHRONIC EFFECTS. The interest in the specificity of action of capsaicin derives from the observation that the acute exposure to capsaicin, usually associated with sustained excitation of the sensitive sensory neurons, is followed by a sustained refractoriness ("desensitization"), a refractoriness not limited only to capsaicin but that extends to a wide variety of apparently chemically unrelated irritants and excitants as well. Tolerance to the heat and pain-producing effects of capsaicin is well-known to those who use hot peppers in their diet—and to those naive individuals inadvertently exposed to high concentrations. One of the mechanisms of this tolerance and refractoriness results from the capsaicin-induced depletion of substance P and the antagonism of nerve growth factor. This specific desensitization implies inactivation of the cellular transduction mechanism used by capsaicin; however, desensitization can occur in the absence of an excitatory action on sensory nerve endings.

Even more intriguing, when capsaicin is administered in high concentration or to neonatal rats, it results in degeneration and permanent loss of the majority of afferent C fibers. These observations were the initial starting points for extensive research endeavors that continue to the present time. To date none of the fascinating projects have realized improvements in therapy. However, there remains great potential for the application of capsaicin or analogs in new types of management of troublesome chronic pain syndromes as well as the elucidation of the pathophysiological roles mediated by peptides and local nerve activity.

CAUTION. Cautions that apply to all these agents are that they are **only to be used externally**; some of them can be extremely toxic if ingested. In addition, some individuals are known to be especially sensitive; allergic sensitization can also occur.

• Drug Effects on Sensory Receptors of Skeletal Muscle and Skeletal Muscle Function

In contrast to fibers that mediate pain, the large, rapidly conducting, afferent fibers from the muscle spindles can be dissected from the largely parallel fiber bundles in dorsal roots entering the spinal cord. Each skeletal muscle spindle is a complex organ with usually 2 or more afferent endings and 4 to 12 intrafusal muscle fibers on and around which the sensory endings terminate (or from which the activity takes origin, depending on the point of view). The sensory endings function physiologically to signal muscle length in response to stretch or the contraction of the long polar portions of the intrafusal muscle fibers.

Spindle Afferent Excitants

Succinylcholine and other depolarizing neuromuscular blocking agents, in addition to their depression of neuromuscular transmission, can produce truly dramatic excitation of muscle spindle afferents. Because one of the reflex consequences of this excitation is an excitation of motor neurons innervating the same muscle, the muscle spindle afferent stimulation is one of the causes of the transient fasciculations, twitches, and exaggerated stretch reflexes that are observed immediately following the intravenous injection of succinylcholine (see Chapter 8). Note that this excitation of spindles, like stretch of the muscle itself, is largely not perceived, even though information from these afferents reaches both the cerebellum and the cerebral cortex.

In addition to succinylcholine, a variety of quaternary nitrogen compounds as well as nicotine also produce muscle spindle afferent excitation. This excitation is due conceivably to direct effects on the sensory endings, but it is more likely the result of contraction and contracture of the specialized intrafusal muscle fibers. The pharmacology of these endings is illustrative of many sensory systems, in that they have unique cholinergic structure-activity relationships for stimulation (agonism) as well as for antagonism. In general, the more nicotinic [as opposed to muscarinic] the cholinergic agents are, the more potent they are, the more excitation they produce, and the more selectively they act on primary endings.

In addition, there are differential sensitivities of the primary and secondary endings, as indicated by marked effects of both nicotine and succinylcholine on the primary endings but only moderate effects on the secondary endings. The specificity of the receptors on the sensory receptor is evident not only from the actions of cholinergic agonists, but also with the selective block of most agents by tubocurarine but not by the antimuscarinic agent atropine.

OTHER AGENTS. A few agents other than cholinergic drugs are known to excite these muscle spindle receptors, including ethanol in blood concentrations associated with ataxia, as well as capsaicin and high potassium levels. (A stimulatory effect of potassium at most sensory endings would be anticipated in view of the membrane depolarization it would be expected to produce.)

The excitatory action of cholinergic agents is also selective for muscle spindle afferents, in that tendon organs in the same muscle are not excited even though they have large afferent fibers of the same size and conduction velocity as many spindle afferents.

Muscle Relaxants

Some of the so-called centrally acting muscle relaxants (**methocarbamol**, **dantrolene**, and **agents with some muscle relaxing actions such as phenytoin**, **chlorpromazine**) act, at least in part, on or through the peripheral sensory systems of muscle (see Chapter 22). Agents with actions on other sensory systems also have the potential for acting on muscle afferents. Benzonatate, a drug used therapeutically because of its cough suppressant action, experimentally depresses muscle spindle afferent activity analogous to its depressant, "local anesthetic," effect on receptors in the lung and bronchi.

Other Endings in Muscle

In addition to spindles and tendon organs, there are other muscle afferent nerve fibers in the Group III and IV categories. In contrast to the muscle spindles, almost nothing is known of the actions of drugs on their terminal receptors except that bradykinin is probably an excitant, a fact consistent with one function of kinins is to mediate muscle pain.

TABLE 13–3. Potentials for Therapy Utilizing Drug Action on Afferent Systems

Potential or Other Action	Some Examples
Antiepileptic for the reflex epilepsies	
Treatment of disorders of taste and smell	For phantageusia, clonazepam, thioridazine, haloperidol, pimozide have been reported to be effective
Altered odors, tastes, sound, and heat (more aversive or less aversive)	Sodium lauryl sulfate in toothpaste makes orange juice more bitter, less sweet
Alteration of appetite or consumption of foods or beverages, food flavors, or conversely, conditioned food aversion	Sweeteners, salt substitutes, glutamic acid, food and beverages mixtures, lithium
Antieating	
Antismoking	
Antidrinking	Acetazolamide abolishes the taste tingle due to carbonation, and alters sweet taste
Diuresis and antidiuresis	Drinking or oral exposure to hypotonic and hypertonic solutions, respectively
Modification of trophic influences of sensory verves	
Modification of the excitation of injured peripheral nerves to α-adrenergic surfaces	
Muscular dystrophy	Amiloride blocks the stretch-activated channel in muscle and muscle in muscular dystrophy; it may be useful as investigatory tool
Drugs as conditioned stimuli—drugs as discriminative stimuli, and possibly as one basis of placebo responses to drugs or other chemicals	Nicotine, alcohol, beverages, hallucinogens, opioids, amphetamines, sedative/hypnotics, psychotropic drugs, disulfiram alcohol reaction
Aromatherapy—fragrances that relieve anxiety	
Anesthetic states	Possibly dissociative conditions or new anesthetics
Anti-itch	Use of organoclay, as in IVYBLOCK, and in antiperspirants to prevent the itching and blistering resulting from exposure to the 3-n-alkyl-catechols produced by poison ivy
Production of itch, pain, unpleasant sensations	Itch powder, tear gases
Detection of toxic levels	Yellow vision with digitalis, diuretics
Use of drugs for esthetic purposes to enhance or modify senses and perception	Perfumes, food seasonings and flavor additives, cannabinols, lysergic acid diethylamide (LSD)

Among other therapeutic drugs acting on sensory endings are

- Phenytoin and muscle relaxants used to modify afferent activity from skeletal muscle (see Chapter 22);
- Benzonatate (TESSALON), antitussive used as a moderately useful cough remedy acting on receptors in the lungs;
- Ipecac and apomorphine, agents used for emesis that probably act on sensory receptors;
- Alprazolam, terfenadine or antiepileptic agents (phenytoin, carbamazepine), which may be helpful in relieving otherwise intractable tinnitus;
- Amitriptyline, carbamazepine, and mexiletine, each of which has been found to be effective in some patients with various painful neuropathic conditions.

Other known therapeutic uses of sensory drugs are listed in Table 13–1. Table 13–3 identifies a number of sites and mechanisms of potential drug development or application that involve actions on sensory systems, including drug effects on appetite generally or for specific flavors (also see Chapter 26 on anorexics and appetite stimulants).

SENSORY EFFECTS AS SIDE EFFECTS

Most drugs have side effects; many side effects consist of sensory disturbances of GI function, vision, taste, smell, and pain. Some drugs and drug classes have prominent or widespread effects on many sensory systems. As would be expected, all drugs that are local anesthetics or have local an-

TABLE 13–4. Drug Classes Having Potential for Effects on Many Sensory Systems

Drug Classes	Unique Sites or Effects
Local anesthetics (on systemic administration)	
eg, lidocaine, tocainide, encainide, amiodarone	
Quinine, quinidine	Tinnitus, peripheral neuropathy, blurred vision
Nonsteroidal anti-inflammatory drugs	Tinnitus, peripheral neuropathy, blurred vision, hearing impairment
Aspirin	
Indomethacin	
Naproxen	
Butazolidin	
Agents that alter calcium or calcium permeability	
Nifedipine	
Mexiletine	
Copper- or vitamin-deficient state	
Penicillamine	
Etidronate	
Cholinergic agonists	Skin, polymodal C nonciceptive fibers, carotid body, muscle spindles
Nicotine, acetylcholine, succinylcholine	
Histamine	C nociceptive, pain, itch, vagal afferents, cough
Adenosine	C nociceptive, pain, itch, cardiac, sympathetic (antagonized by caffeine or theophylline); probably activates peripheral endings, whereas in spinal cord suppresses nociceptive processes
Bradykinin	C nociceptive, pain, itch
Serotonin	C nociceptive, pain, itch
Caffeine	Blocks adenosine's peripheral actions
Substance P	Blocks adenosine's peripheral actions
Interleukins	Blocks adenosine's peripheral actions
Lithium	
Drugs altering NA^+, K^+ levels	Xanthopsia, vertigo, headache, paresthesias
Diuretics, thiazides	
Reserpine	Deafness, dizziness, headaches, pruritus
Tricyclic antidepressants	Numbness, tingling, paresthesias, neuropathy, tinnitus
Retinoids	Numerous side effects on visual auditory, and muscle as well as other major systems—CNS, GI, cardiovascular, neural

CNS = central nervous system; GI = gastrointestinal.

esthetic properties, such as cardiac antiarrhythmics, can produce a variety of sensory disturbances, among which are paresthesias, numbness, vertigo, dizziness, postural hypotension including slowing of the responses of blood pressure to changes in posture, visual disturbances, abnormal taste or smell, loss of appetite, and tinnitus (Tables 13–4 and 13–5). Many of these effects are of particular relevance to geriatric medicine — falls, changes in appetite, restrictions or abnormalities of visual and auditory functions.

The knowledge about side effects of drugs derives largely from alert, astute clinicians or from reports from patients, many of whom are receiving multiple drugs. For some

TABLE 13–5. Examples of Side Effects Attributable to Actions of Drugs on Sensory Systems*

Alterations In	Drug
Vision and Hearing	
Color vision (usually yellow)	Digitalis, pheniramine, thiazide diurectics
Visual acuity	Toxic amblyopia with nicotine, nicotinic acid
Blurred vision	Anticholinergic, atropinic compounds, phenothiazines, tricyclic antidepressants, urinary antispasmodics, enalapril, ranitidine, guanabenz, diphenidol, digoxin, nadolol, hydrochloroquine, amiodarone, diuretics, ACE inhibitors, β-adrenergic blocking agents, many others
Audition	
Tinnitus	Aspirin, quinine, quinidine, ibuprofen, naproxen, bupropion, numerous others
Hearing loss	Streptomycin, amikacin, kanamycin, chloroquine, erythromycin, tocainide, quinine, NSAIDs, naproxen, ketoprofen, indomethacin, bumetanide, ethacrynic acid, reserpine, erythromycin, antihistaminics, antiarrhythmic drugs, tricyclic antidepressants, phenothiazines, allopurinol, cholestyramine, and reported for many others
Skeletal Muscle Systems	
Ataxia, incoordination	Phenytoin, ethanol
Muscle pain postoperatively	Succinylcholine
Tremor	Lithium, phenothiazines, nicotine
Gastrointestinal System	
Nausea and vomiting	Lithium, aspirin, morphine, opioids, alcohol, digitalis, antibiotics, levodopa, NSAIDs, ergotamine, metronidazole, triazolam, guanadrel, baclofen, meclofenamate, methocarbamol, antineoplastic agents, yohimbine
Taste or Smell	
Reduced	Amebicides and anthelminitics (metronidazole, others)
	Anesthetics, local (benzocaine, procaine, cocaine, tetracaine, encainide)
	Anticholesteremic (clofibrate)
	Anticoagulants (phenindione)
	Antihistamines (chlorpheniramine)
	Antimicrobial agents (amphomycin, ampicillin, cefamandole, griseofulvin, ethambutol, lincomycin, sulfasalazine, streptomycin, tetracyclines, tyrothricin)
	Antiproliferative, including immunosuppressive agents (doxorubicin and methotrexate, azathioprine, carmustine, vincristine)
	Antirheumatic, analgesic-antipyretic, anti-inflammatory agents (allopurinol, colchincine, gold, levamisole, D-penicillamine, phenylbutazone, 5-thiopyridoxine)
	Antiseptics (hexetidine)
	Antithyroid agents (carbimazole, methimazole, methylthiouracil, propylthiouracil, thiouracil)
	Diuretics and antihypertensive agents (captopril, diazoxide, ethacrynic acid, acetazolamide, diltiazem, nifedipine)
	Hypoglycemic drugs (glipizide, phenformin and derivatives)
	Muscle relaxants and drugs for treatment of Parkinson's disease (baclofen, chlormezanone, levodopa, cyclobenzaprine)
	Opioids (codeine, hydromorphone, morphine)
	Psychopharmacologic, including antiepileptic drugs (carbamazepine, lithium carbonate, phenytoin, trifluoperazine, amitriptyline [effects of amitriptyline and/or symptom of depression])
	Autonomic drugs (amphetamines, phenmetrazine/phenbutrazate, anticholinergic)
	Vasodilators (oxyfedrine, bamifyline, nitroglycerin, dipyridamole)
Altered	Captopril, minoxidil, griseofulvin, histidine, lithium, benzonatate, trialkyl tin, phytonadione, diethylpropion, fenfluramine, pentoxifylline, phentermine, amoxapine, perphenazine, tricyclic antidepressants, mazindol, diltiazem, nifedipine, sodium lauryl sulfate (toothpaste)
Bitter	Carbamazepine, levodopa, phenylbutazone, organophosphate insecticides, azelastine
Metallic	Allopurinol, ethambutol, metals including gold, metronidazole, methocarbamol, lithium, azelastine, deodorants
Pain	
Headache	Numerous substances including aspirin, NSAIDs, vasodilators, sulfonamides, clonidine, buprenorphine, aminoglutethimide, benzodiazepines, cephalosporin antibiotics, ranitidine, piroxicam, antihistamines, terfenadine, guanadrel, antiarrhythmics, digoxin, lithium, amiloride, tricyclic antidepressants, baclofen, famotine, enalapril, butorphanol, meclofenamate, nifedipine, verapamil, diltiazem, maprotiline, mexiletine, acebutolol, naltrexone
Paresthesias	
	Many drugs, including verapamil, probucol, buspirone, tocainide, amiodarone, nadolol, pindolol, guanadrel, cephalosporins, dronabinol, phenytoin, ergotamine

Adapted and expanded from Schiffman, 1991.
*Partial list grouped roughly by class.
ACE = angiotensin-supporting enzyme; NSAIDs = nonsteroidal anti-inflammatory drugs.

drugs, the sensory side effects may occur so frequently that the majority of individuals receiving the drug will experience the effect. For others, the sensory effects may reproducibly appear only with large doses and/or in only a small percentage of patients. In addition, for drugs commonly used clinically together, such as diuretics and digitalis, it may be difficult to ascertain which drug is responsible for a given side effect, for example, the yellow vision or disturbed vision reported relatively frequently both with digitalis and with thiazide diuretics (Tables 13–4 and 13–5).

The haphazard way in which the data on side effects have been collected over the years, plus the varied terms used to describe such side effects, makes it difficult to draw precise comparisons of agents or to ascertain the actual probability of a given drug or drugs causing a certain sensory side effect. The Interactions and Side Effects Index to the Physicians' Desk Reference (PDR) allows ready access to lists on the side effects of drugs, at least as they are now tabulated in response to requirements of the FDA; the FDA approved package inserts that constitute most of the content of the PDR. Grossly underrepresented in these lists are both generic and older drugs, for example, such agents as aspirin or digoxin.

- *Side effects listed as frequent (eg, greater than 3–5% of a population) can generally be assumed to be associated with the drug or the disease for which it is being used.* Sensory side effects reported at lower frequencies could well be due to the drugs, but might also be due to other causes. Although sensory disturbance side effects may be due to a specific drug, they could also be due to the disease for which the drug is being prescribed. In the case of antihypertensive drugs such as guanadrel or methyldopa, both the drugs and the hypertension itself can cause headaches and paresthesias; either could be the result of drug effects or symptoms of hypertension. In the absence of good placebo-controlled studies, a distinction between two such possible causes is frequently impossible to make.
- *A special population at risk of sensory side effects of drugs is the elderly.* With aging there is frequently a deterioration in sensory function, as well as the taking of many drugs. Both of these result in aggravation of the very functions critical to the maintenance of healthy elders—awareness of their environment and active participation. Flavor enhancement can improve the nutritional status of the elderly (Schiffman et al, 1990). Among the common drug side effects are alterations of vision, hearing, taste, or smell. Decreased visual acuity and blurred vision may be of endogenous origin, but they are frequently contributed to by many drugs—perhaps most commonly by the many drugs with anticholinergic actions.
- *Tinnitus and hearing loss are frequent with aspirin, NSAIDs, a wide variety of antibiotics, and psychotropic drugs.* A change in hearing acuity in a patient mandates a major review of all medications received over past weeks and months.
- *Alterations in taste and smell are a frequent complaint of patients.* Such symptoms usually have an identifiable organic cause and are an indication for the review of medications in a search for a possible culprit. Drug effects include reduction in sensitivity or altered and specific tastes, most commonly bitter or metallic tastes (Table 13–5).

  A curious and instructive observation is provided by drug-induced decrease in craving for chocolate. Bupropion reportedly decreased the craving for chocolate in two patients (Michell, 1989).
- *Headaches are experienced by almost everyone at one time or another.* Yet drugs are a frequently overlooked cause of such headaches. Moreover, some of the most frequent causes are agents that are used commonly to treat headaches, such as aspirin and the NSAIDs. The number of possible perpetrators is extensive, as the partial list in Table 13–5 illustrates.

Patients are most often truthful, and their reports deserve to be accepted in the search for possible causes. Unfortunately, all too often the causes of such symptoms are the very drugs prescribed to alleviate disease and distress. As indicated in the tables, one of the following symptoms related to sensory disturbances could be caused by any of *hundreds to thousands of drug products*:

- Anorexia (see also Chapter 26)
- Nausea
- Vomiting
- Diarrhea
- Constipation
- Abdominal pain or cramps
- Headache
- Paresthesias, tingling
- Pruritus
- Numbness
- Dizziness
- Blurred vision
- Double vision

Therefore, each of such sensory symptoms deserves an explicit consideration and inquiry regarding the possibility that a drug may be responsible. Table 13–6 presents the sites of drug action on afferent systems.

The remarkable sensitivity for detection and differential discrimination in the olfactory system—more than 10,000 different odors—is now beginning to be understood (Table 13–5). Not only does the olfactory epithelium contain a

TABLE 13–6. Major Sites and Mechanisms of Action of Drugs Altering Taste, Smell, and Other Chemosensitive Systems

Modification of local environment, *eg*, nasal airflow, saliva production, vasodilation, local muscle activity
Taste or smell of drug itself delivered orally or by inhalation
Modification of permeability of receptor cell membrane
Alteration of transduction (receptor binding to nerve action potentials) processes
Induction of new membrane channels
Alteration of ion membrane channels for calcium, potassium, sodium
Interference with neurotransmitter systems (sensory systems contain most of the known neurotransmitter systems)
Alteration in the turnover of chemoreceptors
Modification of second messenger systems of adenylate cyclase or phosphoinositide systems; alteration of phosphodiesterases, interactions with adenosine receptors
Alterations in the afferent nerve conduction and central nervous system, *ie*,
Afferent terminals
Sensory pathways
Perceptual systems
Modifications of the *efferent* regulation that many sensory organs possess

large array of some 50 million or so neurons, the receptor systems for the odorant receptors probably consist of 100 or more gene families; this many gene families involved is strikingly different from, say, neurotransmitter receptor systems. Thus, it appears that a substantial amount of sensory coding occurs at the first stage of olfactory perception in the olfactory epithelium itself (Firestein, 1991).

"What are the structural relationships between chemoreceptors and other receptors? All receptors are chemoreceptors in the sense that they respond to [or bind to] chemicals. The difference resides only in the source of the chemical—endogenous or exogenous" (Max, 1992).

SPECIFICITY AND SPECTRUM OF ACTION OF SENSORY DRUGS

The rationales for classification of drugs with sensory effects involve consideration of various levels of integration, spanning from the molecular characteristics of the chemical substances to their localization and distribution, the specificity and spectrum of the action on specific end-organs, the reflex connections of the sensory systems, and finally the role of these sensory systems in adaptive nervous functions and behaviors. Thus, the spectrum of potential actions and effects is broad and ranges from narrow alteration in a specific sense, such as color vision or sensation of heat, to generalized increases and decreases in sensory functions to the extent that anesthesia and analgesia are encompassed in the topic.

Changes in Afferent Input and Conscious Awareness

It is easy to understand that drugs can alter sensory input from the major exteroceptors, such as ringing in the ears after aspirin, itching with histamine, or warmth with pepper. By contrast, it is difficult to appreciate that the vast majority of afferent nerve activity is not perceived directly; rather it is functionally involved in a variety of rather unconscious autonomic biological regulatory processes. For example, color and taste are usually perceived, whereas the detection of many body functions such muscle stretch, intestinal tone, blood sugar levels, or oxygen tension in blood is not. Essentially all of the visceral (interoceptive) afferent traffic is not consciously perceived or remembered (such as changes in neuroendocrine, cardiac, kidney, and respiratory functions). Nevertheless, the alterations in functions resulting from possible drug-induced effects on the sensory system may well be perceived. For example, alteration in the length detectors in skeletal muscle produces discoordination. Although the change in muscle length signaled by the afferent nerves, for example after succinylcholine or ethanol, is not experienced directly in such a situation, the individual perceives discoordination that results from the mismatch between what one wishes to accomplish and what is accomplished with voluntary muscle activation.

Another example is the drop in blood pressure induced by excitation of baroreceptors, an excitation that is not perceived but that results reflexively in fainting and falling, falling that is perceived. Stimulation of carotid chemoreceptors is not perceived, but hyperventilation and air hunger might be.

The autonomic, unconscious alterations of sensory input that can be produced by drugs can be appreciated only in the context of attention and awareness in which the change in afferent input occurs. As the old proverb goes: "We can look, but not see. See, but not perceive. Perceive, but not think. Think, but not act." More often than not, organisms respond to a change in sensory input yet frequently do not perceive the stimulus; commonly we perceive and become aware of only the responses to the afferent alterations after the fact.

The qualitative and quantitative changes in reflexes or the more indirect responses can be predicted only with difficulty, because the actions are functions of a great number of factors. These factors include route of drug administration, dosage, drug distribution, the degree of excitation or depression of various sensory endings, the numbers and type of sensory endings affected, the anatomical distribution of these endings, and finally, their ultimate destinations in the CNS.

The major practical consequences lie in the utilizing and potential therapeutic applications of drug actions on sensory systems, on the one hand, and the avoidance and recognition of the wide variety of potentially serious sensory side effects on the other.

REFERENCES

Aronson JK, Ford AR: The use of colour vision measurement in the diagnosis of digoxin toxicity. Q J Med (New Series XLIX) 195:273-282, 1980.

Berstein JE, Korman NJ, Bickers DR, et al: Topical capsaicin treatment of chronic postherpetic neuralgia. J Am Acad Dermatol 21:265-270, 1989.

Bevan S, Hothi S, Hughes G, James IF, Rang HLP, Shah K, Walpole CS, Yeats JC: Capsazepine: A competitive antagonist of the sensory neurone excitant capsaicin. Br J Pharmacol 107:544-552, 1992.

Buck SH, Burks TF: The neuropharmacology of capsaicin: Review of some recent observations. Pharmacol Rev 38:179-226, 1986.

Busis SN: Treatment of tinnitus. Questions and answers. JAMA 268:1467, 1992.

Culp WJ, Ochoa J, Cline M, Dotson R: Heat and mechanical hyperalgesia induced by capsaicin—cross modality threshold modulation in human C-nociceptors. Brain 112:1317-1331, 1989.

DeMet E, Stein MK, Tran C, et al: Caffeine taste test for panic disorder: Adenosine receptor supersensitivity. Psychiatry Res 30:231-242, 1989.

Dickenson AH: Capsaicin: gaps in our knowledge start to be filled. Trends Neurosci 14:265-266, 1991.

Eldred E, Yellin H, DeSantis M, Smith CM: Supplement to bibliography on muscle receptors: Their morphology, pathology, physiology and pharmacology. Exper Neurol 55(Part 2):1-118, 1977.

Firestein S: A noseful of odors. Trends Neurosci 14:270-272, 1991.

Getchell TV, Doty RL, Bartoshuk LM, Snow BJ Jr (eds): Smell and Taste in Health and Disease. New York: Raven Press, 1991.

Green BG: Capsaicin sensitization and desensitization on the tongue produced by brief exposures to a low concentration. Neurosci Lett 170:173-178, 1989.

Green BG, Mason JR, Kare MR: Chemical Senses, Vol 2. Irritation. New York: Marcel Dekker, 1990.

Hamill OP, Lane JW, McBride DW Jr: Amiloride: a molecular probe for mechanosensitive channels. TIPS 13:373-376, 1992.

Hartigh J den, Hilders CGJM, Schoemaker RC, Hulshof JH, Cohen AF, Vermeij P: Tinnitus suppression by intravenous lidocaine in relation to its plasma concentration. Clin Pharmacol Ther 54:415-420, 1993.

Hartung M, Leah J, Zimmerman M: The excitation of cutaneous nerve endings in a neuroma by capsaicin. Brain Res 499:363-366, 1989.

Henkin R: Cooling the burn from red peppers. JAMA 266:2766, 1991.

Henkin R: Salty and bitter taste. JAMA 265:2253, 1991.

Holzer P: Capsaicin: Cellular targets, mechanisms of action, and selectivity for thin sensory neurons. Pharmacol Rev 43:143-202, 1991.

Hu H, Fine J, Epstein P, et al: Tear gas—harassing agent or toxic chemical weapon? JAMA 262:660-663, 1989.

Jancso' G, Lawson SN: Transganglionic degeneration of capsaicin-sensitive C-fiber primary afferent terminals. Neuroscience 39:501-511, 1990.

Karrer T, Bartoshuk L: Oral capsaicin desensitization and its effect on taste. Chem Senses 15:597, 1990.

Lammers JWJ, Minette P, McCusker MT, et al: Capsaicin-induced bronchodilation in mild asthmatic subjects—possible role of nonadrenergic inhibitory system. J Appl Physiol 67:856-861, 1989.

Lembeck F: Columbus, capsicum and capsaicin: Past, present and future. Acta Physiol Hung 69:265-273, 1987.

Mattes RD, Cowart BJ, Schiavo MA, et al: Dietary evaluation of patients with smell and/or taste disorders. Am J Clin Nutr 51:233-240, 1990.

Max B: This and that: the essential pharmacology of herbs and spices. Trends Pharmacol Sci 13:15-20, 1992.

Michell GF, Mebane AH, Bilings CK: Effect of bupropion on chocolate craving [letter]. Am J Psychiatry 146:119-120, 1989.

Paintaud G, Alvan G, Berninger E, et al: The concentration-effect relationship of quinine-induced hearing impairment. Clin Pharmacol Ther 55:317-323, 1994.

Rayner HC, Atkins RC, Westerman RA: Relief of local stump pain by capsaicin cream. Lancet 2:1276-1277, 1989.

Ross DR, Varipapa RJ: Treatment of painful diabetic neuropathy with topical capsaicin. N Engl J Med 321:474-475, 1989.

Sawynok J, Yaksh TL: Caffeine as an analgesic adjuvant: A review of pharmacology and mechanisms of action. Pharm Rev 45:43-85, 1993.

Schiffman SS: Drugs influencing taste and smell perception. In Getchell TV, Doty RL, Bartoshuk LM, Snow BJ Jr (eds): Smell and Taste in Health and Disease, 851-862. New York: Raven Press, 1991.

Schiffman SS, Frey AE, Warwick ZS: Nutritional assessment of elderly persons eating flavor-enhanced foods. Chem Senses 15:633, 1990.

Smith CM: The effects of drugs on afferent nervous systems. In Burger A (ed): Chemical Constitution and Pharmacodynamic Action. Vol 1. Drugs Affecting the Peripheral Nervous System. New York: Marcel Dekker, 1967.

Smith CM: Variety of Effects Resulting from Drug Action on Sensory Receptors. Vol 4 of Pharmacology and the Future of Man. Basel: S Karger, 1973.

14 Opioid Analgesics—Agonists and Antagonists

Cedric M. Smith

One of the prime objectives of medicine is the alleviation of suffering. Thus, drugs that relieve pain and suffering are a major (perhaps *the* major) subject in all of pharmacology. The hallmark and standard of all medicines used to relieve suffering and pain are the opiates, specifically morphine. Morphine is the standard; after centuries of use it remains an extremely valuable and useful therapeutic agent to prevent or relieve moderate to severe pain.

Morphine is the major active ingredient in an ancient medicinal plant, the opium poppy. In addition, it is the parent substance for a host of synthetic compounds, some of which share some or all of morphine's actions (**opioids**; hence

opioid agonists), whereas some are complete or partial antagonists (**opioid antagonists**).

The study of the nature of the receptors with which morphine binds and thereby initiates its characteristic effects has led only recently to the remarkable discovery that within the body and the nervous system are a number of naturally occurring substances that bind to the morphine receptors to produce morphinelike effects. These naturally occurring substances—endorphins, enkephalins, and dynorphin—are discussed briefly. Nevertheless, because this chapter discusses drug therapy that results in the prevention or relief of pain, the nature of pain and its measurement are addressed initially.

BOX 14–1

DEFINITIONS

- Analgesic—a substance that reduces or abolishes pain, *ie*, a substance that produces analgesia
- Opiate—a substance derived from opium and possessing opiumlike (*ie*, morphinelike) actions, including but not limited to producing analgesia
- Opioid—a compound with morphinelike effects or that binds to the same receptors as morphine, including but not limited to producing analgesia.
- Narcotic—(1) an opioid agonist with pharmacological effects the same or similar to those of morphine, *ie*, a narcotic analgesic; (2) in old popular literature, any agent that can induce narcosis, a state of drugged sleep; (3) in the legal and law enforcement systems, all substances that the laws in that jurisdiction and time define as narcotics, *ie*, narcotics laws, narcotics police, and so forth (these frequently have included not only opiates but many substances that do not have morphinelike effects).

The knowledge base for rational therapy with analgesics includes

1. All of a drug's acute and chronic actions.
2. Mechanisms of a drug's analgesic actions
3. The relationships between the actions of analgesics actions and their potentially serious side effects
4. The variability among individuals with respect to the pharmacokinetics of the drug
5. The variability among individuals and disease conditions in the magnitude of the analgesic effects and of the side effects

ASSESSMENT AND MEASUREMENT OF PAIN

To relieve pain or to assess drug effects on pain, the nature of pain must be understood.

Pain varies with respect to

1. The stimuli, conditions, and sites of pain; the nature and intensity of the pain experienced vary with the number and types of nerves excited, the tissues involved, the excitability and conduction through central nervous system (CNS) pathways, and the levels of endogenous enkephalins and endorphins.
2. The subjective perception of pain as well as the objective responses to pain stimuli (both constitute nociception).
3. The critically important emotional, psychological, and behavioral counterparts of the perception of pain; concurrent stress or anxiety markedly aggravates any pain.

Stimuli and Conditions Causing Pain

Stimuli and conditions causing pain are varied and depend in part on the specific tissue, the nature of the stimulus (*eg*, heat, cold, cutting, stretching, ischemia), and its duration and intensity. For example, depending on the tissue, pain may be associated with incising the skin, stretching of tissues such as muscle or omentum, hypoxia of contracting skeletal muscle, immobility of extremities, distention (of bowel, bladder, and so forth), inflammation, or neuralgia. In general, the stimuli that are perceived as painful have the potential to damage tissues.

Nociception

Nociception is a subjective phenomenon that can vary along the dimensions of intensity or severity, character (*eg*, sharp, dull, boring, aching, burning, viselike), duration, frequency, recurrence, pattern, and location. The objective counterparts of pain perception include changes in heart rate, blood pressure, respiration, vasoconstriction, pallor, sweating, restlessness, withdrawal, and avoidance.

Emotional and Psychological Responses

The emotional and psychological components of pain are inexorably intertwined with the perceptual and reflex components. Among the more important in relation to treatment is the **meaning of the pain to the individual**. Pain perception and reactions are heavily based on expectations and learned responses, some of which are culturally conditioned. A particularly important factor influencing severe, chronic pain is its significance to the patient as actual or potential loss, with an attendant loss of personal control and autonomy. Pain is commonly accompanied by strong reactions of anger, anguish, fear, sadness, anxiety, depression, or frustration. These reactions need to be assessed on their own merits, but many are mutually interactive with pain. For example, anxiety and depression aggravate and potentiate all kinds of pain. Providing patients with greater control over their lives and medication, or relieving their anxiety, can result in marked decreases in perceived pain.

PREVENTION AND ALLEVIATION OF PAIN

> **BOX 14–2**
>
> **PRINCIPLES IN THE PREVENTION AND ALLEVIATION OF PAIN**
>
> - Remove the cause (treat the etiology).
> - Antagonize the mechanisms of pain and suffering.
> - Relieve anxiety.
> - Relieve depression.
> - Provide information to patient and increase patient's sense of personal control.
> - Promote positive suggestions of well-being; utilize the placebo effect potentially present in every patient.
> - Reduce sensory input that aggravates the pain.
> - Provide the most effective and complete pain relief as is possible, as soon as possible.
> - Prevent anxiety, fear, and learned responses that may augment perceived pain and pain-related behaviors.
>
> Take advantage of all of the drugs that may reduce pain, such as
>
> - Local and general anesthetics
> - Nonsteroidal anti-inflammatory drugs (aspirin, acetaminophen, ibuprofen, and others)
> - "Adjunctive agents" including caffeine, amphetamines, and adrenergic agonists such as clonidine, tricyclic antidepressants, carbamazepine, phenytoin, and hydroxyzine
> - Local agents and procedures such as capsaicin (Chapter 13)
> - Physical therapies

Placebo

A response to a drug that is the result of the act of taking it and not its content is termed a *placebo response*. The placebo response can be either positive, *eg*, pain relief, or negative, *eg*, headache or dizziness. Placebos are commonly used as one of the controls in clinical trials of drug actions and side effects; as the sole medication they have little place in modern therapeutics, although pain relief from placebos can frequently be equivalent to that produced by high doses of morphine. Note that

- There is always a placebo effect for essentially all drug administrations.
- The physician needs to learn which effects are from a placebo response and which are truly predictable pharmacological drug effects and how to keep the two separate in clinical thinking.
- Illness behavior including attracting attention; all illness has some secondary gain.
- A response to a "placebo" permits no diagnostic conclusion! A response after taking a placebo *cannot* be taken to mean that the patient is faking, that the patient's pain is not "real" (who could know but the patient?), or that the patient is "imagining" some illness or symptom.
- Patients usually tell the truth.

Classification of Opioids, Opiates, and Narcotic Analgesics

Prior to discussing the actions and uses of **the type of agent, morphine**, and related compounds, it is useful to provide a frame of reference for all the compounds in this class according to receptor action and specificity. The multiple opioid receptors were the first receptors in the brain to be identified and characterized. The first clues were provided by the study of selective agonists and by the availability of opioid antagonists. Five major classes of molecular opioid receptors have been defined. Three of these general classes (many subclasses exist) are designated mu (μ), kappa (κ), and delta (Δ); although the morphinelike analgesic drugs act primarily as agonists at some mu receptors, the kappa and delta receptors are also involved in pain systems and the actions of some opioid agonists. At each mu receptor, two

TABLE 14–1. Classification of Opioids, Opiates, Narcotic Analgesics—Opioid Agonists (Ag), Partial Agonists (pAg), Mixed Agonist/Antagonists, and Antagonists (Ant)*

Compound	Major Receptor Types: Mu	Delta	Kappa
Agonists			
Morphine (and codeine, oxycodone, meperidine, hydromorphone, fentanyl, etc...)	**Ag**	Ag	
Mixed Agonists/ Antagonists			
Buprenorphine (BUPRENEX)	**pAg**/Ant	—	Ant
Pentazocine (TALWIN NX)	Ant	—	**Ag**
Nalbuphine (NUBAIN)	Ant	—	**Ag**
Butorphanol (STADOL)	(Ant)	—	**Ag**
Antagonists			
Naloxone (NARCAN)	**Ant**	**Ant**	**Ant**
Nalorphine (NALLINE)	**Ant**	—	pAg

**Analgesia is the result of agonist activity at certain of the mu, delta, or kappa receptors.* Note also that drugs binding to the same classes of receptors may have different relative affinities for such receptors. (In the above simplified table, dashes are used because either the information is not available or the results are not quantitatively or selectively pertinent.)

A *partial agonist* is a substance that binds only to a limited degree (*ie*, has limited efficacy) to a population of receptors, *eg*, a drug that can bind to a receptor in two ways, one of which is agonistic and the other not. The apparent end effect of such an agent would be a function of the relative affinities for the two ways of binding. An example is buprenorphine at mu receptors.

A *mixed agonist-antagonist* results when the agent is a partial agonist alone but is antagonistic to a strong agonist. (The same end result of apparent mixed agonism-antagonism could result if the opioid agent acts on one subgroup of receptors as an agonist and on another subgroup as an antagonist.)

subclasses exist. At least the delta receptor class is genetically distinct based on cloning of that receptor (Evans et al, 1992). Theoretically, any drug could act by binding to any or all of these classes of receptors and then act as either an agonist or antagonist, or it could have mixed properties—agonist at some sites and antagonist at others.

Table 14-1 shows the specific receptor classes pertinent to most of the clinically used opioid analgesics. Nevertheless, the specificity (as determined by the specificities of agonists and antagonists in relation to their pharmacological actions and receptor topography) varies both with the species and with the neural locations.

ACTIONS OF OPIOIDS AS TYPIFIED BY MORPHINE

The primary source of morphine is opium obtained from the opium poppy. The pharmacological effects of opium, such as smoked opium, are due to its morphine content. (Thus, an opiate or opioid is a substance that produces the effects of opium, *ie*, morphine; an opioid is a substance not derived directly from opium but possessing the same properties. In modern usage, *opioid* and *opiate* tend to be employed interchangeably.) In addition to morphine, opium contains a number of alkaloids (**nitrogen-containing bases derived from plants**), including the therapeutically useful codeine and two agents not therapeutically significant, papaverine and thebaine.

Central Nervous System "Depressant Effects"

The primary uses of morphine derive from its dose-related effects on the CNS to cause analgesia, sedation, mental clouding, and euphoria. It also depresses respiration and the cough reflex and causes constipation, pupillary constriction, nausea, vomiting, and antidiuretic hormone release. (All of these effects are dose-related and occur after all the usual routes of administration—intramuscular, intravenous, or oral.)

Analgesia

The analgesia following administration of morphine is characterized by a sense of relief and well-being accompanying the decrease in pain—its perception and the reflex responses to the pain stimulus. The decrease in responses to pain applies to almost all kinds and intensities of pain; the depression of nociceptive (*ie*, pain) reflexes occurs even in the body below the level of a complete spinal cord section.

Not only does an increase in the sensory threshold for pain occur after the administration of morphine, but the relief from suffering also may exceed that owing solely to pain reduction. This has given rise to the partially accurate statement that morphine decreases the painfulness without a fully corresponding change in the level of perceived pain; after receiving morphine for pain, patients may describe the effects according to the cliché: "I have just as much pain, but it doesn't hurt as bad."

Although there is relief of pain and a change in nociception, morphine has no effects on other sensory modalities. (Reduced visual acuity may occur because of pupillary constriction.) Yet, the relief of pain can be dangerous.

> *Doses of analgesics which suppress the dysphoric sensations connected with the functions of the protective system do not influence sensory perceptions like touch, taste, vision and hearing and their mental assimilation. In this respect, analgesics contrast with general anesthetics. The invaluable relief given by the analgesics rests on their ability to suppress the protective system with its dysphoric sensations and anxiety. When using analgesics we have to keep in mind that they inactivate this protective system which serves the useful purpose of warning against injury.* Therefore the use of analgesics should be permitted, or indeed ordered, only when the warning has been heeded or the functions of the system have lost their meaning *[italics added] (Schaumann, 1956).*

Thus, opioid analgesics should be avoided until after a working diagnosis is made because opioids would abolish the symptoms and signs necessary for a diagnosis, *eg*, of an acute abdominal emergency. Giving an opioid for abdominal pain in the presence of unrecognized acute appendicitis can have tragic consequences.

Antianxiety

Closely associated with the relief of pain is morphine's effect of relieving anxiety, worry, and tension. In this respect alone morphine has a dramatic, acute effect to relieve anxiety and to induce a feeling of relaxation and tranquility, including the relief of painful memories and frustrations. For some individuals, morphine and other opioids produce an elevation of mood—an outright euphoria. Characteristic of this mood elevation are increased feelings of well-being, energy, and effectiveness. Nevertheless, for most people in the absence of pain, the effects of an opiate are most often perceived as mildly unpleasant and dysphoric, with an increase in anxiety or irritability.

Sedation

Morphine affects higher cortical functions; difficulty in concentrating or maintaining a train of thought may occur. In the absence of external stimulation, morphine induces sedation in the sense of drowsiness and induces a dream-filled sleep. With moderate analgesic doses, the patient may sleep but can be readily aroused. With higher doses, coma or a state of unconsciousness or anesthesia results.

Despite all of these neuronal actions, morphine has neither selective muscle-relaxant effects nor antiepileptic/antiseizure effects. If anything, the threshold for seizures is lowered after the administration of opioids.

Depression of Respiration

After the administration of morphine or any of the opioids, the rate and depth of respiration are decreased; the respiratory minute volume declines correspondingly. This depression of respiration is largely caused by a decrease in responsiveness to carbon dioxide (CO_2); this depression is synergic with sleep. With suppression of the CO_2 drive to respiration, hypoxia by way of the carotid chemoreceptors may be the only remaining drive for respiration. Under such a condition, a sudden increase in oxygen in the inspired air may result in cessation of respiration, resulting in further acidosis and CNS depression. With sufficient doses, respiratory arrest occurs and is followed by cardiovascular failure and death.

Respiratory depression is the major serious dose-related, predictable side effect of opioids. All opioids produce this dose-dependent depression of respiration, and it occurs with the doses used clinically for analgesia. As a general rule, equianalgesic doses (doses that produce equivalent degrees of analgesia) of all opioids produce approximately equivalent degrees of respiratory depression (the only exception may be high doses of codeine). The acute toxicity of all opioids is related primarily to their depression of respiration, an effect that can be fatal.

The increased CO_2 level consequent to decreased respiration results in an **increase in cerebrospinal fluid pressure**.

Depression of Cough Reflex

Independent of the effects on respiration, morphine and many of the opioids decrease or abolish the cough reflex. Depending on the patient's condition, a decreased cough reflex could be either a desirable relief of coughing or an undesirable effect, when it is helpful for the patient to cough actively, *eg*, after inhalation anesthesia. Cough suppression is mediated by unique opiate receptors, which are not stereospecific in contrast to most of the other receptor systems (see Dextromethorphan).

Other Central Nervous System Effects

Constriction of the Pupil

A characteristic effect of morphine and many, but not all, opioids is constriction of the pupil. This constriction is the consequence of central effects on the oculomotor (Edinger-Westphal) nucleus; morphine has little direct effect on pupillary muscles. Although this constriction occurs with most doses of morphine, it is not characteristic of all opioids. Moreover, with asphyxia resulting from morphine overdose, pupillary dilation may be present.

Nausea and Vomiting

Morphine induces nausea and even vomiting in some patients because of its stimulation of the chemoreceptor trigger zone in the medulla. With high doses, the converse, a decrease in vomiting, occurs because of morphine's depression of the vomiting center.

Endocrine Effects

Morphine has a complex cluster of effects on the endocrine system, including the depression of the release of a number of hormones (*eg*, antidiuretic hormone, corticotropin, prolactin, growth hormone, and gonadotrophic hormones).

Characteristically, morphine causes decreases in both libido and sexual activity.

Other Actions

Itching is common after systemic administration of morphine. The pruritus is probably caused by at least two mechanisms — histamine release, which is not mediated via opioid receptors, and CNS effects antagonizable by naloxone. The severe itching that can be associated with liver disease, particularly cholestasis, may be the result of increased levels of endogenous opioids inasmuch as it can be alleviated by opioid antagonists (Jones and Bergasa, 1992).

SITES AND MECHANISMS OF ANALGESIC ACTION OF MORPHINE AND OPIOIDS

Sites

Morphine has actions at a number of sites along the pain-analgesic pathways in the CNS. It has spinal, midbrain, thalamic, and cortical sites of action. Nociceptive spinal reflexes are depressed by morphine by way of the actions in the dorsal horn (substantia gelatinosa). Spinal intrathecal or epidural injections of morphine and other opioids can produce relief of pain, and this route has therapeutic utility in certain patients with severe chronic pain.

The opioid systems of the midbrain (periaqueductal gray matter and medulla) have been extensively studied because this area has both algesic and analgesic systems, as well as ascending and descending modulatory functions. The descending modulation of dorsal horn systems involves direct inhibition of nociceptive neurons, inhibition of excitatory relay interneurons, as well as excitation of an inhibitory interneuron. In the midbrain it appears that acetylcholine, neurotensin, γ-aminobutyric acid, norepinephrine, enkephalins, serotonin, and excitatory amino acids are involved in these pain modulation systems. Morphine also modifies the pain systems of the limbic, hypothalamic, and prefrontal cortical areas.

Until recently, the analgesic actions of opioids were thought to be limited to their effects on the CNS, in contrast with the nonsteroidal anti-inflammatory analgesics (Chapter 15). Recent studies have demonstrated that opioid receptors indeed exist in peripheral tissues and that alleviation of pain by opioids might involve peripheral as well as central actions.

Mechanisms

Opioid Receptors

Morphine binds stereospecifically as an agonist to specific receptors that have unique distributions in the nervous system, including (but not limited to) the sites enumerated earlier. These receptors and the binding have been characterized by studies of a large number of chemical analogs, on receptors from various neural sites, by histochemical mapping, and by receptor cloning. Thus, the receptors and receptor systems can be described by

- Neuronal location
- Correlation of chemical structures with pharmacological effects
- Kinetics of binding
- Interactions among ligands
- Influences of other factors possibly associated with the receptor systems such as ions (Ca^{2+}, Na^{+}) and various neuroamines
- Identification of amino acid sequence of cloned receptor

Figure 14–1 summarizes the complexity and some of the mechanisms underlying the remarkable specificity of different opioid compounds to the different receptor systems. This figure shows a minimal topography necessary to account for much of the structure activity relationships among a series of opioid derivatives. The entire receptor system is most likely a part of the nerve membrane and contains binding sites for the major moieties on morphine such as nitrogen and its substituents, the hydroxyl groups, the planar benzene ring, and the large bulky constituents. Not only can the binding sites be identified, but their approximate size and shape also can be deduced from study of the molecular structures that bind to specific sites as compared with those in which the orientation or the size of the important groups precludes effective attachment.

The cloned opioid receptors exhibit a homology to the G-protein-coupled receptors such as somatostatin, with seven predicted transmembrane domains. Although distinct, genes for the mu, delta and kappa receptors belong to the same family with a high degree of homology.

The steric theory of opioid receptors has several components. It assumes that opioid receptors have nuclear sites that are responsible for initiating the pharmacological action of the drug. Secondary sites play two roles: they determine the affinity of the drug for the receptor, and they define or limit the orientation of the drug on the receptor. Differences in the configuration of these two components (nuclear and secondary) may result in several effects on drug-receptor interactions. Changes in the molecular groups that bind to either the nuclear or the secondary sites result in altered activity. (*Allomorphism* is a term proposed to describe a change in the position of the active moieties of the nuclear part of the receptor, where *allosterism* is a change in the positions of the satellite [secondary] sites. Changes in either can result in altered affinity or orienting properties of the receptor for a drug. In addition, the term *allotaxia* has been suggested for the property whereby a drug can occupy the receptor in several orientations or positions [Martin, 1988].)

Future research will undoubtedly define the protein and peptide sequences of isolated opioid receptors and permit the reconstruction of some of the complete receptors, including detailed definition of their pre- and postsynaptic locations on neuronal membranes. **At present, we know that the opiate receptor systems are complex and are**

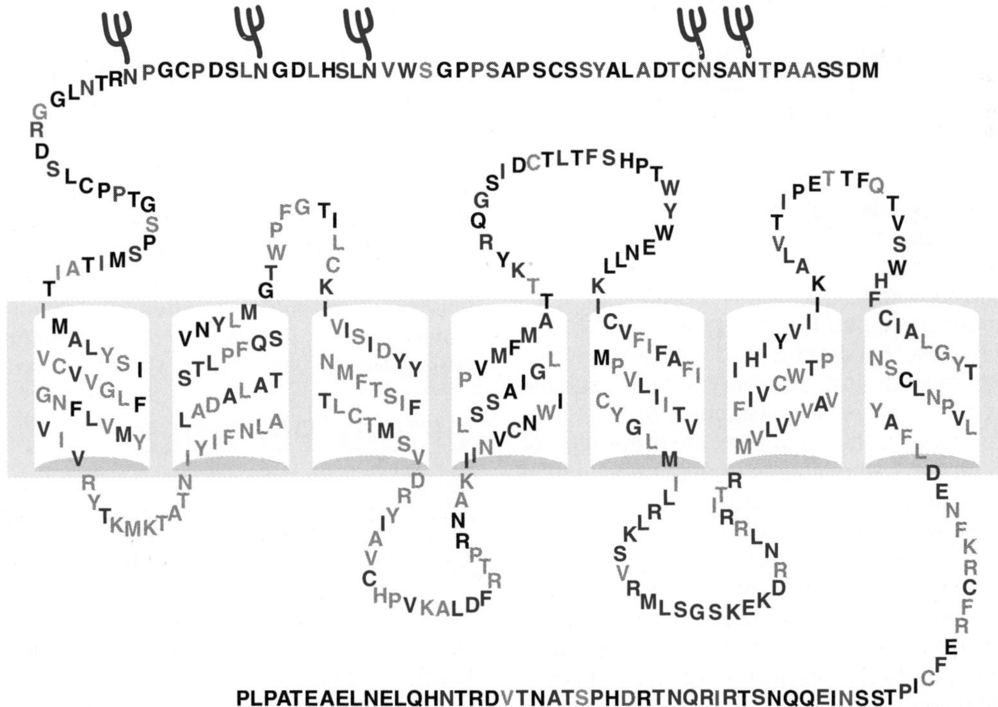

FIGURE 14–1. Cartoon depicting the amino acid sequence of the human mu opiate receptor. *Light blue*, amino acids shared by other neuropeptide and opiate receptors; *dark blue*, amino acids shared with other opiate receptors, remainder in *black*, amino acids not shared by other human opiate receptors. N- and C-terminus portions are found at the left and right sides of cartoon depictions, respectively. Transmembrane domains are indicated by *helices*, although varying alpha-helical contents are contained in each sequence. "Up" is "extracellular" and "down" is "intracellular." Sites for potential mu-receptor N-linked glycosylation are indicated by *branches*. Loop sizes and glycosylation site number vary among members of each family. (Adapted from Uhl GR, Childers S, Pasternak G: An opiate-receptor gene family reunion. Trends Neurosci 17:89–93, 1994.)

located both presynaptically and postsynaptically, that more than one type can be present on a given neuron, and that interaction occurs between different opioid receptors and neurotransmitters.

Depending on how many distinctions are made, from 5 to more than 12 molecularly distinct classes of opioid receptors exist. To understand current therapeutic agents, it is sufficient to identify 4 major classes of opioid receptors whose binding characteristics can be readily correlated with their pharmacological spectra of action. One of these, the cough suppressant receptor, is not stereospecific and is usually not considered among the stereospecific opioid receptors. Three of the most therapeutically relevant stereospecific receptors, as shown in Table 14-1, are the mu, delta, and kappa receptors. The stereospecificity applies both to compounds that are agonists (morphinelike) and to antagonists (such as naloxone). Compounds with pure agonist action at specific sites exist, *eg*, morphine, as do compounds with almost pure antagonist actions, *eg*, naloxone. In addition, many compounds with mixed agonist/antagonist properties are known, and some are clinically useful, *eg*, pentazocine.

The analgesic effects of morphine and the related opioids are the consequence of its binding to mu, delta, and kappa receptors; moreover, only a proportion of these receptors, which are localized at a relatively few specific sites, are actually involved in eliciting analgesia. In addition, mu receptors are involved in the respiratory depression, pupillary constriction, and changes in feeling states of improved self-image, increased energy, and effectiveness produced by opioid agonists. Not only do the opioids act on specific receptors, but neurons differ in their complement of the various receptor subtypes, and not all nociceptive systems contain opioid receptors.

The sigma receptor has relatively little relevance to therapeutics at present inasmuch as it mediates the perceptual, psychotomimetic, and increased irritability effects of certain experimental compounds and may possibly be involved in the actions of phencyclidine (see Chapters 11, 13, and 49). Some of the agonist/antagonists (pentazocine, butorphanol) bind to sigma receptors and have psychotomimetic effects in high doses.

Binding to mu receptors, in addition to producing analgesia, is also responsible in part for feelings of sedation and personal ineffectiveness that can be produced by opioids.

The characterization and discovery of the multiple opioid receptors are major accomplishments of recent research. Advances in the treatment of pain, the prevention of fatal poisoning, and the understanding of drug dependence are direct results of a long search for safe, nonaddicting substitutes for opiates. The evidence for the different receptors came from observations made in prison patients (at the US Public Health Service's Addiction Research Center in Lexington, KY) who were participating in studies on the safety and abuse potentiality of new analgesics. These studies were part of well-integrated efforts—both chemical and analytical studies on animals, human volunteers, and patients—involving the pharmaceutical industry, laboratories at the National Institutes of Health, and experimental studies in animals in academic departments of pharmacology and medicine (Uhl et al, 1994; Martin, 1988). As this chapter and Chapter 11 attest, these goals have been partially but not fully achieved with the availability of potent analgesics with improved safety margins and lesser abuse liabilities.

Receptor-Mediated Mechanisms of Opioid Action

Although receptor research has been remarkably successful in defining receptor structure, locations, and drug specificities, the mechanisms that are set in motion by agonist-receptor binding involved in analgesia are as yet not well defined. Presumably, opioids act to modify ionic permeabilities such as K^+ (and Ca^{2+}) conductance of nerve membranes, which in turn results in hyperpolarization and depression of excitability in the neuronal system. How this is accomplished has not been established. The end results of such actions include alterations in some portions in most, if not all, of the central cholinergic, adrenergic, serotonergic, and dopaminergic neurotransmitter systems.

It is also likely that opioids act by way of modifications of calcium uptake and binding in nerve endings. Electrophysiologically, some of the systems affected by opioids exhibit decreased cell discharge, membrane hyperpolarization, augmentation of hyperpolarization produced by repetitive neuronal firing, decreases in neuronal after-discharges, and decreases in temporal summation. Many appear to be coupled to guanine nucleotide-binding regulatory protein (G-proteins) secondary messengers; moreover, the interactions of receptors with G-proteins determine agonist affinities. The mu receptor may also be coupled to both cAMP and to inhibition of IP_3 (inositol 1,4,5-trisphosphate) turnover. The most relevant action is the ultimate effect of blocking the transmission of nociceptive information in ascending neuronal projections.

Reviewing these many actions emphasizes that the nociceptive systems utilize a number of neurotransmitters: substance P, enkephalin, and serotonin are involved at the spinal cord level, and serotonergic, adrenergic, cholinergic, and dopaminergic systems are involved in the medulla and midbrain pain pathways and reticular activating system, as well as in the periaqueductal gray matter. In general, adrenergic agents, such as amphetamine and dopamine, tend to reduce pain, whereas cholinergic and serotonergic agents tend to exacerbate it. In addition, adenosine or purinergic systems appear to be involved in the augmentation of analgesia produced by caffeine (Sawynok and Yaksh, 1993).

OPIOID PEPTIDES

The discovery and characterization of opioid receptors led directly to searches for endogenous ligands for them. These searches were rewarded with the discovery of a number of peptides that bind to opiate receptors and have morphine-like effects. The availability of the remarkably selective and specific antagonist, naloxone, made much of such research feasible; newer selective agonists and antagonists have permitted remarkable dissections of not only of the pharmacology of new drugs, but also of the physiology and neurochemistry of sensation and pain. A short list of some of the known endogenous compounds includes leucine-enkephalin (H-Tyr-Gly-Gly-Phe-Leu-OH); methionine-enkephalin (H-Tyr-Gly-Gly-Phe-Met-OH); β-endorphin; and dynorphins. (In addition to these peptides, morphine and codeine are present endogenously in low concentrations.)

Leucine-enkephalin (leuenkephalin) is identical to metenkephalin except for the replacement of "met" by "leu." Dynorphin is a 17-amino acid peptide containing the leucine-enkephalin sequence. These peptides are not synthesized directly but rather are the products of the cleavage of larger precursor polypeptides. Their local application to parts of the brain results in effects similar to those of opiates, and the actions are blocked by opioid antagonists. Although a large number of derivatives have been studied, none have yet been found to have clinical utility. But the search is not over. A number of as yet unidentified opioid peptides have been detected in brain extracts, and an opiate receptor ligand (binding agent) different from known endorphins has been reported in cerebrospinal fluid.

The endogenous opioid peptides bind members of the different classes of receptors to varying degrees; for example, dynorphin binds predominantly to kappa sites, whereas metenkephalin binds equally to the mu and kappa receptors.

The functions of these endogenous peptides with opiate actions remain an area of intense research. In general, it appears that they are not elaborated or active as analgesics in the normal state. This is consistent with the fact that the administration of opioid antagonists does not result in pain or other effects opposite to the effects produced by opioids, as would be expected if they antagonized existing opioids in the brain.

On the other hand, these endogenous opioid systems appear to be involved in the modulation of the responses to pain and nociceptive input by way of the extensive neural systems that modulate pain perception and responses. Sustained pain and certain types of stress are associated with the release of endogenous opioids. Consistent with such pain-induced release is the observation that naloxone administration can in certain circumstances increase the intensity of existing pain produced by noxious stimulation.

The troublesome itching associated with cholestasis appears to result from the down-regulation of the opioid receptors or the presence of high levels of opioids endogenously, in that naloxone administration to patients with chronic cholestatic liver disease not only alleviates the itching but it also provokes a syndrome similar to opiate withdrawal.

Thus, the endorphins and enkephalins and related substances probably have specific functions in specific neural systems but not directly as neurotransmitters. Evidence suggests that they may be involved as modulators of the presynaptic mechanisms involved in neurotransmitter synthesis/release in nociceptive pathways, including the descending modulation of nociceptive pathways.

In addition to pain systems, the endorphins are involved in central systems of appetitive drives (*eg*, for food, water, and sex), memory, mood states, mental processes, and traumatic nervous system damage. In experimental animals, naloxone dramatically increases the recovery of neurons damaged by trauma such as spinal cord compression. Other tissues, such as the placenta, are being found to contain endorphinlike peptides and their macromolecular precursors.

In recent years, not only have morphinelike peptides been discovered, but a wide variety of other peptides also have been identified as being involved in the regulation of organ function and behavior. Some examples of these peptides are the octapeptide involved in the control of food intake; pentagastrin; somatostatin; and thyrotropin-releasing factor, luteinizing hormone-releasing factor, and follicle-stimulating hormone.

MORPHINE-RELATED COMPOUNDS USED AS COUGH SUPPRESSANTS

Dextromethorphan

The lack of stereospecificity in the cough suppressant actions of morphine-related compounds was revealed by the discovery and introduction of dextromethorphan—the *d* isomer of a synthetic opioid. Dextromethorphan is an effective cough suppressant essentially devoid of any of the analgesic, respiratory-depressant, or euphorigenic effects of opioid agonists. Dextromethorphan is now widely available in over-the-counter cough and cold remedies; it has largely replaced codeine as a cough suppressant medication.

The rare serious overdose with dextromethorphan can apparently be reversed by naloxone. Although dextromethorphan is relatively devoid of toxic effects at recommended doses, it is not adequately appreciated that it can interact with monoamine oxidase inhibitors such as phenelzine or with fluoxetine to result in the life-threatening "CNS serotonin syndrome." Clomipramine and meperidine have each also been implicated in such adverse drug interactions (see also Chapter 50).

Dextromethorphan has also been found to have neuroprotective properties (see Naloxone), but it is difficult to obtain adequate blood levels in humans.

EFFECTS OF MORPHINE ON OTHER SYSTEMS

Smooth Muscle

Intestine

Many opioids share with opium and morphine the properties of causing constipation and decreasing the propulsive activity in the small and large intestines. This constipative effect has been known and utilized since antiquity. The decrease in motility and propulsion is the consequence of nonpainful, sustained contraction of the smooth muscles of the gut.

This constipating effect of opioids is a common, and sometimes distressing, side effect of all of the opioid agonists. Diarrhea is characterized by persistent propulsion, and morphine, even in doses below those needed for analgesia, provides effective temporary symptomatic relief of diarrhea.

The mechanism of the constipating action of opioids is complex, but it is known to be the result of both central and peripheral actions: actions in the CNS to increase vagal innervation of the bowel, and local actions directly on smooth muscle and on cholinergic neuroeffector transmission. At least a significant portion of the constipative, smooth muscle contractions can be antagonized by atropine, indicating that the opioid actions involve activation of cholinergic systems. (Both central and peripheral opiate receptors are involved in coordinated smooth muscle activity, as evidenced by the fact that naloxone, in experimental investigations, has been shown to increase intestinal motility.) The antidiarrheal actions of opioids are the result not only of changes in motility but also of an enhancement of net water and electrolyte absorption in both the large and the small bowel. This antisecretory action of opioids is stereospecific and blocked by naloxone.

ANTIDIARRHEAL PREPARATIONS. The time-honored antidiarrheal preparation of paregoric (a tincture of opium containing benzoic acid, camphor, and anise oil) is still available as an over-the-counter drug; its active ingredient is morphine.

Newer antidiarrheal agents that act selectively on opioid receptors include diphenoxylate (LOMOTIL is the trade name preparation that also includes atropine) and loperamide (IMODIUM, PEPTO DIARRHEA CONTROL—both are over-the-counter medications). That LOMOTIL contains atropine is not commonly appreciated and has contributed to anticholinergic toxicity, especially in the elderly. Diphenoxylate has morphinelike actions in high doses and, at least potentially, could be abused. Loperamide is essentially free of morphinelike effects outside of those on smooth muscle, yet a patient was reported to have increased the dose chronically to some 40 times the dose used for diarrhea control.

Biliary Tract, Bronchi, Ureters, and Urinary Bladder

Opioids increase biliary tract tone and pressure and can produce biliary colic. Morphine and other opioids can cause bronchoconstriction and ureteral smooth muscle contraction. For most patients these effects do not cause symptoms, but in the face of disease, such as cholelithiasis or bronchial asthma, the benefits and need for analgesia must be weighed against the risk of aggravating pre-existing conditions. For example, although opioids do cause constriction of the ureter, they are commonly administered in spite of this action to relieve the excruciating pain that may be caused by kidney stones.

In addition, morphine causes an increase in the tone of the detrusor muscle, urinary bladder, and vesical sphincter, which may lead to urinary retention or difficulty in urination.

All of these effects on smooth muscles can occur with doses equal to or sometimes less than those needed for analgesia. Thus, they all may be present as side effects when using opioids as analgesics.

Histamine Release

Morphine and many opioid agonists, such as heroin, cause peripheral vasodilation and itching. These effects are mediated at least in part by the release of histamine and can be blocked by the opioid antagonist naloxone.

Cardiovascular Effects

In doses used to produce analgesia, morphine and opioid agonists have little influence on the cardiovascular system. A flush of the skin is not uncommon, and a minor degree of orthostatic hypotension consistent with moderate peripheral vasodilation can be detected. This peripheral vasodilation is caused partly by histamine release.

TIME COURSE OF MORPHINE ACTIONS

After intramuscular or subcutaneous administration of morphine, the onset of action is prompt, yet the peak of analgesia may be delayed for 30 or 40 minutes. This delay appears to be related to the delay in the penetration of morphine to brain sites, because a similar time course for the appearance of peak analgesia is observed upon intravenous administration. Agents with greater lipid solubilities have a more rapid onset of action.

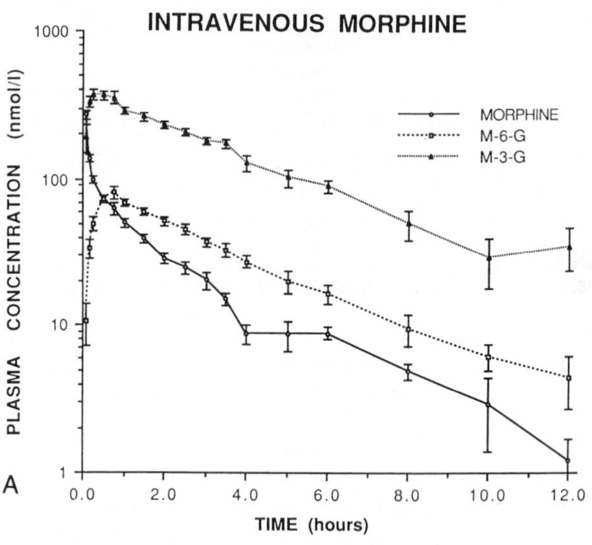

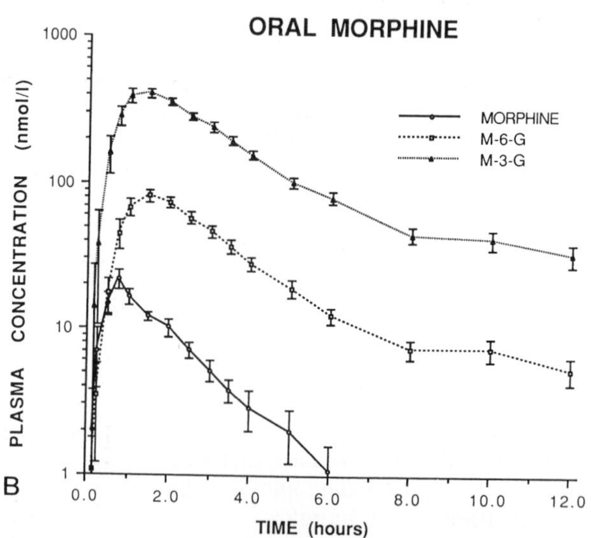

FIGURE 14–2. Plasma concentrations (mean + standard error of the mean [SEM]) of morphine, morphine-6-glucuronide (M-6-G), and morphine-3-glucuronide (M-3-G). (*A*), After intravenous administration of morphine, and (*B*), after oral administration of morphine. Note the logarithmic scale for the plasma concentrations. (From Osborne R, Joel S, Trew D, Slevin R: Morphine and metabolite behavior after different routes of morphine administration: Demonstration of the importance of the active metabolite morphine-6-glucuronide. Clin Pharmacol Ther 47:12–19, 1990.)

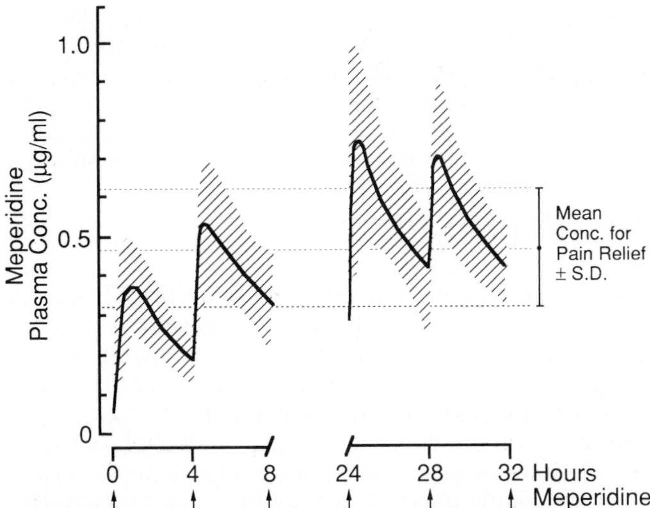

FIGURE 14–3. Practical aspects of blood levels—the importance of regular dosing and cumulation was explicitly examined in patients receiving meperidine (DEMEROL) postoperatively every 4 hours. The intensity of the pain experienced by patients postoperatively was measured at the same time as a blood sample was taken to measure the meperidine level.

The mean blood level of meperidine associated with pain relief (the minimal analgesic level) is plotted on the graph as the *horizontal dotted line* at ~0.48 µg/mL, with the ±1 standard deviation shown by the *horizontal dotted lines*.

The *heavy solid lines* indicate the actual mean blood levels obtained after the first, second, and last two doses; the *shaded areas* depict the standard deviation. Note the apparent absence of tolerance and the cumulation of levels into the analgesic, pain-relieving blood level range. (From Austin KL, Stapleton JV, Mather LE: Relationship between blood meperidine concentrations and analgesic response: A preliminary report. Anesthesiology 53:460–466, 1980.)

All narcotic analgesics are weak bases, moderately ionized at pH 7. Morphine is effective after oral administration, but the degree of first-pass effect differs appreciably among patients; therefore, the dose and frequency of oral administration must be adjusted on an individual basis.

Morphine is metabolized to two glucuronides, at the hydroxyl groups at positions 6 and 3 of the structure. The 6 glucuronide, to the surprise of many, not only has been found to have morphinelike effects but also appears to be many times as potent as morphine. In relation to the relevant kinetics, after intramuscular injection, the active agent is primarily morphine. After single oral doses, both morphine and the 6 glucuronide are present in active levels. With chronic oral administration, the 6 glucuronide accumulates to a greater degree than does morphine; thus, the glucuronide metabolite plays an increasingly significant role with chronic administration (Fig. 14–2).

The glucuronide metabolites are excreted by the kidney along with some free morphine; 90% of administered morphine can be accounted for in urinary excretion products over 24 hours. (As is discussed later, tolerance to an opioid is **not** caused by alterations in its metabolism.)

Not only are the metabolism and excretion of morphine and its active metabolite important in assessing morphine's effects, but they are also important to a discussion of the actions of codeine and heroin, two agents whose actions are caused, at least in part, by their conversion *in vivo* to morphine.

The duration of action of morphine and its metabolite is directly related to blood (*ie*, brain) levels; the analgesic effects are greater with higher blood levels, and the relief of pain decreases in parallel with the decline in blood (*ie*, brain) levels. Thus, no absolute or discretely definable duration of action exists; rather, in the face of continuing pain, the administration of morphine or other agonists such as meperidine results in maximal pain relief within 1 hour, followed by a gradual increase in pain over a period of 2–6 hours (Figs. 14–2 and 14–3). Thus, the time course of the relief of pain depends on the dose and the blood level achieved, the severity of the pain, and the individual patient's threshold for pain and its relief (Fig. 14–4).

TOLERANCE AND DEPENDENCE

With repeated administration of opioids, a tolerance to the effects of the agent develops. (By tolerance it is meant that a higher dose is needed to produce a given effect, or that a given dose produces quantitatively less effect). In general, this tolerance to opioids is limited to the so-called depressant effects of analgesia, respiratory depression, antianxiety effects, and drowsiness. Although individuals may be relatively tolerant to the respiratory depressant actions, suffi-

FIGURE 14–4. Variability among cancer patients with chronic pain with respect to the amount of morphine required for relief of pain. All the patients were receiving doses of morphine sufficient to relieve their pain. The cumulative frequency expressed as percent of patients is plotted against the total 24-hour oral intake of morphine. Note that the median daily dose, the dose that half of the patients were receiving, is relatively low, only 90 mg, whereas some patients required many times that dose level in order to obtain satisfactory analgesia. (Data from McQuay HJ, Caroll D, Faura CC, et al: Oral morphine in cancer pain: Influences on morphine and metabolite concentrations. Clin Pharmacol Ther 48:236–244, 1990.)

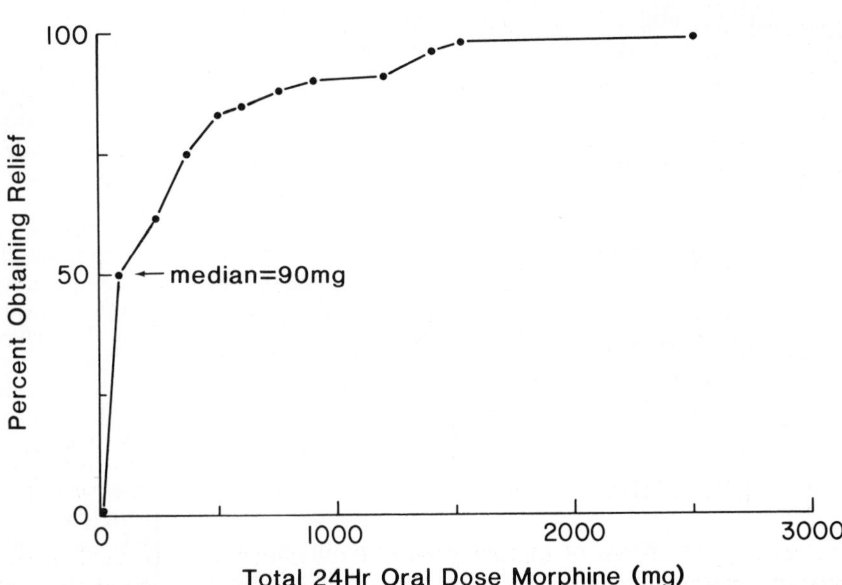

ciently high doses can produce respiratory depression and possibly death. In contrast, little tolerance develops to the constipation or pupillary constriction produced by opioids.

The development of tolerance depends on dose, repetition rate, and regularity of administration. The maximum degree of tolerance with opioids can be large, allowing doses some 10 to 20 times the initial dose to be tolerated.

The mechanism of functional tolerance and physical dependence involves the opioid and the neurotransmitter systems described earlier. In addition, the *N*-methyl-D-aspartate (NMDA) type of glutamate receptors and calcium channels are also known to be involved because blockade of these receptor systems reduces development of tolerance and dependence with chronic opioid administration.

Although marked tolerance can be observed in those dependent on opioids, in the clinical use of analgesics for pain relief, the development of tolerance is rarely a problem. Tolerance development is almost never a problem during the 1 – 3 days of opioid analgesic use commonly needed postoperatively or following trauma (Fig. 14 – 3). Even when opioids are used for the management of chronic pain (*eg*, for those terminal cancer patients who have pain), the tolerance that develops can be readily managed by dosage adjustment. Dosage and frequency of administration must be adjusted individually because patients vary markedly in their sensitivities (Fig. 14 – 4).

Cross-tolerance occurs among all opioid agonists.

With repeated administration of opioids, both habituation and dependence can develop (see Chapter 49). Presumably, the development of the habit of repeatedly taking a drug is related to a drug's potential to produce desirable subjective states such as euphoria, the relief of anxiety, or some other feeling state.

Physical dependence also occurs after chronic administration of progressively larger amounts, so that upon discontinuation of such administration, a characteristic withdrawal, or abstinence, sickness appears. Amounts required to induce such physical dependence can exceed, for example, 60 mg/day of morphine or its equivalent (analgesic intramuscular doses of morphine are 6 – 10 mg, commonly given every 4 – 6 hours).

The signs and symptoms of the abstinence syndrome are as follows: autonomic nervous system — sweating, vomiting, diarrhea, abdominal cramps, runny nose, shivering, goose flesh, increased heart rate and blood pressure, increased body temperature, and mydriasis; CNS — sleeplessness, restless sleep, irritability, tremor, joint and muscle pains, anorexia, yawning, dehydration, ketosis, weight loss, and hypophoria. The peak severity occurs some 36 – 72 hours after the last dose, and the symptoms gradually wane over a period of 2 – 5 weeks. This withdrawal is not life-threatening to an otherwise healthy individual and can be alleviated by any narcotic analgesic of the opiate-opioid class (see Chapter 49). A protracted abstinence syndrome of months in duration has also been identified.

SIDE EFFECTS OF MORPHINE AND OPIOIDS

The major side effects of morphine and opioids are the dose-related predictable effects just described. In addition, allergic reactions do occur; however, the claim of patients that they are allergic to one or another of the opioids must be assessed accurately. These reports can range from outright allergic reactions of potentially serious import, to precipitation of bronchial asthma, to the occurrence of predictable opioid effects such as nausea, vomiting, or constipation.

ACUTE POISONING

Acute poisoning with morphine and other opioids occurs with overdoses relative to the person's sensitivity, accidentally because of misjudgment in clinical settings, because of overdosing by addicts, and in suicide attempts. Among fatal drug poisonings, the narcotic analgesics are among the most commonly encountered, exceeding even alcohol. The signs and symptoms of poisoning are predictable on the basis of a knowledge of the pharmacology of the drug; characteristically, they include coma, pin-point pupils, and respiratory depression. With severe respiratory depression, impairment of cardiovascular function also occurs. Nevertheless, although respiratory depression with pin-point pupils is highly suggestive of opioid intoxication, barbiturate poisoning can present similarly. Conversely, with sustained hypoxia, morphine intoxication can result in pupillary dilation.

The treatment of suspected opioid overdose consists of the support of respiration and cardiovascular functions plus the administration of the definitive antagonist, naloxone. The naloxone administration will probably have to be repeated, inasmuch as naloxone has a shorter duration of action than morphine or of any other opioids that might have caused the poisoning.

CLINICAL USES

BOX 14 – 3
CLINICAL USES OF MORPHINE

Morphine remains a mainstay in the treatment (and prevention) of moderate to severe pain and of the situation and factors associated with such pain. Among the common situations and uses are

1. Preoperatively to relieve anxiety, produce analgesia, and reduce amount of anesthetic required; postoperatively to produce some degree of analgesia
2. To treat severe pain, *eg*, pain of fracture, large areas of soft-tissue trauma, a stone in a hollow viscus (such as ureteral stone), or metastatic carcinoma of bone
3. Postoperatively to relieve pain and discomfort in the immediate post-surgical period. In the absence of complications, postoperative pain requiring opioid medication usually lasts no more than 1 – 2 days.
4. To relieve pain associated with untreatable disease, such as metastatic cancer; for this purpose, orally administered morphine recently has been established as beneficial and useful; tolerance and dependence do occur with months of administration of high doses, but morphine requirement for pain relief disappears if the diseased tissues are removed (note that various oral preparations of morphine are not bioequivalent).

The important principles of use of morphine (and all opioid analgesics) address the classic questions of "who, what, where, when, and how much." These principles, outlined in Box 14-3, are all firmly established by medical research as well as by legal precedent. Failure to adhere to them can have tragic consequences because the opioid drugs have great potential for harm as well as benefit.

The selection of the drug, dose, route, and regimen should be based on the pain being experienced and anticipated; that is, the drug therapy needs to correspond to the pain syndrome. The opioid or any analgesic should be administered only after the diagnosis, even a preliminary diagnosis, has been made because the analgesic can mask the pain that is required for an accurate diagnosis. In severe acute pain, doses should be adequate to effect relief of the pain and then repeated frequently enough to maintain pain relief. **Pain intensities, degree of suffering, and individual sensitivity to opioids vary markedly among different patients. Moreover, adequate pain management requires the regular administration of doses to obtain the requisite accumulation (Fig. 14-3). It is now well established that p.r.n. (*pro re nata*, as needed) orders and prescriptions for management of severe pain are inappropriate and should be avoided. Rather, a specific repetition rate should be prescribed and then modified on the basis of the patient's actual responses. The established best prevention for the development of the chronic pain syndrome is the appropriate and adequate treatment of acute pain.**

Neonates

Neonates have a decreased clearance of morphine, as compared with adults. In addition, wide variability in the pharmacokinetic and pharmacodynamic parameters exists in neonates, including the absence of the active morphine-6-glucuronide. A dose regimen based on two consecutive constant-rate infusions has been proposed to achieve and maintain a steady-state concentration (Chay et al, 1992).

Patient-Controlled Analgesia

Automated intravenous delivery systems are now available that permit intermittent self-administration of opioids, for example morphine or hydromorphone. This technique has been found useful for relief of pain associated with surgery, sickle cell crises, and cancer. The systems operate under two modes—demand dosing of fixed dose injected intermittently, or constant-rate infusion plus demand dosing. The physician or nurse determines the loading dose, rate of background infusion, dose per demand, minimum time between demand doses (the lockout interval), and the maximum total dose over a specified time interval (*eg*, a demand dose of 1 mg of morphine sulfate with a lockout time of 5 to 10 minutes). By avoiding the potentially wide swings in blood levels associated with infrequent intramuscular administration, patient-controlled analgesia can provide more constant and uniform analgesia. In addition, it provides the patient with a sense of control and, more often than not, results in less analgesic drug use than is given in the more conventional intramuscular injections. The potential addictive aspects of opioid infusions have been negligible. Typical opioid side effects can occur, and operator errors can potentially result in continuous or excessive doses.

Another innovation that avoids the fluctuating levels associated with intermittent dosing is the transdermal system developed utilizing a fentanyl transdermal patch (DURAGESIC), which delivers 25-100 μg/hour of fentanyl for a total of 72 hours (see Fentanyl).

The major caution when selecting doses of any opioid is to be certain that excessive depression of the CNS and respiratory gas exchange is avoided. Special caution is in order when an opioid is used with other CNS depressants or in patients who have emphysema, bronchial asthma, or any other limitation of respiratory gas exchange.

OPIOID AGONISTS

Meperidine

A number of different opioids are available for clinical use (Table 14-2). Meperidine (DEMEROL, PETHIDINE) is considered here because it has been one of the most frequently ordered opioids for moderate to severe pain and for pre- and postoperative pain. It is a synthetic congener with a simpler structure than morphine; nevertheless, it has, with a few exceptions, all of the same major properties.

The actions of the opioid agonists are considered with reference to those of morphine. In short, meperidine is approximately one sixth as potent as morphine, and in sufficient doses it can produce equivalent degrees of analgesia and respiratory depression. In equianalgesic doses, meperidine is somewhat shorter-acting and less constipating, and it fails to produce pupillary constriction or cough suppression.

Pharmacological Effects

• **ANALGESIA.** The maximum level of analgesia obtainable with meperidine is equivalent to that obtained with morphine. Meperidine is less potent; 80-100 mg intramuscularly produces analgesia equivalent to that obtained with 10 mg of morphine sulfate.

• **BEHAVIOR AND SUBJECTIVE STATE.** Meperidine produces an affective state similar to that of morphine with feelings of calmness and well-being. Anxiety is relieved, and a dreamy drowsiness is common. High doses result in progressive depression of awareness and cognition and finally, coma. In excessive doses, CNS excitation also occurs with tremor, muscle twitches, and even seizures. (These excitatory effects are caused, at least in part, by a metabolite of meperidine, normeperidine, as described in Time Course of Action.)

• **RESPIRATION.** In acute doses equianalgesic to morphine, meperidine produces equivalent degrees of respiratory depression. Thus, the acute margin of safety is essentially equal to that of morphine.

• **COUGH REFLEX.** In contrast to morphine and codeine, meperidine does not depress the cough reflex. The absence of effects on the cough reflex is neither intrinsically medically beneficial nor harmful. Postoperatively, after inhalation general anesthesia, an active cough reflex is frequently desirable because coughing and deep vigorous respiration help prevent the development of atelectasis.

• **PUPIL.** In analgesic doses, meperidine does not

TABLE 14–2. Selected Opioid Analgesics Listed From Longest to Shortest Duration of Action

Morphinelike	Trade Name	Duration of Action (hours)	Analgesic Doses (mg)* IM	Oral	Used IV
Methadone	DOLOPHINE	4–6+	2.5–10	10	–
Levorphanol	LEVO-DROMORAN	4–6+	1–2	2–4	–
Codeine		4–5	15–60	15–60*	–
Hydromorphone†	DILAUDID	4–5	1–2	1–6	–
Oxymorphone‡	NUMORPHAN	4–5	1	NA	–
Morphine		**4–5**	**8–10**	**60**	+
Meperidine†‡		2–4	75–100	300	+
		IV			
Fentanyl	SUBLIMAZE	<1	0.05–01	NA	+
Sufentanil	SUFENTA	<1	NA	NA	+
Alfentanil	ALFENTA	<1	NA	NA	+
Selected Opioid Combination Oral Products					
Codeine	Many products with aspirin and with acetaminophen		NA	7.5–60	
Oxycodone	PERCODAN with aspirin			5–10	
	PERCOCET with acetaminophen		NA		
Hydrocodone	HYCODAN with homatropine methylbromide		NA	10	
	LORCET 10/650 with 650 mg of acetaminophen		NA	10	

*Lower doses used for cough suppression (*eg*, 10–20 mg for codeine).
†Less constipation.
‡Not antitussive.
IM = intramuscular; IV = intravenous; NA = not applicable.

produce pupillary constriction. (After toxic doses some pupillary constriction may occur, but this is not marked.)

• **SMOOTH MUSCLE.** Meperidine is spasmogenic on gastrointestinal, ureteral, and biliary smooth muscle, but these effects are somewhat less than those obtained with morphine. The clinical significance of this difference from morphine has long been a matter of dispute.

Side Effects

Similar to those of morphine, meperidine's side effects include respiratory depression, mental clouding, dizziness, sweating, nausea, vomiting, dysphoria, and urinary retention. High doses or chronic administration may give rise to seizures because of the normeperidine metabolite.

Time Course of Action

Meperidine, on average, has a shorter duration of action than morphine—approximately 2–4 hours versus 3–4 hours. In severe pain, such as in sickle cell crises, only 1–2 hours of pain relief might be obtained in some patients. Figure 14–3 illustrates the effects that can be predicted with meperidine. The mean blood level of meperidine associated with at least minimal pain relief did not change over a 32-hour period with repeated administration of meperidine (100 mg intramuscularly) every 4 hours. *Thus, no tolerance to the analgesic effects of meperidine was seen, even when it was given regularly on a 4-hour schedule.*

From these investigations it can be concluded that

1. Essentially no tolerance to the analgesic effects of meperidine develops during the immediate postoperative period (2–4 days).

2. The blood levels of meperidine in most of the patients after the first dose did not even achieve a minimal analgesic level, but an analgesic level was achieved with the accumulation occurring with the second and later doses. Thus, better pain relief is obtained when the meperidine is given on a regular basis rather than on the erratic basis of a p.r.n. (as needed) order.

3. Individuals differ markedly with respect to the blood levels obtained after given doses, as well as with respect to the levels needed to produce relief of pain. Hence, a large variation exists in the dose needed to obtain relief of pain; a large individual variability in time course and half-lives with meperidine (and other opioids) also exists. For example, meperidine could well have been given on a shorter schedule, *eg*, every 2.5 to 3 hours, in many patients.

Meperidine is metabolized in the liver to normeperidine. Normeperidine is not only twice as toxic as meperidine, but it has a longer half-life. As might be expected, with chronic administration of meperidine, normeperidine can accumulate. In addition, meperidine metabolism is subject to induction; for example, meperidine given after chronic phenobarbital administration results in increased normeperidine levels. As a consequence, *meperidine should not be used chronically, and it should be avoided in patients who have been receiving phenobarbital or any other drug likely to cause hepatic drug-metabolizing systems to be increased.*

Tolerance and Dependence

Without doubt, the repeated administration of meperidine is associated with habit formation, tolerance, and physical dependence with withdrawal symptoms upon discontinuation. (That is, meperidine [DEMEROL] is an addicting substance; see Chapter 49.)

Methadone

Actions

Methadone is a synthetic agent with effects similar to those of morphine. It has

- The same pharmacological actions as morphine
- A slower onset and longer duration of action
- Effects that are probably more predictable on acute oral administration than those of morphine
- Respiratory depression equivalent to that produced by morphine in equianalgesic doses

Side Effects

The side effects and risks of methadone are similar to those of morphine.

Tolerance and Dependence

Chronic use of methadone results in tolerance and dependence. The withdrawal syndrome may be months in duration.

> BOX 14–4
> **CLINICAL USES OF METHADONE**
>
> Three established uses of methadone exist:
>
> 1. As an analgesic
> 2. For treatment of the acute withdrawal syndrome after stopping any chronically administered opioid
> 3. For long-term management of opioid dependence (for a discussion of methadone maintenance, see Chapter 49).
>
> As an analgesic, methadone is suited especially for oral administration and for when a longer-acting agent than morphine is desired. The use of the shorter-acting morphine or meperidine permits ready dosage and frequency adjustments but frequent dosing. On the other hand, methadone need not be administered as frequently, but dosage adjustment in the event of excessive sedation or inadequate pain relief may be more difficult.

Codeine

Actions

- The chemical structure and effects of codeine are basically similar to those of morphine.
- The pharmacological effects are actually due in large part to the morphine produced by the metabolism of codeine.
- Some 10–20% of the population fail to obtain analgesic effect from codeine because of deficiencies in metabolism via the debrisoquin metabolic pathway.

By tradition, codeine has been used mostly for oral administration in relatively low doses for either cough suppression (antitussive) or for relief of mild to moderate pain. For example, low doses of codeine are combined frequently with aspirin or other nonsteroidal anti-inflammatory compounds for the management of moderate pain when the nonsteroidal agent is not adequate, such as in the management of pain following dental procedures, or for postoperative pain that does not require the usual parenteral doses of morphine. Actually, if a sufficient dose is administered to most individuals, codeine has the potential of producing analgesia equivalent to that produced by morphine.

Side Effects

The side effects of codeine are essentially those described for morphine. When administered in the usual oral doses (30 or 60 mg), the most common complaint is constipation. Some patients are aware of vague peculiar or unpleasant feelings, although some find the feelings pleasant and desirable; codeine, even orally, has a potential of being habit-forming.

Codeine and alcohol are the intoxicants involved in the abuse of **cough syrup**. The abuse potential is considered to be low—probably a reflection of the fact that the preponderance of prescriptions are for oral administration of relatively low doses, but it certainly does occur.

> BOX 14–5
> **CLINICAL USES OF CODEINE**
>
> Codeine is a frequently used analgesic, commonly combined with nonopioid analgesics. Such combinations are, in principle, rational inasmuch as the combination provides more pain relief than either one alone, and the use of low doses of each reduces the potential toxic effects of each.
>
> Codeine is available not only in oral preparations but in parenteral formulations and can be used for the management of mild to severe pain.

Other Opioids

Table 14–2 lists a number of the currently available opioid agonists. Note that many of them are effective analgesics; none has significant advantages over morphine, codeine, methadone, or the mixed opioid agonist/antagonists in the management of most painful conditions.

BOX 14-6

PROPOXYPHENE (DARVON—a drug of limited efficacy and potential for serious toxicity and abuse)

Actions. Propoxyphene has been extensively used as an analgesic for mild to moderate pain in conditions for which low-dose oral codeine has been traditionally prescribed. It is commonly administered in combination with aspirin or caffeine (or both) or acetaminophen. Although the claim is made that the combinations are more effective in relieving mild pain than aspirin or acetaminophen alone, the analgesia produced by propoxyphene alone is probably small. Unlike codeine, propoxyphene is not antitussive. Its limited analgesic efficacy and significant potential toxicity make the benefit-risk ratio so small that its use has doubtful justification.

Toxicity. Propoxyphene has long been viewed erroneously by the public and many physicians as being useful for relatively mild pain and devoid of serious side effects. On the contrary, its acute and chronic potential toxicity places it in doubtful status even as a prescribed drug. In acute overdoses it can be rapidly fatal. Its toxic effects are additive or more than additive with other CNS depressants such as alcohol or muscle relaxants. The CNS depression produced by propoxyphene is complicated by convulsions that are difficult to treat. It is second only to barbiturates as a prescription drug associated with drug fatalities, many of which are suicides or accidental overdoses.

Treatment of acute overdose centers on the maintenance of an adequate airway and assisted or artificial respiration, and the administration of naloxone (0.4–2 mg) intravenously, repeated every 2–3 minutes until an adequate respiratory response is obtained or a total of 10 mg is given.

Not only is acute toxicity a potential problem, but the chronic ingestion of propoxyphene can result in drug dependence with habituation, tolerance, and physical dependence.

Thus, the inclusion of propoxyphene (DARVON and combination preparations DARVOCET and DARVON-N WITH A.S.A.) in this textbook is justified largely on the basis of continuing misuse by some dentists and physicians when medications that are equally or more effective, less hazardous, and frequently less expensive are available.

Patients need to be educated regarding the facts about the drug, as described in the package insert and patient information brochures. They need to know especially about the potential interactions and the potential for abuse. Although the potential for abuse (or abuse liability) of codeine or of propoxyphene is less than that of parenteral morphine or meperidine, it remains a significant liability that deserves attention and prevention.

Heroin

Heroin is the diacetyl derivative of morphine; the sale and manufacture of heroin have been illegal since the 1930s.

The effects of heroin given intramuscularly are indistinguishable from those of morphine given by the same route. It is an effective opioid (narcotic) analgesic when administered in clinical situations.

Upon intravenous injection, heroin has a rapid onset of effects, both objectively and subjectively; this onset is much more rapid than after an equianalgesic dose of morphine, owing probably to its more rapid entry into the brain (see Chapter 49).

Heroin is metabolized extensively to morphine, and most of its pharmacological effects are due to morphine as well as to the heroin itself.

There are many other opioid agonists that could be used clinically; none of these possesses major advantages over those covered here.

SHORT-ACTING OPIOID AGONISTS

Fentanyl

Actions

- Fentanyl is a potent opioid agonist of relatively recent origin; a dose of 100 μg is approximately equivalent in analgesic activity to 10 mg of morphine or 75 mg of meperidine.
- It has a rapid onset, short duration of action, and greater lipid solubility than morphine.
- It is available for intravenous and intramuscular injections and as a sustained-release skin patch (fentanyl transdermal system, DURAGESIC; oral transmucosal lozenge, ORALET).

The major actions are similar to those of morphine. To date, it has been used for its sedative and analgesic effects almost exclusively in the context of anesthesia and operative procedures, as a principal anesthetic agent or as an analgesic in combination with other agents (see Chapter 11).

Side Effects

- Dose-related depression of respiration ranging from decreased sensitivity to CO_2 to outright apnea may occur. Some depression of respiration can persist longer than effective analgesia and is manifested by shallow, slow respiration. The respiratory depression appears 5–15 minutes after intravenous injections and can persist for up to 4 hours after a single dose.
- Caution—in view of the potent, rapidly occurring actions of fentanyl, it should be given only by those trained in its use and when the opioid antagonist naloxone, resuscitative equipment, and properly prepared staff are immediately available.
- Fentanyl may cause skeletal muscle rigidity, which can be especially troublesome when this involves respiratory and trunk muscles. The muscle activity can be so marked that it can interfere with the induction of anesthesia.
- Few direct effects on cardiac function exist except for the production of moderate bradycardia.
- Histamine release is rarely a problem.

Chronic Toxicity

Although fentanyl has not been chronically administered therapeutically, repeated self-administration results in a morphine-type dependence; the availability of the drug presents a significant risk for abuse by anesthesia professionals.

Sufentanil

Actions

- Sufentanil is similar in actions and therapeutic uses to fentanyl.
- It is up to 10 times more potent than fentanyl. (Using doses such as 8 μg/kg intravenously, it produces profound analgesia almost immediately.)
- It has a short onset and duration of action.
- Sufentanil has a distribution time of a few minutes and an elimination half-life of approximately 2–3 hours. More than 90% is bound to plasma proteins.
- Sufentanil is employed as the sole analgesic, as an anesthetic, or in combination with other anesthetics.

Side Effects

- Respiratory depression
- Muscular rigidity, as with fentanyl

The respiratory depression produced by sufentanil or fentanyl can be reversed by naloxone.

Insufficient data exist on the safety of sufentanil during pregnancy or in labor and delivery to support its use in these conditions.

Tolerance and Dependence

Sufentanil, like fentanyl, is a Schedule II controlled drug substance that can produce tolerance and dependence of the morphine type.

Alfentanil

Alfentanil is, like the others in this group, a potent opioid, but it is distinguished by a rapid onset and an even shorter duration of action than those of sufentanil. The rapid and short duration of action allow it to be used not only by intravenous injection but also by intravenous infusion. (Although the time required for recovery, recurrence of pain, and adequate respiration vary markedly according to blood level, individual patient, and the procedure, as a generalization alfentanil is shorter-acting than sufentanil, which is of significantly shorter duration of action than fentanyl, which in turn is much shorter-acting than morphine.) If recovery from morphine required approximately 2 hours, fentanyl would require 1 hour, and sufentanil and alfentanil, 20 minutes or less. The level of analgesia or "anesthesia" obtained with alfentanil can be regulated by close observation of the patient or by blood levels. Thus, alfentanil is currently enjoying wide use (1) as an analgesic adjunct in the maintenance of anesthesia with other agents such as barbiturates/nitrous oxide/oxygen, and (2) as a primary anesthetic for induction of anesthesia for general surgery.

These rapidly acting, short-duration fentanyl derivatives have found widespread use in anesthesia, especially for cardiac surgery. But they have a number of disadvantages or unwanted side effects. In addition to the anticipated respiratory depression, amnesia is not always complete, episodes of hypertension or bradycardia occur, and muscle rigidity is common.

MIXED OPIOID AGONIST/ANTAGONISTS

Pentazocine

Investigation of the subjective effects of the first known morphine antagonist, the *N*-allyl derivative (nalorphine, NALLINE), revealed that it had analgesic effects. The substance also produced unpleasant subjective effects that precluded further consideration as an analgesic. Nevertheless, that observation established that a compound could be, at the same time, both an analgesic and an opioid antagonist, and that it probably would not be abused. This observation set the stage for the discovery decades later of therapeutically useful agents that were mixed agonist/antagonists. The first of these widely marketed as an analgesic was pentazocine.

Actions

- Analgesia is the result of pentazocine's agonistic actions at the kappa class of opioid receptors.
- Analgesia and drowsiness are similar to those produced by morphine.
- A 30-mg dose of pentazocine is approximately equianalgesic with 10 mg of morphine or to 80–100 mg of meperidine.
- The time course and duration of action of 3 hours is similar to those of morphine.

Side Effects

- Respiratory depression, which on a single acute dose is equivalent to that produced by an equianalgesic dose of morphine, may occur.
- Sedation may occur, and some patients experience hallucinations or confusion.
- Nausea, vomiting, and dysphoria are common.
- Cardiovascular effects are similar to those of morphine.
- No antidiuretic effect is seen.
- Gastrointestinal effects are not prominent (and have not been studied extensively).
- Seizures have occurred after administration of pentazocine in patients susceptible to seizures.
- Repeated parenteral injections of pentazocine result in the unsightly and nearly irreversible induration of connective tissues in the skin.

Tolerance and Dependence

Chronic administration of pentazocine results in tolerance and dependence.

Its oral use has low abuse liability, but with injection a small number of cases of abuse (many of them involving medical professionals) have occurred. Pentazocine became a drug of abuse; it was used intravenously in combination with the antihistaminics tripelennamine (PYRIBENZAMINE) or diphenhydramine (BENADRYL). This abuse led to the development of a unique oral preparation, TALWIN-NX, consisting of pentazocine combined with naloxone. If the combination is injected intravenously, the naloxone effectively antagonizes the opioid effects of the pentazocine. On the other hand, when the combination is ingested, the naloxone is rapidly metabolized, leaving only the pentazocine to produce its desired analgesic effects.

Opioid Antagonism

Pentazocine, and potentially all the mixed agonist/antagonists, can antagonize the actions of opioid agonists such as morphine. Obviously, its use should be avoided in anyone who has received an opioid recently or those dependent on any opioid.

Nalbuphine

Actions

- Nalbuphine is an effective analgesic.
- It has approximately the same potency and duration of effect as morphine.
- Analgesia is the consequence of kappa receptor agonism.

Side Effects

- Nalbuphine, as well as butorphanol, has proportionately fewer respiratory depressant effects after high doses than does morphine. Consequently, for possible chronic use or when high doses are used, these agents may have a wider margin of safety and may represent a useful alternative to morphine.

Butorphanol

Actions and Side Effects

- Butorphanol is a potent kappa agonist (*eg*, the usual analgesic dose is 2–4 mg intramuscularly).
- Duration of action is similar to that of morphine.
- Side effects are similar to those of morphine but with less respiratory depression following high doses or overdoses.

Buprenorphine

Buprenorphine is a unique opioid by virtue of its long duration of action and high potency.

- It is a potent analgesic (a dose of 0.3 mg intramuscularly is equivalent to 10 mg of morphine).
- It is long-acting; peak effects occur in approximately 1 hour, and the analgesic action can be sustained for up to 6 hours.
- The actions of buprenorphine are the consequence of its tight binding and partial agonistic actions at the mu and kappa opioid receptors.
- It is effective parenterally but is also well absorbed upon sublingual administration.

Side Effects

- The side effects are similar to those produced by morphine — most common are sedation and drowsiness; nausea and vomiting occur in 10 to 20%.
- Most serious is depression of respiration similar to that with morphine in equianalgesic doses, but relatively lesser increases with increasing doses than obtains with morphine.
- High doses of naloxone are required to reverse the action of buprenorphine.
- It is an antagonist of morphine and other opioid agonists.

Dezocine

Dezocine is a new mixed agonist/antagonist available in a parenteral formulation. It is similar to morphine in time course of analgesic effects and side effects.

General Comments Regarding Mixed Agonist/Antagonists

- Some individuals will probably develop dependence on each of these mixed agonists/antagonists, but the data to date suggest that they are all less likely to be associated with habitual self-administration or physical dependence than morphine. The physical dependence in buprenorphine-maintained patients is of a low order of intensity and long duration. Upon detoxification, the patients exhibit only mild signs of acute abstinence and discomfort (see Chapter 49).
- These agents should be avoided in any patient who might have received or might receive another opioid.

Chronic Pain

This chapter has focused on the treatment of severe to moderate pain in the context of acute pain, such as that occurring postoperatively, or severe pain of malignant disease. Certain opioids are contraindicated for chronic use because of potential toxicity, for example meperidine and propoxyphene. Other opioids have been used with reported efficacy for both pain of some malignancies and of some nonmalignant conditions, for example migraine headaches or rheumatoid arthritis.

The expression "chronic pain" is used ambiguously. On

the one hand it refers simply to the pain associated with chronic disease, whether this is associated with malignant or nonmalignant conditions. On the other hand, chronic pain is used to refer to a somewhat ill-defined condition, "chronic pain syndrome," which consists of persistent complaints of moderate to severe pain, but where the pain reported is inconsistent with the only modest apparent pathology and an overt indifferent, inappropriate affect. In any event, chronic pain associated with prolonged tissue damage or nerve injuries results in extensive changes in the functions of nociceptive pathways.

For certain chronic conditions, opioids appear to be the last option for drug therapy sufficient to provide relief of pain, yet their use poses major problems of potential abuse, difficulty in monitoring, and harassment by regulatory agencies. Rational and reasonable guidelines for the use of opioids in the therapy of chronic nonmalignant pain have only recently been proposed (Portenoy, 1994; Reidenberg and Portenoy, 1994). These guidelines include exploiting all methods of analgesia, close and regular monitoring of all therapies, rational dose adjustments of analgesics, the detection and avoidance of drug hoarding or drug abuse, plus the essential documentation of the patient's condition, responses to drugs, and appearance of untoward effects and behaviors.

OPIOID ANTAGONISTS

Naloxone

Actions

- Naloxone (NARCAN) is the prototype opioid antagonist and the antagonist drug of choice at the present time. It antagonizes opioid-induced euphoria, analgesia, drowsiness, and respiratory depression. It appears to be less effective against the stimulant actions such as pupillary constriction and smooth muscle contraction. (Naloxone, as a selective and specific antagonist at the mu receptor, has been employed extensively as a tool in investigating whether or not opioids are involved in a particular toxic state or physiological function; although selective for the mu receptor, it also has antagonistic actions at the other opioid receptor sites.)
- It has a short duration of action. Therefore, it is critically important to administer adequate doses and repeated doses in cases of suspected opioid toxicity. Recovery usually lasts many more hours than the usual therapeutic effects of the given opioid.
- Avoid its use in individuals who have developed a tolerance from the chronic administration of narcotic analgesics, because naloxone can evoke an acute, severe withdrawal syndrome.
- Use it with caution, if at all, in patients who have recently received an opioid agonist to relieve or prevent pain, because of the possibility of precipitating severe pain and pain-related reflexes consequent to the antagonism of any opioid present (see Chapter 49).

Side Effects

Naloxone is one of the most selectively acting drugs in the pharmacopeia. Its major side effects derive directly from its mechanism of action—antagonism of opioid agonists at all of the known opioid receptors.

Prior to the introduction of naloxone, nalorphine (NALLINE, *N*-allyl normorphine) was available for use as an antagonist. It was a mixed agonist-antagonist, such that if given after an opioid, the opioid effects were reversed; however, when given alone, it produced respiratory depression, cough suppression, miosis, and analgesia. Because many individuals have experienced unpleasant reactions, such as feelings of unreality, dreams, hallucinations, sweating, nausea, or groggy sensations, it was used solely as an antagonist; it is now clinically obsolete.

Future Uses of Opioid Antagonists

- Naloxone has been found experimentally to reduce and reverse the nervous system damage associated with trauma or ischemia. In the future, a number of agents will be routinely used to avoid some of the pathophysiological processes that aggravate the recovery from nervous system damage.
- Naloxone and experimental antagonists have been found to antagonize and relieve the itching of cholestatic liver disease—a troublesome symptom that responds to little else. This observation raises the possibility that the itching produced by a number of opioid agonists such as morphine is a central process and not caused solely by histamine release.
- Oral doses of naloxone have been shown to be capable of relieving the constipation without reducing analgesia in patients receiving oral morphine for alleviation of sustained pain in hospice settings.
- Opioid antagonists with longer durations of action have been tested for the treatment of addiction, *ie*, secondary prevention of relapse to heroin use. Such agents include **naltrexone**, which is longer acting than naloxone, and **cyclazocine**, which is longer acting than naltrexone. Although these are effective antagonists, addict-patients have not generally liked or stayed on these antagonists chronically (see Chapter 49).

To date, no new therapeutic drug has resulted from the recent breathtaking advances in knowledge about pain, analgesia, and addiction. For example, the endorphin structures primarily confirm the structural conclusions from studies of thousands of morphinelike substances. Current limitations on use of the endorphins depend as much as anything on the practical concerns for predictable absorption and appropriate durations of action. Preliminary evidence suggests that given intravenously, the endorphins can relieve narcotic withdrawal symptoms without producing euphoria, and that certain opioid peptides can enter the CNS after their intravenous administration.

REFERENCES

Austin KL, Stapleton JV, Mather LE: Relationship between blood meperidine concentrations and analgesic response: A preliminary report. Anesthesiology 53:460–466, 1980.

Burks TF: Actions of drugs on gastrointestinal motility. *In* Johnson LR (ed): Physiology of the Gastrointestinal Tract, 2nd ed, 723–743. New York: Raven Press, 1987.

Chay PCW, Duffy BJ, Walker JS: Pharmacokinetic-pharmacodynamic relationships of morphine in neonates. Clin Pharmacol Ther 51:334–342, 1992.

Drugs for Pain. Med Lett Drugs Ther 35:1–6, 1993.

Evans CJ, Keith DE Jr, Morrison H, et al: Cloning of a delta opiate receptor. Science 258:1952–1955, 1992.

Evans DAP: Genetic Factors in Drug Therapy, Clinical and Molecular Pharmacogenetics. Cambridge: Cambridge University Press, 1993.

Jaffe JH, Martin WR: Opioid analgesics and antagonists. *In* Gilman AG, Rall TW, Nies AS, Taylor P (eds): Goodman and Gilman's The Pharmacological Basis of Therapeutics, 8th ed, 485–521. New York: Pergamon Press, 1990.

Jones EA, Bergasa NV: The pruritus of cholestasis and opioid system. JAMA 268:3359–3362, 1992.

Kromer W: Endogenous and exogenous opioids in the control of gastrointestinal motility and secretion. Pharmacol Rev 40:121–162, 1988.

McQuay HJ, Caroll D, Faura CC, et al: Oral morphine in cancer pain: Influences on morphine and metabolite concentration. Clin Pharmacol Ther 48:236–244, 1990.

Martin WR: The evolution of concepts of opioid receptors. *In* Pasternak GW (ed): The Opiate Receptors, 3–22. Clifton, NJ: The Humana Press, 1988.

Martin WR: Pharmacology of opioids. Pharmacol Rev 35:283–323, 1983.

Max B: This and that: an artefactual alkaloid and its peptide analogs. TIPS 13:341–345, 1991.

Meltzer HY (ed): Psychopharmacology: The Fourth Generation of Progress. New York: Raven Press (in press).

Meredith TJ, Jacobsen D, Haines JA, Berger J-C (eds): Naloxone, Flumazenil and Dantrolene as Antidotes. Volume 1 of IPCS/CEC Evaluation of Antidotes Series. Cambridge: Cambridge University Press, 1993.

Osborne R, Joel S, Trew D, Slevin R: Morphine and metabolite behavior after different routes of morphine administration: Demonstration of the importance of the active metabolite morphine-6-glucuronide. Clin Pharmacol Ther 47:12–19, 1990.

Portenoy RK: Opioid therapy for chronic nonmalignant pain: Current status. *In* Fields HL, Liebeskind JC (eds): Progress in Pain Research and Management. Vol 1. Pharmacologic Approaches in the Treatment of Chronic Pain: New Concepts and Critical Issues. Seattle, WA: International Association for the Study of Pain, 1994, pp 247–287.

Reidenberg MM, Portenoy RK: The need for an open mind about the treatment of chronic malignant pain. Clin Pharmacol Ther 55:367–369, 1994.

Sawynok J, Yaksh TL: Caffeine as an analgesic adjuvant: A review of pharmacology and mechanisms of action. Pharmacol Rev 45:43–85, 1993.

Schaumann O: Some new aspects of action of morphine-like analgesics. Br Med J 2:1091, 1956.

Turner JA, Deyo RA, Loeser JD, et al: The importance of placebo effects in pain treatment and research. JAMA 271:1609–1614, 1944.

Twycross RG, McQuay HF: Opioids. *In* Wall PD, Melzack R (eds): Textbook of Pain, 2nd ed, 686. New York: Churchill Livingstone, 1989.

Uhl GR, Childers S, Pasternak G: An opiate-receptor gene family reunion. Trends Neurosci 17:89–93, 1994.

Wall PD, Melzack R (eds): Textbook of Pain, 2nd ed. New York: Churchill Livingstone, 1989.

Yaksh TL, Aimone LD: The central pharmacology of pain transmission. *In* Wall PD, Melzack R (eds): Textbook of Pain, 2nd ed, 181. New York: Churchill Livingstone, 1989.

Inflammation and Nonsteroidal Anti-Inflammatory Drugs: Prostaglandin and Non-Prostaglandin Synthesis Inhibitors 15

James B. Lee and Steven C. Lee

INFLAMMATION

Inflammation is a fundamental pathophysiological response designed to eliminate any noxious stimulus introduced into the host, including radiant, chemical, physical, infectious, and immune provocations. The inflammatory reaction is divided into an acute and a chronic response.

The acute reaction, described by Celsus in the first century A.D., is characterized by redness, heat, swelling, and pain (*rubor, calor, tumor,* and *dolor*), with an accompanying loss of function. The pain response may be characterized by hyperalgesia and/or itching, submaximal expressions of the pain phenomenon. The acute reaction is optimally observed in the skin, where provocative stimuli such as caustic chemicals, burns and wounds, infections, and allergens elicit all four classic components of the inflammatory response.

The chronic reaction is characterized by persistent pain, swelling, and cellular proliferation with an accompanying chronic and often major loss of function such as that observed in rheumatoid arthritis. In this instance, redness and heat may be conspicuously absent.

The two most important classes of pharmacological agents that inhibit the acute and/or chronic inflammatory response are:

1. The nonsteroidal anti-inflammatory drugs (NSAIDs, typically carboxylic or enolic organic acids), the prototype of which is aspirin; and
2. The adrenal glucocorticosteroid hormones (SAIDs), the prototype being hydrocortisone (cortisol)

The mechanisms of acute and chronic inflammatory reactions are complex, vary from tissue to tissue, and depend on the etiological agent. Common mechanisms include chemotactic stimuli, phagocytosis, and lysosomal enzyme release as well as activation of the clotting, fibrinolytic, kinin, and complement pathways. Many of the chemical mediators identified so far are listed in Table 15-1.

- Histamine release appears to occur early in the initial stages of inflammation.
- Bradykinin, a nonapeptide, is formed from α_2-globulins by the release of proteases from polymorphonuclear leukocytes after they migrate to an area of inflammation.

TABLE 15–1. Chemical Mediators of Acute Inflammation

Vasoactive amines: histamine; serotonin
Kallikrein and kinins: bradykinin
Hageman, other clotting factors: thrombin
Fibrinolytic system: plasmin
Complement components
Eosinophil, platelet activators
Products from arachidonic acid
  Nonenzymatically: oxidation products of arachidonate
  Via cyclooxygenase: endoperoxides (PGG_2, PGH_2); thromboxanes (TXA_2); prostaglandins (PGE_2, PGI_2)
  Via lipoxygenase: Hydroperoxy acids; hydroxy acids, leukotrienes
Oxygen-derived products
Lysosomal constituents (neutral protease)

TABLE 15–2. Functions of Arachidonic Acid Products in Inflammation

PGE_1, PGE_2, PGI_2
  Fever and local heat
  Vasodilation
  Vasopermeability synergism with bradykinin and histamine
  Hyperalgesia synergism with bradykinin and histamine
Thromboxane A_2
  Platelet aggregation
Leukotriene B_4
  Chemotaxis

- Lipases activate many arachidonic acid byproducts such as prostaglandins (PGs), thromboxanes (Txs), and leukotrienes (LTs).
- Platelet activating factors and oxygen-free radicals are also released as chemical mediators of inflammation.

The initial steps in these reactions involve a number of different cell types and cellular interactions. Most of these chemical mediators appear to have similar effects in that they dilate capillaries in the area of inflammation, increase capillary permeability causing greater transudation, and heighten leukocyte intracapillary adhesiveness and diapedesis into the interstitium, where active phagocytosis occurs (Table 15–2). Recently, it has been disclosed that blood monocytes and tissue macrophages are primary sources of many cytokines. One of the cytokines is the polypeptide hormone termed interleukin-1, which not only has a potent effect on the inflammatory response but also enhances the immune response by supporting B-lymphocyte proliferation and antibody production as well as T-lymphocyte production of lymphokines.

NONSTEROIDAL ANTI-INFLAMMATORY DRUGS

Anti-inflammatory agents may be classified as either steroidal (SAIDs) or nonsteroidal (NSAIDs). NSAIDs may be further subdivided into either prostaglandin synthetase inhibitors (PSIs) or non–prostaglandin synthetase inhibitors (non-PSIs) (Table 15–3). Through convention, the generic term NSAID has come to refer to newer specific PSIs exclusive of aspirin. This has led to conceptual confusion because the NSAID aspirin is in fact a PSI. In addition, many important anti-inflammatory compounds are NSAIDs, but do not act by inhibition of PG synthetase. It is evident that the PSIs are represented by carboxylic or enolic acid compounds, whereas the non-PSIs are a heterogeneous chemically unrelated group of compounds, classified according to their effects on various symptoms and/or diseases (*ie*, the analgesic-antipyretic para-aminophenols, anti–rheumatoid arthritis agents, and antigout preparations). This chapter will therefore refer to NSAIDs as either PSIs (including aspirin) or non-PSIs according to the classification shown in Table 15–3. We will examine the PSIs (including aspirin) and then the non-PSIs (para-aminophenols and the antirheumatoid agent gold). Steroidal anti-inflammatory agents and other antirheumatoid (immunosuppressives, antimalarials, penicillamine) and antigout non-PSIs are described elsewhere in this text.

PROSTAGLANDIN SYNTHETASE INHIBITORS

Because nonsteroidal analgesics and antipyretics are perhaps the most widely prescribed and over-the-counter medications used in medicine today, it is important to thoroughly understand the mechanism of their action, their interactions with other drugs, and potent and at times serious side effects. Serious and at times fatal sequelae have frequently

TABLE 15–3. Nonsteroidal Anti-Inflammatory Drugs (NSAIDs)

Prostaglandin Synthetase Inhibitors (PSIs)		Non–Prostaglandin Synthetase Inhibitors (non-PSIs)		
Carboxylic Acids	***Enolic Acids***	***Para-amino Phenols***	***Anti–Rheumatoid Arthritis Agents***	***Antigout Agents***
Salicylic	Oxicams	Phenacetin	Gold	Colchicine
Acetic		Acetaminophen	Immunosuppressives	Allopurinol
Propionic			Penicillamine	Uricosuric
Fenamic			Levamisole	Probenecid
			Antimalarial	Sulfinpyrazone
			Chloroquine	
			Hydroxychloroquine	

been the result of failure to appreciate these actions of aspirinlike drugs. Inasmuch as, with the exception of the para-aminophenols, all such analgesic-antipyretic preparations exhibit the property of PG synthesis inhibition, the biosynthesis of PGs will be outlined in detail before specifically discussing the pharmacological properties of these agents.

Arachidonic Acid Cascade

Arachidonic acid and its metabolite byproducts (the arachidonic acid cascade) are important mediators of fever and inflammation. The rate-limiting step in the formation of the metabolites of arachidonic acid seems to be the initial step, namely, the calcium-dependent release of free arachidonic acid from the cell membrane phospholipid pool. Noxious proinflammatory agents disrupt the cell membrane, leading to activation of phospholipase A_2 and resultant degradation of the cell membrane phospholipid layer into arachidonic acid and diacyl glycerol moieties. Although this reaction, mediated through phospholipase A_2, is predominant in most tissues and cells including leukocytes, phospholipase C may play another role in arachidonic acid release through liberating a diglyceride, which is then hydrolyzed by another lipase to yield arachidonic acid. The mechanism of release of arachidonate esterified to the glycerol moiety of phospholipids is beyond the scope of this discussion. However, a major action of the anti-inflammatory glucocorticoids appears to be a decrease in arachidonic acid release from phospholipids by corticosteroid inhibition of phospholipases A_2 and/or C. The biosynthesis of PGs and TXs is illustrated in Figure 15-1.

Following the release of arachidonic acid, a sequence of events leads to the formation of the prostaglandins. In the first biosynthetic pathway, PG cyclooxygenase catalyzes the initial step, yielding two PG endoperoxides: PGG_2 and PGH_2. This reaction is inhibited by aspirin, indomethacin, and other PSIs (Ferreira et al, 1971; Smith and Willis, 1971). These intermediates are labile and can be converted into stable PGs such as PGE_2, PGD_2, and $PGF_{2\alpha}$. The PGs, isolated and identified from sheep seminal vesicles and rabbit renal medulla

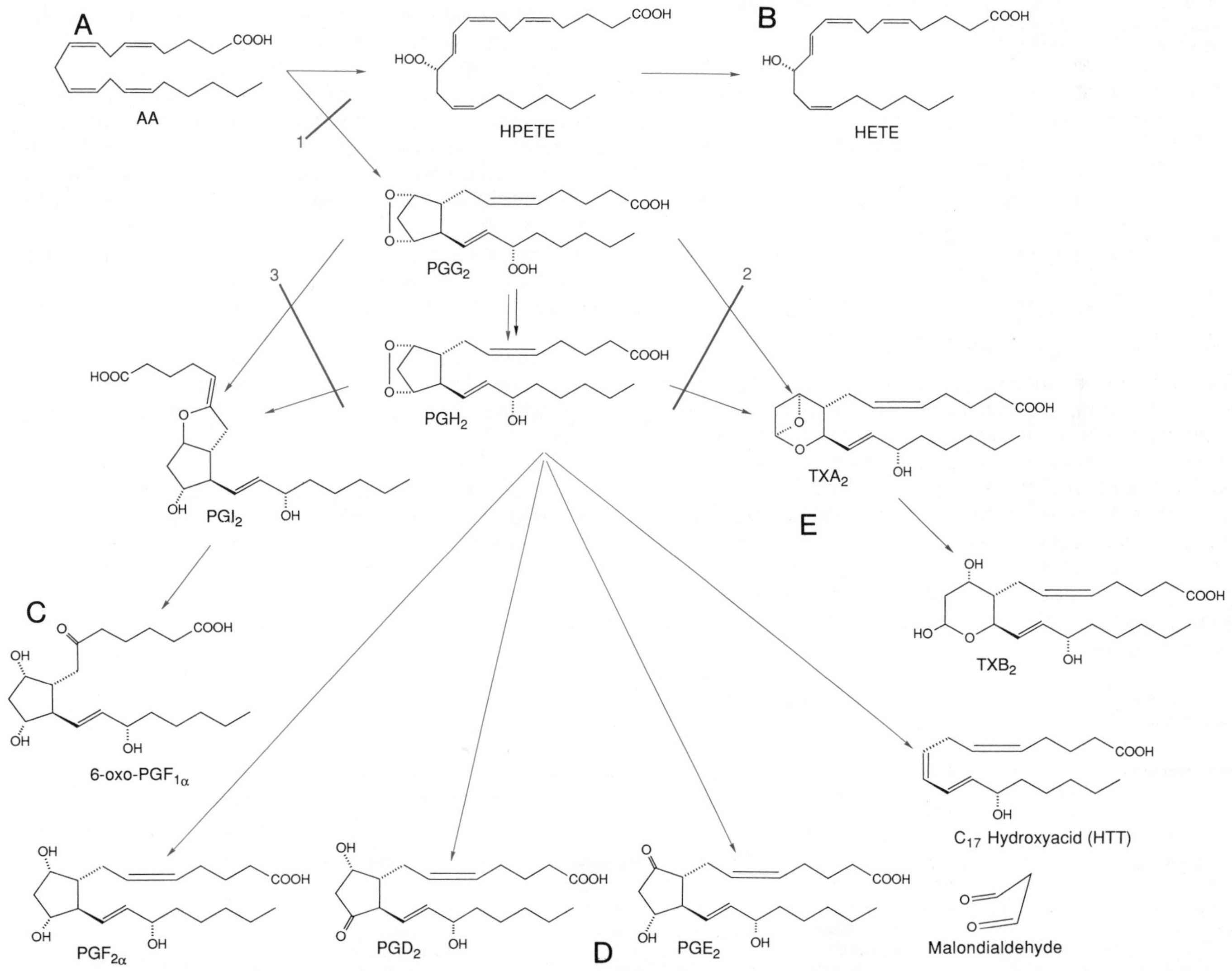

A
COOH
AA
1
HOO
COOH
HPETE
B
HO
COOH
HETE
COOH
PGG2
OOH
3
2
COOH
PGH2
OH
HOOC
PGI2
OH
OH
COOH
TXA2
OH
E
C
COOH
OH
OH
OH
6-oxo-PGF1α
OH
COOH
HO
TXB2
OH
COOH
OH
C17 Hydroxyacid (HTT)
OH
COOH
OH
PGF2α
OH
OH
COOH
PGD2
OH
COOH
OH
PGE2
OH
D
Malondialdehyde

FIGURE 15-1. Metabolic pathways of prostaglandin (PG) synthesis from arachidonic acid (AA). Sites where cyclooxygenase inhibitors (aspirinlike drugs—prostaglandin synthetase inhibitors), thromboxane synthetase inhibitors (imidazole and 1-methyl imidazole), and prostacyclin (PGI_2) synthetase inhibitors (15-hydroperoxyarachidonic acid and 13-hydroperoxylinoleic acid) act are indicated by the numerals 1, 2, and 3, respectively. (HETE = 12-hydroxyarachidonic acid; HPETE = 12-hydroxyperoxyarachidonic acid; TXA_2 = thromboxane A_2; TXB_2 = thromboxane B_2.) (From Moncada S, Vane JR: Unstable metabolites of arachidonic acid and their role in haemostasis and thrombosis. Br Med Bull 34:129-135, 1975.)

in the early 1960s (Bergstrom et al, 1962, 1963; Lee et al, 1962, 1963, 1965), are composed of a basic 20-carbon fatty acid containing a cyclopentane ring, the so-called hypothetical prostanoic acid. The carbons are numbered 1 to 20 from the carboxyl to the terminal methyl group. The designations of PGE_1, PGE_2, and PGE_3 refer only to the number of double bonds in the aliphatic side chains. The PGE_2 class is the most abundant naturally occurring group. For PG_1s, the precursor is 8,11,14-eicosatrienoic acid (dihomo-γ-linolenic acid), and for PG_2 the precursor is 5,8,11,14-eicosatetraenoic acid (arachidonic acid). PG_3 is formed from 5,8,11,14,17-eicosapentaenoic acid. In addition to the classic PGs, unstable PGG_2 and PGH_2 can be metabolized to thromboxane A_2 by thromboxane synthetase and to PGI_2 by prostacyclin synthetase. These labile compounds are rapidly converted to stable but biologically inactive TXB_2 and 6-keto-$PGF_{1\alpha}$, respectively.

Pharmacological Properties of Major Classes of Prostaglandin Synthesis Inhibitors

The major mechanism whereby PSIs exert their therapeutic and toxic effects has been hypothesized to be their ability to inhibit PG synthesis (Ferreira et al, 1971; Smith and Willis, 1971). These drugs block the cyclooxygenase pathway, nonselectively inhibiting the synthesis of PGs. Therefore, the anti-inflammatory effects of these drugs are in general related to inhibition of PG and TX synthesis. A property shared by the PSIs is their chemical relationship of being weak organic acids. Major classes of PSIs are shown in Table 15-4. Some are not universally available and will not be discussed further. Plasma half-life, dosage for treatment of rheumatoid arthritis, and cost analysis of anti-inflammatory therapy are provided in Table 15-5. Specific characteristics for individual PSIs will be discussed initially, followed by an evaluation of some of the major adverse side effects commonly observed with almost all of the PSIs.

Because acetylsalicylic acid (aspirin) has been used empirically for years for its analgesic and antipyretic properties, antedating all anti-inflammatory agents except quinine, it is the prototype with which all other NSAIDs are compared. Indomethacin, in use since 1965, represents the prototype of the newer class of more potent NSAIDs that have appeared in the last 25 years. Because aspirin and indomethacin are classic PG cyclooxygenase inhibitors and have been more extensively studied than other agents, a more detailed description of their effects and side effects will be presented.

It should be emphasized that *all* of the anti-inflammatory drugs discussed provide only symptomatic relief in chronic inflammatory disorders such as rheumatoid arthritis. They do not alter the chronic course of the disease, including pannus formation with bone destruction, joint malformation, and loss of function.

Salicylates

HISTORICAL ASPECTS. One of the earliest analgesic-antipyretics was quinine, derived from the bark of the cinchona tree. The bark of the willow tree also had similar bitter tasting properties and produced relief of pain and fever. Rev. Edmund Stone in 1763 wrote to the president of the Royal Society in England outlining his experience in successfully treating "agues" with a powdered extract of the willow tree bark. The active ingredient of the bark was shown to be salicylic acid derived from salicin, isolated in 1829 by Leroux. Acetylsalicylic acid (aspirin) was discovered as a byproduct of coal tar by a German chemist, Charles Gerhardt, in 1853 and later prepared by another German chemist, Hoffman. The therapeutic effectiveness of acetylsalicylic acid as an anti-inflammatory analgesic-antipyretic was described by Heinrich Dreser in 1899, who helped popularize its usage under the name *aspirin.* Aspirin is believed to be derived from the German word for acetylsalicylic acid, *acetylspirsaure* (from *Spirea,* a plant from which salicylic acid had been prepared for years, and *Saure,* the German word for acid).

CHEMISTRY, METABOLISM, AND EXCRETION. The structures of the salicylates are shown in Figure 15-2. Salicylic acid, the parent derivative closely related to benzoic acid, is believed to be the active component of the salicy-

TABLE 15-4. Major Classes of Prostaglandin Synthetase Inhibitors

Carboxylic Acids				Enolic Acids
Salicylic Acids and Esters	***Acetic Acids***	***Propionic Acids***	***Fenamic Acids***	***Oxicams***
Aspirin	Indomethacin	Ibuprofen	Mefenamic	Piroxicam
Diflunisal	Sulindac	Naproxen	* Meclofenamic	
Salicylates	Tolmetin	Fenoprofen	† Flufenamic	
Sodium	Diclofenac	Ketoprofen		
†Calcium	Etodolac	Flurbiprofen		
†Choline	Nabumetone	Oxaprozin		
*Choline magnesium	Ketorolac			
*Magnesium				
*Salicyl				

*Not available in Japan.
†Not available in the United States.

TABLE 15–5. Plasma Half-Life, Usual Anti–Rheumatoid Arthritis (RA) Dosage, and Cost of Prostaglandin Synthesis Inhibitors

Agent	Plasma Half-Life (hours)	Daily RA Dosage (mg)*	Tablet Strength (mg)	Cost of 100 Tablets (dollars)	Monthly Cost per Mean RA Dosage (dollars)†
Carboxylic Acids					
Salicylates					
Aspirin, generic	9–16‡	3000–5000	325	1.69	6
Diflunisal (DOLOBID)	8–12	500–1000	250	105.40	94
Acetic Acids					
Indomethacin (INDOCIN)	4–5	75–150	25	59.70(G.21.75)	70(G.26)
Sulindac (CLINORIL)	16	300–400	150	104.70(G.78.00)	63(G.47)
Tolmetin (TOLECTIN)	1–2	600–1800	200	78.95(G.62.25)	152(G.112)
Diclofenac (VOLTAREN)	2	75–150	25	55.60	67
Etodolac (LODINE)	7	—§	200	125.10	—
Nabumetone (RELAFEN)	24	1000–2000	500	123.95	112
Ketorolac (TORADOL)	2–9	—§	10	144.20	—
Propionic Acids					
Ibuprofen (MOTRIN, RUFEN)‖	2	1200–3200	400	19.95(G.15.36)	30(G.23)
Naproxen (NAPROSYN, ANAPROX)**	13	500–1000	250	89.70	81
Fenoprofen (NALFON)	2–4	1200–2400	200	65.40	176
Ketoprofen (ORUDIS)	2–4	150–300	50	133.70(G.120.80)	160(G.145)
Flurbiprofen (ANSAID)	3–9	200–300	100	130.85	98
Oxaprozin (DAYPRO)	21	1200	600	147	88.30
Fenamic Acids					
Mefenamic Acid (PONSTEL)	2–4	—§	250	118.25	—
Meclofenamate (MECLOMEN)	2–4	200–400	50	83.30(G.45.25)	150(G.81)
Enolic Acids					
Oxicams					
Piroxicam (FELDENE)	50	20	10	153.90(G.139.00)	92(G.84)

*Daily RA dosage in divided doses 3–4×/day except diclofenac (2–3×/day); diflunisal, sulindac, and naproxen (2×/day), and piroxicam, nabumetone, and oxaprozin (1×/day).

†Monthly cost rounded off to the nearest dollar; G. = generic.

‡At low daily doses (3000 mg), plasma half-life for salicylate is 2–4 hours.

§Not indicated for RA.

‖Available as over-the-counter preparations as 200-mg tablets (ADVIL, NUPRIN, MEDIPREN).

**Available as over-the-counter preparation as 220-mg tablets (ALEVE).

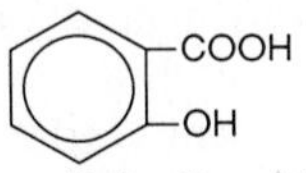

Salicylic acid (COOH, OH)

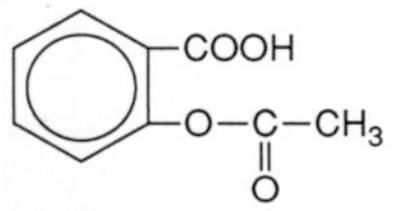

Acetylsalicylic acid (aspirin) (COOH, $O-C(=O)-CH_3$)

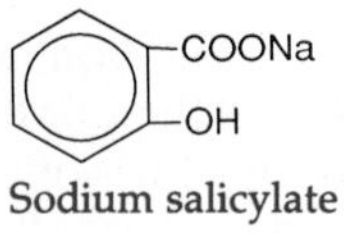

Sodium salicylate (COONa, OH)

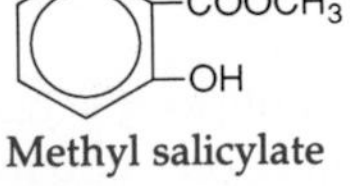

Methyl salicylate ($COOCH_3$, OH)

FIGURE 15–2. Chemical structures of common salicylates.

lates. Acetylsalicylic acid, sodium salicylate, and salicylic acid are all absorbed as the nonionized gastric irritating acid by the acid pH of the gastric juice. Alkalinization of gastric HCl promotes absorption in the buffered salt conformation (*ie*, sodium salicylate), with resultant reduction in gastric irritation. Absorption of salicylates occurs rapidly in the stomach and upper small intestines, although in the alkaline media of the latter, absorption is slower and less predictable. Thus, peak salicylate levels from rapid gastric absorption (1–3 hours) may be slightly blunted and delayed by alkalinization of stomach contents and use of buffered and/or enteric-coated aspirin preparations. However, this does not generally alter clinical effectiveness of these preparations and may significantly reduce gastric irritation.

Following absorption, the salicylates are transported, bound to albumin (90%), and as such compete with and displace a host of similarly transported naturally occurring compounds (*ie*, hormones such as thyroxine and steroids) and drugs (*ie*, penicillin, warfarin, barbiturates, etc.). The salicylates have two major acetylating properties, which are integral to the biochemical effects of salicylates: the acetylation of their plasma albumin by reacting with lysine, and the irreversible acetylation (and consequent inactivation) of PG cyclooxygenase. The salicylates are distributed throughout the body by pH-dependent passive diffusion. The majority (80%) of salicylate is converted to water-soluble conjugates by hepatic glycine conjugation; these conjugates are excreted in the urine together with smaller amounts (5%) of free salicylic acid and gentisic acid. Although differences exist, the majority of organic acid PSIs to be discussed are absorbed, metabolized, and excreted in a similar fashion to aspirin and thus will not be discussed further.

PHARMACOLOGICAL ACTIONS AND THERAPEUTIC INDICATIONS. The major anti-inflammatory analgesic and antipyretic effects of aspirin and other PSIs that result from PG synthesis inhibition have been discussed at length. Obviously, these pharmacological properties are central to the beneficial effects of aspirin and PSI in a variety of inflammatory disorders.

A recent application of low aspirin administration has been proposed to be its potential for prevention of cardiovascular catastrophes (*ie*, coronary thrombosis and cerebrovascular accident) by virtue of its preferential inhibitory action on platelet thromboxane A_2, leading to a prolongation in the bleeding time. In normal hemostasis, after vascular injury such as trauma, plaque formation sets into motion a train of events leading to clot formation and re-epithelialization of vascular endothelium. It is believed that adenosine diphosphate (ADP)-mediated activation of platelet phospholipase A_2 initiates this process, which in turn generates two platelet aggregating pathways, PG-TXA_2 and platelet activating factor (Paf-acether). In the PG pathway, PGG_2 and PGH_2 result in TXA_2 formation, which in turn results in vasoconstriction and platelet aggregation. PGH_2 either from endothelial or platelet arachidonate products results in production of vasodilating and platelet inhibitory PGI_2. Paf-acether derived from liberation of platelet arachidonate also results in platelet aggregation.

It is believed that aspirin at low dosage prolongs the bleeding time by inhibiting platelet TXA_2 and Paf-acether production to a greater extent than vascular PGI_2 synthesis and for the lifetime of the platelet (*ie*, 7–8 days). The net result is a preponderance of anti-platelet aggregating PGI_2 and a prolonged bleeding time. It is premature to state whether daily low-dose aspirin administration (81–325 mg/day) will be beneficial to patients after myocardial infarction or stroke or to patients with incipient tendencies to these phenomena (*ie*, higher risk subjects with abnormal plasma lipids, smokers, and those with positive family histories). However, current data support the beneficial effects of such aspirin treatment. Widespread clinical trials and therapeutic recommendations for this indication are underway. Obviously, aspirin should be avoided in patients with hypoprothrombinemia (*ie*, hepatic disease), on oral anticoagulant therapy (aspirin also displaces anticoagulants such as warfarin from plasma binding sites), hemophilia and other bleeding diatheses, and in patients undergoing surgery where its usage could be hazardous.

DRUG INTERACTIONS. Aspirin displaces a number of drugs from plasma protein binding sites, including the other anti-inflammatory PSIs such as the acetic and propionic acid derivatives, warfarin, methotrexate, tolbutamide, propamide, phenytoin, and probenecid. Aspirin also antagonizes the effect of diuretic therapy such as spironolactone and, by its competitive actions on the organic renal transport system, increases penicillin G concentration and decreases the uricosuric effect of sulfinpyrazone and probenecid. The anti-inflammatory effects of aspirin are affected little by other drugs although its gastrointestinal side effects such as gastritis and bleeding are increased by concomitant use of alcohol. Because the hemorrhagic effects of aspirin are accentuated by its platelet-inhibiting properties and by displacement of the anticoagulant warfarin from plasma proteins, the combination of alcohol and aspirin ingestion in patients on anticoagulant therapy can be lethal.

AVAILABILITY AND DOSAGE. *Aspirin* and *sodium salicylate* are available in 325- and 650-mg tablets (pediatric aspirin as 81-mg tablets and adult aspirin preparations as 975 mg are also available). The route of administration is always oral. Timed release, enteric-coated, buffered preparations, and suppositories are marketed. Therapeutic levels may be blunted or delayed with timed-release and enteric-coated preparations, which, however, have a definite place for use in patients prone to gastric irritation and peptic ulceration (*ie*, the elderly and patients with poor food intake). The buffering capacity of buffered aspirin is often inadequate to neutralize gastric HCl and, even when effective, may enhance renal salicylate elimination by alkalinization of the urine, leading to lower therapeutic levels. Rectal administration by suppository is rarely used because of unpredictable absorption and mucosal irritation.

The analgesic and antipyretic dose for adults ranges from 325 to 975 mg (usual dose, 650 mg) four times per day after meals and with bedtime milk or snack. Self-medication

BOX 15–1
THERAPEUTIC USES

Salicylates are used in a variety of inflammatory disorders, including rheumatic fever, rheumatoid arthritis, osteoarthritis, ankylosing spondylitis, headache, fever, myalgias, and dysmenorrhea. They may also be helpful for the prevention of cardiovascular catastrophes.

Two additional cardiovascular uses for aspirin and other PSIs are to enhance closure of patent ductus arteriosus in the newborn and to treat Bartter's syndrome. Because experience in treating these disorders has been extensive with more potent PSIs, these indications will be discussed in the indomethacin section.

Salicylic acid and its derivatives have two additional properties that have led to their topical use as counter-irritants. These compounds are absorbed by the skin and are highly irritating, at times producing keratolysis. These pharmacological properties have led to the use of salicylic acid (often in combination with benzoic acid) as a keratolytic agent in the treatment of warts, corns, and other localized hyperkeratotic skin disorders. Methyl salicylate, commonly known as oil of wintergreen, has found a therapeutic niche as a counter-irritant. It is effective when applied to the skin adjacent to inflamed tender muscles such as occur in the myalgias accompanying physical exercise and viral infections. It is also used as a topical adjunctive therapy over sites of arthralgias, such as in rheumatoid arthritis. Classic PSI side effects may occur from excessive skin absorption but are rare.

should not exceed 4 – 5 days before physician consultation, and all high fevers in infants and young children demand immediate physician evaluation because life-threatening dehydration may rapidly occur. The usual pediatric dose of aspirin is 60 – 75 mg/kg/day. Such dosage schedules produce blood salicylate levels usually less than 30 mg/dL and are not associated with signs of salicylism (*vide infra*). The dosage regimen for more severe and chronic inflammatory disorders such as rheumatic fever and rheumatoid arthritis is more rigorous and prolonged (Table 15 – 5).

Salicylates are also available as salicyl, choline, magnesium, and combined choline-magnesium compounds. Salicylsalicylic (salsalate) is a dimer of salicylic acid that is insoluble in acidic gastric fluids, but is partially hydrolyzed to two molecules of salicylic acid in the alkaline milieu of the small intestine. Its half-life in plasma is 14 – 18 hours; twice-daily dosage yields satisfactory blood levels. The amount of salicylic acid available from salsalate is 15% that of acetylsalicylic acid (aspirin) on a molar basis but its attenuated side effects in production of gastrointestinal irritation and peptic ulceration make it a desirable choice in patients with rheumatic disorders who are prone to such gastrointestinal disorders. The recommended dosage for rheumatoid arthritis or osteoarthritis is 3000 mg/day given in divided doses.

Diflunisal is a difluorophenyl derivative of salicylic acid that, however, is not metabolized to salicylic acid. Although it exhibits more potent dose equivalency to aspirin in its anti-inflammatory and analgesic properties, its prolonged half-life (Table 15 – 5) allows for twice-daily dosing. Diflunisal, unlike aspirin, is devoid of significant antipyretic activity. Diflunisal appears in the milk of lactating women and in general possesses all side effects common to the PSIs although reportedly to a lesser degree. For instance, diflunisal appears to produce less gastrointestinal and auditory symptoms than aspirin and has therefore found acceptance as a long-acting analgesic for the relief of musculoskeletal pain, including that of osteoarthritis. It has also been employed in the treatment of rheumatoid arthritis. Diflunisal is available in 250 and 500 mg tablets with total recommended daily dosage of 500 – 1000 mg, not to exceed 1500 mg (Table 15 – 5).

TOXIC REACTIONS TO SALICYLATES. Adverse reactions shared by all PSIs including aspirin will be discussed separately. However, there are certain toxic effects following aspirin overdosage or sensitivity that are relatively specific for salicylates. Since these may be serious and life threatening, they will be discussed in detail.

Salicylism is the aggregate term applied to a well-described syndrome resulting from aspirin (and other salicylate) overdosage. The overdosage of aspirin that has resulted in fatalities is extremely variable, depending upon patient's size, rate of absorption, and so forth. In general, mild to moderate toxicity is observed with doses between 150 and 250 mg/kg body weight and severe to lethal toxicity in doses above 250 mg/kg body weight. However, severe intoxication has occurred at the lower ingestion doses and survival at doses far above the higher ingestion amounts. Methyl salicylate (oil of wintergreen) is particularly toxic in low doses, with fatalities reported following ingestion of a single teaspoon (approximately 5 g). Mild salicylate toxicity is usually associated with plasma salicylate levels 40 – 70 mg/dL, moderate 70 – 150 mg/dL, and severe to lethal above 150 mg/dL.

Early symptoms of salicylate intoxication include tinnitus, decreased auditory acuity, headache, sweating, and nausea and vomiting. Hyperventilation is almost always present, attributable to a direct stimulating effect of salicylates on the central nervous system respiratory centers and from CO_2 generated by aspirin's uncoupling of oxidative phosphorylation. This results in an initial respiratory alkalosis that is compensated within 3 days by enhanced renal sodium and potassium bicarbonate excretion. Compensated respiratory alkalosis (normal blood pH, normal or low PCO_2 and low serum bicarbonate) coupled with the aforementioned symptoms is the usual presentation of salicylism in adults and is treated by measures outlined below.

Salicylism in children represents a more ominous picture. At toxic aspirin doses, profound central nervous system effects occur, including respiratory depression, marked hyperthermia, vomiting, diarrhea, and sweating. All combine to produce superimposed respiratory and metabolic acidosis, ultimately leading to convulsions, coma, and death. The metabolic acidosis is the result of organic acid accumulation (salicylates and their derivatives, lactic and acetoacetic acids, sulphuric and phosphoric acids) in the face of already depleted buffer stores from renal bicarbonate loss as a compensation for the initial phases of respiratory alkalosis.

The initial treatment of salicylism is directed to removing unabsorbed gastric salicylate by intubation and/or induction of vomiting (ipecac) as well as immediate intravenous therapy for correction of hypovolemia, dehydration, and acid-base abnormalities. Appropriate intravenous solutions of glucose and electrolytes are dictated by interpretation of laboratory data and invariably include sodium bicarbonate to replenish depleted stores and promote urinary alkalinization to enhance renal salicylate excretion. Immediate initial treatment of hyperpyrexia by environmental cooling (*ie*, alcohol sponges, tepid water) is indicated.

Aspirin hypersensitivity occurs in a small number of patients (0.3%), particularly those with asthma and nasal polyps. Manifestations of hypersensitivity include vasomotor rhinitis, urticaria, bronchial wheezing, and angioneurotic edema, including full-blown lethal anaphylactic reactions with laryngeal edema, generalized edema, vasomotor collapse, and shock. Such reactions constitute a true medical emergency, with immediate treatment directed to relief of airway obstruction, oxygen, and parenteral administration of epinephrine and corticosteroids. Patients with this hypersensitivity should be advised to avoid aspirin and all other PSIs.

Reye's syndrome is a potentially fatal encephalopathy associated with fatty hepatic degeneration and dysfunction in children in association with influenza epidemics and with the varicella virus. Although aspirin may precipitate or accentuate this disorder, no unequivocal proof exists that it is a major causative factor. Nevertheless, prudence suggests abstaining from the use of aspirin in children for the symptomatic treatment of influenza and varicella.

Acetic Acids

INDOMETHACIN

Pharmacological Actions and Therapeutic Indications. Indomethacin has all the classic anti-inflammatory-analgesic-antipyretic actions of aspirin but is 20 – 30 times more potent. It is important to note, however, that not all the effects of indomethacin can be attributed to PG synthesis inhibition. Thus indomethacin decreases production of renin by the juxtaglomerular cells of the kidney cortex, which may result in important blood pressure and salt and water effects independent of the prostaglandins. Similarly, indomethacin may affect cyclic-AMP functions by virtue of its inhibitory effect on phosphodiesterase.

BOX 15–2
THERAPEUTIC USES

The clinical indications for indomethacin include symptomatic relief in osteoarthritis, ankylosing spondylitis, and rheumatoid arthritis (*eg*, alleviation of morning stiffness, increased mobility, increased grip strength), including relief of acute exacerbations with reduction in joint swelling and tenderness. Indomethacin is extremely useful in the treatment of acute gouty arthritis, acute bursitis, and acute tendinitis.

Unique indications for prostaglandin synthesis inhibition with indomethacin (and other PSIs) exist in Bartter's syndrome and patent ductus arteriosus in the newborn. Bartter's syndrome is characterized by hyperplasia of the renal juxtaglomerular apparatus, hyper-reninemia, hyperaldosteronism, hypokalemic alkalosis, and normal blood pressure associated with an elevated excretion of PGs. Indomethacin provides dramatic reversal of the above abnormalities which are probably largely related to increased PG production. Because the hypokalemia is only partially reversed, it has been postulated that a primary deficit in renal tubular potassium chloride transport underlies this disorder and that overproduction of renal PGs is a secondary compensatory mechanism to the related hypovolemia. Nevertheless, indomethacin treatment remains a mainstay of treatment for this disorder.

Intrauterine maintenance of a patent ductus arteriosus is dependent on oxygen tension, gestational age, and PGs. Patent ductus arteriosus in the newborn in the past was corrected by surgical closure, but because patency of this vascular channel is PG-dependent, medical treatment with PSIs such as indomethacin has led to a 60–90% success rate, often obviating the need for surgical intervention. The usual dose is 0.2 mg/kg orally every 12–24 hours to a cumulative maximum of 0.6 mg/kg. Because the plasma half-life of indomethacin in the infant is 3–4 times that of the adult (20 hours) and renal blood flow in the infant is PG-dependent, urine flow usually decreases during treatment. Although renal effect is reversible and well-tolerated in normal infants, acute renal failure may be precipitated in infants with renal disease. In addition to renal failure, indomethacin is also contraindicated in infants with bleeding diatheses and gastrointestinal disease (*eg*, thrombocytopenia, hyperbilirubinemia, enterocolitis).

Absolute contraindications to indomethacin include pregnancy, especially in the last trimester, where indomethacin-induced premature closure of the ductus may occur; hypersensitivity reactions to indomethacin, aspirin, and other PSIs; bleeding abnormalities; and where predisposition to precipitation of indomethacin's serious side effects may occur. Because indomethacin is one of the most potent PSIs, its side effects are very prominent. The most serious side effects include those of the gastrointestinal tract (dyspepsia, nausea and vomiting, abdominal pain, flatulence, diarrhea, and peptic ulceration with and without hemorrhage) and the renal system (interstitial nephritis, papillary necrosis, and acute renal failure). These will be discussed (see Side Effects Common to Prostaglandin Synthetase Inhibitors).

Availability and Dosage. Indomethacin is available as 25- and 50-mg capsules, 75-mg sustained-release (SR) capsules, and as a suspension (25 mg/5 mL), all for oral use. The drug is also available as 50-mg suppositories and as an intravenous preparation (1 mg indomethacin/vial to be reconstituted with 1–2 mL saline or distilled water).

The initial dose is usually 25 mg orally 3 times a day with daily increments of 25–50 mg at weekly intervals up to a daily maximum of 150–200 mg as dictated by therapeutic response and/or side effects. One may substitute 75-mg SR capsules once or twice a day for 25–50 mg capsules three times daily. It is often advantageous to give a large proportion of the daily dose (up to 75 mg) at bedtime with milk to relieve morning stiffness and pain. The use of indomethacin suppositories should be minimized to avoid rectal irritation and bleeding. Similar dose regimens may be used for acute flares of rheumatoid arthritis, osteoarthritis, ankylosing spondylitis, and acute gouty arthritis. In the last condition, an initial daily total of 150 mg in divided doses is recommended.

Initial intravenous dosage to infants with patent ductus arteriosus is 0.2 mg/kg with subsequent doses of 0.1, 0.2, or 0.25 (dependent on age) given at 12–24-hour intervals. Severe oliguria may occur and urinary output must be monitored and further dosages withheld until renal function returns to normal.

SULINDAC

Pharmacological Actions and Therapeutic Indications. Sulindac is a biologically inactive prodrug. Approximately 90% of the drug is absorbed following oral administration. It is rapidly irreversibly oxidized to an inactive sulfone metabolite and reversibly reduced to a sulfide metabolite, which is believed to be the pharmacologically active form. About 95% of the prodrug and its metabolites are bound to plasma proteins, with peak plasma concentrations of the active sulfide metabolite occurring in 2 hours. Because of an extensive enterohepatic circulation, the plasma half-life of the sulfide metabolite is 16 hours, allowing for more prolonged anti-inflammatory activity and a twice-daily dosing schedule.

Although sulindac possesses all the side effects of the PSIs, they may be modified or lessened because sulindac is a prodrug with little renal excretion of the active sulfide metabolite. The gastrointestinal symptoms (nausea and epigastric pain) appear to be of less magnitude and occur with a decreased incidence (approximately 20%) when compared with indomethacin (30–50%). Similarly, evidence suggests a "renal sparing" effect of sulindac, particularly in patients with glomerulonephritis and cirrhosis (Ciabattoni et al, 1980). However, the degree of renal sparing by sulindac has

> **BOX 15–3**
> **THERAPEUTIC USES**
>
> The pharmacological indications for sulindac are identical to those of indomethacin (rheumatoid arthritis, osteoarthritis, ankylosing spondylitis, acute gout, and bursitis and tendinitis). Unlike indomethacin, sulindac has not been utilized to any degree for pharmacological closure of patent ductus arteriosus in the newborn or in Bartter's syndrome.

proven to be controversial particularly in hypovolemic states, where renal blood flow is prostaglandin-dependent and where PSIs (including sulindac) may precipitate acute renal failure. There have been 23 reports following sulindac administration of a rare complication of renal lithiasis with incorporation of sulindac metabolites in the renal stones. This complication has not been reported for other PSIs and may be related to the unique metabolism sulindac undergoes following absorption.

Availability and Dosage. Sulindac is available in 150- and 200-mg tablets. The recommended initial dose is 150 mg twice daily with weekly increments to a maximum of 400 mg as determined by therapeutic response and/or side effects. In acute bursitis or tendinitis and acute gouty arthritis, the recommended starting dose is 200 mg twice daily for approximately 1 week.

TOLMETIN

Pharmacological Actions and Therapeutic Indications. As with all PSIs, tolmetin's pharmacological actions are mediated in large part by PG synthetase inhibition. It is more potent than aspirin but less than indomethacin. Side effects are most frequently gastrointestinal with nausea, abdominal pain and diarrhea, vomiting, and dyspepsia. Central nervous system (CNS) side effects including headache and drowsiness are reportedly less severe and less frequent than with indomethacin. Unlike most other PSIs, tolmetin does not displace anticoagulants such as warfarin from plasma protein-binding sites although it does prolong the bleeding time, presumably due to its inhibiting effect on platelet TXA_2 and prolongation of prothrombin time.

> **BOX 15–4**
> **THERAPEUTIC USES**
>
> The therapeutic indications are identical to all PSIs (rheumatoid arthritis, osteoarthritis, and ankylosing spondylitis), although usage in acute gouty arthritis and other musculoskeletal disorders is not recommended.

Availability and Dosage. Tolmetin is available as 200- and 600-mg capsules for oral use. The initial recommended dosage is 400 mg three times daily for a total daily dosage of 1200 mg, which can be increased or decreased according to the patient's response and tolerance to a daily range between 600 and 1800 mg, not to exceed 2000 mg. It is recommended the drug be administered on arising and at bedtime with milk or meals. The daily pediatric dosage (greater than 2 years) for juvenile rheumatoid arthritis is 20 mg/kg given three times daily with downward or upward adjustments to 15 – 30 mg/kg, not to exceed 30 mg/kg/day.

DICLOFENAC

Pharmacological Actions and Therapeutic Indications. Diclofenac is a potent PSI approximately equal in potency to indomethacin. Although the mechanism of action of diclofenac is by prostaglandin synthetase inhibition, it also results in a decrease in lipoxygenase products (LTs) by enhancing the uptake of arachidonic acid into triglycerides. The most important attribute of diclofenac that differentiates it from other PSIs is its prolonged uptake into synovial fluid, with concentrations persisting above plasma levels for 24 hours. This fact, coupled with the 2-hour plasma half-life of diclofenac and lack of accumulation of the free acid in patients with hepatic and renal disease, allows for once to twice daily dosing, although three times daily dosages are usually prescribed. Thus, diclofenac does not require dosage reduction in patients with compromised hepatic and renal function.

> **BOX 15–5**
> **THERAPEUTIC USES**
>
> As with other PSIs, diclofenac is indicated as an anti-inflammatory agent in the treatment of rheumatoid arthritis, osteoarthritis, and ankylosing spondylitis. It is also effective as an analgesic in the nonrheumatic conditions dysmenorrhea, renal and biliary colic, oral surgery, and chronic musculoskeletal low back pain.

Availability and Dosage. Diclofenac is available as 25-, 50-, and 75-mg enteric-coated tablets. In rheumatoid arthritis, the recommended oral dosage is 150 – 200 mg/day in divided doses (50 mg 3 – 4 times daily or 75 mg twice a day). in osteoarthritis, the recommended dosage is 100 – 150 mg/day (50 mg 2 – 3 times a day or 75 mg twice daily). In ankylosing spondylitis, the recommended dosage is 100 – 125 mg/day (25 mg four times a day with an additional 25-mg bedtime dose if necessary).

ETODOLAC

Pharmacological Actions and Therapeutic Indications. Etodolac is a rapidly absorbed PSI that reaches peak plasma concentrations in about 1 hour with a terminal half-life of 7.3 hours. No significant changes in this pattern distribution are seen in the elderly and in patients with mild to moderate renal impairment. The side effects, contraindications, and drug interactions of etodolac are the same as for other PSIs.

BOX 15-6

THERAPEUTIC USES

Although etodolac is an anti-inflammatory, analgesic, and antipyretic agent, it is not indicated in rheumatoid arthritis because it is less effective than other currently used medications. The principal indication for etodolac is for analgesia and for the treatment of acute and long-term osteoarthritis.

Availability and Dosage. Etodolac is available in 200- and 300-mg capsules. The recommended daily dose for analgesia is 200–400 mg every 6 to 8 hours, not to exceed 1200 mg/day. For osteoarthritis, the recommended initial daily dose is 800 to 1200 mg in divided doses, with subsequent adjustment to 600–1200 mg depending on patient response (400 mg 2–3 times a day, 300 mg 2–4 times a day, 200 mg 3–4 times a day), not to exceed 1200 mg/day.

NABUMETONE

Pharmacological Actions and Therapeutic Indications. Nabumetone is a prodrug that is biotransformed to the potent PSI 6 methoxy-2-naphthylacetic acid (6MNA). Peak plasma concentrations are reached in about 5 hours, with an elimination half-life of 24 hours, allowing single or double daily dosing. Side effects, drug interactions, and contraindications are similar to other PSIs.

BOX 15-7

THERAPEUTIC USES

The principal therapeutic indications are for the treatment of the signs and symptoms of rheumatoid arthritis.

Availability and Dosage. Nabumetone is available as 500- and 750-mg tablets. The recommended daily dosage for osteoarthritis or rheumatoid arthritis is 1000 mg given as a single daily dose increasing to 1500–2000 mg as indicated for relief of symptoms. Double daily dosing may be utilized. Maximum daily dosage is 2000 mg.

KETOROLAC

Pharmacological Actions and Therapeutic Indications. Ketorolac is a pyrrolo-pyrrole PSI used chiefly for the short-term management of acute pain. Ketorolac is available as an oral or intramuscular medication. Pain relief is similar for either preparation. Following either oral or intramuscular administration, peak plasma concentrations are reached in 44–50 minutes, with a terminal half-life of 2.4–9.2 hours. Pain relief with 10 mg of oral ketorolac was comparable to 650 mg aspirin, 500 mg naproxen, or 650 mg aspirin with 60 mg codeine. The side effects are similar to those of other PSIs.

Availability and Dosage. Oral ketorolac is available as 10-mg tablets given 4–6 times a day for the acute management of pain for a period of no longer than 5 days. Ketorolac intramuscularly (IM) is available in a Cortrix syringe or a Tubex cartridge-needle unit as 15 mg/mL, 30 mg/mL, or 60 mg/2 mL. The usual recommended dose is a loading dose of 30–60 mg IM followed by a maintenance dose of half the loading dose (15–30 mg) every 6 hours as needed. The maximum daily dose is 150 mg the first day and 120 mg thereafter. Therapy should not extend beyond 5 days because of appearance of side effects common to other PSIs.

BOX 15-8

THERAPEUTIC USES

Therapeutic indication is for the management of acute pain for a period no longer than 5 days. It is not recommended for preoperative support of anesthesia because it prolongs the bleeding time. It is also not recommended for use in obstetrics because PGs are essential for labor and for patency maintenance of the ductus arteriosus. It is also not recommended for long-term treatment of pain or for concurrent use with other PSIs.

Propionic Acids

IBUPROFEN

Pharmacological Actions and Therapeutic Indications. Ibuprofen was among the first propionic acid PSIs that were introduced in 1974. Like diclofenac and certain other PSIs, it accumulates in synovial fluid for a prolonged time after plasma levels decrease following its peak in 1–2 hours. Although the side effects on the gastrointestinal tract are not uncommon (including peptic ulceration), they reportedly occur with a lesser incidence than with aspirin and indomethacin.

BOX 15-9

THERAPEUTIC USES

Ibuprofen is indicated for treatment of rheumatoid arthritis, osteoarthritis, as an analgesic in the relief of musculoskeletal pain, and in the therapy of primary dysmenorrhea, where it reduces PG levels in menstrual fluid and inhibits uterine contractions. This has led to over-the-counter nonprescription use of ibuprofen for self-medication of dysmenorrhea.

Availability and Dosage. Ibuprofen is available as 300-, 400-, 600-, and 800-mg tablets. For rheumatoid arthritis and osteoarthritis, the recommended divided daily dose is 1200–3200 mg (400-, 600-, 800-mg, 3–4 times a day) tailored to the patient's response and appearance of side effects.

In the treatment of dysmenorrhea, 400 mg every 4 hours is recommended (over-the-counter preparations are available as 200-mg tablets) until symptomatic relief occurs. The same dosage is recommended for analgesic use in conditions other than dysmenorrhea.

NAPROXEN

Pharmacological Actions and Therapeutic Indications. Naproxen is one of the more potent PSIs among the propionic acid derivatives, being 10–20 times more potent than aspirin. Naproxen also possesses two unique characteristics that have been utilized in more effective anti-inflammatory therapy. First, the prolonged half-life of naproxen allows for twice-daily dosing. Second, naproxen has potent inhibitory properties on leukocyte migration (as colchicine), which may explain its success in the treatment of acute gouty arthritis. Naproxen undergoes 6-demethylation and is excreted as conjugates of this metabolite and the free acid. As with other PSIs, a small percentage (<1%) appears in the milk of lactating mothers. Toleration of gastrointestinal side effects and CNS side effects is reportedly better than with indomethacin, but as with other PSIs, the whole spectrum of side effects with naproxen has been observed.

> **BOX 15–10**
> **THERAPEUTIC USES**
>
> Naproxen is indicated in the treatment of rheumatoid arthritis, juvenile arthritis, osteoarthritis, ankylosing spondylitis, acute tendinitis and bursitis, acute gouty arthritis, and as an analgesic such as in dysmenorrhea.

Availability and Dosage. Naproxen is available as the free acid (NAPROSYN) in 250-, 375-, and 500-mg tablets as well as an oral suspension (250 mg/10 mL). Naproxen sodium (ANAPROX) is available as 275-mg tablets (equivalent to 250 mg naproxen). For rheumatoid arthritis, osteoarthritis, and ankylosing spondylitis, the recommended daily dosage is 500–1000 mg naproxen (250–500 mg, twice a day). Dosage is adjusted according to symptom relief and/or side effects at 1–2-week intervals with total dosage not to exceed 1500 mg/day. For juvenile arthritis, the recommended daily dosage is 10 mg/kg given in divided doses twice a day.

For acute gouty arthritis, the recommended dose is 750 mg followed by 250 mg every 8 hours until the attack subsides. As an analgesic such as for dysmenorrhea and acute tendinitis and bursitis, the usual dosage is initially 500 mg followed by 250 mg every 6–8 hours, not to exceed 1250 mg daily. Naprosyn is available as over-the-counter tablets of 220 mg for the treatment of dysmenorrhea and bursitis.

FENOPROFEN

Pharmacological Actions and Therapeutic Indications. Fenoprofen shares the same pharmacological effects and side effects as the other aspirinlike PSIs. However, the incidence of gastrointestinal and other side effects is also reportedly lower than those of aspirin and indomethacin.

Availability and Dosage. Fenoprofen is available as 200-, 300-, and 600-mg pulvules. The recommended daily oral dose for rheumatoid arthritis and osteoarthritis is 1200–2400 mg (300–600 mg 3–4 times a day) not to exceed 3200 mg. Again, adjustments in individual dosage will depend on symptomatic benefit and the occurrence of side effects.

> **BOX 15–11**
> **THERAPEUTIC USES**
>
> Fenoprofen is indicated for acute flares and chronic symptomatic pain relief in rheumatoid arthritis and osteoarthritis. Like ibuprofen, fenoprofen is also effective as an analgesic for musculoskeletal pain and dysmenorrhea.

KETOPROFEN

Pharmacological Actions and Therapeutic Indications. Ketoprofen possesses PG synthesis inhibitory properties common to PSIs but also inhibits LT production and has antibradykinin activity and lysosomal membrane–stabilizing actions. About 60% of the drug is excreted as glucuronide conjugates of hydroxylated metabolites and the unchanged compound.

> **BOX 15–12**
> **THERAPEUTIC USES**
>
> Ketoprofen is indicated for the chronic treatment of rheumatoid arthritis and osteoarthritis.

Availability and Dosage. Ketoprofen is available for oral use in 25-, 50-, and 75-mg capsules. The recommended daily dose is 150–300 mg given in divided doses 3–4 times a day with milk, food, or antacids (as with other PSIs). The recommended dosage for dysmenorrhea is 25–50 mg 3–4 times a day for optimum clinical response with minimal side effects.

FLURBIPROFEN

Pharmacological Actions and Therapeutic Indications. Although used worldwide for years, flurbiprofen is among the most recently introduced PSIs (like etodolac, nabumetone, and ketorolac) in the United States. It exhibits all the classic anti-inflammatory and side effects of other PSIs. Ninety percent of flurbiprofen is excreted as conjugates of hydroxylated metabolites and the unchanged compound.

> **BOX 15–13**
> **THERAPEUTIC USES**
>
> Flurbiprofen is indicated for the long-term management of rheumatoid arthritis and osteoarthritis.

Availability and Dosage. Flurbiprofen is available for oral use in 50- and 100-mg tablets. The recommended total daily dosage is 200–300 mg in divided doses (3–4 times a day) adjusted according to clinical response and/or side effects. The largest recommended single dose is 100 mg in a multidosage regimen.

OXAPROZIN

Pharmacologic Actions and Therapeutic Indications. The most recently introduced PSI is the propionic acid derivative oxaprozin. Like other NSAIDs, oxaprozin is 99% bound to albumin but has a long half-life of 21 hours, allowing single daily dosing. The effects and side effects of oxaprozin are similar to those of other PSIs. Oxaprozin is primarily indicated for the treatment of rheumatoid arthritis and osteoarthritis.

Availability and Dosage. Oxaprozin is available as 600-mg caplets. The usual dosage is 1200 mg (two 600-mg caplets) once daily, not to exceed 1800 mg. Smaller doses of 600 mg may be effective in individual patients.

Fenamic Acids

Pharmacological Actions and Therapeutic Indications. The fenamates are derivatives of N-phenyl-anthranilic acid. Of such compounds, only *mefenamic acid* and *meclofenamate* are available in the United States. The fenamates have not received wide clinical acceptance for chronic treatment of inflammatory disorders because of their high incidence of gastrointestinal side effects, particularly diarrhea that may be protracted and severe. Because of this, the use of mefenamic acid is not recommended for more than one week.

Mefenamic acid and meclofenamate are potent PG-synthesis inhibitors. Meclofenamate possesses the property of $PGF_{2\alpha}$ antagonism, in this case of isolated bronchial smooth muscle contraction. The drugs are excreted in the urine (60%) as glucuronide metabolite conjugates and in the feces (40%) as unconjugated metabolites.

> **BOX 15–14**
> **THERAPEUTIC USES**
>
> Although meclofenamate has an approved indication for treatment of rheumatoid arthritis and osteoarthritis (Table 15–5), the high incidence of diarrhea (10–30%) with bowel inflammation and at times steatorrhea precludes its overall effectiveness in these disorders. Therefore meclofenamate is not recommended as initial treatment for rheumatoid arthritis and osteoarthritis. It is not indicated for use in children. Mefenamic acid is indicated for use as a shortterm analgesic, and as treatment for dysmenorrhea, treatment regimens not to exceed 1 week.

Availability and Dosage. Meclofenamate is available as 50- and 100-mg capsules. Recommended daily dosage for rheumatoid arthritis and osteoarthritis (not initial drug of choice) is 200–400 mg in divided doses (50–100 mg 4 times a day). Mefenamic acid is available as 250-mg capsules. For short-term analgesia and relief of dysmenorrhea, the recommended initial dose is 500 mg followed by 250 mg 4 times a day with antacids, food, or milk, not to exceed 1 week (usually 2–3 days for dysmenorrhea).

Oxicams

PIROXICAM

Pharmacological Actions and Therapeutic Indications. All of the previously mentioned PSIs including the salicylates are carboxylic acids, whereas the oxicams are benzothiazines possessing an enolic 4-hydroxy substituent. Due to an active enterohepatic circulation, piroxicam has a uniquely prolonged half-life (30–85 hours) that permits single daily dosing (20 mg) to achieve plateaued therapeutic blood levels (3–8 μg/mL) after 7–10 days. At this point, daily drug elimination is equal to daily oral intake. Elimination is renal (65%) and fecal (35%) as glucuronide conjugates of the free acid and hydroxylated metabolites.

Piroxicam has potent anti-inflammatory, analgesic, and antipyretic activities derived primarily from its PG-synthetase inhibitory properties. The most prominent side effects are gastrointestinal, occurring in about 20% of treated patients.

> **BOX 15–15**
> **THERAPEUTIC USES**
>
> Piroxicam is indicated for the chronic management of rheumatoid arthritis and osteoarthritis. In this regard, it is therapeutically equivalent or superior to aspirin and indomethacin with reportedly greater tolerance. However, once-a-day dosing results in maximal compliance, which is probably a major reason for its therapeutic effectiveness.

Availability and Dosage. Piroxicam is available in 10- and 20-mg capsules. Recommended daily dosage is 20 mg as a single dose or 10 mg twice daily. Maximum effect is not evident for 1–2 weeks, when steady-state concentrations are reached. Accordingly, therapeutic assessment of efficacy should be delayed for 10–14 days.

Side Effects Common to Prostaglandin Synthetase Inhibitors

Many side effects are common to all PSIs. The most potentially lethal are gastrointestinal, renal, hypersensitivity, and bleeding reactions.

Gastrointestinal Side Effects

Among the most commonly encountered side effects during long-term PSI administration are gastrointestinal symptoms. These include dyspepsia, epigastric pain, nausea, vomiting, flatulence, and abdominal cramps, which can be associated with peptic ulceration and massive gastrointestinal hemorrhage and ulceration. The true incidence of these symptoms with any given PSI is almost impossible to determine, but individual symptoms for all PSIs have been reported to be in the range of 5–10%, with an incidence of total gastrointestinal symptoms of 20–60% for aspirin. A similarly high incidence exists for indomethacin, leading to discontinuance of medication in about 20% of patients on this PSI. Although a somewhat lesser total incidence has been reported with other PSIs (10–25%), individual patients with gastrointestinal symptoms to one PSI tend to show similar symptom vulnerability when placed on a different PSI.

Although symptomatic peptic ulceration with and without gastrointestinal hemorrhage and perforation reportedly occurs in about 1% of all patients during PSI treatment, recent studies indicate the incidence of bleeding is much higher with asymptomatic gastrointestinal ulcers, where bleeding with anemia was as high as 40%. The patients at high risk include the elderly, those taking high and prolonged doses, and those with a history of previous ulcers. In patients presenting with gastrointestinal bleeding, a history of previous ingestion of PSIs is extremely high, approaching 60%. Many practicing gastroenterologists claim that severe gastrointestinal bleeding is almost invariably associated with prior ingestion of PSIs and/or alcohol, the combination of the two being potentially lethal.

Because the anti-inflammatory and toxic effects may be related to cyclooxygenase inhibition, which is shared by all PSIs, similar toxic effects may be seen with all PSIs when administered in doses sufficient to result in anti-inflammatory actions. When tolerance to one PSI develops, another PSI may be substituted but at the risk of losing therapeutic efficacy and/or continuing toxicity. Alternatively, the side effects may be diminished by the use of antacids or a histamine (H_2)-receptor antagonist such as cimetidine while continuing PSI therapy. The use of enteric-coated salicylates or nonacetylated salicylates may also provide satisfactory alternatives. However, in patients who have experienced major gastrointestinal toxicity such as massive bleeding or active peptic ulcers, PSI administration is contraindicated and non-PSI treatment should be instituted.

Misoprostol (CYTOTEC), an orally active analog of PGE_1, has been introduced for prevention of hyperchlorhydria, gastric bleeding, and ulceration. Because PGs normally exert a cytoprotective effect on the gastric mucosa, and because this effect is reduced or abolished following administration of PSIs, the rationale for gastric PGE replacement during PSI treatment is obvious. Studies to date indicate that during chronic PSI treatment, oral administration of misoprostol (100–200 g 4 times a day) reduced gastric ulceration from 22% to 1–5%, which was associated with a significant reduction in fecal blood loss. There was no effect on the efficacy of PSI anti-inflammatory effects. There was also no effect in prevention of duodenal ulceration or abdominal pain. The main side effect of misoprostol is diarrhea (14–40%). The drug is contraindicated in pregnant women because it may induce miscarriage.

Renal Side Effects

The renal side effects of PSI administration include hypertension, azotemia with oliguria progressing to acute renal failure, hyponatremia and hyperkalemia, edema, papillary necrosis, interstitial nephritis, and the nephrotic syndrome. It is important to understand the rationale behind the discovery of the renal PGs and the normal role of the renal PGs in renal function.

The renal prostaglandins (PGA_2, PGE_2, and $PGF_{2\alpha}$) were discovered and identified in the early 1960s (Lee et al, 1962, 1963, 1965) following a search for renal vasodepressor substances that might underlie the "antihypertensive endocrine function" of the kidney. According to this hypoth-

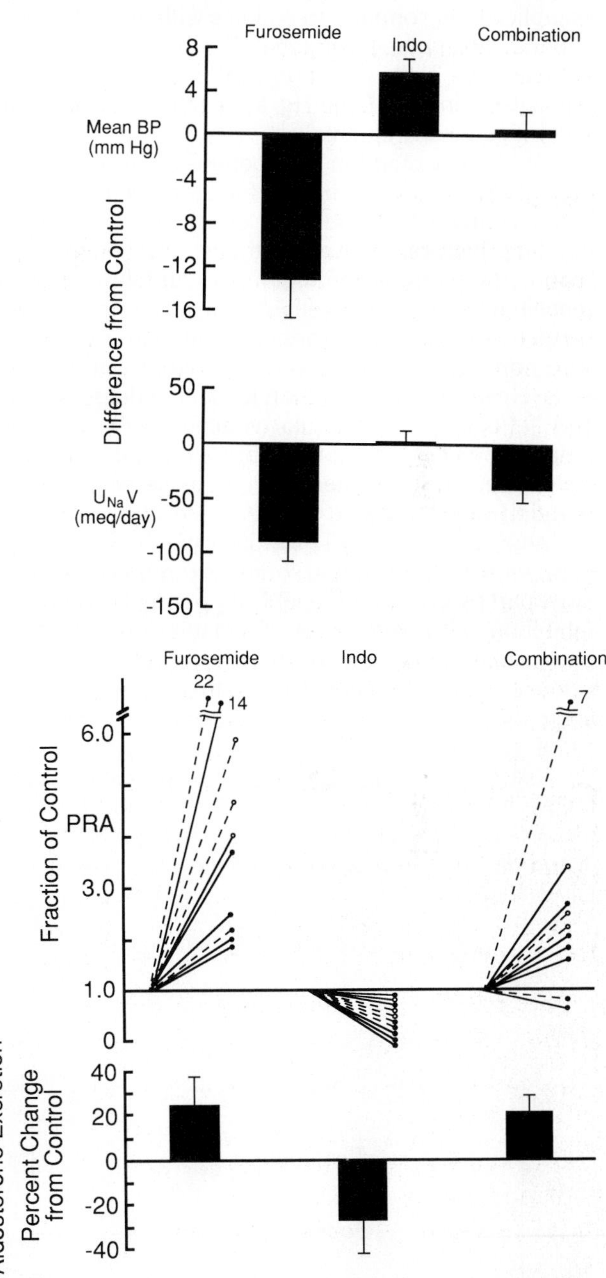

FIGURE 15–3. Effect of furosemide (80 mg every 8 hours × 4 days), indomethacin (Indo; 50 mg every 6 hours × 4 days) and combined furosemide and indomethacin in three normal subjects (*open circles*) and in six patients with essential hypertension (*closed circles*) on blood pressure (BP) sodium excretion ($U_{Na}V$), plasma renin activity (PRA), and urinary aldosterone. *Bar graphs* are the mean of cumulative 4-day periods. Results expressed as mean ± standard error. All results were statistically significant except combined treatment on blood pressure and the effect of indomethacin on daily urinary Na excretion. (From Patak RV, Mookerjee BK, Bentzel CJ, et al: Antagonism of the effects of furosemide by indomethacin in normal and hypertensive man. Prostaglandins 10:649–659, 1975.)

esis, hypertension may reflect a deficiency of vasodepressor compounds, allowing pressor axes (*ie*, renin-angiotensin, sympathetic nervous system) to act unopposed, leading to the development of hypertension with normal levels of pressor activity. It is no surprise therefore that PSI administration may result in blood pressure elevation in susceptible individuals. This can be severe and, if not recognized and PSI treatment decreased or stopped, can lead to cardiovascular complications common to patients with untreated essential hypertension not receiving PSIs. For the most part, as shown in Figure 15-3, the elevation in blood pressure with PSIs is mild, averaging 5-10 mmHg, a rise often overlooked in routine office measurements.

With the exception of hypertension, most of the detrimental effects of PSIs on renal function occur in a setting of hypovolemia with decreased "effective" intravascular volume and high renin levels. Although PGE_2 increases renal blood flow, glomerular filtration rate, and sodium excretion, renal function including renal blood flow is not normally dependent on PGs. PG synthesis inhibition in such individuals with normal kidney function is therefore without renal effects. However, any condition leading to decreased plasma and "effective" intravascular volume results in decreased renal blood flow. This can be illustrated by the hypovolemic state induced by reduced sodium intake when glomerular filtration rate estimated as creatinine clearance or inulin clearance decreases by 12 to 15% respectively. At this point, basal renal blood flow and sodium excretion is supported in large part by continued renal PGE_2 production (Fig. 15-4). Inhibition of PG synthesis by PSIs in this situation can reduce basal renal blood flow to below levels critical for maintenance of normal function, leading to azotemia, oliguria, and acute tubular necrosis. Clinical hypovolemic conditions include sodium restriction, diuretic therapy, posthemodialysis, existing renal disease, and edematous states where effective intravascular volume and renal blood flow is compromised (congestive heart failure, cirrhosis, and nephrotic syndrome). Close monitoring of the cardiovascular states and renal function is imperative in such patients receiving PSIs.

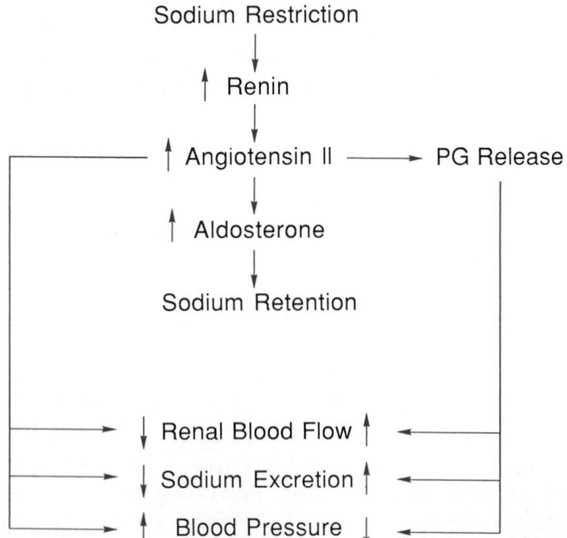

FIGURE 15-4. Hypothetical schema whereby volume depletion may lead to renin-angiotensin release and physiological antagonism of angiotensin II antinatriuretic and hypertensive actions. (PG = prostaglandin.) (From Lee JB: Prostaglandins and the renin-angiotensin axis. Clin Nephrol 14:159-163, 1980.)

An important renal side effect of PSIs is sodium retention associated with edema in 10-25% of patients. Because PGE_2 has a direct inhibitory effect on renal tubular sodium transport, the effect of PSIs has been attributed to increased sodium chloride reabsorption and increased capillary permeability. This effect may occur independently from the decrease in glomerular filtration rate and renal blood flow known to occur with PSIs. Severe hyperkalemia and hyponatremia may also be observed, which is believed to be secondary to PG synthesis suppression leading to hyporeninemia and hypoaldosteronism (Fig. 15-3).

An additional renal effect of PSIs is an increase in maximal urinary concentration and a decrease in free water clearance (PGEs inhibit vasopressin-induced water reabsorption), which is the rationale for use of PSIs in nephrogenic diabetes insipidus. Dilutional hyponatremia may thus be observed in PSI-treated patients.

Other nephrotoxic effects of PSIs that may or may not be related to PG synthesis inhibition are papillary necrosis and interstitial nephritis with and without nephrotic syndrome. Paradoxically, PSI has been employed in the treatment of nephrotic syndrome, which produces a decrease in massive proteinuria, the result of PSI-induced decreases in glomerular filtration rate. However, deterioration of renal function may occur in this instance, with production of irreversible azotemia and renal failure.

Hypersensitivity and Bleeding Reactions

These have been discussed in the section on Salicylates and apply as well to all PSIs.

Drug Interactions with Prostaglandin Synthesis Inhibitors

Diuretics and Antihypertensive Drugs

The first observation that PSIs blunt or abolish the diuretic and/or vasodepressor effects of antihypertensive medications was the observation that indomethacin inhibits the natriuretic and blood pressure lowering effects of furosemide in hypertensive man (Patak et al, 1975). It is evident from Figure 15-3 that furosemide administration alone lowered mean blood pressure by 10-20 mmHg, which was associated with enhanced renal sodium elimination and elevation in plasma renin and aldosterone. Indomethacin alone caused a slight rise in blood pressure, no change in sodium excretion, and marked suppression of plasma renin and aldosterone. The blood pressure lowering effect of furosemide was completely abolished and sodium excretion blunted by 50% with concomitant indomethacin administration. In subsequent animal studies, it was demonstrated that the natriuretic effect of furosemide was the result of a direct effect of furosemide in stimulating renal PGE_2 synthesis (Katayama et al, 1984).

That PSI inhibition of renal PG synthesis produces a drastic reduction in the antihypertensive and natriuretic effects of the loop diuretic furosemide applies to many other antihypertensive drugs and diuretic compounds, including β-adrenergic blocking agents, thiazide diuretics, prazosin, and captopril. The attenuation of natriuretic and hypotensive effects of diuretic and antihypertensive drugs has been demonstrated with aspirin, indomethacin, flurbiprofen, piroxicam, diclofenac, and naproxen.

Because almost any PSI may interfere with the actions of a wide variety of antihypertensive and diuretic agents, patients should be closely monitored as to the effectiveness of these drugs when concomitantly receiving PSIs. Generally, this will include patients with hypertension and diseases associated with edema (congestive heart failure, cirrhosis, and nephrosis).

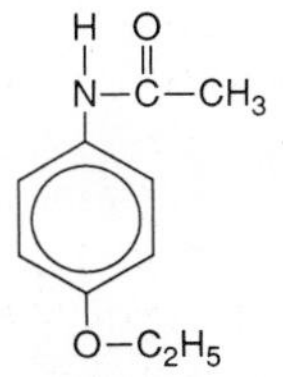

NON-PROSTAGLANDIN SYNTHETASE INHIBITORS

Para-aminophenols

Historical Aspects

The para-aminophenols are aminobenzenes derived from acetanilid, which was originally discovered to have antipyretic activity in 1886 by Cahn and Hepp. However, its extreme toxicity stimulated a search for other structurally similar compounds, which led to the formulation of phenacetin and acetaminophen. Phenacetin was extensively utilized in a wide variety of analgesic mixtures but its causal role in analgesic-abuse nephropathy led to its withdrawal from the market.

Acetaminophen is the active metabolite of both acetanilid and phenacetin. It was first used by von Mering in 1893 and has been available as a nonprescription drug in the United States since 1955.

Chemistry, Metabolism, and Excretion

The chemical structures of phenacetin and acetaminophen are shown in Figure 15-5. Following ingestion, acetaminophen is rapidly and completely absorbed, reaching a peak plasma concentration in 30-60 minutes, with a plasma half-life of 2 hours. Acetaminophen, unlike PSIs, is only slightly bound to plasma proteins. It is extensively metabolized by hepatic microsomal enzymes to glucuronide and sulfate conjugates, which are almost entirely excreted by the kidney within 24 hours. An important (albeit quantitatively minor) metabolite of acetaminophen is the hydroxylated metabolite N-acetyl-benzoquinone, which reacts with and depletes renal and hepatic glutathione following acetaminophen ingestion in toxic doses.

Normally phenacetin is metabolized to acetaminophen, its active metabolite, and many other metabolites, some of which are toxic and produce methemoglobin and erythrocyte hemolysis. Because phenacetin is no longer readily available for analgesic-antipyretic use, it will not be discussed further.

H O
N-C-CH_3
O-C_2H_5
Phenacetin

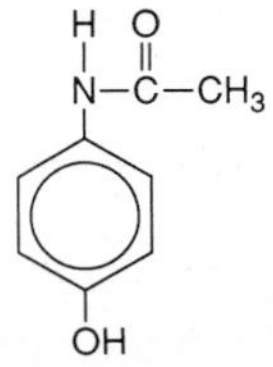

H O
N-C-CH_3
OH
Acetaminophen

Acetaminophen: Metabolism

FIGURE 15-5. Chemical structures of phenacetin and acetaminophen.

Pharmacological Actions, Side Effects, and Therapeutic Indications

Acetaminophen is only a weak prostaglandin synthetase inhibitor. It possesses no anti-inflammatory reaction but displays analgesic-antipyretic activity roughly equivalent to that of aspirin. Little is known of the mechanism of the analgesic properties of acetaminophen, although its major actions are believed to be on the CNS rather than in the periphery.

Acetaminophen produces few side effects at the usual dosage (325-650 mg 3-4 times a day) when taken infrequently and for short durations. However, when taken in massive doses or for prolonged periods (daily or weekly for years), serious hepatic or renal side effects have been reported. With massive overdosage (10-15 g), hepatic toxicity may occur, which becomes potentially lethal in doses of 20-25 g. The onset of acetaminophen hepatitis occurs within 2-3 days and is manifested by nausea, vomiting, fever, and malaise, followed by jaundice and the classic signs of liver failure. Liver function tests are typically abnormal (elevated transaminases, hyperbilirubinemia, and prolonged prothrombin time). Pathologically, biopsy specimens show central lobular necrosis. Hepatic failure may be accompanied by acute renal failure. Minimal hepatic damage can be expected with acetaminophen plasma levels in the range of 120 μg/mL 4 hours after ingestion and severe damage with plasma levels in excess of 200 μg/mL 4 hours after ingestion. Treatment should be immediate with supportive measures, gastric lavage, induction of emesis with ipecac, and a full course of sulfhydryl replacement. All these measures are most effective if performed within 4 hours of treatment. Sulfhydryl replacement with replenishment of glutathione stores may be accomplished by oral administration of N-acetylcysteine (MUCOMYST) with an initial loading dose of 140 mg/kg followed by 70 mg/kg every 4 hours for 17 doses (for emergency information, the Rocky Mountain Poison Center, Denver, CO, may be called at 1-800-525-6115).

> **BOX 15-16**
> **THERAPEUTIC USES**
>
> Acetaminophen is indicated for relief of headache, dysmenorrhea, myalgias, neuralgias, fever, and where aspirin and other PSIs are contraindicated (gastrointestinal side effects, renal symptoms, and bleeding disorders).

Availability and Dosage

Acetaminophen is available over-the-counter under a host of trade names (ANACIN-3, DATRIL, TEMPRA, PANADOL, TYLENOL, *etc.*) in tablets or capsules of 160, 325, 500, and 650 mg. Preparations also include chewable tablets, elixirs, solutions, wafers, and suppositories. Combinations with other analgesic, antihistaminic, and antisecretory agents (*ie,* aspirin, caffeine, phenyltoloxamine, *etc.*) are also available (ANACIN, EXCEDRIN EXTRA-STRENGTH, PERCOGESIC, *etc.*). Combinations with codeine (15, 30, 60 mg) have proven useful for the relief of more severe pain (post dental extraction, post minor surgery, neuralgias, *etc.*) although drug dependence on codeine is a hazard of prolonged usage. The usual adult dose of acetaminophen is similar to aspirin (650 mg 3-4 times a day), with a total daily dose not to exceed 4000 mg. A physician should be consulted if no relief is obtained after 7-10 days.

ANTI-RHEUMATOID ARTHRITIS AGENTS

Gold

Chemistry, Metabolism, and Excretion

Gold salts have been in use for over 60 years in the treatment of rheumatoid arthritis. Their particular value lies in the fact that unlike the other NSAIDs, gold has been shown to retard the progression of bone and articular destruction. Chemically, gold linked to sulfur is rendered water-soluble by linkage to hydrophilic compounds (glucose, sodium malate). The three most commonly utilized preparations are gold sodium thiomalate, aurothioglucose, and auranofin.

Following intramuscular administration of gold sodium thiomalate and aurothioglucose, peak plasma concentrations occur in 2-6 hours with an initial plasma half-life of about 1 week. However, with extended treatment and prolonged accumulation, the plasma half-life is extended for weeks. Gold is bound to plasma protein (95%) during the first 7 days but thereafter may be transported in sizeable amounts by erythrocytes. Gold accumulates in many tissues including synovial membrane, macrophages, skin, and hepatic and renal tubular cells, where it can persist for years. Gold is eliminated by the kidneys (60%) and in the feces (40%). Following oral administration of auranofin, about 25% of the gold is absorbed. The terminal plasma half-life is about 26 days. The renal and hepatic excretion rates are comparable to the intramuscular preparations. It is obvious that the accumulation of gold and its elimination are slow processes that lead to delayed therapeutic responses.

Pharmacological Actions, Side Effects, and Therapeutic Indications

The mechanism whereby gold suppresses the chronic inflammatory response and retards cartilage and bone destruction is unclear. The accumulation of gold in macrophages depresses macrophage activity, migration, and immune responses. Its accumulation in the synovial cells reaches concentrations 5-10 times that of other tissues, probably accounting for its preferential anti-inflammatory activity in chronic rheumatoid arthritis.

> **BOX 15-17**
> **THERAPEUTIC USES**
>
> Gold therapy (chrysotherapy) is indicated in the treatment of rheumatoid arthritis that remains active after a course of PSI treatment for several months.

Side effects of parenteral administration include a host of systemic reactions, the most common of which is dermatitis (15-25%) and skin pigmentation with pruritus, which can lead to exfoliative dermatitis and alopecia. Stomatitis is also a common side effect. Other serious parenteral effects include renal reactions (proteinuria, hematuria, and nephrotic syndrome) and more rarely hematological reactions (anemia, leukopenia, and thrombocytopenia). Hypersensitivity reactions ("nitroid" effects with flushing dizziness and sweating) as well as overt anaphylactic reactions have been reported. Encephalitis, enterocolitis, peripheral neuropathy, hepatitis, and pulmonary infiltrates are more uncommon side effects from gold administration. The oral preparation auranofin exhibits all the above side effects but with lesser incidence and severity. However, with auranofin, gastrointestinal disturbances, particularly diarrhea, are common. Gold treatment is contraindicated in patients with diabetes mellitus, renal disease, enterocolitis, hepatic dysfunction, congestive heart failure, hypertension, blood dyscrasias, recent hepatitis, recent irradiation, or a history of prior gold intolerance and allergic reactions. Gold treatment is not advised in pregnant or lactating mothers.

Examination of the skin, buccal mucosa, and the urine for red blood cells and albumin together with blood counts should be performed before each injection and/or at regular intervals. Treatment of side effects includes gold therapy cessation and the use of glucocorticoids for severe renal, dermatological, and hematological reactions.

Availability and Dosage

Gold sodium thiomalate (MYOCHRYSINE) is available in 25- and 50-mg/mL ampules. Aurothioglucose (SOLGANAL) is available as a 10-mL multiple dose vial (50 mg/mL). Auranofin (RIDAURA) is available as 3-mg capsules.

The usual parenteral dose is 10 mg IM the first week, 25 mg the second and third weeks, followed by 50 mg at weekly intervals for a total dosage of 1000 mg or until symptoms abate at a lower cumulative dose. If a favorable therapeutic response is evident after 1000 mg and side effects are absent or minimal, therapy can be extended indefinitely at intervals of 1 month. A beneficial response may not be evident for months. The weekly dose of gold should not exceed 100 mg in resistant cases. The recommended oral dosage with auranofin is 6 mg/day, increasing to a maximum of 9 mg/day if a favorable response is not evident after 6 months.

REFERENCES

Bergstrom S, Ryhage R, Samuelsson B, Sjovall J: The structure of prostaglandins E, $F_{1\alpha}$ and $F_{2\alpha}$. Acta Chem Scand 16:501–502, 1962.

Bergstrom S, Ryhage R, Samuelsson B, Sjovall J: The structures of prostaglandins E_1, $F_{1\alpha}$ and $F_{1\beta}$. J Biol Chem 238:3555–3564, 1963.

Ciabattoni G, Cinotti GA, Patrono C: Renal effects of anti-inflammatory drugs. Eur J Pharmacol Inflamm 3:210, 221, 1980.

Ferreira SH, Moncada S, Vane JR: Indomethacin and aspirin abolish prostaglandin release from the spleen. Nature (New Biol) 231:237–239, 1971.

Katayama S, Attallah AA, Stahl RA, et al: Mechanism of furosemide-induced natriuresis by direct stimulation of renal prostaglandin E_2. Am J Physiol 247:F555–F561, 1984.

Lee JB, Covino BG, Takman BH, Smith ER: Renal medullary vasodepressor substance, medullin: Isolation, chemical characterization and physiological properties. Circulation Res 17:57–77, 1965.

Lee JB, Crowshaw K, Takman BH, et al: The identification of prostaglandin E_2, $F_{2\alpha}$ and A_2 from rabbit kidney medulla. Biochem J 105:1251–1260, 1962.

Lee JB, Hickler RB, Saravis CA, Thorn GW: Sustained depressor effect of renal medullary extract in the normotensive rat. Circulation Res 13:359–366, 1963.

Patak RV, Mookerjee BK, Bentzel CJ, et al: Antagonism of the effects of furosemide by indomethacin in normal and hypertensive man. Prostaglandins 10:649–659, 1975.

Smith JB, Willis AL: Aspirin selectively inhibits prostaglandin production in human platelets. Nature (New Biol) 231:235–236, 1971.

16 *Histamine and Antihistamines (H_1-Receptor Antagonists)*

F. Estelle R. Simons and Keith J. Simons

HISTAMINE

Synthesis and Storage

Histamine is formed from the decarboxylation of the amino acid histidine by the enzyme L-histidine decarboxylase. Most histamine is stored preformed in cytoplasmic granules of tissue mast cells and blood basophils, in close association with proteoglycans such as heparin or chondroitin 4-sulfates that make up the granule matrix. In humans, mast cells are found in the loose connective tissue of all organs, especially around blood vessels, nerves, and lymphatics of the skin, upper and lower respiratory tract, and gastrointestinal mucosa. Non–mast cell sites of histamine formation and storage include epidermal cells, gastric mucosa, central nervous system (CNS) neurons, and regenerating or rapidly growing tissue.

Histamine plays a central role in the immediate hypersensitivity and allergic responses, in gastrointestinal secretion, and in neurotransmission.

Release

Activation of human mast cells and basophils by antigen bridging of membrane-bound immunoglobulin E (IgE) aggregates IgE receptors and initiates a cascade of metabolic events in the membrane, leading to opening of calcium channels and release of secretory granules containing histamine and other preformed pharmacologically active chemicals.

Some substances stimulate release of histamine from mast cells and basophils directly and without prior sensitization. These include clinically useful materials such as morphine, succinylcholine, tubocurarine, and radiocontrast media; and nontherapeutic substances such as the polypeptides in stinging insect venoms, low–molecular-weight peptides cleaved from complement, basic polypeptides such as bradykinin and substance P, cytokines, histamine-releasing factors from a variety of cells, and polybasic materials such as compound 48/80. Nonspecific tissue injury produced by scratching or by physical factors such as cold can also stimulate release of histamine from mast cells directly.

Once released, histamine diffuses rapidly into the surrounding tissues and appears in the blood within minutes. Histamine concentrations in plasma are normally very low, but transient elevations of plasma histamine are found after experimental challenge with antigen or with physical factors such as exercise in patients with asthma and after challenge with physical factors such as cold, vibration, or pressure in patients with urticaria.

Metabolism and Excretion

Although the turnover of histamine in secretory granules in mast cells and basophils is very slow, epidermal cells, gastric mucosa, CNS neurons, and any tissues undergoing growth or regeneration synthesize and metabolize histamine at a rapid rate.

Only 2 or 3% of histamine is excreted unchanged in the urine. Most is metabolized to *N*-methylhistamine by *N*-methyltransferase (50–70%) or to imidazole acetic acid by diamine oxidase (histaminase) (30–45%).

Histamine Receptors

The types of histamine receptors described to date are H_1-receptors, which play an extremely important role in allergic disorders; H_2-receptors, which are important in gastric acid secretion, in immune system down-regulation, and in feedback control of histamine release; H_3-receptors, which are involved in modulation of cholinergic neurotransmission in human airways, also in CNS functioning, and in the feedback control of histamine synthesis and release; and low-affinity H_{IC} receptors, which may be involved in histamine's role as an intracellular messenger. Histamine receptors have been defined pharmacologically for many years, but their actual structure and method of signal transduction by interaction with G proteins are now being elucidated. The gene encoding the H_1 and H_2 receptors has been cloned.

Pharmacological Actions of Histamine on the H_1-Receptor

Histamine, through its action on H_1-receptors, produces contraction of vascular and bronchial smooth muscle, causes pruritus, activates airway vagal afferent nerves, and stimulates cough receptors.

Histamine works on both H_1-and H_2-receptors to increase the amount (H_2) and the viscosity (H_1) of mucous glycoprotein secretion from goblet cells and bronchial glands in the respiratory epithelium and to increase vascular endothelial permeability, thereby decreasing the blood pressure and causing flushing, headache, and tachycardia.

BOX 16–1
USE OF HISTAMINE IN CLINICAL MEDICINE

The histamine-induced wheal-and-flare response in the skin is widely used in clinical trials to assess the efficacy of H_1-receptor antagonists. When a dilute solution of histamine is introduced into the epicutaneous region or injected intradermally, a characteristic sequence of events known as the *triple response of Lewis* occurs. At the injection site, a small, localized red area appears within minutes, becoming maximal in 1 minute. A wheal then replaces the original red area at the injection site, becoming maximal in 10 minutes. A brighter red flush or flare develops beyond the wheal, also becoming maximal in 10 minutes. The initial red area is due to the direct vasodilator effect of histamine, the wheal reflects histamine's capacity to cause edema, and the flare is due to histamine-induced stimulation of local axon reflexes causing vasodilation indirectly.

Histamine, in a weak isotonic solution administered by inhalation, is used in pulmonary function testing to assess bronchial hyperreactivity in patients with clinically stable chronic asthma.

Histamine is no longer used to test parietal cell function and gastric acid secretion because, in the dose required parenterally for this purpose, it causes flushing and warmth of the skin, a decrease in systolic blood pressure, acceleration of heart rate, headache, and other distressing side effects.

ANTIHISTAMINES

History

Antihistamines have been widely used in clinical medicine since the 1940s, when phenbenzamine, pyrilamine, diphenhydramine, and tripelennamine were synthesized. In the early 1970s, antihistamines with a gastric antisecretory effect were developed; subsequently H_2-receptor antagonists such as cimetidine, ranitidine, and famotidine have revolutionized the treatment of peptic ulcer and related gastric hypersecretory states (see Chapter 33). In 1981, the introduction of the first relatively nonsedating H_1-receptor antagonist, terfenadine, was another important milestone in antihistamine research. Recently, the era of H_3-receptor antagonist investigation has begun.

H_1-Receptor Antagonists

Basic Pharmacology

STRUCTURE AND CLASSIFICATION. H_1-receptor antagonists bear some structural resemblance to histamine; and, like histamine, they contain an ethylamine group. The traditional classification of H_1-receptor antagonists according to chemical structure (*eg*, ethanolamine, ethylene diamine, alkylamine, piperazine, piperidine, and phenothiazine) is becoming anachronistic, because some of the second-generation H_1-receptor antagonists, such as terfenadine and astemizole, do not fit readily into the old classification system. Cetirizine, a piperazine, is the carboxylic acid metabolite of the first-generation H_1-receptor antagonist hydroxyzine (Fig. 16–1).

PHARMACOLOGICAL ACTIVITIES. At low concentrations, H_1-receptor antagonists are reversible, competitive antagonists of the actions of histamine on H_1-receptors. The principal pharmacological actions of H_1-receptor antagonists are to relax vascular and bronchial smooth muscle, decrease pruritus, inhibit activation of airway vagal afferent nerves, and decrease cough receptor stimulation. Like the H_2-receptor antagonists, they also decrease glycoprotein secretion in the respiratory epithelium and decrease vascular endothelium permeability, hypotension, flushing, headache, and tachycardia (Table 16–1).

In addition to their H_1-blocking activity, some of the new H_1-receptor antagonists such as terfenadine, loratadine, and cetirizine have antiallergic properties; that is, they inhibit release of mediators of inflammation such as histamine and prostaglandin D_2 from mast cells and basophils. Cetirizine also has an anti-inflammatory effect and inhibits recruitment of inflammatory cells, including eosinophils, neutrophils, and basophils, to the site of an immediate (type 1) hypersensitivity reaction (Table 16–1; see also Chapter 50). Thus some of the new H_1-receptor antagonists are said to have antiallergic properties.

Drowsiness from antihistamines has been attributed to inhibition of histamine *N*-methyltransferase with consequent elevations of CNS histamine concentrations and blockade of central histaminergic receptors. Antagonism of other CNS receptor sites, such as those for serotonin (5-hydroxytryptamine), acetylcholine, and α-adrenergic stimulation, may also be involved. The *second-generation* H_1-receptor antagonists, terfenadine, astemizole, loratadine, cetirizine, acrivastine and azelastine, do not penetrate into the CNS as well as the first-generation H_1-receptor antagonists do. Also, they are relatively free from antiserotonin effects, anticholinergic effects, and α-adrenergic blocking activity.

Clinical Pharmacology

PHARMACOKINETICS. H_1-receptor antagonists are reasonably well absorbed when administered by mouth,

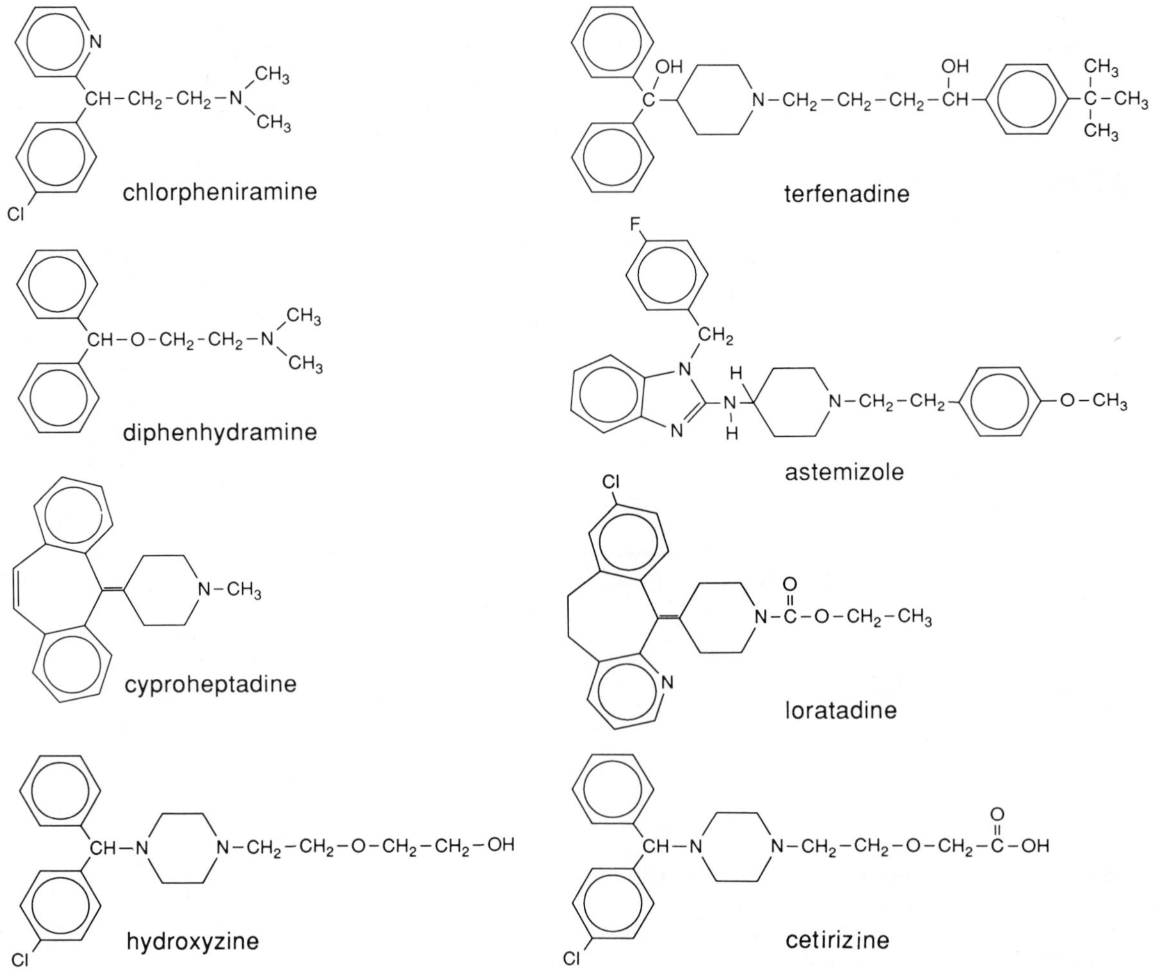

FIGURE 16–1. Chemical formulas of some representative first-generation H_1-receptor antagonists: chlorpheniramine, an alkylamine; diphenhydramine, an ethanolamine; cyproheptadine, a piperidine; and hydroxyzine, a piperazine; and the second-generation H_1-receptor antagonists, terfenadine, astemizole, loratadine, and cetirizine, a piperazine.

with peak serum concentrations reached approximately 2 hours after dosing. All the first-generation H_1-receptor antagonists and most of the second-generation H_1-receptor antagonists available currently are metabolized by the hepatic cytochrome P-450 system. Clearance rates and β-phase serum elimination half-life values are extremely variable, with half-life values ranging from 24 hours or less for chlorpheniramine, brompheniramine, hydroxyzine, acrivastine, terfenadine, and loratadine to 9.5 days for astemizole and its active metabolites. Apparent volumes of distribution tend to be large. They are usually uncorrected for bioavailability because intravenous formulations are available for comparison with oral formulations for only two H_1-receptor antagonists —chlorpheniramine and diphenhydramine (Table 16–2).

TABLE 16–1. Pharmacological Actions of H_1-Receptor Antagonists

Relax vascular and bronchial smooth muscle
↓ Pruritus
Inhibit activation of airway vagal afferent nerves
↓ Cough receptor stimulation
↓ Amount and viscosity of mucous glycoprotein secretion in respiratory epithelium*
↓ Vascular permeability*
↓ Hypotension*
↓ Flushing*
↓ Headache*
↓ Tachycardia*
↓ Release of mediators of inflammation†
↓ Recruitment of inflammatory cells†
↓ Early and late response to antigen†

*These are also H_2-receptor antagonist effects.
†Some, but not all, H_1-receptor antagonists have these effects.

Children have shorter serum elimination half-life values for H_1-receptor antagonists than adults do, and the elderly may have prolonged values compared with those of young adults. Serum elimination half-life values of H_1-receptor antagonists generally increase with the increasing age of the patient. The serum elimination half-life of most H_1-receptor antagonists is prolonged in patients with severe hepatic dysfunction.

Cetirizine, the relatively nonsedating carboxylic acid metabolite of hydroxyzine, has unique pharmacokinetic properties. Unlike other H_1-receptor antagonists, it is not extensively metabolized by the hepatic cytochrome system; rather, 60% of a dose of cetirizine appears as unchanged drug in the urine within 24 hours. It has a mean serum elimination half-life value of 6.6 to 10.6 hours in adults, 7.0 hours in school-age children (Fig. 16–2*A*) and 4.9 hours in children under 4 years of age. In adults with renal insufficiency

TABLE 16–2. Pharmacokinetics and Pharmacodynamics of H_1-Receptor Antagonists

H_1-Receptor Antagonist	β-Phase Serum Elimination Half-Life (Hours)	Significant Wheal Suppression After a Single Dose (Hours)*
First-Generation		
Chlorpheniramine	24.4 (11.0)‖	24
Brompheniramine	24.9	9
Triprolidine	2.1	—
Diphenhydramine	9.2 (5.4)‖	10
Hydroxyzine	20.0 (7.1)‖	36
Second-Generation		
Terfenadine†	17.0	12–24
Astemizole	9.5 days‡	§
Cetirizine	6.6–10.6 (4.9–7.0)‖	24
Loratadine	11.0	12–24
Acrivastine	1.4–2.1	<12

*Dose-dependent; see specific references for doses used.
†Terfenadine metabolite I.
‡Includes $t_{½}$ of hydroxylated metabolites.
§A single dose of astemizole does not suppress the wheal and flare very well, but after a short course of treatment (7 days) suppression may last for weeks.
‖Serum elimination half-life in children.

the half-life may be increased. Acrivastine is also eliminated primarily unchanged via the kidneys.

Breast milk concentration versus time curves parallel serum concentration versus time curves in single-dose studies of H_1-receptor antagonists.

PHARMACODYNAMICS: RELATIONSHIP OF EFFICACY TO SERUM CONCENTRATIONS. Maximal antihistaminic effects of the H_1-receptor antagonists occur several hours after peak serum concentrations have passed and persist even when serum concentrations of the parent compound have declined to the lowest limits of analytical detection. H_1-receptor antagonists should therefore be given *before* an anticipated allergic reaction, if possible, in order to achieve maximal efficacy. The duration of action of these medications, as assessed objectively by suppression of the histamine- or allergen-induced wheal and flare in the skin or subjectively by suppression of symptoms of, for example, rhinoconjunctivitis or urticaria, is much more prolonged than might be expected from consideration of the serum elimination half-life values (Figs. 16–2 and 16–3).

The degree and duration of wheal-and-flare suppression relate to H_1-receptor antagonist dose as well as to the serum elimination half-life of the drug. Some first-generation H_1-receptor antagonists, such as tripelennamine and triprolidine, in manufacturers' recommended doses, are not very effective in suppressing the wheal and flare. Others, such as chlorpheniramine and hydroxyzine, are more effective and should not yet be discarded from therapeutic use; a single dose of chlorpheniramine or hydroxyzine suppresses the histamine-induced wheal and flare for 24 hours.

A single dose of the second-generation H_1-receptor antagonist loratadine (10 mg) suppresses the histamine-induced wheal and flare for 12 to 24 hours. A single dose of terfenadine (60–120 mg) or cetirizine (10 mg) significantly suppresses the wheal-and-flare response to histamine for 24 hours. A single dose of astemizole (10 mg) is not very effective in suppressing the histamine-induced wheal and flare, but after a short course of astemizole (10 mg daily) has been discontinued, the histamine-induced wheal-and-flare may remain suppressed for 6 to 8 weeks (Table 16–2 and Fig. 16–3).

LACK OF SUBSENSITIVITY. Long-term administration of first-generation H_1-receptor antagonists may be associated with an *apparent* decrease in efficacy. This phenomenon has been attributed to autoinduction of hepatic metabolism and increased hepatic clearance of the H_1-receptor antagonist, with consequent lower serum and, presumably, lower tissue concentrations of the medication. Support for this concept was based on limited data obtained in dogs administered diphenhydramine or chlorcyclizine by mouth for a few weeks. In a study designed to reexamine this issue, however, dogs administered hydroxyzine daily for 150 days (21 weeks), intramuscularly to ensure compliance, had somewhat higher mean serum hydroxyzine concentrations at the end of the treatment course than on the first day of treatment, significantly slower mean clearance rates, and longer mean serum half-life values on days 30, 60, 120, and 150 than after the first dose of hydroxyzine on day 1. No evidence of autoinduction of metabolism was found.

Furthermore, humans do not eliminate chlorpheniramine or terfenadine more rapidly during long-term dosing than during short-term dosing, and the efficacy of chlorpheniramine, loratadine, terfenadine, or cetirizine in suppressing skin tests to histamine or in relieving rhinoconjunctivitis symptoms does not diminish over a period of 4 to 12 weeks, as demonstrated in studies in which compliance was monitored rigorously (Fig. 16–2*B*). The apparent subsensitivity reported years ago with the first-generation H_1-receptor antagonists may have been due, at least in part, to poor compliance because of sedation or lack of efficacy.

Efficacy in Treatment of Allergic Disorders

H_1-receptor antagonists provide relief of allergic rhinoconjunctivitis symptoms. They have a modest bronchodilator effect in patients with asthma. They effectively relieve pruritus, new wheal formation, and duration of whealing in patients with urticaria; and first-generation H_1-receptor antagonists effectively relieve pruritus in patients with atopic dermatitis. The effectiveness of H_1-receptor antagonists in treatment of upper respiratory tract infections and in otitis media is controversial. Formulations and recommended dosages of representative H_1-receptor antagonists are listed in Table 16–3.

ALLERGIC RHINOCONJUNCTIVITIS. In patients with allergic rhinitis, histamine released in the immediate (type 1) hypersensitivity response binds to H_1-receptors on the blood vessels in the nasal mucosa, submucosa, and lamina propria. Histamine produces symptoms by inducing vasodilation through a direct effect on relaxation of the vascular smooth muscle and by increasing secretion from the submucous glands through a vagal reflex.

In studies in which patients with allergic rhinitis are challenged intranasally with antigens to which they are sen-

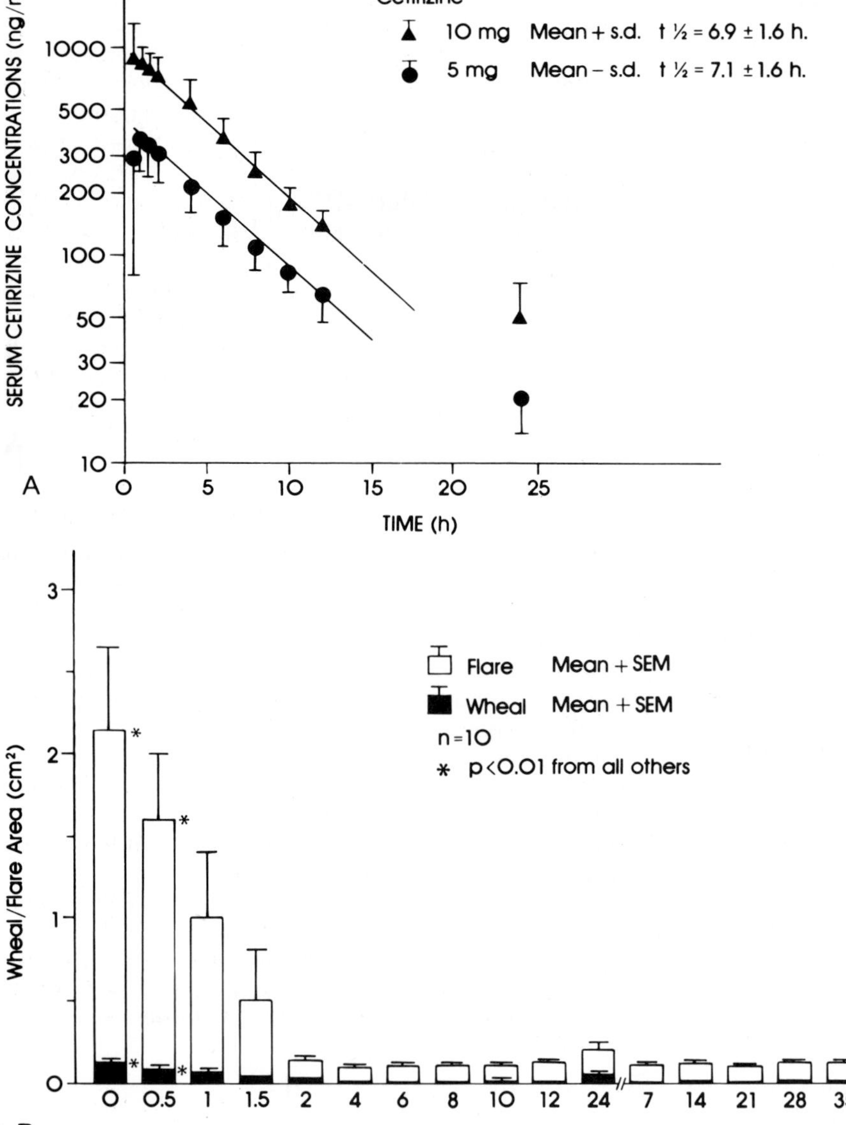

FIGURE 16–2. (*A*) In a double-blind, parallel-group study of a single oral dose of cetirizine 5 mg in 10 children with allergic rhinitis versus a single oral dose of cetirizine 10 mg in 9 children with allergic rhinitis, the serum elimination half-life of cetirizine was approximately 6.9–7.1 hours. (*B*) A single dose of cetirizine 5 mg in children significantly suppressed the mean histamine-induced wheal-and-flare areas resulting from epicutaneous tests with histamine phosphate, 1 mg/ml from 1 to 24 hours postdose. During chronic cetirizine dosing in the subsequent 5 weeks, the wheal-and-flare suppression 12 hours after the cetirizine dose did not differ significantly on days 7, 14, 21, 28, and 35. (From Watson WT, Simons KJ, Chen XY, Simons FE: Cetirizine: A pharmacokinetic and pharmacodynamic evaluation in children with seasonal allergic rhinitis. J Allergy Clin Immunol 84:457–464, 1989.)

sitized, H_1-receptor antagonists given by mouth relieve the sneezing, itching, and nasal discharge of the immediate reaction to allergen. Some second-generation H_1-receptor antagonists decrease release of mediators of inflammation such as histamine in nasal secretions.

In numerous placebo-controlled double-blind studies in which patients have recorded symptom scores over weeks or months, H_1-receptor antagonists have proved to be useful in ameliorating sneezing, itching, and nasal discharge and also for relief of ocular symptoms such as itching, tearing, and erythema (Fig. 16–4). They are not as effective in relieving congestion; hence, decongestants such as pseudoephedrine are sometimes added to the H_1-receptor antagonists in order to provide relief of this symptom.

In studies in patients with seasonal or perennial rhinitis, the second-generation H_1-receptor antagonists have been generally found to be superior to placebo and comparable to a first-generation H_1-receptor antagonist such as chlorpheniramine. The second-generation H_1-receptor antagonists are used increasingly for the treatment of allergic rhinoconjunctivitis because they are relatively nonsedating. Terfenadine, 60 mg twice daily or in some countries 120 mg once daily, astemizole 10 mg daily, loratadine 10 mg daily, cetirizine 10 mg daily, and acrivastine 8 mg three to four times daily are the doses recommended by the manufacturers as providing optimal efficacy with minimal likelihood of causing sedation or other adverse effects (Table 16–3). Terfenadine seems to provide faster onset of symptom relief than that of astemizole, but in long-term studies, astemizole provides greater overall symptom relief than that obtained with terfenadine. Terfenadine, loratadine, and cetirizine appear to be comparable.

Although H_1-receptor antagonists are extremely useful in the treatment of mild or moderate allergic rhinoconjunctivitis, other chemical mediators contribute to the inflammation in the nasal mucosa and conjunctiva in this disorder, and these mediators are not blocked by H_1-receptor antagonists. Patients with severe allergic rhinoconjunctivitis gener-

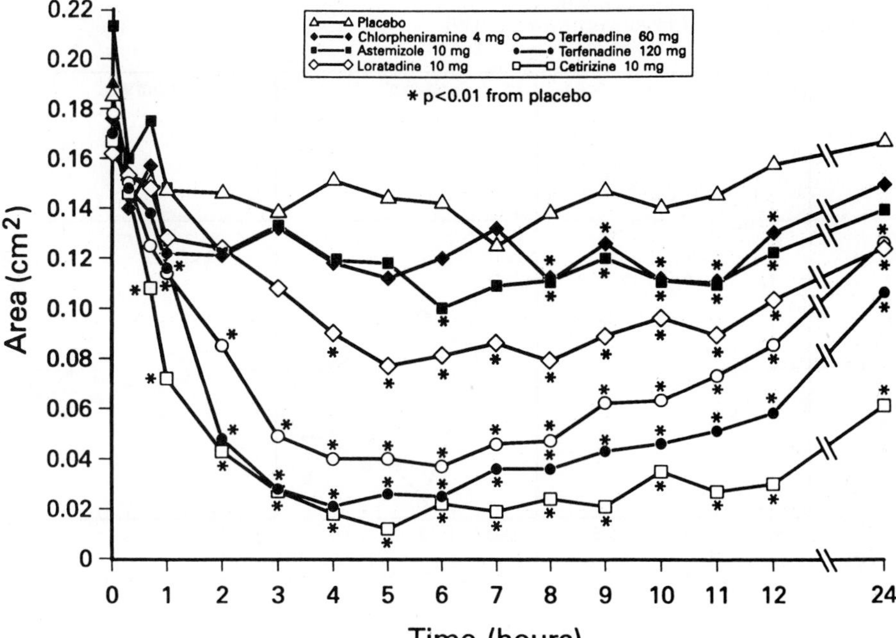

FIGURE 16–3. In a single-dose, double-blind, seven-way cross-over study in 20 healthy men, chlorpheniramine 4 mg, astemizole 10 mg, loratadine 10 mg, terfenadine 60 mg, terfenadine 120 mg, cetirizine 10 mg, and placebo differed significantly in their suppressive effect on the histamine-induced wheal. The rank order of suppression was placebo (*least* suppressive), chlorpheniramine 4 mg, astemizole 10 mg, loratadine 10 mg, terfenadine 60 mg, terfenadine 120 mg, and cetirizine 10 mg (*most* suppressive). (From Simons FE, McMillan JL, Simons KJ: A double-blind, single-dose, cross-over comparison of cetirizine, terfenadine, loratadine, astemizole, and chlorpheniramine versus placebo: Suppressive effects on histamine-induced wheals and flares during 24 hours in normal subjects. J Allergy Clin Immunol 86:540–547, 1990.)

ally require a topical intranasal corticosteroid for complete relief of symptoms.

ASTHMA. Histamine is an important mediator of asthma symptoms. Most of the histamine in the lungs is located in the secretory granules of mast cells in the airway. Specific challenge with allergen or nonspecific challenge with exercise or cold air stimulates the release of this preformed mediator of inflammation and contributes to airflow obstruction. Plasma histamine concentrations increase transiently after bronchoprovocation with inhaled allergen and in association with spontaneous acute asthma episodes. Histamine contributes to asthma symptoms by numerous mechanisms of action: causing bronchoconstriction and stimulation of cough receptors via H_1-receptors; causing increased permeability of the vascular endothelium and increased amount and viscosity of mucous glycoprotein secretion from bronchial glands and goblet cells via H_1- and H_2-receptors; and causing increased permeability of the respiratory endothelium via H_2-receptors.

The *first-generation* H_1-receptor antagonists chlorpheniramine, diphenhydramine, and hydroxyzine have some bronchodilator effect, but in clinically useful antiasthma doses they cause sedation and other adverse effects. The *second-generation* H_1-receptor antagonists ter-

TABLE 16–3. Formulations and Dosages of Representative H_1-Receptor Antagonists

Generic (Trade Name)	Formulation	Recommended Dose
First-Generation		
Chlorpheniramine maleate (many named products)	Syrup, 2.5 mg/5 ml; tablets, 4 mg; time-release, 8, 12 mg; parenteral solution, 10 mg/ml	Pediatric,* 0.35 mg/kg/24 hours; adult, 8–12 mg b.i.d.‡
Diphenhydramine hydrochloride (BENADRYL)	Children's liquid, 6.25 mg/5 ml; elixir, 12.5 mg/5 ml; capsules, 25 or 50 mg; parenteral solution, 50 mg/ml	Pediatric,* 5 mg/kg/24 hours; adult, 25–50 mg t.i.d.‡
Hydroxyzine hydrochloride (ATARAX)	Syrup, 10 mg/5 ml; capsules, 10, 25, 50 mg	Pediatric,* 2 mg/kg/24 hours; adult, 25–50 mg o.d. (h.s.) *or* b.i.d.‡
Second-Generation (Relatively Nonsedating)		
Terfenadine (SELDANE)	Suspension, 30 mg/5 ml;† tablet, 60 mg, 120 mg†	Pediatric, 3–6 years old: 15 mg b.i.d., 7–12 years old: 30 mg b.i.d.; adult, 60 mg b.i.d. *or* 120 mg o.d.‡
Astemizole (HISMANAL)	Suspension, 10 mg/5 ml;† tablet, 10 mg	Pediatric,* 0.2 mg/kg/24 hours; adult, 10 mg o.d.‡
Loratadine (CLARITIN)	Tablet, 10 mg	Adult, 10 mg o.d.‡
Cetirizine (REACTINE)	Tablet, 10 mg†	Adult, 5–10 mg o.d.‡
Acrivastine (SEMPREX)	Tablet, 8 mg	Adult, 8 mg t.i.d.‡

Note: To minimize the potential central nervous system depressive effects of the first-generation H_1-receptor antagonists listed in this table, many physicians now try to give as much as possible of the daily dose at bedtime.

*For patients weighing ≤40 kg.

†Not available in the United States at the time of publication.

‡b.i.d. = twice a day; t.i.d. = three times a day; o.d. = once a day.

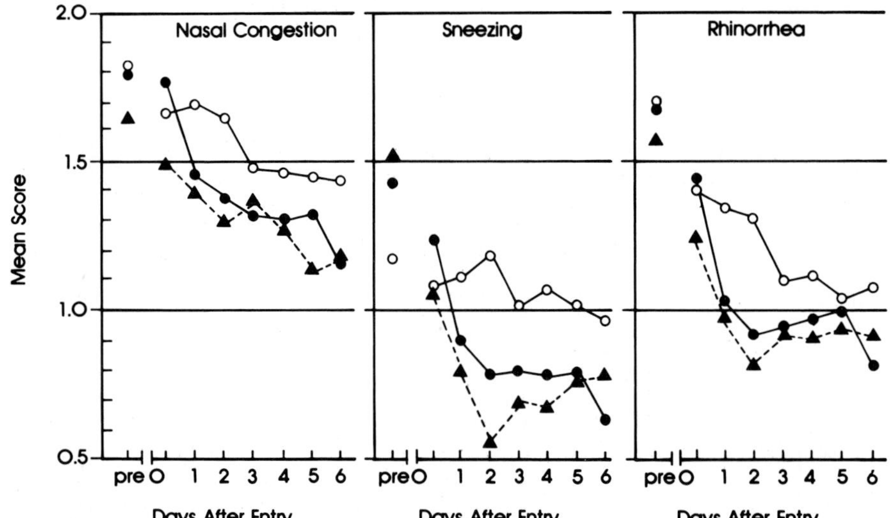

FIGURE 16–4. Efficacy of terfenadine and chlorpheniramine versus placebo in patients with allergic rhinoconjunctivitis. Both H_1-receptor antagonists were effective in reducing sneezing and rhinorrhea but were not significantly more effective than placebo in relieving nasal congestion. The incidence of sedation in the terfenadine-treated group (7.6%) and in the placebo-treated group (2.4%) did not differ significantly. The incidence of sedation in the chlorpheniramine-treated group was 19%, significantly higher than in either the terfenadine- or the placebo-treated group. The physicians' pretreatment severity scores are presented in the upper left corners of each plot because no pretreatment severity of symptoms was obtained from the patients' diaries. (From Kemp JP, Buckley CE, Gershwin ME, et al: Multicenter, double-blind, placebo-controlled trial of terfenadine in seasonal allergic rhinitis and conjunctivitis. Ann Allergy 54:502–509, 1985.)

fenadine, astemizole, loratadine, and cetirizine clearly have dose-related bronchodilator activity and a protective effect against histamine-, and allergen-, exercise-, hyperventilation-, and cold, dry air–induced bronchospasm; like their predecessors, they do not protect against methacholine-induced bronchospasm. In doses higher than required for allergic rhinitis treatment, these medications can provide some relief from mild seasonal or chronic asthma symptoms when taken over weeks or months.

H_1-receptor antagonists are not drugs of first choice for asthma; however, patients with asthma who require H_1-receptor antagonists for treatment of concurrent rhinoconjunctivitis or urticaria will not be harmed by H_1-receptor antagonist treatment and may benefit from the antiasthma effect of the H_1-receptor antagonist (see Chapter 17).

CHRONIC URTICARIA. In placebo-controlled, double-blind studies in adults with chronic idiopathic urticaria, the first-generation H_1-receptor antagonists hydroxyzine, chlorpheniramine, and diphenhydramine and the second-generation H_1-receptor antagonists terfenadine, astemizole, cetirizine and loratadine result in significant remission of symptoms compared with the relief provided by placebo. They reduce pruritus and the number, size, and duration of urticarial lesions. In chronic urticaria treatment, use of first-generation H_1-receptor antagonists is declining in comparison to the use of the nonsedating second-generation H_1-receptor antagonists. Terfenadine and astemizole have been compared directly in patients with chronic urticaria, and astemizole seems to be the more effective of these two medications, although it may have a slower onset of action.

ANAPHYLAXIS. In patients with anaphylaxis, for whom, of course, *treatment of first choice is epinephrine,* first-generation H_1-receptor antagonists such as chlorpheniramine and diphenhydramine, which are available in formulations for intravenous administration, are useful adjunctive treatment for control of pruritus, rhinorrhea, and other symptoms. Second-generation H_1-receptor antagonists are not currently recommended for use in anaphylaxis because they are not available in formulations for intravenous administration and there are no published studies of their efficacy in anaphylaxis.

ATOPIC DERMATITIS. The mechanism of itching associated with atopic dermatitis remains unknown, but histamine is almost certainly involved to some extent because histamine concentrations are increased in the skin and in the plasma of patients with this disorder. First-generation H_1-receptor antagonists, which may have a CNS sedative effect, seem to relieve itching in atopic dermatitis better than second-generation H_1-receptor antagonists do, leading some investigators to conclude that the second-generation H_1-receptor antagonists should not replace the first-generation H_1-receptor antagonists in the treatment of this condition.

OTHER. H_1-receptor antagonists are widely used for symptomatic treatment of upper respiratory tract infections, although there is limited evidence from double-blind, placebo-controlled studies to support this practice. Similarly, H_1-receptor antagonists have been widely prescribed for patients with acute otitis media and for those with chronic otitis media with effusion, despite studies demonstrating that these medications do not significantly hasten the resolution of otitis media. The second-generation H_1-receptor antagonists have not been adequately studied in otitis media.

The first generation H_1-receptor antagonists dimenhydrinate and promethazine are still used for prophylaxis in treatment of motion sickness; dimenhydrinate is also used in patients with vestibular disturbances. Second-generation H_1-receptor antagonists, acting either at the peripheral vestibular end-organ or at CNS structures *outside* the blood-brain barrier, may also be effective in the treatment of these disorders, but further studies are required.

Adverse Effects

FIRST-GENERATION H_1-RECEPTOR ANTAGONISTS. First-generation H_1-receptor antagonists may cause sedation, impairment of cognitive function, diminished alertness, slowed reaction times, confusion, dizziness, and tinnitus or anticholinergic effects such as dry mouth, blurred vision, and urinary retention. These symptoms, to which elderly patients and patients with hepatic dysfunction may be more prone, correlate with peak serum concentrations. Some first-generation H_1-receptor antagonists, such as diphenhy-

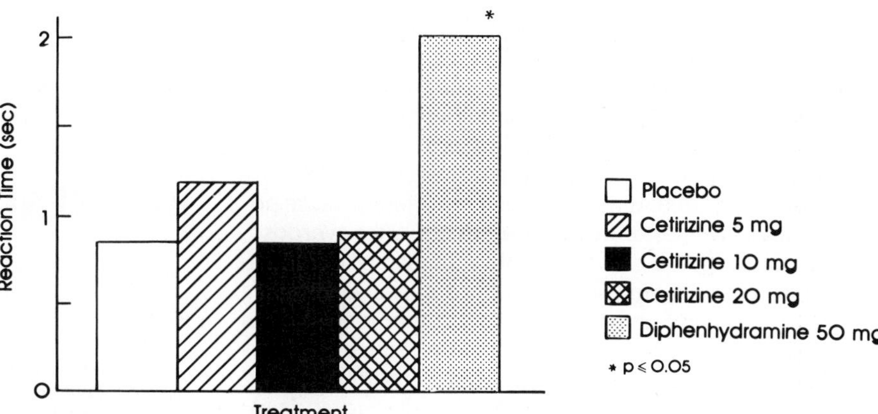

FIGURE 16–5. Double-blind, five-way cross-over study in 15 male volunteers, mean age 23.8 years, who ingested placebo, cetirizine 5, 10, or 20 mg, and diphenhydramine 50 mg. Numerous subjective measurements of drowsiness and objective measurements of mental performance were made 2 hours after dosing. During simulated accident avoidance in a simulated automobile-driving situation, diphenhydramine 50 mg slowed the reaction time significantly compared with placebo and with cetirizine 5, 10, and 20 mg. (From Gengo FM, Gabos C, Mechtler L: Quantitative effects of cetirizine and diphenhydramine on mental performance measured using an automobile driving simulator. Ann Allergy 64:520–526, 1990.)

dramine, in ordinary therapeutic doses occasionally cause unusual adverse effects such as dystonic reactions. (Paradoxically, diphenhydramine may produce dramatic relief of acute dystonic reactions produced by antipsychotic drugs [see Chapter 23].)

Fatal or near fatal intoxication has been reported rarely following ingestion of massive overdoses of first-generation H_1-receptor antagonists such as tripelennamine, chlorpheniramine, cyproheptadine, dimenhydrinate, diphenhydramine, or hydroxyzine. Toxic encephalopathy or psychosis may occur and has even been reported after topical application of an H_1-receptor antagonist such as diphenhydramine; patients with epidermal breakdown are particularly susceptible to this adverse effect. Adults usually manifest lethargy, extreme drowsiness, or coma after first-generation H_1-receptor antagonist overdose, but young children may suffer from excitation, irritability, hyperactivity, insomnia, visual hallucinations, and seizures. Patients generally exhibit anticholinergic effects such as dryness of the mucous membranes, fever, flushed facies, pupillary dilatation, urinary retention, decreased gastrointestinal motility, and hypotension. Tachycardia, conductance disturbances, dysrhythmias, and occasionally, myocardial depression refractory to vasopressor support have been reported. Cardiorespiratory arrest and death may occur.

Treatment of a patient who has overdosed on a first-generation H_1-receptor antagonist consists of general supportive measures, such as evacuation of stomach contents, use of anticonvulsants, and hemodialysis. Shortly after ingestion of an H_1-receptor antagonist with strong antiemetic effects, gastric lavage may be more effective than a centrally acting emetic such as ipecac. There are no specific antidotes for H_1-receptor antagonist poisoning. Histamine itself is not helpful because the signs and symptoms of an H_1-receptor antagonist overdose are *not* related to histamine H_1-receptor blockade.

SECOND-GENERATION H_1-RECEPTOR ANTAGONISTS. Although many of the *first-generation* H_1-receptor antagonists produce sedation or other CNS system symptoms in approximately 20% of users, the incidence of sedation or other CNS impairment in patients receiving a *second-generation* H_1-receptor antagonist such as terfenadine, astemizole, loratadine or cetirizine in manufacturers' recommended doses is comparable to the incidence of sedation in patients receiving placebo and is not clinically important in most patients (Fig. 16–5). The incidence of sedation is not zero, however; therefore, from time to time, physicians may encounter patients who complain of sedation after ingestion of a second-generation H_1-receptor antagonist. Also, when manufacturers' recommended doses of these medications are exceeded, the frequency of sedation may increase.

The relative lack of sedation produced by the new H_1-receptor antagonists has been documented in numerous double-blind, placebo-controlled studies. Methods of assessment of sedation have been subjective (*eg*, a diary card on which the patient records daytime sleepiness) and objective (*eg*, multiple sleep-latency tests, in which the investigator obtains an electroencephalographic record of the length of time a patient takes to fall asleep during the day, under standardized conditions). Some of the different types of tests used for assessment of sedation and other CNS adverse effects of H_1-receptor antagonists are summarized in Table 16–4.

Investigators do not always find a strong correlation between subjective symptoms of sleepiness and objective measurements of CNS dysfunction such as prolongation of reaction time, indicating that patients may not necessarily recognize reduction in alertness and functioning produced by H_1-receptor antagonist ingestion.

Fixed-dose combinations of second-generation H_1-receptor antagonists with decongestants such as pseudoephedrine are associated with a higher incidence of insomnia and other CNS adverse effects than first-generation H_1-receptor

TABLE 16–4. Some Tests Used for Assessment of Sedation and Other Central Nervous System Adverse Effects of H_1-Receptor Antagonists

Subjective
Diary cards to record daytime sleepiness
Visual analog scales to record daytime sleepiness
Self-rating of sleepiness, impairment, and fatigue, using Stanford Sleepiness Scale or Profile-of-Moods questionnaire

Objective
Multiple sleep-latency test
Latency of P3 evoked electroencephalographic potentials (measure of sustained attention and cerebral processing speed)
Dynamic visual acuity
Pupillary light responses
Critical flicker fusion
Simple reaction time
Choice reaction time
Digit-symbol substitution
Monitoring of computer-simulated driving errors
Monitoring of actual driving errors

antagonist/decongestant fixed-dose combinations, in which the CNS stimulation of the decongestant is counteracted by the sedation produced by the H_1-receptor antagonist.

Other adverse effects of second-generation H_1-receptor antagonists have been reported. Astemizole may cause appetite stimulation and inappropriate weight gain. Rarely, astemizole and terfenadine have been reported to cause potentially fatal adverse cardiovascular effects. After overdose, or when administered concomitantly with macrolide antibiotics such as erythromycin or clarithromycin, antifungals such as ketoconazole or itraconazole or other medications that inhibit the hepatic mixed-function oxygenase cytochrome P-450 system, they may cause a prolonged QTc interval, polymorphic ventricular tachycardia (*torsade de pointes*) and other cardiac dysrhythmias by blocking the delayed rectifier potassium current in ventricular myocytes.

INTERACTION OF SECOND-GENERATION H_1-RECEPTOR ANTAGONISTS WITH CENTRAL NERVOUS SYSTEM—ACTIVE SUBSTANCES. The first-generation H_1-receptor antagonists enhance the adverse psychomotor effects of ethanol, diazepam, and other CNS-active chemicals. The second-generation H_1-receptor antagonists, in manufacturers' recommended doses, have not been found to potentiate the CNS effects of these substances.

Safety in Pregnancy and Lactation

Although teratogenic effects of first-generation H_1-receptor antagonists (piperazines) have been noted in animals, fetal anomalies in humans have not been proved to be due to any H_1-receptor antagonists. A neonatal withdrawal syndrome has been described in infants born to mothers receiving large therapeutic doses of hydroxyzine or diphenhydramine immediately before parturition.

Embryo toxicity, fetal wastage, fetal anomalies, or other problems in pregnancy in humans have not been attributed to any of the second-generation H_1-receptor antagonists to date. The number of pregnant patients who have received these medications is small, however; and in most countries they are classified as Schedule C drugs or equivalent—that is, although there is no evidence that they are unsafe, they should be used only if expected benefits outweigh the unknown potential risks of toxicity. H_1-receptor antagonists are excreted in breast milk.

SUMMARY

H_1-receptor antagonists differ considerably from one another in some aspects of basic pharmacology and in pharmacokinetics and pharmacodynamics. An understanding of these differences will facilitate their optimal clinical usage.

The second-generation H_1-receptor antagonists do not penetrate into the CNS as readily as the first-generation H_1-receptor antagonists do. In manufacturers' recommended doses, they cause no more sedation than a placebo does.

Because of their more favorable benefit/risk ratio, the second-generation H_1-receptor antagonists are replacing the first-generation H_1-receptor antagonists in the symptomatic treatment of allergic rhinoconjunctivitis and in relieving pruritus in patients with urticaria. They have a mild beneficial effect in patients with chronic asthma. They have *not* supplanted the first-generation H_1-receptor antagonists in atopic dermatitis treatment or as adjunctive treatment of pruritus and other symptoms in patients with anaphylaxis.

REFERENCES

Arrang JM, Garbarg M, Lancelot JC, et al: Highly potent and selective ligands for histamine H_3-receptors. Nature 327:117–123, 1987.

Birnbaumer L, Brown AM: G proteins and the mechanism of action of hormones, neurotransmitters, and autocrine and paracrine regulatory factors. Am Rev Respir Dis 141:S106–S114, 1990.

Campoli-Richards DM, Buckley MMT, Fitton A: Cetirizine: A review of its pharmacological properties and clinical potential in allergic rhinitis, pollen-induced asthma, and chronic urticaria. Drugs 40:762–781, 1990.

Clissold SP, Sorkin EM, Goa KL: Loratadine. A preliminary review of its pharmacodynamic properties and therapeutic efficacy. Drugs 37:42–57, 1989.

De Backer MD, Gommeren W, Moereels H, et al: Genomic cloning, heterologous expression and pharmacological characterization of a human histamine H_1 receptor. Biochem Biophys Res Commun 197:1601–1608, 1993.

Gantz I, Schaffer M, DelValle J, et al: Molecular cloning of a gene encoding the histamine H_2-receptor. Proc Natl Acad Sci 88:429–433, 1991.

Garrison JC: Histamine, bradykinin, 5-hydroxytryptamine, and their antagonists. *In* Gilman AG, Rall TW, Nies AS, Taylor P (eds): Goodman and Gilman's The Pharmacological Basis of Therapeutics, 8th ed, 575–588. New York: Pergamon Press, 1990.

Gengo FM, Gabos C, Mechtler L: Quantitative effects of cetirizine and diphenhydramine on mental performance measured using an automobile driving simulator. Ann Allergy 64:520–526, 1990.

Howarth PH: Histamine and asthma: An appraisal based on specific H_1-receptor antagonism. Clin Exp Allergy 20:31–41, 1990.

Ichinose M, Barnes PJ: Inhibitory histamine H_3-receptors on cholinergic nerves in human airways. Eur J Pharmacol 163:383–386, 1989.

Kemp JP, Buckley CE, Gershwin ME, et al: Multicenter, double-blind, placebo-controlled trial of terfenadine in seasonal allergic rhinitis and conjunctivitis. Ann Allergy 54:502–509, 1985.

McTavish D, Goa KL, Ferrill M: Terfenadine: An updated review of its pharmacological properties and therapeutic efficacy. Drugs 39:552–574, 1990.

McTavish D, Sorkin EM: Azelastine. A review of its pharmacodynamic and pharmacokinetic properties, and therapeutic potential. Drugs 38:778–800, 1989.

Richards DM, Brogden RN, Heel RC, et al: Astemizole. A review of its pharmacodynamic properties and therapeutic efficacy. Drugs 28:38–61, 1984.

Rimmer SJ, Church MK: The pharmacology and mechanisms of action of histamine H_1-antagonists. Clin Exp Allergy 20:3–17, 1990.

Saxena SP, Brandes LJ, Becker AB, et al: Histamine is an intracellular messenger mediating platelet aggregation. Science 243:1596–1599, 1989.

Simons FER: H_1-receptor antagonists. Comparative tolerability and safety. Drug Safety 10:350–380, 1994.

Simons FER: H_1-receptor antagonists: Clinical pharmacology and therapeutics. J Allergy Clin Immunol 84:845–861, 1989.

Simons FER: Loratadine, a non-sedating H_1-receptor antagonist (antihistamine). Ann Allergy 63:266–268, 1989.

Simons FER, McMillan JL, Simons KJ: A double-blind, single-dose, crossover comparison of cetirizine, terfenadine, loratadine, astemizole, and chlorpheniramine versus placebo: Suppressive effects on histamine-induced wheals and flares during 24 hours in normal subjects. J Allergy Clin Immunol 86:540–547, 1990.

Simons FER, Simons KJ: The pharmacology and use of H_1-receptor antagonist drugs. N Engl J Med 330:1663–1670, 1994.

Simons FER, Simons KJ: Second-generation H_1-receptor antagonists. Ann Allergy 66:5–19, 1991.

Watson WTA, Simons KJ, Chen XY, Simons FER: Cetirizine: A pharmacokinetic and pharmacodynamic evaluation in children with seasonal allergic rhinitis. J Allergy Clin Immunol 84:457–464, 1989.

Drugs Used in the Treatment of Asthma 17

David A. Stempel

Asthma is a respiratory disease characterized by a distinctive form of bronchial hyperresponsiveness linked to a unique form of airway inflammation. Both of these processes result in a variable degree of obstruction of respiratory airflow. They are not exclusive to asthma, but this combination constitutes the disease complex. Asthmatic respiratory obstruction may be triggered by allergen exposure, common respiratory infections, exercise, cold air exposure, medications, and airway irritants. Respiratory airway obstruction occurs only in the individual with a predisposed hyperresponsive airway.

The airway of the untreated asymptomatic asthmatic patient with mild disease is remarkable for the presence of eosinophilic infiltration, actively degranulating mast cells, epithelial disruption, hypertrophy of airway smooth muscle, and hypersecretion of mucus. The fluid obtained with bronchial alveolar lavage reveals increased numbers of T lymphocytes that release cytokines, which orchestrate the inflammatory process. The illness may frequently go unrecognized or is undertreated because it is usually only identified from a detailed history that includes questions about physical activity and quality of sleep.

Biopsy and bronchial alveolar lavage studies have increased our understanding of the disease mechanisms. Significant gains in the pharmacotherapy of asthma also have been made during the last decade. Perplexing is the realization that the morbidity and mortality of asthma have been increasing, although these advances would suggest the opposite. Explanations include

- The increase in asthma due to poor air quality, inability of physicians to adequately deliver health care especially to the indigent patient
- The possibility that the therapy for the disease is adversely affecting its outcome
- The possibility that the true incidence of the disease is actually increasing

Allergy is a common component of asthma in children and young adults. Although the mode of inheritance is controversial, ample evidence exists to support a genetic mode of transmission. Environmental exposure, especially in early childhood, predisposes to the development of allergic reactivity and clinical expression of asthma. In the sensitized individual, repeated low-level exposure may lead to airway inflammation. When this inflamed airway is exposed to viral infections, allergens, exercise, or airway irritants, deterioration of lung function and evidence of airflow obstruction occur (see Fig. 17 – 1).

Allergic asthma provides a model for understanding the mechanisms that produce the inflammatory process and the bronchial hyperresponsiveness. The sensitized airways of the asthmatic undergo an immediate bronchoconstriction 15 – 20 minutes after allergen exposure, which may resolve by 1 hour. This is the **immediate phase** and reflects the secretion of mediators from activated mast cells. Leukotrienes C_4 and D_4, prostaglandin D_2, and histamine are the mediators that are recovered in bronchioalveolar lavage. The late-phase reaction starts at 2 – 4 hours and reaches its maximum at 6 – 8 hours. This late phase response is evidenced by the migration of neutrophils followed by eosinophils into the airway; this inflammatory phase of asthma results in more pronounced and prolonged disease activity.

The hallmark of asthma is airflow obstruction combined with inflammatory processes involving mucosal edema, mucus production, and increased vascular permeability. The mast cell and surface basophils, fundamental in the immediate phase, are the result of the interaction of a specific allergen with immunoglobulin E (IgE) antibodies bound to receptors on these cell surfaces. The bridging of IgE receptors leads to modification of the receptor and causes a complex sequence of biochemical events to occur, resulting in cellular activation, arachidonic acid metabolism, and mediator release. The observation that even in the mild asymptomatic asthmatic evidence of mast cell degranulation exists suggests an ongoing inflammatory state that may precede allergen exposure.

Precipitating factors in allergic asthma include perennial as well as seasonal allergens. Several of these allergens induce perennial symptoms as a result of their persistence in the indoor environment. Dust mites feed off dried skin debris and represent a significant indoor allergen burden in the

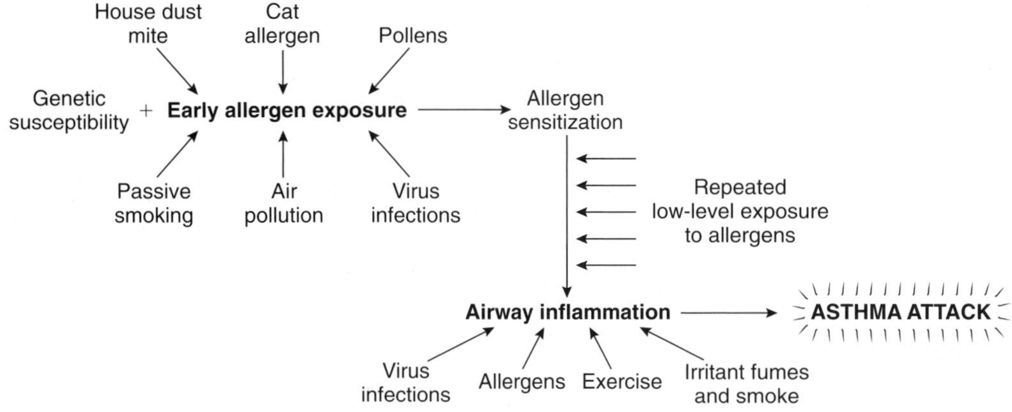

FIGURE 17–1. Schematic representation of early and later life events leading to airway allergen sensitization and asthma. (Redrawn from Holgate S: Mediator and cytokine mechanisms in asthma. Thorax 48:103–109, 1993.)

home. Mites are present in mattresses, pillows, stuffed animals, carpeting, and upholstery. Mites do not circulate in the air unless they are disturbed, and attention to decreasing exposure needs to focus on areas where the nose and mouth are in close contact with the mite source. Simple environmental controls that emphasize encasing mattresses and pillows in watertight coverings and washing all bedding in hot water (hotter than 130°F) are an important aspect of treating the inflammatory process by preventing the development of airway inflammation. A concept under consideration is whether the at-risk child might be treated with environmental control, thereby preventing the development of disease.

Viral respiratory infections also have been identified as major factors in producing acute airflow obstruction and inflamed airways. IgE antibodies to specific respiratory viruses have been identified during acute wheezing symptoms. Similar release of inflammatory mediators has been identified in conjunction with virus-induced asthma. Late-phase airway reactivity has been demonstrated after rhinovirus infection. Although allergic reactivity is a common component of asthma, it is equally important to recognize the significance of viral infections in the pathophysiology of asthma.

DIAGNOSTIC APPROACH

The evaluation of the patient with asthma should include a thorough patient history that investigates environmental factors that are important in the disease process. The prevalence of allergic reactivity in asthma is high enough to warrant selected allergy evaluation for essentially all patients who use regular asthma medications. Dust mite allergy is ubiquitous and often missed when a patient history is being taken. This knowledge allows the patient to institute appropriate environmental control measures, important in reducing the inflammatory component of asthma. Identification of specific triggering factors and environmental manipulation can have a dramatic impact. Epicutaneous skin testing provides accurate data on clinical sensitivity. Quality radioallergosorbent testing also can provide useful data when skin testing is not available. Lung function testing is an essential part of the diagnosis of asthma and is important in monitoring the disease activity. It is analogous to recording blood pressure in the hypertensive patient and blood glucose levels in the diabetic. Lung function testing should be accessible and affordable to allow its being routinely performed in the patient with asthma. The extent of the diagnostic evaluation of the asthmatic should reflect the disease severity.

The grading of the severity of asthmatic disease by levels one through four provides a useful rubric for both the diagnostic and therapeutic management. Level one consists of individuals with limited illness who are readily treated, allowing them to be essentially disease-free and to experience no adverse effects of therapy. At the other extreme, level four consists of seriously ill patients for whom therapy can be lifesaving and can provide acceptable but limited function and reductions of exacerbations; it is likely that patients with level four asthma will experience some adverse effects from therapy (Tables 17–1 and 17–2).

TABLE 17–1. Asthma Symptom Scores

	Level 0	Level 1	Level 2	Level 3	Level 4
Frequency	Rare	1–2/month	1–2/week	3–7/week	>1/day
Daily activity limitation	None	1–2/month	1–2/week	3–7/week	Daily
Aerobic activity limitation	None	Weekly	3/week	Daily	Unstable
Sleep disruptions	None	1/month	1/week	2/week	>2/week
School/work absences	None	<1/month	<2/month	4/month	>4/month
β-agonist dosage	<4/month	<4/week	<2/day	<3/day	4/day
Anti-inflammatory	None	None	Low dose	Moderate dose	High dose

TABLE 17–2. Asthma Algorithm Diagnostic Approach for Chronic Management

	Level 1	Level 2	Level 3	Level 4
Pulmonary Functions				
Home peak flow	Consider	Daily	Twice daily	Twice daily
Assess peak flow variability	Consider	Yes	Yes	Yes
Spirometry	Consider	Yes	Yes	Yes
Lung volumes	No	No	Yes	Yes
Methocholine testing	No	Rarely	Not needed	Not required
Assess Allergic Reactivity				
By history	Yes	Yes	Yes	Yes
Limited skin testing	If indicated	Yes	**Important**	Yes
Complete skin testing	Occasional	Occasional	Recommended	**Important**
Serologic testing	Infrequent	Infrequent	Infrequent	Infrequent
Radiographic Imaging				
Chest radiograph	If indicated	If indicated	Suggested	Recommend
Sinus imaging	If indicated	If indicated	Consider	Recommend
Follow-up Examination	Annual	1–2/year	2–4/year	6–12/year
Consultation				
Based on disease level	Rarely	If indicated	Recommended	Assumes care
ER or hospital visit	Consider	Suggest	Recommended	Recommended

TREATMENT STRATEGIES

In view of its pathophysiology, the management of allergic asthma has evolved into the strategy of

- Patient education with an emphasis on prevention
- Normalization of airway function
- Reduction of inflammation
- Improvement of the patient's quality of life

The first aspect of asthma care is **patient education**. Asthmatics must understand the nature of the disease and how to prevent and treat its symptoms. Management should begin with **prevention**. Emphasizing the avoidance of allergens that result in airway inflammation is essential. Although it is frequently overlooked in patients with less severe disease, avoidance of allergens may have important clinical significance in limiting disease severity. Avoidance of dust mites and other indoor allergens should be considered in all patients with specific reactivity. Environmental irritants such as cigarette smoke need to be eliminated. Treatment of seasonal allergic rhinitis also may be helpful in reducing exacerbations of asthma.

The **monitoring of disease activity** in asthma is important for effective therapy. Peak flow monitoring (peak expiratory flow rates [PEFRs]) and symptom diaries, used properly, permit early recognition of symptoms and can prompt initiation or modification of therapy. Patients need to be cognizant of early signs of asthma and to have a therapeutic plan if symptoms increase. Individuals with asthma should strive for normal exercise tolerance, and sleep should not be interrupted by coughing or wheezing.

The 1980s saw significant swings in drug therapy of asthma. There have been profound changes in the selection of primary and secondary medications. The arc of the pendulum seems to be diminishing as understanding of the pathophysiology of asthma and the therapeutic effect of the drugs increases. Asthma is clearly not a "one-drug" disease, and the physician must be familiar with the relative advantages and disadvantages of the available medications. Combination therapy is generally the rule rather than the exception (Table 17–3).

The steps of asthma therapy are multiphasic:

- The immediate need is to provide a bronchodilator effect to relieve airway obstruction.
- Second is the need to resolve the inflammatory process in the airways, with consequent improvement in pulmonary function and reduced airway hyperresponsiveness.
- Third is the need to protect the airways from the inflammatory response to allergens and to irritant stimuli.

The major medication groups are those that are primarily bronchodilators (β-adrenergic agonists, theophylline) and those that are considered antiasthma drugs (cromolyn, inhaled glucocorticoids, and nedocromil); in addition, immunotherapy and a diverse group of alternative medications are used, mostly in the patients who have not responded well to other treatments.

The treatment of asthma in the United States is currently changing to reflect the importance of inflammation in the disease pathogenesis. The use of agents to treat inflammation has become the nucleus of therapy in asthmatics with persistent symptoms. Bronchodilators are important for

TABLE 17–3. Asthma Stepwise Care

	Level 1	Level 2	Level 3	Level 4
Avoidance	Yes	Essential	Essential	Essential
Albuterol	<Daily	PRN <BID	PRN <TID	As needed
Cromolyn, Nedocromil	0	Mild symptoms? Children	Synergy with IC?	0
Inhaled Corticosteroids (IC)	0	300–500 μg/day	600–1200 μg/day	1200–2400 μg
Salmeterol	Short-term, limited illness	Maintain IC, improve QOL	Symptom control	Recommend
Theophylline	0	Alternative	Alternative	Trial
Prednisone	<2 × /year	<3–4/year	Acute flares	Lowest dose

b.i.d. = twice a day; p.r.n. = as needed; QOL = quality of life; t.i.d. = three times a day.

acute care, whereas in chronic illness they are used for adjuvant therapy.

Asthma is a diverse disease. Each patient's case varies in severity and in the triggering factors. Several pathways of disease activity exist, although airway inflammation appears to be evident in all phases of the illness. The treatment approach thus varies depending on the patient's disease severity and on the etiology of acute episodes. Therapy needs to be individualized but should emphasize treatment of inflammation. Although broad classifications of mild, moderate, and severe asthma (levels one to four) permit a simple categorization for therapeutic intervention, they do not adequately reflect the complexity of the disease. Asthma severity is a composite of a patient's symptoms and the medications that are required to achieve the goals of therapy.

Role of Bronchodilators

• β-Adrenergic Agonists

The advantage of β-adrenergic medications is their rapid onset of effect in relief of acute bronchospasm. This action is achieved via smooth-muscle relaxation and increased mucociliary clearance. This group of medications (albuterol, terbutaline, and pirbuterol; see Chapter 8) has evolved from those that are relatively short-acting (epinephrine and isoetharine). The newer available agents have selectivity for bronchodilatation with minimal cardiac side effects. Two of the newer compounds, salmeterol and formoterol, appear to extend the duration of action to 10–12 hours and to maintain β-2 selectivity.

In addition to having excellent bronchodilator properties, this class of medications provides an excellent bronchoprotective effect for pretreatment of exercise-induced asthma. Administered prior to allergen exposure, these drugs are useful in blocking the early pulmonary response; however, in standard doses, they fail to prevent the late-phase reaction. Recent studies suggest that higher doses of albuterol not only provide a bronchodilator effect and improve bronchial hyperreactivity but also block late-phase reactions. These studies also support the concept that bronchodilators are not only effective when treating active bronchospasm but may provide some protection against subsequent attacks by blocking the fall in prostaglandins after allergen exposure.

Inhaled bronchodilators are the primary drugs used to treat acute bronchospasm and to prevent exercise-induced bronchospasm. For more persistent symptoms, these drugs are now viewed as supplementary to the antiasthma medications. The frequency of bronchodilator use may be applied as a criterion for implementing or increasing anti-inflammatory therapy. Although no definite criteria exist, it has been suggested that bronchodilators be used on a regular basis once a day while anti-inflammatory treatment is indicated.

Salmeterol is a new, longer-acting member of this class of medications. Its place in routine asthma therapy is not yet well defined. It is clearly advantageous for the patient with nocturnal asthma and for patients whose symptoms are not well controlled by the use of anti-inflammatory agents. This drug is of value in patients who have frequent symptoms and peak flow variability despite adequate therapy with inhaled corticosteroids. Further, it may reduce the amount of inhaled steroids in patients who require higher dosing schedules. Salmeterol also may have a role in the treatment of the patient who requires short-term bronchodilators for self-limited asthma that occurs after viral infection and during allergen seasons.

The most effective route of administration of β-adrenergic agents is by inhalation. Oral preparations may be of some use in young children, in individuals who cannot master proper inhalation techniques, or, in long-acting forms, to treat nocturnal symptoms. Successful use of inhaled β-agonists is obtained only after the proper inhalation technique is taught and repeatedly reviewed. All too often it is assumed that patients who have used an inhaler in the past know the proper skills of inhalation. Studies indicate that the proper *metered dose inhaler (MDI)* technique may be difficult to teach. The key components of proper technique include simultaneous actuation of the canister at the beginning of a slow, deep inspiratory effort. The inhalation is followed by 5–10 seconds of breath holding. The sequence is then repeated. The inhaler may be placed in the mouth or 2 inches in front of an open mouth. The most common mistake is not executing the timing of inhalation and the depression of the canister concurrently. The use of a spacer device, such as an Aerochamber (Mona) or Inspiraease (Key Pharmaceuticals), may help a patient to overcome the difficulty with coordination. Large-volume spacers (500–750 mL) actually may improve deposition of the drug in the lungs. Spacing devices may enable younger children to use MDIs. Delivery system depends on the patient's age and coordination and on the activity of the asthma symptoms.

Inhaled bronchodilators are important in all phases of asthma. They are useful just prior to the administration of inhaled anti-inflammatory drugs if cough or wheeze symptoms are present, as pretreatment before exercise or prior to allergen exposure, and during acute flares of asthma. During exacerbations, the inhaled β-adrenergics can be used up to every 4 hours. If PEFRs have fallen significantly or there is an increase in coughing, the first and second inhalations of the drugs should be separated by 5 – 10 minutes. If a nebulizer is used, the therapy can be split with a similar break. This allows for airway bronchodilation and then better deposition of the subsequent treatment.

The safety of routine use of inhaled bronchodilators as maintenance medications recently has been questioned. A double-blind crossover study compared the regular use of fenoterol with "as-needed" inhaled β-agonist (Sears et al, 1990). Fenoterol is a potent but less β_2 selective drug than albuterol or terbutaline. Overall, asthma control was better in 70% of patients on intermittent as-needed bronchodilator drugs compared with patients on the regularly administered fenoterol. Moreover, epidemiological studies suggest that all bronchodilators, and especially fenoterol, are associated with a modest increase in the risk of death from asthma, an increased risk not observed with cromolyn or with inhaled steroids. More recently, Suissa interpreted the Canadian population study to conclude that the increased morbidity and mortality was confined to those patients who used excessive amounts of these drugs. The current National Heart Lung and Blood Institute guidelines advise early institution of antiasthma therapy, with inhaled bronchodilators serving primarily in rescue or bronchoprotective situations. Clearly the answer to the safety of routine bronchodilators is still open. With these variable results, individualized therapy is important. One suggestion might be to follow PEFR and to adjust the dose of inhaled bronchodilator, depending on this measure of lung function. If the PEFR is greater than 85%, consider omitting the bronchodilator and limiting treatment to an antiasthma agent such as cromolyn or inhaled glucocorticoid. (This important topic is discussed by Nelson et al, 1991 and by Burrows and Lebowitz, 1992.)

Several possible explanations for the poor outcome with routine use or with overuse of beta-agonists exist. Some feel that these drugs might adversely affect the airway receptors and intrinsically permit damage to the airway. Another hypothesis for poor long-term responses to the regular use of inhaled β-2 bronchodilator therapy is that a patient who feels better tolerates higher levels of allergen exposure. If the β-agonists do not block the inflammatory response, this may serve as a pathway for chronic inflammation. Alternatively, chronic use of β-agonists may desensitize a patient to the effect of this drug and decrease its duration of action. At present, agreement exists that the appearance of an increased use of such drugs probably reflects inadequate control of asthma and suggests the need for re-evaluation of therapy, specifically addressing a possible inflammatory focus.

Nevertheless, inhaled β-agonists are an integral part of all phases of asthma care. Although some may suggest that more conservative use of these drugs is warranted in chronic care, it is clear that β-agonists are a very important component of acute intervention.

• Theophylline

Theophylline is a xanthine, closely related structurally to caffeine (Table 17 – 4). Although it is a weak bronchodilator when compared with β-adrenergic agents, theophylline's main advantage is its long duration of action. This is especially useful in the management of nocturnal asthma. Theophylline has a moderate bronchoprotective effect in pretreatment before exercise and histamine challenge. It also attenuates the early- and late-phase responses to allergen exposure, possibly as the result of anti-inflammatory properties.

Theophylline's role in the treatment of chronic asthma has been evolving over decades. In the early 1980s, long-acting theophylline preparations were the foundation of asthma care. A recent decline in the use of theophylline is related to several possibilities. The recent focus of asthma pathophysiology suggests that anti-inflammatory agents are more appropriate first-line drugs. In addition, the increase in side effects noted with the use of a higher dosage of theophylline led to physician apprehension.

The initial enthusiasm for long-acting theophylline was caused by the belief that serum levels could be easily titrated to achieve maximal efficacy. Unfortunately, the theophylline levels, rather than the patient response, became the driving focus of attention. *Theophylline dosing needs to be individualized to account for patient variability in absorption and elimination.* A tendency for absorption to be slower at night than during the day exists. In the past, the perception that constant theophylline levels could be maintained throughout the day often reflected the summation of average data for patients in the studies rather than that for individual patients.

TABLE 17 – 4. Structure of Xanthine, Caffeine, and Theophylline

Agent	Structure
Xanthine	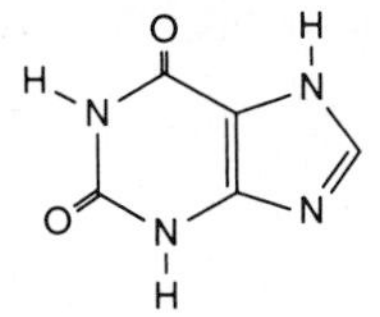
Caffeine	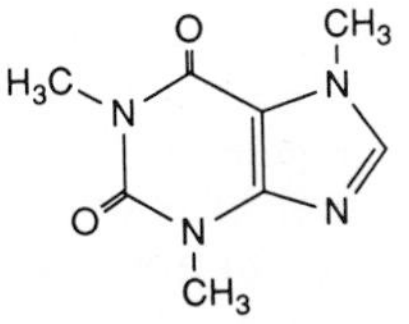
Theophylline	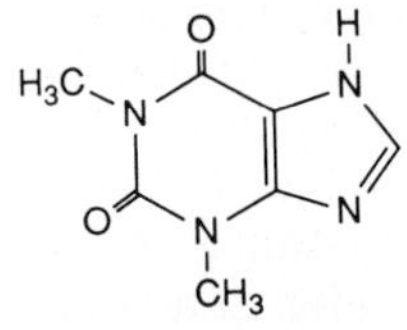

Minor side effects of theophylline are frequently tolerated if serum levels are within the therapeutic range. Behavioral changes analogous to those seen with caffeine, a drug with similarities in structure and bronchial effect, are occasionally noted. Theophylline's effect on cognitive skills appears to be limited. Adverse behavioral effects are usually attributable to increased motor activity in certain patients. The most common adverse effects are headache, insomnia, tremor, nausea and vomiting, abdominal discomfort, restlessness, diuresis, and increase of gastric secretion. At high blood levels, cardiac arrhythmias or seizures may occur.

Another source of concern is the potential effect of viral respiratory illness or fever on theophylline metabolism. Decreased clearance of theophylline during viral infection and/or fever may result in increased serum theophylline concentrations and the possibility of serious side effects. Patients at risk appear to be those who receive high-dose theophylline treatment. Higher dosages of theophylline should be avoided. Theophylline levels should be maintained in the 7 – 15 μg/mL range to minimize the risk of adverse effects. Behavior changes, enuresis, nausea, vomiting, and headache should alert the physician to monitor serum levels and to adjust dosage.

A large variety of drugs and foods, as well as smoking, significantly modify the clearance of theophylline; therefore, it is of critical concern to monitor levels, as well as response, other drugs, and exposure to smoke (Table 17 – 5). Moreover, different theophylline preparations may have different pharmacokinetics.

Despite these limitations, theophylline has an important place in asthma care:

- It is easy to use when compliance with inhaled medications is difficult.
- It is effective in treating nocturnal symptoms because of its long duration of effect.
- It is a useful adjunct to inhaled anti-inflammatory medications.
- It reduces the need for frequent courses of oral glucocorticoids.
- Clinical response should be the primary indicator for dosage adjustment.
- Serum concentration should be used as a guide for safety.

• Anticholinergics

This group of medications has limited application in the treatment of chronic asthma. Although they would empirically seem to be beneficial, their actual application is limited to a small subclass of patients. These drugs as MDIs add little to inhaled β-adrenergics, although newer agents with a longer duration of action administered in sufficient bronchodilator doses may result in the increased use of this class of medication. Some patients with severe asthma treated with a combination of nebulized β-adrenergic agonist and anticholinergics may exhibit an increased duration of bronchodilator action.

To summarize, patients with asthma need a bronchodilator and an antiasthma medicine. Any anticholinergic is in third position after anti-inflammatories and β-adrenergics.

TABLE 17 – 5. Factors Affecting Theophylline Blood Levels

Conditions Increasing Theophylline Blood Levels

Older age (>50 years)
Obesity
Liver disease
Congestive heart failure
Chronic obstructive pulmonary disease
Acute viral infections
High-carbohydrate, low-protein diet
Influenza A vaccine
Drug use
- Troleandomycin
- Erythromycin preparations
- Allopurinol
- Cimetidine
- Propranolol

Conditions Decreasing Theophylline Blood Levels

Young age (1 – 16 years)
Cigarette smoking
Eating charcoal-broiled meat
Low-carbohydrate, high-protein diet
Drug use
- Phenobarbital
- Phenytoins
- Isoproterenol

From Kaliner M, Eggleston PA, Mathews KP: Primer on allergic and immunologic diseases. Chapter 3: Rhinitis and asthma. JAMA 258:2851 – 2873, 1987. Copyright 1987, American Medical Association.

Treatment of Inflammation

• Cromolyn Sodium

This antiasthma medication (cromolyn sodium [GASTROCROM, INTAL, NASALCROM]) blocks both the early- and late-phase pulmonary response to allergen bronchial challenge. It also prevents the development of airway hyperresponsiveness that follows single-allergen challenge in a sensitized patient. Cromolyn's primary advantage lies in its low frequency of adverse effects, thus making it a safe medication for use in children.

Cromolyn is effective in controlling persistent symptoms when given on a daily basis. It must be given chronically; maximum effects require up to 2 weeks to appear. It can be used as follows:

- To prevent exercise-, cold air –, sulfur dioxide –, and allergen-induced asthma
- For chronic administration to reduce overall symptom scores.

Because viral infections are a common trigger for asthma in children, cromolyn also may prevent inflammation during these illnesses, although no studies to support this hypothesis exist.

Cromolyn can be delivered in a nebulizer to the young infant and child or by MDI for older patients. Initial dosing of cromolyn should be three to four times a day, with either 20 mg by nebulizer or two inhalations (~7 mg per actuation) by MDI. After a positive clinical response and stabilization of lung function, this dose can frequently be reduced to two to three times a day.

• Nedocromil

Nedocromil (TILADE) drug inhibits allergen-induced early- and late-phase reactions. Long-term therapy also may reduce nonspecific bronchial hyperreactivity. Nedocromil also appears to have an additive effect with inhaled steroids. It can be dosed two to three times a day and needs to be used as a preventive medication. Its onset of action appears only several days after initiating therapy, as compared with cromolyn, which requires a couple of weeks before its major therapeutic effects are achieved. Both cromolyn and nedocromil appear to be effective in patients with milder disease.

• Glucocorticoids

Glucocorticoids (see also Chapter 55) represent the most efficacious anti-inflammatory agents available for the treatment of asthma. When administered prior to a bronchial challenge with allergen in a sensitized patient, these drugs block the late-phase pulmonary response and the development of airway hyperresponsiveness. Continuous administration is also effective in reducing the immediate pulmonary response to allergen challenge.

The inhaled glucocorticoids are effective on topical administration, and systemic side effects can be reduced when delivered by this route. Three products are available in the United States (*beclomethasone dipropionate*, *triamcinolone acetonide*, and *flunisolide*) and two others in England (fluticasone and budesonide). Studies comparing the efficacy of these drugs are limited. Of the three preparations available in 1994 in the United States, the limited data would indicate that these drugs are equally efficacious and equally toxic when compared on a microgram dose basis. Because the majority of patients with asthma require a low dosage of these medications (300–400 μg/day), beclomethasone dipropionate is the most convenient and cost-effective preparation. (Fluticasone has greater first-past clearance and thereby has a better efficacy-to-safety relationship.)

The current strategy in asthma therapy includes the early use of anti-inflammatory medications. Anti-inflammatory agents, not including theophylline, improve bronchial reactivity, consistent with the view that airway hyperreactivity is related to the degree of inflammation. Anti-inflammatory agents are important in those patients whose disease activity is not adequately controlled by cromolyn or nedocromil. Inhaled steroids significantly decrease bronchial hyperreactivity.

The power of the inhaled agents, especially the newer agents such as budesonide, can be demonstrated in patients with asthma by improvement of their PC20s. This improvement can be maintained for at least a few months after the dosage is reduced. Moreover, patients treated with inhaled steroids in addition to a β-agonist have better asthma control and a decrease in bronchial reactivity. The improvement in asthma with these combinations is not readily predicted and may be dose-related or compound-specific. Studies of bronchial biopsies of patients using inhaled steroids have demonstrated that the numbers of mast cells and eosinophils are reduced after therapy with inhaled steroids but not with bronchodilators. Furthermore, the epithelial disruption that is noted in mild asthma appears to be repaired after treatment with inhaled glucocorticoids is initiated.

POTENTIAL ADVERSE EFFECTS OF STEROIDS. Concern about the possible effects of inhaled steroids on growth in children has been addressed recently. Data from two studies suggest that linear growth in children may be reduced with the regular use of budesonide or beclomethasone. The short-term growth suppression that originally was reported was not observed when the children were followed for longer periods of time and with standard doses of budesonide (Pederson, Personal communication, 1993). Earlier studies that were carried out over longer periods showed no adverse effect on linear growth with the regular use of either inhaled beclomethasone or budesonide. Interestingly, budesonide has the best topical-to-systemic ratio of the agents available at present.

Other potential adverse effects of steroids are alterations in diurnal cortisol secretion reported for beclomethasone and a reduction in serum osteocalcin (a protein secreted by osteoblasts) levels with the use of budesonide. These recent data about potential adverse systemic effects need to be put in proper perspective. Asthma is a serious disease with life-threatening consequences if not appropriately treated. Growing children need medications with the least potential for side effects that adequately control disease. Moreover, children with poorly managed chronic asthma may exhibit decreased growth. In the more recent studies on growth suppression, the children investigated had very mild symptoms. Inhaled steroids, when used appropriately in the treatment of asthma, have a good risk-benefit ratio and result in less morbidity than does either untreated asthma or frequently used oral steroids. In fact, asthmatic children receiving prednisone can have growth acceleration—probably because of improvement in pulmonary function. No evidence exists that indicated use of inhaled steroids should be avoided.

In adults with asthma, concerns have been raised as to whether the use of inhaled steroids may predispose to the development of osteoporosis. Although the data are still not conclusive, it appears that inhaled steroids might have the advantage of reducing the dosage of systemic steroids, thereby decreasing the likelihood of osteoporosis.

Recently, higher doses of inhaled steroids have been suggested for *refractory asthma*. This therapy appears to be successful in many patients. With higher doses of inhaled corticosteroids, more evidence of systemic absorption is noted; however, absorption is still less than that with oral administration. Newer inhaled agents, such as budesonide and fluticasone propionate, should have fewer systemic effects as the result of their more rapid metabolism once absorbed. Higher doses of inhaled steroids could be used in patients with disease that is more difficult to control. The dose should be reduced once the clinical response is established.

Oral steroids are used in the treatment of acute flares of asthma that have not responded to treatment with bronchodilators or cannot be controlled with antiasthma medications. Their use may be necessary at the initiation of treatment with inhaled antiasthma medications to improve lung function, to reduce inflammation, and to allow for proper deposition of these medications in the airway. Outpatient treatment with 2 mg/kg/day of oral steroids divided into two equal doses or with a maximum of 40 mg twice a day is suggested. Therapy should be continued for 4 – 7 days, depending on the clinical response. Clinicians vary in their opinions regarding a possible need to taper the dose reduction following such short-burst therapy.

• Immunotherapy

Immunotherapy is suggested in patients with allergen-induced asthma that is not controlled with avoidance and with the use of standard doses of inhaled bronchodilators and antiasthma medications. Patients should have a clinical history of asthma flares consistent with allergen exposure, and a prick-puncture skin test should confirm the allergy. Standardized allergen extracts should be used when available. With the increasing emphasis on treating inflammation, it might be questioned whether earlier use of immunotherapy is warranted to prevent allergen-induced asthma in situations where avoidance is not possible.

The use of immunotherapy to block inflammation appears to be rational and is now gaining experimental support. Evidence now exists that immunotherapy decreases the number of eosinophils observed in the bronchial lavage fluid of allergic asthmatics when they are exposed to seasonal allergens. It is exciting to observe pathological evidence that supports the use of a therapeutic regimen that has been employed for decades and was invented before the disease pathophysiology was understood or the mechanism of the therapy was known.

• Alternative Therapies

If drug therapy, environmental control, immunotherapy (if appropriate), or investigation of social situation does not yield improvement, an "alternative therapy" for the refractory patient should be considered These therapies include medications such as troleandomycin, low-dose methotrexate, gold, intravenous gamma globulin, hydroxychloroquine, dapsone, or cyclosporine. The use of any of these drugs is still quite controversial and should be considered in only carefully selected cases and administered by physicians knowledgeable in the pharmacological properties of each agent. Further studies need to be performed before any of these drugs become generally accepted means of medical management of asthma.

• Strategies for the High-Risk Patient

Recognition and diagnosis of the high-risk patient are important. With the increasing mortality of asthma it is imperative to identify and then develop strategies to address this population. High-risk patients include those with frequent emergency room visits, intensive care unit admissions, or a history of requiring assisted ventilation. Socioeconomic problems and dysfunctional family situations may contribute to the risk. Denial and noncompliance are associated problems. These factors need to be addressed in managing these patients. Psychiatric intervention is sometimes required.

COMMENT

Significant advances have been made in understanding the pathophysiology of asthma. Guidelines for treatment have now been developed based on the recognition of the importance of bronchodilation and of the control of inflammation. Goals for therapy should include allowing the patient to enjoy full participation in physical activities, good school attendance or work, and uninterrupted sleep; these goals should be achieved with minimal side effects. Achievement of these goals requires effective patient education and self-monitoring. Implementation of appropriate drug administration, patient education, and monitoring should lead to a reduction in mortality from asthma. Nevertheless, both timely access to appropriate health care and the availability of new medications and new information remain essential conditions.

The importance of asthma, with its high prevalence and serious morbidity, is very likely to lead to the development of new potential therapies; these, in turn, will require demonstration that outcome is improved with treatment, *ie*, demonstration of efficacy. Too often therapies have been justified in isolation and combined with other medications because of their apparent reasonableness without actual tests of efficacy or safety. It is now important to examine total asthma care, which includes patient education, avoidance of triggering factors, monitoring of disease activity, and therapeutic interventions by assessing outcome, including symptom scores, physiological parameters, quality of life issues, and total cost of therapy. The examination of these factors will make it possible to judge whether new treatments really have or have not improved a patient's outcome.

REFERENCES

Beasley R, Roche WR, Roberts, WR, Holgate, ST: Cellular events in mild asthma and after bronchial provocation. Am Rev Respir Dis 139:806–817, 1989.

Booth H, Fishwick K, Harkawat R, Devereux G, Hendrick DJ, Walters EH: Changes in methacholine induced bronchoconstriction with long acting B_2 agonist salmeterol in mild to moderate asthmatic patients. Thorax 48:1121–1124, 1993.

Burrows B, Lebowitz MD: The β-agonist dilemma. N Engl J Med 326:560–561, 1992.

Cockcroft DW: Therapy for airway inflammation in asthma. J Allergy Clin Immunol 87:914–919, 1991.

Creticos PS: Drug Therapy of Asthma. *In* CM Smith, AR Reynard (eds): Textbook of Pharmacology, Philadelphia: WB Saunders Co, 1051–1066, 1992.

Dutoit JI, Salome CM, Woolcock AJ: Inhaled corticosteroids reduce the severity of bronchial hyperresponsiveness in asthma but oral theophylline does not. Am Rev Respir Dis 136:1174–1178, 1987.

Guidelines on the management of asthma. Thorax 48:s1–s24, 1993.

Holgate S: Mediator and cytokine mechanisms in asthma. Thorax 48:103–109, 1993.

International consensus report on the diagnosis and treatment of asthma. Eur Respir J 5:601–641, 1992.

Laitinen LA, Laitinen A, Haahtela T: Airway mucosal inflammation even in patients with newy diagnosed asthma. Am Rev Respir Dis 147:697–704, 1993.

Laitinen LA, Laitinen A, Haahtela T: A comparative study of the effects of an inhaled corticosteroid, budesonide, and a beta 2-agonist, terbutaline, on airway inflammation in newly diagnosed asthma: a randomized, double-blind, parallel-group controlled trial. J Allergy Clin Immunol 90:32–42, 1992.

National Asthma Education Program Expert Panel Report. Guidelines for the diagnosis and management of asthma. Washington DC: National Asthma Education Program; August, 1991. US Department of Health and Human Services publication 91-3042.

Nelson HS, Szefler SJ, Martin RJ: Regular inhaled beta-adrenergic agonists in the treatment of bronchial asthma: Beneficial or detrimental? Am Rev Respir Dis 144:249-250, 1991.

Sears MR, Taylor DR, Print CG, Lake DC, Li Q, Flannery EM, Yates DM, Lucas MK, Herbison GP: Regular inhaled beta-agonist treatment in bronchial asthma. Lancet 336:1391-1396, 1990.

Sporik R, Holgate ST, Platts-Mills TAE, Cogswell JJ: Exposure to house-dust mite allergen and the development of asthma in children. N Engl J Med 323:502-507, 1990.

Suissa S, Ernst P, Bolvin J-F, Horwitz RI, Habbick B, Cockroft D, Bials L, McNutt M, Buist AS, Spitzer WO: A cohort analysis of excess mortality in asthma and the use of inhaled β-agonists. Am J Respir Crit Care Med 149:604-610, 1994.

Szefler SJ: Glucocorticoid therapy for asthma: clinical pharmacology. J Allergy Clin Immunol 88:147-165, 1991.

Szefler SJ: Anti-inflammatory drugs in the treatment of allergic disease. Clin Allergy Med Clin N Am 1994, in press.

18 Treatment of Headache; Ergot Alkaloids

Cedric M. Smith

CLASSIFICATION OF HEADACHES

Headache is one of the most common symptoms and disease syndromes, affecting people of both sexes and of all ages. More than 90% of the adult population has experienced at least a few or many headaches. Although the majority of headaches are infrequent, of minor consequence, time-limited, and discontinue after modest therapy of aspirin or its equivalent, or with no medication at all, some can be incapacitating and can recur as often as every day. In a large sample of young adults, 57% of the males and 76% of the females had experienced a headache within 4 weeks of being interviewed (Linet et al, 1989). Moreover, they are a frequent presenting medical complaint; for example, they were found to be the seventh leading presenting complaint in ambulatory care centers. Usually self-limited, persistent headache is a symptom worthy of attention because it occurs in two thirds of those who are found to have brain tumors; however, a persistent headache is caused by a brain tumor in only approximately 1 in 1000 patients.

Classification of headaches provides a convenient frame of reference for the consideration of drugs used in their treatment, either to prevent headaches from occurring or to relieve them once they have begun (Table 18–1). Rational therapy of headaches rests on an understanding of the pathophysiology of the syndromes and the factors that aggravate or trigger them. Many of the drugs discussed in this chapter have already been presented in some detail in chapters dealing with nonsteroidal anti-inflammatory drugs (NSAIDs), adrenergic blockers, and calcium channel blockers.

The focus of this chapter is on the drug treatment of the most frequently occurring headache syndromes:

- Vascular headaches, including migraine and cluster headaches
- Tension, or common, headaches
- Both common and migraine headaches (most patients have both)
- Trigeminal and postherpetic neuralgia, which can manifest with facial and head pain; effective therapies for neuralgia are different from those for other headaches
- Drug- and intoxicant-induced headaches

Some ergot alkaloids, such as ergotamine, have essentially unique uses in medicine in the treatment of migraine headaches. Thus, a short section of this chapter is devoted not only to ergot alkaloids used for headache but also to those used for other purposes.

COMMON HEADACHES

Syndromes and Pathophysiology

The mechanisms underlying tension, or common, headache are currently under some dispute. The names used in the past reflect the differences of opinion. Since the 1950s it has been assumed that such headaches were caused by sustained contraction of the neck muscles—hence the name "muscle contraction headache." However, sustained muscle contraction cannot be demonstrated in most patients studied, and muscle relaxants are generally ineffective in treating these headaches. The other common name has been "tension headache," referring to the fact that headaches appear to accompany psychological tension and stress. Given the absence of compelling data on the mechanisms of these headaches, the term "common headache" is used in this chapter to refer to such recurrent nonspecific headaches, the type of headache suffered occasionally by the majority of people.

There are, as Table 18–1 indicates, a variety of headache syndromes. Note that many headaches have been found to be associated with certain drugs or intoxicants.

TABLE 18–1. Overview of Clinical Classification of Headache

- I. Migraine
  - A. Migraine headache: some examples of the various types of migraine headache are
    1. Classic (with aura)
    2. Common (without aura)
    3. Ophthalmoplegic and hemiplegic
    4. Basilar artery migraine
    5. Many other varieties (also included in some classifications are migraine equivalents such as aura without headache or attacks of pain in the abdomen or other sites)
  - B. Triggers, predisposing factors for migraine, or similar mechanisms
    1. Familial
    2. Stress—afterward
    3. Change in blood glucose, fasting
    4. Hormonal—premenstrual more frequent than other times in the menstrual cycle
    5. Oversleeping
    6. Dietary factors—high tyramine, chocolate, nuts, citrus juice, aged cheese
    7. Depression
    8. Panic and anxiety disorders
    9. Alcoholic drinks, certain red wines
    10. Bright sunlight
    11. Hypoxia
    12. Carbon monoxide
    13. Drugs—nitroglycerin, marijuana, estrogen, oral contraceptives, benzodiazepines, numerous others
    14. Drug withdrawal/rebound—ergotamine, NSAIDs, benzodiazepines, MAOI, caffeine
    15. Collagen disease
    16. Fever
- II. Common (tension, chronic recurring undifferentiated headache, muscle contraction)
  - A. Frequently occur in same patients who have migraine
  - B. Etiology, predisposing, or confounding factors; see also all the other varied causes of headaches, including
    1. Depression
    2. Primary sleep disorder—*eg*, central or peripheral sleep apnea with periods of hypoxia
    3. Panic and anxiety disorders
    4. Caffeine withdrawal
    5. Benzodiazepine withdrawal
    6. Stress, emotional and psychodynamic factors
    7. Cervical osteoarthritis
    8. Muscle tension
    9. Temporomandibular joint dysfunction
- III. Cluster headaches and chronic paroxysmal hemicrania
  - A. Cluster headaches: 70–90% in men; precipitated by alcohol, histamine, or nitroglycerin
  - B. Chronic paroxysmal hemicrania: ~80% in women; alleviated specifically by indomethacin
- IV. Miscellaneous without structural lesion
  - A. Cold stimulus headache, benign exertional, and headaches associated with sexual activity
- V. Headache associated with head trauma
- VI. Headache associated with vascular disorders and hypertension
- VII. Headache associated with nonvascular intracranial disorder
- VIII. Headache associated with substances or their withdrawal
  - A. Headache induced by acute substance use or exposure
    1. Nitrate- or nitrite-induced headache
    2. Monosodium glutamate-induced headache
    3. Carbon monoxide-induced headache
    4. Alcohol-induced headache
    5. Other substances
  - B. Headache induced by chronic substance use or exposure
    1. Ergotamine-induced headache
    2. Analgesic abuse headache
    3. Other substances
  - C. Headache from substance withdrawal (acute use)
    1. Alcohol withdrawal headache (hangover)
    2. Other substances
  - D. Headache from substance withdrawal (chronic use)
    1. Ergotamine withdrawal headache
    2. Caffeine withdrawal headache
    3. Narcotics abstinence syndrome
    4. Other substances
  - E. Headache associated with substances but with uncertain mechanism
    1. Birth control pills or estrogen
    2. Other substances, such as a benzodiazepine
- IX. Headache associated with noncephalic infection

(*Continued*)

TABLE 18–1. Overview of Clinical Classification of Headache *Continued*

X. Headache associated with metabolic disorder
   A. Hypoxia
      1. High altitude headache
      2. Hypoxic headache (low-pressure environment, pulmonary diseases causing hypoxia)
      3. Sleep apnea headache
   B. Hypercapnia
   C. Mixed hypoxia and hypercapnia
   D. Hypoglycemia
   E. Dialysis
   F. Headache related to other metabolic abnormality
XI. Headache or facial pain associated with disorder of cranium, neck, eyes, ears, nose, sinuses, teeth, mouth, or other facial pain or cranial structures
XII. Cranial neuralgias, nerve trunk pain, and deafferentation pain including trigeminal neuralgia (tic douloureux)
XIII. Headache not classifiable

Adapted and reduced from Olesen J: Classification of headache disorders, cranial neuralgias and facial pain; and diagnostic criteria for primary headache disorders. Cephalalgia 8(Suppl 7):35–38, 1988. For many of the classifications, only the major heading is reproduced here. Some of the trigger and etiological factors have been added to this classification.

MAOI = monoamine oxidase inhibitor; NSAID = nonsteroidal anti-inflammatory drug.

Diagnosis is critical for rational therapy of these headaches; drugs or other intoxicants obviously should be ruled out in the process of management (see also Chapter 50).

Among the more common of the headaches produced by intoxicants are the caffeine withdrawal headaches (see Chapter 25) and the headache frequently associated with the hangover that may be experienced by the majority of individuals the morning after a night of overindulgence in alcoholic beverages. To illustrate the complexity of headaches, headache is perhaps the most common symptom of hangover, but also frequent are nausea, vomiting, tremor, dry mouth, anxiety, depression, guilt, diarrhea, photophobia, sweating, and chills. Hangover headaches are frequently pulsatile and aggravated by movement or by bearing down; however, they may be generalized, steady, and aching in nature. Thus, this and many other headache syndromes are complex and occur as a function of individual differences and, in the case of hangover, the amount of alcohol consumed and the level of methanol reached as a consequence of alcohol metabolism (Smith and Barnes, 1983; Jones, 1987).

Drugs Useful in Treatment

Abortive Treatment

• **NONSTEROIDAL ANTI-INFLAMMATORY DRUGS.** The well-known, established drugs that alleviate headache are the NSAIDs, notably the old agent aspirin (Chapter 15); some of the newer agents, such as ibuprofen, have been found to produce a rapid onset of relief in as little as 15 minutes. In addition to the NSAIDs, acetaminophen has been found to have efficacy essentially equivalent to that of aspirin. For severe headaches, parenteral administration of ketorolac (TORADOL) can be quite effective (see Chapter 15).

• **THE CAFFEINE CONNECTION.** Many of the over-the-counter preparations for headache are combinations of an NSAID or acetaminophen with caffeine. The caffeine combinations may have somewhat greater effectiveness. The origin of the inclusion of caffeine, along with a wide variety of headache nostrums that have fallen out of use, is lost in the history of the varied and complex pharmaceutical preparations; however, it is possible that its inclusion began when it was discovered inadvertently that some headaches were caused, at least in part, by a reduction or withdrawal from the usual caffeine consumption (*ie*, a caffeine withdrawal headache). In addition to the side effects of NSAIDs discussed in Chapter 15 is the paradoxical occurrence of headache during the chronic use of NSAIDs. Recurrent headache can be caused by chronic use of two major classes of headache medications: NSAIDs or ergot alkaloids.

• **SUMATRIPTAN (IMITREX).** Sumatriptan is a new agent used primarily for migraine headaches (see later in this chapter); it has been reported to be effective in approximately 30% of patients with common headaches.

• **AVOID MOST COMBINATION PRODUCTS.** Caution should be exercised in the use of **combination products** (many of which are heavily advertised and promoted) that contain barbiturates, codeine, or so-called muscle relaxants. **Such combinations may be truly hazardous**. The first hazard is that most consumers are not aware of their ingredients. For example, the administration of a combination product that contains aspirin to patients with aspirin-sensitive asthma can result in near-fatal consequences. A second hazard is that the so-called **antianxiety**, **barbiturate**, or **muscle relaxant agents** have significant potential for causing acute or chronic toxicity. In short, headache is one condition that needs not only short-term management for relief of the immediate symptoms but also long-term management in combination with patient education regarding agents to use and those to avoid.

• **AVOID THE USE OF OPIOIDS.** Severe headaches, whether common or migraine, can be alleviated by opioids. However, a more appropriate therapy for severe unrelenting headache may be the intravenous (IV) administration of chlorpromazine or prochlorperazine; such treatment is warranted only in patients who have severe, incapacitating headaches that do not respond to oral preparations.

Preventive Prophylactic Treatments

Drugs to treat headache can be divided according to their use into those that are taken to relieve an ongoing headache, those for abortive treatment, and those that are taken chronically to prevent the recurrence of the headache. In fact, the primary concern of management of the patient with headache is the determination of the triggers of the headache, the avoidance of such triggers, and the procedures that can serve to decrease the individual's sensitivity to such triggers. Table 18–1 presents a long list of conditions, situations, or drugs that are rather well-established as triggers of headache and predisposing conditions. Prominent among these triggers are specific foods and underlying physiological conditions, including notably the biopsychiatric affective disorder of depression. For example, depressive mood disorder is present in some 40% of those with migraines, and a prominent symptom of depression is common headache and disordered sleep; however, which comes first is difficult to determine.

Given that common headache syndromes and migraine syndromes may constitute a continuum, the triggers listed for migraines may well be operative also in individuals who fail to exhibit the full migraine syndrome.

In view of the association of headache with sleep disorders, affective disease, panic disorders, anxiety disorders, and substance abuse, including the chronic taking of analgesic drugs, all patients with recurrent headaches need not only a thorough diagnostic work-up but also counseling and periodic follow-up that addresses at the least all of the factors and conditions listed in Table 18–1. Approximately 90% of patients with headaches can be helped significantly by appropriate therapy; however, at present, most patients fail to receive an adequate evaluation and appropriate therapy.

MIGRAINE AND OTHER VASCULAR HEADACHES

Syndromes and Treatment of Migraine Headaches

Migraine headaches are frequently classified among the primary vascular headaches because of (1) the symptoms of throbbing and tenderness along vessels and (2) the sequence of vasoconstriction followed by vasodilation that figures prominently in theories of the migraine pathophysiology.

Probable Mechanisms

- The central nervous system is involved in establishing pattern and recurrence, including blocking of central 5-hydroxytryptamine 2 (5-HT2) receptors.
- Migraine headaches involve both efferent and afferent autonomic nerves.
- Constriction (usually nonpainful) of cerebral and cranial vessels usually precedes the headache itself (corresponds to time of aura and to some of the visual disturbances).
- Following the period of arterial constriction, vessels dilate, and neurogenic-induced plasma extravasation occurs.
- Nitric oxide may be a key molecule in migraine and other vascular headaches.
- Increased platelet aggregation occurs.
- Vasconstriction and plasma extravasation involve calcitonin gene-related peptide, 5-HT, 5-HT_2, and 5-HT_{1D} receptor.
- Plasma 5-HT drops during the attack.

Migraine disease involves a complex sequence of neurogenic, vascular, neuroendocrine, and fluid balance interactions. Sensory nerves innervating cranial blood vessels are the ultimate source of the pain. These vessels are subject to serotonergic and adrenergic actions, prostaglandin release, alterations in calcium movements involved in the vascular muscle function, alterations in platelet aggregation, and inflammation and edema of vessel walls. In addition, migraine may be associated with systemic retention of water followed by diuresis. Major neural systems participate in the pathophysiology of the attack, the response to triggering factors, and the cyclic natural history of the disease. A variety of endogenous neuroeffective substances have been demonstrated to be involved in the migraine syndrome; a partial list includes serotonin, norepinephrine, histamine, prostaglandins, substance P, and enkephalins.

Abortive Treatment

It is the clinical impression that the earlier the treatment for a migraine attack is started, the more effective it will be.

NSAIDs

The primary initial therapy for migraine headaches includes the same drugs used for common headaches—aspirin, acetaminophen, and NSAIDs (such as naproxen or ibuprofen)—given alone or perhaps with caffeine. Ketorolac, the new NSAID, can produce greater pain relief than other NSAIDs and thus is potentially useful for relief of severe headaches—both common and migraine types.

ERGOT ALKALOIDS

• **ACTIONS.** Ergot alkaloids have long-standing credentials as one of the standard types of drugs used in the abortive treatment of the migraine attack. The most extensively used of the alkaloids is ergotamine, but dihydroergotamine and ergonovine are also probably effective.

In prescribing ergot preparations, it is useful to keep the patient's situation in mind. Most patients will have had prior attacks and are aware of the aura, if any, as well as their characteristic initial symptoms. Frequently occurring with the onset of migraine are visual disturbances and nausea that can progress to brief or protracted vomiting. Under such circumstances, the possible gastrointestinal (GI) side effects of any agent and the route of administration take on important dimensions. Oral administration may not be feasible, or if undertaken, might be followed by vomiting, thus confusing the treatment even further. Hence, most agents are available not only for oral administration but also for sublingual, inhalational, intramuscular (IM), or rectal administration.

The mechanism of the headache-relieving action of the ergot alkaloids is complex and continues to be disputed. For many years it was assumed that the efficacy of ergot alkaloids was due to vasconstriction, which is consistent with the knowledge that the headache phase of the migraine attack is accompanied by vasodilation, whereas the aura and initial visual disturbances are associated with vasconstriction in the extracranial and retinal vessels. However, direct vasoconstriction may be a partial but insufficient explanation.

The ergot alkaloids have multiple and complex effects on blood vessels and neurons. These actions include direct effects on smooth muscle, as well as agonist and antagonist effects on receptors for serotonin, tryptamine, dopamine, and norepinephrine (illustrated in Table 39 – 2 in Rall, 1990). At present it is not possible to state which of these actions is most relevant to the alleviation of migraine and other vascular headaches produced by ergotamine; nevertheless, *the preponderance of current observations favors an effect on serotonergic systems.*

• PREPARATIONS. Ergot alkaloids available and useful for abortive treatment of migraine headaches are as follows:

• Ergotamine. Oral, sublingual, inhalation, rectal, or IM preparations (frequently combined with caffeine for increased effects) of ergotamine are available. For example, ergotamine tartrate, a 1-mg tablet, is given orally, and the dose is repeated every ½ hour if necessary to a maximum of six tablets per attack (and a maximum of 10 tablets per week).

• Dihydroergotamine mesylate (DHE 45 injection). This form of the drug is given exclusively through the IM or subcutaneous routes. DHE is a serotonin agonist at 5-HT_{1A} and 5-HT_{1D} receptors. The combined use of IV metoclopramide followed by dihydroergotamine appears to be an effective treatment for the chronic intractable migraine (Raskin, 1986).

• Ergonovine. Ergonovine is less effective orally than ergotamine but is thought to produce less nausea and vomiting.

• ADVERSE EFFECTS OF ERGOT ALKALOIDS. Ergotamine preparations have an unpleasant taste, and their toxicity includes symptoms of nausea, vomiting, abdominal cramps, diarrhea, painful uterine contractions, vasoconstriction, coldness, and numbness and tingling in the fingers and toes. High dosages cause thirst, confusion, hallucinations, and unconsciousness; with chronic use, gangrene of the extremities and valvular heart disease have been reported. Ergot alkaloids have an interesting history as agents of mass poisonings and hallucinations (see Chapters 49 and 50).

Another problem associated with the use of ergotamine is the appearance of ergotamine rebound headaches that occur in individuals who use ergotamine on a regular basis. This can be avoided if 2 days are allowed to elapse between repeated uses of ergotamine.

Any of the ergot alkaloids, including ergotamine, are contraindicated during pregnancy and in patients with hypertension, occlusive vascular disease, and liver or kidney disease.

SUMATRIPTAN

Sumatriptan (IMITREX) is a new drug with great promise for relief of attacks as well as for prevention of migraine headaches. To date, it appears to be quite effective and to have few serious side effects.

• ACTIONS. Sumatriptan is a selective 5-HT_{1D} agonist that acts

1. To constrict large intracranial blood vessels
2. To decrease inflammation around sensory nerves
3. To decrease neurogenic plasma extravasation from vessels

Sumatriptan is much more effective and more likely to be effective than any prior medication. In addition to relieving headache, it reverses the photophobia, phonophobia, nausea, and vomiting of migraine. (What its effectiveness might be for relieving hangovers and other headache syndromes remains to be determined.)

• ADVERSE EFFECTS. The following negative side effects may occur:

- Nausea or vomiting is the most common complaint with oral sumatriptan tablets.
- Angina occurs in some patients; thus, the drug is contraindicated in patients with coronary heart disease because of possible constriction of coronary vessels.
- There have been reports of cerebrovascular accidents in patients taking sumatriptan, but the actual risk factor has yet to be established.
- Transient pain may be present at the subcutaneous injection site.
- Tingling, flushing, burning of the skin, a feeling of heaviness, or a sense of tightness in the chest may occur.

• PHARMACOKINETICS AND ROUTES OF ADMINISTRATION. Sumatriptan is only available as a subcutaneous preparation. Peak serum concentrations are maintained for 5 to 20 minutes, with an overall half-life of approximately 2 hours.

Oral preparations of sumatriptan also have been found to be effective. Peak serum concentrations occur in 1½ hours; extensive first-pass clearance is performed by the liver, with only about 15% of an oral dose reaching the systemic circulation.

One of the limitations in the use of sumatriptan for treating headache has been the recurrence of headache within 24 hours following its treatment.

• CAUTIONS. The following cautions should be kept in mind when considering the prescription of sumatriptan:

- Do not prescribe sumatriptan for patients with coronary heart disease or with high risk factors for stroke.
- Do not administer sumatriptan until 24 hours after the last dose of ergotamine has been given.
- Although there is evidence for prophylactic efficacy, sumatriptan is not currently recommended for prophylaxis.
- Because sumatriptan is a new drug, its long-term safety has not been established.

OTHER DRUGS

Other drugs that may have utility in aborting the migraine attack include the following:

- Phenothiazines — IV chlorpromazine or prochlorperazine can be given for severe headache that is unresponsive to other medications (see Chapter 23).
- Isometheptene mucate (MIDRIN) — a nonselective α-adrenergic blocking agent given at the onset of an attack. It has not been studied in detail. Its side effects include drowsiness, nausea, and vomiting.
- Propranolol — given at the onset of migraine headaches but used more frequently as a preventive drug. Note that propranolol is contraindicated in the presence of ergotamine and vice versa.
- Verapamil — has been reported to be effective in treating acute headache (see Chapter 32).

For severe nausea and vomiting, metoclopramide (REGLAN) has been employed with some success; metoclopramide is an antidopaminergic agent with the side effect of causing increased GI absorption of many drugs. It possesses the extrapyramidal and dystonic effects of other dopamine antagonists.

Prophylactic Treatment

Chronic administration of propranolol is the therapy of choice for prevention of migraine (see Chapter 10); this preventive efficacy may be related to the blockade of vasodilation. Another β-adrenergic blocking agent, Timolol (BLOCADREN), has been approved recently by the Food and Drug Administration.

The chronic administration of NSAIDs has been established as effective prophylactic therapy for migraine. Physicians who took one aspirin tablet (325 mg) every other day in the double-blind Physician's Health Study (Buring et al, 1990) were found to have 20% fewer recurrences of migraine headaches than those who received the placebo.

The following also have been found to be effective prophylactic therapies in certain patients:

- Calcium channel blockers (Chapter 32)
- Cyproheptadine
- Ergotamine
- Amitriptyline (Chapter 24)
- Clonidine (Chapter 9)
- Methysergide (SANSERT; see Preventive Treatment)
- Sodium valproate (DEPAKENE)
- Naproxen or flurbiprofen
- Fluoxetine

An herbal remedy, feverfew, has been found to be effective in migraine prevention, but it is not available commercially in standardized formulations (Murphy et al, 1988).

Cluster Headaches and Chronic Paroxysmal Hemicrania

Abortive Treatment

Cluster headache attacks can be cataclysmic in intensity and in the incapacitation that they can produce. Treatment is directed generally toward prophylaxis and prevention. Drugs used to treat migraine are also used to treat cluster headache, with the emphasis on obtaining the most rapid onset of action possible (*eg*, sumatriptan subcutaneously or IM dihydroergotamine).

Cluster headaches may be aborted in some 50–70% of cases by the inhalation of 100% oxygen administered through a facemask at the rate of 8–10 L/minute for 5–10 minutes. Interestingly, oxygen is a potent vasoconstrictor of the carotid vascular bed.

Indomethacin has been reported to be almost specific for relieving this cluster-related headache. The very fact that cluster headache responds more frequently to this NSAID than to others suggests that cluster headache has a syndrome and mechanisms somewhat different from those of other types of headache (Sjaastad, 1992). Nevertheless, this syndrome does respond to a certain degree to aspirin and to a variety of the NSAIDs. Sumatriptan may prove to be effective and a significant advance, but information is not yet available.

Preventive Treatment

Methysergide (SANSERT) is the drug of choice when preventive therapy is indicated. Although methysergide is effective, it has serious potential toxicity; it is thought to act by blocking both the vasoconstriction and inflammatory effects of serotonin.

Adverse effects of methysergide include the potentially serious side effect of retroperitoneal fibrosis, a generally irreversible fibrous infiltration around the kidneys and ureters. Less serious but sometimes troublesome side effects include dizziness, GI disturbances, hallucinations, anxiety, weight gain, and hair loss.

In severe cases of frequent cluster headaches, methysergide is still used, but the chronic therapy is interrupted every 4 months or more often for a drug holiday of 4–6 weeks. Such intermittent therapy appears to produce appreciable periods of relief without increasing the risk of retroperitoneal fibrosis.

Methysergide represents an apt example of the therapeutic dilemma presented by a drug that, although uniquely effective, has the potential for unpredictably causing a serious side effect.

Treatment of cluster headaches can be a therapeutic challenge. Most common among the drugs for such treatment are lithium (Chapter 24) and indomethacin. A variety of agents, such as those mentioned for the treatment of migraine, have been found to be effective for treating cluster headaches in some patients.

Lithium is noteworthy for its effectiveness in treating chronic paroxysmal hemicrania. It is reportedly much more effective against this syndrome than it is against the recurrence of cluster headaches. Other therapies include prednisone with all of its potential problems, chronic ergotamine, and indomethacin.

OTHER USES OF ERGOT ALKALOIDS

Ergonovine and Methyl Ergonovine

Two ergot alkaloids, ergonovine maleate (ERGOTRATE) and methylergonovine maleate (METHERGINE), are administered postpartum (by IM or sometimes IV routes) with or immediately after the delivery of the placenta. The drugs cause prompt, sustained contraction of the uterine muscle and thereby reduce the extent of blood loss during the postpartum period. Side effects of such use of ergot alkaloids are infrequent but may include nausea, vomiting, and increased blood pressure.

Treatment with ergot alkaloids is strictly prohibited during pregnancy or labor. (For the induction of labor, oxytocin can be used [Chapter 52]. The prostaglandins $PGF_{2\alpha}$ and PGE_2 produce uterine contractions, but they are not approved for use to induce labor or for therapeutic abortion.)

Agents related to ergot alkaloids include bromocriptine, a dopaminergic agonist that has been found to be useful in the treatment of Parkinson's disease (Chapter 21).

Lysergic acid diethylamide (LSD) is a semisynthetic ergot alkaloid with a history of experimental and nonmedical uses (see Chapters 49 and 50).

OTHER HEADACHES

Many of the headaches associated with fever, head trauma, and vascular disorders are responsive, at least to some degree, to the NSAID analgesics. If the headache is excessively severe, opioids may be required (see Table 18-1, sections V, VI, and VII).

A variety of drugs can be associated with causing, triggering, or exacerbating headaches. The drug effects range from acute action (such as the effects of vasodilators like nitrates or histamine) and an acute rebound (such as hangover due to alcohol) to those associated with chronic use and with drug withdrawal, such as the effects of the cessation of chronic intake of caffeine, benzodiazepines, or ergotamine (see Table 18-1, section VIII).

Headaches and facial pain, such as trigeminal neuralgia, are characterized by chronically recurring attacks of severe lancinating pain. Carbamazepine (TEGRETOL) or phenytoin (DILANTIN) has been found to provide moderate relief in some, but not all, patients. For patients who cannot obtain adequate relief, microneurosurgery is sometimes dramatically effective in providing relief by alleviating nerve compression caused by a blood vessel.

Neuralgia also can be the result of infection with herpes or herpes zoster. Carbamazepine is employed frequently to relieve such pain. Amitriptyline has been reported to be moderately effective in such patients. Studies of desipramine demonstrated its utility and probable superiority over amitriptyline, particularly in view of its lesser degree of anticholinergic and sedative effects. Amitriptyline and other tricyclic drugs have analgesic effects that appear to be independent of their antidepressant actions.

USE OF OPIOIDS FOR SEVERE HEADACHES

The principal strategy for the rational use of analgesics to relieve pain is to progress from the use of low dosages of aspirin or acetaminophen, to higher dosages, to higher dosages with adjuncts, and eventually to preparations that contain low doses of codeine or its equivalent if the milder options do not provide adequate relief. Codeine-containing combination preparations are dispensed rather freely by some physicians, with the predictable result of their chronic use and escalation of dose by some patients. Although some headaches and pains experienced may truly be unrelieved by nonopioid medications, caution is warranted regarding the use of codeine, meperidine (DEMEROL), or other opioids. Once such therapy is initiated, its continuation is likely to be required over months and years because of the recurrent nature of headache syndromes with serious risk of dependence and toxicity (see Chapter 14). A better management strategy is to perform a thorough initial diagnostic study, including the detection of triggers and psychiatric conditions; this can lead to adequate treatment initially. Such an approach would reduce significantly the inappropriate and excessive administration of codeine or meperidine.

REFERENCES

Abramowicz M (ed): Sumatriptan for migraine. Med Lett 34:91-93, 1992.

Blau JN: Migraine: Clinical and Research Aspects. Baltimore: Johns Hopkins University Press, 1987.

Buring JE, Peto R, Hennekens CH: Low-dose aspirin for migraine prophylaxis. JAMA 264:1711-1713, 1990.

Diamond S: Head pain. Clin Symp 46:1-34, 1994.

Diamond S, Dalessio DJ (eds): The Practicing Physician's Approach to Headache. Baltimore: Williams and Wilkins, 1992.

Diamond S, Freitag FG: Do non-steroidal anti-inflammatory agents have a role in the treatment of migraine headaches? Drugs 37:755-760, 1989.

Drexler ED: Severe headaches: When to worry, what to do. Postgrad Med 87:164-180, 1990.

Edmeads J: Four steps in managing migraine. Postgrad Med 85:121-134, 1989.

Ekbom K, Waldenlind E, Levi R, Andersson B, Boivie J, et al: Treatment of acute cluster headache with sumatriptan. N Engl J Med 325:322-326, 1991.

Ferrari MD, Saxena PR: Clinical and experimental effects of sumatriptan in humans. Trends Pharmacol Sci 14:129-133, 1993.

Ferrari, MD, The Subcutaneous Sumatriptan International Study Group. N Engl J Med 325:316-321, 1991.

Fozard JR, Gray JA: 5-HTIC receptor activation: A key step in the initiation of migraine? Trends Pharmacol Sci 10:307-309, 1989.

Glover V, Sandler M: Can the vascular and neurogenic theories of migraine be reconciled. Trends Pharmacol Sci 10:1-3, 1989.

Jones AW: Elimination half-life of methanol during hangover. Pharmacol Toxicol 60:217-220, 1987.

Jones J, Sklar D, Dougherty J, White W: Randomized double-blind trial of intravenous prochlorperazine for the treatment of acute headache. JAMA 261:1174-1176, 1989.

Kishore-Kumar R, Max MB, Schafer SC, et al: Desipramine relieves postherpetic neuralgia. Clin Pharmacol Ther 47:305-312, 1990.

Kunkel RS: Cluster headache. Pain Management 3:44-51, 1990.

Kunkel RS: Management of migraine. Pain Management 2:156-161, 1989.

Linet MS, Stewart WF, Celentano DD, et al: An epidemiologic study of headache among adolescents and young adults. JAMA 261:2211-2216, 1989.

Moskowitz MA: Neurogenic versus vascular mechanisms of sumatriptan and ergot alkaloids in migraine. Trends Pharmacol Sci 13:307-311, 1992.

Murphy JJ, Heptinstall S, Mitchell JRA: Randomized double-blind placebo-controlled trial of feverfew in migraine prevention. Lancet 2:189-192, 1988.

Olesen J: Classification of headache disorders, cranial neuralgias and facial pain, and diagnostic criteria for primary headache disorders. Cephalalgia 8(Suppl 7):35-38, 1988.

Olesen J, Thomsen LL, Iversen H: Nitric oxide is a key molecule in migraine and other vascular headaches. Trends Pharmacol Sci 15:149-153, 1994.

Rall TW: Oxytocin, prostaglandins, ergot alkaloids, and other drugs; tocolytic agents. *In* Gilman AG, Rall RW, Nils AS, Taylor P (eds): Goodman and Gilman's The Pharmacological Basis of Therapeutics. New York: Pergamon Press, 1990.

Raskin N: Repetitive intravenous dihydroergotamine as therapy for intractable migraine. Neurology 36:995-997, 1986.

Sjaastad O: Cluster Headache Syndrome. Philadelphia: WB Saunders Co, 1992.

Smith CM, Barnes GM: Signs and symptoms of hangover: Prevalence and relationship to a alcohol use. Drug Alcohol Depend 11:249-269, 1983.

Solomon GD: Therapeutic advances in migraine. J Clin Pharmacol 33:200-209, 1993.

Stewart WF, Lipton B, Celentano DD, Reed ML: Prevalence of migraine headache in the United States. JAMA 267:64-69, 1992.

Drugs Used in the Treatment of Gout 19

Margaret A. Acara

Gout is a disease that is caused by hyperuricemia. Elevated uric acid levels in the blood result in the deposition of urate crystals, which leads to acute inflammatory reactions. Tophi, inflamed swellings in subcutaneous tissue, are observed most frequently in the large toe, ankle, or heel but also may be found in other areas such as the wrist, fingers, earlobes, and elbows. Episodes of acute gouty arthritis are excruciatingly painful, requiring prompt treatment. Although only a minority of patients with hyperuricemia ever develop gout, all patients with gout have hyperuricemia. When gout does occur, it is usually after 20–30 years of hyperuricemia and, if primary in nature, requires a lifetime of commitment to therapy.

Primary gout occurs through a direct defect in uric acid production or excretion. Most patients with primary gout exhibit a renal defect, and 10–25% of patients with primary gout have renal stone formation. Secondary gout is associated with hyperuricemia that results from another disorder. Neoplastic disease, such as leukemia, leads to the breakdown of cellular nucleoproteins and excess formation of uric acid. Lead nephropathy and glycogen storage disease result in the decreased elimination of uric acid. Hyperuricemia also may be induced by drugs that interfere with uric acid excretion.

When the blood uric acid level reaches the saturation concentration of 7–8 mg/dL, the crystals are phagocytosed by granulocytes; this is accompanied by a release of lysosomal enzymes and acidic substances into synovial fluid. The result is a slightly more acidic environment that promotes further crystal precipitation. Because the joints in the extremities have a more acidic environment, they are susceptible areas for deposition.

The pKa of uric acid is 5.75, and at the plasma pH of 7.4, it is 98% dissociated. When the pH of the environment favors dissociation, monosodium urate crystals are formed. At a pH of 4.75, uric acid is 91% undissociated, and uric acid crystals form. Thus, in the renal tubule with its more acidic environment, the possibility of the formation of uric acid stones and the development of renal failure exists.

> BOX 19–1
>
> **THREE PHARMACOLOGICAL APPROACHES TO THE TREATMENT OF GOUT**
>
> - Decrease the synthesis of uric acid.
> - Increase the excretion of uric acid.
> - Terminate the inflammatory response.
>
> Whether or not (and when) to treat hyperuricemia itself is controversial, but a blood uric acid level higher than 7 mg/dL may warrant treatment.

URIC ACID SYNTHESIS

Uric acid is the end product of purine metabolism in humans. Humans and great apes do not have the enzyme uricase that converts uric acid to the more water-soluble allantoin. Figure 19–1 shows the final step in the pathway of purine metabolism, which is the conversion of hypoxanthine and xanthine to uric acid by the enzyme xanthine oxidase.

An average person produces approximately 600–700 mg of uric acid per day. The most common metabolic defect that leads to overproduction of uric acid is a deficiency in the enzyme hypoxanthine-guanine phosphoribosyltransferase (HGPRTase). When this occurs, hypoxanthine is not cycled back through inosinic acid; instead, production of xanthine and thereby uric acid increases.

Inhibitor of Xanthine Oxidase—Allopurinol

One major drug is used to inhibit the production of uric acid: allopurinol (XYLOPRIM). Allopurinol is a competitive inhibi-

hypoxanthine — xanthine oxidase → xanthine — xanthine oxidase → uric acid

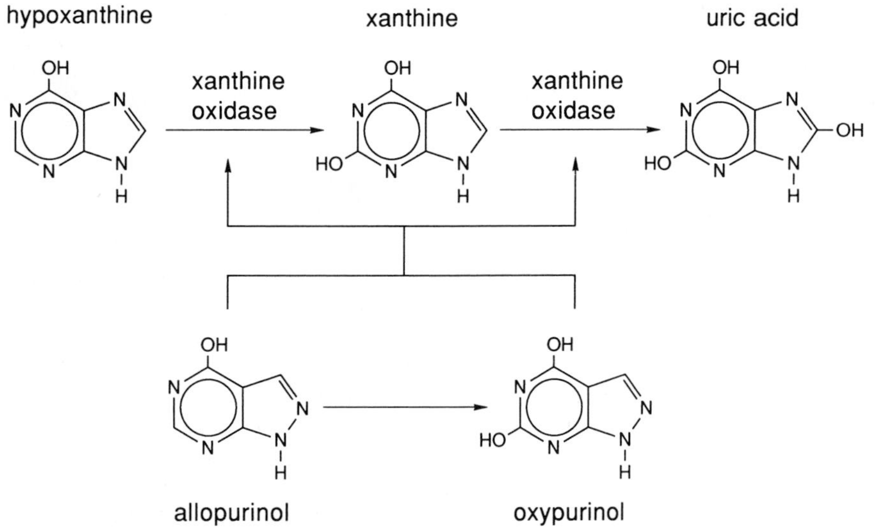

allopurinol → oxypurinol

FIGURE 19–1. Pathway of purine metabolism.

tor of xanthine oxidase. It decreases the level of uric acid and increases the level of its precursors, hypoxanthine and xanthine. Allopurinol is metabolized by xanthine oxidase to oxypurinol, which is an active metabolite that inhibits the same enzyme by forming a reversible complex with it. Chronic administration of allopurinol leads to accumulation of oxypurinol and contributes to its long-term therapeutic use.

- Treatment with allopurinol results in a decrease in the plasma level of uric acid and, concomitantly, its urinary excretion. Because of xanthine oxidase inhibition, an increase in plasma levels and in urinary excretion of the precursors hypoxanthine and xanthine occurs. Precipitation of these oxypurines as crystals appears not to be a problem because they are more soluble than uric acid.
- Allopurinol is well absorbed and not well bound to plasma proteins. It is eliminated mainly by metabolism, and its half-life is 2–3 hours. On the other hand, its active metabolite oxypurinol is reabsorbed, and it has a much longer half-life of 18–20 hours.
- Patients who are overproducers of uric acid and those with excessive tophi are candidates for allopurinol therapy. In addition, patients who do not respond to uricosuric agents and those with high uric acid levels who have developed renal stones are treated successfully with allopurinol.
- The side effects of allopurinol include skin rash, fever, gastrointestinal (GI) upset, and liver toxicity. Therapy with allopurinol, as with the uricosurics, should not be initiated during an acute attack. The initial decrease in plasma uric acid levels causes the mobilization of urate from deposits in the body in sufficient amounts to aggravate the acute attack of gout.
- The most important drug interaction with allopurinol therapy is that resulting from coadministration with mercaptopurine or azathioprine. The oxidation of these drugs is inhibited by allopurinol, and it is necessary to decrease their dosage by as much as 75% when these agents are administered concomitantly. Allopurinol interferes somewhat with the hepatic microsomal drug-metabolizing enzymes, and caution is required for the administration of drugs metabolized by this system.

RENAL EXCRETION OF URIC ACID

The kidney is the major organ involved in the elimination of uric acid. Two thirds of uric acid cleared from the blood appears in the urine. The remaining third appears in intestinal secretions. The binding of uric acid to plasma proteins is small — less than 10% — and the remainder is filtered freely at the glomeruli. Fractional excretion of uric acid is 0.1, indicating net reabsorption.

Mechanisms for the renal handling of uric acid involve a complex system that includes filtration, reabsorption, and secretion. Bidirectional transport systems are present in the proximal tubule and operate simultaneously. A transporter for uric acid reabsorption is present on the brush border membrane, and one for secretion is situated in the basolateral membrane. Entry of uric acid into the cell is active and saturable and can be competed for by other organic acid molecules. Competition for the secretory transport carrier can result in increased uric acid blood levels, whereas competition for the reabsorptive carrier can result in decreased uric acid blood levels. Because the major direction of uric acid movement is reabsorptive, adequate dosages of drugs that compete for the uric acid transport carriers have the predominant effect of decreasing uric acid reabsorption, increasing its excretion, and lowering the blood level.

Uricosuric Agents

Uricosuric agents enhance uric acid excretion by inhibiting filtered urate reabsorption in the proximal tubule. Initial treatment with uricosuric agents may be associated with mobilization of uric acid deposits, increased amounts of uric acid reaching the kidney, and the danger of papillary necrosis. Also, as with all drugs that occupy the organic anion transport system, low doses may raise blood levels. Until drug levels build up to a sufficient concentration to decrease reabsorption, a risk of acute gouty attack exists. Therefore, an agent that prevents the acute attack may be administered before the uricosuric. In addition, a high fluid intake of 3–4 L/day and, in some cases, alkalization of the urine may be useful to prevent uric acid precipitation in the kidney.

Probenecid

- The most widely used uricosuric agent is probenecid (BENEMID). It is the prototypical inhibitor of organic anion secretion but when given in sufficient amounts it interferes with uric acid reabsorption.
- Probenecid is bound to plasma proteins, but it also is secreted by the organic acid transport system and thus has a relatively short half-life (6–12 hours). Its occupation of the organic acid transporter may result in interference with the excretion of other drugs that are organic acids and may lead to longer half-lives and higher concentrations of these drugs when they are administered simultaneously. In fact, probenecid is used to maintain levels of certain agents whose regular half-lives may be short.
- Probenecid is effective in increasing uric acid excretion and lowering hyperuricemia, except in patients with renal failure. Some GI irritation and hypersensitivity reactions occur with probenecid, but in general it is well tolerated.

Sulfinpyrazone

Sulfinpyrazone (ANTURANE) is another frequently used uricosuric agent. It is an active metabolite of the anti-inflammatory agent phenylbutazone and, as such, has some anti-inflammatory action. Sulfinpyrazone has the same mechanism of action and characteristics as probenecid, but it is longer-acting and more potent. Sulfinpyrazone has become available as an inhibitor of platelet aggregation in the prophylactic treatment of myocardial infarction.

In general, salicylates antagonize the uricosuric effects of these agents, and they should not be used with uricosuric agents.

BOX 19-2
COADMINISTRATION OF ALLOPURINOL AND A URICOSURIC AGENT

Because uricosuric agents and allopurinol produce decreased uric acid levels by different mechanisms, their coadministration leads to a more effective therapy to decrease uric acid levels. However, the combined therapy is complicated by the resulting changes in pharmacokinetic profiles. Uricosuric agents increase the urinary clearance of oxypurinol but decrease the excretion of xanthine and hypoxanthine.

TREATMENT OF GOUTY INFLAMMATION

Drugs used to treat the inflammation associated with gout are administered not only during the acute attack but also are used prophylactically to prevent the acute attack and in combination with uricosuric agents or allopurinol at the initiation of therapy to decrease the risk of an acute attack of gouty arthritis. Colchicine and indomethacin are the major anti-inflammatory agents used in the treatment of gout, and they differ in their mechanisms of action. They are not effective in decreasing uric acid synthesis or reabsorption.

Colchicine

- Colchicine decreases the release of lactic acid and the movement of granulocytes into the inflamed area, breaking the cycle that leads to the inflammatory response. Colchicine is specific for the treatment of gout, and its relief of pain in this disease contributes to the diagnosis. It is not used to treat other inflammatory disorders.
- Therapy with colchicine is begun at the first sign of the acute attack and is continued until relief is obtained or until GI reactions appear. A maximal dosage is 6–7 mg per day. Adverse GI side effects have been observed in 80% of patients treated with colchicine and are the most common cause for changing to another anti-inflammatory agent.
- Because of its toxicity, the prophylactic use of low doses of colchicine is more common today than the use of the drug to treat the acute attack.

Indomethacin

- Indomethacin (INDOCIN) is anti-inflammatory, antipyretic, and analgesic.
- It is useful for the management of the acute attack of gouty arthritis.
- Indomethacin inhibits the cyclooxygenase enzyme that is involved in the production of prostaglandins. For this reason, it is contraindicated in patients with renal disease, in whom the prostaglandins are important mediators of renal function. Indomethacin has no effect on uric acid synthesis or excretion.
- Central nervous system effects (*eg*, headache, vertigo, and confusion) and GI effects (*eg*, nausea, indigestion, and vomiting) are included in the adverse effects of indomethacin. Ocular effects such as blurred vision and corneal deposits have also been reported.

OTHER FORMS OF TREATMENT

Other nonsteroidal anti-inflammatory drugs, including naproxen, fenoprofen, and ibuprofen, are also effective in the treatment of acute gouty arthritis. Initial dosages should be near maximal and gradually tapered as symptoms subside (see Chapter 15).

Occasionally adrenal corticosteroids and corticotropin are used to treat the inflammation associated with acute gouty attacks. However, these drugs are reserved for severe cases and are then administered by intra-articular injection for brief periods (a maximum of 3 days).

A diet low in purines may be of some benefit in decreasing hyperuricemia. However, available drugs are so effective that dietary restrictions may not be necessary. Low-purine diets can decrease the serum uric acid level by 1 mg/dL.

REFERENCES

Insel PA: Analgesic-antipyretics and antiinflammatory agents; drugs employed in the treatment of rheumatoid arthritis and gout. *In* Goodman AL, Rall TW, Nies AS, Taylor L (eds): The Pharmacological Basis of Therapeutics, 8th ed. New York: Pergamon Press, 1990.

Star VL, Hochberg MC: Prevention and management of gout. Drugs 45:212–222, 1993.

Wortmann RL: Uric acid and gout. *In* Seldin DW, Giebisch G (eds): The Kidney: Physiology & Pathophysiology, 2nd ed. New York: Raven Press, 1992.

PART IV

DRUG TREATMENT OF EXCESSIVE OR INAPPROPRIATE MUSCLE ACTIVITY

Antiepileptic Agents 20

Arthur W. K. Chan

"**Epilepsy**" refers to a group of central nervous system disorders characterized by sudden, transitory, and recurring seizures that are accompanied by elementary or complex impairment of one or more of the following functions: motor (convulsion), sensory, autonomic, and psychic. The seizures are nearly always associated with abnormal and excessive neuronal discharges that are discernible in the electroencephalogram (EEG).

Idiopathic or **primary** epilepsy is the term for seizures that have no identifiable cause, whereas **symptomatic** or **secondary** epilepsy denotes those seizure dis-

> **BOX 20–1**
>
> **EEG TERMINOLOGY**
>
> EEG discharges recorded during the occurrence of seizures are termed **ictal** EEGs. **Postictal** EEG discharges are those recorded immediately after the termination of a seizure, and **interictal** (interseizure) EEG discharges are those recorded at any other time between seizures.

orders that have known causes, such as neoplasm, metabolic imbalances, cerebrovascular disease, infection, or developmental abnormalities. Some seizures are not classified as epilepsy (*eg*, those elicited by alcohol or drug withdrawal or by electrolyte imbalance and those caused by high fever [febrile seizures]).

Most studies report the **prevalence** of epilepsy to be 4 to 8 cases per 1000; however, some studies report lower (1.5/1000) or higher (>40/1000) prevalence figures (Hauser et al, 1991).

CLASSIFICATION OF EPILEPTIC SEIZURES

The Classification Commission of the International League Against Epilepsy adopted an international classification of seizure types in 1981 and proposed the classification of epilepsies and epileptic syndromes in 1985. The classification of seizure types is primarily focused on clinical manifestations and their neurophysiological basis, the main purpose being to facilitate the choice of drug treatment. The classification of epilepsies is concerned with groupings of seizures or syndromes and their underlying causes. Table 20 – 1 summarizes the essential features of the different types of seizures. Because different drugs are used to treat different types of seizures, rational drug therapy requires a basic understanding of the seizure types and a comprehensive diagnosis.

MECHANISMS OF EPILEPSY

The pathophysiological mechanisms of epilepsy are still not completely understood. Because of the complexity of brain functions and the diversity of seizure types, it is unlikely that a single mechanism can explain the initiation and spread of the sustained synchronous neuronal discharges during an epileptic seizure. Rather, it is likely that more than one mechanism for seizure disorders exists.

Some suggested mechanisms for seizure disorders are as follows:

- Synchronous firing of neurons may require specifically timed inhibitory and excitatory neuronal activity, but the specific mechanism for sustaining the synchronous firing is unknown.
- Most seizures begin with the firing of a relatively localized group of neurons, the seizure focus, perhaps caused by a reduction in inhibitory neurons in the focus. The seizure focus may be formed or originated by factors such as hypoxia at birth, local biochemical changes, head trauma, ischemia, or endocrine disorders. It is not known how a dormant focus can be transformed to one that can initiate the spread of synchronous firing to neighboring areas.
- Alterations in the membrane or in the metabolic properties of individual neurons may induce neuronal hyperexcitability. These changes may in turn affect Ca^{2+} and Na^{+} conductances.
- Biochemical abnormalities affecting the synthesis, storage, release, reuptake, and receptor binding characteris-

TABLE 20 – 1. Classification of Epileptic Seizures

	Seizure Type	Features
I. Partial seizures (focal, local seizures)*	A. Simple partial seizures	Consciousness not impaired. Convulsions involving only the motor (jacksonian motor epilepsy) or sensory system (jacksonian sensory epilepsy): also may occur with autonomic or psychic symptoms, depending on the local contralateral EEG discharge in the cortical area.
	B. Complex partial seizures	Impairment of consciousness either at onset or following simple focal onset. Manifestations are varied and complex, involving confused behavior. Interictal EEG generally shows unilateral or bilateral focal discharges in the temporal or frontal region. Ictal EEG shows diffuse discharges.
	C. Partial seizures leading secondarily to generalized seizures	Progression of A or B to generalized seizures, or from A → B → generalized seizures.
II. Generalized seizures (convulsive or nonconvulsive)*	A.1. Absence seizures	Brief (a few seconds to half a minute) attack with sudden onset and termination; impairment of consciousness. Ictal EEG usually shows bilateral and synchronous 3-Hz spike-and-wave pattern but may be 2 – 4 Hz. Symptoms may include blank stare and eye movement, with or without jerking of the limbs or body.
	A.2. Atypical absence seizures	Slower onset and cessation than usually seen for absence seizures. EEG more heterogeneous.
	B. Myoclonic seizures	Brief, single, mild-to-violent jerks of arms or head with brief bursts of multiple spikes in ictal or interictal EEG.
	C. Clonic seizures	Rhythmic, multiple jerks of all parts of the body, with loss of consciousness.
	D. Tonic seizures	Rigid, violent muscular contractions, fixing the limbs in some strained position. Loss of consciousness.
	E. Tonic-clonic seizures (*grand mal*)	Generalized tonic muscle contractions with flexion of the upper extremities and forced extension of the lower extremities, followed by rhythmic contractions of the limbs. Usually lasts several minutes. Loss of consciousness.
	F. Atonic seizures	Sudden loss of muscle tone, leading to a head drop or slumping to the ground.
III. Unclassified seizures		Incomplete data.

*The term *status epilepticus* denotes seizures that are repeated frequently enough that recovery between attacks does not occur. Status epilepticus may be focal or generalized.

EEG = electroencephalogram.

tics of amino acid neurotransmitters such as the inhibitory γ-aminobutyric acid (GABA) and the excitatory glutamic acid may enhance neuronal excitability.

- A reduced level of $Na^+ + K^+$ATPase in the synaptosomal membrane may lead to elevated extracellular potassium, which has been shown to be associated with seizure activity.
- Genetic factors may play a role in some forms of epilepsy.
- The kindling process — a progressive increase in the motor seizures elicited by a series of periodic convulsive treatments (*eg*, electrical brain stimulation or chemical treatment) — may contribute to the genesis of epileptic seizures.

DRUGS USED IN THE TREATMENT OF EPILEPSY

General Features

- Before the initiation of drug treatment, **it is essential to have an accurate and comprehensive diagnosis**. Underlying causes such as hypoglycemia, infection, or tumor need to be treated. An accurate medical history is not only a *sine qua non* but also may alert doctors to possible seizure-inducing factors.
- **Antiepileptic drugs suppress but do not cure seizure disorders.** Drug therapy is often protracted, which can cause problems related to compliance with taking medications and to chronic drug toxicity.
- **An initial therapeutic aim is to use only one drug (monotherapy).** Advantages of monotherapy include a decreased likelihood of adverse drug-drug interactions; fewer side effects; better compliance by patients; lower cost; and better seizure control in some patients. However, for a minority of patients such as those with severe, difficult-to-treat epilepsy, a multidrug regimen may occasionally be superior to monotherapy. Risks of multidrug therapy include exacerbation of seizures and inability to evaluate the effectiveness of individual drugs.
- When a total daily dose is increased, **sufficient time (about five half-lives) should be allowed for the serum drug level to reach a new steady-state level** before an evaluation of the drug's efficacy at the new level can be determined. Likewise, dose-related toxicity cannot be fully evaluated until the new steady-state level is reached.
- **The drugs are usually administered orally.** The intravenous (IV) route is reserved for emergency treatment of status epilepticus and certain neonatal and infantile seizures. Rectal suppositories of diazepam (VALIUM) are sometimes used for treatment of febrile seizures.
- **The drugs are metabolized in the liver.** Metabolites of some drugs also possess antiepileptic activities. The unmetabolized drugs and their metabolites are excreted in the urine, usually as conjugates of glucuronic or sulfuric acid.
- **Several classes of antiepileptic drugs share some common chemical structures** (Fig. 20–1). Examples of individual drugs are phenytoin, ethosuximide, and trimethadione. **However, other antiepileptic drugs exist that differ widely in their chemical structures**: *eg*, valproic acid and carbamazepine.
- **The monitoring of plasma drug levels is very useful** in determining compliance, kinetic drug interactions, and inadequate or excessive drug dosage.
- **Precipitating or aggravating factors can affect seizure control by drugs.** Some examples of such factors include stressful situations, sleep deprivation, progressive neurological disease, and excessive alcohol intake.
- **The sudden withdrawal of drugs should be avoided.** Seizures or status epilepticus may be triggered by the abrupt cessation of drug treatment.
- **Some drugs may have teratogenic actions.** About 0.5% of all pregnancies occur in women with epilepsy. Approximately one third of pregnant epileptic women have

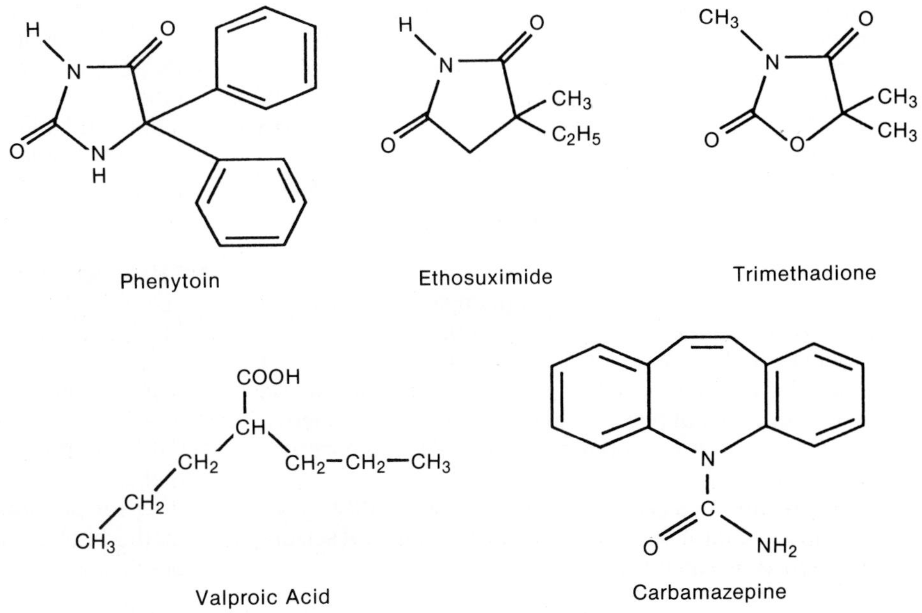

Phenytoin

Ethosuximide

Trimethadione

Valproic Acid

Carbamazepine

FIGURE 20–1.

an increase in seizure frequency relative to their nonpregnant state. The increase in seizures could be the result of either noncompliance or of altered disposition of antiepileptic drugs during pregnancy; hormonal, metabolic, respiratory, and psychological factors may also play a role. On the other hand, antiepileptic drugs have been implicated in causing a twofold increase in a variety of birth defects. Thus, clinicians are faced with the dilemma of the need to prevent seizures in pregnant women and the need to minimize fetal exposure to drugs. Ideally, epileptic women of childbearing age need to be counseled about the risks of pregnancy associated with the use of antiepileptic drugs before conception. **Trimethadione is absolutely contraindicated in epileptic women planning to have children.** Other drugs such as valproate, carbamazepine, and phenytoin also may cause fetal malformations. In spite of the potential hazards, **antiepileptic drugs should not be discontinued in pregnant women** for whom the medication is essential for seizure control. Risks can be minimized by using monotherapy with the lowest effective dose, but the decision to reduce dosage or to change to another drug should be made on an individual basis, taking into account the patient's history of frequency and severity of seizures. Neonatal hemorrhage caused by drugs (*eg*, from phenytoin or phenobarbital) can be prevented by vitamin K supplementation beginning in the third trimester. With proper management, more than 90% of women with epilepsy can have successful pregnancies and healthy children.

Phenytoin

- Phenytoin (DILANTIN) has a broad range of action against most types of seizures except absence seizures.
- Its antiepileptic actions result from its numerous effects on neuronal tissue, such as its ability to regulate sodium transport across neuronal membranes and to inhibit sodium channels during seizure discharges and its effect on post-tetanic potentiation.
- When used intravenously, phenytoin (50 mg/minute) is effective in controlling tonic-clonic status epilepticus, but there is a lag time of 15–20 minutes before the occurrence of seizure reduction. For this reason, the simultaneous IV administration of both phenytoin and diazepam has been suggested.
- The therapeutic plasma concentration of phenytoin is 10–20 μg/mL, but this level varies widely among individuals. The initial adult dosage is 3–5 mg/kg/day, with a maintenance dose of 4–6 mg/kg/day, not to exceed 500 mg.
- The concurrent administration of phenytoin with another drug can result in pharmacokinetic interactions, with a rise or decline in the plasma level of phenytoin or of the other drugs. For example, chloramphenicol and isoniazid can cause elevations of plasma phenytoin levels, and phenytoin often causes a decrease in plasma carbamazepine levels.
- Mephenytoin (MESANTOIN) and ethotoin (PEGANONE) are the other hydantoins. Their use in the treatment of seizure disorders still remains limited.

Side Effects

Central nervous system toxicity (*eg*, ataxia and nystagmus) occurs at the high end of or above the therapeutic range of plasma phenytoin levels; nausea, gingival hyperplasia, sedation, gastrointestinal disturbances, rash, folate deficiency, anemia, and vitamin K deficiency (particularly in pregnant epileptic patients) may occur.

Phenobarbital

- Phenobarbital is widely used in the treatment of generalized tonic-clonic seizures as well as simple and complex partial seizures but is not indicated in the treatment of absence seizures. Compared with carbamazepine, it has a lower success rate in the management of partial seizures.
- It is also effective in treating status epilepticus by IV administration (100 mg/minute up to 10 mg/kg) but may cause respiratory depression, excessive sedation, and hypotension. Another disadvantage is its relatively long response time and the fact that it may take up to an hour to reach peak brain levels. Nevertheless, it has been shown that effective brain concentrations of phenobarbital can be achieved within 3 minutes.
- The prophylactic treatment of febrile seizures with phenobarbital is not recommended unless the seizures are associated with transient or permanent neurologic deficits, prolonged (>15 minutes) or focal seizures, or a family history of nonfebrile seizures.
- The therapeutic range has been reported as being 10 to 40 μg/mL.
- Instead of the sedative effect that commonly is seen in adults taking phenobarbital, a paradoxical effect in children and the elderly may be manifested as hyperkinetic activity and insomnia. Tolerance to the sedative effect of the drug usually develops after 1 to 2 weeks of treatment.
- Pharmacokinetic interactions with other drugs such as phenytoin depend on a balance between phenobarbital's ability to induce phenytoin's metabolism and its action as a competitive inhibitor of phenytoin's metabolism because both drugs undergo parahydroxylation and glucuronidation. Valproate levels are often lower in patients taking it with phenobarbital than in patients taking valproate alone, but valproate is known to elevate serum levels of phenobarbital by as much as 40%.
- **Physical dependence** can develop after chronic use of phenobarbital. Discontinuation of phenobarbital therapy should progress slowly to avoid withdrawal seizures. Other side effects include skin rashes, ataxia, nystagmus, and possible teratogenic effects.
- Other barbiturates include methylphenobarbital and metharbital, the former being regarded merely as a prodrug for phenobarbital but more expensive. The role of metharbital as an antiepileptic drug in contemporary practice is debatable.

Primidone

- Primidone (MYSOLINE) is effective against partial and secondarily generalized tonic-clonic seizures but is not useful for absence seizures.
- **It has two active metabolites**—phenobarbital and phenylethylmalonamide. Ample evidence that primidone has antiepileptic properties independent of phenobarbital now exists; however, some portion of its antiepileptic activity is assumed to be caused by the derived phenobarbital.
- No generally accepted therapeutic range of primidone exists, but levels between 8 and 12 μg/mL seem appropriate.

Side Effects

Drowsiness, weakness, dizziness, nausea, nystagmus, and problems of folate and vitamin D disturbance may occur.

Ethosuximide

- Ethosuximide (ZARONTIN) is specifically indicated for the control of absence (*petit mal*) seizures. If tonic-clonic seizures also occur, ethosuximide can be combined with carbamazepine, phenytoin, or other antiepileptic drugs. However, valproate, which protects against both absence and tonic-clonic seizures, should be considered instead.
- Its mechanisms of action are still not well defined. Possible mechanisms include its ability to reduce the low-threshold calcium current in thalamic neurons and to increase the influence of inhibitory neurotransmitters.
- The maintenance dosage is 15–40 mg/kg/day once daily or with meals. The effective plasma levels are 40–100 μg/mL, but levels of up to 150 μg/mL may be required and are well tolerated.
- Other drugs of the same class (succinimides) are methsuximide (CELONTIN) and phensuximide (MILONTIN). Methsuximide is used to treat absence seizures only when less-toxic drugs fail to produce adequate control. Phensuximide is seldom used because of its low efficacy and serious side effects.

Side Effects

Minor side effects occur in 25–40% of patients who take ethosuximide, including drowsiness, nausea, vomiting, gastric distress, anorexia, dizziness, lethargy, headache, fatigue, photophobia, and behavioral changes. Serious toxic effects are uncommon.

Trimethadione

- Trimethadione (TRIDIONE) is effective against absence seizures; however, it has become less popular than ethosuximide and valproic acid, partly because of its toxicity.
- It is rapidly and almost completely metabolized by demethylation to form dimethadione, which has antiepileptic activity and a long elimination half-life (10–20 days). The therapeutic effect of long-term trimethadione treatment is a result of the action of dimethadione.
- The mechanism of action is not known but may be caused by the ability of trimethadione and dimethadione to raise the threshold for repetitive activity in the thalamus and to inhibit corticothalamic transmission.
- **Paramethadione** (PARADIONE), another member of the oxazolidinedione family, is effective primarily against absence seizures. However, it appears to have less consistent efficacy than trimethadione.

Side Effects

Hemeralopia (light blindness) and photophobia occur in about 30% of subjects. Other common side effects include sedation, fatigue, loss of concentration, and incoordination. About 10% of patients have rash, exfoliative dermatitis, and erythema multiforme. Neutropenia can develop in about 20% of patients. The so-called **fetal trimethadione syndrome** has been described in children whose mothers took trimethadione during pregnancy and is characterized by a combination of physical anomalies, growth retardation, and mental retardation.

Valproic Acid

- Unlike most antiepileptic drugs, **valproic acid (DEPAKENE) has a broad spectrum of antiepileptic activity**, being highly effective against absence seizures, tonic-clonic seizures, and myoclonic seizures. It is also useful in the treatment of partial seizures and febrile seizures.
- Coadministration of valproic acid with other drugs such as phenobarbital or ethosuximide can cause a rise in their serum levels. Conversely, valproate can decrease plasma levels of carbamazepine when the two drugs are taken together.
- A pharmacodynamic interaction between valproic acid and clonazepam has been reported in children, resulting in drowsiness in some patients or status epilepticus in others.
- The exact mechanism(s) of action of valproate are still unknown, despite suggestions that it may enhance GABA-ergic tone in the substantia nigra, limit sustained repetitive firing, or modulate excitatory amino acid neurotransmission.
- Neural tube defects may occur in the offspring of women who took valproate during pregnancy.

Side Effects

The most common side effects of valproic acid are nausea, vomiting, and gastrointestinal distress, particularly during the early phase of therapy. These can be minimized by the use of enteric-coated tablets and by the administration of the drug with or after meals. Sedation is another common side effect. Although dose-related elevations in liver enzymes may occur in over 40% of patients, most cases are asymptomatic. The primary risk of fatal hepatic dysfunction occurs in children under 2 years of age who are receiving valproate as polytherapy. Other rare toxic effects are pancreatitis and hyperammonemia.

Carbamazepine

- Carbamazepine (TEGRETOL) is used for the treatment of complex partial seizures, generalized tonic-clonic seizures, and other partial seizures, but it is not useful for absence seizures. Because it possesses a lower level of psychological and behavioral toxicity than either phenytoin or phenobarbital, carbamazepine is now considered a major antiepileptic drug and is increasingly prescribed.
- It is metabolized into carbamazepine-10, 11-epoxide, a pharmacologically active metabolite.
- Carbamazepine tends to decrease the plasma level-to-dose ratio of other drugs, but it is very sensitive to induction by other antiepileptic drugs; this results in a decrease in its own plasma level-to-dose ratio. Drugs such as propoxyphene, erythromycin, verapamil, and isoniazid can cause carbamazepine intoxication.

Side Effects

Rashes, usually transient, occur in about 5% of patients who take carbamazepine. Other common side effects include drowsiness, headache, gastrointestinal upset, diplopia, and blurred vision. Hematologic monitoring has been recommended because of carbamazepine's rare side effects in causing aplastic anemias and benign leukopenias.

Benzodiazepines

Diazepam

Diazepam (VALIUM) is the drug of choice for the emergency treatment of status epilepticus and prolonged seizures and is administered intravenously (5 – 10 mg, repeatable up to 30 mg). However, repeated IV doses of diazepam are not recommended because of the risk of respiratory depression and hypotension. For this reason, a loading dose of another long-acting antiepileptic drug such as phenytoin or phenobarbital is usually administered in addition. Rectal diazepam is sometimes used for the prophylaxis of febrile seizures. Oral diazepam is not recommended for long-term treatment of epilepsy because of poor efficacy and development of tolerance and dependence. One of its metabolites, *N*-desmethyldiazepam, also has antiepileptic actions.

Clonazepam

Clonazepam (CLONOPIN) is very effective against absence, myoclonic, and atonic seizures. It is less effective for treating infantile spasms and partial seizures. The simultaneous administration of clonazepam and valproate may exacerbate absence attacks, with the possibility of continuous absence seizures. The most common **side effects** are drowsiness, ataxia, and behavior changes.

Clorazepate

- This antianxiety agent (clorazepate [TRANXENE]) is effective in selected patients with generalized or partial seizures. It is most effective in patients with partial seizures who have psychic symptomatology and frequent seizures (more than 20 per month).
- It is a **prodrug**, being metabolized to the pharmacologically active *N*-desmethyldiazepam; the latter is responsible for the antiepileptic actions of clorazepate.
- The primary side effect is lethargy, to which tolerance frequently develops. Occasionally, adverse behavioral changes can occur, especially in children.
- Sudden withdrawal of the drug may trigger withdrawal psychosis and/or seizures.

Other Benzodiazepines

The following drugs are not currently approved by the Food and Drug Administration for treatment of epileptic seizures:

Nitrazepam, which is effective in the treatment of infantile spasms, myoclonic seizures, and Lennox-Gastaut syndrome

Clobazam and its active metabolite, *N*-desmethylclobazam, which are effective against partial and generalized seizures and in epilepsy of widely differing etiologies in patients of all ages

Lorazepam, which can be used for the treatment of status epilepticus.

Miscellaneous Antiepileptic Drugs

Acetazolamide

Acetazolamide (DIAMOX) and other sulfonamide carbonic anhydrase inhibitors have been shown to be effective against most types of seizures — generalized tonic-clonic, absence, and complex partial seizures. However, their value is limited because of the rapid development of tolerance to their antiepileptic effects. They are more useful as adjuncts to other antiepileptic drugs such as phenytoin, carbamazepine, and ethosuximide.

Bromides

Potassium, sodium, and ammonium bromides have major historical significance as the prototypes of modern antiepileptic drugs. However, their use has been superseded by less toxic drugs.

Adrenocorticotropic Hormone

Adrenocorticotropic hormone (ACTH) is useful in the management of infantile spasm and, to a lesser extent, other severe, intractable, mixed seizures in children. The mechanism of action is still unknown, and controversy exists about the dose, duration of therapy, and long-term benefits of therapy with this drug.

Lidocaine

Lidocaine (XYLOCAINE) is useful for the treatment of refractory status epilepticus but is not approved for the treatment of epilepsy.

OTHER TREATMENTS FOR EPILEPSY

Surgery

It has been estimated that in the United States about 360,000 patients with uncontrolled partial complex seizures exist, at least 75,000 of whom would be suitable candidates for surgery. However, far fewer surgeries for this condition are performed each year.

Two methods of surgical treatment exist. In the first, surgery is conducted to resect a focal and accessible lesion. The second method involves surgical removal of selected brain regions to alter seizure activity or to modify the spreading of neuronal discharges. The outcome is better for the first method, with one study reporting about 55% of patients becoming seizure-free and another 28% having a decrease in the frequency of seizures.

Cerebellar Stimulation

Cerebellar stimulation involves the surgical implantation of an electrical stimulator in the cerebellum; however, the initial reports of its success in controlling intractable seizures have not been confirmed. Currently, this procedure is of more theoretical than practical importance.

NEW DRUGS

At least 25% of epileptic patients have seizures that are resistant to available antiepileptic drug therapies. Therefore, a need to develop and test new drugs exists. The following list describes several of the nearly 20 new agents that are currently undergoing clinical evaluation.

- Several new drugs were developed based on the premise that compounds that can enhance the activity of the inhibitor neurotransmitter GABA might decrease abnormal excitation and control seizures. **Progabide** is essentially a GABA prodrug but has not fared well in clinical studies. **Vigabatrin (gamma-vinyl GABA)**, an irreversible inhibitor of the enzyme that metabolizes GABA (GABA aminotransferase), has been shown to be effective in long-term therapy in approximately one third of patients with previously drug-resistant epilepsy. Initial reports showed the development of brain lesions in animals that were given vigabatrin, but recent investigations indicate that such lesions do not occur in humans. **Gabapentin** is an amino acid that is structurally related to GABA but freely crosses the blood-brain barrier. It has been shown to be clinically effective in controlling partial and secondarily generalized seizures as add-on-therapy, and studies have reported that some patients with refractory epilepsy can be maintained on gabapentin alone.
- **Lamotrigine** is believed to act mainly by inhibiting excitatory amino acid release, hence stabilizing neuronal membranes via blockade of voltage-sensitive sodium channels. Several clinical trials have shown that it has efficacy against partial and generalized tonic-clonic seizures.
- **Felbamate** is a dicarbamate that is related to meprobamate. It was recently approved by the Food and Drug Administration as an antiepileptic agent. It is effective in the treatment of partial-onset seizures with or without generalization and has a favorable safety profile.

REFERENCES

Beghi E, Mascio RD, Tognoni G: Drug treatment of epilepsy. Outlines, criticism and perspectives. Drugs 31:249–265, 1986.

Brodie MJ: Established anticonvulsants and treatment of refractory epilepsy. Lancet 336:350–354, 1990.

Brodie MJ: Status epilepticus in adults. Lancet 336:551–552, 1990.

Chadwick D: Diagnosis of epilepsy. Lancet 336:291–295, 1990.

Chan AWK: Drugs used in the treatment of epilepsy. *In* Smith CM, Reynard AM (eds): Textbook of Pharmacology, 320–339. Philadelphia: WB Saunders, 1990.

Classification Commission: Proposal for classification of epilepsies and epileptic syndromes. Epilepsia 26:268–278, 1985.

Classification Commission: Proposal for revised clinical and electroencephalographic classification of epileptic seizures. Epilepsia 22:489–501, 1981.

Devinsky O: Seizure disorders. Clin Symposia 46:1–34, 1994.

Fariello RG: Biochemical approaches to seizure mechanisms: The GABA and glutamate systems. *In* Porter RJ, Morselli PL (eds): The Epilepsies, 1–19. Boston: Butterworths, 1985.

Hauser WA, Annegers JF, Kurland LT: Prevalence of epilepsy in Rochester, Minnesota: 1940–1980. Epilepsia 32:429–445, 1991.

Levy RH, Dreifuss FE, Mattson RH, et al (eds): Antiepileptic Drugs, 3rd ed. New York: Raven Press, 1989.

Meldrum BS, Porter RJ (eds): New Anticonvulsant Drugs. Vol 4 of Current Problems in Epilepsy. London: John Libbey & Co, 1986.

Porter RJ: New antiepileptic agents: Strategies for drug development. Lancet 336:423–426, 1990.

Porter RJ, Morselli PL (eds): The Epilepsies. Boston: Butterworths, 1985.

Rylance GW: Treatment of epilepsy and febrile convulsions in children. Lancet 336:488–491, 1990.

Trimble MR (ed): Chronic Epilepsy: Its Prognosis and Management. New York: John Wiley & Sons, 1990.

Wada JA, Seino M: Recent classification of seizures and epilepsies. *In* Wada JA, Ellingson RJ (eds): Clinical Neurophysiology of Epilepsy: Handbook of Electroencephalography & Clinical Neurophysiology, 3–36, No. 4. New York: Elsevier Science Publishers BV, 1990.

Wallace SJ: Childhood epileptic syndromes. Lancet 336:486–488, 1990.

Yerby MS: Pregnancy and epilepsy. Epilepsia 32(Suppl 6):S51–S59, 1991.

21 Antiparkinson Drugs

Linda A. Hershey

PARKINSON'S DISEASE

Tremor, rigidity, and bradykinesia form the symptom complex known as "parkinsonism." When James Parkinson first described this syndrome in 1817, he included other symptoms such as facial masking, drooling, postural instability, gait disorder, and slurred speech. We now realize that depression and dementia are also commonly seen in Parkinson's disease. About 1% of the population over the age of 50 is affected by idiopathic Parkinson's disease, while another 2 to 3% have one of the secondary forms of parkinsonism.

Secondary Forms of Parkinsonism

Drugs that block central dopamine receptors (antipsychotic agents and metoclopramide) and drugs that deplete dopamine from nerve endings (reserpine) cause a reversible syndrome, drug-induced parkinsonism.

- Vascular parkinsonism usually presents with gait disorder, rigidity, and bradykinesia (tremor is rare). It develops in patients with vascular risk factors, such as hypertension, diabetes, and coronary artery disease.
- Progressive supranuclear palsy usually begins like the akinetic-rigid form of Parkinson's disease and may respond initially to levodopa. When ophthalmoplegia and early dementia appear, the diagnosis is clarified.
- Alzheimer's-type dementia patients develop memory disorder and personality change before they manifest signs of parkinsonism. In contrast, the dementia of idiopathic Parkinson's disease is seen many years after the onset of motor symptoms and signs.
- The dementia and parkinsonism of pugilism usually begin concurrently. This syndrome is seen in professional boxers and is thought to be the result of multiple head injuries.
- Shy-Drager syndrome usually presents with some form of autonomic disturbance (impotence, syncope, or urinary retention). Another name for this form of parkinsonism is multisystem atrophy.
- Carbon monoxide poisoning can produce a syndrome of mild parkinsonism that may resolve over weeks to months.

Neuropathology

Selective degeneration of dopamine-containing neurons in the substantia nigra develops in patients with idiopathic Parkinson's disease. There may also be loss of norepinephrine-containing neurons in the locus ceruleus. There is currently no good explanation for the selective vulnerability of pigmented brainstem neurons in this disease. A good animal model of Parkinson's disease uses a byproduct of opiate synthesis, 1-methyl-4-phenyl-1,2,3,6-tetrahydropyridine (MPTP).

Clinical Stages of Idiopathic Parkinson's Disease

- *Stage I* patients have unilateral, while *Stage II* patients have bilateral symptoms and signs. Neither of these groups has postural instability.
- *Stage III* patients complain of occasional postural instability, gait disorder, or both. They do not yet require the use of an assistive device to ambulate.
- *Stage IV* patients need assistance in many activities of

daily living, including the use of a cane or a walker to help with ambulation.

- *Stage V* patients are bedbound or wheelchair bound. They require assistance in almost all daily activities.

Antiparkinson Therapies

Levodopa is the most effective drug for treating functionally disabled patients with Parkinson's disease (Stages III–V). Low doses of levodopa also provide mild symptomatic relief for some patients with various secondary forms of parkinsonism. Deprenyl, amantadine, and anticholinergic agents are useful alone or in combination in early stages of idiopathic Parkinson's disease (Stages I and II). All three of these drugs work synergistically when given in combination with carbidopa/levodopa. Bromocriptine and pergolide are usually added to carbidopa/levodopa in Stage III or IV to maximize function and to minimize levodopa-induced motor fluctuations.

LEVODOPA

Mechanism of Action

Levodopa, the immediate precursor to dopamine, stimulates dopamine synthesis. Dopamine, in turn, acts as an inhibitory neurotransmitter at both D_1 and D_2 dopamine receptor sites. Activity at both receptor sites is necessary for optimal relief of the symptoms of Parkinson's disease. The standard therapeutic formulation of levodopa with carbidopa (SINEMET) is better tolerated than levodopa alone, because carbidopa blocks the systemic amino acid decarboxylase and minimizes synthesis of dopamine in the periphery (Table 21 - 1).

TABLE 21 – 1. Levodopa and Dopamine Agonists

Generic Name	Brand Name	Dosage Forms	Daily Dosage
Carbidopa/ levodopa	SINEMET	Tablets (25/100) (25/250)	Start: 25/100 b.i.d. Maximum: 25/250 q4h
Carbidopa/ levodopa	SINEMET-CR	Tablets (25/100) (50/200)	Start: 25/100 b.i.d. Maximum: 100/400 t.i.d.
Benserazide/ levodopa	MADOPAR	Capsules (125/250)	Start: 1/2 tab b.i.d. Maximum: 250/500 t.i.d.
Bromocriptine	PARLODEL	Tablets (2.5 mg) Capsules (5 mg)	Start: 1/2 tab h.s. Maximum: 10 mg t.i.d.
Pergolide	PERMAX	Tablets (0.05 mg) (0.25 mg) (1.0 mg)	Start: 0.05 mg h.s. Maximum: 1.0 mg t.i.d.

q4h = every four hours; b.i.d. = twice daily; h.s. = at bedtime; t.i.d. = three times daily.

> **BOX 21 – 1**
> **THERAPEUTIC EFFECTS**
>
> Carbidopa/levodopa is usually initiated when patients lose responsiveness to one or more of the less potent antiparkinson drugs, or when a patient develops gait or balance problems. Failure to respond to levodopa after a month or more should suggest one of the secondary forms of parkinsonism. In idiopathic Parkinson's disease, the best results of carbidopa/levodopa are seen within the first 2 to 5 years of therapy. As the disease progresses, there is an apparent shortening of levodopa's duration of action ("wearing-off" effect). This is explained by the progressive reduction in dopamine storage capacity as nigral neurons degenerate. The controlled-release preparation of carbidopa/levodopa (SINEMET-CR) can reduce the "wearing-off" effect and increase the time that a patient remains able to function ("on" time).

Acute Adverse Effects

Peripheral adverse effects of carbidopa/levodopa (nausea, anorexia, and vomiting) can be avoided by the addition of extra doses of carbidopa (available free of charge from the manufacturer). Central adverse effects of carbidopa/levodopa (dyskinesias, vivid dreams, hallucinations, confusion, and orthostatic hypotension) can be minimized by dosage reduction. Sudden discontinuation of carbidopa/levodopa should be avoided, however, because this can produce a symptom complex similar to that of neuroleptic malignant syndrome (fever, rigidity, and confusion).

Chronic Adverse Effects

After about 5 years of carbidopa/levodopa therapy, many Parkinson's patients develop either the "wearing-off" effect or sudden fluctuations between mobility and immobility (the "on-off" effect). Paradoxically, these motor fluctuations are more likely to appear in early-onset Parkinson's patients who are good responders to carbidopa/levodopa.

Food Interaction

Levodopa is an aromatic amino acid that competes with other amino acids in the gut for intestinal absorption and with circulating amino acids for transport across the blood-brain barrier. Patients are initially advised to take carbidopa/levodopa with meals in order to minimize nausea and vomiting. As tolerance develops to these peripheral adverse effects, they can take the drug on an empty stomach in order to facilitate absorption and maximize bioavailability. When the "wearing-off" effect develops, patients are counseled to limit the amount of protein in their diet to 40 g/day.

Contraindications

Demented patients with Parkinson's disease, Alzheimer's disease, or progressive supranuclear palsy are more likely than nondemented patients to develop drug-induced confusion with levodopa. Similarly, schizophrenic patients with drug-induced parkinsonism are at higher risk of central adverse effects. Patients with known melanoma should not take levodopa, because of the risk of acceleration of tumor growth.

DEPRENYL

Mechanisms of Action

Deprenyl or selegeline (ELDEPRYL) is a selective inhibitor of monoamine oxidase type B (MAO-B). It slows the catabolism of dopamine and reduces the formation of oxygen-free radicals. It also blocks the conversion of MPTP to its neurotoxic metabolite, MPP^+.

> **BOX 21-2**
> **THERAPEUTIC EFFECTS**
>
> Deprenyl produces mild symptomatic relief in patients with Stage I or II Parkinson's disease. At a dose of 5 mg twice daily, it delays the need for carbidopa/levodopa by 6 months to a year. It is not clear whether this effect is symptomatic (by increasing synaptic dopamine) or protective (by reducing formation of free radicals), or both.

Adverse Effects

Deprenyl can cause insomnia (possibly because methamphetamine and amphetamine are among its metabolites). It is therefore recommended that the two daily doses be taken early in the morning and before the noon meal. When taken in combination with carbidopa/levodopa, deprenyl can exacerbate central dopaminergic adverse effects such as chorea, confusion, and hallucinations. Reducing the daily carbidopa/levodopa dosage by 10 to 30% can minimize these side effects. Giving deprenyl with meals can usually eliminate nausea.

Drug Interactions

Both fluoxetine (PROZAC) and meperidine (DEMEROL) interact adversely with deprenyl, just as they interact with MAO-A inhibitors. Nevertheless, there is no risk of tyramine-rich foods producing hypertension, as long as the daily deprenyl dose is kept at 10 mg or less. Only at higher doses does deprenyl behave as a nonselective MAO inhibitor.

Contraindications

Chronic liver disease is a contraindication to the use of deprenyl because the drug can occasionally cause hepatotoxicity. Patients with advanced Parkinson's disease who no longer respond to carbidopa/levodopa and those who experience the "on-off" effect are unlikely to benefit from the addition of deprenyl.

AMANTADINE

Mechanisms of Action

Amantadine (SYMMETREL) was originally developed as an antiviral agent. Its antiparkinson effects are mediated primarily by enhancement of dopamine release, but amantadine is also a weak dopamine agonist and a mild blocker of dopamine re-uptake.

> **BOX 21-3**
> **THERAPEUTIC EFFECTS**
>
> Amantadine, like deprenyl, produces symptomatic relief in patients with early Parkinson's disease (Stages I and II). Two or three daily doses of amantadine (100 mg each) are enough to postpone the need for carbidopa/levodopa by a year or more. Patients who lose their therapeutic response to amantadine may notice symptomatic improvement with the addition of small doses of carbidopa/levodopa, deprenyl, or both.

Adverse Effects

Ankle edema and livedo reticularis (a skin rash) disappear with the discontinuation of amantadine, as do central dopaminergic side effects such as confusion and hallucinations. Nervousness, anxiety, and insomnia are side effects that can be minimized by taking two daily doses, instead of three.

Contraindications

Amantadine is usually contraindicated in patients with renal failure because its clearance depends upon normal kidney function. It should be used with caution in patients with epilepsy because it is known to lower the seizure threshold.

ANTICHOLINERGICS

Mechanism of Action

Overactivity of striatal cholinergic neurons develops in Parkinson's disease because of reduced inhibitory (dopaminergic) input from the substantia nigra. Anticholinergic drugs can counteract excessive central cholinergic activity to some extent.

BOX 21–4
THERAPEUTIC EFFECTS

Tremor, dystonia, and drooling are the symptoms of Parkinson's disease most amenable to anticholinergic therapy (Table 21–2). Drug-induced parkinsonism, vascular parkinsonism, and striatonigral degeneration are also likely to respond to these agents to some extent.

Adverse Effects

The most common anticholinergic side effects are dry mouth, constipation, blurred vision, and urinary retention. Patients with dementia are likely to notice increasing confusion or worsening of their memory disorder. Excessive daytime sedation is sometimes an unwelcome side effect of diphenhydramine.

Contraindications

Glaucoma is usually an absolute contraindication to the use of anticholinergic agents. Patients with benign prostatic hypertrophy are at greater risk for developing urinary retention. As mentioned above, demented patients usually tolerate these agents poorly.

BROMOCRIPTINE

Mechanisms of Action

This ergot alkaloid derivative was initially developed to simulate prolactin inhibitory factor (dopamine) and to suppress hypothalamic overactivity that is manifested as amenorrhea and galactorrhea. In the striatum, bromocriptine works as an agonist at D_2 dopamine receptors and as a mild antagonist at D_1 receptors.

TABLE 21–2. Anticholinergic Agents

Generic Name	Brand Name	Dosage Forms	Daily Dosage
Trihexiphenidyl	ARTANE	Tablets (2, 5 mg)	Start: 2 mg b.i.d. Maximum: 5 mg q.i.d.
Benztropine	COGENTIN	Tablets (0.5, 1, 2 mg)	Start: 0.5 mg b.i.d. Maximum: 2 mg q.i.d.
Diphenhydramine	BENADRYL	Capsules (25, 50 mg)	Start: 25 mg h.s. Maximum: 50 mg q.i.d.

b.i.d. = twice daily; h.s. = at bedtime; q.i.d. = four times daily.

BOX 21–5
THERAPEUTIC EFFECTS

Monotherapy with bromocriptine in Parkinson's disease is not usually recommended, because it is less effective, more costly, and more toxic than monotherapy with carbidopa/levodopa. Bromocriptine is effective, however, as an adjunct to carbidopa/levodopa in patients with Stage III or IV Parkinson's disease. It is especially helpful in patients who have developed levodopa-induced chorea. These movements are thought to be mediated primarily through D_1 dopamine receptor sites, and bromocriptine is a mild antagonist at these sites. If the dose of carbidopa/levodopa is reduced while the dose of bromocriptine is increased, the chorea can often be eliminated.

Adverse Effects

One percent of Parkinson's patients develop symptomatic orthostatic hypotension after their first dose (1.25 mg) of bromocriptine. This is mediated by a partial blockade of both central and peripheral α-adrenergic receptors. Patients should be advised to take bedtime doses of bromocriptine during the first week or two of therapy. The drug can then be gradually increased to 10 mg/day, taken in four divided doses (the ideal therapeutic range for adjunctive bromocriptine is 10–20 mg/day). Other adverse effects such as nausea, hallucinations, and delusions can be avoided by tapering the dose of carbidopa/levodopa. Patients who develop Raynaud's phenomenon (cold-induced discoloration of the extremities) should taper, then discontinue their bromocriptine.

Contraindications

Patients with underlying orthostatic hypotension, peripheral arterial disease, or coronary artery disease are particularly vulnerable to the alpha-blocking side effects of bromocriptine. Demented patients are more likely to develop hallucinations or confusion.

PERGOLIDE

Mechanisms of Action

This ergoline derivative is different from bromocriptine in that it is an agonist at *both* D_1 and D_2 dopamine receptor sites. It is about 10 times as potent a D_2 agonist as bromocriptine. Like bromocriptine, it also inhibits prolactin release.

BOX 21-6
THERAPEUTIC EFFECTS

Pergolide is used as an adjunct to carbidopa/levodopa and is usually initiated in patients with Stage III or IV Parkinson's disease. Like bromocriptine, it is useful in patients who have developed levodopa-induced chorea. In one study, the addition of pergolide allowed for an average reduction of 46% in the dose of carbidopa/levodopa.

Adverse Effects

Orthostatic hypotension can be seen with pergolide, just as it is seen with bromocriptine. Therefore, the first dose (0.05 mg) should be given at bedtime. Because tolerance to this adverse effect usually develops over several weeks, the dose must be increased slowly. In order to avoid hypotension, nausea, and hallucinations, it is best to simultaneously taper the dose of carbidopa/levodopa. Nasal congestion, ankle swelling, and Raynaud's phenomenon are other side effects of pergolide.

Contraindications

Just as with bromocriptine, pergolide should be used with caution in those with peripheral arterial disease, coronary artery disease, and orthostatic hypotension. As with bromocriptine, demented patients are more likely than nondemented patients to develop hallucinations and confusion with pergolide. Unlike bromocriptine, however, pergolide is teratogenic and is contraindicated for use in women in their childbearing years.

REFERENCES

Abramowicz M (ed): Drugs for Parkinson's disease. Med Lett 35:31-34, 1993.

Ahlskog JE, Muenter MD: Pergolide: Long-term use in Parkinson's disease. Mayo Clin Proc 63:979-987, 1988a.

Ahlskog JE, Muenter MD: Treatment of Parkinson's disease with pergolide: A double-blind study. Mayo Clin Proc 63:969-978, 1988b.

Birkmayer W, Knoll J, Reiderer P, et al: Increased life expectancy resulting from addition of L-deprenyl to Madopar treatment in Parkinson's disease: A long-term study. J Neural Transm 64:113-127, 1985.

Butzer JF, Silver DE, Sahs AL: Amantadine in Parkinson's disease. Neurology 25:603-606, 1975.

Cotzias GC, VanWoert MH, Schiffer LM: Aromatic amino acids and modification of parkinsonism. N Engl J Med 276:374-378, 1967.

D'Amato RJ, Alexander GM, Schwartzman RJ, et al: Evidence for neuromelanin involvement in MPTP-induced neurotoxicity. Nature 327: 324-326, 1987.

Davis GC, Williams AC, Markey SP, et al: Chronic parkinsonism secondary to intravenous injection of meperidine analogues. Psychiatry Res 1:249-254, 1979.

Duvoisin RC: Cholinergic-anticholinergic antagonism in parkinsonism. Arch Neurol 17:124-136, 1967.

Elizan TS, Yahr MD, Moros DA, et al: Selegiline as an adjunct to conventional levodopa therapy in Parkinson's disease: Experience with this type B monoamine oxidase inhibitor in 200 patients. Arch Neurol 46:1280-1283, 1989.

Fabbrini G, Juncos J, Mouradian MM, et al: Levodopa pharmacokinetic mechanisms and motor fluctuations in Parkinson's disease. Ann Neurol 21:370-376, 1987.

Jankovic J: Pergolide: Short-term and long-term experience in Parkinson's disease. *In* Fahn S, Marsdon CD, Jenner P, Teychenne P (eds): Recent Developments in Parkinson's Disease, 339-345. New York: Raven Press, 1986.

Jankovic J, Fahn S: Physiologic and pathologic tremors. Ann Intern Med 93:460-465, 1980.

Klawans HL, Weiner WJ: Parkinsonism. *In* Nausieda PA, Goetz CG (eds): Textbook of Clinical Neuropharmacology, 1-35. New York: Raven Press, 1981.

LeWitt PA, Ward CD, Larsen TA, et al: Comparison of pergolide and bromocriptine therapy in parkinsonism. Neurology 33:1009-1014, 1983.

Nutt JG, Woodward WR, Anderson JL: The effect of carbidopa on the pharmacokinetics of intravenously administered levodopa. Ann Neurol 18:537-543, 1985.

Nutt JG, Woodward WR, Hammerstad JP, et al: The "on-off" phenomenon in Parkinson's disease: Relation to levodopa absorption and transport. N Engl J Med 310:483-488, 1984.

Parkes D: Bromocriptine. N Engl J Med 301:873-878, 1979.

Parkinson Study Group: DATATOP: A multicenter clinical trial in early Parkinson's disease. Arch Neurol 46:1052-1060, 1989a.

Parkinson Study Group: Effect of deprenyl on the progression of disability in early Parkinson's disease. N Engl J Med 321:1364-1371, 1989b.

Rinne UK: Combined bromocriptine-levodopa therapy early in Parkinson's disease. Neurology 35:1196-1198, 1985.

Schwab RS, England AC, Poskanzer DC, Young RR: Amantadine in the treatment of Parkinson's disease. JAMA 208:1168-1170, 1969.

Spencer SE, Wooten GF: Altered pharmacokinetics of L-dopa metabolism in rat striatum deprived of dopaminergic innervation. Neurology 34:1105-1108, 1984.

Skeletal Muscle Relaxants 22

Cedric M. Smith

Drugs covered in this chapter are commonly included in the category of "centrally acting muscle relaxants," which refers to a heterogeneous group of drugs used to produce muscle relaxation, with the exception of the neuromuscular blocking agents such as tubocurarine used in anesthesia. The most frequent clinical uses of these skeletal muscle relaxants are as adjuncts in the therapy of muscle spasticity, muscle spasm, and the immobility associated with strains, sprains, and injuries especially of the back and, to a lesser degree, injuries to the neck. They have been used also for the treatment of a variety of neurological conditions that have in common the presence of skeletal muscle hyperactivity, for example, the muscle spasms that can occur in multiple sclerosis.

These skeletal muscle relaxants are a heterogeneous group not only in terms of their chemistry and sites of actions but also in terms of their mechanisms of action as well as their clinical uses. Some of them are discussed in other sections of the book, for example, diazepam (VALIUM) in the antianxiety chapter (see Chapter 25). General pharmacology and organ system pharmacology of such agents are not repeated in this chapter; the reader is referred to those chapters in which the drugs are discussed in greater detail.

The agents are discussed in order of their sites of action, starting in the ultimate periphery, the skeletal muscle itself, and ending with the agents that have actions at the cortical and midbrain levels in the central nervous system (CNS). Drugs used strictly in the treatment of Parkinson's disease that may have rigidity as one of its components as well as tremor are covered in Chapter 21.

AGENTS ACTING DIRECTLY ON SKELETAL MUSCLE—INTRACELLULAR IN MUSCLE FIBERS

Dantrolene

Actions

Dantrolene (DANTRIUM) is a unique drug in terms of its effects and site of action. Dantrolene's action is restricted to the intracellular space inside skeletal muscle fibers; specifically, it interrupts the sarcoplasmic excitation-contraction coupling responsible for muscle contraction. This intracellular action in skeletal muscle is associated with a reduction of the release of calcium ions that initiate muscle contraction.

In addition to having effects on extrafusal muscle fibers responsible for developing muscle contractions, shortening, and force, dantrolene's effect on muscle intrafusal fibers results in a relaxation of these fibers and thus a decrease in the activity from muscle spindles. The possible relaxant effects from this action are discussed more in Box 22-1.

BOX 22-1
THERAPEUTIC USES

- **Spasticity and muscle spasms**. Dantrolene has found its greatest utility in the treatment of spasms and spasticity associated with cerebral palsy and of the spasticity and mass reflex movements that can occur in paraplegic and hemiglegic patients. Although it produces relaxation, in larger doses and in certain muscles it can, produce muscle weakness—an extension of its therapeutic effect.

  Muscle spasm and spasticity is only one of the reasons why individuals with cerebral palsy have disordered, uncoordinated muscle function. To the degree that the excessive activity of muscle spasticity impairs normal muscle coordination and strength, its relaxation is therapeutically beneficial. However, in muscle groups in which the major functional defect is primarily inadequate coordination, relaxation and weakness frequently further impair functional capabilities. The major problem in cerebral palsy is most often a defect in the coordination of muscle activity rather than excessive tone or muscle spasticity. Although reducing spasticity may be useful therapeutically and functionally when that is impairing movement, there are limits to the numbers of individuals for whom it is helpful and to the magnitude of beneficial effects that can be achieved by any muscle relaxant.
- **Malignant neuroleptic syndrome and malignant hyperthermia**. A unique use of dantrolene is in the management of the malignant neuroleptic syndrome and in the syndrome of malignant hyperthermia. These syndromes are described briefly in Chapter 23 where the antipsychotic drugs—the agents that have been associated most closely with the malignant neuroleptic syndrome—are covered. The major objective of the use of muscle relaxants in these conditions is the rapid reduction in the excessive muscle activity, resulting in decreased hyperthermia and avoidance of the damage to muscle that can result in myoglobinemia, myoglobinuria, and possible kidney damage.

  Although dantrolene can be used in other syndromes such as low back spasm, it is not commonly used for that purpose.

Adverse Effects

The most frequent adverse reactions to dantrolene are drowsiness, dizziness, and weakness. It can also result in a wide variety of side effects, including insomnia, gastrointestinal (GI) disturbances, mental confusion, myalgia, and abnormal hair growth.

The major limitation to the chronic use of dantrolene is the possible occurrence of severe liver toxicity or pleural effusion. Both of these serious side effects warrant close monitoring of all patients receiving this drug. The individuals at higher risk of such side effects are those with pre-existing liver damage, females, and patients over 35 years of age; it also appears that long-term use increases the risk.

AGENTS ACTING ON SKELETAL MUSCLE MEMBRANE

Quinine (QUINAMM)

BOX 22-2
THERAPEUTIC USES

The old drug quinine (QUINAMM), which has a long time-honored use as an antipyretic, analgesic, and antimalarial drug, remains in medicine for its unique ability to stabilize the muscle membrane against repetitive activity. It is used in two specific disease conditions. One is **myotonia congenita** (Thomsen's disease), a congenital condition in which there are repetitive action potentials generated in the muscle fibers following a single or brief excitation/contraction. In this condition, there appears to be a failure in the ability to relax a previously contracted muscle. Another condition of repetitive muscle activity is the nocturnal muscle cramp, which can be particularly distressing in the elderly. Quinine is effective in these disease states because it decreases the repetitive generation of action potentials along membranes and especially along the membranes of skeletal muscle fibers.

Site and Mechanism of Action

A muscle contraction is initiated by an action potential that travels down the axon from the motor neuron to the neuromuscular junction, and the release of the neurotransmitter followed by the generation of a single propagated action potential along the muscle fiber. In myotonia a single action potential generated from the neuromuscular junction along the muscle membrane is associated not with just a single potential but with a burst of repetitive action potentials that results in a short-lasting tetanus; with many muscle fibers these repetitive action potentials give rise to a muscle cramp. This repetitive activity occurs not only in a single motor unit in single muscle fibers but in a number of muscle fibers at approximately the same time. The action of quinine is quite similar to the action and mechanism of action of its optical isomer quinidine, which has an antiarrhythmic effect on the heart. The mechanism of action of quinine is similar to that of quinidine in three ways: a membrane-stabilizing action, interference with the voltage-dependent sodium permeability, and increased threshold for action potential generation (see Chapter 29).

Adverse Effects

For the most part the side effects of quinine are similar to those of quinidine. These side effects have received the time-honored name of *cinchonism*, which derives from the fact that quinine is obtained from the bark of the cinchona tree.

CINCHONISM—SIDE EFFECTS OF QUININE OR QUINIDINE:

- Disturbances of hearing and vision (tinnitus, deafness, vertigo, blurred vision, photophobia, and even retinal ischemia)
- Disturbances of GI function (nausea, vomiting, or diarrhea)
- Disturbances of skin (rashes, pruritus, angioedema, and hypersensitivity)
- Disturbances of cardiac rhythm (cardiac irregularities or bradycardia)

The chronic use of quinine as treatment of headaches and fever was popular 25 or more years ago. (Quinine is also mentioned as an example of a drug that affects sensory systems in Chapter 13.)

Calcium/Calcium Channel–Blocking Agents

The intravenous administration of calcium salts in the form of calcium gluconate has been used in the past for the treatment of muscle cramps. However, this therapy has been largely discontinued. There are also clinical reports of the effectiveness of verapamil, the calcium channel-blocking agent, for the treatment of muscle cramps (verapamil is discussed in greater detail in Chapter 32).

DRUGS ACTING ON MUSCLE SPINDLES

Muscle spindles are a major source of afferent input from skeletal muscle. Each muscle spindle has at least 1 primary ending or 1 or more afferent endings wrapped around a complex of 8 to 12 intrafusal muscle fibers; the intrafusal fibers serve to regulate the sensitivity of the stretch receptors to stretch and velocity of stretch. At the risk of oversimplification, the primary endings sense rate of stretch of the muscle, whereas the secondary endings are much more exclusively involved in sensing only the static length of the muscle. Thus, the primary and secondary endings are each under selective regulation by the contractions of intrafusal muscle fibers; the individual intrafusal fibers are specialized so that some of them primarily regulate the sensitivity to the dynamic rate of change of length, whereas others are more involved in regulating the static length sensitivity of the muscle spindle afferents.

The muscle spindle system as well as the tendon organs are complex components of the even more complex motor control system; they are involved in spinal regulation of motor control as well as midbrain and cerebellar coordination of muscle activity, both postural tone as well as movements. In addition, the spindle afferents project to the cerebral cortex; however, the function of these extensive cortical projections is not well understood.

Clinically, spasticity is characterized by exaggerated stretch reflexes, the reflexes mediated over the muscle spindle system. For understanding the uses of the drugs discussed in this chapter, it is sufficient to note that the muscle spindle system is intricately involved in maintenance of muscle tone, the occurrence of muscle spasm and muscle rigidity, and disturbances of muscle coordination. (Agents that excite muscle spindle afferent endings are discussed in Chapter 13 on sensory actions of drugs.)

The clinically useful drugs that have actions on the muscle spindles also have other sites of action (see Table 22–1).

Methocarbamol

Mephenesin (ROBAXIN) was the first compound with selective muscle relaxant actions that did not act directly on muscle; it is obsolete therapeutically because of its short duration of action. Another drug of the same chemical class and with many of the same actions is methocarbamol.

- Mephenesin, and probably methocarbamol, depresses muscle spindle afferent activity, presumably by a direct effect on the muscle spindle ending; this effect occurs with doses that are associated with muscle relaxation. These and related compounds also have spinal cord sites of action and are discussed further later.

Phenytoin

Phenytoin (DILANTIN), the well-known antiepileptic drug, has been shown experimentally and in clinical studies to have a relaxing effect, especially when it is combined with chlorpromazine. One of phenytoin's actions is to decrease the excitability of the sensory ending of muscle spindles to stretch; this effect has been found to occur in experimental preparations of rigidity in concentrations consistent with those obtained clinically.

DRUGS ACTING SOLELY OR IN PART ON SPINAL CORD REFLEXES

Methocarbamol

Actions

Methocarbamol (ROBAXIN) is the prime agent of this class that remains in the clinical armamentarium. Methocarbamol and mephenesin were shown in the early 1950s to have selective effects on spinal cord reflexes that were mediated over multineuronal pathways, as compared with their effects on monosynaptic reflexes. When the mono- and polysynaptic reflexes of a given segment of the spinal cord were tested with barbiturate or with ether anesthesia, the two types of reflexes were depressed to approximately equivalent degrees; a 50% depression of the monosynaptic reflex would be accompanied by approximately 50% depression of the polysynaptic reflex. In contrast, mephenesin and methocarbamol selectively depressed the polysynaptic spinal reflexes to a greater degree than the monosynaptic. This simple observation led to the categorization of a class of agents that were assumed to act as muscle relaxants by blocking interneurons in multisynaptic reflex chains.

Other agents frequently included in this category of interneuron blocking agents, and presumed to act in a similar fashion, are chlorzoxazone (PARAFLEX), metaxalone (SKELAXIN), and carisoprodol (SOMA). As a matter of fact, however, these agents are not exclusively selective in their effects on interneurons; in larger doses they actually depress motor neurons as well. Their actions on interneurons are not the sole site or mechanism of their muscle relaxant actions. They also depress reflexes that impinge on fusimotor neurons (those neurons that innervate intrafusal muscle fibers) and thereby depress muscle spindle afferent activity indirectly. In addition, these agents have a number of other actions that are plausibly associated with their clinical utility as muscle relaxants in cases of spasticity and rigidity, such as depression of repetitive activation of neurons and depression of posttetanic potentiation, as tested with spinal monosynaptic reflexes.

Adverse Effects

Like many of the various muscle relaxants, CNS sedation with drowsiness is the most common side effect. In larger than therapeutic doses, ataxia and ultimately coma result.

Diazepam

Actions

Diazepam (VALIUM) is unique among the benzodiazepines in having a clinically useful selective effect to produce muscle relaxation in doses equal to or below those that cause a reduction in anxiety or sleep. The muscle relaxant activity of diazepam is in part related to its action at the spinal cord level, where it augments presynaptic inhibition; diazepam increases the γ-aminobutyric acid (GABA)-mediated actions presynaptically on the excitatory boutons on the motor neuron. In fact, it was the demonstration of the site of this action that helped define the unique action of the benzodiazepines, first on presynaptic inhibition and second on GABA-mediated inhibition. (The site and mechanism of action of diazepam is discussed further in the chapter dealing extensively with benzodiazepines, Chapter 25.)

The major limitations in the therapeutic use of most of the muscle relaxant drugs including diazepam are the dose-related side effects of sedation, drowsiness, and muscle incoordination; sufficient doses of the agents result in ataxia or sleep, or ultimately coma, especially in combination with alcohol or other CNS depressants.

Baclofen

Actions

Baclofen (LIORESAL) has unique actions at the spinal, and probably supraspinal, levels to reduce the excitatory synaptic influences on the motor neuron and other neurons in the descending excitatory pathway to skeletal muscle. Baclofen reduces the release as well as the efficacy of the excitatory amino acid transmitters. In this connection it probably acts to block the release and action of both aspartate and glutamate at least at the spinal cord level. Interestingly, the drug is a structural analog of GABA, and it was synthesized originally with the idea that it would interact with the GABA system. It acts, at least in part, as an agonist on GABA receptors at spinal and supraspinal sites in the substantia nigra (Turski et al, 1990). Thus, it decreases the reflex excitation of the motor neuron as well as the influence of descending excitation inasmuch as these depend upon an adequate level of excitability of the motor neuron in order to evoke muscle contraction or sustained muscle activity.

> **BOX 22-3**
> **THERAPEUTIC USES**
>
> Baclofen has found its greatest use in muscle spasm associated with neurological disease, such as multiple sclerosis and spinal cord injury.

Adverse Effects

The side effects of baclofen, in addition to the predictable weakness and fatigue, include nausea, GI disturbances, confusion, headache, insomnia, urinary frequency, and mania. A variety of neurological symptoms following baclofen have been reported, but it may be difficult to interpret whether they are due to the drug, the underlying disease, or a combination of the two.

Cyclobenzaprine

Actions

Cyclobenzaprine (FLEXERIL) is a close chemical relative of amitriptyline. Somewhat unexpectedly it was found to produce relaxation of experimentally produced rigidities and, subsequently, the muscle spasms in human disease conditions. Cyclobenzaprine appears to have a unique profile of action in the CNS. Its site of action is in the midbrain and at the spinal level, resulting in a depression of repetitive motor neuron activity. It produces a selective depression of the experimental rigidity following spinal cord ischemic damage with a wider margin of safety than most other relaxants. In addition, in larger doses cyclobenzaprine has sedative and sleep-inducing activity and has a side effect profile quite similar to amitriptyline.

Adverse Effects

In addition to causing drowsiness, cyclobenzaprine has the same side effects as amitriptyline, including the cardiac and atropine-like effects. It has all of the characteristic effects of anticholinergic agents, including drowsiness and mental confusion, as well as the peripheral autonomic effects of dry mouth, paralysis of accommodation, and changes in GI function.

> **BOX 22–4**
> **THERAPEUTIC USES**
>
> Evidence to date suggests that cyclobenzaprine is much more effective as a muscle relaxant than is amitriptyline or any other tricyclic antidepressant. (The complexity of clinical low back syndromes and drug actions can be illustrated by the fact that psychiatric depression itself predisposes individuals to low back syndromes. Depression also augments and aggravates pain. In addition, the tricyclic antidepressants have a limited analgesic effect and are used in the management of a variety of chronic pain conditions.)

DRUGS AND DRUG ACTION AT SUPRASPINAL AND CEREBELLAR LEVELS

As might be anticipated, the muscle relaxant drugs already mentioned act not only at the spinal level but also at the supraspinal level. To the degree that they have been investigated, most have actions at supraspinal, midbrain, or higher levels that may be more important quantitatively than their actions at the spinal cord level. This general conclusion is not based on extensive research of all available agents; those that have been examined and found to have midbrain and supraspinal actions are diazepam, methocarbamol, orphenadrine, cyclobenzaprine, baclofen, phenytoin, and chlorpromazine.

Orphenadrine

Actions

Orphenadrine (NORFLEX) has been shown to act supraspinally to decrease experimental rigidity, at least in part by decreasing the excitation of fusimotor neurons and the fusimotor outflow to muscle spindles and, thereby, depressing stretch reflexes.

> **BOX 22–5**
> **THERAPEUTIC USES**
>
> Orphenadrine has some clinical efficacy as an adjunct to rest and physical therapy in the relief of painful musculoskeletal disorders. It produces relaxation of skeletal muscle hyperactivity, notably that associated with strains and sprains of the low back muscles, ligaments, and tendons.

Adverse Effects

Most of the side effects of orphenadrine are the consequence of its anticholinergic actions — dry mouth, tachycardia, urinary retention, blurred vision, mental confusion, drowsiness, constipation, or hallucinations.

Chlorpromazine

Actions

Chlorpromazine (THORAZINE) has been long known to depress the fusimotor system at some site(s) between the cerebellum and midbrain to the spinal cord level. In conditions in which there is hyperactivity of fusimotor neurons, chlorpromazine depresses fusimotor neuron outflow and thereby depresses muscle spindle sensitivity and the associated stretch reflexes.

> **BOX 22–6**
> **THERAPEUTIC USES FOR MUSCLE RELAXATION**
>
> The combination of phenytoin with chlorpromazine has been found to be effective in reducing muscle spasm and spasticity. It appears that the muscle spindle activity is effectively suppressed by combining an agent that acts directly on the afferent ending with an agent (chlorpromazine) that decreases fusimotor outflow. (The possibility of using other agents, such as methocarbamol or cyclobenzaprine in combination with phenytoin or other spindle afferent depressants, has not been explored; there are few data by which one could predict what such a combination might accomplish. It is theoretically possible that the combination would be appreciably more effective and less toxic than any single agent.)

THERAPEUTIC MANAGEMENT OF MUSCLE SPASM

Table 22–1 summarizes various sites of action of the different drugs mentioned. Inasmuch as skeletal muscle hyperactivity is an end result of a variety of pathophysiological mechanisms, relaxation of skeletal muscle can be achieved by drug actions at many different sites. Moreover, the muscle spasm and spasticity, such as are associated with acute strains or repeated strains of the lower back, are made worse by anxiety or depression. Poor posture and generally inadequate muscle tone are primary risk factors for the occurrence of muscle and fascial strain syndromes.

The recovery from an acute low-back insult requires the individual to avoid further strain and stress and to limit motion until the inflammation and reflex hyperactivity resolves. Thus, thorough diagnostic assessment of the individual and the disorder, bed rest, the use of nonsteroidal anti-inflammatory agents, and application of physical therapy interventions are essential components of the overall management of an acute back strain. Drugs are appropriately viewed as adjuncts to the overall management of the disease condition, and not as the primary or definitive therapy.

TABLE 22–1. Primary Sites of Action of Skeletal Muscle Relaxants

Drug or Class	Muscle	Muscle Membrane	Neuro-muscular Junction	Muscle Spindle		Spinal Cord: Presynaptic	Motor Neuron	Inter-neurons	Mid-brain	Basal Ganglia	Cortex (Antianxiety, Sedation)
				Afferent	*Fusimotor*						
Dantrolene	+										
Quinine		+									
Phenytoin				+							?
Chlorpromazine					+						+
Tubocurarine/ succinylcholine (and related)			+		+						
Methocarbamol				+	+	+	(+)	+	+		+
Diazepam					+	+			+	S.N.	+
Baclofen						+	+			S.N.	
Cyclobenzaprine									+		+
Antiparkinsonian Agents											
Amantadine										+	
Biperiden, trihexyphenidyl (and related)										+	

S.N. = substantia nigra.

Overall, any drug that promotes bed rest or restful sleep will tend to be beneficial for acute back strains, and any drug that tends to decrease the level of anxiety or depression will also be potentially beneficial. The complexity of back injuries and their reflex consequences has made it difficult to ascertain the specific sites of drug action. It is generally accepted that the drugs presented in this chapter have some limited efficacy and when used appropriately as adjuncts, they can provide some benefit. Nevertheless, their effects are not profound, and other influences may be equally or more important than the drug therapy itself.

BOX 22–7
THERAPEUTIC USES OF MUSCLE RELAXANTS

Essential to rational therapy with any of the "muscle relaxants" is an explicit therapeutic objective:

1. Reduction of unwanted muscle spasm or movements
2. Improved muscle coordination
3. Reduction of pain
4. Improved mobility and range of motion
5. Modification of precipitating factors such as depression, anxiety, muscle weakness

The therapeutic management of many patients with low back and other syndromes in which muscle spasm is a feature remains far from satisfactory. Drugs are not uniquely useful, in part because the primary objectives of therapy may be to increase range of motion or to abolish pain, whereas these so-called relaxant drugs in fact may have little effect on mobility or pain as such.

Some clinicians suggest that the drug against which they would compare other drugs would be cyclobenzaprine, whereas others would select diazepam or an adequate dose of one of the nonsteroidal anti-inflammatory drugs. These differences in clinical opinion reflect the paucity of studies and the fact that these agents, although effective, are only to a limited degree. A useful strategy would be to use a given agent and increase the dose until benefit or side effects occur. If no useful effect is obtained and the condition persists, an alternative drug could be tried using a similar approach.

In addition to the low-back syndromes, there are a number of conditions that are associated characteristically with skeletal muscle hyperactivity in which drug therapy may be beneficial. These include the hand-shoulder syndrome, the temporomandibular joint syndrome, stiff neck or wry neck, stiff man syndrome, black widow spider bites, nocturnal muscle cramps, the neck pain associated with the use of new eyeglasses, as well as the muscle spasms that accompany arthritis, spinal cord injury, and multiple sclerosis.

DRUG THERAPY OF ESSENTIAL TREMOR

Essential tremor affects about 5% of the general population, whereas Parkinson's disease affects less than 1%. The frequency of this postural tremor is usually faster (4 - 11 cps) than that of the parkinsonian rest tremor (3 - 6 cps). Essential tremor is referred to as *familial tremor* when a positive family history is elicited. Essential tremor is uniquely relieved by alcoholic beverages.

Propranolol

Actions

Propranolol (INDERAL) was the first β blocker to be used in the treatment of essential tremor. Although it may not abolish essential tremor, propranolol can reduce tremor amplitude in 50 - 70% of patients so affected.

Peripheral adrenergic mechanisms are intact in essential tremor and thus it has either sensory or central actions to reduce essential tremor.

Adverse Effects

Because propranolol can induce bronchospasm, it is contraindicated in patients with chronic obstructive lung disease or asthma. A selective β_1 antagonist, such as metoprolol, is preferable for these patients. Propranolol is contraindicated also in patients with brittle diabetes, because it may mask the symptoms of hypoglycemia (tremor, tachycardia, and diaphoresis). It can lower blood pressure, so it should be used cautiously, or not at all, in patients whose blood pressure is lower than normal (see Chapter 10).

> **BOX 22-8**
> **THERAPEUTIC USES**
>
> Propranolol is useful in the treatment of not only essential tremor, but also drug-induced postural tremors such as those unmasked by tricyclic antidepressants or lithium. Lower doses than those used in essential tremor are usually effective in the treatment of drug-induced tremors. Essential tremor patients who are not compliant with taking three or four doses of propranolol each day should take nadolol, a β blocker with a 24-hour half-life that can be given once daily.

Primidone

Actions

In 1981, O'Brien and colleagues noted that a patient with both epilepsy and essential tremor experienced reduction in tremor amplitude while being treated with the anticonvulsant primidone. They treated 20 other essential tremor patients and found a good clinical response in 12 (six could not tolerate the drug's adverse effects). Primidone produces more acute toxicity than does propranolol, but is slightly more effective in treating essential tremor.

Primidone, whose half-life is 10 hours, is converted to two active metabolites: phenylethylmalonamide (PEMA) with a half-life of 24 - 28 hours, and phenobarbital with a half-life of 50 - 120 hours. The mechanism for primidone's antitremor action is unknown, although it appears that it is due to primidone itself and not to either of its metabolites (see Chapter 20).

Adverse Effects

Vertigo, nausea, and unsteadiness are early adverse effects of primidone that are often dose-limiting. Patients should be warned that they may experience a flu-like syndrome (headache, nasal congestion, and nausea), but this is usually short-lived.

REFERENCES

Basmajian JV: Acute back pain and spasm. A controlled multicenter trial of combined analgesic and antispasm agents. Spine 14:438 - 439, 1989.

Bennett RM, Gatter RA, Campbell SM, et al: A comparison of cyclobenzaprine and placebo in the management of fibrositis. A double-blind controlled study. Arthritis Rheum 31:1535 - 1542, 1988.

Borenstein DG, Wiesel, SW: Low Back Pain: Medical Diagnosis and Comprehensive Management. Philadelphia: WB Saunders Co, 1989.

Delwaide PJ: Electrophysiological analysis of the mode of action of muscle relaxants in spasticity. Ann Neurol 17:90 - 95, 1985.

Deyo RA, Rainville J, Kent DC: What can the history and physical examination tell us about low back pain? JAMA 268:760 - 765, 1992.

Eldred E, Yellin H, Desantis M, Smith CM: Supplement to bibliography on muscle receptors: Their morphology, pathology, physiology and pharmacology. Exp Neurol 55(Part 2):1 - 118, 1977.

Guan XM, Peroutka SJ: Basic mechanisms of action of drugs used in the treatment of essential tremor. Clin Neuropharmacol 13:210 - 223, 1990.

Kirkaldy-Willis WH (ed): Managing Low Back Pain, 2nd ed. New York: Churchill Livingstone, 1988.

Meredith TJ, Jacobsen D, Haines JA, Berger J-C: Naloxone, flumazenil and dantrolene as antidotes. Volume 1 EPCS/CEC Evaluation of Antidotes Series. Cambridge University Press, Cambridge, 1993.

O'Brien MD, Upton AR, Toseland PA: Benign familial tremor treated with primidone. Br Med J 282:178 - 180, 1981.

Raines A: Centrally acting muscle relaxants. In Pradhan SN, Maickel RP, Dutta SN (eds): Pharmacology in Medicine: Principles and Practice, 184 - 188. Bethesda, MD: SP Press International, 1986.

Smith CM: The pharmacology of sedative/hypnotics, alcohol, and anesthetics: Sites and mechanisms of action. In Martin WR (ed): Drug Addiction I, 413 - 587. Vol 45/1 of Handbook of Experimental Pharmacology. Heidelberg: Springer-Verlag, 1977.

Smith CM: Relaxants of skeletal muscle. In Root WS, Hoffman FG (eds): Physiological Pharmacology. Vol. II. New York: Academic Press, 1965.

Ward A, Chaffman MO, Sorkin EM: Dantrolene: A review of its pharmacodynamic and pharmacokinetic properties and therapeutic use in malignant hyperthermia, the neuroleptic malignant syndrome and an update of its use in muscle spasticity. Drugs 32:130 - 168, 1986.

Ward NG: Tricyclic antidepressants for chronic low-back pain. Mechanisms of action and predictors of response. Spine 11:661 - 665, 1986.

Young RR: Treatment for spastic paresis. N Engl J Med 320:1553 - 1555, 1989.

PART V

DRUG TREATMENT OF PSYCHIATRIC DISORDERS

23 Antipsychotic Drugs (Neuroleptics)

Jerrold C. Winter

The discovery in the mid-1950s of the clinical efficacy of chlorpromazine can truly be said to have revolutionized the practice of psychiatry. Prior to that time no regularly efficacious treatment was available for the most common psychotic disorders. Discovery of the neuroleptics made possible the release to their homes and to their communities of many thousands of patients who previously faced the prospect of lifetime institutionalization.

Unfortunately, the early hope that psychotic patients would be cured by antipsychotic drugs has not been realized; amelioration of the signs and symptoms of the disorders better characterizes the usual course of drug therapy. In addition, despite the dozens of neuroleptics marketed since chlorpromazine, none represents a quantum advance beyond that prototypical agent. Nonetheless, there is at the present time considerable optimism that one or more of the "atypical" neuroleptics (see below) will offer significant advantages.

There is a tendency among students of medicine to regard psychotherapeutic drugs in general, and neuroleptics in particular, as the province of psychiatry. In fact, surveys have indicated that two thirds of all prescriptions for antidepressants and neuroleptics are written by physicians other than psychiatrists. Even those physicians who do not themselves prescribe neuroleptics will certainly encounter patients who are maintained on these drugs. It is therefore essential that all physicians have a working general knowledge of the indications, adverse effects, and drug interactions of the neuroleptics.

INDICATIONS FOR USE

Psychosis is the condition most often treated with neuroleptics. Although psychosis has been variously defined, the essential feature is partial or complete separation from reality. The origins of psychosis are multiple and may include factors that are not amenable to treatment with neuroleptics. For example, a number of drugs of abuse may produce acute departure from reality that may be aggravated by the use of antipsychotic drugs. Therefore, careful medical evaluation is essential prior to the initiation of neuroleptic therapy.

The most common forms of psychosis for which neuroleptics are indicated are the **schizophrenic disorders**. These disorders are characterized by chronicity, impaired function, and disturbances of thinking and affect. The American Psychiatric Association's Diagnostic and Statistical Manual of Mental Disorders, third edition, Revised (DSM-III-R), provides the following specific criteria for the diagnosis of schizophrenia: (1) one or more psychotic symptoms such as delusions, hallucinations, illogical thinking, or disorganized behavior; (2) deterioration from a previous level of functioning; (3) continuous signs of the illness for at least 6 months; (4) a tendency toward onset before age 45; (5) symptoms not due to affective disorders; and (6) symptoms not due to organic mental disorder or mental retardation.

Although psychosis is the primary indication for the use of neuroleptics, they are widely prescribed as well for a variety of aberrant behaviors of nonspecific origin including aggression, hostility, and self-destructive behavior. These drugs play a significant, albeit ill-defined and sometimes controversial, role in the treatment of disturbed children. Delusions and hallucinations in the demented elderly are often treated with neuroleptics, as are the manic and delusional symptoms of manic-depressive psychosis. In a nonbehavioral application, the antiemetic properties of certain of the neuroleptics are made use of to reduce nausea and vomiting associated with cancer chemotherapy. This and other minor uses of the neuroleptics are not discussed in this chapter.

HISTORY AND NOMENCLATURE

Phenothiazine is a tricyclic chemical long known to have anthelmintic properties. In 1950, **chlorpromazine**, a simple derivative of phenothiazine, was synthesized by Paul Charpentier and his colleagues at the Rhone-Poulenc Laboratories in France (see the structures later in this chapter). Chlorpromazine was initially examined by the French surgeon Henri Laborit as a part of his studies of the role of histamine in surgical shock. Noting that the drug produced a state of calmness and indifference ("ataraxia"), Laborit suggested possible uses in psychiatry. Confirmation of that suggestion was provided by Jean Delay and Pierre Deniker in Paris in 1952. Thirty-eight psychotic patients treated with chlorpromazine by Delay and Deniker became less aggressive and agitated and suffered fewer delusions and hallucinations.

Reserpine, a drug derived from the Indian shrub Rauwolfia serpentina, is best known to today's students of medicine as an antihypertensive agent. However, there is also reason to regard it as the first antipsychotic drug. As a part of traditional Indian medicine, rauwolfia was used for a variety of conditions including insanity. Although reserpine's effects in mental disturbances were reported by Indian psychiatrists as early as 1931, it was work by the American psychiatrist Nathan Kline that brought reserpine to worldwide attention. Because of a range of adverse effects, including disturbances of the extrapyramidal motor system (EPMS), and questions as to its efficacy, reserpine was quickly eclipsed for psychiatric use by the phenothiazines. Among reserpine's legacies is the word **tranquilizer**, coined by F. F. Yonkman to characterize its pharmacological effects in animals.

In this chapter, the terms **antipsychotic agent** and **neuroleptic** are used interchangeably. The former has the advantage of simplicity and obvious meaning, whereas the latter has the virtue of brevity. Some continue to use the word ataractic, but there is little to recommend it. Least desirable of all is reference to neuroleptics as tranquilizers. Distinction between major tranquilizers, the neuroleptics, and the so-called minor tranquilizers, the anxiolytics, does not help. Phenothiazines and other neuroleptics are pharmacologically and therapeutically distinct from anxiolytics such as the benzodiazepines (see Chapter 25). The implication of a continuum of therapeutic or pharmacological activity by use of a common term, tranquilizer, contributes to patient misunderstanding as well as to the possibility of inappropriate prescribing by physicians.

POTENCY AND EFFICACY

Each of the drugs illustrated is of proven **efficacy** in the treatment of psychosis. However, as noted earlier, none can be considered curative. In most patients, there is rapid improvement in the most florid signs of psychosis followed by a plateau. Whatever the degree of improvement that is maintained, there seldom is doubt as to the continued presence of the disease, which is indicated either by residual impairment of function during neuroleptic treatment or by relapse upon discontinuation of treatment.

As was discussed in Chapter 2, **potency** is defined as the quantity of a drug, usually expressed as milligrams per patient or milligrams per kilogram, required to produce a given therapeutic effect. With respect to the neuroleptics illustrated there is a wide range of acceptable doses for any given drug and an even wider range between drugs. For example, when haloperidol was first introduced for use, dosages of a fraction of a milligram per day were not uncommon, whereas patients have sometimes been treated with as much as 2 g/day of chlorpromazine. Representative doses are given in Table 23–1.

Haloperidol (HALDOL) F–C₆H₄–C(=O)–$(CH_2)_3$–N(piperidine)(OH)–C₆H₄–Cl

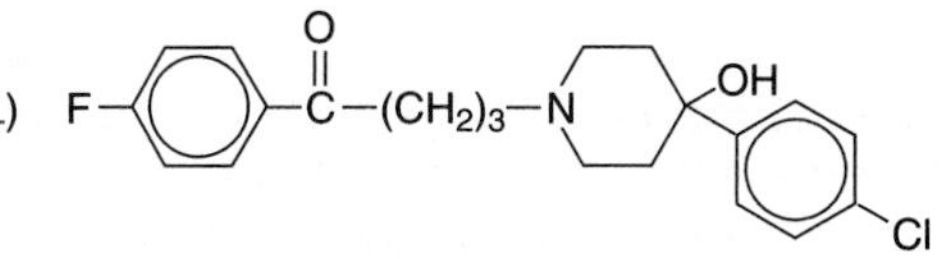

Chlorpromazine (THORAZINE) S, N, Cl, $(CH_2)_3-N(CH_3)_2$

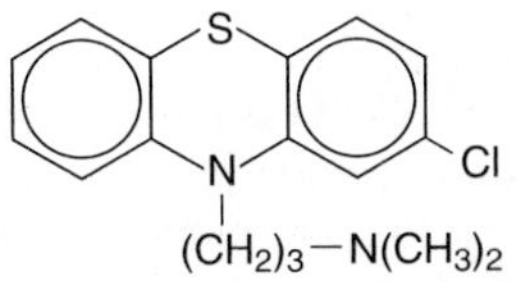

A portion of the high degree of variation in doses both within and between neuroleptics is no doubt due to characteristics inherent to each drug. In addition, however, this variability is a reflection of the fact that (1) antipsychotic drugs as a group have a high therapeutic index, at least with

TABLE 23–1. Relative Potency of Neuroleptic Drugs

Drug	Equivalent Dose (mg)	Daily Dose Range (mg)
Chlorpromazine	100	50–1200
Thioridazine	100	50–800
Trifluoperazine	2	2–80
Haloperidol	2	2–100
Clozapine	79	75–700

respect to lethal effects, (2) antipsychotic drugs do not always produce completely satisfactory therapeutic results, and (3) individual patients appear to differ widely in their sensitivity to these drugs.

As is true for other classes of drugs, neuroleptics are sometimes classified on the basis of their **relative potencies**. For example, within the phenothiazine family of antipsychotics, the typical dose of a piperazine-type drug such as trifluoperazine is significantly less than that of chlorpromazine, an aliphatic, or of thioridazine, a piperidine. Thus,

Thioridazine (MELLARIL)

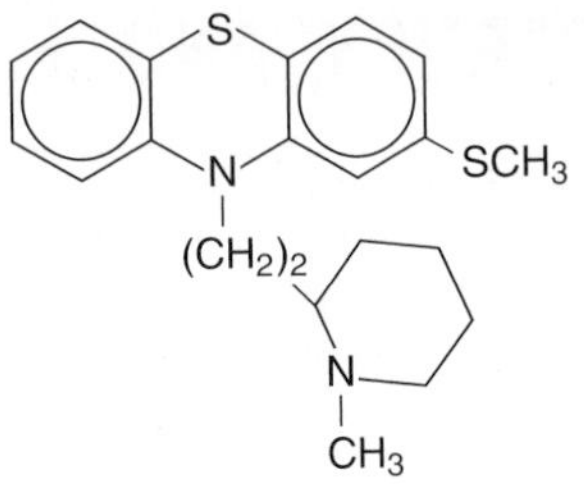

S, N, SCH_3, $(CH_2)_2$, N, CH_3

Fluphenazine (PERMITIL; PROLIXIN)

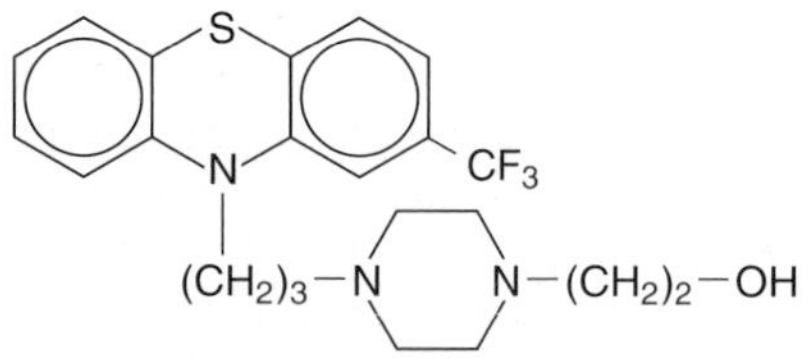

S, N, CF_3, $(CH_2)_3-N$, $N-(CH_2)_2-OH$

fluphenazine is a high-potency phenothiazine. Although it is true that certain adverse effects are correlated with potency, the pattern of correlation is not consistent; trifluoperazine is, for example, less likely to produce sedation than is chlorpromazine but more likely to cause disturbances of the EPMS. Potency *per se* is for the phenothiazines, as for most other drugs, of little importance in the selection of the most appropriate therapeutic agent.

MECHANISM OF ACTION

The precise pharmacological mechanisms by which neuroleptics exert their beneficial effects are unknown. The explanation for this state of ignorance is simple: the etiology of the major psychotic disorders, including schizophrenia, is unknown. However, consideration of the pharmacological properties of the drugs may provide some clues.

The 12 neuroleptics available for use at present in the United States represent five distinct chemical classes. The largest group is the phenothiazines, currently represented by seven drugs. There are two thioxanthenes, and each of the remaining three chemical classes has but a single representative. Despite their variety of chemical structures, the antipsychotic drugs share certain effects, particularly with respect to the neurotransmitter dopamine.

It was noted earlier that reserpine sometimes causes disturbances of the EPMS, a peculiar effect not previously produced by any pharmacological agent. However, similar effects soon were observed following treatment with chlorpromazine and, subsequently, with every other neuroleptic. A portion of the syndrome produced by neuroleptics closely resembles Parkinson's disease, a disorder caused by loss of dopaminergic neurons in the substantia nigra and their axonal projections to the striatum. It is now thought likely that neuroleptic-induced extrapyramidal disturbance is due to antagonism of striatal dopamine function.

There is little reason to believe that activity in the EPMS is related to psychosis. However, with the discovery of other aspects of dopamine function, the notion that dopaminergic antagonism is responsible for the therapeutic effects of antipsychotics became more plausible. In particular, the rhinencephalon or limbic lobe was found to receive projections from dopaminergic neurons of the mesencephalon. The limbic system, composed of the limbic lobe and associated areas of the thalamus, epithalamus, and hypothalamus, has long been associated with emotional functions.

The **dopamine hypothesis of schizophrenia** states that hyperactivity in dopaminergic systems causes the signs and symptoms characteristic of the disease. Primary support for the hypothesis comes from the observation that all clinically effective antipsychotic drugs block one or another aspect of dopaminergic function. Further evidence is provided by the fact that chronic treatment with amphetamine, a drug believed to interact with dopaminergic systems, causes a syndrome that closely resembles paranoid schizophrenia.

Despite widespread acceptance of the dopamine hypothesis of schizophrenia, recent discoveries suggest a more complex picture. For example, multiple dopamine receptors have now been cloned but the precise role of each in psychosis remains to be established. "Typical" antipsychotics such as haloperidol and the phenothiazines have high affinity for the D_2 dopamine receptor and induce dysfunction of the EPMS. In contrast, clozapine, an "atypical" antipsychotic, has a relatively low affinity for the D_2 dopamine receptor and produces minimal disturbance of motor function but has high affinity for serotonin receptors. It is hoped that further refinement of our knowledge will permit truly rational drug discovery and significant advances in the pharmacotherapy of the psychoses.

Clozapine (CLOZARIL)

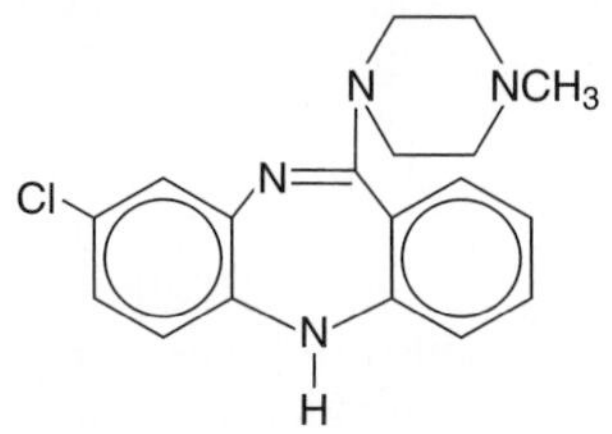

N, NCH_3, N=, Cl, N, H

ADVERSE EFFECTS

The fact that there are no consistent, generally agreed upon differences in efficacy among the 12 neuroleptics illustrated in this chapter has led to major emphasis being placed upon their relative adverse effects. With reference to the whole spectrum of these possible effects, significant differences between individual agents do exist. Therapeutic advantage may sometimes be gained by taking these differences into consideration. For example, the elderly are particularly prone to orthostatic (postural) hypotension, dizziness, and life-threatening falls. In the elderly, one may wish to choose a neuroleptic with minimal hypotensive activity even if the drug has a rather high incidence of another unwanted action. In the sections that follow, the adverse effects of neuroleptics are discussed first in general terms and then with respect to individual agents.

The antagonism of dopaminergic activity by neuroleptics has already been noted. In addition, there is clinically significant interaction of these drugs with a number of other chemical messengers. Of particular importance are functions mediated by acetylcholine and by norepinephrine. Although it is sometimes useful to group together those adverse effects that are related to one chemical transmitter or another, the present scheme of classification is according to organ system.

Central Nervous System

Sedation

In general, neuroleptics depress activity in the central nervous system (CNS). The resulting drowsiness and sedation are sometimes useful in agitated and assaultive patients but more often are regarded as undesired properties. This is especially true during maintenance therapy. There appears to be no relationship between the degree of sedation produced and the actual antipsychotic effects. Although multiple mechanisms are probably involved, activity of neuroleptics at histaminergic and cholinergic receptors in the CNS seems a likely factor.

Neuroleptics are unlike ethanol and the barbiturates in that their depressant effects are not accompanied by disinhibition of behavior akin to drunkenness. Nonetheless, driving and other psychomotor skills may be impaired; this is of particular concern early in treatment. Although effects on respiration are usually modest, particular caution must be exercised in treatment of patients with respiratory infections or chronic respiratory disorders.

The depressant effects of antipsychotic drugs are at least additive with those of ethanol, barbiturates, opiates, and other depressants of CNS activity. Although it is difficult to prove that antipsychotic drugs truly potentiate the effects of these agents, it should be assumed to occur and appropriate adjustments in dosage should be made when neuroleptics are combined with such drugs.

Sedation is most often associated with chlorpromazine and the piperidine phenothiazines, but its occurrence should be anticipated with all the neuroleptics. Potentiation of the effects of depressant drugs is not peculiar to a particular class of antipsychotic drug. Haloperidol is the neuroleptic most often chosen for the acute control of aggressive and assaultive behavior.

Seizures

Neuroleptics decrease the convulsive threshold and may precipitate seizures in persons with pre-existing CNS pathology. This effect is best documented with respect to chlorpromazine but should be anticipated with all neuroleptics. Potentiation of the depressant effects of barbiturates does not extend to their anticonvulsant properties. For this reason, doses of barbiturates and other antiepileptic agents should not be reduced routinely on initiation of antipsychotic drug therapy. Furthermore, neuroleptics are contraindicated in the treatment of conditions such as ethanol and barbiturate withdrawal, in which there is an increased probability of seizures.

Hypotension

The effects of antipsychotic drugs on blood pressure appear to result from a combination of depression of activity in medullary cardiovascular centers and blockade of peripheral adrenergic receptors. Changes in resting blood pressure usually are minimal, but significant postural (orthostatic) hypotension may occur. Dizziness and transient loss of consciousness may result. Particular caution must be exercised in the use of these drugs in the elderly and in those with pre-existing impairment of the cerebrovascular circulation.

In the periphery, neuroleptics appear to be selectively active at α-adrenergic receptors, and epinephrine reversal may occur. This is a phenomenon in which doses of epinephrine that usually produce pressor effects result in hypotension owing to unopposed stimulation of β-adrenergic receptors. The pressor agent of choice in neuroleptic-induced hypotension is levarterenol (norepinephrine). Although antipsychotic drugs in general have higher affinities for the α_1-adrenergic receptor compared with the α_2 subtype, antagonism of the antihypertensive effects of α_2 agonists such as clonidine has been reported.

The available clinical data do not permit precise comparison of neuroleptics with respect to their hypotensive properties. However, it generally is assumed that hypotension is less likely to occur following the uses of piperazine-type phenothiazines and nonphenothiazine neuroleptics. The claim that molindone is without clinically significant hypotensive effects remains to be substantiated. For any given agent, the risk of hypotension is increased by parenteral administration.

Temperature Regulation

An early use of chlorpromazine was to facilitate the lowering of body temperature prior to cardiac surgery. However, it is now recognized that neuroleptics are not specific hypothermic agents but instead serve to loosen in general the homeostatic mechanisms that normally maintain body temperature. Thus, patients maintained on neuroleptics may become hyperthermic when exposed to high environmental temperatures, and several deaths have been reported. Although disordered temperature regulation is thought to be mediated by neuroleptic blockade of muscarinic acetylcholine receptors in the hypothalamus, any tendency toward hyperthermia may be further enhanced by peripheral cholinergic blockade that results in decreased sweating.

Antiemetic Properties

Nausea and vomiting are profoundly influenced by dopamine-sensitive receptors of a medullary center called the chemoreceptor trigger zone (CRT). The antiemetic properties of neuroleptics are believed to arise from dopaminergic blockade in the CRT. Thus, neuroleptics, especially chlorpromazine and prochlorperazine, often are used to control nausea and emesis in a variety of disease states as well as that associated with cancer chemotherapeutic agents. However, the antiemetic effects of neuroleptics may obscure the diagnosis and treatment of conditions characterized by nausea and vomiting. These include intestinal obstruction, brain tumor, and Reye's syndrome as well as a variety of drug intoxications.

Extrapyramidal Motor System

Neuroleptics are believed to act as antagonists of dopaminergic components of the EPMS. The functional consequences of neuroleptic-induced disturbance of the EPMS may be divided into four distinct syndromes: dystonia, akathisia, parkinsonian syndrome, and tardive dyskinesia. The first three occur soon after initiation of neuroleptic therapy and usually are amenable to treatment. In contrast, tardive dyskinesia may first appear only after years of neuroleptic use and may then be irreversible.

DYSTONIA. These effects may appear shortly after initiation of neuroleptic therapy and are often referred to as acute dystonic reactions. Dystonias are particularly common following parenteral administration. Hypertonicity of the muscles of the neck and back may progress to torticollis and opisthotonos, respectively. Difficulty in swallowing and spasms of the muscles of the jaw, tongue, and eyes may occur.

Withdrawal of the neuroleptic at the first appearance of dystonia usually results in complete relief within 24 to 48 hours. Reassurance of the patient as to the essentially benign nature of the condition is also helpful. In those instances when neuroleptic withdrawal is not possible due to the nature of the psychosis, or when the dystonia is especially severe, intravenous or intramuscular administration of an anticholinergic agent can be expected to reduce symptoms within minutes. Oral administration of an anticholinergic agent may then be added to the treatment regimen.

AKATHISIA. The literal meaning of this term is "without sitting." It refers particularly to motor restlessness and a desire on the part of the patient to be in constant motion. An anxietylike subjective state may also be present. Because of the distinctly unpleasant nature of neuroleptic-induced akathisia in normal subjects, it is reasonable to conclude that this syndrome may contribute to noncompliance by some patients. Reduction of dosage may be of value.

PARKINSONIAN SYNDROME (PSEUDOPARKINSONISM). As is implied by its name, this condition closely resembles idiopathic Parkinson's disease. It is characterized by an unchanging facial expression, drooling, tremors, disturbances in posture and gait, and rigidity, especially of the upper limbs. Akinesia, a state of decreased motor activity, is often a major sign of the parkinsonian syndrome. Anticholinergic antiparkinsonian drugs are of value in treating the neuroleptic-induced condition. In contrast with true Parkinson's disease, therapy with levodopa has been found to be ineffective and, in some instances, to worsen the syndrome.

It is generally assumed that among the phenothiazines, extrapyramidal disturbances are least likely following the piperidines and most likely with the piperazines; chlorpromazine and the thioxanthenes are intermediate. There is, however, a tradeoff in that the piperidines tend to be most troublesome in terms of anticholinergic effects and disturbances of cardiac rhythm. Among the nonphenothiazines, a full spectrum of tendencies to produce extrapyramidal disturbances is seen. Haloperidol is most likely to produce extrapyramidal disturbances; more limited experience suggests that loxapine is intermediate in frequency of these effects, whereas molindone is relatively inactive.

Clozapine deserves special mention with respect to neuroleptic-induced extrapyramidal disturbances. As was noted above, clozapine is an atypical antipsychotic. Clinical trials of the drug conducted in the early 1970s demonstrated antipsychotic efficacy and a very low incidence of EPMS disturbance. However, reports of agranulocytosis caused clozapine to be withheld from the US market until 1989. The decision to approve the drug was based on evidence that clozapine may be effective in some schizophrenics resistant to other neuroleptics and on the provision of a surveillance program to detect agranulocytosis. Current estimates of incidence of clozapine-induced agranulocytosis range from 1.1 to 1.5%, with nearly all cases arising within the first 5 months of treatment.

TARDIVE DYSKINESIA. As is implied by its name, tardive dyskinesia has a delayed onset, sometimes becoming apparent only after years of treatment. Among the more prominent signs of tardive dyskinesia are involuntary movements of the tongue, face, mouth, and jaw. However, essentially all aspects of EPMS dysfunction have now been recognized as possible tardive effects. Thus, tardive dystonia, parkinsonism, and akathisia have been reported.

Tardive dyskinesia differs in a number of respects from the EPMS disturbances that appear in the first several weeks to months of neuroleptic therapy. Most important is the apparent irreversibility of the condition. It responds poorly if at all to antiparkinsonian agents and may worsen rather than improve with discontinuation of neuroleptic treatment. Whereas the early-onset extrapyramidal disturbances are thought to be due to the direct effects of dopaminergic blockade in the striatum, tardive dyskinesia has many of the features of a supersensitivity phenomenon.

No consensus exists regarding treatment of tardive dyskinesia. The hypothesis that a low tendency to produce acute extrapyramidal disturbance is correlated with fewer tardive effects is unproved, and all neuroleptics are suspect. It is hoped that clozapine will prove to be an exception to this rule. Principles of prevention include the use of the lowest possible doses of antipsychotic drugs for the shortest periods of time consistent with a therapeutic effect. Regular assessment of the continued efficacy of neuroleptics is essential. At the first signs of tardive dyskinesia, neuroleptic therapy should, if possible, be stopped.

NEUROLEPTIC MALIGNANT SYNDROME. An unusual and sometimes fatal reaction to antipsychotic drugs that combines features of disordered temperature regulation and extrapyramidal reactions is called the neuroleptic malignant syndrome (NMS). Since the syndrome was first described in 1960, fewer than 200 cases have been reported in the world literature. Concern is not with numbers but with the fact that about 10% of patients with NMS die. The hallmarks of NMS are hyperthermia and rigidity, presumably of extrapyramidal origin. In addition, delirium and increased blood pressure often occur. The most common laboratory finding is an elevated level of creatine phosphokinase.

Treatment of NMS is uncertain but should include termination of all neuroleptics and use of general supportive measures including body cooling and rehydration as needed. A variety of drugs with activity on dopaminergic systems have been tried. Among those claimed to have some beneficial effects are bromocriptine, amantadine, levodopa, and the anticholinergic antiparkinsonian agents. However, no consensus has emerged as to the efficacy of these agents. Attempts to control rigidity have most often employed benzodiazepines or dantrolene. The latter drug has been found to be of value in treating malignant hyperthermia, a condition that shares several of the features of NMS. It is not possible to attribute NMS to any particular neuroleptic at this time.

Cardiovascular System

Neuroleptic-induced tachycardia is mediated by a combination of reflex activity triggered by hypotension and a direct antimuscarinic effect on the myocardium. The clinical significance of these actions in healthy patients is uncertain. However, in those with coronary atherosclerosis, sustained tachycardia increases the probability of overt arrhythmias and myocardial infarct.

Of all the neuroleptics, the arrhythmogenic effects of thioridazine have been best documented. Even relatively modest doses may be associated with prolongation of the QT interval, decreased amplitude of the T wave, the appearance of U waves, and a widening of the QRS complex. Although it is generally assumed that neuroleptics as a group have a high therapeutic index, there is no doubt that overdose of thioridazine and possibly others can be fatal. In addition, it is suspected that sudden unexplained death in patients maintained on antipsychotic drugs may often be due to cardiac dysfunction.

Those physicians who prescribe neuroleptics must take into account possible untoward effects on the myocardium, especially by the piperidine phenothiazines and particularly in those patients with pre-existing coronary atherosclerosis or disturbances in cardiac rhythm. In addition, combination of antipsychotic drugs with sympathomimetics should be avoided. Outpatients maintained on neuroleptics should be cautioned against the concurrent use of amphetamines, cocaine, and nonprescription products such as cold remedies and aids to weight loss that contain sympathomimetic agents.

Endocrine Systems

Dopamine released by the hypothalamus passes through the hypothalamicoadenohypophyseal portal system to the pituitary, where it functions to inhibit the release of prolactin. The antidopaminergic effects of neuroleptics thus account for the increase in serum prolactin that is consistently seen in patients treated with these drugs. Neuroleptic-induced hyperprolactinemia is sometimes associated with galactorrhea, menstrual changes, and gynecomastia. A theoretical hazard of elevated levels of prolactin is an increase in incidence of hormonally mediated cancers, especially cancer of the breast. However, several studies have failed to detect an increased incidence of breast cancer in patients maintained on phenothiazines.

A number of other adverse effects of antipsychotic drugs may have an endocrine component. These include sexual dysfunction and undesired weight gain. Both have most often been associated with the piperidine phenothiazines. Chlorpromazine-induced fluid retention has been reported, and a number of neuroleptics cause an increase in appetite possibly through antihistaminergic or antiserotonergic effects.

Miscellaneous Adverse Effects

Peripheral Antimuscarinic Actions

The use of antipsychotic drugs is often associated with one or more signs of an atropinelike syndrome. Thus, blurred vision, exacerbation of narrow angle glaucoma, dry mouth, sinus tachycardia, constipation, urinary retention, and decreased sweating may occur.

Jaundice

Shortly after the introduction of chlorpromazine, liver dysfunction, usually in the form of cholestatic jaundice, was associated with its use. Because this is a relatively rare condition, the risk imposed by individual agents is not known with certainty. The condition usually is reversible on discontinuation of neuroleptic use. If treatment is to continue, an agent from another chemical class should be chosen. Periodic liver function tests are indicated in patients chronically treated with phenothiazines. Reversible changes in liver function tests are commonly observed with initiation of phenothiazines.

Hematological Disorders

Blood dyscrasias, including agranulocytosis, eosinophilia, leukopenia, hemolytic or aplastic anemia, thrombocytopenic purpura, and pancytopenia, are rare. However, because of the possibly fatal outcome of these disorders, patients and their families should be warned to report sore throat or other signs of infection.

Dermatological Disorders

The skin is the site of several toxic effects of the neuroleptics. Earliest in onset and presumed to have an immunological basis is an urticarial reaction. With long-term treatment, unusual sensitivity to the sun and discoloration of the skin may occur. A possibly related condition is deposition of fine particulate matter in the lens and cornea of the eye. Ocular changes have most often been associated with long-term, high-dose therapy with thioridazine. Under these circumstances, regular examinations of the eye are indicated.

Tolerance and Physical Dependence

It is generally assumed that some measure of tolerance develops to the sedative and hypotensive effects of neuroleptics. Nonetheless, particular care must be exercised in the use of these drugs in the elderly. Physical dependence on antipsychotic drugs is seldom reported. However, a withdrawal syndrome including vomiting and movement disorders has been described. For this reason, gradual reduction in dosage following long-term treatment is prudent.

REFERENCES

Andreason NC, Flaum M, Swayze VW, et al: Positive and negative symptoms in schizophrenia. Arch Gen Psychiat 47:615-621, 1990.

Baldessarini RJ: Drugs and the treatment of psychiatric disorders. *In* Gilman AG, Rall TW, Nies AS, Taylor P (eds): Goodman and Gilman's The Pharmacological Basis of Therapeutics. New York: Pergamon Press, 1990.

Fleischhacker WW, Roth SD, Kane JM: The pharmacological treatment of neuroleptic-induced akathisia. J Clin Psychopharmacol 10:12-21, 1990.

Hollister LE, Czernansky JG: Clinical Pharmacology of Psychotherapeutic Drugs, 3rd ed. New York: Churchill Livingstone, 1990.

Jacobsen E: The early history of psychotherapeutic drugs. Psychopharmacology 89:138-144, 1986.

Roberts GW: Schizophrenia: The cellular biology of a functional psychosis. Trends Neurosci 13:207-211, 1990.

Rosenberg MR, Green M: Neuroleptic malignant syndrome. Arch Intern Med 149:1927-1931, 1989.

Drugs Used in the Treatment of Mood Disorders 24

Jerome A. Roth

MOOD DISORDERS

The major mood (or affective) disorders of endogenous origin are characterized by changes in mood and behavioral states, and are generally classified into two polar conditions, mania and depression episodes or syndromes. In actuality these are likely to be overly simplistic terms to describe the variety of behavioral and mood changes, but they do represent relevant clinical states that often require drug intervention. Disorders of mood can be debilitating if the magnitude of the disorder prevents one from functioning with a "normal" daily existence.

As with all major behavioral disorders, it is now assumed that the affective disorders of endogenous origin result from specific biochemical changes in the brain. It is highly unlikely that depression originates from only a single biochemical alteration in all patients. It is more likely that it is caused by any one of a number of neurological changes that have, as an end result, a similar alteration in behavioral state. A variety of theories have been proposed for the cause of depression, and these are presented below.

Criteria for Major Depressive Syndrome

Episodes of depression are rather common moods that many individuals (~ 15% over a lifetime) have experienced in their lives. The diagnostic criteria for a major depressive episode are primarily based on the American Psychiatric Association's Diagnostic and Statistical Manual of Mental Disorders, third edition, Revised (DSM-III-R) classification and include at least four of the following symptoms (not associated with schizophrenia or other psychotic disorders): depressed mood; weight loss or gain; insomnia or hypersomnia; psychomotor agitation or retardation; loss of interest in pleasure or usual activities; fatigue or loss of energy; feeling of worthlessness; diminished ability to concentrate; or recurrent thoughts of suicide. Drug intervention is warranted if the intensity of the depression is severe enough to interfere with normal daily function and the duration is in the order of weeks or months. In most episodes of depression, the depression is self-limiting and spontaneous recovery is likely even if no drug is administered. The other common feature of unipolar depression is that it often recurs, in that many individuals experience more than one episode of depression. Depression is also a frequent concomitant of other syndromes such as stroke and Parkinson's disease, and can be due to a variety of drugs (Chapter 22). Approximately 20% of all depressed patients also experience psychotic symptoms.

Etiology of Major Depression

Depression is a heterogeneous disorder probably resulting from a number of different biochemical changes in the brain. The one theory that has withstood the test of time and is consistent with responses to many therapeutic drugs is the "biogenic amine" theory of depression. This theory can be divided into two parts.

- Catecholamine theory: depression is associated with an absolute or relative deficiency of neuronal catecholamines, particularly norepinephrine, at functionally important adrenergic receptor sites in the brain.
- Indoleamine theory: depression is associated with an absolute or relative deficiency of indoleamines, specifically 5-hydroxytryptamine (5-HT), at functionally important receptor sites in the brain.

The biogenic amine hypothesis for depression is based on the following observations: (1) Drugs that deplete norepinephrine and/or 5-HT promote depression; and (2) drugs that increase the levels of norepinephrine or 5-HT in the brain have been shown to have a mood elevating effect and are used in the treatment of depression.

Although the biogenic amine hypothesis has proved to be a useful model for the development of drugs for the treatment of depression, it does not adequately explain why the clinical effects of antidepressant drugs require approximately 2 to as long as 6 weeks before a therapeutic response is observed. Because of this delayed onset of response to the antidepressants, current theory suggests that a down-regulation of either the norepinephrine or 5-HT receptors is ultimately responsible for the therapeutic actions of these drugs. This idea of down-regulation is supported by experimental data demonstrating a correlation between the response of the down-regulation of these receptors and the therapeutic response.

TREATMENT OF MAJOR DEPRESSION

Electroconvulsive Therapy

Electroconvulsive therapy (ECT) is considered to be an effective treatment for depression, especially in those depressed patients who do not respond to drug treatment. The major advantages of ECT are:

- Because drug treatment takes 2 to 6 weeks before a therapeutic response is observed, ECT may be the treatment of choice in cases of severe depression in which suicide attempts have occurred.
- It also may be the preferred treatment in cases where drug treatment is hazardous or contraindicated.

The major disadvantages of ECT are:

- Patients very often will choose the drug treatment in preference to ECT because of the fears and anxieties associated with this latter treatment. Patients may view pills as an easier means of treatment even though the drugs may have to be administered for prolonged periods of time and may have serious potential side effects.
- ECT can cause memory loss. Most of the memory loss associated with ECT is transient; however, this treatment has been reported to cause some permanent memory loss as well in some patients.

Drug Treatment

There are basically four classes of drugs used clinically for treatment of unipolar depression:

- Tricyclic antidepressants
- Monoamine oxidase inhibitors
- Second-generation antidepressant drugs
- Selective serotonin re-uptake inhibitors (SSRIs)

Tricyclic Antidepressant Drugs

The tricyclic antidepressant drugs are generally considered the drug of first choice for the treatment of unipolar depression; however, they have limited efficacy in that only about two thirds of the depressed patients will respond favorably. They are structurally related to the phenothiazines but may exacerbate the psychotic symptoms when administered to schizophrenic patients. Table 24 – 1 lists seven tricyclic antidepressants used clinically in the United States.

The first tricyclic drug used clinically was imipramine. The chemical structure of imipramine is similar to that of the antipsychotic phenothiazines. Imipramine was not designed originally for use in the treatment of depression but was synthesized as an analog of phenothiazine for possible use as an antipsychotic agent. However, it displayed only modest antipsychotic properties and could exacerbate schizophrenic psychosis. Surprisingly, some depressed patients improved, and clinical trials demonstrated ultimately that imipramine had a mood-elevating effect. Thus, it became one of the first so-called tricyclic antidepressant drugs.

When administered to normal nondepressed individuals, the tricyclic antidepressant drugs have little behavioral effects beyond mild sedation although it has been reported that they may produce psychotic symptoms or manic behavior in some predisposed individuals.

As a general rule, all tricyclic antidepressant drugs are equally effective in alleviating the symptoms of depression. Amitriptyline and doxepin are reported to be the most sedating of the tricyclic drugs and therefore are preferentially used for treatment of agitated depression or where sedation or improved sleep is desired.

Also commercially available are two tricyclic antidepressant formulations in combination with other psychoactive drugs. TRIAVIL and ETRAFON are trade names for products composed of a combination of amitriptyline plus perphenazine, principally designed for treatment of depression characterized by agitation or psychotic behavior. The other combination drug (LIMBITROL), composed of amitriptyline and chlordiazepoxide, is designed for treatment of depression characterized by anxiety. Whether these combinations are any more effective than the individual drugs for treatment of these disorders is questionable.

MECHANISM OF ACTION. The probable mechanism of the antidepressant actions of the tricyclic antidepressant drugs has been attributed to their inhibition of the neuronal re-uptake of either norepinephrine or 5-HT. Presumably, the increased levels of these neurotransmitters resulting from this process within the synaptic cleft is ultimately responsible for the down-regulation of their respective postsynaptic receptors.

METABOLISM. The two major routes for the metabolism of the tricyclic antidepressant agents are via the mixed-function oxidase enzyme system. These include hydroxylation of either or both of the aromatic rings and *N*-demethylation of one or both of the methyl groups associated with the side-chain amine. In both cases the end products are pharmacologically active. The hydroxylated aromatic rings can be conjugated with glucuronic acid or sulfate and this process ultimately inactivates the drug.

HALF-LIFE. The tricyclic antidepressant agents are highly lipid-soluble and tightly bound to serum proteins, and half-lives for the tricyclic antidepressants are generally in excess of 20 hours. Although often administered in multiple daily doses, the tricyclic drugs can also be given once a day, preferably at bedtime because of the sedating properties of the drugs.

Appreciable partial tolerance appears to develop over time to both the sedating and anticholinergic side effects.

TABLE 24–1. Tricyclic Antidepressants Currently Used Clinically in the United States

Drug	Structure	Therapeutic Dosage (mg/day)*
Imipramine (TOFRANIL, others)	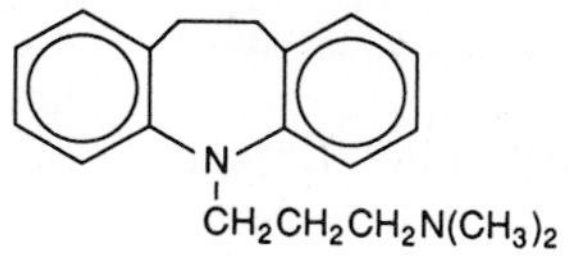 N–$CH_2CH_2CH_2N(CH_3)_2$	50–150 (300†)
Desipramine (NORPRAMIN, others)	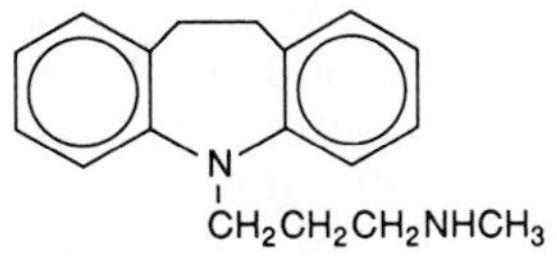 N–$CH_2CH_2CH_2NHCH_3$	50–150 (300†)
Amitriptyline (ELAVIL, others)	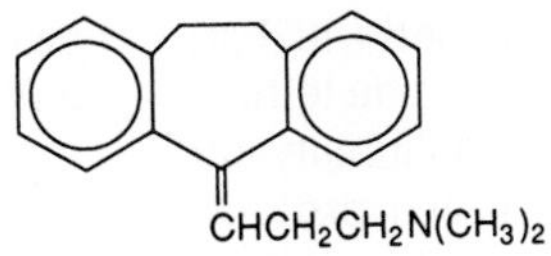 $=CHCH_2CH_2N(CH_3)_2$	50–150 (300†)
Nortriptyline (AVENTYL, others)	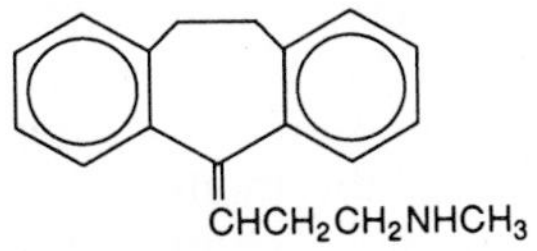 $=CHCH_2CH_2NHCH_3$	20–100
Protriptyline (VIVACTYL, others)	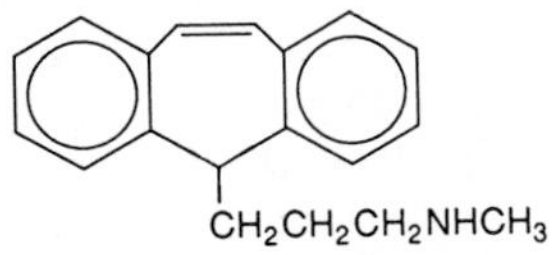 $CH_2CH_2CH_2NHCH_3$	10–40
Doxepin (SINEQUAN)	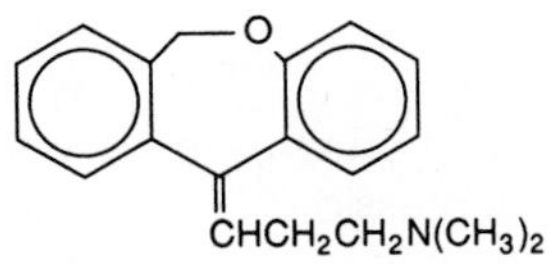 O; $=CHCH_2CH_2N(CH_3)_2$	40–150
Trimipramine (SURMONTIL)	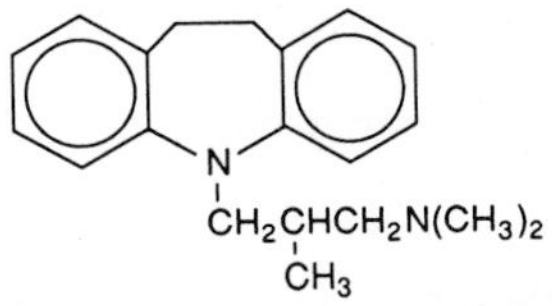 N–$CH_2CH(CH_3)CH_2N(CH_3)_2$	20–50

*Doses are given as examples only.
†Maximum "permissible" dose.

ADVERSE REACTIONS

- The most common adverse effect of the tricyclic antidepressant drugs is cholinergic blockade, including dry mouth, constipation, blurred vision, and tachycardia. The anticholinergic effects observed with the tricyclic antidepressant drugs are, in general, more severe than are encountered with the phenothiazine antipsychotic drugs. Amitriptyline displays the greatest anticholinergic effects, desipramine the least. Because of the anticholinergic side effects and because they inhibit the re-uptake of catecholamines, the tricyclic drugs are, as a general rule, contraindicated in individuals with any cardiac complications.
- The tricyclic antidepressant drugs frequently produce postural hypotension. Less common, but possible, cardiac effects include atrial fibrillation, atrioventricular (AV) block or ventricular tachycardia, and quinidinelike effects.
- Although rare, patients can develop an allergy to the tricyclic antidepressants. As with any other drug class, if a patient develops an allergy to any one of the tricyclic antidepressant drugs, a different class of antidepressant has to be employed.
- Tricyclic antidepressant drugs can potentiate the pressor effects of sympathomimetic agents.
- The tricyclic antidepressants can antagonize the antihy-

pertensive effects of guanethidine by preventing its uptake into the neuron.

- Tricyclic antidepressants can induce a hypertensive crisis when taken in conjunction with or administered sequentially before or after a monoamine oxidase inhibitor. The combination of a tricyclic antidepressant drug and a monoamine oxidase inhibitor should be avoided because it is a potentially lethal combination.
- Drug toxicity and overdose: The lethality of the tricyclic antidepressant drugs is primarily the result of their effect on cardiac rhythmicity, although the central nervous system (CNS) depressant effects can contribute to toxicity. The depressant activity of the tricyclic drugs is additive with other CNS depressant agents. In general, they are more toxic than the phenothiazine antipsychotic drugs, and the frequency of toxicity is also greater because they are administered to a patient population that is at risk of suicide attempts; thus, they should be dispensed with caution and in total quantities that are not likely to be lethal if taken all at once. Because of their high lipid solubility and the fact they are extensively bound to plasma proteins, treatment of an overdose of the tricyclics necessitates support of the vital functions and usually requires a prolonged period to fully eliminate the drug. Small doses (1 to 2 mg) of physostigmine can be carefully administered to patients who have overdosed on the tricyclics; this treatment produces a very rapid recovery but for only a short period of time because of the short duration of action of physostigmine.
- Measurements of blood levels are of value not only in the event of possible toxicity but also when the patient fails to respond to usual dose regimens.

Monoamine Oxidase Inhibitors

The monoamine oxidase inhibitors were the first drugs used clinically in the 1950s for the treatment of depression. The use of monoamine oxidase inhibitors for treatment of depression stemmed from the observations that isoniazid, a hydrazine derivative used for the treatment of tuberculosis, had a mood-elevating effect in patients hospitalized in sanitariums for this disease. Although many monoamine oxidase inhibitors were clinically tested as antidepressants, only three drugs are currently employed in the Untied States for the treatment of depression.

Because the drugs listed in Table 24 – 2 all possess similar pharmacological activities, the selection is based largely on a physician's experience with a particular agent. The three drugs are nonselective, irreversible inhibitors of the two forms of monoamine oxidase, type A and type B. As discussed in Chapter 4, the A form of monoamine oxidase is localized within the neuron and is responsible for the deamination of norepinephrine and 5-HT. Recent studies have demonstrated that it is the inhibition of the A form of monoamine oxidase that imparts the antidepressant effects of these drugs. Because these drugs irreversibly inhibit monoamine oxidase, it takes up to 10 days to 2 weeks for the body to resynthesize new enzyme. Thus, if a patient has to be switched from a monoamine oxidase inhibitor to a tricyclic antidepressant agent, a 2-week period is required to allow monoamine oxidase levels to return to normal and prevent a potentially lethal drug interaction with the tricyclics.

The major limitations for the widespread use of the monoamine oxidase inhibitors for the treatment of depression has been the potential for serious side effects. The minor adverse effects include:

- Excessive stimulation: May produce euphoria and unwanted behavioral excitement. Decreasing dosage can possibly prevent the excessive stimulation, and changing the class of antidepressant can correct these deficiencies.
- Allergic reactions: If an allergic reaction develops, patient must be switched to a different class of antidepressant.
- Orthostatic hypotension: The mechanism for hypotension is unknown but is presumed to be centrally mediated.
- The monoamine oxidase inhibitors can potentiate the action of opioids such as meperidine by interfering with their metabolism.
- The major reason why the monoamine oxidase inhibitors are not widely used is their potential lethal interaction with sympathomimetic amines, leading to a severe hypertensive crisis. Any food or cold medication that contains any

TABLE 24 – 2. Monoamine Oxidase Inhibitors

Drug	Structure	Therapeutic Dosage (mg/day)
Phenelzine (NARDIL)	$C_6H_5-CH_2-CH_2-NH-NH_2$	30 – 90
Tranylcypromine (PARNATE)	$C_6H_5-CH-CH-NH_2$ (CH–CH bridged by CH_2)	10 – 60
Isocarboxazid (MARPLAN)	$C_6H_5-CH_2-NH-NH-C(=O)-$ (isoxazole ring, N, O, CH_3)	10 – 30

sympathomimetic amine such as tyramine, phenylethylamine, phenylephrine, and the like is contraindicated in patients receiving monoamine oxidase inhibitors. These include foods such as bananas, red wines, aged cheeses, chocolate, yeast, and so forth. In the event of severe hypertensive crisis, short acting β-adrenergic blocking agents can be administered. Of interest is the fact that isoniazid overdose can be reversed by pyridoxine (Brent et al, 1990).

In the future, new monoamine oxidase inhibitors are likely to be introduced that reversibly inhibit the A form of the enzyme. It is worth noting that the new highly selective monoamine oxidase inhibitors currently being developed do not produce a hypertensive crisis when used in the presence of foods containing sympathomimetic amines.

Second-Generation Antidepressant Drugs

The name second-generation antidepressant inhibitors implies that these newer drugs represent a different class of agents. Initially it was thought that some of these agents worked by a different mechanism than the two classes of drugs described above. In actuality, this term is now used to describe a structurally diverse group of agents that apparently do not have exactly the same actions as the tricyclic antidepressant agents or monoamine oxidase inhibitors. Yet, for the majority of these agents, their mechanisms of action appear to be similar at least in part to the tricyclic drugs. None of these drugs should be used in combination with the monoamine oxidase inhibitors.

- Maprotiline (LUDIOMIL): Maprotiline is a tetracyclic antidepressant agent structurally and chemically similar to the tricyclic drugs as illustrated by the structure below. Mechanistically and functionally, this drug is also similar to the tricyclic antidepressant agents, including the side effects associated with its use. Although this agent is therapeutically effective, there is little advantage of its use over the tricyclic agents.

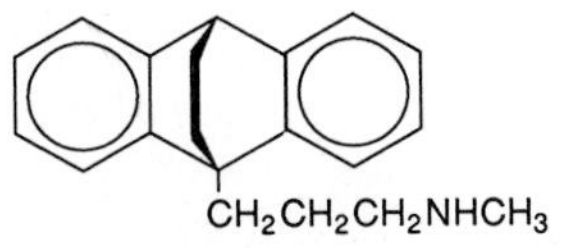

$CH_2CH_2CH_2NHCH_3$

Maprotiline

- Amoxapine (ASENDIN): This compound is the *N*-demethylated derivative of the antipsychotic drug loxapine. Mechanistically, it blocks the neuronal re-uptake of both norepinephrine and 5-HT and thus provides a little additional benefit over the tricyclic antidepressant drugs. In addition, it blocks dopamine receptors and therefore may have the potential to cause tardive dyskinesia upon prolonged use.

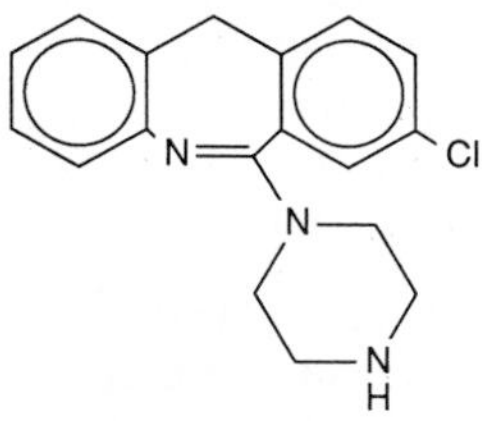

N Cl N N H

Amoxapine

- Trazodone (DESYREL): Trazodone represents one of the new class of drugs that, at therapeutic concentrations, apparently inhibits neither monoamine oxidase nor the re-uptake of the catecholamine neurotransmitters. It is reported to have less anticholinergic action and is less cardiotoxic than any of the other antidepressant agents and appears to produce fewer side effects than the other antidepressant agents. It is at least as sedating as amitriptyline or doxepin. Trazodone, however, can cause priapism, and prolonged use can lead to permanent impotency. The mechanism of action of trazodone is not fully understood but may involve a down-regulation of either norepinephrine or 5-HT receptors.

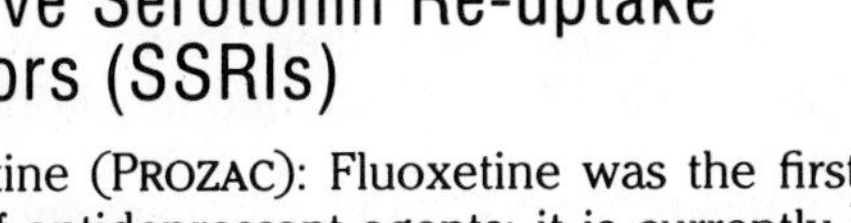

N $NCH_2CH_2CH_2N$ N N O

Trazodone

- Bupropion (WELLBUTRIN): Bupropion represents a new chemical class of antidepressants introduced in the hope that it would avoid the drawbacks of the tricyclics. The drug's antidepressant effects are equivalent to those of amitriptyline. Its neurochemical effects differ from the other agents in that it primarily inhibits dopamine uptake. (This illustrates the fact that three neurotransmitter systems are involved in mood disorders—catecholaminergic, serotonergic, and dopaminergic.) Although bupropion lacks the cardiac toxicity of the tricyclics, it carries the potential of causing restlessness and agitation, insomnia, and seizures; it has been associated with psychotic reactions in some patients. The prevalence of seizures is 0.4%, with high dosages and other predisposing factors contributing to the risk.

The use of bupropion is limited by the wide variety of side effects and potentially serious drug interactions (MAO inhibitors, levodopa, drugs affecting hepatic drug metabolizing enzymes, and agents that lower seizure threshold), although fatalities from overdoses have yet to be reported.

Adequate blood concentrations are achieved within 2 hours following oral administration. The half-life ranges from 8 to 24 hours; several of the metabolites have even longer elimination half-lives.

Selective Serotonin Re-uptake Inhibitors (SSRIs)

- Fluoxetine (PROZAC): Fluoxetine was the first of a new class of antidepressant agents; it is currently one of the most widely used agents for the treatment of depression. It appears to function by selectively inhibiting neuronal re-uptake of 5-HT (serotonin), which ultimately leads to a down-regulation of the receptors. It is a highly lipid-soluble compound and has a half-life of approximately 2 to 3 days. It is metabolized to the *N*-demethylated derivative by

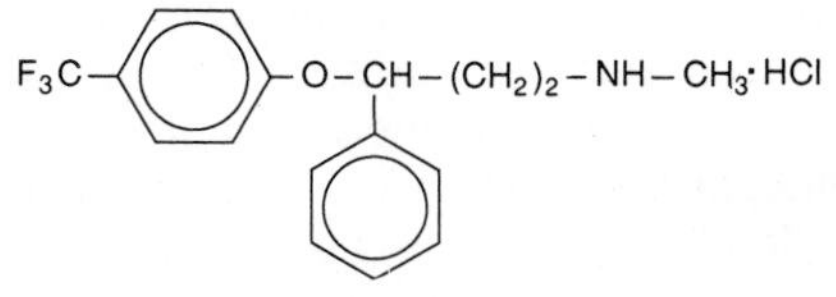

F_3C – O – CH – $(CH_2)_2$ – NH – $CH_3 \cdot HCl$

Fluoxetine

the mixed-function oxidase, and this metabolite is also pharmacologically active, with a half-life of approximately 8 days.

Fluoxetine inhibits cytochrome P-450 enzymes, which are involved in metabolism of many drugs. The most common adverse effects associated with fluoxetine are nervousness, anxiety, and insomnia. Other less common side effects include amnesia, arrhythmias, headaches, hypo- or hypertension, decreased appetite, allergic reactions, gastritis, constipation, dry mouth, and fatigue.

- Paroxetine (PAXIL): Paroxetine is a new highly selective 5-HT neuronal re-uptake blocker with a half-life of approximately 1 day. Unlike the other selective 5-HT blockers, the metabolites of paroxetine are inactive. Many of the side effects associated with the other selective 5-HT uptake inhibitors are also observed with this drug, including nausea, somnolence, sweating, tremor, ejaculatory disturbances, and hyponatremia. Paroxetine inhibits P-450 enzymes but to a lesser degree than fluoxetine.
- Sertraline (ZOLOFT): Sertraline is the third of the new SSRIs with properties quite similar in action and efficacy to paroxetine and fluoxetine. Of the three it has the least effect on cytochrome P-450 enzymes.
- Choice among SSRIs: The three SSRIs, in general, do not have the anticholinergic, antihistaminic, or adrenergic blocking activity of the tricyclic antidepressants. Thus, they are less likely than tricyclics to cause orthostatic hypotension, cardiac effects, seizures, dry mouth, or blurred vision. They also are less likely to cause weight gain. The possibility of overdose remains a serious problem in any treatment of patients with depression, but these serotonin uptake inhibitors are not as likely to cause lethal cardiac effects. New SSRIs are likely to be introduced in the near future.

For the treatment of mild to moderate depression, fluoxetine, sertraline, paroxetine, or bupropion is currently preferred over a tricyclic antidepressant because all are generally equally efficacious and the tricyclics cause more side effects. For the seriously depressed patients, tricyclics are still preferred by many.

All studies have found a small group of patients who do not respond to initial medication. In such refractory patients the following is recommended: (1) the dose should be increased if possible in view of side effects; (2) obtain a blood level to ensure compliance and adequate absorption; and (3) if there is still no response, taper the present medication and dose and then initiate a substitute medication—with great caution and monitoring for potential interactions.

- Chlorimipramine (ANAFRANIL): Chlorimipramine is the 3-chloro analog of imipramine and functions primarily by selectively inhibiting the neuronal re-uptake of 5-HT. Although it functions in much the same manner as that of fluoxetine discussed above, chlorimipramine is effective in the **treatment of obsessive-compulsive disorders**. Essentially all of the side effects discussed above for the tricyclic antidepressant drugs are also associated with chlorimipramine, including the anticholinergic, increased susceptibility to seizures, and sexual dysfunctions. It is extensively metabolized to the antidepressant desmethylimipramine, and is ultimately inactivated by conjugation. The half-life of the parent drug is approximately 1 day and that of the pharmacologically active metabolite approximately 3 days. A useful alternative in obsessive-compulsive disorders is fluoxetine—especially in depressed patients.

BIPOLAR DISORDERS

Etiology

Bipolar disorder (or manic-depressive syndrome) is characterized by cyclical changes in affective state between the manic and depressive phases of behavior. Bipolar patients cycle between the two affective states, and similar to those with major depression, require treatment when the mood changes are of sufficient magnitude to disrupt their lives or the lives of people closely associated with them. There is considerable evidence that bipolar disorder is genetically linked; however, the etiology for this disorder is not fully understood.

Treatment

Lithium

The major drugs for treatment of manic phase bipolar disorder are the antipsychotic drugs and lithium. Psychotic behavior usually requires active treatment with antipsychotic drugs as well as lithium, whereas lithium is the central agent for long-term management. Since the late nineteenth century, lithium has had a long history of various medical uses but it wasn't until the studies of Cade in 1949 in Australia that lithium was used for treatment of bipolar disorder. Although the European scientific community started using lithium for the mania of bipolar disorder in the 1950s, it wasn't until over a decade later that this drug was accepted for use in the United States for treatment of this affective disorder.

Although lithium has been used extensively for treatment of mixed bipolar disorder, the mechanism of its actions remains almost totally unknown. Recent studies have demonstrated that lithium inhibits the phosphatase responsible for the conversion of inositol monophosphates to inositol, but how or whether this inhibitory process leads to suppression of the manic behavior is still a mystery.

Lithium is used primarily to suppress recurrences of the manic phase of bipolar disorder. It is not useful for the acute manic episodes, where the more classic antipsychotic drugs or benzodiazepines appear to be more effective in quelling the extreme mania and psychotic behavior. Lithium is employed as maintenance therapy and appears to modulate the cycling. Lithium can prevent the occurrence of both the depressive as well as the manic episodes in some but not all patients. In those patients whose depressive episodes do not respond to ongoing lithium treatment, an appropriate antidepressant drug can be administered along with lithium, although care should be taken to prevent recycling of the patient back into a manic state.

- **Lithium has an extremely low therapeutic index, and blood levels have to be monitored and main-**

tained to prevent toxicity. When patients are initially treated with lithium, their blood levels are carefully monitored to ensure that the blood levels fall within the therapeutic range.

- Acceptable therapeutic blood levels of lithium range between 0.8 and 1.2 mEq/liter of blood. Between 1.6 and 2.0 mEq/liter, toxic manifestations are observed, which include gastrointestinal disturbances, weakness, thirst, and hand tremors. Blood levels above 2.0 mEq/liter of blood are associated with severe toxicity, including coma, convulsions, and death.

The toxic effects of lithium may vary widely in a given patient at various times. About 95% of ingested lithium is eliminated via the kidney. Lithium is reabsorbed in the kidney by the same transport system associated with the reuptake of sodium. Thus, changes in sodium concentrations in blood can greatly alter lithium levels. During periods of excessive sodium loss in the summer due to sweating, lithium reabsorption may increase and its blood concentrations rise to toxic levels. Under these conditions sodium intake has to be adjusted to meet the loss of excreted sodium. Lithium has a long half-life of approximately 20 hours and is normally administered in multiple daily doses or twice a day in slow-release capsules.

Chronic treatment with lithium that maintains plasma concentrations at the higher end of the therapeutic scale has been reported to lead to polyuria and impairment of renal function manifested by glomerular necrosis. In a few individuals, lithium has been reported to cause thyroid enlargement, which may lead to the development of goiter. In either of these cases, lithium treatment must be discontinued.

Other Drugs Used for Treatment of Bipolar Disorders

- The anticonvulsant carbamazepine (TEGRETOL) has been shown to be effective for the treatment of bipolar depression and is effective against both the manic and depressive phases of the disorder. The mechanism of action is unknown but implies that the initiating events in the brain provoking seizures may also elicit the mood swings characteristic of mixed bipolar disorder.
- Currently, valproic acid is also being evaluated as a therapeutic agent for treatment of this disorder.

REFERENCES

Brent J, Vo N, Kulig K, Rumack BH: Reversal of prolonged isoniazid-induced coma by pyridoxine. Arch Intern Med 150:1751–1753, 1990

Cade JFJ: Lithium salts in the treatment of psychotic excitement. Med J Aust 2:349–352, 1949.

Choice of an antidepressant. Med Lett 35:24–26, 1993.

Cooper JR, Bloom FE, Roth RH: The Biochemical Basis of Neuropharmacology. 6th ed. New York: Oxford University Press, 1991.

Frommer DA, Kulig KW, Marx JA, Rumack B: Tricyclic antidepressant overdose: A review. JAMA 257:521, 1987.

Hollister LE: Psychiatric Disorders. Chapter 13 in Clinical Pharmacology: Basic Principles in Therapeutics, Third Edition, Melmon KL, Morrelli HF, Hoffman BB, Nierenberg DW (eds). McGraw-Hill, New York, 1992, pages 338–380.

Kaplan HI, Sadock BJ (eds): Comprehensive Textbook of Psychiatry IV. 4th ed. Baltimore: Williams & Wilkins, 1985.

Kramer PD: Listening to Prozac. Viking-Penguin Group, New York 1993.

Meltzer HY (ed): Psychopharmacology—The Third Generation of Progress. New York: Raven Press, 1987.

Montgomery SA: Advances in the pharmacology and clinical applications of serotonin. International Clinical Psychopharmacology Volume 8, Supplement 2:1–94, 1993.

Montgomery SA: Antidepressants in long-term treatment. Annu Rev Med 45:447–457, 1994

Paroxetine for treatment of depression. Med Lett 35:24–25, 1993.

Veith RC, Raskind MA, Caldwell JH, et al: Cardiovascular effects of tricylic antidepressants in depressed patients with chronic heart disease. N Engl J Med 306:954, 1982.

Ward MEd, Musa MN, Bailey L: Clinical pharmacokinetics of lithium. J Clin Pharmacol 34:280–285, 1994.

25 Drugs Used in the Treatment of Anxiety

Cedric M. Smith

ANXIETY SYNDROMES

Anxiety is a complex of subjective feelings and characteristic behaviors: tension, apprehension, fear, worry, and difficulty thinking or concentrating. It is usually accompanied by behavioral signs and symptoms of trembling, tremors, muscle tension, restlessness, and fatigue with autonomic hyperactivity in the respiratory, cardiovascular, urinary, and gastrointestinal systems.

The intensity of anxiety ranges from normal, beneficial responses to threatening or tragic situations to anxiety that is harmful when inappropriate to the situation or functionally disabling.

Diagnosis of the source of anxiety is essential because inappropriate drug selection presents potential for great harm.

Anxiety can be the result of:

- Threatening environment or situation, such as anticipating life-threatening surgery
- One of the psychiatric disorders, such as generalized anxiety disorder, panic disorder, agoraphobia, social phobia, simple phobias, post-traumatic stress syndrome, or obsessive-compulsive disorder; each of these is treated differently
- The acute effects of many drugs, including notably caffeine, theophylline, ephedrine, amphetamines, cocaine, thyroid hormones, digitalis, imipramine, indomethacin, baclofen, levodopa, and propranolol (see Chapter 50)
- Rebound or withdrawal effect after chronic alcohol, benzodiazepine, or other sedative drug use
- A variety of medical or psychiatric conditions including hypoglycemia, anemia, vitamin B_{12} deficiency, hyperthyroidism, coronary heart disease, mitral valve prolapse, personality disorders, mood disorders, or schizophrenia

INSOMNIA AND SLEEP DISORDERS

Anxiety frequently causes insomnia, which is a symptom, not a diagnosis. Difficulty falling asleep or staying asleep is relatively common, but not life-threatening. In addition to anxiety, insomnia may have other causes; among the most common are disturbances of sleep-wake cycles, noisy or disruptive environment, drug effects as described above for anxiety, drug/alcohol abuse, medical disease, and psychiatric mood disorders. Nighttime insomnia can also occur in individuals with other sleep disorders such as narcolepsy or sleep apnea syndromes.

DRUGS USED IN THE TREATMENT OF ANXIETY

In the past the drugs used to treat anxiety and insomnia have been referred to as "sedative/hypnotics." Sedative (and sedation) in this context refers to any of a variety of calming or nervous system depressant effects as determined subjectively by the individual or by observation of the demeanor or behavior. However, although the terms "sedation" and "sedative" lack precise definitions, they commonly refer to an "anxiolytic" action or a mild depression of central nervous system (CNS) function, for example, as an undesirable side effect.

The benzodiazepines are now the major class of drugs used therapeutically for antianxiety and hypnotic (sleep-inducing) actions. Traditionally, the "sedative/hypnotic" drugs have included a large variety of other agents as well: barbiturates; meprobamate (MILTOWN, EQUANIL); and a diverse group of substances that possess actions similar to the barbiturates. Of these the following are still on the market: glutethimide; methyprylon (NOLDAR); ethchlorvynol (PLACIDYL); and chloral hydrate (NOCTEC and others). In addition, many drugs used primarily for other purposes have sedative or hypnotic effects. These include phenothiazines; tricyclic antidepressants; diphenhydramine and many other antihistamines; opioids; propranolol; and clonidine. Antidepressants such as imipramine may be as useful in generalized anxiety disorder as benzodiazepines.

The term "hypnotic agents" specifically refers to substances that produce or promote sleep; "hypnosis," on the other hand, is a general term usually used in reference to the phenomenon of hypnosis and hypnotic trances. Thus, in common parlance, benzodiazepines are sedative/hypnotic, antianxiety or anxiolytic agents, some of which are used therapeutically for the temporary relief of anxiety or insomnia.

Benzodiazepines

The first benzodiazepine studied and marketed was chlordiazepoxide (LIBRIUM). Although the benzodiazepines were developed after the discovery of their unique structures and actions, some of the compounds were later found to be endogenous in the brain and cerebrospinal fluid.

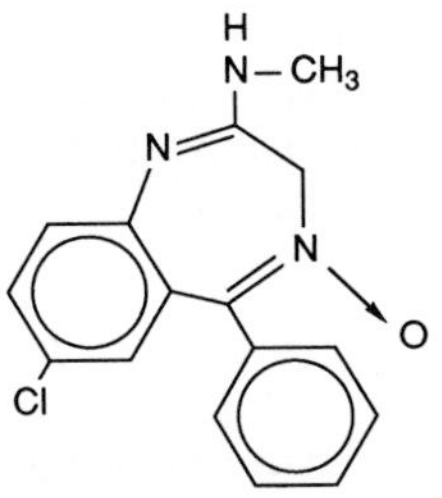

Chlordiazepoxide (LIBRIUM)

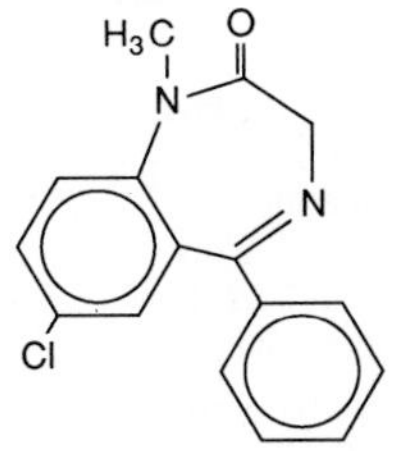

Diazepam (VALIUM)

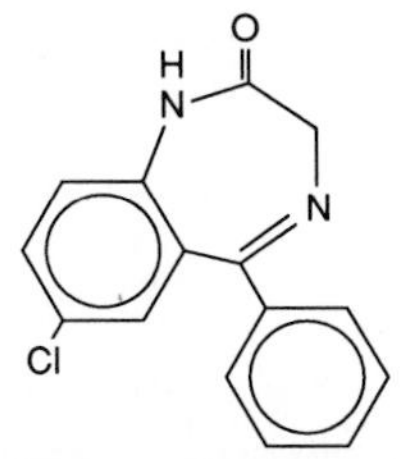

Desmethyldiazepam

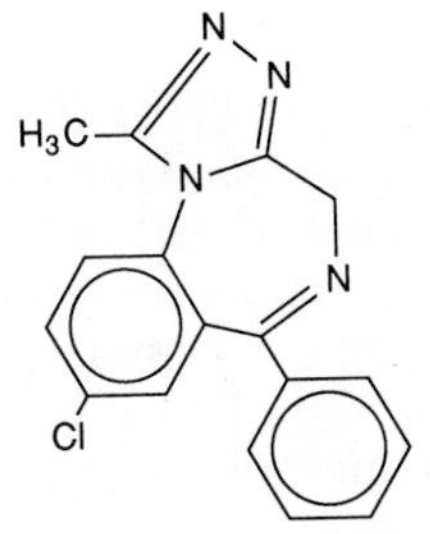

Alprazolam (XANAX)

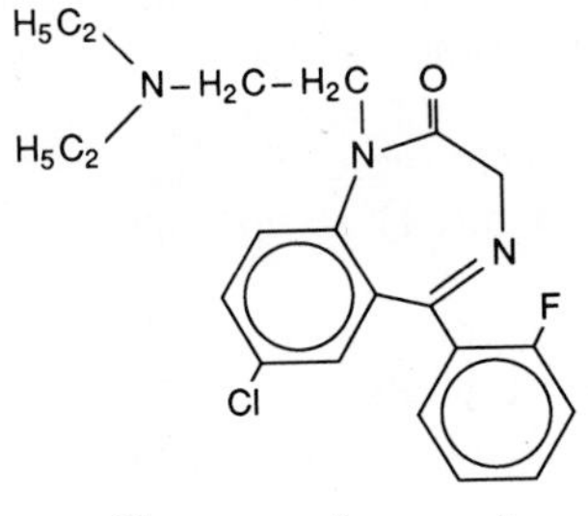

Flurazepam (DALMANE)

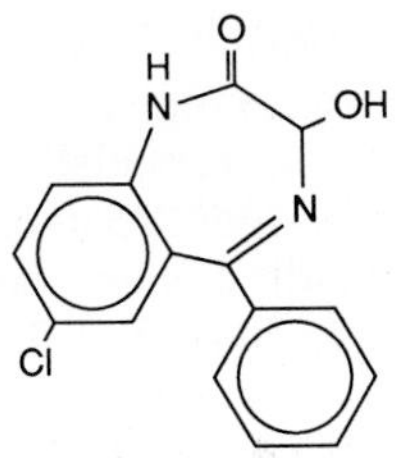

Oxazepam (SERAX)

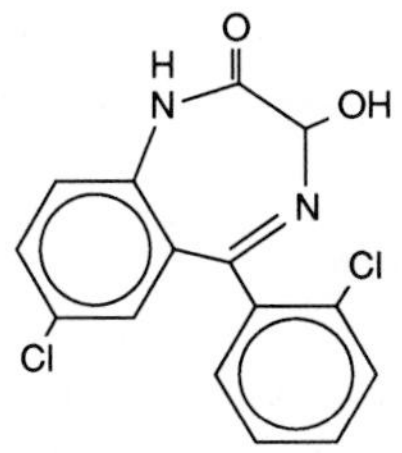

Lorazepam (ATIVAN)

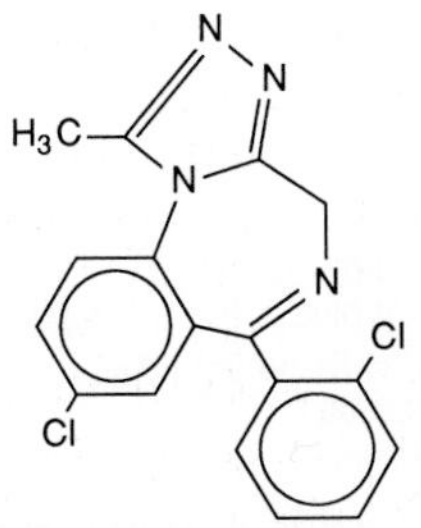

Triazolam (HALCION)

Actions and Effects

ACUTE DOSE-RELATED EFFECTS. Following is a list of the more important dose-related effects produced by all the benzodiazepines in clinical use. These *similarities* are important. However, the *differences* among agents in the spectra of their predominant effects and the variations in pharmacokinetics constitute the rational bases for their different therapeutic uses, for example, as anesthetics, as antianxiety agents, as hypnotic agents, or as muscle relaxants.

- Relief of anxiety and feelings of relaxation; some individuals like the feeling they perceive after taking a benzodiazepine, others do not
- Sedation, calming, drowsiness, sleep (after a benzodiazepine taken at bedtime, there is, on average, an increase in total sleep time, a decrease in sleep latency, a decrease in awakenings, an increase in stage 2, and a decreased time in stages 3 and 4); sleepwalking can occur
- Amnesia
- Impairment of cognitive functioning, confusion, and difficulty in coherent thinking
- Slurred speech, muscle incoordination, nystagmus, and ataxia
- Skeletal muscle relaxation that is clinically useful is obtained with only one compound, diazepam
- Dizziness, headache, nausea, and nervousness
- Paradoxical, behavioral "disinhibition," as manifested by aggressiveness and hostility, may occur
- Effects are additive or synergistic with all CNS depressants
- Respiratory depression, especially in combinations with other agents that produce CNS depression (deaths due to alcohol and sedative drug interactions, most of which are benzodiazepines, exceed 2500 per year in the United States, and such interactions are involved in more than 47,000 emergency room admissions annually)

TAKEN OR GIVEN CHRONICALLY. These agents have a number of characteristic properties when they are taken for extended periods of time.

- Accumulation of the drug and its metabolites in blood and tissue levels appears as a function of its half-life (Table 25-1).
- Tolerance develops during the course of a single dose of long-acting compounds such as diazepam. For example, although sedation initially appears 30 to 60 minutes after an oral dose of diazepam it wears off and disappears after some 4 hours; however, the blood and brain levels have declined only to a very small degree over this time period (excretion half-life in blood is more than 30 hours; Table 25-1). This type of functional tolerance is frequently referred to as "acute tolerance" and may be seen with many CNS depressants such as ethanol and the barbiturates, as well as the benzodiazepines (see Chapters 48 and 49).
- Tolerance also occurs with chronic administration; it appears to develop more rapidly with short intervals between doses. The tolerance to the sedative effects occurs earlier and to a greater extent than to the antianxiety actions, but some tolerance to the latter can occur. This is consistent with the general observation that the time course of development and the magnitude of functional tolerance to the different drug effects (*eg*, sedation, antianxiety, or muscle relaxation) are not the same.
- Habituation and physical dependence can occur with both therapeutic and "excessive" doses to a degree equivalent to pentobarbital. The withdrawal symptoms include anxiety, paresthesias, headache, nervousness, irritability,

TABLE 25-1. Benzodiazepines: Duration of Action and Potential for Accumulation After Oral Administration*

Class/Agent	Half-Life (Range—hours)	Onset of Action (t ½—minutes)	Rebound Insomnia/Anxiety
Short Duration of Action			
Triazolam (HALCION)	1-5	Fast 2-30	++++
Medium Duration of Action			
Lorazepam (ATIVAN)	8-24	Intermediate 30-55	+
Oxazepam (SERAX)	3-20	Slow 45-90	+
Temazepam (RESTORIL) (plus active metabolite, oxazepam)	6-20	Slow 45-50	+
Alprazolam (XANAX)	6-27	Fast-intermediate 30-45	
(and metabolite)	(20-200)		
α-Hydroxyalprazolam			
Halazepam (PAXIPAM)	14 (medium)	Intermediate 45	
Estazolam (PROSOM)	10-24	Intermediate	
Long Duration of Action			
Agents acting directly and as desmethyldiazepam (nordazepam)	20-200		
Clorazepate (TRANXENE)		Fast 15-45	
Prazepam (CENTRAX)		Slow	
Halazepam (PAXIPAM)		Slow	
Diazepam (VALIUM)		Fast	
Chlordiazepoxide (LIBRIUM)		Intermediate	
Quazepam (DORAL) (directly plus active metabolites)	27-53 (~70-195)	Fast 30	
Flurazepam (DALMANE), plus its longer-lasting	1.5	Fast 15-45	
metabolite, desalkylflurazepam	30-200		

*Note that the range of values observed from samples of given population increases as the size of sample is expanded, *ie*, the likelihood of having a patient possessing a very long or very short half-life increases as the number of patients observed increases (sample size). The ranges in this table were individual values from reported relatively small samples of patients, and in actual practice even larger and smaller individual values are to be expected.

insomnia, gastrointestinal upset, tremor, and seizures. **It is important to know that many of these withdrawal symptoms are the very same ones that the drug was being used to alleviate.** The time course of the withdrawal can be especially protracted, appearing only after 4 to 5 days or a week (!) after the drug is discontinued, and lasting for weeks. The management of the withdrawal involves tapering the dose over weeks and months, depending on the initial level of the specific agent (Chapter 49).

Sites and Mechanisms of Action

The benzodiazepines appear to act directly on those CNS systems that mediate the functions they modify. Thus, the mood and emotional effects of the benzodiazepines result, most probably, from their actions on limbic systems (amygdala and hippocampus). Spontaneous and evoked neuronal activity in these areas is decreased; the long feedback networks in these systems appear especially vulnerable, such as the loop from limbic forebrain to reticular system and back to cortex. Effects on the limbic system include depression of repetitive after-discharges, an action consistent with their antiseizure and antiepileptic actions.

The mental confusion and amnesia are also consistent with effects on hippocampus and cortical association areas. The sleep-promoting properties of benzodiazepines appear to arise from their cortical effects or their effects on the neuronal sleep-wakefulness clocks. They do not, in contrast to the barbiturates, have selective effects on the reticular activating system.

The effects of benzodiazepines (specifically diazepam) on muscle function and motor control are the result of effects on the supraspinal, reticular, and cerebellar systems. Although there are demonstrable spinal effects of diazepam, such as to increase presynaptic inhibition, these are of less importance in producing muscle relaxation than the supraspinal actions. In addition to direct effects on motor control systems, relaxation of tense skeletal muscles is one of the consequences of the supraspinal antianxiety effects.

The subjective and behavioral manifestations of fear and anxiety are decreased, along with the usual concomitants of fear, anxiety, and escape behaviors, such as blood pressure, heart rate, respiratory rate, piloerection, gastrointestinal motility, and the like. One of the characteristic effects of these agents in animal behavioral studies is an increase in learned behaviors that had been suppressed by prior punishment of that behavior.

Electrophysiological studies have demonstrated the following actions:

- Increased presynaptic inhibition at both spinal and supraspinal sites
- Augmented effects of endogenously released γ-aminobutyric acid (GABA)
- Increased GABA-mediated neuronal inhibition
- Decrease in the potentiation of synaptic transmission that occurs after a period of repetitive activity, that is, a depression of posttetanic potentiation (PTP).

Benzodiazepines bind stereospecifically with receptors that are widely distributed in the nervous system. Many of these receptors are associated with the GABA receptor and chloride channels. The receptors that bind the benzodiazepines have been characterized as "heterogeneous" or as "multiplicity of binding" to summarize the fact that there is a wide variation in the specificities of binding with respect to neural sites, molecular specificity, affinities, agonist versus antagonist actions, and neuronal synaptic consequences of binding.

Benzodiazepines can be classified according to their "agonist" or "antagonist" effects on specific receptors. All of the benzodiazepines prescribed for their antianxiety, sleep-promoting, muscle relaxant, and antiseizure actions appear to be pure agonists. (The antagonist, flumazenil, is discussed later.)

A proposed model of the benzodiazepine receptor systems can serve to summarize the complex relationships of the benzodiazepine binding site(s) with other receptor systems for GABA, the primary gating ligand for transmembrane chloride ion channels. Figure 25–1 illustrates a generic GABA receptor protein sequence and a possible topological structure. The GABA receptor system is a hetero-oligomeric protein consisting of several distinct polypeptide types (α, β, γ, δ). The arrangement of some of the major allosteric relationships established experimentally follows:

- The receptor is associated with and modulates the transmembrane chloride ion channel that is gated by the primary ligand, GABA; the chloride channel can exist in an open and a closed configuration. The channel is composed of a number of protein subunits.
- The GABA site on this receptor complex is associated primarily with the β subunit, whereas the α subunit contains the binding site for benzodiazepines. The γ subunit appears to be required for the benzodiazepine receptor–mediated modulatory effects.
- The benzodiazepine binding site appears to be able to modulate allosterically the affinity and availability of GABA-binding sites in either direction. It may also modulate the coupling of the GABA receptor with the chloride channel.
- The receptor complex is ultimately connected to intracellular protein kinases and cyclic adenosine monophosphate (cAMP) sites.
- Kinetic and binding studies have led to the conclusion that each channel may have two or more benzodiazepine (BZ) binding sites, each of which can bind either an agonist or an antagonist. At one site, binding with benzodiazepine agonists results in a "depressant" effect (*ie*, an augmentation of GABA binding and an increase in chloride conductance), whereas binding at the other, a "convulsant" or "inverse agonist" site, results in a decrease in chloride conductance. (This is one theory to explain the fact that similar substances with similar binding characteristics can actually have opposite effects.)
- Each channel receptor system also has related but molecularly different sites that bind barbiturates (agonist) and picrotoxin (antagonist and convulsant). Binding at such sites also modifies GABA effects on chloride permeability; in high concentrations binding at these sites directly affects the chloride channel.
- The presence of GABA enhances the affinity of agonists to benzodiazepine receptors; conversely, benzodiazepine agonists enhance GABA-receptor binding.

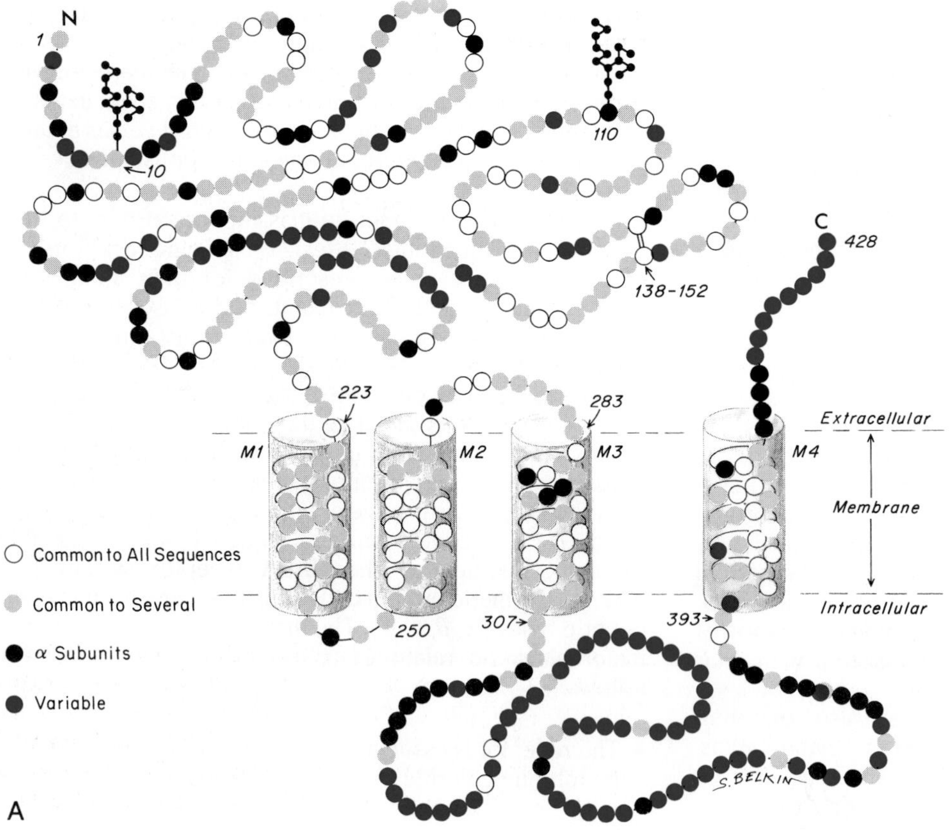

FIGURE 25–1. *(A)* Generic $GABA_A$ receptor protein subunit sequence and putative topological structure. The numbering follows that of the rat α_1 sequence used by Khrestchatisky M, MacLennan AJ, Chiang MY, et al: A novel alpha-subunit in rat brain $GABA_A$ receptors. Neuron 3:745–753, 1989. Note the NH_2 terminal (labeled N, residue 1) presumed extracellular domain, with probable sites for asparagine glycosylation (polymeric black circles at positions 10 and 110), and the cystine bridge (solid line connecting 138 and 152). Four putative membrane-spanning α-helical cylinders M1, M2, M3, and M4 are shown. The COOH-terminus (labeled C, residue 428) is again extracellular. A large intracellular cytoplasmic loop between M3 and M4 is present. The color code indicates the degree of variability within the family of rat polypeptides published to date: α_1, α_2, α_4, β_1, β_2, β_3, γ_2, and δ. Those amino acids identical in all the clones are shown in white, those identical in two or more types are gray, those identical in all α but not in β, γ, or δ are black, and those that vary between types are in color.

Illustration continued on following page

- Barbiturates, ethanol, and other agents can enhance agonist binding to the benzodiazepine receptor.
- Benzodiazepine antagonists, such as flumazenil, primarily bind to the benzodiazepine receptors and have little effect on GABA-induced chloride fluxes.
- At least three subclasses of benzodiazepine receptors exist in the brain based on structural and functional diversity; the subclasses have different regional distribution in brain sites, with different distributions between GABA and benzodiazepine binding and between different benzodiazepines.

Benzodiazepine binding is regulated and influenced by a variety of factors, including the prior occurrence of seizures or the administration of benzodiazepines. A decrease in benzodiazepine receptor concentration (down-regulation) that accompanies chronic administration of a benzodiazepine is one factor, but not the only factor, responsible for the development of tolerance.

Time Course of Action

It is important to remember the large variability among patients with respect to drug sensitivity as well as the time course of onset and duration of action.

ABSORPTION. Benzodiazepines can be administered orally, intramuscularly, and intravenously. However, not all can be administered by all routes.

- Oral: Although the benzodiazepines are orally effective, there are significant differences among them. Diazepam, flurazepam, and desmethyldiazepam (the active metabolite formed in the stomach after administration of the prodrug clorazepate) are among the most rapidly absorbed; on the other hand, oxazepam is one of the more slowly absorbed (Table 25–1).
- Intramuscular: The intramuscular route should be avoided for diazepam and chlordiazepoxide because they are poorly and erratically absorbed after intramuscular injection. Midazolam and lorazepam are marketed for both intravenous and intramuscular use.
- Intravenous: Most of the benzodiazepines are poorly soluble in water and are not available for intravenous use. Agents useful for intravenous administration are diazepam and midazolam, the two agents used for conscious sedation techniques (see Chapter 11). Intravenously administered diazepam may be painful and is occasionally followed by phlebitis, but this route is quite useful in the management of seizures, for conscious sedation techniques, and as a component of anesthesia.

DISTRIBUTION. All the benzodiazepines in use are bound 50% or more to plasma proteins, and their distribution to tissues such as brain is correlated with lipid solubility. For example, diazepam has not only a more rapid absorption from the intestine than chlordiazepoxide, it has a higher lipid solubility and a more rapid distribution to the CNS. There is selective localization first in gray matter, followed by white matter, including even the myelin of peripheral nerves. Diazepam accumulates in fat, as does its metabolites, desmethyldiazepam and oxazepam.

METABOLISM AND EXCRETION. The benzodiazepines are metabolized, via *N*-dealkylation or hydroxylation by liver microsomal systems, followed by conjugation to form inactive glucuronides, which are excreted in the urine. Duration

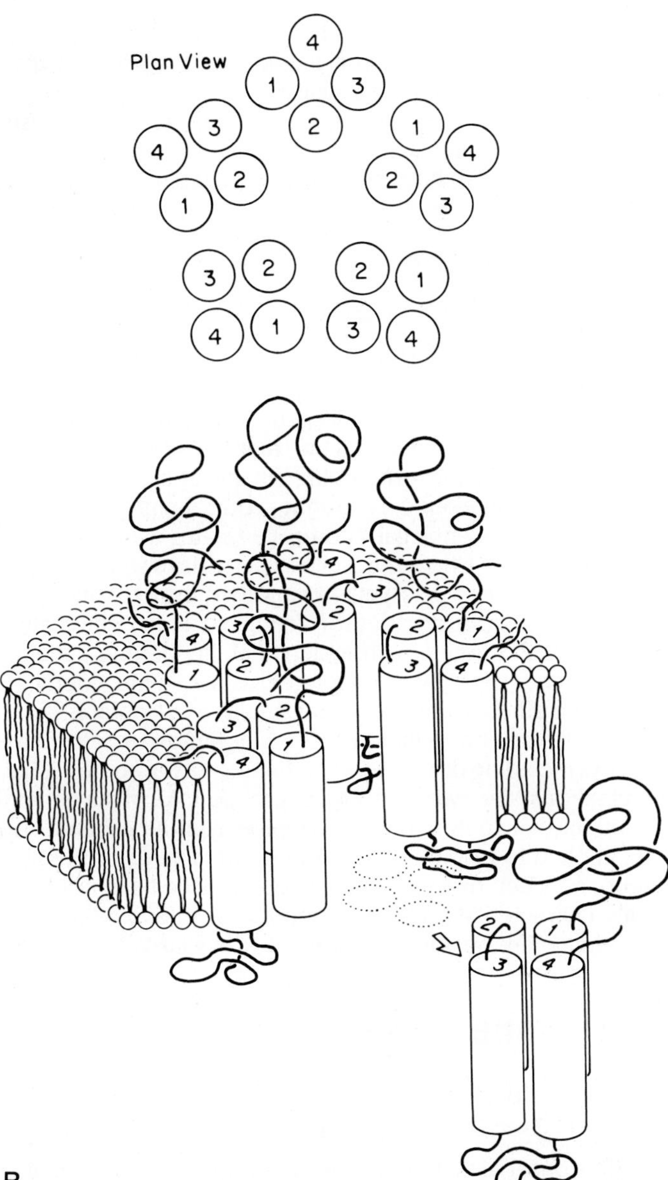

FIGURE 25-1. *Continued* (*B*) Model of the $GABA_A$ receptor-chloride channel protein complex. The ligand-gated ion channel is proposed to be a hetero-oligomer composed of five subunits of the type shown in *A*. Each subunit has four membrane-spanning domains (cylinders numbered 1-4), one or more of which contribute to the wall of the ion channel. The structure is patterned after the well-characterized nicotinic acetylcholine receptor, another member of the same gene superfamily. The naturally occurring oligomers are composed of some of the α, β, γ, and δ polypeptides, but the exact subunit composition, stoichiometry, and number of subunits are not known at this time. (*Panels A* and *B* from Olsen RW, Tobin AJ: Molecular biology of $GABA_A$ receptors. FASEB J 4:1469-1480, 1990.)

of action of the different compounds are functions of three interactive processes:

1. Appearance of acute and chronic functional tolerance
2. Kinetics of the metabolism of all of the compounds (except oxazepam and lorazepam) to active metabolites with longer durations of action than the parent compounds
3. Metabolism to the inactive metabolites

Note the very long half-lives (Table 25-1), except for triazolam, and the inevitable accumulation that will occur with chronic administration. Note also the striking variations among patients in both the rates of onset and the durations of action; these values are from individual controlled trials; the variations will be even larger in actual patients. Moreover, there is considerable variability in the plasma levels attained for given doses.

TABLE 25-2. Hazards and Contraindications of Benzodiazepines

- If mental alertness is required, for example for driving or operating dangerous machinery
- In depressive mood disorders or psychosis
- As hypnotic in patients with sleep apnea or snoring
- In individuals who may have the potential to develop drug dependence (*ie*, 20% of the general population and all moderate to heavy drinkers!)
- With concomitant alcohol use or combined with other central nervous system (CNS) depressants
- In pregnant women, and possibly in all women of childbearing age
- Prior to checking for potential adverse drug interaction with previous, current, or future medications
- In the elderly, inasmuch as drug effects (acute and chronic) may be indistinguishable from or contribute to organic brain disease
- For chronic use (>2-4 weeks) for most cases of anxiety or insomnia

Adverse Effects

The benzodiazepines given alone are remarkable in their intrinsic safety; there is a large margin of safety between the doses effective therapeutically and doses that produce serious respiratory depression. Their safety derives from the fact that, when given orally, they have essentially no effect on cardiovascular or other functions important to life. However, when given intravenously or given when other CNS depressant drugs are present, which is frequently the case, they can produce potentially serious respiratory depression. The major acute adverse effects are simply extensions of the pharmacodynamic actions described earlier; the major limitations to their use are listed in Table 25-2.

Thus, a major potential for adverse reactions stems from drug interactions, both pharmacokinetic and pharmacodynamic in origin. Any substance that alters liver microsomal metabolism can potentially alter benzodiazepine metabolism. Thus, possible interactions should be assessed *prior* to initiating therapy (Table 25-2; Olkkola et al, 1994).

Benzodiazepine Antagonist—Flumazenil

Benzodiazepine antagonists are under active investigation. The first agent clinically available is flumazenil (MAXICON). It effectively antagonizes the CNS effects of benzodiazepines, including the depression of respiration. It acts as a selective, competitive antagonist of benzodiazepines, and clinical reports of effective reversal of poisonings have included a number of benzodiazepines, including diazepam, lorazepam, midazolam, and temazepam. It has little, if any, ability

BOX 25–1
THERAPEUTIC USES

- **Antianxiety:** Benzodiazepines can relieve the anxiety of generalized anxiety disorder and, in some patients, panic attack syndromes; the anxiety associated with the trials and tribulations of "everyday life" can also be reduced.
- **Sleep promotion:** All of these agents can result in relief of insomnia, especially sleep that is difficult because of anxiety, such as in preoperative or grief situations. The drugs commonly used for sleep promotion are triazolam, temazepam, quazepam, estazolam, and flurazepam. The shortest acting compound, triazolam (HALCION), when given at bedtime has the potential for actually causing increased wakefulness early in the morning or increased insomnia the next day, so-called rebound insomnia (Table 25–1). The sleep-promoting actions are time-limited and decrease over days of daily use. Thus, the agents are useful only for periods of 1 to 2 weeks, unless the dose is increased, an undesirable action. It is extremely important to realize that insomnia is a symptom, not a diagnosis, and that the most common causes of insomnia are drug/alcohol abuse, psychiatric mood disorders, and medical illness. Benzodiazepines are contraindicated in individuals who snore or have sleep apnea.
- **Conscious sedation procedures:** Commonly used are diazepam (VALIUM) and midazolam (VERSED). They are used as one of the many components in anesthesia for emergency management of seizures (diazepam, see Chapter 20).
- **Skeletal muscle relaxation:** Diazepam (VALIUM) is the only one used (see Chapter 22).
- **Alleviation of the withdrawal syndrome upon discontinuation of alcohol or a benzodiazepine:** Diazepam and oxazepam are the most frequently used agents (see Chapter 48).
- **Sedation and calming of manic or unmanageable patients:** Lorazepam (ATIVAN) is often used in place of or in addition to haloperidol.
- **Other disorders possibly responding to benzodiazepines:** panic disorder (alprazolam), depression (alprazolam), bipolar (clonazepam, lorazepam), convulsive disorders (see Chapter 20).

to antagonize barbiturates, inhalation anesthetics, or alcohol (although some reports of antagonism have appeared). It is likely to become a routinely available antidote for coma due in part or solely to a benzodiazepine. In addition, flumazenil will probably prove useful for diagnostic purposes in poisoning, in the management of cognitive disorders including hepatic encephalopathy, and in the provocative diagnosis of panic disorder.

Flumazenil can be administered intravenously. Its duration of action of 1 to 4 hours is relatively short, and thus treatment of poisoning usually requires continuous monitoring of the patient's vital signs and the repeated administration of flumazenil. Although the short duration of action may lead to undermedication of benzodiazepine poisoning, the brief duration allows for ready adjustment of dose and frequency as well as its use for diagnosis of possible benzodiazepine accumulation or toxicity.

As might be expected, benzodiazepine antagonists, such as flumazenil, can precipitate an abstinence syndrome in individuals who have taken benzodiazepines chronically.

Zolpidem, the Nonbenzodiazepine "Benzodiazepine"

Zolpidem (AMBIEN) is a new agent that binds selectively to benzodiazepine receptors (but that on strictly chemical grounds is not a benzodiazepine but an imidazopyridine derivative). It is marketed as "nonbenzodiazepine" and hence escapes the present legally controlled status of many benzodiazepines (see Chapter 61). It is said to have weak anxiolytic and sedative effects, yet is a rapidly acting hypnotic agent of relatively short duration of action. Its mean elimination half-life is 2.5 hours, with wide variability among patients, and a higher peak level and longer half-life in the elderly. Its hypnotic efficacy appears to be similar to triazolam.

Adverse effects include effects common to benzodiazepines including drowsiness, dizziness, ataxia, amnesia, hallucinations, sleepwalking, and depression. All of the general cautions that apply to benzodiazepine hypnotics should also be applied to zolpidem. The long-term hazards or possible rebound sleep disturbances or dependence have not been fully characterized, although reports of tolerance and dependence are beginning to appear (Cavallaro et al, 1993).

Buspirone

Buspirone (BUSPAR) is a unique compound with antianxiety efficacy. It has a number of special characteristics:

- Slow onset of action; requires a week or more for antianxiety response; has at least one active metabolite
- Different mechanism of action than either barbiturates or benzodiazepines; probably acts as a partial agonist on certain 5-hydroxytryptamine (5-HT) 1A receptors
- Demonstrates the feasibility of new treatments of anxiety and related syndromes
- Generally fewer side effects; less sedation than benzodiazepines
- Low abuse potential; those previously taking benzodiazepines don't especially "like" buspirone; no withdrawal or dependence reported
- No potentiation of alcohol effects; not useful for management of alcohol withdrawal
- Drug of choice for the severe anxiety that can occur in those recovering from alcohol or sedative drug dependence, after the acute withdrawal

Barbiturates

Barbiturates have been divided traditionally into long-acting, short-acting, and ultra-short-acting agents. This division is consistent with their major therapeutic uses. Phenobarbital, a long-acting agent, has had a long history of use as a long-acting sedative and antianxiety agent, but these uses have been essentially completely supplanted by benzodiazepines and other drugs. Phenobarbital is now used solely in treatment of epilepsy and is covered in Chapter 20.

At the other end of the spectrum are the ultra-short-acting agents, the thiobarbiturates that are used exclusively for anesthesia (discussed in Chapter 11).

The remaining short-acting barbiturates have been used therapeutically primarily as hypnotic agents. Two of the more widely prescribed were secobarbital (SECONAL) and pentobarbital (NEMBUTAL and others). These agents were effective in promoting or causing sleep. Although they and related compounds remain on the market, they have been supplanted by benzodiazepines. As used to promote sleep at bedtime the usually recommended doses of the barbiturates are effective and present by themselves little risk except sedative hangover; that is, the drug effects persist into the next day with grogginess and difficulty in thinking and concentrating. In children and some individuals the barbiturates have a paradoxical excitatory action.

In larger doses the barbiturates produce a dose-related depression of CNS function ranging from mild sedation and mental clouding — to sleep — to coma — to coma with respiratory depression and eventually death. Their potential lethality is well demonstrated by the fact that until the last few years barbiturates were one of the most commonly employed drugs in completed suicides.

In addition, chronic consumption of doses two to four times the hypnotic dosage leads to tolerance and physical dependence. Experimental studies of these short-acting barbiturates led to the definition of the barbiturate-alcohol class of dependence syndromes. They exhibit both cross-tolerance and cross-dependence with alcohol (see Chapter 49).

For occasional use for short periods of insomnia due to situational anxiety, the benzodiazepines are at least as effective in promoting useful sleep as the barbiturates and have a much larger safety margin. The decline in use of the barbiturate hypnotics is mostly due to the availability of less toxic agents.

Miscellaneous Antianxiety Agents

Adrenergic Blockers

Other agents known to modify anxiety are propranolol and other β-adrenergic blockers, which have been used to prevent performance anxiety or stage fright; they suppress both the peripheral autonomic and motor symptoms of anxiety and the feelings of anxiety (see Chapter 10).

Antidepressants

The tricyclic antidepressants may be useful not only in the relief of insomnia but also as treatment of anxiety accompanied by depression or for panic attacks, or as adjuncts in treatment of pain (see Chapter 14). The major limitations of antidepressants center on the delay in onset of effects and the possible cardiovascular effects of orthostatic hypotension or arrhythmias.

Neuroleptics

Low doses of antipsychotic agents, such as haloperidol, have been used in treatment of anxiety, especially in the elderly. A major limitation in their use is the possible development of extrapyramidal syndromes or tardive dyskinesia.

Antihistamines

A common side effect of antihistamines (H_1-blocking agents) is sedation, drowsiness, and sleep. Among the most sedating of these substances is one of the first antihistamines discovered, diphenhydramine (BENADRYL and others). At the present time it is perhaps the most widely used medicine for sleep by prescription as well as over the counter. Depending on dose, it does increase sleep quality and duration.

Hydroxyzine (VISTARIL, ATARAX, and others) is an antihistamine that has been used as an antianxiety agent and as an adjunct to analgesics. These agents have not been the subject of well-controlled clinical trials in comparison with benzodiazepines. The place of these antihistamines in the therapy of anxiety is uncertain (see also Chapter 16).

Chloral Hydrate

Chloral hydrate is a relatively safe, rapidly effective, reliable hypnotic for short-term use. It has an unpleasant taste and odor so it has to be dispensed as chilled capsules or administered rectally. The active moiety is the metabolite, trichloroethanol, with 4 to 10 hours' half-life. It is potentially more toxic than benzodiazepines. Large doses cause coma, respiratory depression, hypotension, arrhythmias, and myocardial depression; obviously it is contraindicated in patients with hepatic, cardiac, or renal impairment. Chronic use can result in dependence.

A number of possible interactions with other drugs have been reported in addition to additive effects with all CNS depressants: transient potentiation of oral anticoagulants; flushing, tachycardia, and anxiety with intravenous furosemide.

Obsolete "Sedative/Hypnotics" Still Currently in Some Use

Meprobamate

Meprobamate (MILTOWN), which has many of the properties of the barbiturates, remains on the market but is largely of historical interest as one of the early tranquilizing drugs developed and introduced in the 1950s. It was promoted as different from phenobarbital or other barbiturates, in that it produced alleviation of tension and anxiety, and that it was less hazardous than the barbiturates. Although these touted differences in therapeutic efficacy were never thoroughly established, the agent enjoyed extensive popularity. One reason for its good safety record was the fact that the recommended dosages that were usually prescribed were relatively small, and these produced few side effects (or drug-induced therapeutic effects either). This compound is described frequently as having skeletal muscle-relaxing effects, but there is no basis for such claims (see Chapter 22).

Ethchlorvynol

An essentially obsolete agent used in the past to promote sleep, ethchlorvynol (PLACIDYL) has recently experienced a resurgence in use by practitioners trying to avoid the trouble of controlled drug laws. It has a variety of toxicities and its use is probably not warranted. Although it can facilitate sleep, it has a long duration of action, 10 to 25 hours' half-life. It can cause hypotension, nausea, vomiting, urticaria, facial numbness, toxic amblyopia, and in large doses prolonged unconsciousness; blood dyscrasias have also been reported. Chronic use can produce physical dependence with serious withdrawal symptoms upon discontinuation of the drug.

Glutethimide

Glutethimide has essentially all of the actions of short-acting barbiturates used as hypnotics. It has a history of extensive prescription, as well as abuse and toxicity. Overdosages were frequently fatal. There is no rational clinical basis for its use at present.

REFERENCES

American Medical Association: Drug Evaluations. Vol 1. Chicago: American Medical Association, 1993.

American Psychiatric Association Task Force on Benzodiazepine Dependence: Benzodiazepine Dependence, Toxicity and Abuse. Washington, DC; American Psychiatric Association, 1990.

Ankier SI, Goa KL: Quazepam: A preliminary review of its pharmacodynamic and pharmacokinetic properties and therapeutic efficacy in insomnia. Drugs 35:42-62, 1988.

Bailey L, Ward M, Musa MN: Clinical pharmacokinetics of benzodiazepines. J Clin Pharmacol 34:804-811, 1994.

Barnett A, Iorio LC, Billard W: Novel receptor specificity of selected benzodiazepines. Clin Neuropharmacol 8(Suppl 1):S8-S16, 1985.

Busto U, Sellers EM, Naranjo CA, et al: Withdrawal reaction after long-term therapeutic use of benzodiazepines. N Engl J Med 315:854-859, 1986.

Cavallaro R, Regazzetti MG, Covelli G, Smeraldi E: Tolerance and withdrawal with zolpidem [letter]. Lancet 342:374-375, 1993.

Ciraulo DA, Sands BF, Shader RI: Critical review of liability for benzodiazepine abuse among alcoholics. Am J Psychiatry 145:1501-1506, 1988.

Eison AS, Temple DL Jr: Buspirone: Review of its pharmacology and current perspectives on its mechanism of action. Am J Med 80(Suppl 3B):1-9, 1986.

Enna SJ, Mohler H: γ-aminobutyric acid (GABA) receptors and their association with benzodiazepine recognition sites. *In* Meltzer HY (ed): Psychopharmacology: The Third Generation of Progress, 265. New York: Raven Press, 1987.

Hauri P (ed): Case Studies in Insomnia. New York: Plenum Medical Book Company, 1991.

Hallström C (ed): Benzodiazepine Dependence. Oxford: Oxford Medical Publications, 1993.

Hindmarch I, Beaumont G, Brandon S, Leonard BE (eds): Benzodiazepines: Current Concepts. New York: John Wiley & Sons, 1990.

Hollister LG, Müller-oerlinghauser B, Richels K, Shader RI: Clinical uses of benzodiazepines. J Clin Psychopharmacol 13(Suppl 1), 1993. [Note: Does not assess safety or risk; review funded by three pharmaceutical company sponsors.]

Janicek PG, Davis JM, Preskorn SH, Ayd FJ Jr: Principles and Practice of Psychopharmacotherapy. Baltimore: Williams & Wilkins, 1993.

Kudo Y, Kurihara M: Clinical evaluation of diphenhydramine hydrochloride for the treatment of insomnia in psychiatric patients: A double-blind study. J Clin Pharmacol 30:1041-1048, 1990.

Labbate LA, Pollack MH, Otto MW, et al: The relationship of alprazolam and clonazepam dose to steady-state concentration in plasma. J Clin Psychopharmacol 14:274-276, 1994.

Lasagne L, Shader RI: A white paper on the appropriateness of proposals by the FDA to modify labeling of benzodiazepine sedative-hypnotics. J Clin Pharmacol 34:812-815, 1994.

Mandema JW, Tuk B, van Steveninck AL, Breimer DD, Cohen AF, Danhof M: Pharmacokinetic-pharmacodynamic modeling of the central nervous system effects of midazolam and its main metabolite α-hydroxymidazolam in health volunteers. Clin Pharmacol Ther 51:715-728, 1992.

Mendelson WB: Human Sleep—Research and Clinical Care. New York: Plenum Medical Book Co, 1987.

Meredith TJ, Jacobsen D, Haines JA, Berger J-C: Naloxone, flumazenil and dantrolene as antidotes. Vol 1. EPCS/CEC evaluation of Antidotes Series. Cambridge: Cambridge University Press, 1993.

Mody I, DeKoninck Y, Otis TS, Soltesz I: Bridging the cleft at GABA synapses in the brain. Trends Neurosci 17:517-525, 1994.

Olkkola KT, Backman JT, Neuronen PJ: Midazolam should be avoided in patients receiving the systemic antimycotics hetoconazole or intraconazole. Clin Pharmacol Ther 55:481-485, 1994.

Willcox SM, Himmelstein DV, Woolhandler S: Inappropriate drug prescribing for the community-dwelling elderly. JAMA 272:292-296, 1994.

Zolpidem for insomnia. Med Lett 35:35,36, 1993.

Drug Therapy in Obesity and in Attention-Deficit Disorder 26

Cedric M. Smith and Jerrold C. Winter

The two topics discussed in this chapter are combined because of the frequent use of the same medications for two entirely different objectives: (1) for weight reduction and (2) for the reduction of the symptoms of attention-deficit disorder. In both instances, the drugs are adjuncts, not definitive therapy. Both conditions occur in people of all ages from childhood to mature adulthood, and the medications can be used to treat most of these patients. In both conditions, the reasonable objective of treatment is modest improvement in symptoms, and in both, an appreciable percentage of patients exist that do not find the drug therapy useful, either because they are not benefited or because they experience excessive side effects.

Nevertheless, in spite of the emotional atmosphere surrounding the amphetamine group of drugs and the complexity of the clinical syndromes, present evidence based on clinical trials suggests that in a limited but significant number of patients, drug adjuncts can contribute to clinical improvement. Thus, we focus narrowly on the actions and side effects of the use of drugs as adjuncts in therapy for these conditions.

The very fact that drug therapy can have beneficial consequences, by its own merits, demonstrates that more effective and safe therapies can be developed in the future.

DRUGS USED IN WEIGHT CONTROL

Weight-Control Programs

Obesity is a condition of excessive body weight, much of which is fat. In the absence of organic disease, obesity is the result of the oral intake of energy that exceeds the expenditure of energy. Effective programs for weight control include

1. Exercise, for aerobic function and strength — this regulates and increases energy expenditure and helps to improve physical status and appearance.
2. Diet — this restricts total energy intake and ensures that nutritional needs are met.
3. Medication — this should be used as a well-controlled adjunct to exercise and dietary controls.
4. Behavior modification — this augments and facilitates exercise, diet, and medication programs.

It is assumed that any anorexiant drug adjuncts in a weight-loss program are being prescribed and administered as part of a coherent comprehensive weight-reduction program. Among the comprehensive initial medical assessments in such programs must be the determination of whether the possibility exists that any drugs might serve as a contributing factor for alterations in taste and appetite (see Tables 13 – 5, 50 – 11). The many interesting therapeutic opportunities for use of the large number of different agents with effects on appetite control systems is comprehensively reviewed by Blundell (1993).

Amphetamine and Related Compounds (Table 26 – 1)

Treatment of excessive weight and the frequently associated programs designed to improve physical fitness and appearance involve two critical aspects.

1. Reducing appetite (with an "anorexiant") and reducing food consumption in humans and animals, probably through adrenergic and dopaminergic mechanisms (see Chapter 9)
2. Modifying energy expenditures, food preferences, activity, and sleep patterns

Given that the exercise and behavior needs of the patient are being addressed, diet and medication can be considered. Many, although not all, of the drugs that have been found to be useful in weight reduction are *d, l* amphetamine and its chemical congeners; the major pharmacodynamic activity resides in the dextro isomer, dextroamphetamine.

TABLE 26–1. Amphetamine and Related Drugs That Have Had Some Use in the Treatment of Obesity

Amphetamine (*d, l* amphetamine) (BIPHETAMINE—cation complex of dextroamphetamine and amphetamine)
Dextroamphetamine (DEXEDRINE tablets; DEXEDRINE SPANSULES)
Benzphetamine (DIDREX)
Diethylpropion (TENUATE)
Mazindol (SANOREX)
Methamphetamine (DESOXYN, "speed")
Phendimetrazine (PRELU-2 timed-release capsules, PLEGINE)
Phentermine (ADIPEX-P, FASTIN, IONAMIN)
Phenylpropanolamine (PPA; in a variety of forms and combination products, *eg*, various DEXATRIM products, COMTREX, and many others)

Fenfluramine (PONDIMIN)

Many of the drugs share the properties of amphetamine to increase alertness, decrease drowsiness or sleep, increase stamina, and reduce mental and physical fatigue. Most people experience an increased sense of energy and well-being with the drugs, but some become manic, and others may find that they are more anxious than usual. A fine tremor in hands or fingers may be present. Blood pressure and heart rate may be slightly elevated. In relatively large amounts, amphetamine produces anxiety, mania, paranoia, psychosis, and cardiac arrhythmias. Amphetamine effects are perceived to be desirable by some; these people can develop significant abuse and dependence (see Chapters 9 and 49).

The anorexiant effects of these drugs are associated with

- Decrease in appetite
- Less interest in food
- Less pleasure from eating
- Increasing satiety with eating
- Decrease in total energy intake

The actions of amphetamine in the central nervous system (CNS) are complex but can be summarized as increasing the release of catecholamines, especially dopamine, and of secondary importance, increasing the release of norepinephrine. The actions are dose-related and include decreased uptake of both active and passive dopamine presynaptically (via increased exchange diffusion and passive diffusion and via increased membrane transporter activity), resulting in increased release from the terminals and from storage vesicles. In high concentrations, amphetamine also inhibits monoamine oxidase (MAO), potentially further increasing the synaptic concentrations of catecholamines. How these synaptic actions are translated into the central neurophysiological systems of appetite and mood is the subject of current active research.

Fenfluramine

Although most anorexiants in current use have actions and side effects similar to those of amphetamine, the side effects of some of them, notably fenfluramine (PONDIMIN), differ considerably. Fenfluramine, although as efficacious as amphetamine in reducing appetite and food consumption, produces CNS sedation rather than excitation as a side effect.

Fenfluramine does share the effects of amphetamines in decreasing appetite and food consumption in double-blind controlled studies; it has analogous effects in some animal models. Interestingly, in experimental models it suppresses hunger (increases satiety) but has little effect on the perceived pleasantness (hedonic) response to sweet foods. It probably acts on serotonergic systems, in contrast to amphetamines, which appear to act on dopaminergic (and adrenergic) systems.

The half-life of fenfluramine after oral administration is about 10 to 20 hours. The side effects include sedation, drowsiness, diarrhea, dry mouth, and confusion. A conventional dose regimen is 20 mg three times a day or 60 mg of extended-release formulation. Overdoses of more than 300 mg have been associated with convulsions, coma, and cardiac arrhythmias.

Fenfluramine is contraindicated in patients with a history of drug abuse (although little evidence exists that fenfluramine is positively reinforcing or that it produces desirable subjective effects), glaucoma, alcohol abuse or dependence, psychosis, or hypertension.

Dexfenfluramine, the dextrostereoisomer of fenfluramine, is also effective in producing weight loss, although it is not yet available in the United States.

Phenylpropanolamine

Phenylpropanolamine (PPA) is available over the counter in a variety of forms and combination products such as DEXATRIM capsules, DEXATRIM EXTRA STRENGTH, DEXATRIM PLUS VITAMINS, DEXATRIM PLUS VITAMIN C, MAXIMUM STRENGTH DEXATRIM, DEXATRIM, MAXIMUM STRENGTH CAFFEINE-FREE caplets, DEXATRIM PRE-MEAL caplets, DIMETAPP, ACUTRIM, APPEDRINE, AYDS, COMTREX, ORNADE, and many others.

ACTIONS. Phenylpropanolamine is similar to amphetamine with respect to

- Weight loss only shown in short-term controlled studies
- Cardiovascular effects of increased blood pressure and cardiac arrhythmias

Phenylpropanolamine is different from amphetamines with respect to

- Little CNS stimulation
- Little concrete evidence of dependence

SIDE EFFECTS AND HAZARDS. Although capable of producing short-term weight loss, PPA does *not* have an established place in rational weight-loss therapy. Moreover, it has a number of recognized hazards. First is a potentially serious interaction with caffeine. *Concomitant ingestion of caffeine and PPA results in significantly increased PPA levels; this is associated with an augmentation of the cardiovascular effects of PPA.* Second is its usual use over the counter without the requisite program of regular and limited dosage, exercise, and the essential diet. Thus, as presently marketed and used, PPA is unlikely to be a useful weight-reduction agent and presents significant hazards of overdosage and adverse drug interactions.

Current Opinion on the Use of Medications

Weintraub and associates (1992) have reported in detail a series of studies sufficiently well designed and controlled

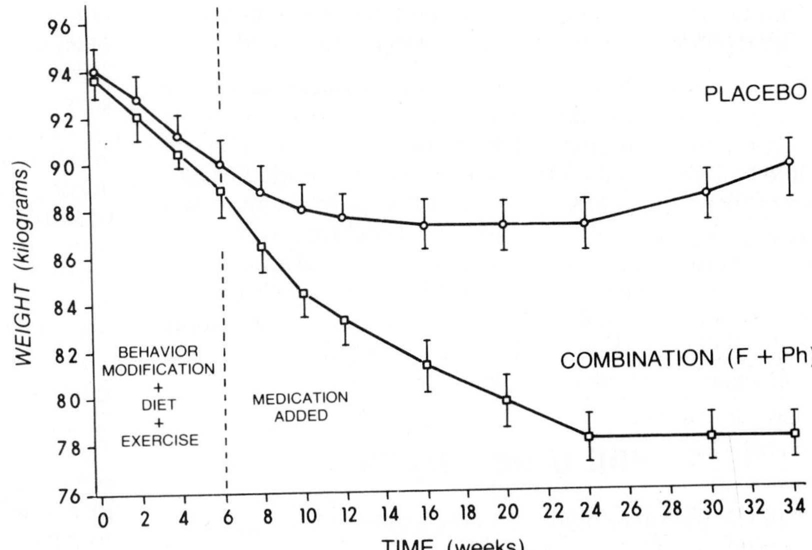

FIGURE 26–1. Participant body weight (in kilograms) by study week. *Open circles* represent placebo group mean ± SEM (n = 54). *Open squares* represent fenfluramine plus phentermine group mean ± SEM (n = 58). (From Weintraub M, Sundaresan P, Madan M, et al: Long-term weight control study I (weeks 0 to 34): The enhancement of behavior modification, caloric restriction, and exercise by fenfluramine plus phentermine versus placebo. Clin Pharmacol Ther 51:586–594, 1992.

and carried through over a sufficient period of time to permit rational assessment of the appropriate and effective use of anorexiants in weight-loss programs. Their conclusions deserve to be widely known and present the single best summary in this sometimes controversial area. Two figures are taken from those reports (Figs. 26–1 and 26–2).

Most important among their conclusions were

- ". . . *anorexiant medications do help many people to lose weight and maintain weight loss. . . .*" The medication used was a combination of phentermine (resin, IONAMIN, 15 mg) and fenfluramine (60 mg extended-release, PONDIMIN). Dry mouth was the most common side effect, in comparison with placebo; less frequent were gastrointestinal complaints (abdominal pain, metallic taste, diarrhea, constipation) and CNS complaints (drowsiness, sleep disturbances, dizziness, sadness). Most of these side effects decreased or disappeared after 4 weeks on the program. Blood pressure, on average, decreased significantly.
- The medication program enhanced ". . . *weight loss more than behavior modification, exercise, and caloric restriction alone. . . . Weight loss [was] . . . maintained for several years if medications [were] used in conjunction with other interventions*" (exercise, diet, behavior modification). Even greater efficacy would have been obtained if dosage regulation and maintenance had been possible in the trial.
- ". . . *no evidence of nontherapeutic use or any type of abuse of anorectic medications*" was found. Although the investigators sought to obtain such information, no evidence of drug seeking, reports of pleasurable effects of

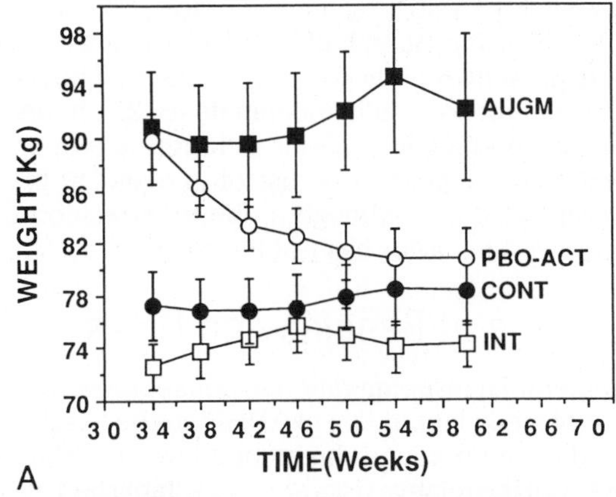

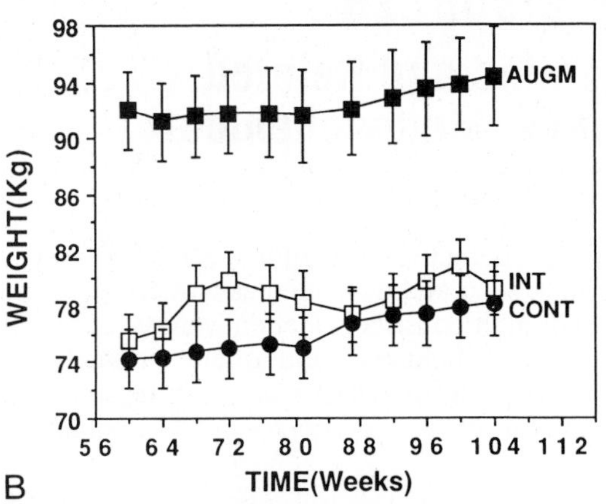

FIGURE 26–2. (*A*), Participant body weight (in kilograms) in the period from weeks 34 to 60 in different treatment groups. Weights from all participants were included in the calculation up to the point when they left the study. Results shown are mean values ± SEM. The number of participants in the treatment groups at weeks 34 and 60 were as follows: placebo to active, $n = 54$ and $n = 52$; active and continuous, $n = 23$ and $n = 21$; active to intermittent, $n = 12$ and $n = 20$; and active to augmented, $n = 12$ and $n = 7$. Participants in the active to intermittent group did not take medication in the period from weeks 34 to 46 and did take medication in the period between weeks 46 and 60. (*B*), Participant body weights (in kilograms) in the period from weeks 60 to 104 in different treatment groups. Weights from all participants were included in the calculation up to the point when they left the study. Results shown are mean values ± SEM. The number of participants in the treatment groups at weeks 60 and 104 were as follows: continuous, $n = 37$ and $n = 33$; intermittent, $n = 36$ and $n = 30$; and augmented, $n = 27$ and $n = 20$. Participants in the intermittent group did not take medication between weeks 60 and 72 and between weeks 87 to 100, and they did take medication between weeks 72 and 87 and between weeks 100 and 104. (*Panels A* and *B* from Weintraub M, Sundareson P, Schuster B, et al: Long-term weight control study II (weeks 34 to 104): An open-label study of continuous fenfluramine plus phentermine versus targeted intermittent medication as adjuncts to behavior modification, caloric restriction, and exercise. Clin Pharmacol Ther 51:595–601, 1992.) (AUGM = augmented group; CONT = continuous group; INT = intermittent group; PBD-ACT = placebo to active group.)

the drugs, or evidence of any withdrawal symptoms with gradual taper on the crossover designs was found.

In spite of these very positive, encouraging results using a rational design of drug selection and dosage, two major negative results were found. First, some individuals received little benefit from the medications, even when the dosages were increased (although some did respond to increased doses). Second, few solo practitioners could reconstruct the program reported; however, similar multimodal approaches would be practical in group practice or in health maintenance organization settings. Third, the study results imply that long-term (years) maintenance of weight loss by some patients may require continued medication.

Caffeine and Other Drugs

Caffeine and other diuretics frequently have been included in weight-control programs in combination drug products. Little evidence exists that these drugs have any beneficial effect other than to produce a transient decrease in body weight associated with diuresis. To the degree that caffeine increases activity and energy expenditure, it could conceivably contribute positively to a weight-loss program. However, to date, essentially no evidence exists to support its inclusion in, or exclusion from for that matter, such programs. In view of the unexpected interaction between caffeine and PPA, caffeine combinations with amphetaminelike compounds would best be avoided altogether.

Thyroid hormone has also been prescribed when the major problem was excess weight. There is no rational place for thyroid hormone in weight-loss programs except in individuals who are demonstrably hypothyroid.

DRUGS THAT IMPROVE SYMPTOMS OF ATTENTION-DEFICIT DISORDER

Amphetamine and Related Compounds, Methylphenidate, and Pemoline

Attention-deficit/hyperactivity disorder (ADHD) is a syndrome most often seen and described as a developmental disorder of children. It consists of inattentiveness, easy distractability, impulsive behavior, and often hyperactivity. High rates of comorbidity of ADHD with antisocial conduct, anxiety, and mood disorders have been amply documented.

Actions

The amphetamines (including dextroamphetamine) and methylphenidate (RITALIN) have a calming effect on many aspects of the behaviors characteristic of ADHD; attention span is increased, impulsiveness is decreased, classroom disruptions are decreased, academic performance is improved, motor activity is decreased, and the children are less distractable. Despite a great deal of controversy, amelioration of symptoms in a major proportion of the subjects has been overwhelmingly documented in hundreds of studies. The benefits are frequently evident not only to teachers and parents but also to the children themselves.

Clearly, some patients benefit much more than others. In addition, the clinical effects of the different compounds do not appear to be identical, which would be consistent with experimental animal data. Thus, it is conceivable that some individuals may respond to one compound differently, or better, than to another. These differences probably relate both to minor qualitative differences in the drugs and to differences in actual doses and pharmacokinetics.

Side Effects

The side effects of the amphetamines are for the most part predictable. Anorexia and insomnia are common; weight loss, headache, and abdominal pain can occur but are less frequent. The suggestion has been made that long-term use may be associated with suppression of growth, but the data are mixed; questions remain concerning that aspect of long-term effects of continued treatment with amphetamines, methylphenidate, and pemoline.

Although they are feared, no clear-cut evidence of long-term effects on mood and affect have been documented. Part of the problem is the fact that children with ADHD are more likely to also have some other cognitive or neurological disorder than control groups.

Although some expected it, methylphenidate therapy does not appear to depress creativity; however, further studies are warranted.

Time Course of Effects

The effects of these agents are apparent within the time course of a single dose. The ameliorating behavioral effects are most pronounced during the absorption phase, *ie*, 1–4 hours after oral administration. In fact, the beneficial effects decline more rapidly than the blood levels would predict, *ie*, the effects exhibit "acute tolerance" (Brown et al, 1979).

The elimination half-life of amphetamine and pemoline in hyperactive children is approximately 7 hours. In contrast, the half-life of methylphenidate is 2.5 hours. Sustained-release preparations result in longer elevations of plasma levels and appear to be useful in avoiding the need for a noontime dose, although a direct correlation of level with improved behavior has not been documented.

Critique of Benefits and Risks

Rather than inspiring rational, collaborative assessment, the use of methylphenidate in ADHD has been subject to critical media attention and threatened lawsuits. The benefits and many of the relative risks are well established. It is hoped that the decision to use medication will be based on a rational assessment of benefits and risks by the subjects and their parents in cooperation with teachers and school nurses.

One of the questions of this "stimulant" therapy centers on how severe the behavior has to be to warrant medication in relation to the consequences of treatment.

A second and perhaps the most difficult issue is how long the treatment should be continued. Even in adults with this syndrome, evidence exists that these drugs may have beneficial effects. To date, studies of alternative therapies of adult ADHD are lacking.

In view of the ready access of these patients to the amphetamines used as therapy, the question of possible abuse of stimulants has been raised, with mixed answers. A few children are known to abuse their medications. More often, however, they tend either to be noncompliant or to recognize the benefits and continue the therapy. The associations with other psychiatric disorders are common and complex. First, a large overlap exists between ADHD and substance abuse disorders as well as conduct and mood disorders; nevertheless, children with no comorbid conduct disorder are at negligible risk for substance abuse disorders. Children whose ADHD symptoms persist into adulthood are at high risk for concomitant substance abuse, especially if antisocial personality characteristics are also present. Thus, assessment and long-term management require multimodal diagnosis and intervention, focusing on both the mood and conduct disorders, and the ADHD.

Alternative Therapies

A number of behavioral and drug therapies have been promoted. However, none has been demonstrated in controlled studies of sufficient duration to have beneficial effects equal to those of the "stimulants." As has been demonstrated in weight-loss studies, drugs that are not stimulants, such as fenfluramine, may exist that might be capable of ameliorating the attention-deficit behavior.

REFERENCES

Barkley RA, DuPaul GJ, McMurray MB: Attention deficit disorder with and without hyperactivity: Clinical response to three dose levels of methylphenidate. Pediatrics 87:519–531, 1991.

Brown GL, Hunt RD, Ebert MH, Bunney WE, Kopin IJ: Plasma levels of D-amphetamine in hyperactive children. Psychopharmacology 62:133–140, 1979.

Blundell J: Pharmacological approaches to appetite suppression. TIPS 12:147–157, centerfold illustration, 1993.

DuPaul GJ, Rapport MD: Does methylphenidate normalize the classroom performance of children with attention deficit disorder? J Am Acad Child Adolesc Psychiatry 32:190–198, 1993.

Funk JB, Chessare JB, Weaver MT: Attention deficit/hyperactivity disorder, creativity and the effects of methylphenidate. Pediatrics 91:816–819, 1993.

Kruesi MJP, Rapaport JL: Psychoactive agents. *In* Yaffee SF, Aranda JV (eds): Pediatric Pharmacology: Therapeutic Principles in Practice, 2nd ed, 413–424. Philadelphia: WB Saunders Co, 1992.

Lafreniere F, Lambert J, Rasio E, Serri O: Effects of dexfenfluramine treatment on body weight and postprandial thermogenesis in obese subjects. A double-blind placebo-controlled study. Int J Obes 17:25–30, 1993.

Martin RJ, White BD, Hulsey MG: The regulation of body weight. Am Scientist 79:528–541, 1991.

Pelham WE, Greenslade KE, Vodde-Hamilton M, et al: Relative efficacy of long-acting stimulants on children with attention deficit–hyperactivity disorders: A comparison of standard methylphenidate, sustained-release methylphenidate, sustained-release dextroamphetamine, and pemoline. Pediatrics 86:226–237, 1990.

Safer DJ, Krager JM: Effect of a media blitz and a threatened lawsuit on stimulant treatment. JAMA 268:1004–1007, 1992.

Seiden LS, Sobol KE, Ricaurte GE: Amphetamine: Effects on catecholamine systems and behavior. Annu Rev Pharmacol Toxicol 32:639–677. 1993.

Yaffee SJ, Aranda JV (eds): Pediatric Pharmacology: Therapeutic Principles in Practice, 2nd ed. Philadelphia, WB Saunders Co, 1992.

Weintraub, Michael: Long-term weight control study: Conclusions. Clin Pharmacol Ther 51:642–646, 1992.

Wilens TE, Spencer T, Biederman J: Role of medication in the treatment of adult attention deficit disorder. *In* Nadeau KG (ed): Attention Deficit Hyperactivity Through the Lifespan. New York: Brunner/Mazel, 1994.

Wilens TE, Biederman J, Spencer TJ, Frances RJ: Comorbidity of attention-deficit hyperactivity and psychoactive substance abuse disorders. Hosp Clin Psychiatry 45:421–435, 1994.

Winter, Jerrold: True Nutrition, True Fitness. Clifton, NJ: Humana Press, 1991.

PART VI

CARDIOVASCULAR SYSTEM PHARMACOLOGY

27 Treatment of Congestive Heart Failure—Digitalis Glycosides

Claire M. Lathers

TREATMENT OF CONGESTIVE HEART FAILURE

Although this chapter focuses on digitalis glycosides, substances that have had more than 200 years of medical use, in recent years the glycosides have no longer been the primary drug of choice for congestive heart failure. The current approach to drug therapy for patients with heart failure due to left ventricular dysfunction is an angiotensin-converting enzyme (ACE) inhibitor (discussed in Chapters 29 and 35), frequently combined with a digoxin and a diuretic (Chapter 35). Patients who do not respond to or tolerate an ACE inhibitor may benefit from a combination of hydralazine and isosorbide dinitrate (Chapters 29 and 30).

Digitalis glycosides are among the most frequently prescribed drugs in the United States. In 1987 more than 12 million prescriptions were written for digoxin (Gheorghiade, 1992). The recognition of the variability in clinical responses resulting from the pharmacokinetics and drug interaction complexities, in the face of frequent occurrence of digitalis toxicity, makes the therapeutic use challenging indeed. The unusually narrow margin between therapeutic and toxic dosages and serum levels of digitalis mandates that the physician be both knowledgeable about, and attentive to, early symptoms of digitalis toxicity to achieve the best risk-benefit ratio. Recognition of toxicity is imperative because a high mortality ensues when digoxin is continued after the appearance of toxic symptoms.

TABLE 27–1. Cardiac Glycoside Preparations

Agent	GI Absorption	Onset (IV—minutes)	Peak (hours)	Half-Life (days)	Metabolic Path	Digitalizing Dose (IV)	Maintenance Dose (Oral)	Therapeutic Concentration (Serum)
Digoxin	55–75%	15–30	1½–5	1½–2	Renal	0.75–1.0 mg	0.25–0.5 mg	0.2–2.0 ng/mL
Digitoxin	90–100%	25–120	4–12	4–7	Liver	1.0 mg	0.10 mg	10–25 ng/mL
Ouabain	Unreliable	5–10	½–2	<1	Renal, some GI	0.3–0.5 mg	—	0.4–0.6 ng/mL

Adapted/condensed from Antman EM, Smith TW: Pharmacokinetics of digitalis glycosides. *In* Smith TW (ed): Digitalis Glycosides, Chapter 15, 241–275. Orlando: Grune & Stratton, 1986. Adapted from Smith JW: Drug therapy: Digitalis glycosides. Reprinted with permission from the New England Journal of Medicine, vol 28, pp 719–722, 1973.

GI = gastrointestinal; IV = intravenous.

DIGITALIS GLYCOSIDES—DIGOXIN

The structure of each digitalis glycoside consists of an aglycone or genin conjugated with one to four molecules of sugar. The aglycone or genin moiety contains the pharmacological activity, whereas the sugar molecules enhance water solubility and cell penetrability. Thus, the sugar portion of the structure influences glycoside potency and the dose response relationship. The combination of an unsaturated lactone ring and the steroid ring imparts cardiotonic activity to the structure.

Digoxin is the most often used glycoside; over recent years digitoxin has been less and less prescribed. Both of these have an aglycone with three molecules of digitoxose and 2,6-dideoxyhexose joined in the glycoside linkage.

PHARMACOKINETICS

Differences in the pharmacokinetics and pharmacodynamic properties among the various digitalis glycosides are due to variations in water or lipid solubility and polarity caused by both the diversity in the chemical structure (Table 27–1) and the formulation of the product. These pharmacokinetic differences influence the onset of the pharmacodynamic action, that is, the inotropic effect, of the various glycosides (Lewis, 1992). Digoxin possesses a half-life of 1 to 1½ days. It is relatively well absorbed after oral administration but tablet preparations vary in the degree to which they are absorbed, varying from 60 to 80%, compared with a standard of 100% after intravenous dosing. Improved bioavailability from 90 to 100% has been achieved with an encapsulated gel preparation. The various digitalis preparations exhibit different degrees of binding to plasma proteins: digitoxin 86%; acetyldigitoxin 81–90%; digoxin 10–15%; and ouabain is not bound. (Ouabain is mentioned in this chapter not because it is used clinically, which it is not, but because its solubility and pharmacokinetic properties have resulted in its extensive use in research on the mechanisms of action of digitalis.)

Differences in protein binding in blood probably do not account for the differences in onset or speed of action among the glycosides, but protein binding in cardiac tissue may be involved in determining the duration of action. Table 27–1 summarizes the onset of action, the peak effect, and the therapeutic serum concentration for the clinically important glycosides. Figure 27–1 illustrates the relationship between tissue and plasma digoxin concentration after its IV administration, and Figure 27–2 depicts its distribution in human tissue 5.5 hours after its administration.

Digoxin is primarily excreted by the kidney; its half-life is increased in patients with renal disease. Because there is, in most patients, a positive correlation between the decrease in creatinine clearance and in the plasma digoxin concentration, pharmacological agents such as vasodilators that change renal perfusion will change the rate of elimination of digoxin. (In contrast, digitoxin is extensively metabolized and its half-life is increased in the presence of liver disease.) Thus, when using glycoside preparations, patient management requires assessment of renal and liver function.

Digoxin is also metabolized to a number of metabolites that may exhibit cardioactivity (Table 27–2). An additional and important problem associated with the use of digoxin is that different brands of the preparation have significantly different bioavailability characteristics (absorption, metabolism, time course of effects). These differences have caused problems in **digitalizing (establishing a steady level of digitalis effects or blood level)** and maintaining patients properly. These differences in product, in association with the low therapeutic index of this class of agents, necessitate constant patient surveillance.

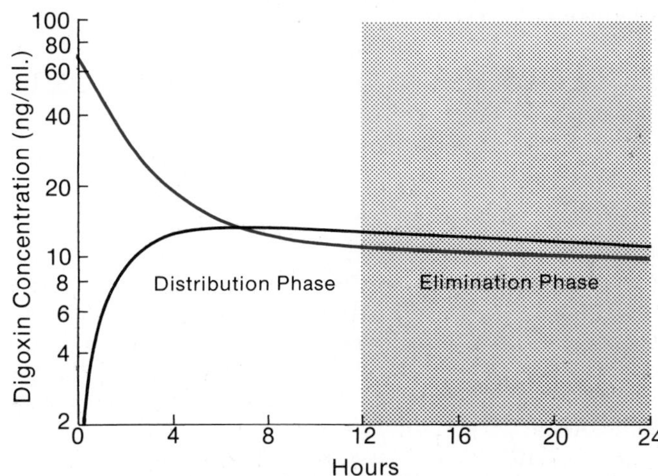

FIGURE 27–1. Relationship between tissue and plasma digoxin ion concentration after administration of an intravenous dose of the drug. Concentration in plasma is shown in red; concentration in tissue, in black. (Redrawn from Soldin SJ: Digoxin—Issues and controversies. Clin Chem 32:5–12, 1986.)

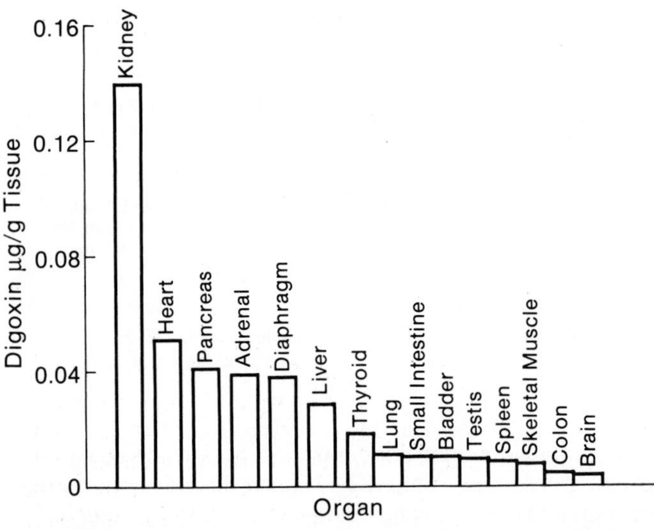

FIGURE 27–2. Tissue digoxin in a patient who received 1.0 mg of tritium-labeled digoxin 5.5 hours before death. Note the concentration in the kidney, the major organ of excretion, and that in the heart, diaphragm, and liver. (Redrawn from Doherty JE: Clinical use of digitalis glycosides: An update. Cardiology 72:225–254, 1985. By permission of S. Karger AG, Basel.)

TABLE 27–2. Cardioactivity of Digoxin Metabolites

Metabolite	Activity Relative to Digoxin (%)
Dihydrodigoxin	2–6
Dihydrodigoxigenin	2
Digoxigenin	4–21
Digoxigenin mono-digitoxiside	66
Digoxigenin bis-digitoxiside	77

Data from Soldin SJ: Digoxin—Issues and controversies. Clin Chem 32:5–12, 1986.

Actions and Mechanism of Action

Increased Force of Contraction

The major features of the pathophysiology of congestive heart failure are depicted in Figure 27–3. The failing heart manifests decreased myocardial contractility and catecholamine content; the catecholamine deficit is thought to be due to the inability of synthesis to follow the increased sympathetic activity involved in the compensatory responses to the decreased cardiac output.

Digitalis increases the force of contraction at a given fiber length or tension when added to an isolated papillary muscle preparation. When administered *in vivo* it increases ventricular contractility in normal and in failing hearts. This increase in myocardial contractility is referred to as its **positive inotropic effect** (Fig. 27–4).

In the normal heart the peak rate of rise of intraventricular pressure and intramyocardial tension during isovolumic contraction is increased by digitalis. The period of isovolumic left ventricular contraction is shortened, whereas the mean systolic ejection rate is increased. In the failing heart, the ability of digitalis to increase myocardial contractility results in an improvement of the impaired circulatory dynamics. Generally, but not always, the stroke volume and cardiac output will be increased and the elevated left ventricular end-diastolic pressure (Fig. 27–5) and volume will be decreased. In addition, the contractility of atrial tissue is increased by the administration of digitalis. The increased atrial contractility increases ventricular filling and thus also contributes to the increased cardiac output.

Increased Cardiac Output in Presence of Congestive Heart Failure

Digitalis has no effect on, or only slightly decreases, cardiac output in the normal heart. No change results in reflex adjustments in the force of cardiac contraction to prevent the decrease in cardiac output that would otherwise occur when digitalis increases afterload by increasing vasoconstriction

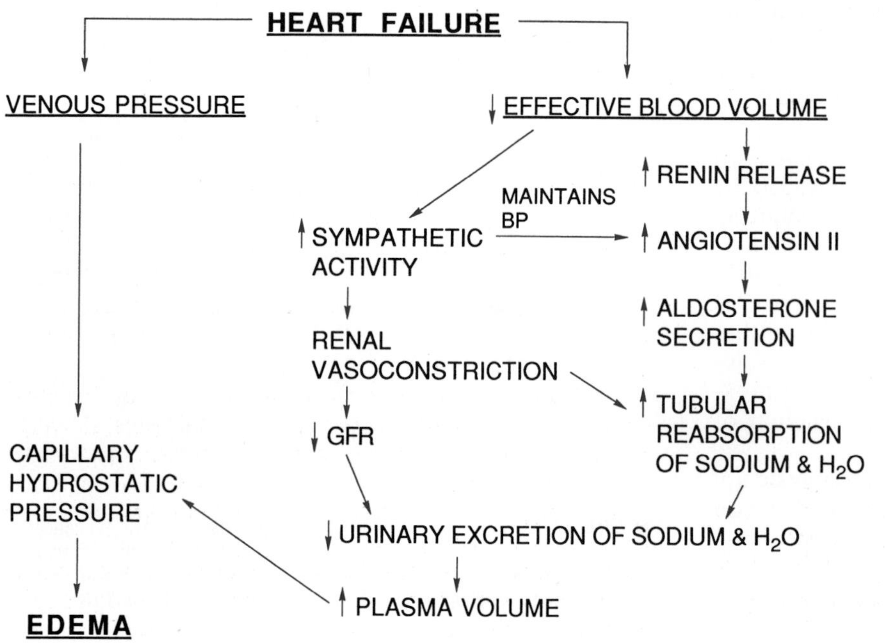

FIGURE 27–3. Major pathophysiological features of congestive heart failure. (BP = blood pressure; GFR = glomerular filtration rate; H_2O = water.)

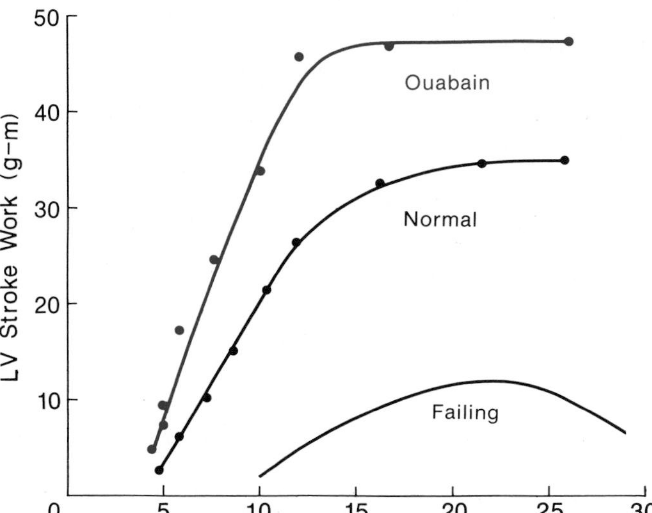

FIGURE 27–4. The effect of a digitalis glycoside (ouabain) on myocardial function obtained in a normal dog before and after administration of ouabain, 0.05 mg/kg. Left (L) atrial pressure was increased by infusion of blood into the atrium at appropriate rates. The curves labeled *normal* and *ouabain* were obtained experimentally. For comparison, a hypothetical curve for a failing heart has been added. Note that a reduction of atrial pressure from 30 to 10 cmH_2O would increase the work output of the failing heart. The glycoside, by increasing contractility of the heart, shifts the function curve, permitting greater work output at any given atrial pressure. (LV = left ventricle.) (Redrawn from Cotten MD, Stopp PE: Action of digitalis on the nonfailing heart of the dog. Am J Physiol 192:114, 1958.)

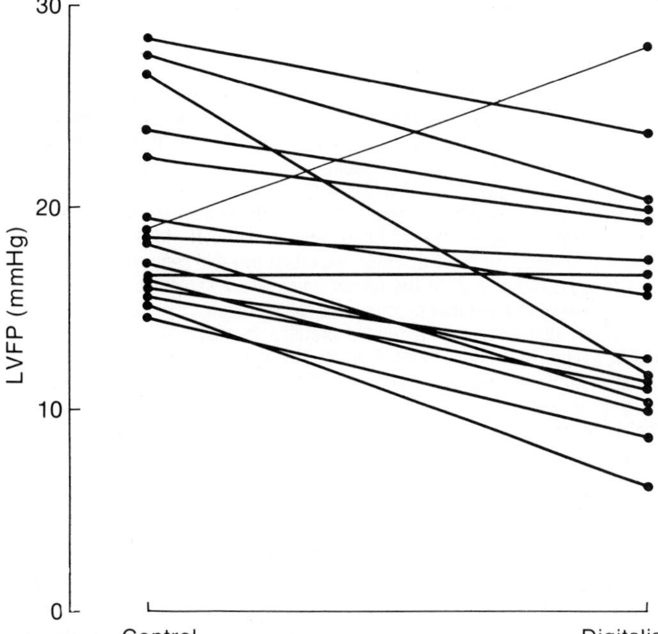

FIGURE 27–5. Effects of intravenous digitalis on left ventricular end-diastolic pressure (LVFP) in patients with acute myocardial infarction in whom the preglycoside LVFP was above normal (greater than 12 mmHg). All patients had congestive heart failure without cardiogenic shock. (Redrawn from Mason DT, Amsterdam EA, Lee G: Digitalis glycosides: Clinical pharmacology and therapeutics. *In* Mason DT [ed]: Congestive Heart Failure: Mechanism, Evaluation, and Treatment, 321. New York: Dun-Donnelley, 1976.)

of the arterial tree (below). When digitalis is given to an individual in congestive heart failure, the direct myocardial action increases the stroke volume and results in an increase in cardiac output, overcoming the peripheral vasoconstriction action on the arterial vessels. Digitalis induces a reflex decrease in sympathetic activity also, thus reducing afterload, increasing ventricular ejection, and decreasing venoconstriction.

Oxygen Consumption

Myocardial oxygen consumption is increased after digitalis because of the enhanced contractility. In the normal heart there is no change in the physical size of the heart, but wall tension is increased, resulting in increased energy and oxygen requirements. In the failing heart digitalis induces an increase in the stroke volume that results in a decrease in the size and wall tension of the myocardium. The consequence is a decrease in oxygen consumption that compensates for the increase in oxygen consumption associated with the digitalis-induced increase in myocardial contractility.

Postulated Cellular Explanation of Positive Inotropic Action

The positive inotropic action of digitalis results from its effects on the sodium/potassium-activated adenosine triphosphatase (ATPase) and the functional increase in the availability of calcium to the myocardial troponin-tropomyosin actomyosin system. Inhibition of the ATPase enzyme results in an inhibition of the Na^+ pump and results in an increase in the intracellular sodium concentration. This increase in intracellular sodium is thought to displace calcium from the sarcoplasmic reticulum and increase the concentration of intracellular calcium available for excitation-contraction coupling. The resultant increased calcium binding to troponin-tropomyosin activates the actomyosin system and increases myocardial contractility. The proposed mechanisms are shown in Figures 27–6 and 27–7 (see Smith [1988] for an in-depth discussion).

Electrophysiological Properties

Sinoatrial and Atrioventricular Nodes

In therapeutic concentrations, digitalis has little effect on the resting transmembrane potential. Nontoxic doses of digitalis exert their effects on cardiac rhythm primarily by modifying autonomic neural discharges that impinge on atrial and atrioventricular (AV) nodal tissues. Usually, these indirect actions of digitalis on the autonomic nervous system result in a decrease in the rate of impulse formation by the sinoatrial (SA) node.

On the other hand, toxic levels of digitalis may be associated with partial depolarization of SA nodal fibers, slowing or stopping the generation of action potentials. High concentrations also depress conduction of the impulses through the AV node by first decreasing conduction velocity and then increasing the effective refractory period. The conduction changes are associated with decreases in the maximal diastolic potential, in the rate of rise of the action potential, and in the amplitude of the action potential at the AV node.

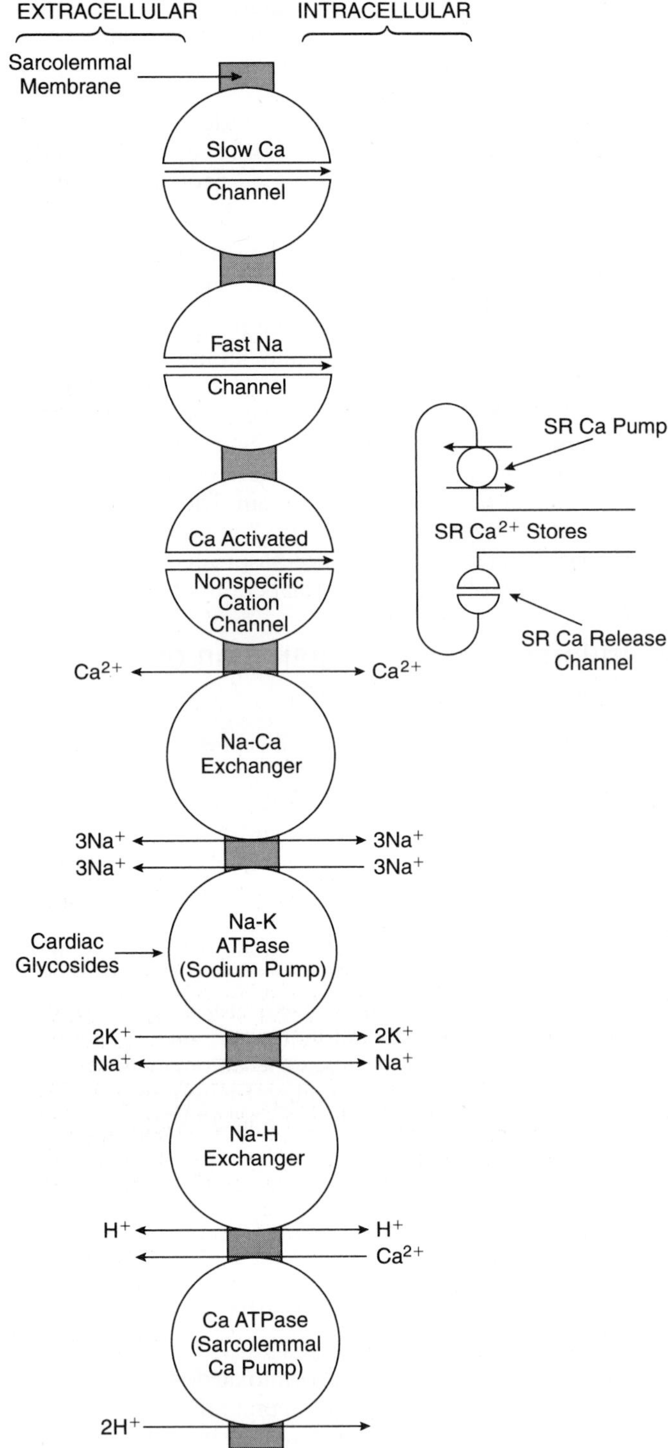

FIGURE 27–6. Selected components regulating cellular calcium homeostasis in myocardial membrane systems. (1) The slow calcium channel, a voltage-sensitive protein complex that carries the slow inward calcium current during Phase 2 of the cardiac action potential, provides the pulse of intracellular calcium (Ca^{+}) that triggers calcium-induced release of a much larger amount of activator calcium from stores in the sarcoplasmic reticulum (SR). The *arrow* indicates the principal direction of ion movement when the channel is activated. (2) The fast sodium channel, another voltage-sensitive structure, mediates the upstroke of the cardiac action potential; this depolarization event results in activation of the slow calcium channel. (3) A putative intracellular calcium-activated nonspecific cation channel, less well characterized than the preceding components (1 and 2), is thought to account for the transient depolarizing (and hence, arrhythmogenic) inward current that occurs in response to toxic doses of cardiac glycosides. (4) The sodium-calcium exchanger is a membrane component that mediates the facilitated, bidirectional exchange of sodium for calcium across the sarcolemmal membrane. This process is sensitive to membrane potential because of the asymmetry of charge movement inherent in the stoichiometry of the process (three sodium ions for every calcium ion). (5) The sodium pump (Na^{+}-K^{+} ATPase)—the cardiac glycoside-binding site—is located on the outward-facing surface of the alpha subunit of this enzyme, which mediates the active transport of sodium and potassium ions against their respective concentration gradients. (6) The sodium-hydrogen exchanger, an amiloride-sensitive protein, mediates the electroneutral exchange of sodium for hydrogen ions and helps to facilitate the accumulation of intracellular sodium (and hence, intracellular calcium) in response to cardiac glycosides. (7) The sarcolemmal calcium pump has a relatively low-capacity but high-affinity ATP-dependent ion-transport protein that extrudes calcium from cardiac cells against a large electrochemical gradient and helps to maintain the low levels of intracellular calcium ions that prevail during diastole. To the right of the sarcolemmal membrane are represented (8) the sarcoplasmic-reticulum ATP-dependent calcium pump that is responsible for diastolic relaxation by rapid sequestration of calcium at end systole, and (9) the ryanodine-sensitive sarcoplasmic-reticulum calcium-release channel that accounts for calcium-induced release of most of the calcium that activates contractile proteins in mammalian myocardium. (ATP = adenosine triphosphate.) (Reprinted by permission of *The New England Journal of Medicine*. Redrawn from Smith TW: Digitalis. Mechanisms of action and clinical use. N Engl J Med 318:358–365, 1988. ©1988 Massachusetts Medical Society.)

Atrial and Ventricular Muscle Fibers

After digitalis there is an increase in automaticity due to an enhanced Phase 4 depolarization and the generation of ectopic impulses due to the initiation of delayed after-depolarizations. The response in the specialized atrial fibers is similar to that observed experimentally in Purkinje fibers (below).

The duration of the action potential is moderately decreased after digitalis. Although this decrease is not marked, it is thought to explain the decrease in the QT interval in the electrocardiogram (ECG). Ventricular transmembrane action potentials exhibit an increase in the slope of the plateau and a decrease in the slope of Phase 3. These changes are associated with alterations in the ST segment and in the T wave.

High concentrations of digitalis decrease the resting potential and the amplitude of the action potential in both atrial and ventricular fibers and decrease the maximal rate of depolarization during Phase 0. As conduction velocity de-

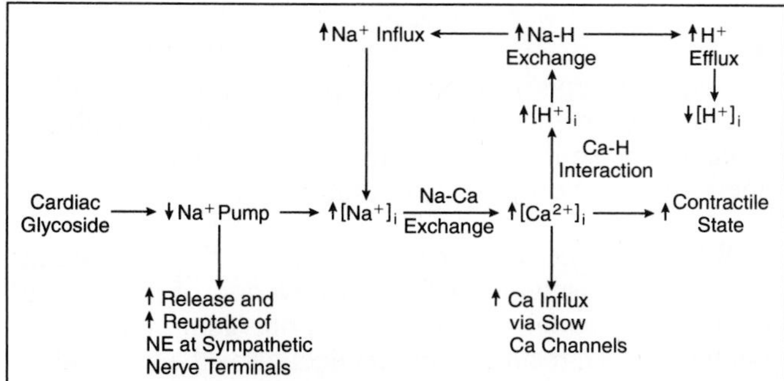

FIGURE 27–7. Mechanisms of modulation of myocardial function by cardiac glycosides. In addition to the horizontal sequence leading from cardiac glycoside-induced inhibition of the sodium-ion pump to enhanced myocardial contractile state, three ancillary processes are shown: enhanced norepinephrine (NE) release and reduced reuptake at cardiac sympathetic-nerve terminals, which may occur in experimental circumstances but have doubtful clinical relevance; an enhanced slow inward calcium current with increased calcium influx through slow calcium channels in response to an increased concentration of intracellular calcium ions over a limited range of values for these ions; and decreased intracellular pH (increased $[H^+]_i$) in response to increased intracellular calcium, leading to enhanced sodium-hydrogen exchange and hence, augmentation of the rise in intracellular sodium ($[Na^+]_i$) caused by sodium-pump inhibition. (Reprinted by permission of *The New England Journal of Medicine*. Redrawn from Smith TW: Digitalis. Mechanisms of action and clinical use. N Engl J Med 318:358–365, 1988.©1988 Massachusetts Medical Society.)

creases, inexcitability occurs (Fig. 27–8). Although depolarization in Phase 4 does not occur in atrial or ventricular muscle fibers, delayed after-depolarizations may develop.

Purkinje Fibers

Much of the experimental evidence used to explain the toxic effects of digitalis on the electrical activity of the heart is based on studies using Purkinje fibers. The time of exposure to the glycoside and the concentration used determine the effect on the transmembrane action potential and on the resting potential (Fig. 27–9). With low, but not high, rates of stimulation, a small increase in the action potential duration occurs with digitalis. This is followed by a decrease in the action potential duration due mostly to a shortening of the duration of the Phase 2 plateau; this change is associated generally with an increase in the slope of Phase 4 depolarization and a subsequent decrease in the resting potential or maximal diastolic potential and a further decrease in the action potential duration. Eventually, the maximal rate of rise of Phase 0 (V_{max}) and the amplitude of the action potential decrease; these changes may be due to the less negative resting potential or because Phase 4 depolarization causes the upstroke of the action potential (Phase 0) to start at a less negative potential.

With high levels of digitalis, V_{max} and conduction velocity decrease; eventually the Purkinje fibers become inexcitable.

The nature of the action of glycoside on Phase 4 depends on the concentration of extracellular potassium. Low concentrations of potassium generally cause an increase in the slope of Phase 4, resulting in increased automaticity. At high levels of potassium, the time course of the change in the membrane potential is altered and is associated with the appearance of "delayed after-depolarizations" (Fig. 27–10). "After-depolarizations" have been described either as a transient depolarization, initially subthreshold, early during

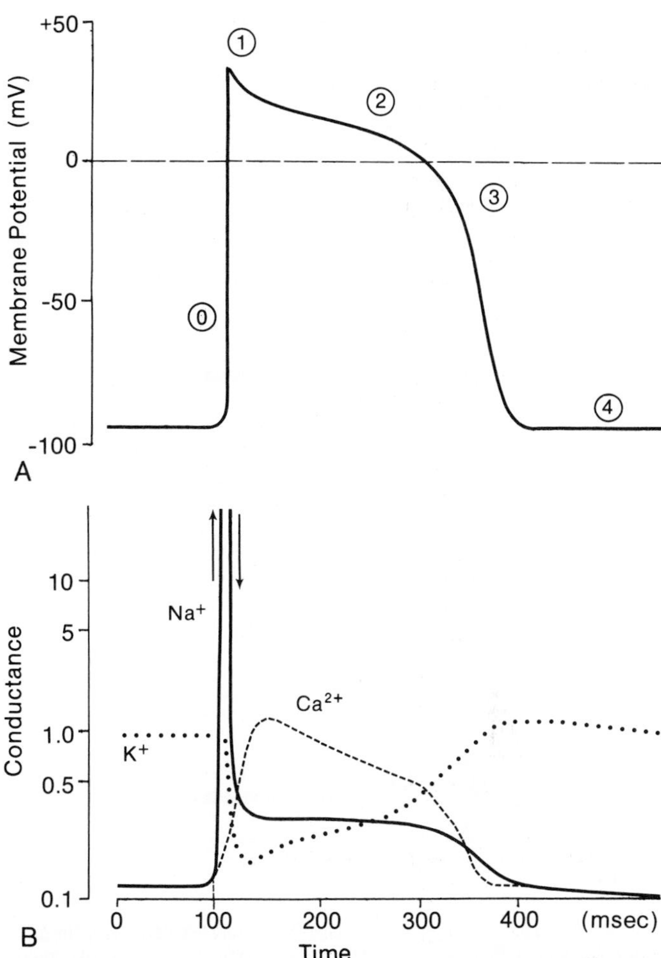

FIGURE 27–8. (*A*), A schematic diagram of a cardiac transmembrane action potential. Vertical axis is membrane potential in millivolts (mV). Cardiac cells have an electronegative resting membrane potential, which is maintained until a stimulus of sufficient magnitude occurs to lower the resting membrane potential to its threshold potential, which then results in an action potential. Phase 0, or rapid depolarization, results from a rapid influx of sodium into the intracellular space. This is followed by three phases of repolarization. The first (Phase 1) is a short rapid repolarization, followed by a plateau (Phase 2), and finally by a return to its resting membrane potential (Phase 3). (*B*), Ionic conductances (mmho/cm^2) for sodium (Na^+), potassium (K^+), and calcium (Ca^{2+}) during these phases.

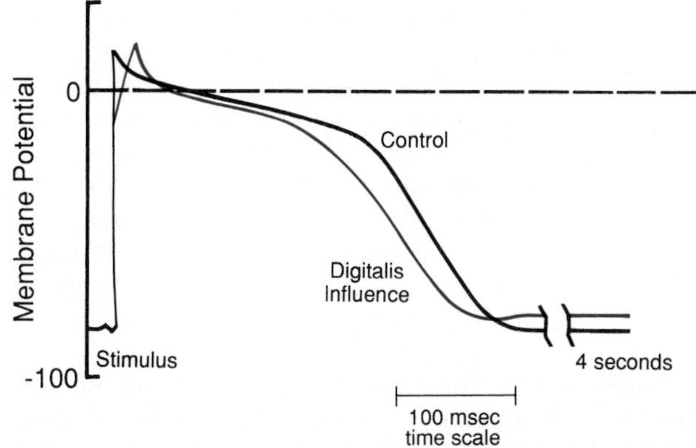

FIGURE 27–9. Effects of a digitalis glycoside (ouabain) on the cardiac action potential. The transmembrane potential was determined using conventional 3-M potassium chloride (KCl) intracellular microelectrodes. Although Phase 3 was accelerated by the glycoside, the maximal diastolic potential after repolarization was less than in the control. (Redrawn from Miura DS, Biedert S: Cellular mechanisms of digitalis action. J Clin Pharmacol 25:490–500, 1985.)

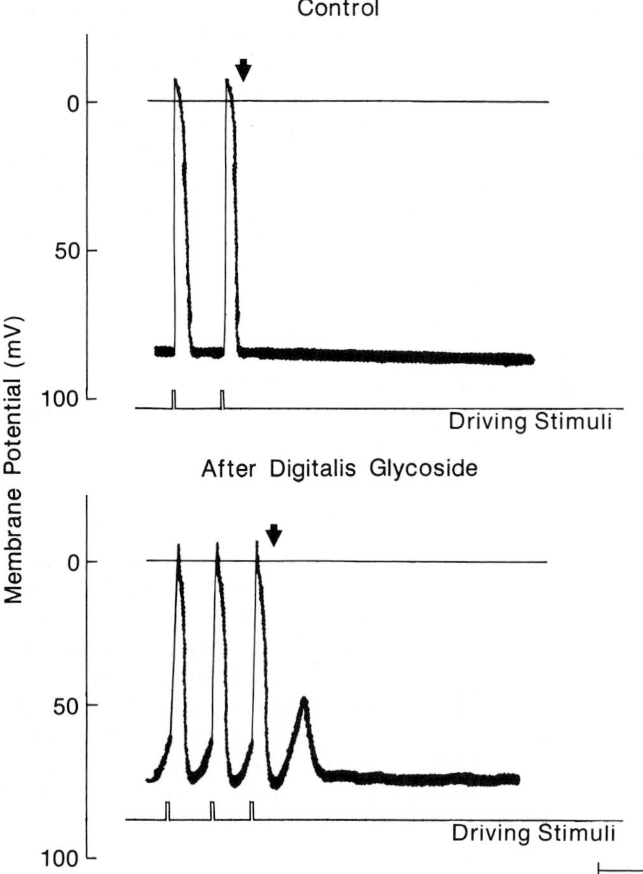

FIGURE 27–10. Digitalis-induced changes in Phase 4 depolarization. The *top panel* is the control Purkinje fiber superfused with Tyrode's solution. The drive stimuli are discontinued at the *arrows*, and electrical quiescence follows. The *bottom panel* was recorded after 35 minutes of superfusion with 2×10^{-7} M ouabain. Phase 4 depolarization is occurring, and discontinuation of the driving stimuli (*arrow*) is followed by a delayed after-depolarization and subsequent electrical quiescence. (Adapted from Rosen MR, Wit AL, Hoffman BF: Electrophysiology and pharmacology of cardiac arrhythmias. IV. Cardiac antiarrhythmic and toxic effects of digitalis. Am Heart J 89:391, 1975.)

Phase 4 or as a damped train of after-depolarizations. The amplitude of the after-depolarization increases as digitalis toxicity develops until the threshold for the initiation of an action potential is reached. At this point the delayed after-depolarization initiated by the extra response is also likely to reach the threshold, because the amplitude of the delayed after-depolarization increases as the interval between the action potentials decreases. Thus, digitalis can trigger ectopic beats by two different mechanisms: (1) the development of delayed after-depolarizations, and (2) the exaggeration of the normal depolarization that constitutes Phase 4.

The precise mechanisms and sequence of events underlying the effects of the glycosides on cardiac transmembrane potentials are complex and thus remain subjects of continuing research. The glycosides have no appreciable effect on the fast inward sodium current; thus, the other factors probably involved include, in this approximate sequence:

- Inhibition of sodium/potassium ATPase and increased duration of the action potential
- Increase in extracellular potassium locally
- Increased permeability to potassium
- Decrease in outward sodium current
- Modest decrease in resting membrane potential
- Increase in slope of diastolic depolarization (Phase 4)
- Small increase in conduction velocity associated with the small decrease in resting membrane potential
- Increase in action potential duration

With higher concentrations of digitalis, the decrease in pump activity results in additional lowering of the resting membrane potential, and both the potassium equilibrium potential and the resting potential decline as the extracellular potassium concentration increases. The internal sodium concentration increases the sodium equilibrium potential and prolongs the action potential amplitude decrease. The increase in the slow inward current shifts the action potential plateau to more positive potentials and prolongs the action potential duration. It is assumed that toward the end of the plateau the total outward current is increased enough to offset the change in the slow inward current, because the action potential actually becomes shortened; three contributory factors are thought to be involved:

1. An elevation of the internal calcium concentration speeds up the inactivation of the slow inward current and increases the outward current carried by potassium.
2. As the pump is further inhibited, the external potassium concentration increases even more during each action potential and thus speeds the onset of repolarization.
3. As toxicity develops, Phase 0 is depressed because of
   a. a greater loss of the resting potential and the voltage-dependent inactivation of the sodium channels;
   b. the greater increase in the internal sodium concentration; and
   c. the direct action of the glycoside to modify the voltage dependence of sodium channel inactivation.

Conduction velocity decreases because of the reduction in the excitatory currents associated with smaller than normal action potentials and because of the decrease in the extracellular spread of current produced by calcium at the gap junctions between cardiac fibers. The overall result of these changes is a reduction in the amount of cardiac tissue that can be excited by an action potential at any one time.

Multiple factors are involved in the complex cellular electrophysiological changes associated with arrhythmias induced by digitalis toxicity. Among these factors are the likelihood that different areas of the Purkinje and ventricular fibers respond differently, that is, the digitalis effects are not uniform over the heart. Moreover, the manifestations of the toxicity depend on the rate at which the fibers are stimulated. In addition, the effects vary with potassium and calcium concentration: an increase in external potassium concentrations inhibits the development of toxic effects; an increase in extracellular calcium facilitates the occurrence of toxicity. The increase in the extracellular potassium may reverse digitalis toxicity by stimulating the sodium/potassium ATPase-related membrane pump or by decreasing the binding of digitalis to the sodium/potassium ATPase enzyme.

Electrocardiographic

The primary effects on the ECG of therapeutic dosages and levels of digitalis are:

- PR interval prolongation
- QT shortening
- ST depression
- T-wave depression.

The effect of digitalis on the ST segment has been referred to as the hockey-stick appearance or as an inverted correction mark and may be quite characteristic, especially in the absence of pre-existing T-wave abnormalities (Fig. 27–11).

Organ/System Pharmacology

The Cardiovascular System

The effects of a digitalis glycoside are the result of multiple actions, including changes in the force of ventricular contraction, heart rate, vascular smooth muscles, reflex hemodynamic status, activity of the autonomic nervous system, and the presence or absence of congestive heart failure. Measurements of the effect of digitalis on arterial blood pressure, cardiac output, heart size, and end-diastolic and venous pressures vary with the presence or absence of anesthesia, exercise, and stress.

Blood Pressure

The intravenous (IV) injection of cardiac glycosides, especially aglycones, increases arterial pressure as a result of a direct vasoconstrictive action on peripheral vessels plus a central or reflexly induced increase in sympathetic nerve activity. The vasoconstriction that occurs through an action on the α-adrenergic receptors occurs in a dose-response fashion. Thus, an IV bolus dose may cause an immediate contraction of the smooth muscle vasculature through the direct action of the glycoside followed by a more prolonged vasoconstriction that can be blocked by α-blocking agents. In a normal individual, mean arterial blood pressure, systemic vascular resistance, and venomotor tone may be moderately increased and forearm blood flow decreased by glycosides. Patients with congestive heart failure respond with reduced peripheral resistance and vasomotor tone. Usually there is no increase in arterial pressure, although it may increase if there is an increased stroke volume.

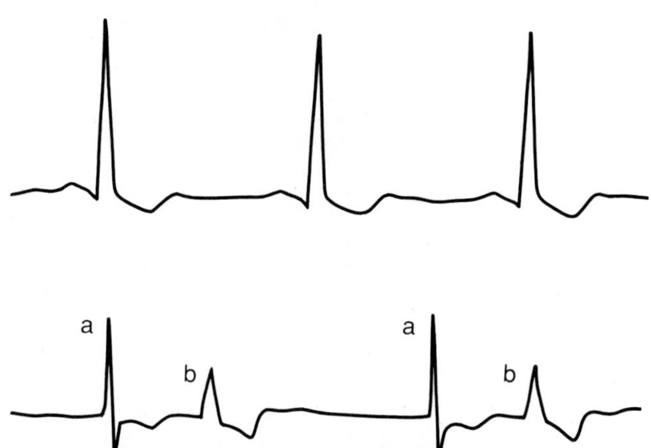

FIGURE 27–11. Electrocardiographic effects of digitalis glycoside. *Top tracing* has been copied from an electrocardiogram in a patient receiving digitalis, showing the typical "hockey-stick" appearance of the ST segment. *Bottom tracing* shows coupled ventricular extrasystole. (a = normal Q, R, and S wave complex; b = ventricular extrasystole.) (Redrawn from Joubert PH: Digitalis in clinical practice. S Afr Med J 50:146–152, 1976. This figure has been redrawn from the South African Medical Journal vol 50 dated 31 January 1976, with permission.)

Smooth Muscle of Veins

Digitalis acts directly on the smooth muscles of veins to induce constriction. This action is prominent in the hepatic veins and may cause venous pooling in portal vessels.

Heart

Contractility increases as a consequence of the direct positive inotropic action of digitalis. Heart rate may decrease moderately, stroke volume increase, and end-systolic ventricular volume decrease slightly. The increase in contractility is countered by the combined effect of increased systemic vascular resistance and decreased heart rate; thus cardiac output generally remains constant or decreases slightly. The decrease in the heart rate is primarily due to a reflex action mediated through arterial baroreceptors to the increase in arterial pressure.

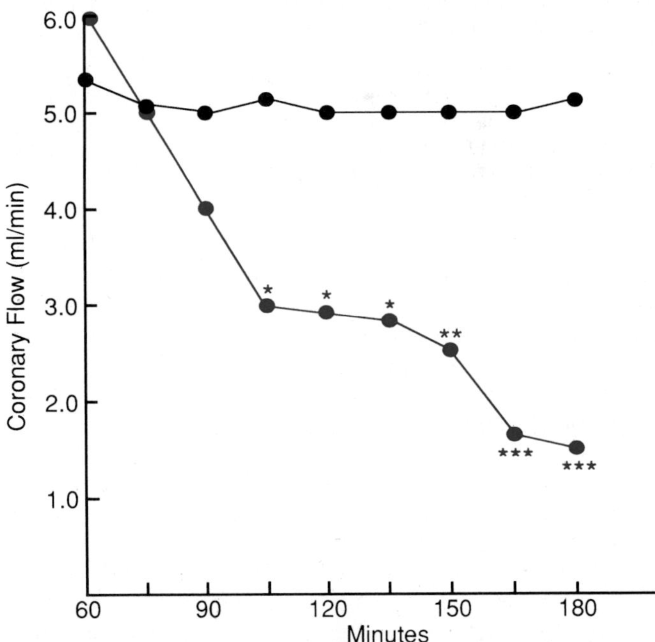

FIGURE 27–12. Effects of digitalis glycosides on flow in coronary vessels. Coronary flow (mL/min) was measured in isolated perfused guinea pig Langendorff's heart preparations. Hearts were equilibrated for the first 60 minutes following mounting. At 62 minutes, ouabain (1.37×10^{-6} M) was added to the reservoir bottle containing perfusing media. Untreated controls (n = 14) are shown in black; ouabain-treated hearts are in color. (*Single asterisk* represents p = 0.02; *double asterisk* represents p = 0.005; and *triple asterisk* represents p = 0.001.) (Redrawn from Tanz RD, Russell NJ, Banerian SP, Sharp VH: Ouabain-induced tachyarrhythmias and cell damage in isolated perfused guinea pig hearts. I. Protection by propranolol. J Mol Cell Cardiol 14:655, 1982.)

Coronary Circulation

Therapeutic dosages of digitalis induce little or no direct action on coronary circulation, but after toxic dosages coronary vessels are constricted with a decrease in coronary flow (Fig. 27-12). The autonomically mediated constriction is a dose-related effect that is centrally mediated and that can be blocked by α-blocking agents.

Adverse Effects

In 1785 Withering estimated the prevalence of digitalis toxicity to be 18-25%. In the 1970s reports suggested that it varied between 20 and 30%; the incidence reported in 1988 was lower, with a prevalence of 5-15%. The detection of digitalis toxicity is confounded by the fact that *digitalis serum levels in patients exhibiting good control of cardiac failure with no toxicity significantly overlap with those obtained in patients manifesting digitalis toxicity (Fig. 27-13). Thus, determining the serum level is important but insufficient; it is also essential to monitor the patient's electrocardiogram and clinical condition.*

Digitalis Toxicity

Digitalis toxicity induces arrhythmias through mechanisms involving both direct actions on the heart and through modifications of the neural activity of both divisions of the autonomic nervous system (Table 27-3).

The more common and most serious forms of digitalis toxicity are those related to alterations in cardiac rate and rhythm. Extrasystoles are the most common cardiac effect and generally originate in the ventricle (Table 27-4; Figs. 27-11 and 27-14; Table 27-5 summarizes the factors that may increase sensitivity and tolerance to digitalis). Bigeminy and pulsus trigeminus may develop. Younger patients, in particular, may exhibit sinus arrhythmia. Paroxysmal atrial or ventricular tachycardia may be observed. Although the occurrence is unusual, atrial flutter or atrial fibrillation may be associated in individuals with congestive heart failure who previously exhibited a normal sinus rhythm. Other arrhythmias associated with toxicity may include AV block, AV junctional tachycardia, pulsus alternans, and atrial standstill (Table 27-4). Death associated with digitalis toxicity is most often due to ventricular fibrillation.

CHANGES IN THE AUTONOMIC NERVOUS SYSTEM. After digitalis administration, activity in the vagus nerves to the heart increases, resulting in a slowing of the heart rate and the possible initiation of atrial fibrillation or AV block. Digitalis also alters the activity of the sympathetic nervous system. In the early stages of digitalis toxicity the discharge of the postganglionic cardiac sympathetic branches be-

TABLE 27-3. Mechanisms of Digitalis Toxicity

Site of Action of Digoxin	Toxic Electrophysiological Effect
Sinus node	Antiadrenergic, direct drug effect
Atrium	First-degree direct drug effect, increased automaticity, triggered activity
AV node	First-degree direct effect, cholinergic
Purkinje fibers and ventricular muscle	Increased automaticity, delayed after-depolarizations, reentry mechanism

Reprinted by permission of the Western Journal of Medicine. Bhatia SJS: Digitalis toxicity—Turning over a new leaf? West J Med 145:74-82, 1986.
AV = atrioventricular.

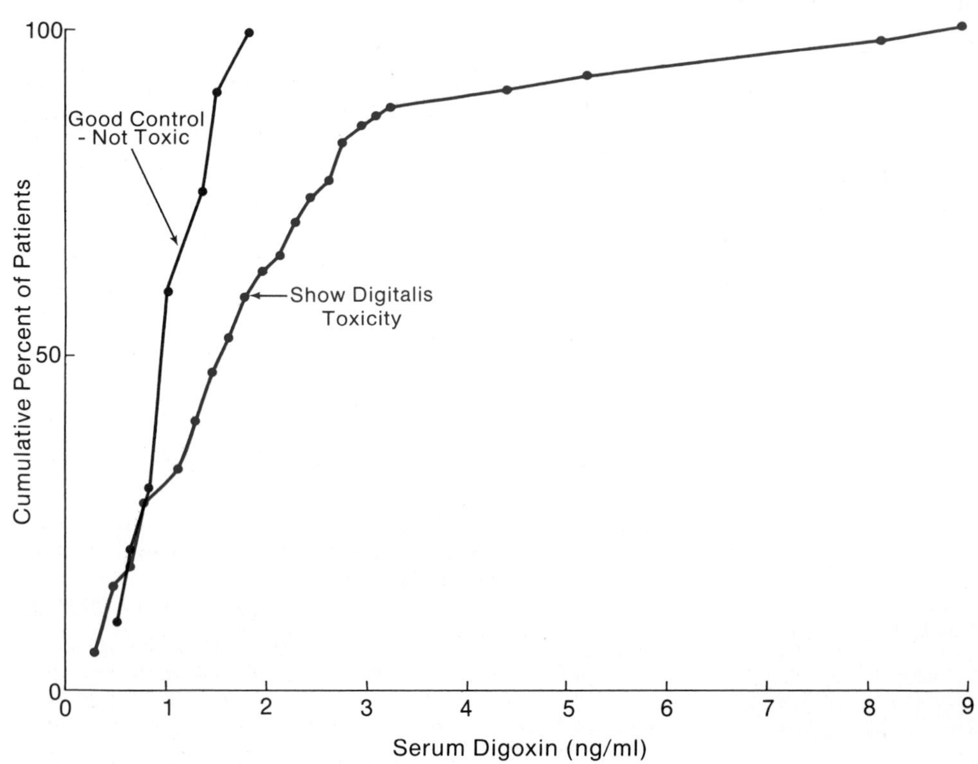

FIGURE 27-13. Relationships between serum digoxin level (abscissa) and digitalis toxicity (ordinate). The "good control—not toxic" curve is a plot of the cumulative percent of patients in good control of their congestive failure and their respective digoxin blood levels. The cumulative frequency plot of the blood levels of those patients who exhibited toxicity is on the right. Note that some patients exhibited toxicity even at very low levels of digoxin, whereas all those in good control without toxicity had levels below 2 ng/mL. (Data from Joubert PH: Digitalis in clinical practice. S Afr Med J 50:146-152, 1976.)

TABLE 27–4. Occurrence of Digitalis-Induced Arrhythmias ($n = 926$)

Type of Arrhythmias	N	Percent of All Arrhythmias*
Ventricular arrhythmias	567	62
Ventricular premature beats	481	
Ventricular tachycardia	85	
Ventricular fibrillation	1	
AV block	314	34
Atrial arrhythmias	248	27
Fibrillation, tachycardia, premature beats, flutter		
Junctional rhythms	138	15
SA arrhythmias	106	12
Tachycardia, bradycardia, arrest, block, wandering pacemaker		
AV dissociation	92	10

Adapted from Fisch C, Stone JM: *In* Fisch C, Surawicz B (eds): Digitalis, 162–173. Orlando: Grune & Stratton, 1969.

*The percentages add up to more than 100% because a given individual or study may have more than one type of arrhythmia.

AV = atrioventricular; SA = sinoatrial.

comes nonuniform, that is, activity in some fibers is increased while simultaneously there are decreases or no changes in others. These nonuniform discharges are probably the result of glycoside action at multiple sites within the adrenergic nervous system (pre- and postganglionic fibers, the postganglionic adrenergic nerve terminal, adrenal catecholamines, baroreceptors, and the central nervous system [CNS], including brain stem regions of the area postrema and the nucleus tractus solitarius). The nonuniform neural discharge imposes a nonuniform increase in excitability within the various parts of the myocardium, predisposing it to the development of arrhythmias. As toxicity progresses, an enhanced sympathetic cardiac discharge contributes to the maintenance of arrhythmias; agents such as reserpine, guanethidine, or bretylium that prevent the actions of the adrenergic neural discharge on the heart can protect against arrhythmias induced by digitalis (see Chapter 28).

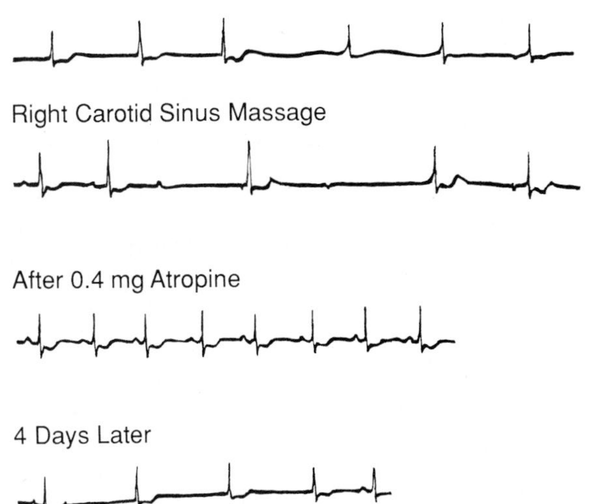

FIGURE 27–14. Electrocardiogram of a 17-year-old female after she attempted to commit suicide by ingesting 3.0–4.0 mg (30–40 tablets) of digitoxin. The *upper strips*, recorded on the day of ingestion, demonstrate depression of sinoatrial (S-A) node activity and supraventricular rate after right carotid sinus massage. The *next strip*, recorded on the same day, shows regular sinus rhythm with a rate of 90 beats/minute and a normal PR interval after intravenous administration of 0.4 mg of atropine sulfate. *Bottom strip*, recorded 4 days after digitoxin ingestion, demonstrates persistent depression of S-A node activity and supraventricular escape complexes. (From Surawicz B, Mortelmans S: Factors affecting individual tolerance to digitalis. *In* Fisch C, Surawicz B [eds]: Digitalis, 127–147. Orlando, FL: Grune & Stratton, 1969.)

TABLE 27–5. Factors Affecting Myocardial Tolerance to Digitalis

Possible Reasons for Increased Sensitivity	Possible Reasons for Increased Tolerance
Cardiac	
Increased automaticity of ectopic pacemakers	Decreased automaticity of ectopic pacemakers
Heart disease*	High potassium*
Heart surgery*	Antiarrhythmic drugs†
Low potassium*	Vagal stimulation
Chronic lung disease	Decreased vagal or increased sympathetic activity
Catecholamines and sympathetic stimulation†	Fever, infection, hypoxia
Impaired SA function and AV conduction	Hyperthyroidism*
Increased vagal activity	Normal infants and young children
Decreased sympathetic activity	Decreased absorption or unusual losses
Heart disease*	Malabsorption
Heart surgery*	Dialysis (?)
Low potassium*	Cardiac bypass (?)
High potassium	
Low magnesium	
Impaired degradation or excretion	
Hypothyroidism*	
Renal disease*	
Liver disease	
Premature infants*	
Old age	
Interaction with drugs	
Extracardiac	
Allergy and hypersensitivity	
CNS disorders, such as CVAs	
Low body weight	

Adapted from Surawicz B: Factors affecting tolerance to digitalis. Reprinted with permission from the American College of Cardiology (Journal of the American College of Cardiology, vol 5, 1985, 69A–81A).

*Factors that appear to be of greatest practical importance.

†Variable effects.

AV = atrioventricular; CNS = central nervous system; CVA = cerebrovascular accident; SA = sinoatrial node.

DIRECT CARDIAC TOXICITY. The ventricular arrhythmias induced by digitalis are the result of the impaired automaticity and the lowered membrane potential at pacemaker sites, plus the slower conduction through such sites and along Purkinje fibers. The presence of both slowed conduction and increased automaticity may result in potentially lethal ventricular fibrillation.

Agents such as manganese and verapamil that block the calcium current through the slow channels decrease or eliminate digitalis-induced arrhythmias. It has been suggested that the loss of potassium, due to inhibition of sodium/potassium ATPase, may be the basis of digitalis toxicity consistent with the fact that potassium may be antagonistic to digitalis

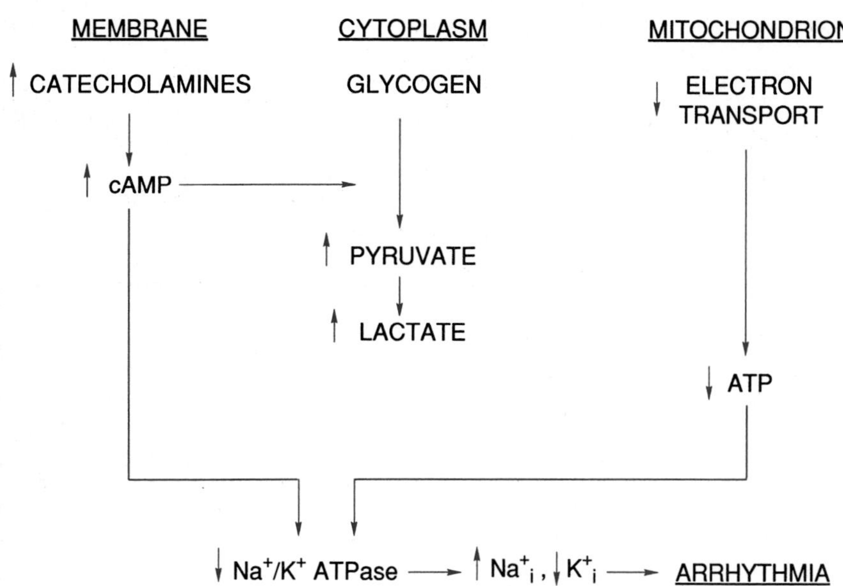

FIGURE 27–15. Proposed mechanism(s) whereby digitalis-induced coronary constriction may contribute to the formation of toxic arrhythmias. (ATP = adenosine triphosphate; cAMP = cyclic AMP; Na^+/K^+ ATPase = sodium pump.) (From Tanz RD: Possible contribution of digitalis-induced coronary constriction to toxicity. Am Heart J 111:812–817, 1985.)

intoxication, especially if serum potassium is low. Low levels of potassium enhance oscillating after-potentials whereas high levels reduce the calcium-induced after-potentials. Thus, the ionic movement of both potassium and calcium is involved in digitalis-induced toxicity.

Coronary Constriction and Toxicity

Figure 27–15 depicts a suggested contribution of digitalis-induced coronary constriction to digitalis toxicity. The resultant ischemia/hypoxia induces a number of changes that may ultimately result in an arrhythmia.

Central Nervous System

EYE. Digitalis toxicity includes a variety of visual disturbances including blurred vision, white borders or a halo around dark objects, transitory amblyopia, and changes in color vision. The last most often includes chromatopsia for yellow and green but occasionally for red, brown, and blue. Data obtained in human subjects indicate that differences in the pharmacokinetic parameters of digitalis preparations may influence the degree to which these agents produce visual disturbances. The error scores in color vision testing increased as the digitalis glycoside plasma levels increased (Table 27–6). It was suggested that these differences among glycosides may be due to the higher uptake of some glycosides into the retina or to a difference in the concentration of the glycoside within the retina. Of the three glycosides, digoxin would be present in the retina in the highest concentration. Nevertheless, patient complaints of disturbed or yellow vision, or actual tests thereof, provide another warning sign of possible toxicity.

BRAIN. Patients intoxicated with digitalis may complain of headache, fatigue, malaise, and drowsiness. These complaints are often noted in the early stages of intoxication. *Mental confusion and disorientation generally precede the more serious signs of cardiac toxicity and they are a significant hazard, all too frequently unrecognized, in the elderly.*

GASTROINTESTINAL. *In some, but not all, patients the earliest symptoms of digitalis overdosage include anorexia, nausea, and vomiting due to a central action on the chemoreceptor trigger zone.* Anorexia is usually observed first, followed several days later by episodes of nausea and vomiting that may begin and end abruptly and then recur with greater severity. Other reported gastrointestinal (GI) effects include diarrhea and abdominal discomfort or pain that subside several days after the digitalis glycoside is discontinued.

TABLE 27–6. Frequencies of Error Scores in Color Vision

Drug	Plasma Digitalis Level		Volume (L)	Extent of Plasma
	Therapeutic	*Toxic*	Distribution	Protein Binding (%)
Digoxin	17/28	5/5	840	10–25
Digitoxin	0/13	7/13	38	86
Acetyldigitoxin	0/8	3/8	57.5	81–90

From Haustein KO, Oltmanns G, Rietbrock N, Aiken RG: Differences in color vision impairment caused by digoxin, digitoxin, or pengitoxin. J Cardiovasc Pharmacol 4:536–541, 1982.

Management of Patients Exhibiting Digitalis Toxicity

As noted earlier, the diagnosis of digitalis intoxication cannot be made solely on the basis of glycoside plasma levels, because a great overlap exists among the levels associated with toxic and nontoxic conditions (Fig. 27–13). Management includes:

- ECG to monitor digitalis-induced toxicity
- Determination of plasma potassium level—and repeat (low potassium levels enhance the likelihood of intoxication, Table 27-5); maintain level of 4 mEq/L
- Discontinuation of digitalis and of diuretics
- Reversal of myocardial ischemia
- Monitoring magnesium levels and acid-base balance
- Administration of antiarrhythmics for ventricular arrhythmias (phenytoin, lidocaine, procainamide, or propranolol may be effective but can make heart block worse, Table 27-7)
- Possible use of temporary pacemaker
- Administration of atropine for sinus bradycardia, SA arrest, or second- or third-degree heart block
- Using Fab fragments of anti-digoxin antibodies, DIGIBIND (Kelly and Smith, 1992)

If IV potassium is given, the ECG must be monitored frequently and plasma potassium levels measured before and after the administration of potassium. The use of potassium may be dangerous if the patient has AV block because potassium depresses AV conduction, an action synergistic with that of digitalis. Also, if the administration of potassium results in hyperkalemia, this will have a direct depressant action on AV conduction, contribute to the initiation of arrhythmias, and may produce complete AV block and cardiac arrest. The administration of potassium may also mask warning signals normally detected by the occurrence of less ominous arrhythmias; thus, lethal arrhythmias such as ventricular fibrillation may occur with no initial warning change in the ECG.

Cardioversion is used infrequently in digitalis toxicity because fatal ventricular fibrillation may develop in the presence of digitalis-induced arrhythmia. Defibrillation is frequently unsuccessful because the myocardium is extremely irritable. In this situation, IV amiodarone has been used (see Chapter 28).

In life-threatening digitalis toxicity, the monoclonal digoxin-specific antibodies, Fab fragments, may be administered. Digoxin has a greater affinity for the antibody and thus binds to the Fab fragment rather than binding to the sodium/potassium ATPase receptor. Thus, digoxin is removed from the receptor site, enters the general circulation, and is readily excreted. Antibodies to the Fab fragments have not been detected in serum, and hemodynamic instability does not develop. The use of the digoxin-specific antibodies reverses its positive inotropic action and eliminates its toxic effects on Purkinje fibers and the AV node. Once the Fab fragments have been used, it is necessary to re-establish therapeutic effects by retitrating the patient with digitalis.

CLINICAL USES

BOX 27-1
THERAPEUTIC USES

The clinical uses for digitalis are changing with the advent of newer pharmacological agents that are less likely to initiate life-threatening toxicity (Smith, 1988; Antman and Smith, 1989; Gheorghiade, 1992). Digitalis therapy is appropriate in carefully selected patients with one or more of the following:

- Congestive heart failure complicated by arrhythmias such as atrial fibrillation, atrial flutter, and atrial and AV nodal paroxysmal tachycardia
- Dilated, failing hearts and impaired systolic function, often manifested as S_3 gallop
- Management of supraventricular arrhythmias

Digitalis is not generally used for patients with elevated filling pressures due to reduced ventricular compliance but with preserved systolic function at rest, unless supraventricular tachycardia is a concomitant problem.

Congestive Heart Failure

The most common therapeutic use for digitalis glycosides is in the management of heart failure complicated by supra-

TABLE 27-7. Potential Uses and Toxicity of Second-Line Drugs for Digoxin Toxicity

Drug	May Increase AV Block	May Increase Ventricular Ectopy	Negative Inotropic Effect	Potential Indications
Procainamide hydrochloride or quinidine	Yes	No	Yes	Ventricular ectopy, ventricular tachycardia, atrial tachycardia with block, AVT
β blockers	Yes	No	Yes	Ventricular ectopy, ventricular tachycardia, atrial tachycardia with block
Verapamil	Yes	No	Yes	Atrial tachycardia with block, AVT, ventricular ectopy, ventricular tachycardia
Amiodarone	Yes	No	Yes	Ventricular tachycardia (refractory dysrhythmia)
Isoproterenol	No	Yes	No	Bradycardia (refractory dysrhythmia)
Bretylium tosylate	No	Yes	No	Ventricular tachycardia, ventricular fibrillation (refractory dysrhythmia)

Reprinted by permission of the Western Journal of Medicine. Bhatia SJS: Digitalis toxicity—Turning over a new leaf? West J Med 145:74-82, 1986.
AV = atrioventricular; AVT = nonparoxysmal atrioventricular junctional tachycardia.

ventricular tachyarrhythmias such as atrial fibrillation. The management of congestive heart failure is designed to decrease sodium and water intake and reduce the work of the heart; it employs such pharmacological agents as digitalis, diuretics, vasodilators, and catecholamines.

Patients with mild heart failure may be treated acutely with synthetic catecholamines and diuretics. Mild heart failure may respond to digitalis. Moderately severe heart failure may respond to digitalis and a diuretic.

Some patients, such as those exhibiting advanced ischemic heart disease, may not respond to this regimen or may become refractory to treatment. Moreover, patients with heart failure due to valvular, coronary artery, or congenital heart disease, even if corrected surgically, may continue to have severe disorders of contractility.

USE OF VASODILATORS AND ANGIOTENSIN-CONVERTING ENZYME INHIBITORS. Treatment of symptomatic patients with dilated ventricles and impaired contractile function should undergo correction of abnormalities of preload with vasodilators acting on the venous bed as well as with diuretics. Vasodilators reduce arteriolar resistance and improve ventricular emptying; such vasodilators include the *ACE inhibitors captopril and enalapril.* These agents serve as adjuncts to diuretics and digitalis in the management of congestive heart failure in those with impaired systolic function. One-year survival of patients with heart failure improved by 38% with a combination of hydralazine and isosorbide dinitrate and by 31% with enalapril and placebo (CONSENSUS Trial, 1986).

One advantage of the combination of an ACE inhibitor with a diuretic, but no digoxin, is that hypokalemia and ventricular arrhythmias occur less frequently. Unfortunately, one disadvantage of this combination is that hypotension and impaired renal function may develop. In contrast, digitalis glycosides tend to improve renal perfusion.

WHEN CAN DIGITALIS BE DISCONTINUED? The use of digitalis in the treatment of chronic heart failure is complicated by the fact that it is not possible to predict which patients may safely have their digoxin discontinued despite continuation of diuretic therapy. It is known that digitalis exhibits a long-term inotropic action in those with a normal sinus rhythm. The withdrawal of digoxin was associated with clinical deterioration in many patients. However, some studies have concluded that chronic digoxin therapy is of no clinical benefit, because substitution of a placebo for 3 months was not associated with clinical deterioration. Thus, the identification of patients with chronic failure in whom digitalis may safely be discontinued is the critical issue. Gradual, cautious discontinuation of digitalis should be seriously considered if:

- The digitalis was initially given to treat acute heart failure associated with myocardial infarctions, pneumonia, or surgery-induced failure and clinical signs of failure have not reappeared.
- Failure was due primarily to diastolic dysfunction because digitalis is not likely to induce an improvement in patients with failure in the presence of a normal left ventricular ejection fraction.
- Heart failure is not present and history is vague regarding prior symptoms.

FOR MYOCARDIAL INFARCTION. The use of digitalis in patients with myocardial infarction is controversial. Digoxin has been shown to produce a minimal but significant improvement in the ejection fraction without compromising left ventricular perfusion or regional wall motion. However, the benefit of the digitalis-induced increase in contractility may be offset by the resulting bulging of the infarcted and ischemic myocardium. Furthermore, the digoxin-induced increase in peripheral resistance may produce an increase in the afterload, which may counter the inotropic action. Different responses to digitalis may result in different patients with infarctions due to the fact that the overall hemodynamic response is a result of several factors: the direct inotropic action on the myocardium; the consequence of the inotropic action on nonresponsive myocardium; and the variable action on systemic vascular resistance. Pulmonary edema may occur as a result of the increased systemic vascular resistance due to the direct arteriolar vasoconstriction. In any event, it is generally held that digitalis should not be used in the patient with infarction if there is no evidence of heart failure.

Cardiogenic Shock

Although digitalis may be used in patients with a normal rhythm and cardiogenic shock due to myocardial infarction, it generally is not because it increases the force of contraction in both normal and hypoxic myocardial tissue.

Antiarrhythmic Actions

SUPRAVENTRICULAR ARRHYTHMIAS. Digitalis is often used to manage supraventricular arrhythmias including paroxysmal atrial tachycardia and atrial flutter, and to shift the atrial or AV junctional tachycardia to a normal sinus rhythm, primarily through its effects to increase cholinergic neural activity.

SLOWING OF VENTRICULAR RATE IN ATRIAL FIBRILLATION OR FLUTTER. Digoxin has been a mainstay of therapy for rate control in the treatment of all varieties of atrial fibrillation, including paroxysmal, chronic, acute, and postoperative (Sarter and Marchlinski, 1992). However, it is less effective than the calcium antagonists or β blockers with respect to AV nodal blockade. Digoxin induces a positive inotropic action whereas the other classes of agents suppress left ventricular function. Consequently, digoxin is the drug of choice when treating atrial fibrillation in the setting of significant left ventricular dysfunction.

Digitalis also controls ventricular rhythm in patients exhibiting atrial flutter or fibrillation by an indirect autonomic effect that slows conduction and prolongs the effective refractory period in the AV node; sometimes the atrial flutter or fibrillation is converted to normal sinus rhythm. When this occurs it is most likely that the underlying congestive heart failure with atrial load has initiated the arrhythmias.

Premature atrial contractions may be suppressed. In general digitalis does not exhibit an antiarrhythmic action in the ventricles; this is predictable because there is no significant vagal innervation of the conducting system in the ventricles.

In recent years, verapamil (Chapter 28) has replaced digoxin as the drug of choice in the immediate management of paroxysmal reentrant supraventricular tachyarrhythmia.

Digoxin has an ancillary role, particularly in patients with impaired ventricular function. Verapamil or diltiazem and beta-adrenergic-blocking agents are used to slow, in an additive manner, the ventricular response in patients with atrial fibrillation or atrial flutter with a rapid ventricular response. In addition, electrical cardioversion is effective in abolishing a variety of tachyarrhythmias, and other antiarrhythmic agents and implantable devices offer alternatives or supplements to digoxin use.

EFFECT OF AGE ON THE ACTION OF DIGITALIS GLYCOSIDES

Pediatric Patients

BOX 27-2

THERAPEUTIC ASPECTS

Oral or parenteral digoxin controls congestive heart failure or arrhythmias in children. The feeding schedule does not appear to complicate the absorption of digoxin from the GI tract. However, drug administration should be at times other than just before or after feeding because regurgitation or vomiting may cause unpredictable loss of drug. Although digoxin is used to manage infants and children, IV *lanatoside C* is often used for rapid digitalization, because the rapid onset of action and time to peak effect are similar to those of digoxin. The use of the intravenous route with digoxin in an emergency situation has the advantage of allowing a smoother transition to parenteral or oral maintenance dosages of digoxin after the emergency situation has been controlled. It is more difficult to make the transition to digoxin maintenance after initial IV lanatoside C because it is excreted more rapidly than digoxin and is marketed only in a parenteral dosing form.

Premature and immature infants require lower dosages of digoxin because of decreased renal function. The dosage regimen must be individualized according to the degree of maturity of the infant. (For a detailed description of dosage regimens for the premature newborn, the full-term neonate, infants, and children, see Wettrell and Andersson, 1986.)

Adverse Effects

With digitalis intoxication pediatric patients may exhibit seizures, coma, and respiratory arrest, yet the ECG may reveal only rather innocuous changes. Visual disturbances similar to those observed in adults have been reported.

Infants often manifest changes in AV conduction and atrial ectopic beats and may demonstrate paroxysmal atrial tachycardia with a variable ventricular response. Rarely do ventricular ectopic beats and tachyarrhythmias occur. Sinus slowing, with a rate less than 100 beats/minute due to increased vagal activity, may develop in premature and newborn infants. Vomiting should be taken as a warning of possible digitalis toxicity.

Geriatric Patients

BOX 27-3

THERAPEUTIC ASPECTS

The geriatric population in general has reduced renal function, necessitating a reduction in the dosage of digoxin. Patients on digitalis entering a nursing home may also receive a diuretic or potassium supplement, or both; *thus, they must be followed and examined regularly to ensure the maintenance of a therapeutic level and to avoid the occurrence of unrecognized toxicity, such as gradually increasing dementia.* Blood levels of digoxin and metabolites after a single dose have been reported to be almost twice as high in the geriatric patient as in younger patients; correspondingly, the digoxin half-life can be 50% greater in the elderly than in younger adults.

Toxic Effects

The elderly patient often takes several other drugs in addition to digitalis, so the possibility of adverse drug interactions with both prescription and over-the-counter preparations must be considered. Digitalis toxicity may develop in the geriatric patient given dosages of digoxin that are well tolerated in younger patients. Suggested explanations for this effect include an age-induced increase in myocardial sensitivity to the normal dosages, higher myocardial levels, hypokalemia due to diuretic or laxative use, a smaller body size, or decreased renal function resulting in an increased half-life for plasma levels of digitalis.

Drug Interactions (see Chapters 50 and 58)

The single most frequent cause of digitalis toxicity arises from the concomitant use of digitalis and diuretics that cause the loss of potassium; these include thiazide diuretics, ethacrynic acid, furosemide, bumetanide, and acetazolamide. (Diuretics that do not cause the loss of potassium include spironolactone, triamterene, and amiloride.)

The concomitant use of digoxin and quinidine increases serum digoxin levels in more than 90% of patients. The average serum increase is twofold, with a range from zero to sixfold. The increase in digoxin levels is due to a decrease in renal and nonrenal clearance and in the volume of distribution. Some digoxin is thought to be displaced from working myocardial-binding sites, but not from Purkinje fibers. The major portion of increased digoxin originates from nonspecific binding sites in skeletal muscle.

Current clinical approaches to the quinidine-digoxin interaction vary, although most physicians lower the amount of digoxin given when quinidine is started and then follow this with a plasma digoxin level within 24 to 48 hours; the follow-up digoxin dosage is adjusted on the basis of the level. When digoxin is used to control the ventricular response in atrial fibrillation, the reduction of the ventricular rate is used as a clinical guide.

The simultaneous use of digoxin and the calcium channel blockers is associated with variable effects on the digoxin levels. In more than 90% of patients, verapamil increases the digoxin levels by decreasing its clearance and, possibly, its volume of distribution. Nifedipine does not appear to alter the digoxin levels, whereas diltiazem induces a small increase. In general, the dosage of digoxin does not need to be adjusted when calcium channel blockers are administered concurrently.

The use of digoxin and *amiodarone* increases the digoxin level twofold by decreasing clearance; the volume of distribution is not altered. Signs of digoxin toxicity may appear as the plasma digoxin levels increase. In general, the dosage of digoxin is not reduced when amiodarone therapy is started.

Spironolactone inhibits active tubular digoxin secretion, causing an increase in plasma digoxin levels. Likewise, antihypertensive agents may decrease renal blood flow and glomerular flow rate to increase the digoxin serum concentrations.

BOX 27-4

ABSORPTION OF DIGOXIN—REDUCED BY:

Antacids, bran, kaolin pectate, cholestyramine resin, cholestipol hydrochloride, activated charcoal, sulfasalazine, neomycin, para-aminosalicylic acid, anticholinergic drugs, metoclopramide, cathartics, cytotoxic agents, and drugs that increase intestinal motility

(If given concomitantly with digoxin and then stopped, dosage of digoxin should be decreased to avoid toxicity.)

NEW DEVELOPMENTS

Since 1785 when William Withering first recognized the benefit of digitalis, it has been the therapeutic basis for the treatment of congestive heart failure. This role has been questioned recently because its action on left ventricular end-diastolic pressure and cardiac output may be modest or of little value. Studies have yet to demonstrate that overall cardiac performance, that is, left ventricular filling pressure and cardiac output, is improved, even though ventricular contractility is consistently improved. Ongoing research is attempting to develop better inotropic agents. The effort to develop a chronically and orally administrable agent to replace or supplement digitalis has been disappointing (Leier, 1992).

Much effort has been invested in the development of newer inotropic agents that possess a better therapeutic index than digitalis. The *phosphodiesterase III inhibitors amrinone, milrinone, and enoximone* are examples of newer positive inotropic agents that have recently been evaluated. Amrinone (INOCOR) is currently available only as an injectable and has been used in the critical care setting for the short-term treatment of patients with severe congestive heart failure who are refractory to cardiac glycosides and diuretics. It has been used also as supportive therapy in coronary bypass and surgical transplant patients. Clinical trials have now shown that the phosphodiesterase III inhibitors offer variable effectiveness, a serious adverse effect profile, and do not improve clinical status or exercise capacity beyond that achieved by digoxin when given long term, either separately or in combination with digoxin (Leier, 1992). Moreover, repeated administration of milrinone is associated with increased mortality. Thus, these agents are not currently generating the clinical use that had been anticipated.

Investigational agents have been developed to "sensitize" the contractile apparatus to calcium and to act in very precise sites of actions. These agents include *forskolin* (directly stimulates sarcolemmal adenylate cyclase to bypass the β-adrenergic receptor in the generation of cyclic adenosine monophosphate [AMP] and thus may not be susceptible to β-adrenergic receptor down-regulation), as well as agents that sensitize the contractile apparatus to calcium or that enhance myocardial contractility by phosphodiesterase inhibition, increasing intracellular sodium ions and enhancing opening of Ca channels.

In the early 1980s digoxin immunoreactivity was noted in dog and human plasma and urine even though no digoxin had ever been administered. This factor has been termed *endoxin* because it is an endogenous substance that binds to digoxin antibodies. This postulated hormone can cross react in digoxin immunoassays, inhibit Na^+/K^+-ATPase, and cause natriuresis and diuresis. A cardiac glycoside inhibitory site has been detected on Na/K-ATPase in species spanning the phylogenetic spectrum from earth-worms to humans, suggesting that an endogenous ligand exists and may have a specific biological function, perhaps as a regulatory substance in the nervous system. Thus the search for endogenous ligands with digitalislike properties is ongoing (Haddy, 1987).

REFERENCES

Antman EM, Smith TW: Current concepts in the use of digitalis. Adv Intern Med 34:425-454, 1989.

Baker DW, Koustam MA, Bottorff M, Pitt B: Management of heart failure: 1. Pharmacologic treatment. JAMA 272:1361-1366, 1994.

Bigger JT: Digitalis toxicity. J Clin Pharmacol 25:514-521, 1985.

The Captopril-Digoxin Multicenter Research Group. JAMA 259:539, 1988.

CONSENSUS Trial Study Group: Effects of vasodilator therapy on mortality in chronic congestive heart failure: Results of a Veterans Administration Cooperative Study. N Engl J Med 314:1547-1552, 1986.

Drugs for chronic heart failure. Med Lett 35:40-42, 1993.

Gheorghiade M (ed): A symposium: Management of heart failure in the 1990s: Assessment of the role of digoxin therapy. Am J Cardiol 69:1G-154G, 1992.

Haddy FJ: Endogenous digitalis-like factor or factors. N Engl J Med 316:621-623, 1987.

Haustein KO, Oltmanns G, Rietbrock N, Aiken RG: Differences in color vision impairment caused by digoxin, digitoxin, or pengitoxin. J Cardiovasc Pharmacol 4:536-541, 1982.

Kelly RA, Smith TW: Recognition and management of digitalis toxicity. Am J Cardiol 69:108G-119G, 1992.

Lathers CM, Kelliher GJ, Roberts J, Beasley AB: Nonuniform cardiac sympathetic nerve discharge: Mechanism for coronary occlusion and digitalis-induced arrhythmia. Circulation 57:1058-1065, 1978.

Lathers CM, Lipka LJ, Klions HA: Controversies in the actions of digitalis substances: Are all digitalis derivatives alike? J Clin Pharmacol 25:501-506, 1985.

Lathers CM, Lipka LJ, Klions HA: Digitalis glycosides: A discussion of the similarities and differences in actions and existing controversies. Rev Clin Basic Pharm 7:1-108, 1988.

Lathers CM, Roberts J: Digitalis toxicity revisited. Life Sci 27:1713-1733, 1980.

Lathers CM, Roberts J, Kelliher GJ: Correlation of ouabain-induced arrhythmia and nonuniformity in the histamine-evoked discharge of cardiac sympathetic nerves. J Pharmacol Exp Ther 203:467-479, 1977.

Leier CV: Current status of non-digitalis positive inotropic drugs. Am J Cardiol 69:120G-129G, 1992.

Lewis RP: Clinical use of serum digoxin concentrations. Am J Cardiol 69:97G-107G, 1992.

Newman TJ, Maskin CS, Dennick LG, et al: Effects of captopril on survival in patients with heart failure. Am J Med 84(Suppl 3A):140-144, 1988.

Roberts J, Kelliher GJ, Lathers CM: Minireview. Role of adrenergic influences in digitalis-induced ventricular arrhythmia. Life Sci 18:665-678, 1976.

Sarter BH, Marchlinski FE: Redefining the role of digoxin in the treatment of atrial fibrillation. Am J Cardiol 69:71G-81G, 1992.

Smith TW: Digitalis. Mechanisms of action and clinical use. New Engl J Med 318:358-365, 1988.

Smith TW (ed): Digitalis Glycosides, 1-348. Orlando: Grune and Stratton, 1986.

Smith TW, Butler VP Jr, Haber E, et al: Treatment of life-threatening digitalis intoxication with digoxin-specific Fab fragments; experience in 26 cases. N Engl J Med 307:1357-1362, 1982.

Soldin SJ: Digoxin — Issues and controversies. Clin Chem 32:5-12, 1986.

Wettrell G, Andersson KE: Cardiovascular drugs II: Digoxin. Ther Drug Monit 8:129-139, 1986.

Withering W: An account of the Foxglove and some of its medicinal uses with practical remarks on dropsy and other diseases. Printed by M Swinney for GGJ and J Robinson, London/Birmingham, 1785.

28 Drugs for Cardiac Arrhythmias

Claire M. Lathers

A variety of pharmacological agents with differing mechanisms of action have been discovered that can aid in restoring the physiological rhythm of the heart. This chapter provides the foundation for understanding the clinical use of current as well as new drugs when they are introduced. Nevertheless, the drugs currently available rarely restore the heart to its fully normal condition. Because none of the agents that are discussed repair the diseased state, the objective is a change of the disturbed rhythm to one that has an improved functional capability. However, the antiarrhythmic drugs may themselves cause life-threatening arrhythmias, as well as a variety of mild to severe central nervous system (CNS), dermatological, gastrointestinal, and hematological side effects (Sun et al, 1994).

CLASSIFICATION OF ANTIARRHYTHMIC AGENTS: A GUIDE FOR THEIR CLINICAL USE

In view of the different actions on the heart of the numerous antiarrhythmic agents, attempts have been made to classify them into rational and clinically useful groups. In 1970 Vaughn Williams published a four-part classification for antiarrhythmic drugs (Table 28–1). Although this classification has received recent minor challenges (Working Group, 1991) it remains generally useful. In addition to the four classes, Harrison (1986) subdivided class I agents into three subcategories (Table 28–2). When referring to these classifications, three points need to be remembered.

1. Drugs are placed in these categories based on their predominant electrophysiological actions, and the classification may not entirely encompass all the mechanisms involved in a given drug's antiarrhythmic effects.
2. Drugs within a class do differ, so that one may be effective in a given patient whereas another drug in the same class may not produce a therapeutic action. Furthermore, drugs included within the same class do not necessarily share the same clinical indications nor do they necessarily share common side effects, especially those that have an extracardiac site of origin. Thus, it cannot be categorically stated that because a given patient has "this type of arrhythmia" that a particular drug or class must be used.
3. The presence of heart disease and arrhythmias may, in turn, modify a drug's antiarrhythmic effects because of the changed actions on ischemic myocardium, altered metabolism, hemodynamics, or on the central and autonomic nervous systems.

TABLE 28–1. Vaughn Williams Classification of Antiarrhythmic Drugs

Class	Actions	Prototype Agent
I	Inhibits Na^+ transport Reduces dV/dt* of phase 0	Quinidine
II	β-adrenergic receptor blockade	Propranolol
III	Prolongs repolarization Alters membrane response	Amiodarone
IV	Calcium channel blockade	Verapamil

From Harrison D: Current classification of antiarrhythmic drugs. Drugs 31:93–95, 1986.

*dV/dt expresses the change in membrane potential as a function of time, *ie*, dV/dt is the rate of rise of action potential. V_{max} is the maximum rate of depolarization, *ie*, the rise in the action potential.

TABLE 28–2. Harrison Modification of Class I Antiarrhythmic Agents

Class	Actions	Agents
IA	Slow dV/dt* of phase 0; moderate prolongation of repolarization; prolong PR, QRS, and QT intervals	Quinidine, procainamide, disopyramide
IB	Limited effect on dV/dt of phase 0; shorten repolarization; shorten QT in clinical dosages; elevate fibrillation thresholds	Lidocaine, tocainide, mexiletine
IC	Markedly slow dV/dt; little effect on repolarization; markedly prolong PR and QRS on ECG	Flecainide

Adapted from Harrison D: Current classification of antiarrhythmic drugs. Drugs 31:93–95, 1986.

*See Table 28–1 for a description of dV/dt.

ECG = electrocardiogram.

Class I Antiarrhythmic Agents—Sodium Channel Blockers

(Tables 28–1 and 28–2)

The Class I antiarrhythmic agents act on receptors in the cardiac sodium channels to reduce sodium entry during cardiac membrane depolarization, decrease the rate of rise of phase 0 of the cardiac action potential, necessitate a greater or more negative membrane potential to allow propagation to adjacent cells (ie, increase threshold), increase the repolarization time, decrease conduction velocity, prolong the effective refractory period of fast response fibers, and decrease automaticity. In general, higher plasma concentrations, that is, higher than those levels usually employed clinically, of class I agents exhibit local anesthetic actions and depress myocardial contractility. Class I drugs suppress normal automaticity in Purkinje fibers and the His bundle and abnormal automaticity in damaged myocardial tissue. Abnormal automaticity is suppressed selectively, allowing the SA node to become or remain the driving pacemaker.

More specifically, although **class IA drugs (quinidine, procainamide, disopyramide,** with quinidine being the prototype drug) do alter conduction velocities and dV/dt (V_{max}), they exhibit relatively more pronounced effects on the absolute and effective refractory periods of Purkinje and ventricular tissue.

The class IA agents are clinically effective in the treatment of atrial and ventricular arrhythmias.

Drugs included in **class IB (lidocaine, phenytoin, tocainide, and mexiletine)** exert little effect on conduction velocities and may improve refractoriness, especially in ischemic areas. They also elevate the threshold for the appearance of fibrillation.

Agents in the **IC class (flecainide)** have a profound effect on His-Purkinje conduction in normal and abnormal myocardium and exhibit a mild to moderate effect on refractoriness.

Electrophysiological observations of the voltage and rate dependency of drug action suggest that classification of class I agents may be based also on the time constants for inactivating Na^+ channels in the cell membrane and on the recovery time once the channels are inactivated. The kinetics

CLASS IA

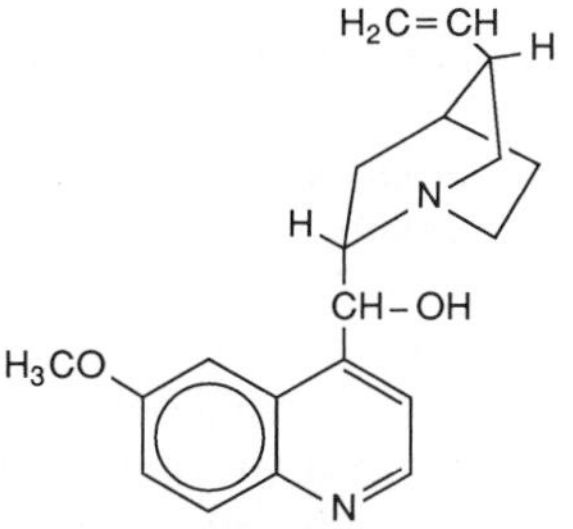

Quinidine

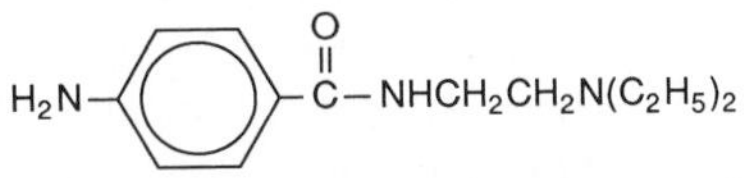

Procainamide: $H_2N-C_6H_4-C(=O)-NHCH_2CH_2N(C_2H_5)_2$

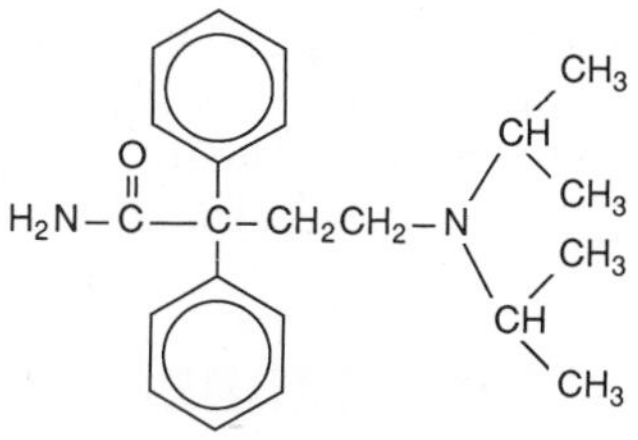

Disopyramide

CLASS IB

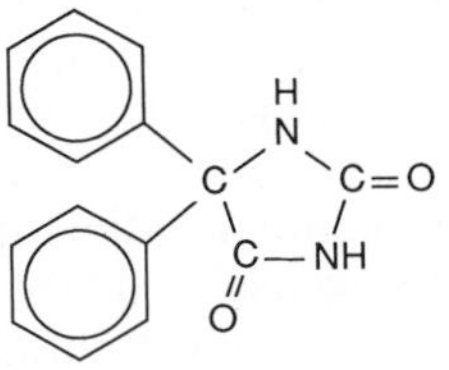

Phenytoin

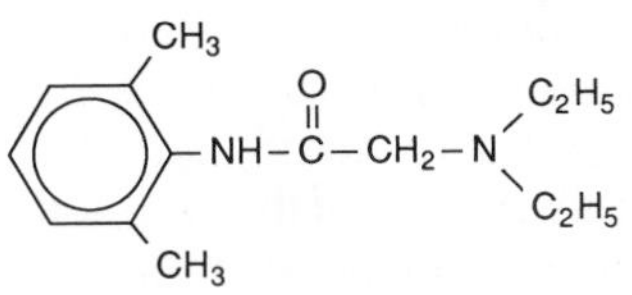

Lidocaine

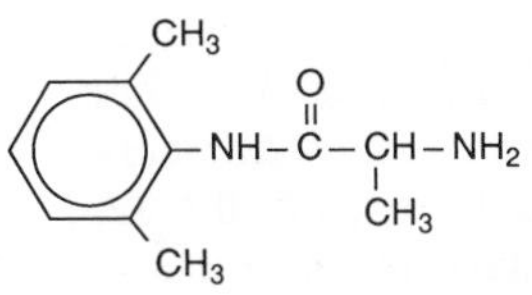

Tocainide

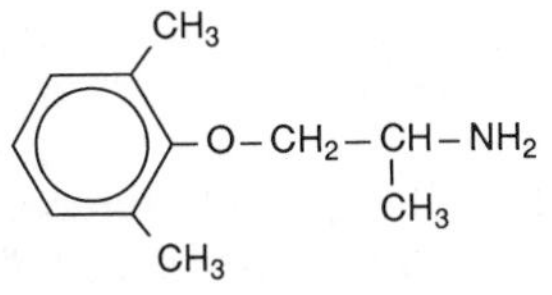

Mexiletine

CLASS IC

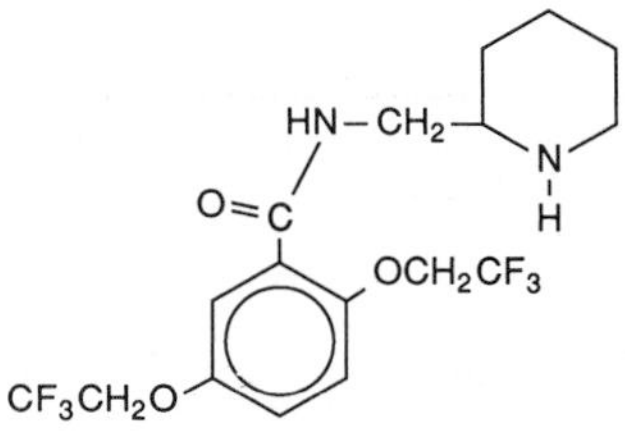

Flecainide

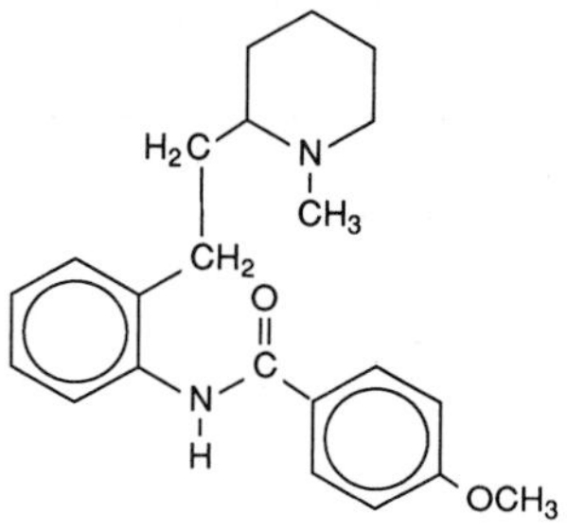

Encainide

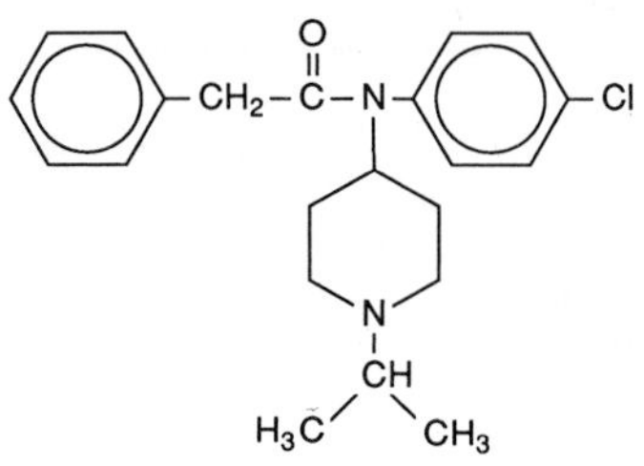

Lorcainide

of the speed of onset of rate-dependent depression of the maximal rate of depolarization (V_{max}) and the action potential duration allow three subgroups to be formed with titles of fast (lidocaine, tocainide, and mexiletine), intermediate (quinidine, disopyramide, and procainamide), and slow (flecainide and encainide) kinetics (Harrison, 1986). This classification is consistent with the IB, IA, and IC subgroups of Vaughn Williams (1992a,b).

Class II Antiarrhythmic Agents—Beta-Adrenergic Blocking Agents

Propranolol is a prototype drug in this class. These agents competitively block β adrenoceptors and inhibit catecholamine-induced stimulation of cardiac β receptors (see Chapter 10). Some class II drugs—propranolol and acebutolol—also produce electrophysiological changes in Purkinje fibers that are similar to those produced by class I agents. Labetalol blocks both α and β adrenoceptors.

Sotalol is a β-blocking agent that possesses electrophysiological actions similar to drugs in class III; thus, it may be categorized as both a class II and a class III agent. The dual actions of sotalol support the concept that the β-blocking property of class II agents may not be the sole mechanism underlying their antiarrhythmic action.

Class III Agents—Sotalol, Bretylium, and Amiodarone

Each of these agents *prolongs the duration of the cardiac action potential* without changing phase 0 of depolarization or the resting membrane potential as well as alters the function of sympathetic innervation of the heart. (Sotalol is a β-blocking agent and as such also possesses class II actions.)

Class IV—Calcium Channel Blockers (see Chapter 32)

These agents block the slow inward calcium current occurring during phases 0 to 2 of the cardiac action potential. Their greatest effects are exerted on slow-response cardiac action potentials in the sinus and AV nodes. They decrease conduction velocity and increase refractoriness in the AV node; thus, conduction of supraventricular impulses through the AV node to the ventricle is decreased.

Combination Therapy

The design of combination antiarrhythmic therapy is possible using this classification. Patients unable to tolerate high dosages of some antiarrhythmic agents may respond to a combination of lower dosages of drugs from different subgroups to produce additive electrophysiological effects while decreasing unwanted side effects. Thus, a combination of a drug from classes IA and IB may induce a maximal decrease in the likelihood of fibrillation while inducing minimal prolongation of repolarization or alteration in the refractoriness.

The combination of drugs in classes IA and IC is contraindicated because of a high incidence of heart block or impaired intraventricular conduction.

CLASS IA ANTIARRHYTHMIC AGENTS

General Characteristics

The class IA drugs contain some of the oldest antiarrhythmics, but their attributes are valuable enough that they are still widely used, and new class IA agents are being developed. Class IA agents are used in the treatment of atrial and ventricular arrhythmias.

Quinidine

Quinidine is effective for prophylaxis against atrial fibrillation and for the treatment of atrial and ventricular premature contractions and of ventricular tachycardia. (Drugs of current choice are discussed in the following sections and in Table 28-3.)

ACTIONS. Quinidine works by two separate mechanisms: a direct action of the drug on myocardial cells, and through its indirect anticholinergic actions (atropinelike). This dual mechanism of action is a characteristic of all the antiarrhythmic agents in this class.

Effects on the SA Node and Atrial Myocardium. The effect of normal vagal nerve activity on the SA node is blocked by quinidine, resulting in an increased rate of depolarization in the cells of the SA node. In opposition to these effects, quinidine acts directly on atrial myocardium, including the specialized cells of the SA node, to decrease excitability and membrane responsiveness. These actions result in an increase in the threshold for excitation (*ie*, a larger stimulus is

TABLE 28–3. Drugs of Choice for the Management of Arrhythmias

Arrhythmia	Acute: First Line	Acute: Alternatives	Chronic: First Line	Chronic: Alternatives
Atrial premature beats	Usually no treatment		Quinidine	Disopyramide Procainamide
Atrial flutter/fibrillation	Cardioversion Verapamil	Verapamil Propranolol Class IA	Verapamil, diltiazem	Amiodarone Digitalis ± quinidine
Paroxysmal atrial tachycardia	Verapamil	Digitalis Propranolol	Digitalis Verapamil	Quinidine Amiodarone
AV nodal tachycardias	Verapamil	Diltiazem Adenosine	Digitalis or propranolol or esmolol	Verapamil Class IA, IC, II
Ventricular premature beats	Class II (β blocker)	Procainamide Quinidine Disopyramide	Class II	Procainamide Disopyramide Amiodarone
Ventricular tachycardia	Cardioversion Lidocaine	Procainamide Disopyramide Quinidine Bretylium	Sotalol Procainamide or disopyramide or quinidine	Amiodarone Flecainide Propranolol Mexiletine

AV = atrioventricular.

required to cause excitation); a decrease in V_{max} (because it relates directly to conduction velocity); and an increase in the effective refractory period. The direct effects on the atrial tissue result in a decreased rate of SA node action potentials, but the net effect on the SA node is negligible; there may occasionally be a slight increase in the rate. The atrial tissue has a net decreased conduction velocity and increased refractory period. Automaticity is reduced throughout the atrial tissues, making quinidine effective in relieving atrial tachyarrhythmias.

AV Node. The actions of quinidine on the AV node are due to its anticholinergic actions; because the AV node is normally under tonic vagal influence, the atropinelike effects of quinidine increase AV nodal conduction. For this reason quinidine is not used alone in treating atrial arrhythmias with fast rates, because increasing the AV nodal conduction would increase the ventricular rate to possibly dangerously high levels. This problem is overcome by prior treatment with digitalis (digitalization), which counters the AV nodal effects of quinidine. (The direct effects of quinidine on the AV node are just the opposite of its anticholinergic actions. The direct effects include an increase in the effective refractory period and a decrease in the conduction velocity.)

Ventricular Myocardium and Specialized Conduction Tissue. All the effects of quinidine on the ventricles are accounted for by the direct effects of the drug: decreased automaticity; decreased conduction velocity; and increased effective refractory period. Automaticity is decreased as evidenced by a decrease in the slope of phase 4 depolarization.

By decreasing conduction velocity and increasing the refractory period, unidirectional blocks of conduction are converted to two-way or bidirectional blocks, thus abolishing reentry loops.

Another action of quinidine that affects both the atria and the ventricle has been termed postrepolarization refractoriness, probably a consequence of the failure of the sodium fast-gate channel to reset itself after the membrane potential has returned to the resting level.

Electrocardiographic Changes. The PR, QRS, and QT intervals are increased. The PR interval, which reflects the speed of the action potentials through the AV node and represents the sum of three processes, is lengthened with quinidine administration. The second process, the AV node delay, is decreased. The third process, the His-Purkinje interval, increases after quinidine.

The QRS interval represents the time needed for depolarization of the ventricles. Its increase in duration following quinidine administration is dose-dependent and provides a good measure of therapeutic effects. The QT interval is lengthened more with quinidine than with any of the other class IA agents. Lengthening of the QT interval represents a slowing of the repolarization of the ventricles. (Nevertheless, an abnormally lengthened QT interval is an ominous sign because it is a sign of quinidine toxicity and is sometimes followed by a rhythm known as torsades de pointes, a dangerous arrhythmia that can lead to ventricular fibrillation and death; Table 28–4.)

ACTIONS ON OTHER ORGAN SYSTEMS. The antimalarial and antipyretic properties of quinine, although retained in quinidine, are not of clinical relevance. The anticholinergic effects of quinidine on the AV node are not confined to the heart inasmuch as it blocks the effects of vagal stimulation or acetylcholine. Quinidine also has substantial α-adrenergic blocking activity, which leads to a significant hypotension when administered intravenously (IV). The combination of the cholinergic blockade and the relative increase in β-adrenergic activity can increase the sinus rate and enhance AV nodal conduction in some patients. It is for this reason, and because there is increased risk of toxicity, that quinidine is seldom given IV.

TIME COURSE OF ACTION—PHARMACOKINETICS. Quinidine is well-absorbed when taken orally (Table 28–5). Approximately 70–95% of the drug is bound by albumin,

TABLE 28–4. Effects and Toxicities of Antiarrhythmic Agents

Drug	Electrophysiological Effects				Hemodynamic Properties	Toxicity
	Automaticity	*APD*	*ERP*	*QRS*		
CLASS IA						
Quinidine	−	+	+	+	Negative inotropism Vasodilation Hypotension	Impaired conduction/asystole Ventricular arrhythmias GI intolerance Cinchonism Thrombocytopenia Drug fever
Procainamide	−	+	0, +	+	Negative inotropism Vasodilation Hypotension	Impaired conduction and ventricular arrhythmias Nausea, vomiting Agranulocytosis Drug-induced systemic lupus erythematosus
Disopyramide	−	+	+	+	Negative inotropism Vasodilation Hypotension AV block	Anticholinergic effects: dry mouth, constipation, urinary retention, blurred vision, psychosis Ventricular arrhythmias Agranulocytosis
CLASS IB						
Lidocaine	−	−	+	0	No impairment of normal contractility Bradycardia	Drowsiness, coma Respiratory arrest Convulsions Heart block
Phenytoin	−	−	0, −	0	Hypotension and altered heart rate	Nystagmus, ataxia Lethargy GI intolerance Gingival hyperplasia Hirsutism
Mexiletine	−	−	0, +	0	Prolonged conduction Bradycardia Hypotension Cardiac depression	CNS: psychosis, convulsions GI: nausea and vomiting Dermatological: photosensitive dermatitis Hepatitis, blood dyscrasias
CLASS IC						
Flecainide	−	−	0	+	Arrhythmias Chest pain Bradycardia Heart failure	Neurological: dizziness, visual impairment, headache, tremor, paraesthesia GI: nausea, constipation, diarrhea, abdominal pain Asthenia, fatigue
Propafenone	−	−	0	+	Bradycardia Arrhythmias	Dizziness, lightheadedness GI upset, bronchospasm
Moricizine	−	−	0	+	Bradycardia Ventricular tachycardia	Dizziness, headache GI upset
CLASS II						
Propranolol	0, −	0, −	0, +	0	Negative inotropism Hypotension Heart failure	Impaired AV conduction/asystole Bronchospasm Nightmares, insomnia
Acebutolol	−	−	0, +	0	Hypotension Bradycardia	Arthralgia, lupus syndrome Bronchospasm Pulmonary syndrome
Esmolol	−	−	0, +	0	Bradycardia Hypotension Heart block	Bronchospasm Pain at infusion site
Sotalol	−	+	0	0	Hypotension Bradycardia Heart blood Torsades de pointes	Bronchospasm Fatigue, arrhythmias
CLASS III						
Bretylium	0, +	+	0	0	Bradycardia Hypotension Torsades de pointes	GI intolerance Parotid swelling
Amiodarone	−	+	+	0	No impairment of normal contractility Hypotension and increased coronary blood flow on IV administration Bradycardia Arrhythmias	Photosensitivity Pigmentation Thyroid function abnormalities Corneal microdeposits Pulmonary fibrosis

TABLE 28–4. Effects and Toxicities of Antiarrhythmic Agents *Continued*

Drug	Electrophysiological Effects				Hemodynamic Properties	Toxicity
	Automaticity	*APD*	*ERP*	*QRS*		
CLASS IV						
Verapamil	—		+	0	Negative inotropism Vasodilation Hypotension	Impaired conduction/asystole GI intolerance Constipation

Adapted from Siddoway LA, Roden DM, Woosley RL: Clinical pharmacology of old and new antiarrhythmic drugs. *In* Josephson ME (ed): Sudden Cardiac Death. Brest AN (ed-in-chief): Cardiovasc Clin 15:199–248, 1985; and Muhidden KA, Turner P: Is there an ideal antiarrhythmic drug? A review with particular reference to Class I antiarrhythmic agents. Postgrad Med J 61:665–677, 1985; Sotalol for cardiac arrhythmias. Med Lett 35:27–28, 1993.

APD = action potential duration; AV = atrioventricular; CNS = central nervous system; ERP = effective refractory period; GI = gastrointestinal; IV = intravenous; — = decreased; + = increased; 0 = no change.

other plasma proteins, and hemoglobin in erythrocytes principally in the uncharged state. The chief elimination route of quinidine is through metabolism in the liver and elimination through the kidneys, although up to 20% of the parent drug may be eliminated directly through the kidney. Most of the urinary metabolites are hydroxylated at a single site on the quinoline ring or on the quinuclidine ring. Some metabolite is in the form of the dihydroxy compound. The therapeutic blood level of quinidine is well-established (2–4 μg/mL), although slightly higher levels are sometimes necessary; clinical signs of toxicity occur at levels of approximately 8 μg/mL. The pharmacokinetics of the major antiarrhythmics are compared in Table 28–5.

BOX 28–1
THERAPEUTIC USES

Quinidine is used primarily to suppress ventricular ectopic areas and to prevent these areas from causing paroxysmal ventricular tachycardia. It may be used for the maintenance of a regular sinus rhythm after atrial fibrillation has been converted, and although no longer indicated for this purpose, it alone may convert atrial fibrillation. Further, quinidine may be used to prevent the development of paroxysmal supraventricular tachycardia. However, in the AV nodal form of paroxysmal supraventricular tachycardia, digitalis is tried usually before quinidine because of the significant toxicity of quinidine. (Although the actions of quinidine and procainamide are similar, quinidine is generally preferred for long-term therapy because of a drug-induced lupus syndrome that can develop with procainamide.)

EFFECT OF AGE ON PHARMACOKINETIC PARAMETERS. Liver disease significantly increases the half-life of the drug, as would be expected; the effect of renal disease on quinidine levels is less clear (Table 28–6). It appears that the normal decrease in renal function that accompanies aging should be accompanied by a decrease in the dosage. However, in states of decreased renal function, including congestive heart failure, there is little change in the quinidine levels. Some of the metabolites of quinidine are thought to be cardioactive.

ADVERSE EFFECTS, DRUG INTERACTIONS, AND CONTRAINDICATIONS (Table 28–4). The adverse effects of quinidine therapy involve the gastrointestinal (GI) system, CNS, immune-mediated responses, cardiac toxicity, and interactions with other drugs. The GI side effects of quinidine can occur after usual therapeutic dosages; these include nausea, vomiting, diarrhea, vague abdominal pain, and loss of appetite.

A unique complex of side effects associated with toxicity of both quinidine and quinine has received a specific name, **cinchonism**. It is particularly likely to appear after rapid administration or large doses; headaches, tinnitus, visual disturbances, and vertigo characterize cinchonism. The symptoms of cinchonism are so characteristic that every physician should be able to recognize them in a patient being treated with quinidine and should suspect intoxication when they appear. Toxicity may be associated also with diplopia, photophobia, altered color perception, confusion, hallucinations, and delirium. Immune-mediated responses are less common with quinidine than with procainamide, but they do occur and include blood dyscrasias, rashes, fevers, and rarely, anaphylactoid reactions. A hypersensitivity response mounted against quinine is active against quinidine also.

The cardiac toxicity of quinidine has already been mentioned, including the potentially fatal rhythm of torsades de pointes, myasthenia gravis can be aggravated by the actions of quinidine at the neuromuscular junction.

Quinidine interacts with many drugs; only a few are presented here (see also Chapter 50). Quinidine directly displaces digoxin from its binding sites on the heart and perhaps sites in skeletal muscles; there is also a reduction in the renal clearance of digoxin. Consequently, the dose of digoxin can be reduced by as much as 50% when administered with quinidine. Thus, if a full dose of quinidine is given to a chronically digitalized patient, serious and even life-threatening arrhythmias can occur. Also, if a patient is already toxic to digoxin and presents with arrhythmia for which quinidine would otherwise be given, it is dangerous to use quinidine as the antiarrhythmic agent.

The anticoagulant warfarin is displaced from its plasma protein-binding sites by quinidine and, therefore, has an in-

TABLE 28–5. Pharmacokinetics of Antiarrhythmic Drugs

Drug	Inactivation or Route of Elimination (%)	Active Metabolites	Protein Binding (%)	Elimination Half-Life (hour)	Oral Bioavailability (%)
Class IA					
Quinidine	Liver 50–90 Kidney 10–30	Probable	70–95	7–18	70
Procainamide	Kidney 30–60 Liver 40–70	Yes	15	2.5–4.7	75
Disopyramide	Kidney 36–77 Liver 11–37	Yes	20–60	7–9	80
Class IB					
Lidocaine	Liver 90	Yes	40–70	1.5–4	35
Phenytoin	Liver 95	No	85	24	70–100
Mexiletine	Liver 90	No	70	8–24	90
Tocainide	Liver 50–60	No	50	12–15	100
	Kidney 40–50		95	3–4	30–40
Moricizine*	Liver >70	?			
Class IC					
Flecainide	Liver 70	No	40	11–30	95
Propafenone	Liver ?	?	97	5–32†	3–40†
Class II					
Propranolol	90+	No	90+	2–6	~30
Sotalol	Kidney 90	No	0	10–20	100
Class III					
Bretylium	Kidney 70–80	No	?(Low)	4–16	20
Amiodarone	Liver 99	Unknown	?(High)	25–55 days	20–50

*Mixed Class IA and IB pattern of effects.
†Long half-life in slow metabolizers.

creased action to prevent clotting. This may result in excessive bleeding or even hemorrhage.

Both quinidine and propranolol exert a negative inotropic action on the heart; because of the possibility of combined cardiac depressant effects, caution is recommended when using both drugs concurrently.

Electrolyte and Acid-Base Imbalance on Arrhythmia and Drug Actions. Potassium is the major electrolyte that must be monitored when administering quinidine. Hypokalemic patients taking drugs such as the thiazides are prone to rhythm disorders and are resistant to therapy with quinidine. Hyperkalemia increases the local anesthetic properties of

TABLE 28–6. Representative Cardiovascular Drugs Exhibiting Age-Related Alterations in Disposition or Response

Drug	Principal Age-Related Factor	Pharmacokinetic Changes V_d	$t_{1/2}$	Cl	Comments
Digoxin	Renal clearance	↓	↑	↓	Reduce dosage
Lidocaine	Liver clearance	↑	↑	0	Reduce dosage
Procainamide	Renal clearance	—	—	↓	Reduce dosage with compromised renal function and congestive heart failure
Quinidine	Liver and renal clearance	0	↑	↓	Individualize dosage
Disopyramide	Renal clearance: anticholinergic side effects	—	↑	↓	Reduce dosage with compromised renal function; check bowel and bladder function
Tocainide	Renal clearance	—	↑	↓	Reduce dosage with compromised renal function
β blockers, lipid-soluble	Liver clearance	0	↑	↓	Decreased response; individualize dosage
β blockers, water soluble	Renal clearance	—	↑	↓	Decreased response; individualize dosage

Adapted from Rocci ML, Vlasses PH, Abrams WB: Geriatric clinical pharmacology. Cardiol Clin 4:213, 1986.
V_d = volume of distribution; $t_{1/2}$ = half-life; 0 = no significant change; — = no information or not relevant; ↑ = increased; ↓ = decreased.

quinidine, so that the decrease in membrane responsiveness is exacerbated.

Quinidine is excreted as a weak base, and its excretion is reduced when urinary pH is increased. Thus, the concomitant administration of acetazolamide or sodium bicarbonate may result in increased serum levels of quinidine. It should be remembered that electrolyte imbalances are common causes or accompaniments of cardiac arrhythmias. Thus, electrolyte imbalances should not only be suspected as causes of arrhythmias but should be corrected before giving most antiarrhythmic drugs, especially in a chronic dose regimen or at unusually high doses.

Contraindications in Heart Block or Congestive Heart Failure. Third-degree heart block (complete) is a contraindication to quinidine therapy because of its intrinsic ability to decrease automaticity; abolishing a ventricular or AV node pacemaker could result in asystole. Quinidine is also usually not administered in the presence of congestive heart failure because its negative inotropic effect would have disastrous effects on an already depressed heart. In addition, most patients with congestive heart failure are already taking digoxin and thus would be at greater risk for toxicity.

Procainamide

ACTIONS. The direct effects of procainamide (PRONESTYL) do not differ from quinidine enough to be clinically significant. Both agents are local anesthetics; they decrease membrane responsiveness, the slope of phase 0, and automaticity, while increasing the effective refractory period.

The drugs differ significantly in their indirect effects, pharmacokinetics, and untoward effects. The indirect effects of procainamide are much less significant than are those of quinidine. There is a much weaker anticholinergic effect and there is almost no α-adrenergic blockade; thus it can be given IV with much less risk of hypotension.

Electrocardiographic Changes. The effect of procainamide therapy on the electrocardiogram (ECG) is similar to that of quinidine because of the similarities in their electrophysiological effects. The PR, QRS, and QT intervals are each lengthened. The QRS and QT intervals are increased in a dose-dependent fashion but are somewhat less affected by quinidine. Furthermore, torsades de pointes is seen in procainamide therapy, albeit much less commonly than with quinidine therapy. Severe toxicity is manifest usually in the ECG as widening of the QRS, third-degree heart block, and ventricular tachyarrhythmias. Procainamide has a more modest effect on the QT and QRS intervals than quinidine, and the sinus rate is usually unchanged (Table 28–4).

ACTIONS ON OTHER ORGAN SYSTEMS. Like quinidine, procainamide causes GI side effects (nausea, vomiting, anorexia, and diarrhea), although they are usually much less pronounced. The CNS effects include mental confusion, giddiness, psychosis with hallucinations, depression, and insomnia.

TIME COURSE OF ACTION—PHARMACOKINETICS. Procainamide is almost entirely absorbed when taken orally, except when it is administered in a sustained-release formulation. The lower bioavailability of the sustained-release preparations is associated with delayed absorption and a duration of action that exceeds 8 hours. The liver metabolizes procainamide by an acetylation process to N-acetyl procainamide (NAPA). The rate at which this process occurs varies markedly, and the population falls into a **bimodal distribution of slow and fast acetylators**. In fast acetylators the concentrations of NAPA in the plasma may equal or exceed those of the parent compound. The ratio of liver metabolism to direct excretion of the parent drug by the kidney is approximately 50:50.

NAPA is a cardioactive metabolite that is being investigated for its own antiarrhythmic properties. Its characteristic action on the heart puts it in the antiarryhthmic class III. That is, conduction is not affected when NAPA is administered alone, but the refractory periods of both the atria and the ventricles are prolonged, as is the time required for repolarization, represented by the QT interval. NAPA has a longer half-life than does the parent compound and is eliminated primarily by the kidney. In states of renal failure the plasma concentration of NAPA may rise to dangerously high levels.

BOX 28–2
THERAPEUTIC USES

Procainamide can be used IV, which makes it a more convenient drug to use than quinidine; IV titration can be followed by oral administration for continued use. A major problem with this drug is its potential to produce a syndrome resembling systemic lupus erythematosus with long-term therapy. Nevertheless, it can be given IV for ventricular tachyarrhythmias resistant to lidocaine therapy. It is an excellent drug for the treatment of tachyarrhythmias in the Wolff-Parkinson-White syndrome.

EFFECT OF AGE ON PHARMACOKINETIC PARAMETERS. Because renal function declines with age, the dosage of procainamide may need to be decreased or the dosage interval increased (Table 28–6). Of class IA drugs, procainamide is the drug of choice in the elderly because quinidine has a higher propensity to cause diarrhea in this population. Diarrhea can be serious in this age group, especially in view of the effects of hypokalemia on antiarrhythmic drug actions.

ADVERSE EFFECTS, CONTRAINDICATIONS, AND DRUG INTERACTIONS. Procainamide is contraindicated in complete heart block; decreasing the automaticity of a ventricular or AV nodal pacemaker, when that is the only pacemaker the patient has, only compounds the problems.

Procainamide can cause an exacerbation of myasthenia gravis because of its ability to decrease the release of acetylcholine at skeletal muscle motor nerve endings. Thus, procainamide administration may be hazardous without optimal adjustment of anticholinesterase medications.

Known hypersensitivity to the drug or similar compounds, including the local anesthetic procaine, is a contraindication. Because hypersensitivity reactions are the most common side effect noted with the use of procainamide, fever occurring within the first days of therapy may necessitate discontinuance of the drug. Moreover, agranulocytosis may develop within a few weeks.

Procainamide should not be given to patients with supraventricular tachycardias without first pretreating them with digitalis, as in the case with quinidine.

A principal adverse effect of procainamide therapy can develop with its long-term use. There is a high percentage of **drug-induced lupus, a syndrome similar to authentic lupus erythematosus**. Procainamide-induced lupus presents with arthralgias followed by a rash and resolves spontaneously when the drug is withheld. It can be monitored (diagnosed) by performing an assay for antinuclear antibodies (ANA). These can be detected in 80% of patients on long-term procainamide therapy. It is not known whether slow acetylators have an increased risk of developing the systemic lupus erythematosus–like syndrome; they may be in that they are more susceptible to hydralazine-induced lupus.

More recently, reports have made an association between neutropenia and long-term procainamide administration. The occurrence of neutropenia is rare and usually resolves upon discontinuation of the drug. It is recommended that routine complete blood counts (CBCs) with differential white counts be done regularly, as well as close follow-up on any complaints, even if they may seem as insignificant as cold symptoms. Because neutropenia is also a rare side effect of quinidine and disopyramide therapy, other alternatives are not necessarily readily available.

Concurrent use of procainamide with quinidine or disopyramide may produce enhanced prolongation of conduction or depression of contractility and hypotension. Anticholinergic agents used concurrently may produce an additive antivagal action on the AV nodal conduction. Because procainamide reduces acetylcholine release, lower amounts of neuromuscular blocking agents are required for muscle relaxation.

CARDIAC AND EXTRACARDIAC EFFECTS OF TOXICITY. Kidney, liver, and heart failure can precipitate toxicity if the dosage is not adjusted. Heart failure decreases perfusion to all organs, including the kidney and the liver. The principal cause for the toxicity is the decreased glomerular filtration rate that accompanies renal failure.

Disopyramide

Disopyramide (NORPACE and others) was developed in an attempt to find a class IA agent with fewer side effects than quinidine or procainamide. With this drug there is a tradeoff by avoidance of some of the untoward effects of the other class IA agents for some of its own.

ACTIONS. The mechanism of action of disopyramide is the sum of its direct and anticholinergic effects. The direct effects are similar to those of quinidine and procainamide except that it has a large negative inotropic effect that can be quite profound in congestive heart failure. The anticholinergic effects of disopyramide are the most prominent of all the agents in the IA class.

ACTIONS ON OTHER ORGAN SYSTEMS. The principal actions on other organ systems are secondary to the anticholinergic effects. In addition, disopyramide acts as a vasoconstrictor and therefore significantly increases the afterload on the heart. This effect is much greater than any similar effects noted with quinidine or disopyramide. This effect on the heart, combined with the negative inotropic effect of the drug, can produce frank heart failure in uncompensated or marginally compensated heart failure.

BOX 28–3
THERAPEUTIC USES

Disopyramide is effective in suppressing premature ventricular complexes and the potential ventricular tachycardia associated with such ectopic foci. It is not as effective in treating supraventricular tachyarrhythmias as quinidine or procainamide. The anticholinergic side effects and significant negative inotropic effect make it a poor choice in the elderly.

TIME COURSE OF ACTION—PHARMACOKINETICS. Disopyramide is well absorbed when taken orally; however, malabsorptive disorders, diarrhea, and myocardial infarction may significantly decrease the absorption of the drug. The great variability in levels currently being observed may be managed in the future by assay of free disopyramide plasma levels. Elimination of the drug is achieved partly by metabolism in the liver, producing a number of metabolites, at least one of which is cardioactive; about half of the parent drug is excreted directly by the kidney.

EFFECT OF AGE ON PHARMACOKINETIC PARAMETERS. Disopyramide is eliminated at a decreased rate in the elderly as a result of the decreased renal function in this population (Table 28–6). Also, disopyramide has a relative contraindication in the elderly because of its prominent negative inotropic effect and because its anticholinergic actions may cause urinary retention in elderly men with benign prostatic hypertrophy.

ADVERSE EFFECTS AND CONTRAINDICATIONS. The major adverse reactions to disopyramide come from its anticholinergic side effects; these may be severe enough to mandate discontinuation of the drug. Among the more prominent of these adverse effects are dry mouth, blurred vision, mydriasis, and possible exacerbation of glaucoma, constipation, and urinary retention. Upon initiation of therapy, ventricular extrasystoles and arrhythmias may be produced. Close observation for these effects in the early stages of therapy are appropriate.

CARDIAC AND EXTRACARDIAC EFFECTS OF TOXICITY. Congestive heart failure in uncompensated and marginally compensated cases can result from the vasoconstrictive and negative inotropic effects of the drug.

Conduction disturbances may be produced as with the other class IA antiarrhythmics as a result of their local anesthetic effects.

INTERACTIONS WITH OTHER DRUGS. Disopyramide does not alter the blood levels of digoxin. However, it interacts with negative inotropic agents such as β blockers to compound their cardiac depressant effects. Moreover, anticholinergic agents should be used with great caution with disopyramide because of its marked cholinergic blocking activity.

Contraindications include complete heart block, congestive heart failure, and other drugs that have a negative inotropic effect such as calcium channel blockers and β blockers.

CLASS IB ANTIARRHYTHMIC AGENTS

General Characteristics

Type IB agents exert little or no effect on V_{max} of phase 0 of normal fibers but depress conduction in fibers with a fast response, decrease the action potential duration, and to a lesser degree, decrease the effective refractory period.

Phenytoin

ACTIONS (Table 28–4)

Sinoatrial Node. Phenytoin (DILANTIN) produces little direct change in SA nodal function. Hypotension can occur with its IV administration, followed by reflex increase in sympathetic activity and an increased sinus heart rate.

Atria. The action potential duration and effective refractory period are not altered until high concentrations are used. The frequency of stimulation and the extracellular K^+ concentration determine the action of phenytoin on membrane responsiveness. At a normal extracellular K^+ concentration (3–5 mM), phenytoin depresses the rate of phase 0 depolarization. Conduction velocity is unaltered or slightly depressed.

Atrioventricular Node. Phenytoin decreases the effective refractory period of the node and increases the conduction velocity. In a patient intoxicated with digitalis, phenytoin can normalize transmission and decrease the ventricular automaticity associated with intoxication.

His-Purkinje System. Phenytoin shortens the action potential duration and the effective refractory period. At normal extracellular K^+ concentrations, phenytoin does not alter or produces a slight decrease in V_{max} of phase 0 depolarization. When membrane responsiveness has been decreased by digitalis toxicity or by hypoxia, phenytoin increases the maximal rate of phase 0 depolarization. The rate of phase 4 depolarization in Purkinje tissue is decreased, as is the rate of discharge of ventricular pacemakers.

Electrocardiographic. Phenytoin may decrease the PR and QT intervals as a result of improved AV conduction and a shortened action potential duration in ventricular muscle.

Organ/System Pharmacology. Rapid IV administration may induce a transient hypotension, the result of a direct action on the vascular bed and heart to produce peripheral vasodilation and depression of cardiac contractility. The slow administration of larger dosages produces a dose-related decrease in the left ventricular force, the rate of force development, and cardiac output. Left ventricular end-diastolic pressure increases.

TIME COURSE—PHARMACOKINETICS. Phenytoin is absorbed completely from the GI tract. It may take up to 12 hours to reach peak plasma levels after the initial oral dose; thus a loading dose is usually given. The relationship between dose and steady state plasma concentrations is not linear, and thus, it is difficult to maintain a consistent plasma concentration (see also Chapter 20).

ADVERSE EFFECTS (see Table 28–4 and Chapter 20). In spite of phenytoin being widely prescribed, only a few deaths have been reported from an overdose of it. The deaths that have occurred have been due to idiosyncratic reactions or hypersensitivity or have occurred during a rapid IV injection. Overdose with phenytoin is treated by focusing on symptomatic and supportive care. Charcoal hemoperfusion, diuresis, and hemodialysis are generally of no benefit.

> BOX 28–4
> **THERAPEUTIC USES**
>
> The primary clinical application of phenytoin for arrhythmias is in the treatment of atrial and ventricular arrhythmias induced by digitalis toxicity. Phenytoin is used also as a prophylactic agent to prevent position version arrhythmias, especially in a digitalized patient. It may also be effective in the treatment of ventricular arrhythmias occurring in acute myocardial infarction, open-heart surgery, anesthesia, cardiac catheterization, cardioversion, and angiographic studies.
>
> Nevertheless, phenytoin, like lidocaine, is much more effective in the treatment of ventricular than supraventricular arrhythmias.

DRUG INTERACTIONS. These are important and are covered in Chapters 20 and 50.

Lidocaine

First used as an antiarrhythmic agent in the 1950s, lidocaine (XYLOCAINE and others), a local anesthetic discussed in Chapter 12, is the mainstay in the treatment of ventricular arrhythmias in intensive care units. One limiting feature is bioavailability after oral dosing, with only one third reaching the circulation because of extensive first-pass hepatic metabolism. Consequently, it is always given parenterally (and almost always IV). This has led to the development of newer, orally effective lidocaine congeners, such as tocainide.

ACTIONS

Sinoatrial Node. Therapeutic concentrations of lidocaine have no effect on sinus rate.

Atria. Actions on atria are similar to those of quinidine. Membrane responsiveness, the amplitude of the action potential, and excitability of atrial muscle are decreased by lidocaine, producing a decrease in the conduction velocity. The effective refractory period is slightly increased or unaltered.

Atrioventricular Node. Conduction velocity and the effective refractory period are altered to a minimal extent by the usual therapeutic dosages of lidocaine.

His-Purkinje System. The amplitude of the action potential and membrane responsiveness are both decreased. If myocardial ischemia has reduced the resting membrane potential to −70 to −60 mV, blood levels on the high side of the therapeutic range of lidocaine may depress phase 0 depolarization in the Purkinje fibers, which can result in complete blockade of conduction. The action potential duration and effective refractory period are shortened at lower levels of lidocaine than required to alter the same parameters in ventricular muscle. Phase 4 depolarization and the spontaneous discharge rate are decreased by lidocaine; high levels suppress automaticity and eliminate phase 4 depolarization.

Ventricular Muscle. Action potential duration and the effective refractory period are decreased.

Electrocardiographic. Lidocaine may shorten the QT interval but usually does not alter the PR, QRS, and QT intervals.

EFFECTS ON ORGANS AND SYSTEMS. When lidocaine is used in therapeutic dosages, it rarely induces hemodynamic changes.

TIME COURSE OF ACTION—PHARMACOKINETICS. Exponential plasma concentration time curves occur after the IV administration of lidocaine. The initial rapid decline represents the distribution phase and has a half-life of 20 minutes. This initial phase is followed by a slow decline associated with elimination and has a half-life of 2 hours. Five to 7 hours are required to achieve steady state plasma concentrations with a constant infusion of lidocaine (Table 28-5).

ADVERSE EFFECTS. Therapeutic plasma concentrations range from 1 to 5 μg/ml. As plasma levels of lidocaine rise above a level of 5 μg/ml, drowsiness, muscle twitching, paresthesias, speech disturbances, vertigo, tinnitus, and disorientation may be observed (Table 28-4). Levels twice that, of 9 μg/ml or more, may be associated with psychosis, respiratory depression, or seizures. Patients receiving lidocaine should be monitored closely because potentially fatal status epilepticus may develop quickly. Such convulsions are dose-related and can be prevented by using a rate of infusion to keep plasma concentrations below 5 μg/ml. Toxic levels may also cause severe bradycardia, sinus arrest, and AV block.

Treatment of lidocaine overdosage should focus on the management of the serious cardiovascular effects, the seizures, and the possibility of methemoglobinemia. Seizures may be relatively refractory to therapy, but phenytoin can be employed. There is a likelihood that seizures may still be present after the lidocaine serum levels have fallen below 5 μg/ml, because the metabolite monoethylglycine xylidide is also a convulsant. If the methemoglobin level is greater than or equal to 30% and is associated with dyspnea, metabolic acidosis, or altered mental status, methylene blue and oxygen should be administered. Severe toxic methemoglobinemia is treated with methylene blue (2 mg/kg, repeat if needed). Within an hour the methemoglobin level is usually reduced by at least 50%. Hemodialysis is not effective.

> **BOX 28-5**
>
> **THERAPEUTIC USES**
>
> Lidocaine is used almost exclusively to treat ventricular arrhythmias; it is ineffective in the treatment of most supraventricular arrhythmias. In the acute myocardial infarction patient, lidocaine will control ventricular arrhythmias and prevent ventricular fibrillation with little risk, because it lacks significant depressant effects on the cardiovascular system and because the toxic side effects are of short duration. Either lidocaine or phenytoin may be used to treat ventricular arrhythmias associated with digitalis intoxication.

PRECAUTIONS AND CONTRAINDICATIONS. The elimination of lidocaine in individuals with congestive heart failure will be delayed. Renal failure does not alter its clearance. Contraindications to the use of lidocaine include severe hepatic dysfunction, a previous history of grand mal seizures following lidocaine, hypersensitivity to amide local anesthetics, or the presence of second- or third-degree heart block. Lidocaine may increase the degree of pre-existing heart block and can depress an idioventricular pacemaker that may be maintaining cardiac rhythm.

Lidocaine plasma concentrations may be increased in the elderly because of increased binding to acid-1-glycoprotein. These concentrations may not produce toxic effects because unbound drug produces the effect. Nevertheless, the use of lidocaine in patients 70 years of age or older is contraindicated (Table 28-6).

DRUG INTERACTIONS. Because lidocaine is metabolized by hepatic microsomes, any drug increasing or decreasing liver microsomal enzyme activity will alter its metabolism, such as cimetidine. Agents that induce or inhibit the liver P-450 system will also alter lidocaine metabolism. Hepatic blood flow is probably the primary determinant of lidocaine disposition.

Tocainide

Tocainide (TONOCARD) and mexiletine are newer class IB antiarrhythmic agents designed in the hope of finding a lidocaine analog that possesses an antiarrhythmic action when given orally, a long duration of action, and a large therapeutic index.

Tocainide hydrochloride (2-amino-N-2,6-dimethylphenyl-alaninamide hydrochloride) is a primary amine analog of lidocaine; tocainide does not undergo appreciable first-pass metabolic degradation in the liver, in contrast to lidocaine. Approximately 10-50% of the tocainide administered is bound to protein. Overall, 50% of tocainide is metabolized in the liver and 40% is excreted in urine.

ACTIONS. Tocainide exhibits most of the electrophysiological effects of lidocaine (Table 28-4). It reduces phase 0 and shortens the effective refractory period of the cardiac action potential.

Atrioventricular Node and Atrial and Ventricular Muscle. The effective refractory period is shortened; the predominant effect is observed in the AV node.

Sinoatrial Node. Tocainide exerts little effect on SA nodal automaticity or intracardiac conduction.

Purkinje Fibers. The slope of phase 4 depolarization is reduced. The rate of rise of phase 0 is decreased, and a depression of the amplitude of the action potential occurs.

Electrocardiographic. Tocainide has minimal effects, although the QT interval is shortened.

ORGAN AND SYSTEM EFFECTS. Tocainide exhibits only a minor effect on cardiac hemodynamics even in patients with cardiac dysfunction.

TIME COURSE OF ACTION—PHARMACOKINETICS. Tocainide is well absorbed after oral administration (Table 28-5). The plasma concentration is related directly to the dosage unless administered with food; food decreases the peak plasma concentration but does not decrease the overall bioavailability. To prevent high initial levels, it is recommended that tocainide be taken with meals.

> BOX 28-6
> **THERAPEUTIC USES**
>
> Tocainide suppresses the presence of premature ventricular contractions in 50% of patients exhibiting them chronically and is of benefit in the treatment of ventricular ectopy associated with the early stages of acute myocardial infarction and those associated with postmyocardial infarction. Tocainide is effective for the short-term suppression of ventricular arrhythmias; it appears to be the logical agent to use for chronic oral dosing of patients in whom IV lidocaine resulted in suppression of ventricular tachycardia and ventricular ectopic activity. The majority of patients exhibiting drug-resistant ventricular arrhythmias, including recurrent sustained ventricular tachycardia or fibrillation, respond positively to the administration of tocainide.
>
> The efficacy of tocainide is approximately that of other drugs in class I, such as quinidine, procainamide, and disopyramide. Although the side effects associated with the use of tocainide are similar in frequency to those reported for quinidine, the unwanted actions of tocainide are often milder and better tolerated, and patients respond well to a change in the dose.

ADVERSE EFFECTS. Tocainide has a wider margin of safety than lidocaine, particularly when actions on the CNS are compared. The most common side effects are GI symptoms and include nausea, vomiting, abdominal pain, anorexia, and constipation. Administration of smaller dosages or concomitant intake with food may minimize these actions. Headaches, dizziness, paresthesias, and tremor are considered more closely correlated with the doses. Hypersensitivity reactions, including rash, induction of arrhythmias, and fatal agranulocytosis, are uncommon, but can occur. Because agranulocytosis, bone marrow depression, leukopenia, hypoplastic anemia, neutropenia, and thrombocytopenia have also been reported and sequelae such as septicemia and septic shock have been reported with doses in the recommended range, periodic CBCs, especially during the first 6 months of use, are recommended.

CAUTIONS. The plasma half-life is 12-15 hours and may be increased twofold in patients with renal failure or hepatic disease.

DRUG INTERACTIONS. No serious adverse interactions have been reported with cimetidine, propranolol, verapamil, digoxin, or warfarin.

Mexiletine

ACTIONS. Mexiletine (MEXITIL) shares many of its electrophysiological effects with lidocaine and tocainide (Table 28-4). Thus, mexiletine decreases V_{max} and the depolarization threshold of both atrial and ventricular myocardium. AV nodal conduction time and refractoriness and His-Purkinje conduction time (HV interval) are increased or unchanged. The ventricular effective refractory period is increased; mexiletine differs from lidocaine in that it has a relatively greater effect at slower pacing rates.

ADVERSE EFFECTS. Like other antiarrhythmic drugs, mexiletine has a narrow therapeutic margin, yet a direct correlation with the concentration of mexiletine and observed toxic effects has not been established. Neurological side effects are generally observed at plasma levels greater than 2.0 μg/ml but occasionally develop at levels less than 1.0 μg/ml. Side effects have been reported for a mean of 30% of the patients taking it (range 10-60%), and the drug may have to be discontinued in from 5 to 30% of the patients. The most common side effects are related to the CNS, are dose-related, and occur with both IV and oral dosages. The initial symptom is a fine hand tremor. Ataxia, dizziness, lightheadedness, nystagmus, paresthesias, blurred vision, diplopia, dysarthria, confusion, drowsiness, psychosis, and seizures have been reported.

Sinus bradycardia or conduction abnormalities have

> BOX 28-7
> **THERAPEUTIC USES**
>
> Mexiletine is effective in the treatment of premature ventricular contractions not associated with acute myocardial infarction as well as in the prevention of ventricular ectopy in the acute infarction patient or postinfarction. Studies combining quinidine and mexiletine demonstrated a better response in treating ventricular tachycardia, whereas the combination of amiodarone and mexiletine controlled drug-refractory ventricular tachycardia. Used alone, mexiletine is effective in a small number of patients with recurrent ventricular tachycardia; in combination with other antiarrhythmic agents it is more effective in drug-refractory patients.

been noted in patients with pre-existent conduction disease such as sick sinus syndrome. The rapid IV bolus administration of mexiletine may produce hypotension, QRS widening, and bradycardia. Aggravation of underlying ventricular arrhythmia and mexiletine-induced torsades de pointes have been observed.

PRECAUTIONS AND CONTRAINDICATIONS. Because mexiletine is primarily (90%) eliminated hepatically, with only 10% of a dose excreted unchanged in the urine, its dose requires adjustment only in patients with severe renal dysfunction — those with a creatinine clearance less than or equal to 10 mL/min.

CLASS IC AGENTS

General Characteristics

Class IC agents depress V_{max}, but unlike class IA drugs, they do not cause a significant change in refractoriness or the action potential duration. Unlike class IB drugs, they do not depress V_{max} in a potassium-dependent manner.

Flecainide

ACTIONS AND PHARMACOKINETICS (Table 28–4). Flecainide (TAMBOCOR) was developed through a systematic study of structural analogs of the procainamide and lidocaine molecules.

Sinoatrial Node. The mean sinus cycle length is usually decreased only slightly; however, it can have unpredictable actions on sinus node automaticity and conduction.

Atria. The maximal rate of depolarization is decreased. The membrane responsiveness curve is shifted to the right. Conduction velocity is decreased.

Atrioventricular Node and His-Purkinje Conduction. AV (AH interval) and His-Purkinje (HV interval) conduction are prolonged by flecainide.

Electrocardiographic. The PR and QRS intervals are prolonged.

ORGAN SYSTEM PHARMACOLOGY. Myocardial contractility is decreased slightly after the administration of flecainide. Ejection fraction and the velocity of circumferential fiber shortening decrease after IV dosing, although not all echocardiography studies confirm this slight negative inotropic action. Blood pressure and the working capacity of patients with heart failure are not modified. Thus flecainide has minimal negative hemodynamic actions.

ADVERSE EFFECTS. It has been suggested that the main consideration when using flecainide is its potential to produce arrhythmias (Table 28–4). Flecainide should be used with caution in the following situations:

- Congestive heart failure, such as in patients with low ejection fraction and ventricular tachycardia
- Sinus node abnormalities
- His-Purkinje conduction defects
- In presence of second- or third-degree AV or bifascicular heart block
- History of myocardial infarction, or an episode of cardiac arrest
- Excessively rapid administration of an IV loading dose

Flecainide treatment should be initiated in the hospital with rhythm monitoring for patients with sustained ventricular tachycardia, symptomatic congestive heart failure or sinus node dysfunction, or those with significant myocardial dysfunction.

Other adverse reactions associated with the use of flecainide include visual disturbances, abdominal cramps and distention, flatulence, headache, drowsiness, dry mouth, nausea, and vomiting. Tremors, hot and cold sensations, shortness of breath, and constipation occur less frequently. With continued use of flecainide, most of these side effects disappear.

> BOX 28–8
> **THERAPEUTIC USE**
>
> Flecainide is beneficial in the treatment of ventricular arrhythmias, including repetitive episodes of ventricular tachycardia and those occurring after acute myocardial infarction and in patients with supraventricular reentry tachycardia and supraventricular extrasystoles. Atrial flutter and atrial fibrillation in patients with Wolff-Parkinson-White syndrome have also responded.
>
> (A comprehensive study [Ruskin, 1989] concluded that for patients with a history of myocardial infarction, the class IC agents be reserved for use in those patients in whom other antiarrhythmic agents are poorly tolerated or not effective. Any IC agent, including propafenone, should be considered to have a similar risk to that of flecainide. Their use is generally unacceptable in patients without life-threatening ventricular arrhythmias, even if the patients are experiencing unpleasant symptoms or signs.)

DRUG INTERACTIONS. When flecainide and amiodarone are used together, the dosage of flecainide should be decreased by 50% and the patient should be monitored for adverse effects. Flecainide can induce a transient elevation of the steady-state digoxin plasma levels. Concurrent dosing with flecainide and propranolol appears to induce less of a decrease in the heart rate than when only propranolol is given, presumably because of an anticholinergic action of flecainide.

Propafenone

ACTIONS. Actions of propafenone (RYTHMOL) include sodium channel blocking, β-adrenoreceptor antagonism, and weak calcium receptor antagonism.

Sinus Node and Atrium. Little or no effect.

Atrioventricular Node and His-Purkinje Conduction. Conduction is prolonged.

Electrocardiographic. PR and QRS intervals are prolonged.

ORGAN SYSTEM PHARMACOLOGY. Propafenone is devoid of pronounced cardiodepressant activity, although negative inotropic effects have been reported in patients with impaired ventricular function (less than 50%), as well as a reduction in systolic blood pressure.

ADVERSE EFFECTS. Like essentially all antiarrhythmic agents, it may aggravate or induce cardiac arrhythmias. The most commonly reported side effects are neurological (dizziness, taste disturbances, blurred vision, headache, and paresthesias) and gastrointestinal (nausea, vomiting, anorexia, and constipation). Rarely reported adverse effects include elevated transaminase levels, cholestatic hepatitis, aggravation of myasthenia gravis, hyponatremia, lupus erythematosus, seizures, paranoia, and/or agranulocytosis.

Use of propafenone in children is well-tolerated, with a spectrum of adverse effects similar to those reported for adults. Its use during pregnancy should be limited but no harm to the fetus occurred when it was given from the 17th week of pregnancy. Direct fetal administration of propafenone in combination with other antiarrhythmic agents during the third trimester did not affect neonatal growth or development in two infants (Gembruch et al, 1988).

PRECAUTIONS AND CONTRAINDICATIONS. Note the large individual differences in kinetics. Its use is contraindicated in the presence of uncontrolled congestive heart failure; cardiogenic shock; sinoatrial, atrioventricular, and intraventricular disorders of impulse generation and/or conduction (*ie*, sick sinus node syndrome, atrioventricular block) in the absence of an artificial pacemaker; bradycardia; marked hypotension; bronchospastic disorders; electrolyte imbalance; and known hypersensitivity to the drug.

DRUG INTERACTIONS. Any drug that is metabolized by hepatic cytochrome systems, as is propafenone, has the potential to alter propafenone's metabolism. Interactions between propafenone and phenobarbital, metoprolol, propranolol, warfarin, digoxin and quinidine have been reported. Increased plasma concentrations of cyclosporine, theophylline, cimetidine, and desipramine have occurred when given with propafenone. Decreased levels of propafenone have occurred when given with rifampicin.

> BOX 28-9
> **THERAPEUTIC USES**
>
> Propafenone pharmacokinetics are complex and individualized dosage titration is necessary. In addition, hepatic dysfunction decreases clearance and increases the elimination half-life.
>
> Propafenone has been effective in the treatment of premature ventricular complexes, ventricular couplets, and nonsustained ventricular tachycardia, and in treatment of malignant ventricular arrhythmias (preliminary mortality data have been encouraging [Bryson et al, 1993] in patients with ventricular fibrillation and sustained ventricular tachycardia). It also may be effective against supraventricular arrhythmias, Wolff-Parkinson-White syndrome, or with rapid anterograde conduction.
>
> Like flecainide, propafenone has the potential to induce arrhythmias; thus, it should not be used in patients with potentially malignant arrhythmias.

Moricizine

ACTIONS. Moricizine (ETHMOZINE), like other class I antiarrhythmic agents, reduces the fast inward sodium current of the action potential. It is a phenothiazine but it lacks the dopamine antagonist activity and the behavioral and autonomic actions characteristic of the neuroleptic phenothiazines. It does not readily fit into any of the subclasses of sodium channel-blocking drugs and thus has proved difficult to subclassify within the group of class I antiarrhythmic agents.

Sinoatrial Node and Atria. No effect on SA recovery time if patient has normal sinus node function.

Atrioventricular Nodal and Intraventricular Conduction. Conduction is slowed.

Electrocardiographic. PR and QRS intervals are increased.

ORGAN SYSTEM PHARMACOLOGY. Congestive heart failure may occur during moricizine therapy, generally in those with reduced left ventricular ejection fractions and a history of congestive heart failure.

PHARMACOKINETICS. Moricizine has a phenothiazine structure chemically unrelated to any currently used antiarrhythmic agent.

After oral administration it is almost completely absorbed from the gastrointestinal tract; however, bioavailability is limited to 30-40% because of a first-pass effect. Hepatic biotransformation involves sulfur oxidation, ring hydroxylation, *N*-dealkylation, acetylation, amide hydrolysis, *N*-oxidation, and glucuronide or sulfate conjugation to yield at least 40 metabolites.

ADVERSE EFFECTS. Cardiovascular effects include the worsening of arrhythmias, conduction disturbances, and heart failure. Nausea and dizziness sufficient to discontinue the drug have been reported. In a few patients drug-related fever, elevation of serum aminotransferase or bilirubin, or thrombocytopenia has been detected. The discontinuation of the moricizine phase of the cardiac arrhythmic suppression trial (CAST) study due to a lack of benefit emphasizes that physicians should use moricizine only after a careful evaluation of the potential benefits and risks (Clyne et al, 1992).

PRECAUTIONS AND CONTRAINDICATIONS. Because the effect of moricizine in patients with abnormal sinus node function is unknown, caution is advised. Significant liver dysfunction reduces plasma clearance and increases the half-life of moricizine. Use with caution in presence of renal disease or pregnancy.

> BOX 28-10
> **THERAPEUTIC USES**
>
> Moricizine is indicated only for treatment of patients with life-threatening ventricular arrhythmias, such as sustained ventricular tachycardia or ventricular fibrillation. In some patients with these disorders who are resistant to other antiarrhythmic agents, short-term dosing with moricizine will suppress the induction of ventricular arrhythmias.

DRUG INTERACTIONS. Given with digoxin, the plasma levels of digoxin are not altered. However, due to its effect on AV nodal conduction, it may further prolong the PR interval in patients taking digoxin or other drugs acting at this site. Cimetidine, but not ranitidine, decreases the clearance of moricizine, increases its mean plasma elimination half-life, and increases plasma concentrations. Theophylline plasma levels are increased and the elimination half-life decreased.

CLASS II AGENTS: BETA-ADRENOCEPTOR BLOCKING AGENTS

General Characteristics

Class II drugs antagonize the effect of sympathetic stimulation on the heart.

Propranolol

ACTIONS AND PHARMACOKINETICS. The antiarrhythmic action of propranolol (INDERAL; Table 28–4) is generally attributed to a combination of β-adrenergic blockade (thus removing the adrenergic modulation of the heart), an increase in the outward potassium current, and, in higher dosages, a depression of sodium permeability, that is, a local anesthetic affect. (Propranolol has a short half-life of 2–6 hours and is usually administered three or four times a day; Fig. 28–1.)

Sinoatrial Node. Propranolol blocks the β receptors in the SA node and thus prevents adrenergic stimulation from increasing the slope of phase 4 depolarization and increasing the spontaneous firing rate in the sinus node. In general, the resting heart rate is only slightly decreased, but increases in heart rate induced by exercise or emotion are decreased. If the patient has pre-existing sinus node disease, the heart rate may be greatly decreased by propranolol.

Atria. Propranolol exhibits a local anesthetic and a quinidinelike action on the atrial membrane action potential in addition to its β-blocking actions. Membrane responsiveness, action potential amplitude, excitability, and conduction velocity are all decreased.

Atrioventricular Node. The conduction velocity through the AV node is decreased, and the AV nodal refractory period is increased after propranolol. This increase in the effective refractory period is thought to explain the antiarrhythmic actions of propranolol.

His-Purkinje System. Therapeutic concentrations of propranolol depress catecholamine-induced automaticity. Membrane responsiveness, the action potential amplitude, and tissue excitability are decreased by propranolol. Conduction velocity is subsequently decreased. All these actions occur at dosages higher than therapeutic concentrations and higher than the dosage required to establish β-adrenoceptor blockade.

Ventricular Muscle. Membrane responsiveness and myocardial excitability are decreased by propranolol. The duration of the action potential is increased only at high plasma concentrations.

Electrocardiographic. The PR interval may be increased, the QT interval is shortened, and the QRS complex duration prolonged only after large doses of propranolol have been administered.

Autonomic Nervous System. The establishment of β-adrenoceptor blockade with propranolol does not affect the α-adrenergic receptor or the parasympathetic division of the autonomic nervous system. Experimental data show that some β blockers, such as practolol and metoprolol, depress spontaneous discharge in the cardiac sympathetic nerves whereas others — timolol or sotalol — do not (Lathers et al, 1986b).

ORGAN SYSTEM PHARMACOLOGY. Propranolol blocks the cardiac β-adrenergic receptor, decreasing the influence of cardiac sympathetic nerves and catecholamine-induced inotropic and chronotropic actions. Systolic ejection periods at rest and during exercise are increased, tending to increase myocardial oxygen consumption. The decrease in heart rate and decrease in force of contraction cause a decrease in myocardial oxygen consumption; this last effect is the dominant action.

ADVERSE EFFECTS AND DRUG INTERACTIONS. The unwanted effects associated with the use of any β-blocking agent are the consequence of their blocking β receptors. The use of a β-blocking agent to control an arrhythmia in the presence of enhanced sympathetic activity may result in hypotension or left ventricular failure. The concomitant use of diuretics, vasodilators, or digitalis may allow the use of chronic oral propranolol in patients with ventricular failure. Interestingly, propranolol-induced heart failure can be reversed immediately by the administration of glucagon.

Amrinone, an inotropic agent, will also increase cardiac contractility in the presence of β blockade established by propranolol. It has been noted that propranolol can precipitate left ventricular failure in individuals previously free of heart failure.

The ability of propranolol to decrease AV conduction may result in bradycardia, AV block, or asystole. Atropine, IV, may reverse propranolol-induced bradycardia. Ventricular asystole associated with the use of propranolol will respond to mechanical or electrical stimulation but does not respond to the administration of exogenous catecholamines.

The rapid IV infusion of propranolol produces vasodilation and results in hypotension. Cardiac β-adrenergic receptor blockade and the direct myocardial depression also contribute to the precipitation of hypotension.

If propranolol is discontinued abruptly in individuals with angina pectoris, cardiac arrhythmias, a worsening of the angina symptoms, or acute myocardial infarction may appear. These effects of discontinuation may be related to the increased cardiac receptor density associated with chronic dosing with β-blocking agents (Lathers et al, 1988b). (For the other important side effects, see Chapters 10 and 30.)

Acebutolol

ACTIONS. Acebutolol (SECTRAL) is a cardioselective β-adrenoreceptor blocking agent possessing mild intrinsic sympathomimetic activity.

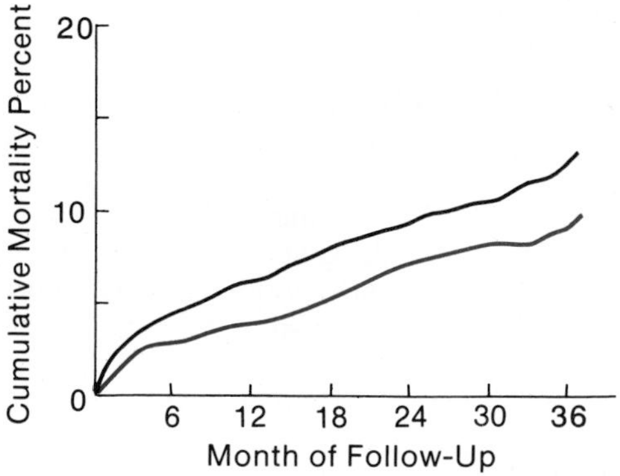

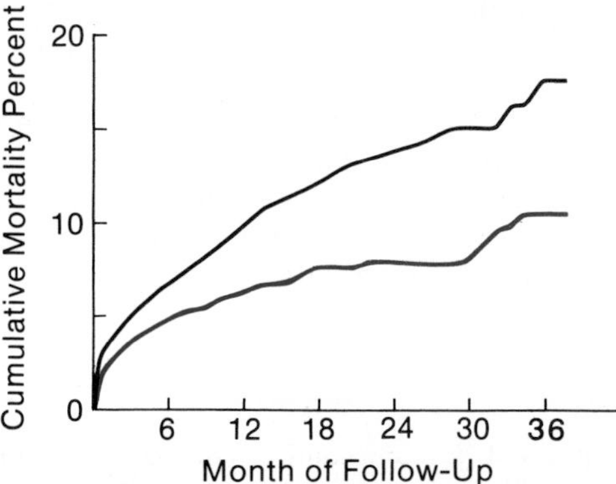

FIGURE 28–1. Survival rates with *β*-blocking agents. Results from two different studies are redrawn to be on the same scale. The *top graph* shows survival results of the *β* Blocker Heart Attack Trial. A total of 3837 patients were randomized to treatment with propranolol (*color*) or a placebo (*black*). After a 3-year follow-up, a significant reduction in mortality occurred in those treated with propranolol. (From National Institutes of Health *β* Blocker Heart Attack Study Group: A randomized trial of propranolol in patients with acute myocardial infarction. JAMA 247:1707–1714, 1982.) The *bottom graph* shows results from a multicenter trial with timolol. A total of 1884 patients with myocardial infarctions were randomized to placebo (*black*) or timolol (*color*) therapy. After an average follow-up of 33 months, a significant reduction in mortality was seen in the timolol group. (From Timolol-induced reduction in mortality and reinfarction in patients surviving acute myocardial infarction. Reprinted with permission from The New England Journal of Medicine, 304:801–807, 1981.)

BOX 28–11
THERAPEUTIC USES

- **Supraventricular Arrhythmias.** The supraventricular tachyarrhythmias of atrial fibrillation, atrial flutter, and paroxysmal supraventricular tachycardia are the chief indications for the use of propranolol as an antiarrhythmic agent. Propranolol decreases the ventricular rate by eliminating β-adrenergic stimulation of receptors in the AV node and thus increasing refractoriness of the AV node. Thus, the therapeutic goal is to decrease the ventricular rate rather than to abolish the arrhythmia; propranolol usually does not achieve the latter. Propranolol is often added to digitalis for atrial fibrillation or flutter not controlled by digitalis alone. A combination of the mechanisms of action of the two drugs, that is, the increased vagal activity induced by digitalis and the establishment of β blockade at the AV node by propranolol, may explain the beneficial effect of the combination (see Table 28–8).

  The combination of propranolol and quinidine increases the probability of converting atrial fibrillation to a normal sinus rhythm. In the treatment of paroxysmal supraventricular tachycardia of the Wolff-Parkinson-White syndrome, when propranolol alone has failed to control the arrhythmia, the addition of quinidine increases the refractoriness in AV tissue, while propranolol increases AV nodal refractoriness. Propranolol alone is not effective in preventing atrial fibrillation after cardioversion, but a combination with quinidine can be more effective than quinidine alone.
- **Ventricular Arrhythmias.** Propranolol is usually not effective in the treatment of ventricular arrhythmias. However, it may be effective in the treatment of ventricular premature depolarizations in patients with no structural heart disease. Propranolol will also suppress the ventricular arrhythmias associated with exercise, anxiety, pheochromocytoma, or thyrotoxicosis. In the presence of ischemic heart disease, propranolol prevents ventricular arrhythmias by decreasing or preventing ischemia.

  Numerous clinical trials have shown that chronic treatment with β blockers, including propranolol, timolol, metoprolol, or atenolol, reduces the incidence of reinfarction and the mortality in individuals who have survived a myocardial infarction (Fig. 28–1). The precise mechanism of the protection afforded by chronic dosing with β-blocking agents has yet to be determined. The possible occurrence of tachyarrhythmias, angina pectoris, or hypertension in the postinfarction period would also justify the chronic use of β-blocking agents.
- **Digitalis-Induced Arrhythmias.** Propranolol can abolish digitalis-induced ventricular arrhythmias. This action is attributed to its direct action on the heart and to suppression of central and peripheral sympathetic neural activity. Nevertheless, phenytoin or lidocaine is the drug of choice for treatment of digitalis-induced arrhythmias because the occurrence of adverse effects, including bradycardia, is greater when propranolol is used.
- **Anesthetic-Induced Arrhythmias.** The inhalational anesthetic halothane sensitizes the heart to the arrhythmic effects of exogenous catecholamines and the catecholamines released during surgery in response to stress, increased pCO_2, or hypotension. The cardiac arrhythmias associated with the use of halothane can be effectively suppressed by propranolol.

Atrioventricular Node Conduction. Conduction is delayed with increased refractoriness without significant alterations in sinus node recovery time, atrial refractory period, or the HV conduction time.

PHARMACOKINETICS. Acebutolol is well absorbed from the GI tract but undergoes extensive first-pass metabolism, resulting in 40% bioavailability of the parent compound. The major N-acetyl metabolite, diacetolol, is active and more cardioselective than its parent. Renal dysfunction decreases elimination of the metabolite, diacetolol, causing a two- to threefold increase in its half-life of some 8–13 hours. Elimination is 30–40% via renal mechanisms and 50–60% via nonrenal mechanisms, including excretion into the bile and direct passage through the intestinal wall.

ORGAN SYSTEM PHARMACOLOGY. Significant reductions in resting and exercise heart rates and systolic blood pressures occur within 1.5 hours after dosing. Exercise-induced tachycardia is reduced for 24–30 hours after dosing. Significant correlations exist between plasma levels of acebutolol, the reduction in resting heart rate, and the percent of β blockade of exercise-induced tachycardia.

ADVERSE EFFECTS. Patients with coronary artery disease should be warned against interruption or discontinuation of acebutolol without a physician's supervision. Cardiac failure rarely occurs but those on β-adrenergic blockers should be observed for the development of impending congestive heart failure (CHF) or unexplained respiratory symptoms.

Most adverse effects have been mild, have not required discontinuation of therapy, and have tended to decrease as duration of treatment increased. The following have been reported: hypotension, bradycardia, heart failure, anxiety, hyper/hypoesthesia, impotence, pruritus, vomiting, abdominal pain, dysuria, nocturia, and a small number of cases of liver abnormalities with increased serum glutamic-oxaloacetic transaminase (SGOT), serum glutamic-pyruvic transaminase (SGPT), and lactate dehydrogenase (LDH). Increased bilirubin or alkaline phosphatase, fever, malaise, dark urine, anorexia, nausea, and/or headache have also occurred. Back pain, joint pain, pharyngitis, wheezing, conjunctivitis, dry eye, eye pain, and, rarely, systemic lupus erythematosus have also been reported.

PRECAUTIONS AND CONTRAINDICATIONS. Daily dose of acebutolol should be decreased by 50% and by 75% when the creatinine clearance is less than 50 and 75% mL/min, respectively, because its major metabolite is eliminated via the kidney. Acebutolol should also be used with caution in those with hepatic dysfunction. Lower maintenance doses may be necessary in the geriatric patient because the bioavailability of both the parent and major metabolite is approximately doubled. Its effects in pregnancy are unknown; it has been shown to cross the human placenta, causing reduced birth weight, decreased blood pressure, and decreased heart rate.

Use in nursing mothers is not recommended because both the parent compound and its major metabolite appear in breast milk. Acebutolol is contraindicated in patients with persistently severe bradycardia, second- and third-degree heart block, overt cardiac failure, and cardiogenic shock.

DRUG INTERACTIONS. Concomitant administration of α-adrenergic agonists (such as the nasal decongestants in over-the-counter [OTC] cold preparations and nasal drops) can result in a severe hypertensive reaction.

> BOX 28–12
> **THERAPEUTIC USE**
>
> In the management of ventricular premature beats, it reduces the total number of premature beats and the number of paired and multiform ventricular ectopic beats and R-on-T beats. It is also used in the management of hypertension in adults.

Esmolol

ACTIONS. Esmolol (BREVIBLOC) is a β_1 cardioselective adrenergic blocking agent. Higher doses will block β_2 receptors located primarily in the bronchial and vascular musculature. It possesses no significant intrinsic sympathomimetic or membrane stabilizing activity at therapeutic doses.

Sinus Node. The sinus node recovery time is prolonged with an increase in the sinus cycle length.

AH Interval. This interval is prolonged during normal sinus rhythm and during atrial pacing, with an increase in antegrade Wenckebach cycle length.

ORGAN SYSTEM PHARMACOLOGY. The heart rate at rest and during exercise is slowed in normal subjects.

PHARMACOKINETICS. Esmolol has a very short duration of action, with an elimination half-life of approximately 9 minutes. It is rapidly metabolized by hydrolysis of the ester linkages, chiefly by the esterases in the cytosol or red blood cells and not by plasma cholinesterases or red cell membrane acetylcholinesterase. Metabolism is not limited by the rate of blood flow to metabolizing tissues such as the liver or affected by hepatic or renal blood flow. It is primarily excreted unchanged by the kidney.

> BOX 28–13
> **THERAPEUTIC USE**
>
> Esmolol is uniquely useful for the rapid control of ventricular rate in patients with atrial fibrillation or atrial flutter in perioperative, postoperative, or other emergent circumstances where short-term control of ventricular rate with a short-acting drug is needed. It is also useful in noncompensatory sinus tachycardia where the rapid heart rate requires intervention.
>
> The IV administration of a β-blocking agent during the acute phase of myocardial infarction achieves plasma concentrations within the therapeutic range almost immediately, circumventing the lower and less predictable levels associated with oral dosing. The short duration of action offers increased safety when the importance of sympathetic stimulation in maintaining cardiac output may be uncertain.

ADVERSE EFFECTS. Intravenous infusion may be associated with hypotension, diaphoresis, dizziness, peripheral ischemia, pallor, flushing, bradycardia, chest pain, syncope, pulmonary edema, and heart block; thrombophlebitis can also occur. Somnolence, confusion, headache, agitation, grand mal seizures, and fatigue have been reported in some patients. A few may exhibit respiratory symptoms of bronchospasms, wheezing, dyspnea, and nasal congestion. Gastrointestinal symptoms of nausea, vomiting, dyspepsia, constipation, dry mouth, and abdominal discomfort occur rarely.

PRECAUTIONS AND CONTRAINDICATIONS. Esmolol should be used with caution in diabetics because it may mask tachycardia occurring with hypoglycemia and in patients with renal failure because its elimination half-life has been shown to increase, increasing its plasma levels. It is contraindicated in patients with sinus bradycardia, heart block greater than first degree, cardiogenic shock, overt heart failure, or bronchospastic disease. Its effects in pregnant females, nursing mothers, and children are not known.

DRUG INTERACTIONS. Catecholamine-depleting drugs such as reserpine may have additive effects. Digoxin levels may be increased. Steady-state levels of esmolol are increased in the presence of morphine. The duration of neuromuscular blockade by succinylcholine is prolonged after esmolol administration.

CLASS III AGENTS

General Characteristics

Class III antiarrhythmic agents prolong the action potential duration and increase the effective refractory period.

Sotalol

ACTIONS. Sotalol (BETAPACE) possesses both β adrenoreceptor blocking action (Class II) and cardiac action potential duration prolongation (Class III) properties. Sotalol is a racemic mixture of d- and 1-sotalol; both isomers exhibit similar Class III antiarrhythmic actions, whereas the 1-isomer initiates almost all of the β blocking actions. The β-blocking action is noncardioselective; it does not exhibit partial agonist or membrane stabilizing actions.

Atria. The atrial action potential and effective refractory periods are prolonged, along with increases in the effective refractory period in bypass tracts (anterograde and retrograde).

Atrioventricular Node. Nodal conduction is decreased and refractoriness is increased.

Ventricular Muscle. Ventricular action potential and effective refractory period are prolonged.

ORGAN SYSTEM PHARMACOLOGY. Congestive heart failure is worsened. Exercise- and isoproterenol-induced tachycardia is antagonized. In hypertensive patients, systolic and diastolic blood pressures are decreased.

PHARMACOKINETICS. Sotalol is rapidly and nearly completely absorbed; its mean elimination half-life is 12 hours, and it is excreted primarily via the kidney. It does not bind to plasma proteins and is not metabolized. Age does not alter the pharmacokinetics but impaired renal function in geriatric patients may increase the terminal elimination half-life, resulting in increased drug accumulation.

ADVERSE EFFECTS. Like other antiarrhythmics, sotalol may initiate arrhythmias. There is a suggestion that it may cause early sudden death in a postinfarction patient population.

Most commonly observed effects leading to its discontinuation include fatigue, bradycardia, dyspnea, proarrhythmia, asthenia, and dizziness. Rarely elevated serum liver enzymes have been observed, but a cause and effect has not been proven.

PRECAUTIONS AND CONTRAINDICATIONS. Sotalol is used almost exclusively to treat ventricular arrhythmias, such as sustained life-threatening ventricular tachycardia. Because it possesses proarrhythmic actions, its use in those with ventricular arrhythmias that are not life-threatening is not recommended.

It is contraindicated in those with sinus bradycardia, second- and third-degree AV block unless a functional pacemaker is present, in congenital or acquired long QT syndrome, cardiogenic shock, uncontrolled congestive heart failure, bronchial asthma, and hypersensitivity to sotalol.

It crosses the human placenta and can be detected in the amniotic fluid; one report of subnormal birth weight was found. It is secreted into mother's milk. Its use in a pediatric population has not been established.

DRUG INTERACTIONS. Because sotalol has the potential to prolong refractoriness, it should not be used in combination with class IA drugs such as disopyramide, quinidine, and procainamide and other class III drugs such as amiodarone; possible interactions with class IB or IC antiarrhythmics has not been well explored.

Proarrhythmic effects of sotalol have been reported more often when given with digoxin; it is unknown if this is an interaction or if it is due to the presence of congestive heart failure, a risk factor for proarrhythmia. Any drug, such as class I antiarrhythmics, phenothiazines, tricyclic antidepressants, terfenadine, and astemizole, that prolongs the QT interval should be given with caution in patients receiving sotalol; caution is also warranted in patients receiving calcium blocking agents because possible additive effects on atrioventricular conduction, or ventricular function, or blood pressure may occur.

> BOX 28–14
> **THERAPEUTIC USE**
>
> Sotalol is used in the treatment of ventricular arrhythmias, such as sustained life-threatening ventricular tachycardia.

Bretylium

Bretylium (BRETYLOL and others), a benzylammonium compound, was marketed initially as an adrenergic neuronal blocking agent to be used in the treatment of hypertension, but the development of tolerance to its antihypertensive effects and its unpredictable oral absorption ultimately precluded its use for hypertension. It is currently used only to suppress ventricular fibrillation occurring during clinical emergencies, such as a myocardial infarction, or when other antiarrhythmic agents have failed.

ACTIONS. Bretylium has two actions. It directly modifies the electrical properties of the myocardium, and it depresses adrenergic neuronal transmission following a brief initial period of increased adrenergic amine release.

Autonomic Nervous System (see Chapters 9 and 10).

Sinoatrial Node (Table 28–4). Only a brief increase in sinus automaticity occurs with the initial release of catecholamines induced by bretylium; this brief effect can transiently worsen arrhythmias. This increase in automaticity is followed by no change or a decrease in automaticity.

Atria. The atrial action potential is prolonged, causing a prolongation of the effective refractory period in the atrial muscle.

Atrioventricular Node. Conduction velocity may be increased and the AV nodal refractory period may be decreased. The initial catecholamine release improves AV transmission to the extent that acceleration of the ventricular rate may develop; thus bretylium cannot be used to treat atrial flutter or fibrillation.

His-Purkinje System. Bretylium increases the firing rate of Purkinje fibers *in vitro* and may induce firing in quiescent fibers. The conduction rate in Purkinje fibers is not altered. The duration of the Purkinje action potential is prolonged.

Ventricular Muscle. The ventricular fibrillation threshold is increased significantly in both normal and ischemic hearts to a greater extent than by other antiarrhythmic agents. The electrical threshold for successful defibrillation is lowered by bretylium, whereas the success rate for defibrillation is increased. The duration of ventricular muscle fiber action potential is prolonged, whereas conduction is not altered.

The membrane responsiveness of Purkinje fibers or ventricular muscle is unaltered.

Electrocardiographic. In normal humans, bretylium administration results in an increase in the sinus rate that is followed by a return to normal or even a decrease. The PR and QT intervals are increased, but the duration of the QRS complex is not altered. If there is an initial increase in the force of myocardial contractility initiated by the catecholamine release, it is followed usually by a decrease in the force of contraction as adrenergic neuronal blockade is established.

ORGAN SYSTEM PHARMACOLOGY. An increase in catecholamine activity, manifested by phase 4 depolarization, an increase in automaticity, and a transient increase in arterial pressure, occurs immediately following its administration. This is followed by a decrease in arterial blood pressure consistent with adrenergic neuronal blockade. The hypotensive effect develops between 1 and 2 hours after the administration of bretylium. Standing upright increases the magnitude of the hypotension, and it is maximal during exercise in an upright position.

PHARMACOKINETICS. Bretylium exhibits poor and unpredictable absorption after oral administration.

ADVERSE EFFECTS. The major adverse effects associated with the use of bretylium relate to its modification of adrenergic function. The catecholamines released not only cause increased blood pressure and heart rate but also may cause anxiety, excitement, flushing, substernal pressure sensation, headache, or angina pectoris. Nasal congestion and conjunctival suffusion may be observed 1 - 2 hours after its acute administration.

The IV use of bretylium to treat acute arrhythmias is associated with profound, long-lasting hypotension resulting from the peripheral vasodilation; more than 10% of patients will require discontinuation of bretylium because of hypotension. Rapid IV administration may initiate nausea and vomiting.

The safety of bretylium in pregnant females or in children has not been determined.

> **BOX 28-15**
>
> **THERAPEUTIC USES**
>
> The only clinical use for bretylium is within the intensive care unit to treat life-threatening ventricular fibrillation or other ventricular arrhythmias (especially ventricular tachycardia) that have not responded favorably to lidocaine or procainamide, or to repeated direct current (DC) countershock. Bretylium appears to be effective in up to 70% of patients exhibiting ventricular fibrillation refractory to all other drugs.

PRECAUTIONS. Bretylium should be avoided if possible in patients with a fixed cardiac output, such as those with severe aortic stenosis or pulmonary hypertension. However, because ventricular fibrillation is fatal, bretylium may be required in spite of the presence of other clinical problems.

Amiodarone

Amiodarone (CORDARONE; Tables 28 - 4 and 28 - 5) is an antiarrhythmic that possesses some of the pharmacological properties of bretylium; for example, it slows repolarization in myocardial fibers and increases the ventricular fibrillation threshold. It is unique because of its extremely long half-life of 25 to 55 days. It is used to suppress supraventricular and ventricular tachyarrhythmias.

ACTIONS. SA conduction may be slowed and the sinus rate decreased. Ventricular, atrial, and AV nodal effective refractory periods are lengthened. The ventricular action potential is prolonged, and the ventricular fibrillation threshold is increased. AH and HV intervals are increased (Table 28 - 4).

ORGAN SYSTEM PHARMACOLOGY. Acute administration induces a mild, transient depression in systemic vascular resistance and left ventricular function.

PHARMACOKINETICS. Amiodarone exhibits a slow onset of action. This makes it difficult to evaluate its efficacy, or lack thereof, as well as the efficacy of other drugs that may be used adjunctively. Amiodarone exhibits an oral bioavailability between 20 and 50%, is thought to be highly bound to plasma proteins, possesses an elimination half-life of 25 - 55 days, and is inactivated primarily by the liver (Table 28 - 5). Thus, some of the manifestations of its toxicity or adverse effects may be long-lasting, even after its administration has been stopped.

ADVERSE EFFECTS. Amiodarone has been used widely and in diverse patient populations. Asymptomatic corneal microdeposits have been reported in almost all patients administered amiodarone; peripheral neuropathy and hypothyroidism also have been reported. Other reported side effects include pulmonary fibrosis, slowing of His bundle conduction, lightheadedness, and bluish-gray tint in the skin.

Interstitial pneumonitis, pulmonary fibrosis, and associated changes in pulmonary function, sometimes irreversible, have been associated with the use of amiodarone. It is desirable to carry out pulmonary function tests and chest radiographs prior to initiation of therapy with amiodarone and during follow-up examinations. Amiodarone may impair myocardial contractility; cause symptomatic sinus bradycardia, SA block, or sinus arrest requiring cardiac pacing; or induce ventricular tachycardia or fibrillation. The frequency of these reactions varies considerably in different studies, and the differences among studies cannot be explained on the basis of different dosages or modes of administration. A consensus on the status of amiodarone awaits thorough evaluation of its long-term toxicity.

BOX 28–16

THERAPEUTIC USES

Amiodarone is generally reserved for therapy of life-threatening ventricular arrhythmias refractory to other agents. It appears to be effective in the prevention of sudden death. It may be used in the long-term management of individuals with recurrent ventricular tachycardia or ventricular fibrillation and in those patients with atrial fibrillation associated with the Wolff-Parkinson-White syndrome.

PRECAUTIONS AND CONTRAINDICATIONS. Amiodarone is used only to treat life-threatening arrhythmias because of its substantial toxicity. Even in patients at high risk of arrhythmic death in whom the toxicity of amiodarone is an acceptable risk, its use may be associated with major management problems.

The therapeutic and toxic actions may be present for weeks after the amiodarone has been discontinued. This may be due to its long half-life or to active metabolites. Metabolism occurs in the liver, and the desethyl derivative accumulates with chronic administration; the biological activity of this metabolite is not known.

DRUG INTERACTIONS. Amiodarone can increase the serum concentrations, the pharmacological effects, and the toxicities of digoxin, phenytoin, quinidine, procainamide, felcainide, β-adrenergic blocking agents, oral anticoagulants, and diltiazem.

CLASS IV AGENTS: CALCIUM CHANNEL BLOCKERS

Verapamil and Diltiazem

Although calcium permeability plays a role in regulating membrane stability and arrhythmias, the calcium channel blockers exhibit disparate actions, and no uniform antiarrhythmic effect can be attributed to them as a general class (see Table 28–7 and Chapter 32).

BOX 28–17

THERAPEUTIC USES

Verapamil is the drug of first chice to treat paroxysmal supraventricular tachycardia due to AV nodal reentry or to abnormal AV conduction (Wolff-Parkinson-White syndrome or concealed bypass tracts). Verapamil also decreases the ventricular response to atrial flutter or fibrillation (Table 28–7).

PRECAUTIONS AND CONTRAINDICATIONS. Verapamil should be used with caution or should not be used in patients exhibiting sick sinus syndrome without an artificial pacemaker or in patients with AV conduction abnormalities. The same is true for patients with severe congestive heart failure or those requiring β-blocking agents or disopyramide. The use of verapamil to treat digitalis-induced delayed after-de-

TABLE 28–7. Efficacy of the Calcium Antagonists in Various Cardiovascular Disorders

Drug	Very Effective	Somewhat Effective	Possibly Effective	Ineffective or Deleterious
Verapamil	Paroxysmal supraventricular tachycardia, atrial fibrillation and flutter Hypertrophic cardiomyopathy Variant angina, angina of effort, unstable angina	Mild–moderate systemic hypertension	Ventricular tachyarrhythmias	Pulmonary hypertension Unloading agent in CHF Raynaud's phenomenon or disease
Nifedipine	Mild–moderate systemic hypertension Pulmonary hypertension Variant angina, angina of effort (especially combined with a β blocker), unstable angina	Unloading agent in CHF Raynaud's phenomenon or disease	Selected patients with hypertrophic cardiomyopathy Migraine headache	Supraventricular or ventricular tachyarrhythmias
Diltiazem	Variant angina, angina of effort		Supraventricular tachyarrhythmias Pulmonary hypertension	Untested in systemic hypertension, Raynaud's disease, or hypertrophic cardiomyopathy

From Winniford MD, Hillis LD: Calcium antagonists in patients with cardiovascular disease. Medicine 64(1):61–73. © by Williams & Wilkins, 1985.
CHF = congestive heart failure.

polarizations and triggered activity is risky, because additional AV block may be induced and automaticity in the His-Purkinje fibers may be suppressed.

DRUG INTERACTIONS. Both verapamil and diltiazem can cause an increase in digoxin serum concentrations. Each can interact with many drugs, including disopyramide, quinidine, lithium, carbamazepine, rifampin, phenobarbital, and flecainide. Moreover, verapamil may increase the effects of inhalation anesthetics as well as depolarizing neuromuscular blocking agents (see Chapter 32).

CLASS V AND OTHER AGENTS

Digoxin

The digitalis glycosides are used commonly in the management of congestive heart failure complicated by supraventricular tachyarrthymias such as atrial fibrillation and atrial tachyarrhythmias. The antiarrhythmic effect results from an action on the atria and AV node and a complex interaction of glycosides on the autonomic nervous system and cardiac cells. Table 28–8 summarizes the combination of antiarrhythmic agents such as quinidine, propranolol, or verapamil with digitalis to treat atrial fibrillation/flutter, paroxysmal supraventricular tachycardias, and the sick sinus syndrome.

Adenosine

The inclusion of adenosine (ADENOCARD) in a category as a "Class VI Agent" is speculative at present.

ACTIONS. Adenosine is highly effective in terminating many reentry arrhythmias. It restores normal sinus rhythm in patients with paroxysmal supraventricular tachycardia, including paroxysmal supraventricular tachycardia associated with Wolff-Parkinson-White syndrome.

Conduction through the AV node is slowed and reentrant pathways interrupted.

ORGAN SYSTEM PHARMACOLOGY. Although it can cause transient hypotension or atrial fibrillation, it is probably safer than diltiazem or verapamil.

PHARMACOKINETICS. Adenosine has a rapid onset of action after administration as a bolus given intravenously. It is rapidly taken up by erythrocytes and vascular endothelial cells; its half-life is less than 10 seconds. Adenosine appears to enter the body pool of endogenous nucleosides and is primarily metabolized to inosine and to adenosine monophosphate (AMP).

ADVERSE EFFECTS. The following have been reported: facial flushing, headache, sweating, palpitations, chest pain, hypotension, shortness of breath/dyspnea, chest pressure, hyperventilation, head pressure, lightheadedness, dizziness, tingling arms, numbness, apprehension, blurred vision, burning sensation, heaviness in arms, and neck and back pain, nausea, metallic taste, tightness in the throat, and pressure in the groin. Because of the short half-life, the adverse effects are usually self-limiting.

Inhaled adenosine may induce bronchoconstriction in asthmatic patients. Adenosine may produce a short-lasting first-, second- or third-degree heart block. Rarely, transient asystole may develop. At the time of conversion to normal sinus rhythm, a variety of new rhythms may appear, last only a few seconds without intervention, and may take the form of premature ventricular contractions, atrial premature contractions, sinus bradycardia, sinus tachycardia, skipped beats, and varying degrees of AV nodal block.

The use of adenosine is contraindicated in patients with

TABLE 28–8. Representative Antiarrhythmic Combinations with Probable Clinical Utility

Combination	Uses	Comments
Digitalis and β blocker or verapamil	Resistant supraventricular tachyarrhythmias with rapid AV conduction	Potentiation of AV nodal effects of each drug alone
Digitalis and class I antiarrhythmic	Supraventricular tachycardias; for conversion/maintenance ? Selected efficacy in ventricular arrhythmia	Digitalis antagonizes vagolytic effects of class I drugs on AV node
Mexiletine and quinidine (classes IB and IA)	Refractory ventricular arrhythmias (monitor assessment)	Decreased dosage, toxicity of each drug, increased efficacy Other combinations of class IB (lidocaine, tocainide, or phenytoin) with quinidine or other class IA may be tried
β Blocker and class I drug	Post-MI ventricular arrhythmia (despite β blocker) Other resistant ventricular arrhythmias Conversion of atrial fibrillation and maintenance therapy Other supraventricular arrhythmias Acute MI, IV with lidocaine	Under study for post-MI arrhythmias β Blocker may decrease toxicity of class I drug
Amiodarone and class I drug	Initial management of resistant ventricular arrhythmias during amiodarone loading	Caution with quinidine (QT prolongation, torsades) May discontinue concomitant therapy after 1–2 months
Amiodarone and digitalis, propranolol, or verapamil	Initial management of resistant supraventricular arrhythmias during amiodarone loading	Caution must be used (additive effects) May discontinue concomitant therapy after 1–2 months

From Anderson JL: Rationale of combination antiarrhythmic drug therapy. *In* Dreifus LS (ed): Cardiac Arrhythmias: Electrophysiologic Techniques and Management. Brest AN (ed-in-chief): Cardiovasc Clin 16:307–327, 1985.

AV = atrioventricular; IV = intravenous; MI = myocardial infarction.

second- or third-degree AV block unless they have a functional artificial pacemaker, in those with sick sinus syndrome except when a functioning artificial pacemaker is present, and in those with known sensitivity to adenosine.

Its effects in pregnant and pediatric patients are not known.

DRUG INTERACTIONS. Adenosine is antagonized competitively by methylxanthines such as caffeine and theophylline. Dipyridamole may potentiate the effects of adenosine, such that smaller doses of the latter may be effective. Since the primary effect of adenosine is to decrease conduction through the AV node, higher degrees of heart block may be produced when used with carbamazepine.

The effects of adenosine are not blocked by atropine.

> BOX 28–18
> **THERAPEUTIC USES**
>
> Adenosine is used for conversion to sinus rhythm of paroxysmal supraventricular tachycardia, including that occurring with accessory bypass tracts (Wolff-Parkinson-White syndrome). If clinically prudent, appropriate vagal maneuvers, such as a Valsalva maneuver, should be done prior to giving adenosine.

REFERENCES

Baker DW, Koustam MA, Bottorff M, Pitt B: Management of heart failure: 1. Pharmacologic treatment. JAMA 272:1361–1366, 1994.

Burckhardt D, Hoffmann A, Kiowski W, et al: Effect of antiarrhythmic therapy on mortality after myocardial infarction. J Cardiovasc Pharmacol 17(Suppl 6):S77–S81, 1991.

Bryson HM, Palmer KJ, Langtry HD, Titton A: Propafenone. A reappraisal of its pharmacology, pharmacokinetics and therapeutic use in cardiac arrhythmias. Drugs 45:85–130, 1993.

Campbell TJ: Subclassification of Class I antiarrhythmic drugs: Enhanced relevance after CAST. Cardiovasc Drugs Ther 6:519–528, 1992.

Clyne CA, Estes NAM, Wang PJ: Drug therapy: Moricizine. N Engl J Med 327:255–260, 1992.

Coumel P: Future trends in antiarrhythmic therapy. J Cardiovasc Pharmacol 17(Suppl 6):S95–S100, 1991.

Drugs for cardiac arrhythmias. Med Lett Drugs Ther 33:55–60, 1991.

Follath F: Clinical pharmacology of antiarrhythmic drugs: Variability of metabolism and dose requirements. J Cardiovasc Pharmacol 17(Suppl 6):S74–S76, 1991.

Friedman L, Schron E, Yusuf S: Risk-benefit assessment of antiarrhythmic drugs: An epidemiological perspective. Drug Safety 6:323–331, 1991.

Gill J, Heel RC, Fitton A: Amiodarone: An overview of its pharmacological properties, and review of its therapeutic use in cardiac arrhythmias. Drugs 43:69–110, 1992.

Grant AO: Models of drug interaction with the sodium channel. Clin Invest Med 14:447–457, 1991.

Grant AO: On the mechanisms of action of antiarrhythmic agents. Am Heart J 123:1130–1136, 1992.

Harrison DC: Current classification of antiarrhythmic drugs as a guide to their rational clinical use. Drugs 31:93–95, 1986.

Lathers CM, Levin RM, Spivey WH: Regional distribution of myocardial beta-adrenoceptors in the cat. Eur J Pharmacol 130:111–117, 1986a.

Lathers CM, Spivey WH, Suter LE, et al: The effect of acute and chronic administration of timolol on cardiac sympathetic neural discharge, arrhythmia, and beta adrenergic receptor density associated with coronary occlusion in the cat. Life Sci 39:2121–2141, 1986b.

Lathers CM, Spivey WH, Levin RM, Tumer N: The effect of dilevalol on cardiac autonomic neural discharge, plasma catecholamines, and myocardial beta receptor density associated with coronary occlusion. J Clin Pharmacol 30:241–253, 1990.

Morgan TK, Sullivan ME: An overview of Class III electrophysiological agents: A new generation of antiarrhythmic therapy. *In* Ellis GP, Luscombe DK (eds): Progress in Medicinal Chemistry, 65–108. New York: Elsevier, 1992.

Podrid PJ: Safety and toxicity of antiarrhythmic drug therapy: Benefit versus risk. J Cardiovasc Pharmacol 17(Suppl 6):S65–S73, 1991.

Rankin AC: Adverse effects of antiarrhythmic drugs. Adverse Drug React Toxicol Rev 11:173–191, 1992.

Ruskin JN: The cardiac arrhythmia suppression trial (CAST). N Engl J Med 321:386–389, 1989.

Sheldon RS, Duff HJ, Hill RJ: Class I anti-arrhythmic drugs: Structure and function at the cardiac sodium channel. Clin Invest Med 14:458–465, 1991.

Sun DK, Reiner D, Frishman W, Grossman M, Luftschein S: Adverse dermatological reactions from antiarrhythmic drug therapy. J Clin Pharmacol 34:953–966, 1994.

Tisdale JE, Webb CR: Are antiarrhythmic drugs obsolete? Clin Pharm 49:714–726, 1992.

Vaughn Williams EM: Classifying antiarrhythmic actions: By facts or speculation. J Clin Pharmacol 32:964–977, 1992.

Vaughn Williams EM: The relevance of cellular to clinical electrophysiology in classifying antiarrhythmic actions. J Cardiovasc Pharmacol 20(Suppl 2):S1–S7, 1992.

Working Group on Arrhythmias of the European Society of Cardiology: The Sicilian gambit. Circulation 84:1831–1851, 1991.

29 Drug Treatment of Hypertension

Joseph L. Izzo, Jr., and David B. Case

HYPERTENSION AND ITS TREATMENT

Risks of Hypertension

Hypertension is one of the most significant risk factors in the development and progression of a variety of cardiovascular diseases, including cardiac hypertrophy and congestive failure, stroke, retinopathy, dissecting aneurysm, progressive renal failure, coronary artery disease, peripheral vascular disease, and their related complications.

Benefits of Therapy in Relation to Severity

The benefits of therapy in *severe hypertension* are well established. The initial report of the Veterans Administration Cooperative Study (1967) was the first controlled demonstration that treatment of individuals with diastolic blood pressure of 115 mmHg or higher significantly diminished the prevalence of stroke, congestive heart failure, renal failure, and dissecting aneurysm. In contrast, remarkably little evidence exists from the large-scale clinical trials that treating mild hypertension produces the expected benefits in reducing coronary artery disease, particularly in reducing myocardial infarction rates, or in decreasing renal failure in the absence of other risk factors. Also, men and women may not benefit to the same extent, a distinction that is further confounded by the dramatically increased risk in postmenopausal compared with premenopausal women.

The Concept of Multiple Risk

The Framingham studies defined major cardiovascular risk factors to be hypertension, hypercholesterolemia, diabetes/hyperglycemia, cigarette smoking, and left ventricular hypertrophy. The value of treatment of mild hypertension is best judged in the context of the coexisting risk factors or diseases present in the person to be treated. For example, diabetic patients must be treated aggressively to maintain as low a blood pressure as can be tolerated because this aggressive therapy reduces the rate of decline of renal function.

Certain risk factors must be addressed *independently,* however, for benefit to be achieved. Specifically, cigarette smokers do not derive equal benefits from antihypertensive therapy when compared with nonsmokers. Smoking cessation is a critical element of any public health policy designed to improve cardiovascular health.

Aging and the Relevance of Systolic and Diastolic Pressures

In urban societies, systolic blood pressure rises by about 1 mmHg per year after the fifth decade. The relationship between age and diastolic blood pressure is less predictable.

An elevation of systolic pressure exceeding 140 mmHg with diastolic pressure remaining at less than 90 mmHg, called "isolated systolic hypertension," can occur at any age but is more prevalent over the age of 70. Despite the absence of diastolic hypertension (>90 mmHg), persons at any age with isolated systolic hypertension have increased rates of stroke and heart attack. The previous reliance on elevated diastolic blood pressure for the diagnosis and treatment of hypertension is now being questioned on the basis of pathophysiology and epidemiological studies.

Classifications of Hypertension

Based on Etiology

Hypertension can be defined in terms of its severity, its association with underlying causes or related conditions, and its association with age and racial groups; it can also be defined in terms of possible mechanisms responsible for maintaining the elevated arterial pressure.

ESSENTIAL HYPERTENSION. The most common form of hypertension is primary (or "essential") and is present in over 99% of all cases of hypertension. No specific etiology has been identified for this form.

TABLE 29–1. Therapy in Secondary Forms of Hypertension

Condition	Specific Drug Therapy	Definitive Therapy
Renal artery stenosis	Converting-enzyme inhibitor Angiotensin analog	Angioplasty
Pheochromocytoma	Phenoxybenzamine Labetalol Prazosin, terazosin Metyrosine β Blocker	Surgery
Aldosterone-producing adenoma	Spironolactone Amiloride Triamterene α Blocker	Surgery
Adrenal hyperplasia	Same as for aldosterone-producing adenoma	No surgery
Coarctation of aorta	β Blocker	Surgery

SECONDARY HYPERTENSION. When a clear causal relationship exists, the hypertension is called "secondary." The common forms are shown in Table 29–1 along with the drugs commonly used to treat or stabilize the specific condition.

Several systemic diseases are associated with high blood pressure, including vasculitic diseases such as systemic lupus erythematosus, scleroderma, and polyarteritis; endocrinopathies such as hyperthyroidism, hypothyroidism, and acromegaly; as well as chronic and acute renal glomerular and tubular diseases. Treatment of the underlying condition often corrects the hypertension; in other cases, antihypertensive drug therapy is required.

Based on Severity

The degree of severity is a practical guide to the urgency and impact of therapy.

MILD HYPERTENSION. A blood pressure higher than 140/90 (either systolic or diastolic) is now becoming the international standard for hypertension. Blood pressures in the range of 140–159/90–104 mmHg are found in 80% or more of all hypertensive patients. It is more important to establish the diagnosis (abnormal readings on at least three individual occasions, with at least two abnormal readings per occasion) than to rush into therapy in this group.

MODERATE HYPERTENSION. Moderate hypertension includes average blood pressure levels of 161–179/105–119 mmHg. In these patients, a search for secondary forms of hypertension (such as renal artery stenosis) may be justified. Some target organ damage may be present; if not, treatment may be delayed until diagnostic testing is complete.

SEVERE HYPERTENSION. Severe hypertension corresponds to blood pressure levels above 180/120 mmHg in adults, with lower levels in children. Absent other medical problems, the condition is termed an "urgency" and should be treated within hours to days, usually with oral drugs. If an immediate risk of cardiovascular or central nervous system complications or death exists, the term "emergency" is used, and treatment is begun without delay.

ACCELERATED AND MALIGNANT PHASE. The term *accelerated hypertension* is used for the most serious hypertensive conditions that are associated with organ damage. These conditions are characterized by a recent increase to severe levels of blood pressure, usually higher than 180/120 mmHg in adults. The term *malignant hypertension* is reserved for cases with advanced retinopathy, specifically hemorrhages, exudates, and papilledema; this condition often occurs with associated encephalopathy, congestive heart failure, or stroke. Treatment is begun as soon as possible, often with intravenous drugs.

The clinical management of hypertensive emergencies and urgencies requires considerable skill and experience. As much damage can be done by lowering the blood pressure too quickly as can be done by not treating the high blood pressure at all. Furthermore, hypertensive urgencies are often complications of other medical processes. Knowledge of these other conditions is essential to the correct choice of an antihypertensive drug. Drugs most commonly used to treat hypertensive crisis are shown in Table 29-2.

GENERAL STRATEGY FOR TREATMENT OF HYPERTENSION

Heterogeneity of Hypertension

It is now widely accepted that hypertension is not a uniform process but rather a phenotype made up of several different components (genotypes, environmental influences, and pathophysiologically discrete syndromes) that form an extremely heterogeneous disorder. Optimizing the therapy for a given patient remains the challenge for the expert clinician. *Thus, no single class of antihypertensive drugs produces a satisfactory "curative" result in all cases of hypertension.* This observation is indirect proof of the heterogeneity of mechanisms that lead to hypertension in the broader population.

If each patient is approached as a "one-patient clinical trial," with one single pharmacological manipulation being employed at a given time, a "pathophysiological fingerprint" of that individual can be obtained. For example, chronic response of an individual to angiotensin-converting enzyme (ACE) inhibition strongly suggests that the hypertension in that person was principally angiotensin II-dependent. In contrast, thiazide diuretics are most effective as monotherapeutic agents in individuals with low activity of the renin-angiotensin system, such as the elderly patient.

Blood Pressure Defense Mechanisms

In many cases, antihypertensive drugs do not cause sustained decreases in blood pressure. In many of these, "normal" physiological responses have been mobilized to defend arterial pressure. *For practical purposes, three principal systems exist that act to defend arterial pressure in acute and chronic situations: (1) the sympathetic nervous system, (2) the renin-angiotensin system, and (3) the extracellular fluid volume.* These systems interact with a dynamic balance achieved at any given time between the degree of vasoconstriction and blood volume that is present. These systems also act in concert to restore arterial pressure to baseline levels. Blood pressure defense mechanisms are activated physiologically by such phenomena as hemorrhage or dehydration.

Systemic Pseudotolerance

In hypertension, vasodilator therapy has a very similar impact as does acute hemorrhage. Activation of the neurohumoral and renal fluid conservation mechanisms tends to abolish the antihypertensive effect of an arterial vasodilator. This is the reason why drugs such as hydralazine, monoxidil, and other direct arterial dilators have acute effects that quickly wane. The term "pseudotolerance" was coined to imply that while the drug's pharmacological effect is maintained, the body's compensatory mechanisms overcome the vasodilatory effects and restore arterial pressure.

Renal Pseudotolerance

Another important phenomenon leading to reduced efficacy of antihypertensive drugs is renal salt and water retention. In hypertensives whose blood pressures have been low-

TABLE 29-2. Drugs for Hypertensive Emergencies

Generic Name	Brand Name	Dose/Route Example	Comment
		Parenteral	
Sodium nitroprusside	NIPRIDE	0.5-10 μg/kg/minute	Good for general use in intensive care units
Labetalol	TRANDATE NORMODYNE	20-80 mg boluses; 0.5-2 mg/kg/minute continuous intravenous infusion	
Hydralazine	APRESOLINE	5-10 mg intramuscularly every 2-6 hours	Still used in obstetrics
Methyldopa	ALDOMET	250-500 mg over 0.5-1 hour	Slower, less predictable effect
Enalaprilat	VASOTEC IV	1.25 mg every 4-6 hours	Current use remains limited
		Oral	
Nifedipine	PROCARDIA	10-20 mg orally; repeat in 30-60 minutes	Very commonly used
Clonidine	CATAPRES	0.2 mg orally followed by 0.1 mg every 30-60 minutes (maximum, 0.6 mg)	Effective oral therapy

ered, there is a "resetting" of the pressure-natriuresis relationships within the kidney. Although the hypertensive subject may actually excrete that salt load faster than a normotensive control, the lowering of blood pressure in the hypertensive individual is accompanied by disproportionate salt and water retention. The resultant increases in extracellular fluid volume further blunt the efficacy of antihypertensive drugs. *This phenomenon of "renal pseudotolerance" is a ready explanation for the clinical observation that concomitant diuretics are often required for the action of other antihypertensives to be sustained and optimized.* Renal pseudotolerance occurs with all classes of hypertensive drugs.

Integrated Therapeutic Strategies

Today it is generally accepted that *the physician should try to lower blood pressure by the least-intrusive means possible.* The prognosis in untreated, isolated mild hypertension is good and may not be substantially worse than in age-matched nonhypertensive people unless coupled with other risk factors. Widespread sentiment exists that the optimum treatment in mild hypertension is nonpharmacological treatments (weight reduction, reduced salt diet, reduced alcohol intake, stress reduction, and others), yet the ability of most patients to sustain the complex life style modifications necessary to keep the blood pressure down is limited. If such nonpharmacological measures are not adequate or applicable, single- or double-drug therapy is used.

The maximal benefit of treatment of hypertension can be obtained only with an integrated approach that includes consideration of other medical conditions, risk factors, lifestyle, and other factors (Box 29–1).

Stepped-Care Algorithms

Based on the success of the large-scale clinical trials that established the basis for treatment of mild and moderate hypertension, stepwise schemes were devised starting in the 1970s. The treatment algorithm was based on the initial use of diuretics (step 1), followed by the sequential addition of antiadrenergic agents to thiazide diuretic (step 2), and later the addition of vasodilators and other drugs if pressure failed to respond (step 3). Although this algorithm has been revised several times, the basic premises remain largely the same.

Many of the precepts of stepped care are fundamentally sound and help to provide some general guidelines for therapy. A few additional practical points are listed in Box 29–2. Neither stepped care nor these "clinical pearls" are adequate to guide therapy by themselves and cannot substitute for experienced clinical judgment.

DRUGS USED TO TREAT HYPERTENSION

The drugs used to treat hypertension are shown in Tables 29–2 through 29–6, 29–8, and 29–9. A number of the drugs discussed briefly in this chapter are considered in much greater detail in other chapters, most notably diuretics (Chapter 35), sympathetic system agents (Chapters 9 and 10), and calcium antagonists (Chapter 32).

BOX 29–1

THERAPEUTIC DETERMINANTS IN HYPERTENSION

1. The **profile of systemic disorders present**. In a diabetic patient, for example, it is extremely important to achieve fastidious control of blood pressure to protect the kidneys and other organs.
2. The **degree of target organ damage present**. The presence of left ventricular hypertrophy, decreased vascular compliance, or albuminuria suggests that hypertension has pathological significance and usually mandates pharmacological treatment.
3. The **coexistence of other risk factors**. The risks of hypertension are magnified by the presence of hypercholesterolemia, glucose intolerance, cigarette smoking, left ventricular hypertrophy, high plasma renin activity, android obesity (high waist-hip ratio), and other factors. These other problems mandate a more agressive approach to hypertension.
4. The **individual characteristics and lifestyle preferences**. Any regimen is effective only if the patient can and will actually continue to take the drugs prescribed. In general, once-daily therapy is now the standard because it improves adherence to therapy. On occasion, twice-daily medications are justifiable; dosing three or four times daily is no longer acceptable. Medication side effects, cost, and other practical factors also may limit the choice of medication.
5. The **presence of true chronic hypertension**. Somewhat surprisingly, a correct diagnosis is not established by all clinicians. Presence of true hypertension is established by multiple readings over several encounters, using appropriate cuff methodology.

BOX 29–2

USEFUL THERAPEUTIC PRINCIPLES IN HYPERTENSION

Goals of Therapy

Medical illnesses, other risk factors, target organ damage patterns, lifestyle issues, and cost are important considerations in setting therapeutic goals. (See Box 29–1.) With regard to blood pressure itself, the major goal of therapy is to reduce resting systolic blood pressure to 140 mmHg or less and diastolic blood pressure to 90 mmHg or less. An important exception to this rule is the older patient with isolated systolic hypertension, in whom attempts to reduce systolic blood pressure below 160 mmHg may be met with significant central nervous system and somatic side effects.

Initial Choice of Agent

A single agent should be tried first. The best drugs for initial therapy are those (1) proven to be effective as monotherapy, (2) compatible with the medical condi-

Continued

BOX 29-2

USEFUL THERAPEUTIC PRINCIPLES IN HYPERTENSION (*Continued*)

tions of the patient, and (3) capable of conferring primary or secondary protection of the heart and blood vessels. Once-daily dosing, low rate of side effects, and low cost enhance the opportunities for therapeutic adherence.

Dosages and Titration

Titration of dosage depends on the type of drug used. Thiazides, β blockers, and angiotensin-converting enzyme inhibitors require minimal titration. Central sympatholytics, α-adrenergic blockers, and calcium channel blockers require somewhat more attention and may be best administered in lower doses initially.

Timing of Changes

Several weeks must be allowed for equilibration and homeostatic adjustments (pseudotolerance) to occur before a given therapy can be fully evaluated. Weeks to months may be required for a given patient to be able to tolerate a lower baseline pressure. Advances in dosage should be gradual and monitored carefully.

Dietary Considerations

Low sodium intake, like diuretic-induced sodium depletion, potentiates the effectiveness of most antihypertensive drugs, particularly converting enzyme inhibitors and adrenergic blockers. The combination of potent diuretics with a low-sodium diet increases the risk of excessive extracellular fluid volume depletion, hemoconcentration, azotemia, hyperuricemia, hyperreninemia, hyperaldosteronemia, and hypokalemia.

Substitution vs Addition

Unnecessary multidrug therapy may result from the stepwise addition of drugs (stepped-care approach). An alternative approach is to substitute another drug for an ineffective one instead of adding to it.

Refractory Hypertension

The failure to respond to drugs is usually caused by one of three different problems: (1) failure to adhere to the prescribed therapy (most common), (2) pseudotolerance (particularly severe salt and water retention that is usually remediable with the addition of diuretics), or (3) secondary hypertension.

Diuretics

• Thiazides and Related Compounds

Thiazide (benzothiadiazines) and related compounds (see Table 29-3) have become the most widely used drugs to treat hypertension and have formed the basis for most intervention trials. Although recent attention has been paid to their metabolic side effects (increases in blood glucose and cholesterol levels, reductions in serum potassium level), thiazide diuretics have proved to be generally effective, safe, well tolerated, and relatively inexpensive.

Thiazides may be combined with almost all other classes of antihypertensive drugs. Their principal value is to potentiate an antihypertensive effect by reversing secondary sodium chloride and water retention (renal pseudotolerance). Thiazides are commonly combined with potassium-sparing diuretics to minimize the dosages and side effects of each drug.

ACUTE ACTIONS OF THIAZIDES (see Chapter 35). Thiazide diuretics block sodium, chloride, and water reabsorption in the cortical diluting segment or distal tubule. The net acute effect is salt and water loss; contraction of extracellular fluid volume (ECFV); and decreased cardiac output, glomerular filtration rate, and renal blood flow. Initially, systolic pressure declines somewhat more than diastolic. These acute changes lead to sympathetic nervous activation, increased renin release, and aldosterone secretion, which limit the antihypertensive effects of ECFV depletion and potentiate the urinary loss of potassium.

CHRONIC ACTION OF THIAZIDES. Over the course of continued treatment, blood volume, cardiac index, and glomerular filtration rate tend to return to near-pretreatment levels. The sustained reduction in blood pressure is related to reduced systemic vasoconstriction.

Plasma norepinephrine, plasma renin activity, and aldosterone excretion, sensitive indicators of relative blood volume depletion, remain elevated during diuretic therapy.

Dosages of the diuretic must be considered together with dietary salt intake. The combination of a low-salt diet and a diuretic creates the potential hazard of excessive volume depletion, azotemia, and hemoconcentration. This may be particularly relevant in the elderly, whose total food and salt intake is often relatively low. In general, long-acting diuretics can be administered in the usual daily doses with the expectation that the normal sodium intake can be followed.

Potassium supplements are commonly given with thiazides. A dose of thiazide reaches a plateau effect after 6-12 weeks. Relatively few patients require more than 50 mg of hydrochlorothiazide or 25 mg of chlorthalidone; raising the dose further increases the occurrence of drug-induced hyperglycemia, hypercholesterolemia, hyperuricemia, and hypokalemia.

• Loop Diuretics

Loop diuretics (Table 29-3) are relatively ineffective as antihypertensive drugs except in patients with renal insufficiency or significant elevation of blood volume. This lack of chronic effect is due to their lack of arterial dilator activity and to their tendency to stimulate the sympathoadrenal and renin-angiotensin systems. Multiple daily doses are required to sustain a volume-depleting action in nonazotemic patients. In some patients with advanced renal disease, a dose of 160-320 mg/day of furosemide may be needed to promote adequate diuresis. However, these high doses may lead to damage of the eighth cranial nerve or produce significant metabolic abnormalities. Unlike thiazides, which may raise serum and ionized calcium levels, loop diuretics promote calcium excretion and have been used to treat hypercalcemic states.

• Potassium-Sparing Diuretics

Potassium-sparing diuretics (Table 29-3) are relatively weak and are most often used in combination with hydrochlorothiazide to antagonize the potassium wasting of the

TABLE 29–3. Oral Antihypertensive Diuretics

Group	Brand Name	Dosage (mg/day)	Comments
	Thiazides		Low doses now preferred to achieve reasonable antihypertensive effect with fewer metabolic side effects of hyperglycemia, hypokalemia, hyperuricemia, or hypercholesterolemia
Bendroflumethiazide	NATURETIN	2.5–5	
Benzthiazide	AQUATAG, EXNA, PROAQUA*	25–50	
Chlorothiazide	DIURIL*	250–500	
Cyclothiazide	ANHYDRON	1–2	
Hydrochlorothiazide	HYDRODIURIL, ESIDRIX, ORETIC*	25–50	
Hydroflumethiazide	DIUCARDIN, SALURON*	25–50	
Methylclothiazide	AQUATENSEN, ENDURON*	2.5–5	
Polythiazide	RENESE	2–4	
Trichlormethiazide	METAHYDRIN, NAQUA*	2–4	
	Thiazidelike Diuretics		
Chlorthalidone	HYGROTON, THALITONE*	25–50	
Indapamide	LOZOL	2.5–5	
Metolazone	DIULO, ZAROXOLYN	2.5–5	
Quinethazone	HYDROMOX	50–100	
	Potassium-Sparing Diuretics		Can be used in conjunction with thiazides
Amiloride	MIDAMOR	5–10	
Spironolactone	ALDACTONE*	25–200	
Triamterene	DYRENIUM	50–100	
	Loop Diuretics		Generally reserved for renal failure or hyperkalemia
Bumetanide	BUMEX	0.5–10	
Ethacrynic acid	EDECRIN	25–200	
Furosemide	LASIX*	20–400	

*Available in generic form.

thiazide and to add to the antihypertensive effect. Spironolactone and amiloride have significant antihypertensive effects in certain patients, particularly those with excess mineralocorticoid secretion. (See Chapter 35.)

Sympatholytics

The activity of the sympathetic nervous system can be blocked at five levels, one within the central nervous system (CNS) and the other four in the peripheral nervous system. For the purposes of this discussion, drugs directly interfering with neurotransmission will be referred to as "sympatholytic drugs" (Table 29–4). Blockers of adrenergic receptors will be considered separately.

Central Sympatholytics

Blockade of sympathetic nervous outflow reduces blood pressure in all forms of hypertension, suggesting that the sympathoadrenal system plays at least a permissive role in the maintenance of elevated blood pressure in both primary (essential) and secondary forms of the disorder.

Central sympatholytic drugs have their primary modes of action at the level of the brainstem, where they interfere with the tonic output of CNS vasomotor control centers located primarily in the ventral rostrolateral areas of the brainstem.

Reduction of sympathoadrenal activity produces a balanced hemodynamic effect that includes arterial and venous vasodilation as well as reduced cardiac responses to exter-

TABLE 29–4. Oral Sympatholytic Drugs

Generic Name	Brand Name	Usual Dose (mg)/Frequency	Comments
	Centrally Acting Drugs		Because of sedative tendency, the bulk of the dosage is usually given in the evening; for example, clonidine 0.1 mg in the morning and 0.2 mg at bedtime. Imidazolines may precipitate rebound hypertension if abruptly withdrawn
IMIDAZOLINES			
Clonidine	CATAPRES	0.1–0.3 b.i.d.	
Clonidine transdermal	CATAPRES-TTS	0.1–0.3 every week	
Guanfacine	TENEX	0.1–0.3 q.d.	
Guanabenz	WYTENSIN	4–16 b.i.d.	
OTHERS			
Methyldopa	ALDOMET	250–750 b.i.d.	Also available parenterally
	Neuronal Depleting Agents		Also affect central nervous system directly
Reserpine	SERPASIL, and others	0.1–0.25 q.d.	
Guanethidine	ISMELIN SULFATE	10–100 q.d.	Postural hypotension common
Guanadrel	HYLOREL	10–100 q.d.	Postural hypotension common

b.i.d. = twice a day; q.d. = every day.

nal stimuli. Central sympatholytic drugs do not tend to cause orthostatic hypotension (greater reduction of blood pressure when the patient is seated and standing compared to when he or she is supine). Drugs that reduce venous tone and cardiac preload might theoretically reduce cardiac output and lead to postural hypotension. In reality, the reduction in afterload (arterial pressure) more than adequately offsets these effects. Central sympatholytics permit renal afferent arteriolar dilation and also reduce plasma renin activity, so that salt and water retention does not always occur.

Sympatholytic drugs tend to be an effective complementary therapy to diuretics and vasodilator drugs, which tend to cause reflex activation of the sympathoadrenal system. In some individuals, pseudotolerance may develop as a result of expansion of extracellular volume, and concomitant diuretics may be needed to maintain reduction of blood pressure.

Imidazolines

CLONIDINE. The imidazoline clonidine (CATAPRES) was developed as a nasal decongestant and was later discovered to cause reduced blood pressure. It acts on imidazoline and α_2 receptors to lower sympathoadrenal outflow. It may also act on postganglionic presynaptic nerve terminals to stimulate α_2 receptors, thereby inhibiting neural norepinephrine release. Clonidine may aggravate bradycardia in patients with sinus node dysfunction and may prolong atrioventricular (AV) conduction when given with digitalis preparations.

Clonidine is used to treat mild, moderate, or severe hypertension, usually in combination with a diuretic. Because of the possible withdrawal syndrome, poorly compliant patients should be treated with other agents. Clonidine may be used to reduce pressure promptly in hypertensive urgencies. A clonidine suppression test has been used in screening for pheochromocytoma to reduce background nonadrenal norepinephrine (NE) release. Clonidine has also been used to treat other withdrawal syndromes such as those from opiates or nicotine.

Clinical Pharmacology. Clonidine is rapidly and nearly completely absorbed after oral administration and is more than 75% bioavailable. Peak plasma concentrations occur in 1–3 hours, although the antihypertensive effects may be noticed within 30 minutes. There is a correlation between blood pressure reduction and plasma drug levels under 2.0 ng/mL. The volume of distribution is 1.2 L/kg, and the plasma half-life is about 9 hours. Clonidine is lipid soluble and enters the CNS. Approximately one half of an oral dose of clonidine is metabolized in the liver to inactive metabolites; the remainder is excreted unchanged by the kidneys. Thus, the dual route of excretion permits the use of lower doses in patients with renal failure.

Dry mouth (xerostomia) and drowsiness occur in at least half of all patients treated with clonidine but diminish somewhat over time. A variety of other side effects have been reported to occur relatively infrequently, including constipation, dizziness, nausea or gastric upset (5%), fatigue, weight gain, gynecomastia, pruritus, pruritic or allergic rash, thinning of hair, sexual impotence, urinary retention, sleep disturbances (insomnia, nightmares), anxiety, depression, congestive heart failure, ventricular arrhythmias, parotid pain, chemical hepatitis, edema and fluid retention, and others.

Drug Interactions. Clonidine combines favorably with diuretics and direct vasodilators to reduce severe refractory hypertension, particularly when β-adrenergic blockers cannot be used. Tricyclic antidepressants, naloxone, tolazoline, and monoamine oxidase (MAO) inhibitors may reverse the antihypertensive effects of clonidine. Additive depressant effects were reported when clonidine was combined with barbiturates, ethanol, and various tranquilizers.

Dosage. Clonidine is available orally and in a transdermal patch that is programmed to deliver 0.1–0.3 mg per day over 7 days. The usual initial tablet dosage is 0.1 mg given once daily at bedtime to patients with mild hypertension, with dose increments of 0.1 mg/day at weekly intervals. If needed, two unequal daily doses can be given, with the larger dose being given at bedtime; the usual clinical range is below 0.6 mg/day.

Withdrawal Syndrome. Abrupt withdrawal of clonidine and related drugs can produce a rebound hypertensive crisis similar in clinical characteristics to pheochromocytoma. The precise mechanisms for the effect are unknown. Approximately 12–24 hours after the last dose, blood pressure rises, often to levels much higher than pretreatment and into the range of moderate to severe hypertension in association with tachycardia, headache, abdominal pain, sweating, anxiety, and occasionally angina or palpitations. The most severe symptoms usually subside in 24 hours, but the syndrome may persist for a week. Similar withdrawal syndromes have been described for each of the other central agonists, with time courses proportional to the half-lives of the drugs. Although the syndrome is uncommon, it can be life-threatening. The manifestations are more pronounced in individuals with underlying moderate or severe hypertension on higher doses of clonidine. However, severe cases have been reported with doses as low as 0.6 mg/day. Concurrent treatment with a β-adrenergic blocker may potentiate the withdrawal syndrome because of the net vasoconstrictive effects of the endogenous catecholamines released during the withdrawal phase. Clonidine withdrawal can be prevented by gradually tapering the dose down over several weeks to doses as low as 0.05 mg/day. Beta blockers should be discontinued before withdrawing clonidine. Selection for clonidine therapy should be based on the patient's potential for adhering to a drug regimen. Peripheral blockers such as prazosin, terazosin, or doxazosin or the β blocker labetalol may also be given as clonidine is withdrawn or to blunt the withdrawal syndrome.

GUANFACINE. Guanfacine (TENEX), a guanidine derivative, lowers blood pressure by a mechanism similar to that of clonidine, inhibiting central sympathetic outflow through the activation of central α_2-adrenergic and probably imidazoline receptors. Its therapeutic uses and effectiveness, adverse effects, and drug interactions are, for practical purposes, the same as those of clonidine. Its advantage over other central sympatholytics is its longer duration of action.

Clinical Pharmacology. Guanfacine has a plasma half-life of 16–20 hours, thereby allowing once-daily dosing. Guanfacine is eliminated both as unmetabolized drug and partially after hydroxylation by renal excretion. However, plasma concentrations and antihypertensive actions are not potentiated in patients with renal insufficiency. Because part of guanfacine is metabolized by the hepatic microsomal system, chronic phenobarbital use results in a shortened plasma half-life. Like other central agonists, guanfacine has been associated with a rebound or withdrawal phenomenon. However, because of the long duration of action of the drug, the onset of the imidazoline withdrawal syndrome tends to occur later than with clonidine (2 – 7 days after cessation of therapy).

Dosages. Guanfacine is usually administered once daily at bedtime. Most of the studies done with this drug were carried out in patients already or subsequently treated with diuretics as well. Most patients respond to a dose of 2 mg/day or less.

GUANABENZ ACETATE. Guanabenz acetate (WYTENSIN) is a guanidine derivative whose principal mechanism of action is similar to clonidine. In addition, it has a slight peripheral ganglioplegic action similar to that of guanethidine. Guanabenz is about 75% bioavailable and about 90% protein-bound. Nearly all of the drug is metabolized; less than 1% unchanged drug is found in the urine. Peak action of the drug occurs 2 – 4 hours after oral ingestion. The plasma half-life varies from about 6 – 12 hours; the antihypertensive effect usually wanes gradually over 10 hours. Side effects, as well as the potential for the development of the imidazoline withdrawal syndrome, are similar to those with clonidine. Daily dosages of 4 – 16 mg are most commonly used.

METHYLDOPA. Methyldopa (L-isomer of alpha-methyldopa; ALDOMET) is a synthetic phenylalanine derivative first developed as an inhibitor of L-aromatic amino acid decarboxylase. Currently, most evidence supports the idea that α-methyl norepinephrine (NE) formed in the brain from α-methyldopa acts principally as an α_2-adrenergic agonist, thereby reducing sympathoadrenal activity by its action on the brainstem vasomotor control centers (ventral rostrolateral neurons).

Methyldopa has been used extensively to treat hypertension associated with renal disease, renal failure, and pregnancy; a desirable hypotensive effect can be achieved without further compromise of renal function and without significant orthostatic fall in pressure.

Clinical Pharmacology. Methyldopa is eliminated as an active drug (63%) or its conjugates by excretion in urine. Some of the active metabolites are excreted slowly in patients with renal failure. Therefore, the dose is reduced in conditions of hepatic and renal dysfunction. Some assays for urinary metanephrines, a screening test for pheochromocytoma, are artifactually increased by methyldopa. Plasma catecholamines and urinary vanillylmandelic acid are not affected, however.

The most frequent side effects reported are sedation, postural hypotension, dizziness, nasal congestion, sexual impotence, dry mouth, depression, and headache. Although these may abate somewhat over time, the availability of newer agents with fewer unpleasant side effects has led to a trend away from initiating therapy with this agent. A series of other less-common side effects may also occur: a reversible malabsorption syndrome (with abnormal biopsy) of the small bowel, positive Coombs' test results with and without hemolytic anemia, increases in liver enzyme levels (chemical hepatitis), and a severe febrile reaction with fevers up to 104°F.

Drug Interactions. Tricyclic antidepressants and MAO inhibitors may blunt or prevent the antihypertensive effects of methyldopa. Sympathomimetic amines in cold remedies, asthma preparations, and amphetaminelike drugs may reverse the antihypertensive effects. Methyldopa may undermine the effectiveness of levodopa in Parkinson's disease, and a paradoxical rise in blood pressure has been observed when phenothiazines and methyldopa were used together. The toxicities of lithium and haloperidol are increased when used with methyldopa, whereas barbiturates increase the metabolic clearance of methyldopa and shorten its half-life. Finally, the combination of methyldopa with other antihypertensive drugs and diuretics may produce hypotension.

Dosages. The initial dose in adults is 250 mg two or three times daily; the dose may be increased at weekly intervals, although a diuretic is usually added after the initial dose if not already present. The usual daily dose ranges between 500 and 1500 mg/day. More recent studies have suggested that the drug can be given as a single dose at bedtime to obviate problems with sedation and orthostasis seen with morning administration.

Ganglionic Blockers

Trimethaphan (ARFONAD)

Although oral ganglionic blocking agents, or the veratrum alkaloids, are no longer used as antihypertensive drugs, the ganglion blocker trimethaphan camsylate is occasionally administered intravenously. Like nitroprusside, trimethaphan always lowers blood pressure, but unlike nitroprusside, some degree of patient head-up position is needed to achieve maximal orthostatic effect. This phenomenon is characteristic of drugs with predominantly venodilatory effects. Trimethaphan can be given by continuous IV infusion for dissecting aortic aneurysm, acute hypertensive pulmonary edema, subarachnoid hemorrhage, and other critical hypertensive conditions.

Catecholamine Synthesis Inhibitors

Metyrosine

Metyrosine (α-methyl tyrosine; DEMSER) inhibits tyrosine hydroxylase, the rate-limiting step in catecholamine biosynthesis, thereby blocking the conversion of tyrosine to dihydroxyphenylalanine. Its use has been restricted to patients with pheochromocytoma because of its demonstrated efficacy in suppressing urinary catecholamine and catecholamine metabolite excretion while controlling the clinical expression of the underlying condition. Generally, phenoxybenzamine is used concurrently. At the time of surgery, phentolamine or sodium nitroprusside is used to modulate swings in blood pressure when the tumor is manipulated. If the tumor produces arrhythmias, β blockers or other specific antiarrhythmic drugs are given.

Neuronal Depleting Agents

Reserpine and Rauwolfia Alkaloids

The medicinal use of plants similar to rauwolfia dates back to ancient Hindu culture. It was not until the 1950s that the potential use for the root of the plant was explored, despite reports 20 years earlier detailing its previous application in psychoses and hypertension. Reserpine became widely used as one of the few available antiadrenergic drugs, despite its well-recognized adverse effects. It is the popular wisdom (though unproven scientifically) that reserpine's side effects are no longer tolerable in an era when "quality of life" is a major concern. In developing nations, however, the low cost of reserpine makes it a therapeutic mainstay.

Reserpine produces a prompt, slowly reversible depletion of catecholamine and 5-hydroxytryptamine stores in postganglionic nerves, the brain, and to a lesser extent, in the adrenal medulla. Reserpine prevents the uptake of NE into storage granules in neurons by inhibiting an adenosine triphosphate-dependent vesicular proton-amine exchange. Impairment of adrenergic neuronal function becomes significant after a 30% depletion of normal stores. Because tissue catecholamines are restored slowly, only small daily doses are required to produce long-term NE depletion. Although reserpine has prominent CNS side effects, the antihypertensive action is attributed principally to depletion of catecholamines from peripheral sympathetic nerve terminals.

Reserpine produces a characteristic hemodynamic profile: slowed heart rate, reduced cardiac output, and mild orthostatic hypotension. Total peripheral resistance is reduced in the supine position. In addition to these effects, reserpine leads to sedation and an attitude of indifference, much like that described for phenothiazines. Extrapyramidal effects may be observed as the dosage is increased. Other rauwolfia preparations include rauwolfia serpentina, alseroxylon, deserpidine, and rescinnamine.

CLINICAL PHARMACOLOGY. Reserpine is well absorbed from the gastrointestinal (GI) tract and is often taken with food to lessen gastric upset. The drug binds to biogenic amine storage sites and is taken up readily in fat tissue and brain. There is no obvious correlation between blood levels and effects. Peak antihypertensive response may take up to 3 or 4 weeks. The drug is metabolized but is excreted largely in the urine.

The most serious side effect is mental depression; other CNS side effects include nightmares, vivid dreams, drowsiness, sedation, dizziness, vertigo, headache, extrapyramidal movements, and reduced threshold for seizures. Some of the side effects of rauwolfia alkaloids are related to a marked increase in vagal tone, including GI reactions such as anorexia, nausea, vomiting, activation of peptic ulcer (increased gastric acid production and motility), increased salivation, and abdominal cramps. Prominent among cardiovascular effects are slowing of the sinus node, ventricular arrhythmias, salt and water retention, congestive heart failure, hypotension, and syncope. Additional side effects include weight gain, muscular dyskinesias, bronchospasm, and increased prolactin secretion with associated sexual impotence and gynecomastia.

DRUG INTERACTIONS. When combined with diuretics, adrenergic blockers, and other vasodilators, reserpine may induce an additive antihypertensive effect. Reserpine may induce a severe hypertensive response when given to a patient on an MAO inhibitor. Arrhythmias have been described when reserpine was added to digitalis or class I antiarrhythmics. Hypotensive reactions have been observed when patients on reserpine received inhalant anesthetic agents. Concurrent use of reserpine and tricyclic antidepressants nullifies the antihypertensive effects and leads to CNS excitement. Reserpine in levodopa-treated patients may worsen the extrapyramidal movement disorder and lead to orthostatic hypotension. Reserpine may lead to excessive sedation if combined with CNS depressants such as barbiturates or minor tranquilizers.

DOSAGES. The bulk of experience with reserpine in clinical trials has been in combination with diuretics and other drugs. The usual dose of reserpine is 0.1 mg given once daily in combination with a thiazide diuretic or a direct vasodilator such as hydralazine. Doses higher than 0.25 mg/day are more likely to produce significant side effects.

Guanidine Derivatives

GUANETHIDINE. Guanethidine (ISMELIN) reduces blood pressure by inhibiting neuronal NE release and by depletion of neuronal NE stores through interference with granular transport mechanisms. As part of its mechanism of action, guanethidine is taken up and stored in adrenergic nerves, where it causes granular degeneration. Guanethidine reduces cardiac output principally by reducing venous tone and venous return, but it also lowers systemic vascular resistance. Like other peripheral (largely venodilatory) sympatholytic drugs, the antihypertensive effects are seen principally in the upright position. Regional blood flow in the hepatic and renal beds is not reduced unless significant postural hypotension occurs. Retention of salt and water is common with guanethidine, however, and may necessitate concomitant diuretic treatment to maintain effectiveness (pseudotolerance).

Guanethidine is rarely prescribed today. Even when there were few choices of antihypertensive drugs, guanethidine was often considered a last-choice drug in view of its limited antihypertensive effect (supine) and because of the frequency and severity of side effects. The drug is included here because there are still a few patients being treated with it whose therapy has not been updated.

The principal side effect of guanethidine is postural hypotension. In fact, hypertension may persist in the supine position. Severe and symptomatic orthostatic hypotension may occur with the drug used alone, particularly when other stimuli for vasodilation are present such as alcohol, exercise, warm environment, dehydration, or other vasodilator drugs. Serious orthostatic hypotension can occur in patients with autonomic neuropathy as found in diabetes mellitus. Because of its negative effects on cardiac output and its action to promote salt and water retention, guanethidine may worsen congestive heart failure. Weakness, diarrhea, retrograde ejaculation, impotence, fatigue, tremors, and parotid tenderness also have been reported to occur. Guanethidine may trigger a hypertensive crisis in a patient with pheochromocytoma by producing increased sensitivity to circulating catecholamines (a type of denervation hypersensitivity).

DRUG INTERACTIONS. All of the tricyclic antidepressants block the effect of guanethidine by inhibiting the nerve uptake of the drug. Phenothiazines also antagonize the action of guanethidine. Sympathomimetic amines, such as those found in typical cold remedies, used in conjunction with guanethidine may result in a significant pressor effect and should be avoided.

GUANADREL SULFATE. Guanadrel sulfate (HYLOREL) reduces blood pressure by the same mechanism as guanethidine. Like guanethidine, it does not enter or act through the CNS. Guanadrel is rapidly absorbed with peak plasma levels attained in about 2 hours and the maximal hypotensive effect 4–6 hours after oral ingestion. The total half-life of the drug is 10 hours; as a two-compartment system, however, 1–4 hours are required for the first phase and 5–45 hours for the second phase. About half of an oral dose is excreted unchanged in the urine. Adverse effects, dosages, clinical uses, and interactions are for all practical purposes the same as for guanethidine.

ADRENERGIC RECEPTOR BLOCKERS

α-Adrenergic Blockers

Alpha receptors are found in most blood vessels, and the highest concentrations are in the arterioles of the skin, kidney, and mucosal surfaces; they are also widely distributed in the venous system. Alpha receptors have two main subtypes (1 and 2), with further delineation of α_2 subtypes in recent years. Alpha$_1$ receptors are found on postsynaptic membranes, whereas α_2 are found on both the post- and presynaptic membranes and in nonneural tissue such as platelets. In general, the vasoconstrictive effects of NE are mediated by α_1-adrenergic activation.

Alpha$_1$-adrenergic receptors activate phospholipase C, and by increasing inositol triphosphate and diacylglycerol, they promote vasoconstriction. Activation of α_1 receptors is associated with calcium entry into cells and vasoconstriction. Moreover, α_1 blockers have now been found to reduce the urinary hesitancy associated with benign prostate hypertrophy, presumably because of their direct actions on the urethral sphincter. A salutary effect of these agents on low-density lipoprotein (LDL) cholesterol also exists via mechanisms that have not been fully elucidated.

Alpha$_2$-adrenergic receptors are coupled with guanine regulatory proteins that inhibit adenylate cyclase activation, an indirect stimulus to vasoconstriction plus a direct vasoconstrictive effect of α_2 stimulation. However, these actions are overwhelmed by the withdrawal of sympathetic nervous outflow, as was discussed under Central Sympatholytics. Blockade of central or peripheral α_2 receptors (as occurs with yohimbine and similar drugs) actually produces *hypertension* due to enhanced sympathetic nervous activity and enhanced neuronal catecholamine release; such a hypertensive effect is a result of the removal of the tonic α_2 receptor-mediated negative feedback of intrasynaptic NE on ongoing neuronal NE release.

Alpha blockers antagonize the vasoconstrictor effects of neurogenic stimulation and circulating catecholamines and reduce blood pressure by decreasing both venous tone and systemic arterial resistance. *Alpha blockers are most easily understood if they are viewed primarily as venodilators.* As is characteristic of venodilators, blood pressure when the patient is in an upright position is lowered more than when he or she is in a supine position, and relative orthostatic hypotension is quite common. Also characteristic of venodilators is the tendency for a diuretic to be required to retain long-term antihypertensive effectiveness. If, as frequently happens, tolerance to the drug appears, the antihypertensive effects may be restored by the addition of a diuretic. Alpha blockers also tend to cause reflex activation of the sympathoadrenal system, further reducing their chronic antihypertensive efficacy. Of the peripheral blockers, phentolamine and phenoxybenzamine block both α_1 and α_2 receptors, whereas the quinazolines—prazosin, terazosin, and doxazosin—are more selective blockers of the postsynaptic α_1 receptors (Table 29-5).

Quinazolines

PRAZOSIN. Prazosin (MINIPRES), a specific α_1 blocker, is a quinazoline derivative that has little effect on α_2 receptors and therefore has peripheral rather than CNS actions. The drug lowers arterial pressure by balanced arterial and venodilator effects such that cardiac output is not increased. Plasma catecholamines are increased and blood pressure tends to be reduced more effectively in the upright than supine position.

Clinical Pharmacology. Prazosin is absorbed readily after an oral dose, reaching peak blood levels in 1–3 hours. The absorption is not retarded or enhanced by the food. Plasma half-life is 3–4 hours but may be prolonged in patients with liver disease or congestive heart failure and in the elderly. Prazosin undergoes first-pass metabolism in the liver, where about 90% of it is later conjugated and demethylated and excreted into bile.

The most common side effect is *first-dose postural hypotension* due to venodilation and excessive venous pooling that can result in syncope and loss of consciousness. This

TABLE 29-5. α **Blockers**

Generic Name	Brand Name	Usual Dose (mg)/Frequency	Comment
α_1 Blockers			
Prazosin	MINIPRES	2-10 b.i.d.	Act as venodilators; tend to lower blood pressure and increase heart rate more in upright than supine position
Terazosin	HYTRIN	2-20 q.d.	Because of volume venodilation and subsequent retention, often requires addition of diuretic
Doxazosin	CARDURA	2-20 q.d.	Too often used at doses too low to sustain antihypertensive efficacy
Nonspecific α Blocker			
Phenoxybenzamine	DIBENZYLENE	30-60 q.d.	Usually used to treat pheochromocytoma

b.i.d. = twice a day; q.d. = every day.

appears to occur more frequently in patients who have been salt-depleted on diuretics, who are on other antihypertensive agents, or who were given initial doses higher than 1 mg. The first-dose phenomenon may be preceded or accompanied by rapid supraventricular tachycardia. In most patients, symptomatic orthostatic hypotension and dizziness abate over several days but may be persistent in some for long periods. To prevent this, it is recommended that the first dose be limited to 1 mg. The manufacturer has suggested that the first dose is best administered at bedtime. This practice seems unwise, however, because many older patients experience chronic nocturia, which when coupled with the normally expected nighttime fall in blood pressure, may exacerbate the tendency for falls and injury due to postural hypotension. A better suggestion is to begin therapy in the morning on a non-work day. Sinus tachycardia, more prominent in the upright than the supine position, also occurs commonly.

Other side effects include dry mouth, salt and water retention, nasal congestion, headache, palpitations, nightmares, sexual dysfunction, lethargy, drowsiness, nervousness, and constipation. Less common adverse effects include urinary frequency and incontinence, priapism, allergic skin reactions, and polyarthritis. Prazosin lowers total cholesterol and LDLs, raises high-density lipoproteins (HDLs) and does not affect carbohydrate metabolism.

Dosage. Prazosin must be given at least twice daily. The first 1-mg dose is given with instructions about possible postural hypotension and dizziness. Caution is warranted with the elderly or those with angina or cerebrovascular disease. The dose may be titrated until it reaches 10–20 mg daily in two doses.

TERAZOSIN AND DOXAZOSIN. Terazosin (HYTRIN) and doxazosin (CARDURA) are quinazoline α_1 blockers that differ from prazosin only in that their longer half-lives and slower onset of action allow once-daily dosing. Elimination is slow, with a terminal half-life of more than 20 hours. The maximal antihypertensive effects are observed 2–6 hours after an oral dose. Dosages are similar to those for prazosin, and usual maintenance doses of 10 mg or greater can be given once daily.

Nonspecific α Blockers

PHENTOLAMINE. Phentolamine (REGITINE) is a short-acting nonspecific competitive antagonist of both α_1 and α_2 receptors. Intravenous (IV) doses can be given in selected clinical emergencies in which NE-induced vasoconstriction occurs. These situations include pheochromocytoma (preparation for surgery), withdrawal of clonidine or other central α_2 agonists, or hypertensive crisis caused by ingestion of tyramine (from wine or cheese) in patients being treated with an MAO inhibitor.

The antihypertensive action of phentolamine is caused both by its α-blocking properties and by a direct vasodilatory action. Physiological responses include baroreflex stimulation, increased sympathoadrenal outflow, and increased cardiac output and renal blood flow. Supraventricular tachyarrhythmia or angina also can occur.

Dosage. Doses of 5–20 mg are given as IV boluses. Alternatively, an infusion may be given starting at the rate of 1 mg/minute.

PHENOXYBENZAMINE. Phenoxybenzamine (DIBENZYLENE) is an irreversible nonspecific blocker of α_1 and α_2 receptors whose use has been largely limited to preparing patients with pheochromocytoma for surgery. It has also been used to treat inoperable malignant pheochromocytoma and chronic prostatism. Phenoxybenzamine (like phentolamine) increases sympathetic outflow while blocking the effects of circulating NE and may produce reflex tachycardia, orthostatic hypotension, and some salt and water retention. Other side effects such as nasal congestion, nausea, vomiting, diarrhea, impaired ejaculation, and stress incontinence limit the drug's acceptability in the treatment of essential hypertension.

Dosage. The dose must be individualized but is usually in the range of 30–60 mg/day in pheochromocytoma.

Beta-Adrenergic Blockers

(see Chapter 10)

Although originally intended for treatment of cardiac arrhythmias and angina pectoris, β-adrenergic blockers have become widely used in hypertension.

Mechanisms of Antihypertensive Action

The exact mechanisms by which β blockers reduce blood pressure in hypertension remain incompletely understood. There is general agreement, however, that the blood pressure-lowering action is caused by at least one of three major mechanisms: cardiac output reduction, renin inhibition, or CNS inhibition. β blockers antagonize both the cardiac β_1 and the noncardiac β_2 receptors. Blockade of β_1 receptors leads to negative chronotropic (decreased heart rate) and negative inotropic (contractility) effects, producing a sustained reduction of cardiac output of about 15%. Release of renin, the enzyme initiating the generation of angiotensin II, is under direct β_1-adrenergic control. Thus β_1-blockers predictably suppress plasma renin activity and have been shown to be preferentially effective in reducing pressure in hypertensive subjects with elevated or normal renin levels (younger subjects and whites) in contrast to those with low renin levels (older subjects and blacks). Propranolol (but not necessarily all β blockers) produces specific changes in the CNS that may contribute to its antihypertensive actions. Higher drug doses appear to be hemodynamically different from lower doses because upright pressures fall with high doses and rise with lower doses.

Clinical Usage

Beta blockers may be used in mild and severe or even malignant-phase hypertension and are a preferred choice in patients who have another indication, such as concomitant supraventricular or ventricular arrhythmias, angina pectoris, recent myocardial infarction, migraine, hypertrophic obstructive cardiomyopathies, hyperthyroidism, panic attacks, or benign essential tremor. Beta blockers can be effectively combined with vasodilators that might otherwise induce

TABLE 29–6. Oral β Blockers

Generic Name	Brand Name	Solubility	Plasma $t_{1/2}$ (hour)	Quinidinelike Activity	Dose Range (mg)	Usual Dosage (mg)
			Nonspecific ($\beta_1 = \beta_2$)			
Propranolol	INDERAL	Lipid	1–5	Yes	40–80 b.i.d.	40 b.i.d.
Propranolol SR	INDERAL SR	Lipid		Yes	60–160 q.d.	80 q.d
Nadolol	CORGARD	Water	16–20	No	20–80 q.d.	40 q.d.
Timolol	BLOCADREN	Lipid	4–6	Yes	5–10 b.i.d.	5 b.i.d.
Perbutalol	LEVITOL	Lipid	16–20	No	20–40 q.d.	20 q.d.
			"Cardioselective" ($\beta_1 > \beta_2$ *at Low Doses*)			
Metoprolol	LOPRESSOR	Lipid	3–4	No	25–100 b.i.d.	50 b.i.d.*
Atenolol	TENORMIN	Water	6–8	No	50–100 q.d./b.i.d.	50 q.d.†
Betaxolol	KERLONE	Water	14–22	Weak	10–20 q.d.	10 q.d.
			Partial Agonists			
Pindolol	VISKEN	Water, lipid	3–4	Weak	5–10 b.i.d.	5 b.i.d.
Acebutalol	SECTRAL	Water, lipid	3–4	Some	200–800 b.i.d.	400 b.i.d.
Carteolol	CARTROL	Water	6–8	No	2.5–10 q.d.	5 q.d.°
			α/β Blocker			
Labetalol	NORMODYNE, TRANDATE	Water, lipid	3–4	Weak	100–400 b.i.d.	200–300 b.i.d.

*Sometimes given as 100 mg q.d.
†Not fully effective for 24 hours because of half-life.
b.i.d. = twice a day; q.d. = every day; SR = sustained release

tachycardia or increase renin release. Although β blockers do not consistently cause net sodium and water retention, they can be combined with diuretics for added effectiveness.

Clinical Pharmacology

Four major pharmacological characteristics differentiate among β blockers: (1) water solubility, (2) degree of partial agonist activity displayed, (3) selectivity for cardiac β_1 receptors, and (4) membrane-stabilizing activity. The first two of these distinguishing characteristics have greater practical importance in hypertension than the others (Table 29–6). Partial agonist activity, also known as intrinsic sympathomimetic activity, is of interest in that drugs such as pindolol and acebutolol actually stimulate β_2 receptors and cause vasodilation while blocking cardiac β_1 receptors and lowering cardiac output. These partial agonists have less tendency to cause cold extremities and bronchospasm (Table 29–6).

The relative selectivity for β_1 (vs β_2) receptors, also called "cardioselectivity," has been touted by manufacturers to reduce the side effects of β blockade. Although low doses of metoprolol or atenolol produce relatively less β_2 blockade than propranolol, the dosages usually used in hypertension tend to cause side effects very similar to those of propranolol.

Adverse Effects

Side effects are caused by the generalized phenomenon of β-adrenergic blockade and are often dose-related. By far the most common complaint is fatigue, probably caused by reduced cardiac output. Bradycardia and congestive heart failure are the most common cardiac side effects, but AV dissociation and aggravation of AV block may also occur. Symptoms of peripheral vascular disease may worsen with β blockade, particularly Raynaud's phenomenon and claudication. Cold hands are a common side effect; actual gangrene is rare.

Somewhat paradoxically, β blockers may actually raise systolic blood pressure, particularly in elderly subjects with low heart rates and reduced cardiac and vascular compliances, because of the tendency of these agents to cause parallel increases in stroke volume and vascular resistance. Administration of β blockers to patients with pheochromocytoma can aggravate blood pressure surges, presumably because of the removal of β receptor–mediated vasodilation.

All β blockers, even combined α/β blockers, tend to increase airway resistance and can aggravate asthma or bronchospasm.

Beta blockers exert prominent metabolic effects that may be clinically relevant in hypertensive patients. Increases of 20–30% in triglycerides or LDLs and decreases of approximately 5% in HDLs have been described. In contrast, β blockers with intrinsic sympathomimetic activity (partial agonism) may exhibit lesser or no effects on lipoproteins. *Pindolol, for example, may actually raise HDLs. Beta blockers block the adrenergic response (tachycardia, nervousness) to hypoglycemia, leaving diabetics without the usual warning signals of low blood sugar. In addition, insulin resistance may occur on long-term therapy.* A number of other side effects have been described, including nausea, vomiting, and diarrhea. The more lipid-soluble blockers are more likely to produce CNS side effects such as depression, nervousness, lassitude, nightmares, insomnia, and hallucinations. Sexual impotence has also been a reported side effect.

Combined α- and β-Adrenergic Blockade

Labetalol

Labetalol is the prototype complex adrenergic inhibitor, having multiple interactions with adrenergic receptors including both inhibitory and partial agonist effects. Labetalol is a β_1 blocker, a partial-agonist β_2 blocker, an α_1 blocker, and it has some direct vasodilatory properties as well. Because of its combined α- and β-blocking activity, net effects in a given case can reflect a combination of both features. Fundamental to the understanding of the effects of labetalol in a given patient is the idea that *its actions as agonist or antagonist depend heavily on the state of activation of the sympathoadrenal system prior to the institution of the drug*. Unfortunately, the clinical level of sympathetic output can be difficult to judge; heart rate is the usual indicator. In a patient with hypertension and tachycardia, labetalol causes a decrease in heart rate and blood pressure. In a patient with autonomic dysfunction, however, labetalol can cause tachycardia and nervousness.

In essential hypertension, IV labetalol, in contrast with "pure" β blockers, reduces blood pressure immediately, with only a modest reduction in heart rate. Over time, however, labetalol may reduce heart rate further, decrease contractility, and slow AV conduction. Although it is a partial β_2 agonist, labetalol may lead to bronchospasm in sensitive asthmatic patients. Labetalol is effective in angiotensin-dependent and angiotensin-independent forms of hypertension and does not adversely affect the lipid profile. Its antihypertensive effect is attenuated by sodium and water retention and is potentiated by concomitant diuretic treatment.

Intravenous labetalol is a versatile antihypertensive agent useful in treating hypertensive crises and can be given to patients who cannot take medications orally. The drug has been popular in controlling perioperative and intraoperative hypertension and can be particularly useful in patients with myocardial infarction or after coronary bypass surgery or angioplasty. The drug has also been used in patients experiencing withdrawal from clonidine and in pheochromocytoma.

Oral labetalol is effective in a wide variety of forms of hypertension. The drug has been tested successfully in subgroups of hypertensives with chronic lung disease, renal insufficiency, diabetes, and congestive heart failure. Unfortunately, these positive characteristics are counter-balanced by significant side effects, principally fatigue and exercise intolerance.

CLINICAL PHARMACOLOGY. Labetalol undergoes extensive first-pass hepatic glucuronidation. The bioavailability is enhanced in patients with liver disease and those taking cimetidine. The plasma half-life is about 6 hours. Because only 5% of the drug is excreted unchanged in the urine, labetalol is given in the same dosages in patients with renal insufficiency. Because labetalol is falsely identified as a catecholamine in some assays, the drug may need to be withheld until testing for pheochromocytoma is completed.

ADVERSE EFFECTS. In general, labetalol is well tolerated provided that dosing is carried out gradually and carefully. Dry mouth and orthostatic hypotension are relatively common but usually mild if the drug is taken with food to delay absorption. Other side effects, similar to those of other β blockers but somewhat less severe, include fatigue (very common), nausea, sleep disturbances, nervousness, nasal congestion, erectile impotence, muscle cramps, paresthesias of the hands or scalp, alopecia, depression, bronchospasm, disturbed AV conduction, brady- and tachyarrhythmias, and facial flushing. Patients on labetalol have developed antinuclear and antimitochondrial antibodies. Hepatic dysfunction, also noted rarely, is characterized by cholestatic jaundice and elevated liver enzymes.

Dosage. See Table 29–6 for drug dosages. Labetalol can also be used intravenously in emergencies.

TABLE 29–7. Pressor Action of Angiotensin II

Neural Mechanisms
1. Increased central sympathetic outflow
2. Presynaptic augmentation of neuronal norepinephrine release
3. Augmentation of adrenal epinephrine release
4. Postsynaptic augmentation of other pressors
5. Baroreflex blunting

Vascular Mechanisms
1. Direct vasoconstriction
2. Cellular hypertrophy and hyperplasia (chronic)

Other Volume-Related Mechanisms
1. Aldosterone release modulation
2. Vasopressin (antidiuretic hormone) release modulation
3. Increased thirst
4. Increased dietary salt intake ("salt appetite")

ANGIOTENSIN-CONVERTING ENZYME INHIBITORS

The Renin-Angiotensin-Aldosterone System

Renin catalyzes the generation of the decapeptide angiotensin I from a hepatically synthesized substrate called angiotensinogen or renin substrate. Angiotensin I is not vasoactive but acts as a substrate for subsequent actions of angiotensin-converting enzyme (ACE); this peptidyl dipeptidase forms the octapeptide angiotensin II, which exerts strong vasoconstrictive and neurohormonal effects. The actions of angiotensin II can be divided arbitrarily into three types: those affecting neurotransmission, those affecting volume-control mechanisms, and those directly causing vasoconstriction (Table 29–7 and Chapter 35).

Relevance of Hydration Status

Angiotensin-converting enzyme inhibitors do not lower blood pressure in normal individuals who have normal total body sodium content. When normal individuals are sodium depleted, however, ACE inhibitors become hypotensive agents. In this setting, where the renin-angiotensin system has been activated and blood pressure homeostasis is supported principally by circulating angiotensin II (and its multilevel actions; see Table 29-7), the effects of ACE inhibition are maximized. This principle of sodium dependency of ACE inhibitor action is true in all clinical situations in which ACE inhibitors may be used, including the treatment of hypertension and congestive heart failure.

High-renin hypertensives (about 15% of hypertensives) have increased heart rate and sympathetic nervous system activity and a personality type that includes a tendency toward suppressed hostility and anger. Increased renin values are also seen in renovascular hypertension, renal parenchymal disease, and malignant-phase hypertension.

Hypertensives with normal renin activity (about 50% of hypertensives) are not easily distinguished.

Hypertensives with low plasma renin activity (about 35% of hypertensives) generally exhibit a limited response to ACE inhibition whether or not sodium depletion has occurred; typically these are older essential hypertensives, black hypertensives, or hypertensives with advanced diabetes.

> ## BOX 29-3
> ## PRACTICAL USE OF ACE INHIBITORS
>
> ***Target Organ Effects***
> Chronic modes of action of angiotensin-converting enzyme (ACE) inhibitors may include a variety of secondary neurohumoral or hemodynamic effects (see Table 29-7). Cardiac hypertrophy and diminished arterial compliance may be reversed by ACE inhibitors.
>
> ***Hyperkalemia***
> Clinically important hyperkalemia with ACE inhibitors has been described when the drug is used with a potassium-conserving diuretic or potassium chloride supplementation. Addition of a loop diuretic in these patients usually corrects the hyperkalemia.
>
> ***Acute Azotemia: Clinical Relevance***
> The appeance of sudden anuria or azotemia after the administration of an ACE inhibitor is an extremely important sign that may signify renal artery stenosis. An acute dose of ACE inhibitor can be used as a standardized test ("captopril renogram") for an acute decrease in glomerular filtration rate, which is usually indicative of renal artery stenosis.
>
> ***Pregnancy: A Contraindication***
> Pregnancy is considered to be a major contraindication to the use of ACE inhibitors due to fetal loss possibilities.
>
> ***First-Dose vs Chronic Response***
> The first-dose response to ACE inhibition only weakly predicts whether a chronic response to the drug will occur. Thus, individual patients should be observed for 3-4 weeks on a given dose of ACE inhibitor before therapeutic changes are made.
>
> ***Dose-Response: 24-Hour Duration of Effect***
> The dose-response curve for ACE inhibitors is more closely related to duration of effect than to degree of blood pressure decrease. Low doses of ACE inhibitor do not last for 24 hours, whereas higher doses do. The minimal effective 24-hour dose of each ACE inhibitor is roughly twice the starting dose (see Table 29-8).

Clinical Usage (Box 29-3)

Mild to Moderate Hypertension

The functional significance of the degree of renin activation present can be assessed by observing the chronic response to ACE inhibitor monotherapy.

Severe Hypertension

In patients with severe hypertension, the ability of ACE inhibitors to lower blood pressure depends on the degree of vasoconstriction. For example, in malignant hypertension or after vigorous diuretic therapy, marked antihypertensive effects can be seen with the first doses of ACE inhibitor. These marked antihypertensive effects may not be sustained as the patient's sodium balance is restored toward a more normal state, however.

Congestive Heart Failure

Angiotensin-converting enzyme inhibitors are considered by many experts to be the optimal first-line agents in dilated cardiomyopathy of any etiology. Not only do ACE inhibitors improve survival and quality of life, but they also have been shown to protect against overt heart failure in patients with impaired cardiac performance.

Chronic Renal Disease

Although renal failure was originally suggested to be a relative contraindication to the use of ACE inhibitors, newer information suggests that ACE inhibition can slow the progression to end-stage renal disease, at least in diabetics.

Drug Interactions

Thiazide diuretics exhibit consistent potentiating actions in combination with ACE inhibitors and are the most attractive agents to combine with them. Monotherapy with ACE inhibition is efficacious in roughly 40% of hypertensives; addition of thiazide raises efficacy to about 80%. Not only are the antihypertensive effects of the two drug types almost fully additive, but many of the untoward biochemical consequences of thiazide therapy (hypokalemia, hyperglycemia, hyperuricemia, hyperlipidemia) are blunted or eliminated by the concomitant use of ACE inhibitors. Other types of antihypertensive drugs also may be used in combination with ACE inhibitors with slightly less efficacious results. Addition of ACE inhibitor to diuretic is sometimes accompanied by an acute hypotensive response. In contrast, if ACE inhibitors are used as first-line agents, the addition of a diuretic results in a smooth antihypertensive response. If the patient has been treated for a prolonged period with a diuretic, some clinicians recommend a short diuretic "holiday" prior to institution of ACE inhibitor therapy.

The only drugs that are not usually appropriate to use in combination with ACE inhibitors are the potassium-sparing diuretics (triamterene, amiloride, or spironolactone), particularly in patients with renal diseases that impair potassium excretion.

Neurological disturbances have occurred in patients taking captopril and cimetidine together. Nonsteroidal anti-inflammatory agents such as ibuprofen, indomethacin, and aspirin tend to reduce renal blood flow and cause reduced tubular sodium excretion, thereby antagonizing the antihypertensive effect of ACE inhibition. Beta blockers exhibit minimal additive effect with ACE inhibitors, perhaps because both act on the renin-angiotensin system.

Specific Drugs (Table 29–8)

Captopril

CLINICAL PHARMACOLOGY. The prototype ACE inhibitor, captopril, is absorbed rapidly, and its effect does not directly correspond to time of administration. The onset of action occurs within 15 minutes, and a peak action is reached after 60–90 minutes. *The duration of effect is strongly dose-related* but is usually between 2 and 8 hours. After the drug is withdrawn, blood pressure may remain reduced for days to weeks, although no evidence for residual drug stores exists.

Captopril is distributed rapidly in most body tissues except for the CNS. Captopril and its metabolites are excreted principally in the urine; elimination half-life is markedly prolonged with the presence of renal disease.

Although ACE inhibitors are usually well tolerated, their safety was impugned during the development of captopril because of the excessive dosages used in the earliest clinical trials. With the exception of taste disturbance with captopril, side effects of all of the ACE inhibitors are similar but not necessarily dose-related. The most common problem is chronic cough, which may occur in as many as 15% of patients. Rash, which is somewhat more common with captopril, is often self-limited and occasionally pruritic; it may occur during the first few days or after an increase in dosage and may be accompanied rarely by fever, arthralgia, eosinophilia, or urticaria. Leukopenia may develop gradually over the first few months of therapy and is a rare cause of agranulocytosis. In addition, lymphadenopathy, anemia in children, a positive antinuclear antibody test, and a false-positive test for urine acetone have been described. Risk factors for neutropenia and proteinuria are the presence of a collagen vascular disease, dosages of captopril higher than 150 mg/day, and decreased renal function. Proteinuria has been observed in low frequency (less than 2% on high dosages) in patients with and without underlying renovascular disease. The proteinuria may begin after months of therapy and may diminish with or without withdrawal of the drug. Captopril and ACE inhibitors may increase fetal mortality and should not be used during the second and third trimesters of pregnancy.

Esters (Enalapril, Fosinopril, Ramipril, Quinapril, Benazepril)

The mechanisms of action of enalapril (VASOTEC) and its related esters are similar to those of captopril. This group has the same spectrum of uses as captopril, although not all carry approved Food and Drug Administration indications for all conditions in which ACE inhibitors have proved to be useful (Table 29–8).

Angiotensin-converting enzyme inhibitor esters are prodrugs that are absorbed rapidly, even in the presence of food. Each drug is about 40% bioavailable and is hydrolyzed in the liver to an active dicarboxylic acid (enalaprilat, fosinoprilat, and others). Peak plasma concentrations and action typically occur 3–6 hours after oral ingestion. Because of their water solubility, lack of hepatic metabolism, and long duration of action, these drugs should generally be used once daily.

The side effects of the ester ACE inhibitors are similar to those of captopril, except that rash and taste disturbances are somewhat less common.

DOSAGES. Adjustment of dose and frequency requires individualization (Table 29–8).

TABLE 29–8. ACE Inhibitors

Generic Name	Brand Name	Indications (FDA Approved)	Dose Range (mg)	Effective Once-Daily Dose (mg/day)*
		Substituted Dipeptides		
Captopril	CAPOTEN	HTN, CHF, CRF	12.5–75 b.i.d.	—
Lisinopril	PRINIVIL, ZESTRIL	HTN, CHF	10–40 q.d.	20
		Ester Prodrugs (Require Hydrolysis)		
Enalapril	VASOTEC	HTN, CHF	5 b.i.d.–40 q.d.	20
Ramipril	ALTACE	HTN	2.5 b.i.d.–20 q.d.	10
Fosinopril	MONOPRIL	HTN	10–80 q.d.	20–40
Benazapril	LOTENSIN	HTN	5 b.i.d.–40 q.d.	20
Quinapril	ACCUPRIL	HTN	5–20 q.d.	10

*Strongest dose-response relationship is for dose vs duration; low doses of any ACE inhibitor last less than 24 hours, yet peak activity (usually 2 hours after administration) remains similar.

CHF = congestive heart failure; CRF = chronic renal failure; FDA = Food and Drug Administration; HTN = hypertension; q.d. = every day.

TABLE 29–9. Antihypertensive Calcium Channel Blockers

Generic Name	Brand Name	Usual Dose (mg)/Frequency	Comments
	Dihydropyridines		Side effects common to all drugs in this subclass include flushing, edema, headache, palpitations, and dyspepsia
Nifedipine SR	PROCARDIA XL ADALAT CC	60 q.d.	
Nicardipine	CARDENE	30–60 b.i.d.	
Felodipine SR	PLENDIL	5–10 q.d.	
Isradipine	DYNACIRC	2.5–5 b.i.d.	
Amlodipine	NORVASC	5–10 q.d.	
	Phenylalkylamines		Affects atrioventricular nodal conduction; constipation common
Verapamil SR	ISOPTIN SR CALAN SR VERELAN SR	180–240 q.d.	
	Benzothiazepines		Decreases sinoatrial nodal activity
Diltiazem SR	CARDIZEM SR DILACOR	120–180 b.i.d.	

b.i.d. = twice a day; q.d. = every day; SR = sustained release.

VASODILATORS

Calcium Channel Antagonists

Calcium antagonists or channel blockers block the movement of calcium into arteriolar smooth muscle and cardiac cells and may inhibit the mobilization of calcium from within these cells. The pharmacology, adverse effects, general therapeutic uses, and drug interactions of these agents are discussed in greater detail in Chapter 32. *With respect to the treatment of hypertension, all calcium channel antagonists act as arteriolar dilators and reduce systemic vascular resistance.* Several studies have found that calcium entry blockers are particularly effective as monotherapeutic agents in low-renin subgroups (see Angiotensin-Converting Enzyme Inhibitors).

Two other classes of antihypertensives exert additive effects when combined with calcium entry blockers: central sympatholytics and β blockers. These drugs tend to reduce the reflex increases in cardiac output caused by the vasodilator effects of the calcium channel antagonists (see Pseudotolerance above), thereby helping to sustain their antihypertensive effects. Nevertheless, neither ACE inhibitors nor diuretics exert fully additive antihypertensive effects when used in combination with calcium entry blockers.

All calcium entry blockers are negative inotropic agents, although this fact does not necessarily mean that they are contraindicated in heart failure, particularly when hypertension and heart failure coexist. Of the three major subclasses of calcium blockers (Table 29–9), the phenylalkylamine analogs (verapamil) are the most negatively inotropic, followed by the benzothiazepines (diltiazem), and finally, the dihydropyridines (nifedipine, nicardipine, felodipine, isradipine, amlodipine).

Verapamil

Verapamil produces both vascular smooth muscle relaxation and nonspecific sympathetic (α_1 receptor) antagonism; it slows AV nodal conduction, usually reducing heart rate and may abolish certain supraventricular tachyarrhythmias yet it is capable of proarrhythmic effects as well.

Verapamil is useful in mild to moderate hypertension, particularly when there is coexisting angina pectoris or another indication for the drug. Some studies indicate enhanced efficacy in "low renin" subclasses (principally blacks and elderly patients). Verapamil can also be useful in cases of hypertensive heart disease with diastolic dysfunction.

Drug Interactions. Verapamil and β blockers, when used in combination, can have additional negative inotropic effects, which can be worsened by concomitant use of cimetidine (and probably other H_2 blockers as well).

Diltiazem

Diltiazem is similar to verapamil in its vasodilatory properties but differs in its cardiac effects. Whereas verapamil acts to slow conduction preferentially at the AV node, diltiazem has a predisposition to slow the sinoatrial node and is therefore more likely to cause clinically significant bradycardia. There also appears to be somewhat less action on enteric smooth muscle and, therefore, less constipation. Diltiazem preparations are quite short-acting; even in their sustained-release forms, twice daily dosing is generally required.

Diltiazem can be used in mild and moderate hypertension, often as a first-line agent when angina pectoris is also present. Because of the negative chronotropic effects, the drug is not generally suitable for combination with a β blocker.

Dihydropyridines (Nifedipine, Nicardipine, Isradipine, Felodipine, Amlodipine)

Nifedipine (PROCARDIA, ADALAT) and the other dihydropyridines differ from verapamil and diltiazem by producing greater arteriolar vasodilation on a dose-weight basis and generally have fewer direct cardiac actions. Except for bepridil, this class of agents has minimal effects on sinoatrial and AV nodal conduction or on automaticity.

Dihydropyridines can be used to treat all degrees of hypertension but are particularly useful for moderate to severe hypertensives and those with angina pectoris. They may be combined successfully with a β blocker to reduce side effects as well as to amplify the antihypertensive and antianginal effects. Absorption of dihydropyridines occurs in the upper GI tract, principally in the proximal small bowel. Despite the popular notion that nifedipine can be absorbed sublingually, in fact it is gastroduodenal absorption that accounts for the fairly rapid onset of action. If rapid onset of action is necessary, one can extract the gel from the capsule and have the patient swallow it, particularly in hypertensive urgencies and emergencies. If the drug is not swallowed (as in a comatose patient) little antihypertensive effect will occur.

NICARDIPINE. Nicardipine (CARDENE) is similar to nifedipine but does not prolong AV conduction. The drug is rapidly and completely absorbed and begins to act within 20 minutes, reaching a peak action between 30 and 120 minutes. Nicardipine is the only IV dihydropyridine approved for use in hypertension.

AMLODIPINE. In contrast to agents whose duration is extended by the use of sustained-release GI formulations (PROCARDIA XL, PLENDIL), amlodipine (NORVASC) is a drug whose metabolism allows once-daily dosing. Amlodipine is hepatically metabolized to inactive byproducts and is extensively bound to plasma protein. The hemodynamic effects and side effects are similar to those of other dihydropyridines.

Other Direct Vasodilators

Hydralazine

Hydralazine (APRESOLINE) acts directly on arteriolar smooth muscle to induce relaxation, with little or no effect on veins. The cellular mechanism involves the activation of guanylate cyclase and the accumulation of intracellular cyclic guanosine monophosphate. Renal, splanchnic, and coronary arteries dilate more than those in the muscles or skin. Heart rate and contractility increase due to baroreflex stimulation, increased sympathoadrenal discharge, and direct effects on the myocardium. These cardiac reactions, however, along with stimulation of plasma renin activity and sodium and water retention, tend to reverse the antihypertensive action of the drug (systemic pseudotolerance). As a consequence, hydralazine is used usually in combination with an adrenergic blocker (usually a β blocker) and a diuretic. *This "triple therapy" using hydralazine, adrenergic blocker, and diuretic was the basic regimen employed in the first successful intervention trials in hypertension (VA trials).*

CLINICAL PHARMACOLOGY. Although hydralazine is rapidly and almost completely absorbed from the GI system, it is highly protein-bound and is metabolized by *N*-acetylation, glucuronidation, and hydroxylation. Genetically slow acetylators develop higher serum levels than fast acetylators and are more prone to dose-related side effects. Peak concentrations in plasma are found 30–120 minutes after dosing, with a total duration of effect of 6–8 hours. Hydralazine is also available in parenteral form. When given intramuscularly or intravenously, blood pressure begins to fall in about 10–20 minutes, which lasts for 2–5 hours.

Hydralazine given alone often produces unacceptable headache, tachycardia, manifestations of baroreflex stimulation, and marked sodium and water retention. These features tend to aggravate angina pectoris. Other side effects include diarrhea, constipation, nasal congestion, flushing, and rashes. A lupuslike syndrome has been described with doses of hydralazine greater than 200 mg/day; the symptoms consist of fever, myalgias, arthralgias, splenomegaly, and edema in association with a positive antinuclear antibody test result.

DOSAGES. The usual oral dosage of hydralazine is 75–200 mg daily in two to four divided doses.

Minoxidil

Minoxidil (LONITEN), a direct vasodilator whose mechanism of action is believed to be similar to that of hydralazine, is significantly more potent and has a longer duration of action than hydralazine. Current usage is limited to severe or resistant forms of hypertension. Its direct arteriolar vasodilation (in the absence of venodilation) leads to marked increases in reflex sympathetic activity, sodium and water retention, cardiac output, and aggravation of angina. Minoxidil is almost always used in combination with a β blocker (or central sympatholytic) and a loop diuretic.

CLINICAL PHARMACOLOGY. Minoxidil is well absorbed by the GI system. Maximal arteriolar dilation occurs within 2–3 hours, with peak plasma levels in about 1 hour after an oral dose. Although the plasma half-life is estimated to be 4.2 hours, the vasodilation may last 1–3 days. Minoxidil is metabolized extensively by the liver.

Reflex sympathetic cardiac stimulation may precipitate tachyarrhythmias and angina pectoris. Flattening or inversion of T waves with increased QRS wave voltage often is observed on the electrocardiogram. These changes may revert to normal with continued therapy. There are a few reports of myocardial fibrosis and necrosis in papillary muscles in patients on long-term minoxidil treatment. Marked orthostatic hypotension may occur if minoxidil is used in combination with ganglionic blockers.

Hair growth (hypertrichosis) occurs in most patients after a few weeks, presumably because of the regional increase in cutaneous blood flow. A topical form of minoxidil is currently available as a treatment for androgenic alopecia and other forms of baldness. Hair growth related to oral minoxidil is most conspicuous on the face, although it occurs over the entire body. The skin may darken and wrinkle as well. These reversible features are not well tolerated in women and children (even with attentive use of depilatories), and are not related to any known endocrine disorder.

Other side effects include nausea and headache. A small fraction of patients often on chronic hemodialysis may develop pericarditis and pericardial effusions.

DRUG INTERACTIONS. Because marked sodium and water retention leading to weight gain and edema occurs commonly, diuretics such as furosemide, ethacrynic acid, or bumetanide are commonly used in conjunction with minoxidil. When used without a diuretic, minoxidil may precipitate congestive heart failure. However, with the use of these diuretics, hypokalemia, hyperuricemia, hyperglycemia, and other complications of loop diuretics may occur. Because minoxidil (and the diuretic used with it) stimulates plasma renin levels, it has been combined with a converting enzyme inhibitor. A concomitant sympatholytic is also required, as with other arterial dilators.

DOSAGE. The usual starting dose is 2.5 – 5.0 mg, advancing to a maximum of 100 mg daily. The dose may be reduced by the balanced addition of a diuretic, sympatholytic or β blocker, or converting enzyme inhibitor.

Diazoxide

Diazoxide is a parenteral nondiuretic thiazide that acts directly on arterioles. Like other arterial dilators it has a marked antinatriuretic effect. Diazoxide is used only for hypertensive emergencies such as malignant hypertension, encephalopathy, and severe hypertension associated with renal parenchymal disease. *It can produce precipitous declines in blood pressure and is unsuitable in patients with dissecting aneurysms, ischemic coronary artery disease, cerebrovascular disease, pheochromocytoma, or arteriovenous malformations.* Because it stops uterine contractions, it is not a good choice in pregnant women with eclampsia.

CLINICAL PHARMACOLOGY. Peak plasma levels occur 3 – 5 minutes after injection and decline over 4 – 12 hours.

The hemodynamic side-effect profile of diazoxide is similar to that of hydralazine and minoxidil. In addition, diazoxide may produce marked hyperglycemia and hyperosmolarity. Loop diuretics, given concomitantly, may aggravate side effects. Headache, nausea, vomiting, flushing, hypersensitive reactions, altered smell and taste, salivation, local pain or irritation at the site of injection, and hemolytic episodes have been described.

DOSAGES. The drug may be given in small successive IV boluses of 0.5 – 1.0 mg/kg at intervals of 15 – 20 seconds or by slow IV infusion.

Sodium Nitroprusside

Sodium nitroprusside is used in controlled IV infusions for the treatment of hypertensive emergencies. Unlike hydralazine, minoxidil, and diazoxide, nitroprusside produces both arteriolar and venous dilation. The vasodilatory mechanism, which appears to be similar to that of organic nitrates, includes enzymatic degradation to form nitric oxide and subsequent guanylate cyclase – dependent vasodilation. Nitroprusside dilates both resistance and capacitance vessels, causing little net cardiac effect with only minimal increases in heart rate, slight decreases in myocardial workload, and minimal effect on coronary blood flow. With appropriate dosing, nitroprusside can maintain renal blood flow and glomerular filtration despite increased plasma renin activity.

Nitroprusside has become a common choice in the treatment of most life-threatening hypertensive emergencies because it has (1) rapid onset of action, (2) consistent effectiveness, (3) acceptable toxicity that can be monitored, (4) easy and precise titratability, and (5) favorable hemodynamic response patterns. If a dissecting aneurysm or pheochromocytoma is present, adrenergic (usually β) blockade should be added to reduce heart rate and ejection velocity.

SPECIAL SITUATIONS. Rebound or refractory hypertension occasionally occurs during or after treatment with nitroprusside, usually in the setting of head trauma, subarachnoid hemorrhage, craniotomy, cardiac failure, cardiac surgery, or occasionally in renovascular hypertension. In all of these conditions, marked activation of the sympathoadrenal and renin-angiotensin systems occurs. Nitroprusside, although a potent arteriolar and venous dilator, does not fully overcome the effects of these pressor systems. Additional sympatholysis using labetalol or methyldopa can be very effective in this situation. When removing patients from nitroprusside therapy, it has become customary to begin therapy with a β blocker, an ACE inhibitor, or other agent prior to complete cessation of nitroprusside therapy.

CLINICAL PHARMACOLOGY. Nitroprusside has almost an immediate onset of action that becomes maximal in 1 – 2 minutes. The half-life is short; reducing the rate of infusion leads to a rise in pressure within 30 seconds. The most frequent adverse effect is hypotension, which usually is a result of excessive dosages. Nausea, vomiting, headache, sweating, restlessness, chest pain, confusion, and palpitations are not uncommon when blood pressure is lowered too rapidly. These side effects may be avoided by slow and careful titration. Less common adverse effects include hypothyroidism, reduced platelet count, and increase in intracranial pressure in patients with mass lesions or metabolic encephalopathy.

TOXICITY. Understanding the metabolism of nitroprusside is important for the clinician because of its potential toxicity. Cyanide ions, which are potent cytochrome poisons, are metabolic byproducts of nitroprusside metabolism. Under usual circumstances, cyanide ions are inactivated by the enzyme rhodanase, which forms thiocyanate. Thiocyanate is excreted in the urine with a half-life of 4 – 7 days in patients with normal renal function. If nitroprusside is used for several days, particularly in patients with renal failure, existing stores of thiosulfate are depleted and cyanide toxicity may develop. Furthermore, thiocyanate itself can be toxic at high levels and must be monitored carefully. Signs of toxicity include confusion, disorientation, muscle twitching, delirium, or overtly psychotic behavior. Toxicity can be controlled by infusing sodium thiosulfate or hydroxocobalamin.

DOSAGE. Usual rates of infusion are between 2 and 5 μg/kg/minute using an infusion pump and continuous monitoring of arterial pressure. Because nitroprusside in solution is quite unstable, it must be protected from light and changed daily.

REFERENCES

Fifth Report of the Joint National Committee on Detection, Evaluation, and Treatment of High Blood Pressure. Washington DC: US Department of Health and Human Services. 1993. NIH publication 93-1088.

Izzo JL Jr: Treatment of mild hypertension and evolutionary process. *In* Glassock RJ (ed): Current Therapy in Nephrology and Hypertension, 3rd ed, 357 – 373. St. Louis: Mosby – Year Book, 1992.

Izzo JL Jr, Black HR (eds): Hypertension Primer. Dallas: American Heart Association, 1993.

Kaplan NM (ed): Clinical Hypertension, 6th ed. Baltimore: Williams & Wilkins, 1994.

Laragh JH, Brenner BM (eds): Hypertension. Pathophysiology, Diagnosis, and Management. New York: Raven Press, 1990.

Veterans Administration Cooperative Study Group on Antihypertensive Agents: Effects of Treatment on Morbidity in Hypertension. JAMA 202:1028 – 1034, 1967.

30 Drugs Used to Relieve Angina Pectoris

Eli R. Farhi

NITRATES

Mechanisms of Action

Intracellular Effects

Over the past decade, it has become increasingly evident that the vascular endothelium functions as a large and active paracrine system, producing potent vasoactive, anticoagulant, procoagulant, and fibrinolytic substances. One of these is *endothelium-derived relaxing factor* (EDRF), which is (or at least acts like) *nitric oxide* (NO) free radical. Nitric oxide is derived from the amino acid L-arginine and is metabolized to an inactive nitrite. EDRF can be released in response to stimulation of specific endothelial receptors for acetylcholine, thrombin, histamine, vasopressin, oxytocin, and $alpha_2$ agents, as well as by adenosine diphosphate (ADP) and serotonin released from aggregating platelets. EDRF then acts on a receptor, probably the heme moiety of soluble *guanylate cyclase* to increase vascular smooth muscle cell *cyclic guanosine monophosphate* (cGMP), which activates a cyclic GMP-dependent protein kinase. This in turn inhibits release of calcium ions from endoplasmic reticulum and other storage sites, causing relaxation of vascular smooth muscle.

Nitrates are pharmacologic agents that possess the biochemical actions of EDRF but do not require an intact endothelium to demonstrate activity. Most recent evidence indicates that organic nitrates are converted to nitric oxide free radical or *S*-nitrosothiol compounds in the vascular smooth muscle cell. These compounds act via the mechanism described above, stimulating guanylate cyclase to produce cGMP, which in turn triggers smooth muscle relaxation. *Sulfhydryl groups* are required both for the formation of NO and for stimulation of guanylate cyclase, a point to remember for the discussion of nitrate tolerance that appears later in this chapter.

Hemodynamic Effects

Nitrates cause relaxation of smooth muscle in veins, arterioles, and arteries. *Venodilation* occurs at very low doses, with a relatively flat dose-response curve, so that near-maximal venous vasodilation is seen at low plasma concentrations of nitroglycerin, with little additional venodilation induced by increased nitroglycerin dosages. Venodilation causes pooling of blood in the venous system, decreasing venous return to the heart. This reduces preload and ventricular dimensions. The law of Laplace can be summarized as

$$\text{Wall Tension} = \frac{\text{Transmural Pressure} \times \text{Radius}}{\text{Wall Thickness}}$$

Venodilation, which decreases intracardiac pressure and dimensions while increasing wall thickness, can thus decrease wall tension. Because myocardial oxygen demand (MVO_2) is related to wall tension, this reduction in preload can markedly decrease MVO_2. This mechanism is particularly important in patients with congestive heart failure, whose ventricular pressures and dimensions may be significantly increased.

In normal patients, the decrease in intracardiac pressures and volumes may result in a fall in stroke volume and (if heart rate remains constant) a fall in cardiac output (in fact, reflex tachycardia may limit or even prevent any decrease in cardiac output). The hemodynamic and antianginal effects of nitrates are most marked when patients are sitting or standing, when the interaction of venodilation in the lower extremities and normal postural drainage may markedly reduce preload.

Larger doses of nitrates produce *arteriolar vasodilation*, reducing systemic vascular resistance and afterload, which will also decrease MVO_2. Occasionally, this reduction in systemic vascular resistance can be harmful. Because

$$\text{Blood Pressure} = \text{Cardiac Output} \times \text{Systemic Vascular Resistance}$$

the drop in systemic vascular resistance, combined with the decrease in cardiac output that may be induced by venodilation, may reduce central aortic pressure excessively. Reflex tachycardia may result. Uncommonly, increased sympathetic tone may attenuate or even prevent nitrate-induced decreases in systolic pressure; such reflex adrenergic responses may produce side effects such as palpitations or (very rarely) even paradoxical worsening of angina.

The venodilation and arteriolar vasodilation induced by nitrates thus reduce myocardial oxygen (and hence blood) requirements, improving the demand side of the supply-demand relationship for coronary blood flow in patients with coronary insufficiency. Nitrates also cause *arterial vasodilation in coronary arteries*, improving the supply of blood as well. In some lesions in some patients, part of the antianginal effect of nitrates is due to a reduction in stenosis severity. Not all coronary arterial stenoses dilate equally after nitroglycerin; the amount of dilation depends on the severity, geometry, and pathology of the lesion. Our present concept of coronary atherosclerotic disease is that most lesions are not entirely fixed rigid tubes; usually there is also an element of dynamic coronary obstruction due to coronary vasoconstriction superimposed on the underlying coronary atherosclerotic lesion. Although nitrates may not affect the fixed disease, they may be able to cause significant dilation of the dynamic component of the obstruction. Relief of this dynamic component may increase arterial diameter only slightly, but it is important to recall that even a small increase in a narrowed lumen can significantly reduce resistance to blood flow across the narrowing because resistance is proportional to the fourth power of the radius.

Generally, nitrates induce a transient increase in coronary blood flow, followed by a fall in global myocardial blood flow below baseline that parallels nitrate-modulated decreases in myocardial oxygen requirements. Although total blood flow may not increase, nitrates have been shown to increase blood flow to regional zones of ischemia, redistributing flow from normally perfused to ischemic areas (particularly the subendocardium). This may be due to a direct effect of nitrates on stenotic coronary arteries, coronary arterioles, or coronary collaterals. Initially, it was believed that this increase in blood supply was the sole mechanism responsible for the antianginal effects of nitrates. This hypothesis was subsequently abandoned when it was shown that a number of other potent coronary vasodilators (such as dipyridamole) were not effective antianginal agents. In addition, when given systemically in doses that cause arterial vasodilation, nitroglycerin relieves pacing-induced angina, yet it may fail to do so when administered at the same dose directly into the coronary arterial bed. Because of observations such as these, **most experts believe that the dominant action of nitrates in myocardial ischemia is unrelated to the direct coronary effects and that the major antianginal effects are modulated through peripheral mechanisms that decrease myocardial oxygen requirements**.

Antiplatelet Effects

An antiaggregatory action of nitrates on platelets has been documented *in vitro* and in patients at plasma nitrate concentrations that are readily obtainable, particularly during intravenous nitroglycerin infusions. This antiplatelet effect may help explain the demonstrated efficacy of nitrates in acute ischemic syndromes, such as unstable angina or acute myocardial infarction, which are associated with acute intraluminal thrombus formation.

Preparations and Administration

A variety of nitrate preparations are presently in clinical use in the United States. *Nitroglycerin* (NTG) is available in sublingual, oral spray, buccal ointment, transdermal patch, and intravenous formulations. The half-life of nitroglycerin is brief (less than 5 minutes); it is metabolized by the liver and by blood vessels, which appear to be responsible for a considerable proportion of degradation.

- *Intravenous nitroglycerin* has a very rapid onset of action and its effects quickly reverse when the infusion is stopped. Infusions should generally begin at a rate of $\leq 25\ \mu g$/min and can be increased by 5 to 10 μg/min until the desired clinical or hemodynamic effect is achieved or side effects occur.
- *Sublingual* (SL) *nitroglycerin* is the standard of therapy for anginal attacks. Most patients respond within 5 minutes; additional doses can be given every 5 minutes, although if angina persists for more than two rounds of SL nitroglycerin, patients should come to the hospital. SL nitroglycerin is especially useful when taken prophylactically, prior to situations or activities that are likely to induce chest pain; when used in this fashion, SL NTG may prevent anginal attacks for up to 30 minutes. Nitroglycerin tablets tend to lose potency when exposed to light, and should be kept in dark containers. Some patients find sublingual nitroglycerin tablets to be small and quite unwieldy. Two other formulations have been developed for these patients.
- A *nitroglycerin spray* can be easily sprayed onto or under the tongue and may be better absorbed than sublingual tablets in some patients with dry mucosal membranes.
- *Buccal nitroglycerin* is also becoming more popular; this preparation of NTG dispersed in a cellulose matrix has a rapid onset of action combined with sustained hemodynamic and clinical effects.
- The *2% nitroglycerin ointment* is relatively inconvenient for ambulatory patients (it is messy and gets all over clothing), but is extremely useful in hospitalized patients be-

cause it can be readily removed in case of adverse effects. It can also be useful in patients who have nocturnal symptoms of angina or congestive heart failure because it can be easily applied just before bedtime.

- *Transdermal nitroglycerin patches* provide relatively constant NTG delivery across the skin for 24 to 48 hours. Relatively low dose patches (2.5 to 5 mg/day) may not produce sufficient plasma and tissue concentrations to produce effective antianginal effects. On the other hand, higher dose patches are likely to produce tolerance (see below); this can often be readily treated by an intermittent dosing strategy, removing the patch for 10 to 12 hours out of 24.

Isosorbide dinitrate (ISDN) is available in sublingual, chewable, and oral formulations in the United States; intravenous isosorbide dinitrate, topical isosorbide dinitrate cream, and an oral isosorbide dinitrate spray have been clinically tested and are used in other countries. The major problem with any oral nitrate preparation is that bioavailability is unpredictable from one patient to the next as a result of differences in gastrointestinal absorption and hepatic first-pass metabolism. Only 20 to 25% of an oral dose of isosorbide dinitrate is bioavailable, mainly because of metabolism by liver glutathione organic nitrate reductase. Thus, rather than using a fixed oral dose of oral isosorbide dinitrate, patients should be given oral nitrates in increasing doses until symptoms are controlled, tolerance develops, and/or side effects occur.

Some believe that 5-isosorbide mononitrate, a metabolite of isosorbide dinitrate, is responsible for the majority of the nitrate effect following oral administration of isosorbide dinitrate. This drug (*isosorbide mononitrate*) is now available in the United States, and appears to have a vasodilating potency at least equal to isosorbide dinitrate. Because it is not subject to first-pass metabolism in the liver, isosorbide mononitrate has a markedly increased bioavailability and a longer plasma half-life than does isosorbide dinitrate.

Some general information regarding these compounds are listed in Table 30 – 1. It is important to emphasize that this table presents average data; there is a great deal of individual variation between patients, however, and nitrate pharmacokinetics in any one patient are not predictable and must be determined empirically.

Adverse Reactions

Nitrates commonly cause *headache, dizziness, flushing,* and some degree of *hypotension.* Headaches, the most common complaint, frequently attenuate or completely disappear after several days to weeks of daily therapy. Hypotension can be particularly severe in the setting of infarction, right heart failure, vagal reactions, and/or hypovolemia. Arterial O_2 saturation may fall after large doses of nitrates because of ventilation/perfusion imbalances caused by the inability of the pulmonary vascular bed to constrict in areas of alveolar hypoxia and redirect perfusion to less hypoxic tissues. Methemoglobinemia is a rare complication of very large doses of nitrates.

Tolerance

Patients exposed to nitrates for prolonged periods of time develop tolerance to the drug, with higher and higher doses being required to produce an equivalent effect. If isosorbide or nitroglycerin ointment is administered three times a day, the magnitude of the antianginal effect decreases with each successive dose. Similarly, transdermal nitroglycerin patches improve exercise performance soon after administration, but this improvement is demonstrably attenuated after the patch has been in place for 24 hours. This effect, which has been termed *nitrate tolerance,* may be due to *intracellular depletion of the reduced sulfhydryl cofactors* required for formation of NO and/or nitrosothiols as well as for stimulation of guanylate cyclase. If more sulfhydryl groups are made available, either by N-acetylcysteine, an agent that helps replete the pool of reduced sulfhydryl groups, or by giving methionine, nitrate tolerance can be partially reversed and the hemodynamic and coronary vasodilator effects of nitroglycerin can be potentiated.

Partial or complete tolerance develops on any nitrate regimen using frequent doses of long-acting nitrates (greater than 20 to 30 mg three or more times daily), continuous delivery (intravenous or transdermal) or long-acting (sustained release) nitrate preparations. Intermittent doses of sublingual nitroglycerin are effective even in patients who have developed tolerance to long-acting nitrates. One method to avoid the development of tolerance is to institute a 10- to 12-hour nitrate-free interval every 24 hours.

TABLE 30 – 1. Pharmacokinetics of Nitrate Preparations

Preparation	Dosage (mg)	Onset of Action (min)	Peak Action (min)	Duration
Sublingual NTG	0.15–0.4	2–5	4–8	10–30 min
Sublingual ISDN	2.5–10	5–20	15–60	45–120 min
Oral NTG spray	0.4–0.8	2–5	4–8	10–30 min
Buccal NTG	1–3	2–5	4–10	30–300 min
Oral ISDN	10–60	15–45	45–120	2–6 hours
Oral NTG	6.5–19.5	20–45	45–120	2–6 hours
2% NTG ointment	1/2–2 inches	15–60	30–120	3–8 hours
Oral ISMN	20	30	60–240	5–7 hours
Transdermal NTG	10–20 mg	30–60	60–180	Up to 24 hours
Intravenous NTG	25–500 μg/min	1–5	3–5	

ISDN = isosorbide dinitrate; ISMN = isosorbide mononitrate; NTG = nitroglycerin.

Withdrawal of nitrates can intensify angina in patients who have been on large doses of long-acting nitrates. The most extreme form of nitrate withdrawal is seen in individuals exposed to industrial doses of nitroglycerin (such as in the manufacture of dynamite). On starting work, particularly on Monday mornings, these people may notice headaches, hypotension, palpitations, and gastrointestinal disturbance. During prolonged exposure during the work week, tolerance develops and symptoms decrease. Withdrawal from the nitroglycerin, on the weekend, can result in spontaneous angina (*ie*, not provoked by physical or mental stress); coronary vasospasm and even acute myocardial infarction have even been seen under these conditions.

β-ADRENERGIC RECEPTOR ANTAGONISTS (β BLOCKERS)

Mechanisms of Action

Beta blockers are drugs that are structurally similar to beta-receptor agonists and inhibit the effects of endogenously released epinephrine and norepinephrine. Thus, they act predominantly by reducing the increases in heart rate, contractility, and (usually) blood pressure that are mediated by increased sympathetic activity during activity or excitement and associated with increased myocardial oxygen demand. At rest, their effects on myocardial oxygen demand are less because of the lower level of sympathetic activity, but even in this state β blockers lower myocardial oxygen demands by reducing arterial pressure. In addition to decreasing myocardial blood requirements, β blockers also may increase blood supply; slower heart rates are associated with more time spent in diastole, the period when the majority of blood flow occurs. Beta blockers reduce the frequency of anginal episodes and raise the anginal threshold, either alone or when added to other antianginal agents.

Because the major therapeutic effects of all β blockers are mediated by the same mechanism, the various agents have a similar spectrum of activity. If a therapeutic dose of one drug is not effective in a particular patient, trying another is rarely worthwhile. Similarly, it is not useful to combine β blockers to try to improve the therapeutic response. The major differences between the different β blockers are in their side effects and in a few broad categories (Table 30-2).

Selectivity

Myocardium contains primarily β_1 receptors, whereas bronchioles and peripheral arterial vessels contain almost exclusively β_2 receptors. *Nonselective β* blockers act on both β_1 and β_2 receptors; *selective β* blockers predominantly affect β_1 receptors, with less marked effects on β_2 receptors. Because blockade of β_2 receptors may lead to unopposed bronchoconstriction and/or peripheral vascular constriction, nonselective β blockade may worsen symptoms of dyspnea or claudication. In addition, mobilization of liver glycogen (the mechanism by which insulin-induced hypoglycemia is counteracted) depends on β_2 receptor mediation. Thus, one may wish to choose a drug with relative β_1 selectivity (metoprolol or atenolol) in patients with asthma, chronic obstructive pulmonary disease (COPD), diabetes, or claudication. However, selectivity is evident only at lower dosages, and the use of selective β blockers in doses sufficient to prevent angina (*eg*, above 50 to 100 mg of metoprolol per day) may affect both β_1 and β_2 receptors.

Lipid Solubility

Lipid solubility may affect the pharmacokinetics and (perhaps) some of the central nervous system side effects of the β blockers.

Pharmacokinetics

The *lipid-soluble β blockers* (propranolol, metoprolol, pindolol) are readily absorbed from the gastrointestinal tract and are metabolized predominantly and extensively by the liver (the "first-pass effect") before reaching the systemic circulation. Thus, propranolol and metoprolol are much more potent when given intravenously rather than orally. In addition, the lipid-soluble β blockers have a relatively short half-life and usually require administration twice or more daily to achieve optimal β blockade. Metabolism of some of the lipid-soluble β blockers (particularly metoprolol and propranolol) may also be highly variable depending on the patient's genetic phenotype; in patients who are slow hydroxylators (up to 10% of whites), the half-lives of these drugs are markedly increased. Conversely, the more *water-soluble β blockers* (atenolol and nadolol) are not readily absorbed from the gastrointestinal tract, but escape hepatic

TABLE 30-2. Differences Among Various β Blockers

Agent	β_1 Selectivity	Lipid Solubility	Route of Elimination	ISA	Dose (mg)
Atenolol	+	Low	Renal	0	50-100 q.d.
Metoprolol	+	Moderate	Hepatic	0	50 q.d.-100 b.i.d.
Nadolol	0	Low	Renal	0	40-240 q.d.
Pindolol	0	Moderate	Hepatic/renal	+	5 b.i.d.-20 t.i.d.
Propranolol	0	High	Hepatic	0	10-80 q.i.d.
Timolol	0	Low	Hepatic/renal	0	10-30 b.i.d.
Esmolol	+	Low	RBC	0	See text

b.i.d. = twice a day; ISA = intrinsic sympathomimetic activity; q.d. = every day; q.i.d. = four times a day; RBC = red blood cells; t.i.d. = three times a day.

inactivation and are excreted virtually unchanged via the kidneys. Doses of these drugs must therefore be reduced in patients with renal dysfunction. The water-soluble β blockers have relatively long plasma half-lives, allowing once-a-day dosage.

Central Nervous System Effects

Up to 20% of patients who take β blockers complain of fatigue, depression, sleep disturbances (including insomnia and nightmares), and/or sexual dysfunction. Unlike many of the other side effects of β blockers, adverse central nervous system (CNS) reactions are relatively dose dependent. These effects may be related to lipid solubility; less lipid-soluble drugs may not cross the blood-brain barrier and enter the CNS as readily. Propranolol is the most lipid-soluble of the β blockers and readily enters the CNS, whereas atenolol is the least lipid-soluble. It is important to remember, however, that there is no definitive proof that the less lipid-soluble agents produce fewer CNS complaints than other β blockers.

Intrinsic Sympathomimetic Activity

Some β blockers (pindolol and acebutolol) are *partial agonists*, which can interact with β receptors to produce a measurable agonist response but at the same time block the β receptors from the greater agonist effects of endogenous catecholamines. Thus, at low levels of endogenous sympathetic activity, these drugs produce low-grade β stimulation, and cause minimal (if any) negative inotropic or chonotropic effects; the partial agonist activity may even induce bronchodilation. When sympathetic activity is high (under stress and during exercise), partial agonists produce hemodynamic effects similar to those of the conventional β blockers. Beta blockers with intrinsic sympathomimetic activity may thus be indicated to prevent the bradyarrhythmias, conduction system disease, myocardial depression, asthma, and peripheral vascular complications seen with conventional β blockers. These theoretical benefits, however, have never been demonstrated in patients. The β blockers with intrinsic sympathomimetic activity, however, have been shown to reduce the lowering of high-density lipoprotein (HDL) and increases in triglycerides produced by β-blockers without intrinsic sympathomimetic activity.

Adverse Reactions

Most side effects of β blockers are predictable consequences of their β-adrenergic blocking effects. Cardiac effects include bradyarrhythmias, conduction blocks, and myocardial dysfunction; other effects include the worsening of asthma, CNS and/or metabolic effects as described above. More idiosyncratic reactions include skin rash, fever, and gastrointestinal symptoms (nausea, diarrhea, or constipation). In addition, one must be wary of the **withdrawal syndrome**; after abrupt withdrawal of any β blocker, increased sympathetic activity may sometimes manifest itself as unstable angina or even myocardial infarction. This syndrome occurs quite rarely; nevertheless, when discontinuing a β blocker (for any reason) it is prudent to taper the drug over a period of several days.

Contraindications

CONGESTIVE HEART FAILURE. Beta-blocking agents can precipitate congestive heart failure either by decreasing myocardial function directly in conditions in which abnormally high myocardial sympathetic activity is needed to maintain cardiac output, or by decreasing heart rate in conditions in which stroke volume is limited and cannot increase to maintain cardiac output. In general, β blockers rarely produce congestive heart failure in patients without pre-existing left ventricular (LV) dysfunction. Even in patients with decreased ventricular contractility, β blockers are not unequivocally contraindicated; the decision must be tailored to the patient, and depends on the degree of underlying left ventricular dysfunction, the amount of symptoms of ischemia and congestive heart failure, and the amount of ventricular dysfunction attributable to ischemic as opposed to nonviable myocardium.

BRADYARRHYTHMIAS OR CONDUCTION SYSTEM DISTURBANCES. Beta blockers should be used with trepidation and caution in these patients (without a pacemaker), even in patients with only mild atrioventricular block.

ASTHMA OR CHRONIC OBSTRUCTIVE PULMONARY DISEASE. As discussed above, blockade of bronchial β_2 receptors produces bronchoconstriction. As a result, asthma and COPD are relative contraindications to the use of such agents. Selective β blockers at low doses may be less prone to cause complications in patients with these diseases.

HYPERCHOLESTEROLEMIA OR HYPERTRIGLYCERIDEMIA. In general, β-blocker therapy does not change total low density lipoprotein (LDL) cholesterol, but increases triglycerides and decreases HDL cholesterol. As mentioned above, these effects are less in the presence of partial agonist activity; pindolol does not affect triglyceride levels and may actually increase HDL.

DIABETES. The symptoms of hypoglycemia as well as counterregulatory metabolic mechanisms are dependent on the sympathetic nervous system. Diabetics susceptible to hypoglycemia may not be aware of usual warning signals and may not rebound as quickly. Most patients with non-insulin-dependent diabetes can tolerate β blockers, although their diabetes may be exacerbated.

PERIPHERAL VASCULAR DISEASE. Blockade of peripheral arterial β_2 receptors abolishes their vasodilatory effects while leaving constrictive α-adrenergic actions unopposed. This may decrease peripheral blood flow and worsen symptoms of claudication or precipitate Raynaud's phenomenon in some patients.

VARIANT (PRINZMETAL'S) ANGINA. As in the peripheral vessels, blockade of vasodilatory β_2 receptors may produce unopposed α receptor–mediated coronary artery vasoconstriction. In some patients, the duration of episodes of vasotonic angina can be prolonged by propranolol. In general, however, patients with angina from coronary artery spasm have an unpredictable response to β blockade. Some patients, particularly those with coexisting fixed lesions, have a reduction in the frequency of exertion-induced angina due to the decrease in myocardial oxygen demand discussed above.

Dosing

The effective therapeutic dose of β blockers varies widely between patients, and may change in any individual patient depending on alterations in renal and hepatic function and concurrent medications. In general, the heart rate response to β blockers is the best clinical indicator of their effectiveness in an individual patient. A reasonable guideline is to try to lower resting heart rate below 60 beats per minute (bpm) (ideally to 45 to 55 bpm), and to reduce the increase in heart rate associated with modest exercise (climbing one flight of stairs) to less than 20 bpm, or the tachycardia induced by strenuous exercise (on a treadmill) by 70 - 80%. Heart rates will often be even lower (40 to 45 bpm) during sleep, but this degree of bradycardia is generally well tolerated. Particular attention must be paid to the patient's other cardiovascular drugs; some of these (most notably digoxin and verapamil) may also reduce heart rate, and, if combined with a β blocker, may result in profound bradycardia.

When rapid β blockade is required to reduce angina by lowering heart rate and/or blood pressure, intravenous esmolol may be the drug of choice. Esmolol is a β_1-selective agent with a rapid onset of action; after an appropriate loading dose, steady-state blood levels can be reached within 5 minutes. Esmolol is rapidly metabolized (chiefly within red blood cells) by hydrolysis of an ester linkage; its half-life is approximately 9 minutes and resolution of drug effect occurs within 20 to 30 minutes of discontinuing the infusion. Esmolol metabolism is not affected by hepatic or renal blood flow, and its short half-life makes its use relatively simple and safe to titrate even in patients with compromised left ventricular function.

CALCIUM CHANNEL ANTAGONISTS

Mechanisms of Action

Four different classes of calcium channel antagonists — the dihydropyridines, verapamil, diltiazem, and bepridil — are currently being used for the treatment of angina. Despite their chemical heterogeneity, the major action of these drugs is to interfere with the entry of calcium into myocytes and vascular smooth muscle cells. These agents (either alone or in combination with β-adrenoreceptor blockers and/or nitrates) are effective in the treatment of chronic stable angina, unstable angina, and particularly in Prinzmetal's angina (Table 30 - 3; see Chapter 32).

Dihydropyridines

Dihydropyridines are the most potent vasodilators of the calcium channel blockers. The prototype of the dihydropyridines is nifedipine, although a number of newer dihydropyridines are now available (nicardipine, amlodipine, felodipine, isradipine, nisoldipine, and nitrendipine). Their antianginal effects are secondary largely to their vasodilatory properties; peripheral vasodilation lowers afterload and thereby reduces myocardial oxygen demand, while dilation of the coronary vascular bed increases oxygen delivery.

TABLE 30 - 3. Usual Cardiovascular Effects of Nifedipine, Diltiazem, and Verapamil

	Nifedipine	Diltiazem	Verapamil
Blood pressure	↓↓↓	↓	↓
Heart rate	0-↑	↓	↓↓
LV function	0	↓	↓↓

LV = left ventricular.

In vitro, the effects of the dihydropyridines on myocardial cells and on the conduction system (particularly the sinus and atrioventricular nodes) are similar to those produced by the other calcium channel antagonists. However, the negative inotropic and chronotropic effects are seen much less commonly clinically, because the marked vasodilation produced by the dihydropyridines decreases arterial pressure, producing a reflex increase in sympathetic output that tends to increase heart rate; it may also increase ejection fraction and cardiac output while decreasing left ventricular filling pressures. Thus, the major hemodynamic effects of dihydropyridines are a significant reduction in resting blood pressure and an increase in heart rate at rest. However, if sympathetic reflexes are attenuated or abolished by disease or drugs (*eg*, β blockers), a frankly cardiodepressant effect may be seen. Dihydropyridines may be the calcium antagonist of choice in patients with mild LV dysfunction, sinus bradycardia, sick sinus syndrome, and/or atrioventricular block because they have fewer negative effects on myocardial contractility, automaticity, and the cardiac conduction system than either verapamil or diltiazem in the clinical dosage range. Nonetheless, nifedipine may be associated with increased mortality in patients with congestive heart failure; other dihydropyridines (particularly amlodipine) may be less dangerous in this situation.

Adverse Effects

The adverse effects of nifedipine are listed in Table 30 - 4. They occur in 15 to 20% of patients and require stopping of the drug in about 5% of patients. Most of the side effects (dizziness, peripheral edema, flushing, headache, and hypotension) are probably secondary to systemic vasodilation; gastrointestinal reactions, particularly nausea, are also common. Nifedipine can cause worsening angina, probably by increasing heart rate in patients with severe coronary artery disease; in such patients, the combination of nifedipine and a β blocker is often useful.

Contraindications

Because of its potent vasodilator effects, nifedipine is contraindicated in patients who are hypotensive or who have severe aortic stenosis. In addition, it is important to re-

TABLE 30–4. Common Side Effects of Nifedipine, Diltiazem, and Verapamil

Nifedipine	Diltiazem	Verapamil
Dizziness (12%)	Dizziness (2%)	Constipation (6%)
Peripheral edema (8%)	Headache (2%)	Dizziness (4%)
Nausea (8%)	Peripheral edema (2%)	Hypotension (3%)
Flushing (7%)	Nausea (2%)	Peripheral edema (2%)
Headache (7%)	Weakness (1%)	Headache (2%)
Weakness (6%)	Rash (1%)	Nausea (2%)
Hypotension (4%)		Fatigue (1%)
Worsening angina (3%)		CHF (1%)
CHF (1%)		Bradycardia (1%)
		3rd degree AVB (1%)

AVB = atrioventricular block; CHF = congestive heart failure.

member that any calcium channel antagonist, even nifedipine, can precipitate heart failure in patients with underlying LV dysfunction.

Verapamil

Verapamil is available in both short-acting (given three or four times a day) and sustained-release preparations (given once or twice a day). Verapamil is a potent myocardial depressant in isolated muscle preparations, but produces only a mildly decreased contractility in patients with normal cardiac function. The major antianginal effect of verapamil is due to peripheral vasodilation, which decreases afterload and thus decreases myocardial oxygen demand. In addition, verapamil decreases heart rate, increasing the amount of time spent in diastole, when most of coronary perfusion occurs. Verapamil also dilates both normal and diseased cardiac arteries and arterioles, and is a potent inhibitor of coronary artery spasm. It thus increases myocardial oxygen delivery in patients with vasospastic angina and in many patients with unstable angina at rest.

Adverse Effects

In patients with cardiac dysfunction, the negative inotropic effects of verapamil may result in significant congestive heart failure. Verapamil also has the most potent effects of the cardiac conduction system of any of the calcium antagonists, frequently slowing heart rate and atrioventricular conduction (in its most benign manifestation simply causing PR prolongation). In general, adverse effects from verapamil occur in about 10% of patients and relate to gastrointestinal symptoms (constipation, nausea), systemic vasodilation (dizziness, hypotension), worsening cardiac function (peripheral edema or congestive heart failure), or conduction system abnormalities (bradycardia or third-degree atrioventricular block).

Verapamil is synergistic with β blockers, and when combined with these drugs can produce marked negative inotropic, chronotropoc, and dromotropic effects; it may also cause marked bradycardia if given with disopyramide. Verapamil also increases serum digoxin levels.

Contraindications

Verapamil is contraindicated in patients with congestive heart failure, hypotension or cardiogenic shock, sick sinus syndrome, second or third degree intrinsic atrioventricular conduction abnormalities (in the absence of a functioning ventricular pacemaker), and patients with suspected digitalis toxicity.

Diltiazem

Diltiazem is a less potent peripheral vasodilator than the dihydropyridines and a less potent negative inotrope and chronotrope than verapamil. Like verapamil and nifedipine, its major antianginal effect is probably due to peripheral vasodilation, resulting in decreased arterial pressure and afterload at rest and during exertion, with a concomitant reduction in myocardial oxygen demand. Diltiazem is also a potent dilator of both epicardial and subendocardial arteries, and inhibits spontaneous coronary artery spasm as well as spasm induced by ergonovine or exercise, increasing myocardial oxygen delivery in patients with vasospastic angina; it is not clear whether this effect plays any role in its treatment of chronic, effort-induced angina. Diltiazem may also reduce resting heart rate (although generally less than verapamil), which will also increase the time available for coronary perfusion; the magnitude of this effect in the treatment of angina is unclear.

Adverse Effects

A major clinical advantage of diltiazem is that it is well tolerated and generally has minimal side effects; these occur in approximately 4% of patients. Common adverse effects include dizziness, headache, peripheral edema, nausea, weakness, and rash. Nonetheless, diltiazem should be avoided in patients with underlying inotropic, chronotropic, or dromotropic disease.

Bepridil

Bepridil is a relatively new calcium antagonist that has recently been approved for use in the United States. Bepridil decreases resting heart rate and blood pressure, thus reducing myocardial oxygen consumption. It is an effective antianginal agent, but it causes QT prolongation and has been associated with torsades de pointes, a serious ventricular arrhythmia. Because of these life-threatening side effects, bepridil is being recommended for use as a last resort in patients for whom all other attempts to treat their angina have failed.

ASPIRIN

In patients with unstable angina, daily aspirin has been unequivocally shown to lower mortality and morbidity. In the Veterans Administration Cooperative Trial, 1266 men who presented early after the onset of unstable angina were randomized to receive either 324 mg aspirin per day or placebo. After 12 weeks, the frequencies of nonfatal myocardial infarction and of death had both decreased approximately 50% in the aspirin group compared with placebo. These benefits were confirmed in a Canadian multicenter trial that randomized 555 patients (of either sex) to aspirin, sulfinpyrazone, or placebo. After 19 months, the risk of nonfatal myocardial infarction and cardiac death was significantly reduced in patients receiving aspirin but not sulfinpyrazone or placebo. The use of aspirin is thus strongly recommended in patients with unstable angina. Whether this beneficial effect extends to patients with stable angina or to other drugs influencing platelet and prostaglandin pathways remains to be seen.

ANTICOAGULATION

In 1980, De Wood and his colleagues presented convincing evidence that intracoronary thrombus formation was involved in the pathogenesis of acute myocardial infarction. More recently evidence supporting a role for the same mechanism in unstable angina has begun to accumulate. For this reason, a number of investigators have attempted to use anticoagulation in the treatment of patients with unstable angina. Théroux and coworkers randomized 479 patients with unstable angina to treatment with aspirin, heparin, or both. After 6 days, the incidence of myocardial infarction was significantly reduced in all three groups; the combination of the two had no greater beneficial effect than either drug alone. Whether treatment with heparin also reduces mortality, whether its beneficial effect continues for longer than 1 week, whether it is also applicable in patients with stable angina, and whether other anticoagulants (especially warfarin) have similar effects are as yet undetermined (see also Chapter 34).

REFERENCES

Abrams J: Nitroglycerin and long-acting nitrates. N Engl J Med 302:1234–1237, 1980.

Braunwald E (ed): Heart Disease: A Textbook of Cardiovascular Medicine, 4th ed. Philadelphia: WB Saunders Co, 1992.

Cairns JA, Gent M, Singer J, et al: Aspirin, sulfinpyrazone, or both in unstable angina. N Engl J Med 313:1369–1375, 1985.

Coronary heart disease. *In* Andreoli TE, Carpenter CCJ, Plum F, Smith LH Jr (eds): Cecil Essentials of Medicine, 2nd ed. Philadelphia: WB Saunders Co, 1990.

De Wood MA, Spores J, Notske R, et al: Prevalence of total coronary occlusion during the early hours of transmural myocardial infarction. N Engl J Med 303:897–902, 1980.

Flaherty JT: Nitrate tolerance. A review of the evidence. Drugs 37:523–550, 1989.

Goldstein RE, Epstein SE: Medical management of patients with angina pectoris. Prog Cardiovasc Dis 14:360–398, 1972.

Gorlin R, Brachfield N, MacLeod C, Bopp P: Effect of nitroglycerin on the coronary circulation in patients with coronary artery disease or increased left ventricular work. Circulation 19:705–718, 1959.

Lewis HD Jr, Davis JW, Archibald DG, et al: Protective effects of aspirin against acute myocardial infarction and death in men with unstable angina. N Engl J Med 309:396–403, 1983.

Murad F: Drugs used for the treatment of angina: Organic nitrates, calcium-channel blockers, and β-adrenergic antagonists. In Gilman AG, Rall TW, Nies AS, Taylor P (eds): Goodman and Gilman's The Pharmacologic Basis of Therapeutics, 8th ed. New York: Pergamon Press, 1990.

Parmley WW, Chatterjee K (eds): Cardiology. Vol. 1: Physiology, Pharmacology, Diagnosis. Philadelphia: JB Lippincott Co, 1993.

Théroux P, Ouimet H, McCans J, et al: Aspirin, heparin, or both to treat acute unstable angina. N Engl J Med 319:1105–1111, 1988.

31 Antihyperlipidemic Agents

Robert Scheig

The Consensus Development Conference on Lowering Blood Cholesterol to Prevent Heart Disease sponsored by the National Institutes of Health in 1984 (Consensus Development Conference, 1985) and updated in 1993 (Summary of the Second Report of National Cholesterol Education Program, 1993) focused attention on the established risk of hypercholesterolemia, specifically high levels of low-density lipoprotein cholesterol (LDL-C), in the development of atherosclerosis. The need to develop screening programs was emphasized, and indications for therapy were outlined. Low levels of high-density lipoprotein cholesterol (HDL-C) are an independent risk factor for the development of atherosclerosis (Miller, 1980), but unlike LDL-C, it is not known if changing HDL-C levels alters risk. Among the complications of atherosclerosis, coronary artery disease itself causes some 500,000 deaths each year in the United States; over 5 million patients are symptomatic at any one time; and the disease costs over $60 billion annually in direct and indirect costs. Thus, therapy that improves serum lipoprotein levels and that reduces the risk of coronary artery disease has become an important medical concern. Hypertriglyceridemia may be a risk factor in the development of atherosclerosis and is a risk factor in the development of pancreatitis when serum levels rise above 1000 mg/dl (Cameron et al, 1974).

Nicotinic acid, resin therapy and the hydroxymethylglutaryl-CoA (HMG CoA) reductase inhibitors reduce serum cholesterol and LDL-C levels and have been shown to reduce the incidence of coronary events. No drug has been shown to increase longevity in primary prevention trials. However, in secondary prevention trials, lowering elevated levels of cholesterol has been shown to cause regression of atherosclerosis irrespective of whether the reduction is accomplished by rigorous diet and change in lifestyle (Ornish et al, 1990), partial ileal bypass surgery (Buchwald et al, 1990) or various drug therapies (Blankenhorn et al, 1987; Brown et al, 1990). Probucol reduces serum cholesterol and LDL-C levels, but lowers HDL-C levels and has not been shown to alter atherosclerotic events. In one large study, gemfibrozil reduced the incidence of coronary heart disease in patients with hypercholesterolemia, presumably either by increasing HDL-C levels or by lowering triglyceride levels inasmuch as there was little change in LDL-C. Gemfibrozil and nicotinic acid are the drugs of choice for the therapy of hypertriglyceridemia.

This chapter reviews lipoprotein metabolism to establish the basis for a rational approach to therapy for hyperlipidemia. Each drug currently in common use is then discussed.

LIPOPROTEIN FUNCTION AND METABOLISM

Chylomicrons

Chylomicrons are formed in the small intestinal mucosa principally from dietary triglycerides, cholesterol, and fat-soluble vitamins (Fig. 31–1). The triglycerides are hydrolyzed by an enzyme, lipoprotein lipase, found in capillaries supplying striated muscle and adipose tissue. The chylomicron remnant particles are recognized by specific receptors located in hepatocytes. These receptors are different from the LDL receptor and are not regulated by cellular cholesterol concentrations. The triglycerides in the remnant particle are either oxidized or used for very low density lipoprotein (VLDL) formation. The absorbed dietary cholesterol is used by the liver cell for membrane formation, incorporated into lipoproteins, or excreted in the bile. Thus, chylomicrons carry energy from dietary triglycerides to striated muscle and adipose tissue and deliver dietary cholesterol and fat-soluble vitamins directly to the liver.

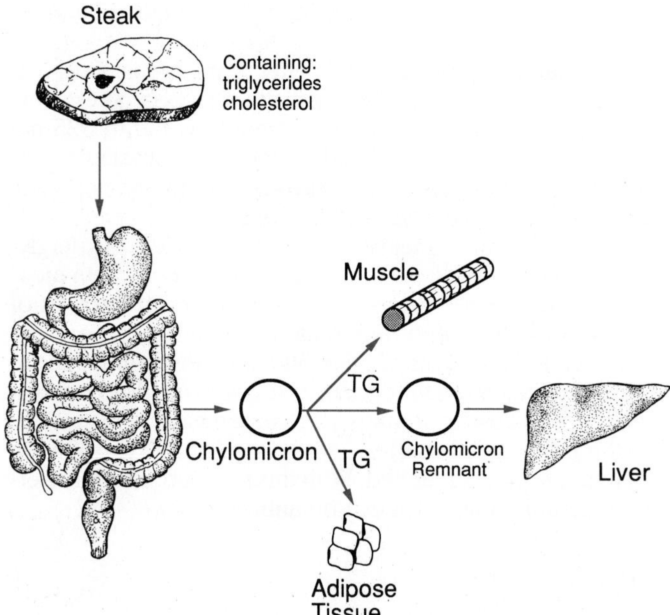

FIGURE 31-1. Dietary triglycerides (TGs) and cholesterol are absorbed from the gut into lymphatics as chylomicrons. Most of the triglycerides are hydrolyzed by lipoprotein lipase, and the fatty acids released are taken up by striated muscle and adipose tissue. The chylomicron remnant is recognized in receptors present only in the liver. Thus, dietary cholesterol goes directly to the liver, as do the remaining dietary triglycerides.

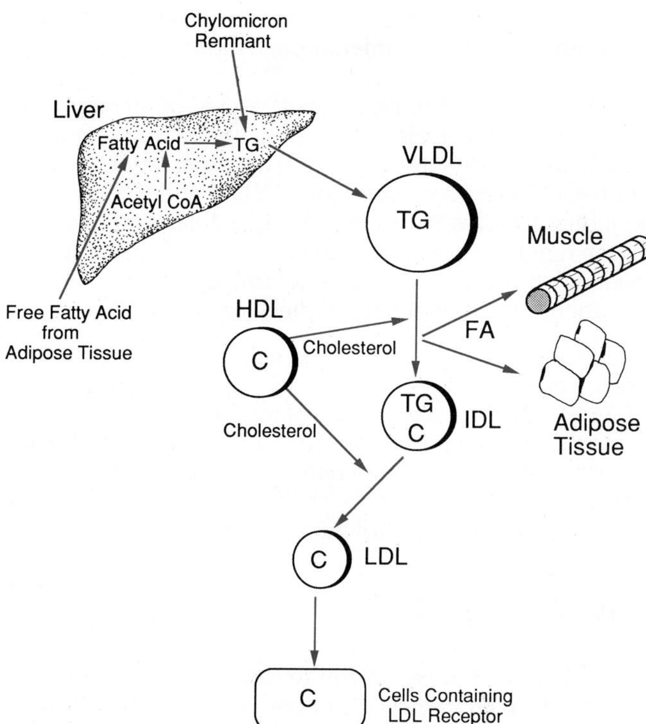

FIGURE 31-2. Very low density lipoprotein (VLDL), made in the liver, consists primarily of triglycerides (TGs) made from fatty acids (FAs) synthesized *de novo* or from adipose tissue or from triglycerides in the chylomicron remnant. Most of the triglycerides are hydrolyzed by lipoprotein lipase, and the fatty acids released are taken up by striated muscle and adipose tissue. In the remodeling, cholesterol is gained from high-density lipoprotein (HDL) with the formation of intermediate-density lipoprotein (IDL) and low-density lipoprotein (LDL). These lipoproteins can then be taken up by any cell containing the LDL receptor. CoA = coenzyme A; C = cholesterol.

Very Low Density Lipoproteins

Very low density lipoproteins (VLDLs) are manufactured in the liver, and triglycerides are their major constituent (Fig. 31-2). The fatty acids in the triglycerides are derived from chylomicron remnants, from circulating free fatty acids released from triglycerides contained in adipose tissue stores, or from fatty acids synthesized by the liver. The liver synthesizes fatty acids from acetyl-CoA derived from the metabolism of carbohydrates, fats, ethanol, and most amino acids. Thus, all calorie-containing foods can be converted to triglycerides, which are secreted by the liver as VLDL. The fatty acids released after hydrolysis by lipoprotein lipase are then taken up by striated muscle and adipose tissue. As the triglycerides are removed from VLDL, considerable remodeling occurs, including the addition of cholesterol from the high-density lipoproteins (HDLs), and LDLs are formed as a consequence. Thus, the two major functions of VLDL are to deliver energy, which may be derived from any calorie-containing source, to striated muscle and adipose tissue and to serve as the precursor of LDLs.

Low-Density Lipoproteins

Low-density lipoproteins (LDLs) are the carriers of cholesterol, which is required by all animal cells for membrane formation. Each cell contains receptors that recognize and bind apoprotein B found in LDL. After binding, parts of the cell membrane pinch off, and the vesicles thus formed deliver cholesterol to the interior. When there is an excess of cholesterol in the cell compared with need, LDL receptor synthesis decreases; and when the intracellular levels of cholesterol fall, more receptors are synthesized such that more cholesterol can enter the cell. Each cell also manufactures its own cholesterol from acetyl-CoA. The rate-limiting step is the conversion of HMG-CoA to mevalonate catalyzed by HMG-CoA reductase. The activity of this enzyme is suppressed when cholesterol accumulates in the cell and increases when there is a paucity of cholesterol.

High-Density Lipoproteins

High-density lipoproteins (HDLs), in addition to being the source of cholesterol for LDL formation, appear to be responsible for reverse cholesterol transport. HDLs are often called the scavenger lipoproteins because they bring cholesterol from cells in the periphery to the liver, where the cholesterol is either excreted in the bile or converted to bile salts, which are then excreted in the bile.

DIET THERAPY

Individuals with total serum cholesterol levels between 200 and 239 mg/dL are considered to be borderline and those over 240 mg/dL at high risk for the development of atherosclerosis (National Cholesterol Education Program, 1988). If

LDL-C measurements are used, levels between 130 and 159 mg/dL are considered borderline, and those over 160 mg/dL are considered high risk.

Diet is deemed to be a critical aspect of therapy in all cases because the major cause of hypercholesterolemia is thought to be the excess calories in the usual American diet. This results in an overproduction of VLDL and LDL. A major additional factor is the excess dietary cholesterol in chylomicron remnants coming to the liver, which results in a continual down-regulation of receptor formation.

Therefore, recommended dietary alterations include:

- Reducing the total number of calories if the patient is overweight.
- Decreasing fat intake to 30% of total calories with about one third derived from polyunsaturated, one third from monounsaturated, and no more than one third from saturated fatty acids.
- Limiting daily cholesterol intake to less than 300 mg.

DRUG THERAPY

When there is failure of diet to lower cholesterol to at least the borderline risk level or when two additional risk factors are present even though the cholesterol level is only borderline, drug therapy is clearly indicated. It has been shown that for each 1% fall in serum cholesterol there is a 2% decrease in the incidence of coronary artery disease (Lipid Research Clinics Program, 1984). Hypertriglyceridemia should be treated if hypercholesterolemia is also present, because by lowering VLDL, LDL may be lowered also. Finally, patients with fasting serum triglycerides above 500 mg/dL in the absence of hypercholesterolemia should be treated in order to prevent pancreatitis. Recommendations regarding altering HDL-C cannot yet be made.

Nicotinic Acid

Nicotinic acid (niacin), the vitamin known to prevent pellagra, has been used in large doses to decrease cholesterol for over 30 years. The mechanism of action is in part due to inhibition of cyclic adenosine monophosphate (AMP) accumulation in adipose tissue, which decreases the activity of triglyceride lipase. This causes a decreased release of free fatty acids from adipose tissue and thereby a decreased formation of VLDL and LDL.

Nicotinic acid

Nicotinic acid is useful, therefore, in the therapy of both hypercholesterolemia and hypertriglyceridemia. It is especially useful in patients with hypercholesterolemia and concomitant hypertriglyceridemia. Nicotinic acid reduces the incidence of recurrent myocardial infarction, decreases the progression of atheroma formation, and increases long-term survival (Canner et al, 1986; Blankenhorn et al, 1987). The drug is readily absorbed and distributed to all tissues.

Its major symptomatic side effects are intense flushing, pruritus, and headache. These usually disappear after a few weeks of therapy and can be alleviated by 160 to 325 mg aspirin/day because these side effects are prostaglandin-mediated. Nausea, vomiting, diarrhea, and, rarely, peptic ulceration are less common side effects.

Because abnormalities of liver function, hyperglycemia, and hyperuricemia occur not infrequently with nicotinic acid treatment, these must be evaluated at the start of therapy and monitored periodically thereafter.

Supplied in tablets of 50 to 500 mg, the starting dosage is 50 to 100 mg three times daily taken with meals to prevent gastritis. The dosage should be increased each week by 100 mg three times daily until a final dosage of 500 to 1000 mg three times daily is reached. With this regimen, a 15% lowering of serum cholesterol can be anticipated.

Resins

Cholestyramine and Colestipol

Cholestyramine (QUESTRAN) and colestipol (COLESTID) are chloride salts of basic anion exchange resins. These resins are not absorbed from the gastrointestinal tract. They avidly bind anions, including bile acids. By interrupting the enterohepatic circulation of bile acids, the liver increases its catabolism of cholesterol to bile acids, and the cholesterol level in the hepatocyte falls. As a consequence, there is both an increase in LDL receptor synthesis and an increase in cholesterol synthesis by the HMG-CoA reductase pathway. Fortunately, the effect on LDL receptor synthesis is the greater of the two. Because of this and because the liver contains about 70% of the body's LDL receptors, serum LDL levels fall.

The major disadvantages of these agents are the difficulty in swallowing the granules and the development of a variety of gastrointestinal (GI) complaints, especially bloating and constipation. Thus, compliance is a problem. Palatability is improved by making a slurry with fruit juice or mixing with applesauce. Rarely, hypoprothrombinemia due to vitamin K deficiency, reduced serum folate levels, and hyperchloremic acidosis have been reported.

It should be noted that the resins commonly cause a further increase in serum triglyceride levels in patients with hypertriglyceridemia. Because the resins can bind many anions, anionic medications such as digitalis, thyroxine, or warfarin should be taken at least 1 hour before, or 4 hours after, the resin.

Cholestyramine is supplied in bulk with a scoop or, for twice the price, premeasured in a packet. Each packet contains 4 g of anhydrous cholestyramine resin. The most common dosage is 8 to 16 g for breakfast, after which the largest concentration of bile salts is discharged into the gut because they have accumulated overnight in the gallbladder, and another 4 to 8 g at lunch.

Colestipol is supplied in bulk with a scoop or in packets, each packet or scoop containing 5 g of the resin. The dosage is 5 to 20 g for breakfast and 5 to 10 g for lunch.

On the average, a 15 to 20% reduction of serum cholesterol can be obtained with resin therapy. When resin is combined with nicotinic acid, a 26% reduction has been obtained, associated with a decreased progression of coronary atherosclerosis (Blankenhorn et al, 1987). Resin alone also decreases the incidence of coronary artery disease (Lipid Research Clinics Program, 1984).

HMG-CoA Reductase Inhibitors

Originally isolated from a strain of *Aspergillus terreus*, the four HMG-CoA reductase inhibitors are now made synthetically. These agents decrease LDL-C by decreasing the hepatic contribution of cholesterol for VLDL and therefore LDL formation; they also increase LDL receptor synthesis by lowering intracellular cholesterol levels. Interestingly, they have no effect on steroidogenesis, presumably because of the extensive first-pass extraction by the liver. Thus, these agents exert their principal effect in hepatocytes, the very cells that contain 70% of the total body LDL receptors and in which all VLDL synthesis occurs.

Single daily dosages are more effective when taken at night rather than in the morning, perhaps because cholesterol is synthesized mainly at night. Plasma concentrations are higher when administration is with a meal rather than when fasting.

Food and Drug Administration (FDA) approval of lovastatin (MEVACOR) occurred in 1987; subsequently, pravastatin (PRAVACHOL), simvastatin (ZOCOR), and fluvastatin (LESCOL) have been approved. These drugs cross the placenta and are excreted in milk. Because their effect on growth is not known, these inhibitors are currently contraindicated during pregnancy and lactation.

Because about 2% of patients develop threefold or more elevation in serum transaminases, serum glutamic-oxaloacetic transaminase (SGOT) or serum glutamate pyruvate transaminase (SGPT) levels should be monitored every 4 to 6 weeks during the first year of therapy. Fortunately, liver function returns to normal on discontinuation of the drug. Myalgia with transient elevations in creatinine phosphokinase has been seen in about 0.5% of the patient population, especially in patients concomitantly receiving gemfibrozil, nicotinic acid, erythromycin, or immunosuppressive therapy. Severe rhabdomyolysis precipitating acute renal failure has been reported.

Lovastatin

Lovastatin is supplied in 10-, 20-, and 40-mg tablets, and the daily dosage is 20 to 80 mg given with the evening meal or twice daily.

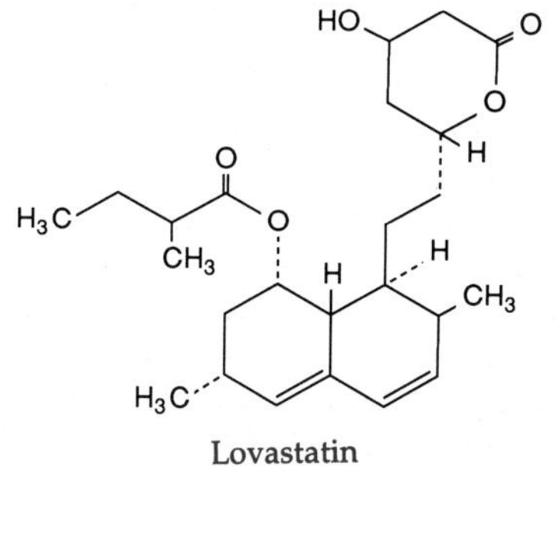

Lovastatin

Pravastatin

Pravastatin comes in 10- or 20-mg tablets, and the recommended dose is 10 to 20 mg daily.

Simvastatin

Simvastatin is packaged as 5-, 10-, 20-, or 40-mg tablets with a suggested daily dose of 5 to 40 mg.

Fluvastatin

Fluvastatin is supplied as a 20-mg tablet and appears to be useful at a dose of 20 mg/day for those with modest elevations of cholesterol.

A 15 to 40% reduction in serum cholesterol can be expected with the first three agents, depending on dose. Maximum effectiveness is achieved in about 4 weeks. If combined with a resin, even greater reductions have been noted (Illingworth, 1984; Thompson et al, 1986).

Probucol

Probucol (LORELCO) is a lipophilic substituted di-t-butylphenol with a chemical structure unlike that of other cholesterol-lowering agents. It appears to increase the fractional catabolic rate of LDL by enhancing nonreceptor-mediated pathways. It prevents oxidation of fatty acids in lipoproteins, which decreases the ability of endothelial cells to take up LDL. Although it decreases HDL-C, it apparently does so by reducing the size of HDL particles. Small HDL particles are capable of enhanced removal of cholesterol from peripheral depots. Supporting evidence for this enhanced reverse transport is the observation that probucol therapy successfully causes the disappearance of tendinous and tuberous xanthomas. Nevertheless, because of its effect on HDL and because its effect on atheroma formation has not been established in humans, probucol is not often used today.

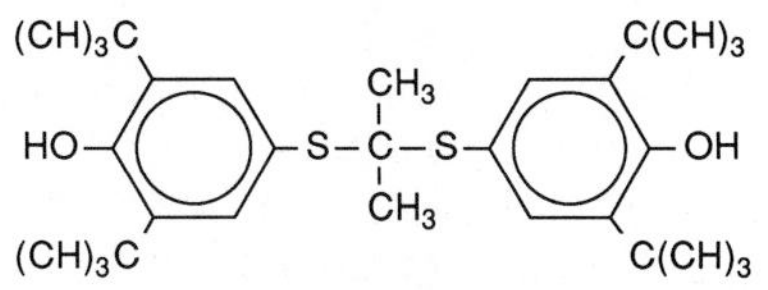

Probucol

Adverse reactions are rare. Diarrhea and flatulence are the most common side effects.

Probucol is supplied as a 250-mg tablet, and the dosage is 500 mg twice daily taken with the morning and evening meals. A 12 to 18% reduction in serum cholesterol can be anticipated, and the effects of long-term administration or combination therapy with a resin may be even better (McCaughan, 1981).

Fibric Acid Derivatives

Gemfibrozil

Gemfibrozil (LOPID) and clofibrate (ATROMID-S) are fibric acid derivatives useful in reducing serum triglyceride levels in patients with high levels of VLDL. Gemfibrozil has been shown also to reduce the mortality from coronary artery disease, presumably by raising the level of HDL-C, because its effect on LDL-C is small and variable (Frick et al, 1987). Gemfibrozil inhibits hydrolysis of triglycerides in adipose tissue and reduces hepatic extraction of free fatty acids. It also lowers VLDL by inhibiting synthesis and increasing clearance of apolipoprotein B.

Gemfibrozil is well absorbed from the GI tract, has a plasma half-life of about 1.5 hours, and does not accumulate with continued use. It is excreted mainly in urine as a glucuronide conjugate.

Severe hepatic or renal disease is a contraindication, and the drug paradoxically causes a pronounced rise in serum lipid levels in primary biliary cirrhosis. Because of structural similarities to clofibrate, which is known to increase gallstone formation, gemfibrozil should be used with caution in patients with biliary tract disease. Occasional liver function abnormalities have been reported, and anticoagulant dosage may have to be reduced. GI side effects are the most frequent symptomatic complications.

Gemfibrozil is supplied as 300-mg and 600-mg capsules, and the usual dosage is 600 mg 30 minutes before the morning and evening meals. A 40 to 45% fall in serum triglyceride level can be anticipated as well as a 20 to 25% rise in HDL-C.

Clofibrate

Clofibrate (ATROMID-S) is used little because it has not been shown to reduce cardiovascular events. In long-term studies, it increases mortality because of noncardiovascular causes, especially malignancy, postcholecystectomy complications, and pancreatitis.

REFERENCES

Blankenhorn DH, Nessim SA, Johnson RL, et al: Beneficial effects of combined colestipol-niacin therapy on coronary atherosclerosis and coronary venous bypass grafts. JAMA 257:3233-3240, 1987.

Brown G, Albers JJ, Fisher LD, et al: Regression of coronary artery disease as a result of intensive lipid-lowering therapy in men with high levels of apolipoprotein B. New Engl J Med 323:1289-1298, 1990.

Buchwald H, Vargo RL, Matts JP, et al: Effect of partial ileal bypass surgery on mortality and morbidity from coronary heart disease in patients with hypercholesterolemia. New Engl J Med 323:946-955, 1990.

Cameron JL, Capuzzi DM, Zuidema GD, Margolis S: Acute pancreatitis with hyperlipidemia. Am J Med 56:482-487, 1974.

Canner PL, Berge KG, Wenger NK, et al: Fifteen-year mortality in coronary drug project patients: Long-term benefit with niacin. J Am Coll Cardiol 8:1245-1255, 1986.

Consensus Development Conference: Lowering blood cholesterol to prevent heart disease. JAMA 253:2080-2086, 1985.

Fluvastatin for lowering cholesterol. Summary of the Second Report of the National Cholesterol Education Program, 1993. Med Lett 36:45-46, 1994.

Frick MH, Elo O, Haapa K, et al: Helsinki heart study: Primary-prevention trial with gemfibrozil in middle-aged men with dyslipidemia. N Engl J Med 317:1237-1245, 1987.

Illingworth DR: Mevinolin plus colestipol in therapy for severe heterozygous familial hypercholesterolemia. Ann Intern Med 101:598-604, 1984.

Lipid Research Clinics Program: The lipid research clinics coronary primary prevention trial results. JAMA 251:351-373, 1984.

McCaughan D: The long-term effects of probucol on serum lipid levels. Arch Intern Med 141:1428-1432, 1981.

Miller GJ: High-density lipoproteins and atherosclerosis. Annu Rev Med 31:97-108, 1980.

National Cholesterol Education Program (Goodman DS, chairman): Report of the Expert Panel on Detection, Evaluation, and Treatment of High Blood Cholesterol in Adults. Arch Intern Med 148:36-69, 1988.

Ornish D, Brown SE, Scherwitz LW: Can lifestyle changes reverse coronary heart disease? The lifestyle heart trial. Lancet 2:129-133, 1990.

Thompson GR, Ford J, Jenkinson M, Trayner I: Efficacy of mevinolin as adjuvant therapy for refractory familial hypercholesterolemia. Q J Med New Series 60 232:803-811, 1986.

Calcium: Hormonal Regulation and Calcium Channel Antagonists

32

David J. Triggle

INTRODUCTION TO CALCIUM

Properties

Calcium, a very abundant element, makes up some 3% of the earth's crust and is similarly abundant in the body. The average individual contains approximately 1 kg of calcium, the majority of which is immobilized as the mineral hydroxyapatite in bones and teeth. Approximately 1 to 2% of the total body calcium is found in ionized form in plasma and the intracellular space. Extracellular calcium is maintained at approximately 2.5 millimolar and free intracellular calcium at less than 10^{-7}M.

The critical calcium-mediated processes of stimulus-response coupling depend upon this small free fraction of intracellular calcium. During cell stimulation or activation the concentration of free ionized intracellular calcium rises to approximately 10^{-6}M.

Additionally, calcium is critical to cellular integrity, to the blood coagulation cascade, and to the activation of phospholipases and proteases.

Abnormal and persistent elevation of intracellular calcium concentrations subsequent to cell damage following a physical or chemical insult may mediate abnormal cell responses, including the hyperreactivity of smooth muscle in hypertension and bronchial asthma, and ultimately cell destruction and death.

To maintain the cellular functions of calcium and to guard against persistent calcium-mediated cell damage, the movements and storage of calcium are regulated in several ways. A major group of drugs in cardiovascular therapy, the calcium channel antagonists, serve to regulate calcium entry into excitable cells.

Requirements

The recommended daily requirements of calcium range between 360 and 1200 mg per day. The adult requirement is between 800 and 1200 mg per day with supplements of 400 mg per day for pregnant and nursing women. Calcium intake, however, varies considerably between 200 and 2500 mg per day. Some concerns exist that dietary calcium deficiencies do exist in segments of the population.

Little evidence suggests that increased dietary intake of calcium can reverse osteoporosis in postmenopausal females, but exercise and adequate bone formation prior to menopause are likely to be ameliorating factors. Other factors, including estrogen levels, are of importance in the prevention of bone resorption (see Chapter 54).

Calcium deficiencies and alterations in calcium-regulating hormones have also been associated with hypertension in some individuals. Calcium supplementation may serve in these individuals to reduce blood pressure.

Defects in Calcium Control

Serum levels of calcium provide a definition of hyper- and hypocalcemic states. Calcium is a controller of cellular excitability, and deficiencies and excesses are associated with increases and decreases respectively in cellular excitability.

Hypocalcemia arises from a chronic calcium deficiency in the diet and from deficiencies of dietary vitamin D or lack of production of parathyroid hormone. Hypocalcemia may also be precipitated by sodium fluoride ingestion or by transfusion with citrated blood. In advanced renal failure associated with hyperphosphatemia, a hypocalcemic state also occurs.

The general signs of hypocalcemia are increased excitability (including paresthesias, tetany, and increased neuromuscular excitability), laryngospasm, and enhanced excitability of other smooth muscles and convulsions.

Hypercalcemia has as principal causes hyperparathyroidism, vitamin D excess, and body immobilization. It may also arise from adrenocortical deficiency, hyperthyroidism, and the use of benzothiadiazide diuretics.

The consequences of hypercalcemia include kidney calcification and loss of function, general deposition of calcium in soft issues including the cardiovascular system and, in the case of hyperparathyroidism, loss of skeletal mass.

THE REGULATION OF CALCIUM

The multiple roles of calcium in cellular function demand that it be a regulated ion. Calcium is regulated at multiple loci by multiple processes (Figure 32 – 1).

Serum Calcium Regulation

Calcium uptake from the diet is regulated actively in the gastrointestinal tract and calcium excretion in the kidney. Bone is the major store of calcium in the body and calcium movement to and from this store is regulated by a triumvirate of hormones — parathyroid, vitamin D, and calcitonin. The levels of these hormones are themselves controlled by plasma calcium levels as part of a self-regulating cycle.

Decreases of serum calcium cause a rise in parathyroid hormone levels leading to a restoration of calcium by enhanced mobilization from bone, increased reabsorption in the kidney, and facilitated absorption in the gut. Similar roles are played by vitamin D metabolites, particularly through enhanced gastrointestinal absorption of dietary calcium.

Increases in serum calcium are associated with increased calcitonin secretion. Calcitonin opposes the actions of parathyroid hormone and vitamin D and mediates enhanced deposition of calcium into bone and increased urinary excretion.

The reciprocal relations between calcium, parathyroid hormone, and vitamin D are indicated in Table 32 – 1. Calcium and phosphate are regulated in coordinate fashion. Through the processes of Figure 32 – 1, the plasma calcium concentration is maintained at approximately 2.5 millimolar (5.0 mEq/liter).

The plasma concentration represents three separate pools: 40% of calcium is bound to plasma proteins, principally to albumin; 10% is complexed to anions including citrate and phosphate; and the remainder represents the free ionized calcium. Distinction between these pools is important because both the total and the ionized calcium levels can be altered independently. Changes in serum albumin

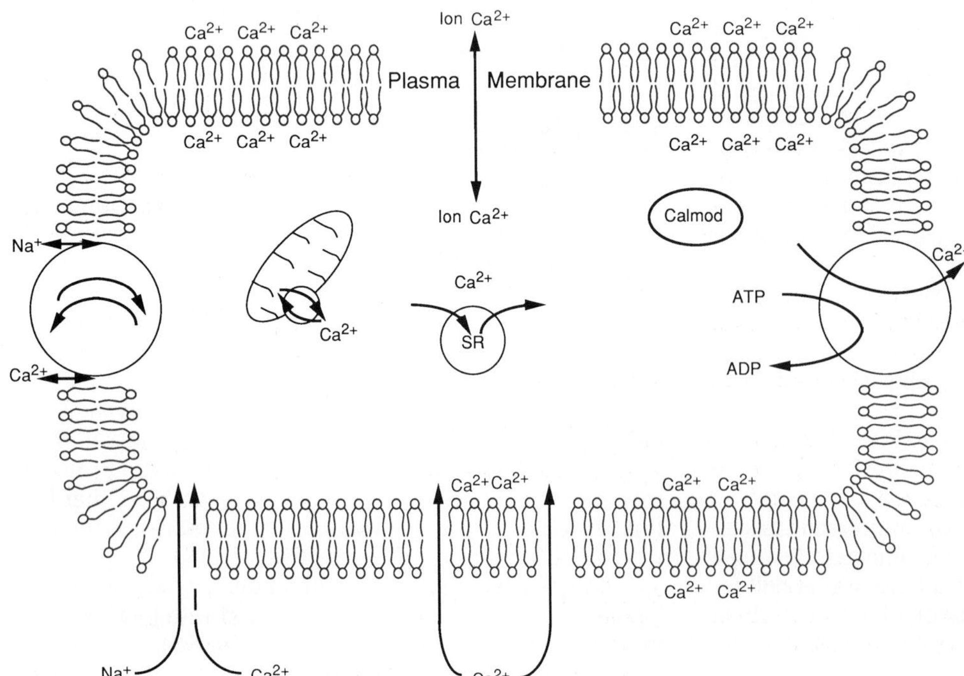

FIGURE 32 – 1. The control of calcium regulation at the cellular level. Depicted are the several calcium mobilization and storage processes operating in many cell types. Not all of the processes indicated may operate in any one cell, and the extent to which any process operates is cell-dependent, stimulus-dependent, and time-dependent. ADP = adenosine diphosphate; ATP = adenosine triphosphate; SR = sarcoplasmic reticulum.

TABLE 32–1. Relationships Between Serum Calcium and Parathyroid Hormone, Calcitonin, and Calcitriol

	Hormone Response		
Plasma Signal	***Parathyroid Hormone***	***Calcitonin***	***Calcitriol***
Ca^{2+} ↓	↑	↓	↑
Ca^{2+} ↑	↓	↑	

Hormone	**Hormone Change**	**Plasma Ca^{2+} Change**
Parathyroid hormone	↑	↑
	↓	↓
Calcitonin	↑	↓
	↓	↑
Calcitriol	↑	↑
	↓	↓

levels change total serum calcium levels, and the increased pH of respiratory acidosis will increase the fraction of ionized calcium without affecting total calcium levels.

Intracellular Calcium Regulation

The concentration of free ionized intracellular calcium is maintained at less than 10^{-7} M in the nonstimulated or resting cell. The large inwardly directed calcium gradient, the availability of internal and releasable stores of calcium, and the presence of intracellular high-affinity calcium-binding proteins, including the ubiquitous calcitonin, confer upon calcium its roles as a cellular messenger.

Cell calcium movements are controlled by several processes (Fig. 32–1). Of particular importance are ligand- and voltage-gated calcium channels through which calcium enters the cell. These channels are regulated by chemical and electrical influences respectively. The voltage-gated channels are the sites of action of the calcium channel antagonists, prominent in cardiovascular medicine.

Calcium is also mobilized from internal stores, notably the sarcoplasmic reticulum or its structural equivalent in nonmotile cells, in response to stimuli. The extent to which internal and external stores of calcium are mobilized depends upon cell and tissue type. Skeletal muscle depends almost exclusively upon internal stores, cardiac muscle employs both sources, and vascular smooth muscle employs dominantly extracellular calcium. Many secretory cells will employ both extra- and intracellular sources of calcium.

Mitochondria represent major depots of intracellular calcium. However, mitochondria are not involved in the physiological availability of calcium for stimulus-response coupling processes. Rather, matrix calcium in the mitochondria controls the activities of the dehydrogenase enzymes. However, under conditions of cellular calcium overload, mitochondria can sequester large amounts of calcium as a protective mechanism.

BONE FORMATION AND RESORPTION

The major mineral of bone is hydroxyapatite with the composition $Ca_{10}(PO_4)_6(OH)_2$. Additionally, there is an organic matrix and the bone cells—osteoblasts, osteoclasts, and osteocytes—that synthesize and resorb bone. Bone undergoes constant remodeling in response to calcium and the levels of vitamin D, calcitonin, and parathyroid hormone and to exercise and stress. A number of agents, hormonal and chemical, affect bone formation and resorption (Table 32–2).

Fluoride enhances bone formation, in part by changing the composition of the mineral to include fluorapatite, and its presence at 1.0 ppm is of considerable practical significance in the reduction of dental caries. However, large doses of fluoride impair mineralization, produce mottling of tooth enamel, and become progressively toxic to the individual.

Bone mineralization is also affected by bisphosphonates, including editronate (ethane-1-hydroxy-1,2-diphosphonic acid, EDHP), which retards bone formation, dissolution, and remodeling by aluminum salts, which complex phosphate, and by strontium, which impairs active vitamin D metabolite formation.

Tetracycline antibiotics have a high affinity for calcium and bone minerals and deposit in bones and teeth to give the latter a cosmetically discoloring appearance.

HORMONAL REGULATION OF CALCIUM

The plasma levels of calcium are regulated by the cooperative actions of vitamin D, parathyroid hormone, and calcitonin.

TABLE 32–2. Agents That Regulate Bone Formation and Resorption

Hormone and Growth Factors	Drugs and Toxic Agents
Activators of Bone Formation	
Vitamin D metabolites	Phosphate
Insulin	Fluoride
Insulinlike growth factors	
Estrogen	
Anabolic steroids	
Thyroxine	
Inhibitors of Bone Formation	
Glucocorticoids	Diphosphonates
Activators of Bone Resorption	
Parathyroid hormone	Endotoxin
Prostaglandins	Retinoids
Transforming growth factor (TGF)	Heparin
Epidermal growth factor (EGF)	
Inhibitors of Bone Resorption	
Calcitonin	Mithramycin
Estrogen	Colchicine

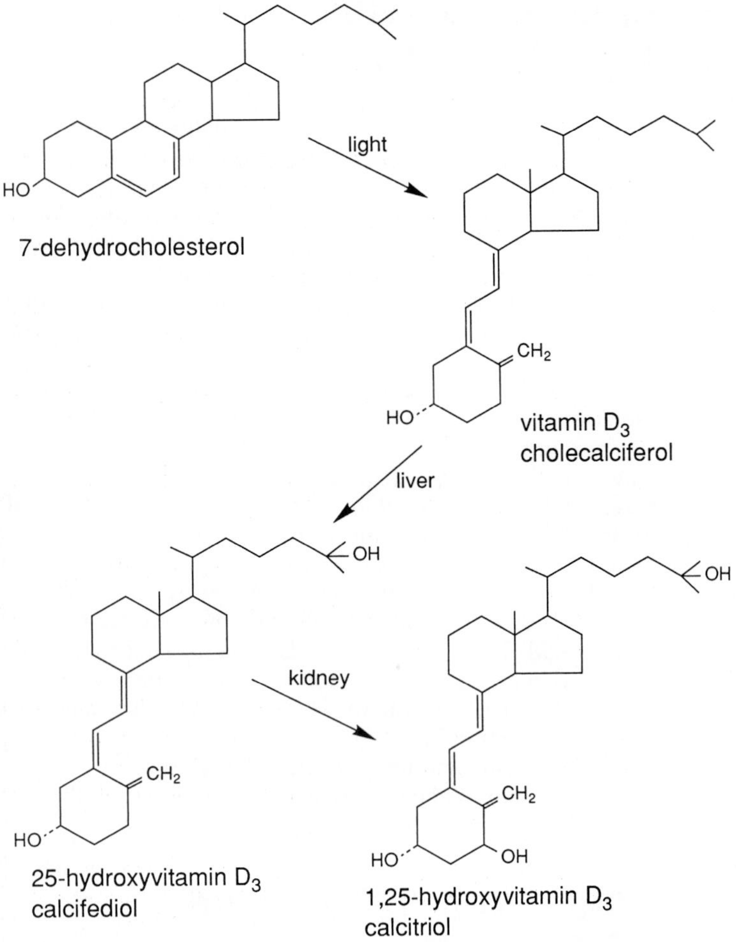

light

7-dehydrocholesterol

vitamin D_3
cholecalciferol

liver

25-hydroxyvitamin D_3
calcifediol

kidney

1,25-hydroxyvitamin D_3
calcitriol

FIGURE 32–2. Pathway of formation of vitamin D from 7-dehydrocholesterol.

Vitamin D

Vitamin D is synthesized in the skin by photochemical reaction from its immediate precursor 7-dehydrocholesterol. The product of this reaction is cholecalciferol or vitamin D_3 (Figure 32–2). Vitamin D_3 is not a calcium mobilizing or antirachitic species, but requires further metabolic activation first in the liver and then in the kidney, at the 25- and 1-positions respectively, to yield 1,25-dihydroxyvitamin D_3 or calcitriol—the active form of vitamin D. A summary of the several forms of vitamin D is in Table 32–3.

Calcitriol belongs to the family of steroid hormones, which includes the sex and thyroid hormones, and exerts its action through a hormone-receptor complex that regulates gene expression. This receptor has a widespread tissue distribution, including intestine, kidney, and bone, but also occurs in glandular and epithelial cells and smooth muscle, suggesting a widespread role for this hormone.

The physiological role of vitamin D is that of a positive regulator of calcium homeostasis. It maintains serum levels of calcium and phosphate by promoting their intestinal absorption, increasing their mobilization from bone, and decreasing their excretion through the kidney.

TABLE 32–3. The Several Forms of Vitamin D

Chemical Name	Abbreviation	Generic Name
Vitamin D_3	D_3	Cholecalciferol
Vitamin D_2	D_2	Ergocalciferol
25-hydroxyvitamin D	25 $(HO)D_3$	Calcifediol
1,25-hydroxyvitamin D_3	1,25 $(HO)_2 2D_3$	Calcitriol

Parathyroid Hormone

Parathyroid hormone is a single-chain peptide of 84 residues that is synthesized as the longer pre-prohormone. The mature hormone is stored in secretory granules of the parathyroid gland.

Release of parathyroid hormone is controlled by plasma calcium levels. A reduction in plasma calcium triggers the release of hormone. If the reduction is persistent, there is accompanying hypertrophy of the parathyroid glands. Conversely, hypercalcemia results in a decreased secretion of hormone and a reduction in glandular mass.

The primary function of parathyroid hormone is to maintain plasma calcium levels. This is achieved by mobilization and conservation of calcium. These effects are mediated principally in the bone, the gastrointestinal tract, and the kidney.

In the bone, parathyroid hormone increases resorption principally from the older and more stable fractions by stimulation of both osteoclasts and osteoblasts. The combined effect of this stimulation is thus the enhancement of bone turnover and remodeling.

In the kidney, parathyroid hormone increases the tubular reabsorption of calcium and inhibits the reabsorption of phosphate. Plasma calcium and phosphate levels increase and decrease, respectively. Additionally, parathyroid hormone enhances the conversion of 25-hydroxycholecalciferol to the active calcitriol. This conversion results in the enhanced absorption of calcium and phosphate from the gastrointestinal tract following an increase in parathyroid hormone levels.

Calcitonin

Calcitonin is a single-chain polypeptide of 32 residues with a disulfide bridge between positions 1 and 7. This bridge is essential for activity. Calcitonin is stored and released from the parafollicular C cells of the thyroid gland.

Release of calcitonin, like that of parathyroid hormone, is regulated by calcium. Secretion is increased or decreased in hyper- and hypocalcemic states respectively. Additionally, calcitriol exerts a direct releasing effect on these C cells. The half-life of calcitonin is brief, approximately 10 minutes.

The primary hypocalcemic and hypophosphatemic effects of calcitonin are exerted on the osteoclasts of the bone. Calcitonin inhibits the bone resorbing properties of these cells by a stimulatory effect on the adenylate cyclase that is inhibited by parathyroid hormone. Long-term effects of calcitonin serve to reduce the number of osteoclasts.

Defects in Hormonal Calcium Regulation

Abnormalities in hormonal calcium regulation are associated with hypo- or hypercalcemic states that have significant effects on both hard and soft tissues.

- Rickets and osteomalacia are well-recognized examples of calcium deficiency in children and adults, respectively, attributable to vitamin D deficiency. The reduced intestinal calcium and phosphate absorption activates the calcium-mobilizing actions of parathyroid hormone. In children this is associated with a failure of bone mineralization and in adults with a decrease in bone density.

  Juvenile dietary rickets is now extremely rare in the United States, but there is evidence for calcium deficiencies in segments of the adult population with low dairy food intake. As a consequence of studies undertaken in the early twentieth century that documented an association between juvenile rickets and inadequate diet and lack of sunshine, foods are routinely enriched with vitamin D.
- Hypercalcemia may be precipitated by excess vitamin D. Prolonged hypercalcemia produces an initially reversible, but subsequently irreversible, renal damage and calcification of soft tissue including the cardiovascular system.

  Hypervitaminosis may be accompanied by growth retardation in children and fetal defects including vitamin D hypersensitivity, reduced parathyroid function, and aortic stenosis.
- Parathyroid gland dysfunction is associated with hyper- and hypocalcemia in hypo- and hyperparathyroidism respectively.

  Hypoparathyroidism may result from loss of the parathyroid gland during thyroid surgery or from defects in glandular secretion. It is accompanied by a reduction in calcitriol levels caused by a reduction in parathyroid hormone-induced calcitriol formation.

  Hyperparathyroidism may arise from hypersecretion of the glands due to hyperplasia or malignancy and may be secondary to other defects in calcium metabolism, including defective intestinal absorption of calcium or renal disease.

BOX 32–1
THERAPEUTIC USES OF PARATHYROID HORMONE, VITAMIN D, AND CALCITONIN

The major uses of vitamin D are in three main areas—nutritional rickets, metabolic rickets, and osteomalacia and hypoparathyroidism. Nutritional rickets, although rare in the United States, can be treated successfully with any one of the available vitamin D preparations. Metabolic rickets is usually treated with calcitriol or dihydrotachysterol or its 25-hydroxy derivative because these agents do not require renal 1-hydroxylation to become activated. Dihydrotachysterol is frequently used in the treatment of hypoparathyroidism because it has a more rapid onset of action than other derivatives.

Calcitonin is effective in reducing calcium and phosphate levels in hypercalcemic individuals with hyperparathyroidism, vitamin D excess, excessive calcium absorption, or malignancies.

Other measures to reduce excess calcium levels include prednisone and other glucocorticoids, phosphates, including sodium editronate, and mithramycin.

Calcitonin is effective in Paget's disease, which is accompanied by extensive skeletal remodeling, but sodium editronate is cheaper and may well be as efficacious. Salmon calcitonin, rather than human or porcine material, is principally used because it has a longer half-life and increased potency. However, resistance may develop due to the formation of antibodies.

Several calcium preparations are available for the rapid treatment of hypocalcemia, particularly in the control of the associated tetany. Calcium chloride, gluconate, and gluceptate can be given intravenously and gluconate, lactate, carbonate, and phosphate are available for oral administration.

Pseudohypoparathyroidism is to be distinguished from idiopathic hypoparathyroidism and reflects a reduction in end-organ sensitivity to parathyroid hormone. There is a deficiency in the guanine nucleotide binding protein Gs. In type 1a deficiency, individuals exhibit unusual physical features termed Albright's hereditary osteodystrophy, and the generalized lack of the G protein leads to hyporesponsiveness to many hormones in addition to parathyroid hormone, including glucagon and thyroid-stimulating hormone (TSH). The deficiency extends also to olfactory dysfunction. In type 1b individuals, the deficiency is confined to the kidney only and such individuals do not display generalized hormone resistance.

DRUG REGULATION OF CELLULAR CALCIUM

Cellular calcium mobilization in response to stimuli is a major component of cellular stimulus-response coupling. These mobilization pathways are the targets of drug action. However, clinically available drugs are available only for one specific pathway — the voltage-gated calcium channel (Figure 32-1).

Cellular Calcium Antagonism

The concept of drug-mediated calcium antagonism was introduced by Albrecht Fleckenstein (1917-1992) when he observed that verapamil mimicked in reversible fashion the effects of calcium withdrawal on cardiac function and that the resultant loss of contractility with minimal effect on action potential configuration could be overcome through increased calcium.

The ability of verapamil and other agents of the phenylalkylamine class to produce coronary and peripheral vasodilation and negative inotropic and chronotropic effects was thus ascribed to this ability to interfere with calcium mobilization for excitation-contraction coupling. Similar effects were subsequently found with agents from other structural classes including the 1,4-dihydropyridine nifedipine and the benzothiazepine diltiazem.

The major therapeutic uses of these agents are in the cardiovascular area, including angina in its several forms, hypertension, and some peripheral vascular disorders and selected cardiac arrhythmias including supraventricular tachycardia (Table 32-4). Nimodipine, a member of the 1,4-dihydropyridine class, is used in the treatment of vasospasm subsequent to subarachnoid hemorrhage. There is current interest in these agents because of their antiatherogenic activities.

TABLE 32-4. Clinical Uses of Ca^{2+} Channel Antagonists

Current Use	Drug*
Myocardial Ischemia	
Exertional angina	D,N,V
Prinzmetal's angina	D,N,V
Unstable angina	D,N,V
Hypertension	D,N,V
Hypertensive emergencies	N
Cardiac Arrhythmias	
Supraventricular tachycardia	N
Atrial fibrillation and flutter	V,D
Hypertrophic Cardiomyopathy	V
Potential Use†	**Drug***
Cardiovascular	
Migraine	V,N
Raynaud's disease	N
Cardioprotection	V,D
Subarachnoid hemorrhage	nimod
Cerebral insufficiency	nimod
Pulmonary hypertension	N?
Congestive heart failure	N?
Noncardiovascular	
Asthma (exercise-induced)	V,N
Esophageal motor disorders	N
Premature labor	N
Urinary incontinence	N
Dementia	nimod

*D = diltiazem; N = nifedipine; V = verapamil; nimod = a 1,4-dihydropyridine analog of nifedipine.

†Only a partial listing of potential uses is provided here. The Ca^{2+} channel antagonists have been suggested to be of potential use in virtually all cases in which hyper- or excessive activity of smooth muscle systems is involved.

Classification, Sites, and Mechanisms of Action

The calcium antagonists are a chemically heterogeneous group of agents with a common ultimate action — blockade of voltage-gated calcium channels.

These several structural groups of agents interact at separate sites on the calcium channel (Figure 32-3). That these agents have discrete sites and mechanisms of actions underscores the relative cardiac: vascular selectivity of these agents.

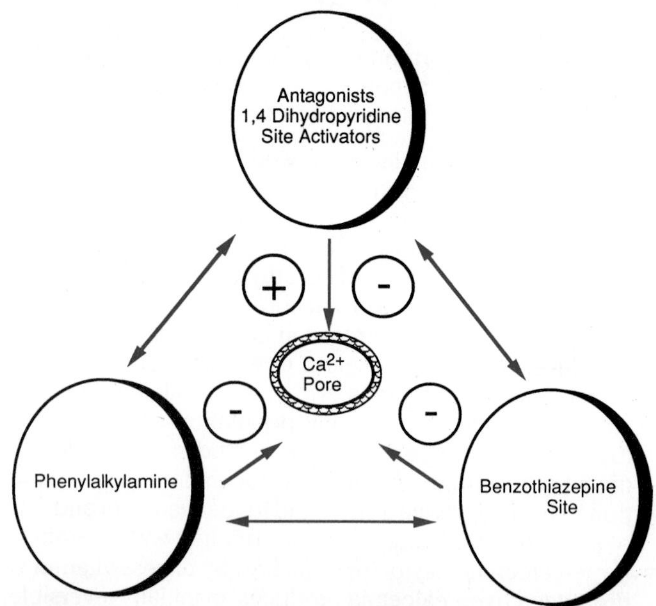

FIGURE 32-3. The organization of the specific binding sites for 1,4-dihydropyridines (antagonists and activators), phenylalkylamine, and benzothiazepine categories of calcium-channel drugs. The binding sites represent an allosteric association linked one to the other and to the gating and permeation processes of the calcium channel.

Nifedipine and second-generation 1,4-dihydropyridines, including amlodipine, nimodipine, and felodipine are vascular selective agents. Their properties are dominated by vasodilating activity. In contrast, verapamil and diltiazem have both vasodilating and cardiac depressant activities. The relative extent to which both properties are exhibited contributes to both the therapeutic and contraindication profiles of these agents (see also Chapters 28–31).

Several factors determine the relative cardiac : vascular selectivity of these agents including the type of calcium channel and the state- or use-dependent characteristics of channel blockade.

Several distinct classes of voltage-gated calcium channel exist. These separate channels are classified by their electrophysiological and pharmacological properties. The L-type channel, sensitive to verapamil, nifedipine, and diltiazem, dominates the cardiovascular system. Other types of channels, N, T, and P, some specific to the central nervous system, exist and have their own distinctive pharmacology. However, therapeutic agents do not exist for these other channel classes.

State- or use-dependent interactions of the calcium antagonists underlie the frequency- and voltage-dependent interactions of these agents. The affinity or access of a drug to the channel is determined by selective interactions with the resting, open, or inactivated states (Figure 32–4). Verapamil and diltiazem interact through an open channel state favored by repetitive stimulation: this underlies their antiarrhythmic properties. In contrast, nifedipine and other 1,4-dihydropyridines interact selectively with the inactivated state of the channel, a state favored by persistent depolarization or tone: this underlies their selective vasodilating properties.

Pharmacological Properties

The major properties of the calcium channel antagonists are directed toward the cardiovascular system. However, they do exhibit several effects in nonvascular smooth muscle and some neuronal systems, and there has been considerable experimental interest in extending their uses (Table 32–5).

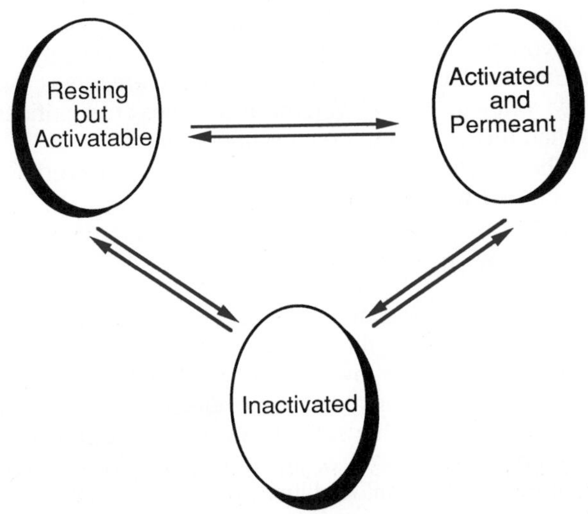

FIGURE 32–4. The calcium channel, shown schematically, cycling through resting, activated (open), and inactivated states.

TABLE 32–5. Additional and Potential Uses of Calcium Channel Antagonists

Cardiovascular	Nonvascular Smooth Muscle	Other
Atherosclerosis	Achalasia	Aldosteronism
Congestive heart failure	Asthma	Epilepsy
Erectile impotence	Chronic obstructive lung disease	Motion sickness
Headache	Urinary incontinence	Tinnitus
Headache: cluster, migraine		Vertigo
Intermittent claudication		
Stroke		

Cardiovascular Effects

All three first-generation calcium antagonists are vasodilators of both the coronary and peripheral arteries. These properties underlie the antihypertensive and antianginal effects of the agents. Nifedipine and other 1,4-dihydropyridines are more potent than verapamil and diltiazem.

Verapamil, nifedipine, and diltiazem inhibit cardiac contractility *in vitro*. The observed potency sequence—verapamil > diltiazem > nifedipine—differs from that for vasodilation. *In vivo*, however, the net effects on cardiac function reflect the balance between direct cardiodepression and cardiostimulation produced by reflex activation (Table 32–6). Nifedipine and other 1,4-dihydropyridines normally produce a net positive chronotropic response because of their powerful vasodilating capacity. This reflex tachycardia is usually short-lived and vanishes on prolonged drug administration, presumably due to resetting of baroreceptors. However, under certain clinical conditions where ventricular function is impaired or where the compensating pathways are lacking, nifedipine can produce cardiac depression.

As antihypertensive drugs, the calcium antagonists contrast with other vasodilators because they exert little chronic activation of the renin-angiotensin-aldosterone (RAA) axis. Additionally, these agents produce a modest diuresis and natriuresis: this also contrasts with other vasodilators. These effects may reflect both changes in renal hemodynamics as well as a direct role for calcium channels in the control of renal ion and water transport (see Chapter 29).

TABLE 32–6. Cardiovascular Profile of Calcium Antagonists

	Nifedipine	Diltiazem	Verapamil
Coronary vessels			
Tone	−−−	−−	−−
Flow	+++	++	++
Peripheral vasodilation	+++	+	++
Heart rate	0,++	−	−
Contractility	0,+	0,−	0,−
AV node conduction	0	−	−
AV node ERP	0	−	−

+ = increase; − = decrease; 0 = no effect; AV = atrioventricular; ERP = effective refractory period.

As antihypertensive agents, the calcium antagonists are appropriate for use in the presence of ischemic heart disease, peripheral vascular disease, left ventricular hypertrophy, diabetes, asthma, chronic obstructive pulmonary disease, and renal failure. These indications reflect the abilities of the antagonists to dilate the coronary vasculature, to not exacerbate peripheral vascular disorders including those of obstructive character, to be without effect on insulin release, to have no detrimental effects on the pulmonary smooth muscle, and to be potent renal vasodilators.

Effects in Other Systems

Although L-type voltage-gated channels are widely distributed, the therapeutic effects of the calcium antagonists are dominantly confined to the cardiovascular system. However, their effects on nonvascular smooth muscle have translated into limited use in achalasia and esophageal motor disorders, urinary incontinence, and uterine contractions.

The calcium antagonists are antiatherogenic in both experimental and clinical situations. The underlying process(es) remain to be defined, but may reflect calcium-dependent effects including smooth muscle cell migration, cell proliferation, and growth factor action.

BOX 32–2
THERAPEUTIC APPLICATIONS

The dominant applications of calcium antagonists are for angina in its several forms, hypertension, some cardiac arrhythmias, and selected vascular disorders. Experimental clinical descriptions are available for many other disorders (Table 32–6).

- **Ischemic heart disease.** Diltiazem, verapamil, and nifedipine are all used acutely and chronically in the several forms of angina—exertional, variant, and Prinzmetal's. Several mechanisms likely contribute to their well-accepted efficacy. These include coronary artery dilation, redistribution of blood flow to ischemic areas, reduction of afterload and a further reduction in oxygen consumption by the heart through reduced contractility. The latter contribution is more important with verapamil and diltiazem (see Chapter 30).
- **Hypertension.** The calcium antagonists are widely employed as antihypertensive agents. All available calcium antagonists are effective in lowering both systolic and diastolic blood pressure. Quite generally, and as with other vasodilators, blood pressure–lowering efficacy increases with increasing pretreatment blood pressure (see Chapter 29).

  The calcium antagonists are also appropriate therapeutic choices for hypertension associated with myocardial ischemia, peripheral vascular disorders, asthma and chronic obstructive pulmonary disease, and diabetes.

  Some evidence suggests that calcium antagonists may be more effective antihypertensive agents in low-renin patients and in elderly individuals.

  Combination therapy of calcium antagonists with β blockers is appropriate and efficacious with nifedipine and other 1,4-dihydropyridines. Considerable caution should be exerted with verapamil and diltiazem in combination. The combination of calcium antagonists and angiotensin-converting enzyme (ACE) inhibitors may be particularly efficacious in severe hypertension.

  Although calcium antagonists, ACE inhibitors, diuretics, and β blockers are all effective in the first-line control of hypertension, only β blockers and diuretics have thus far been shown to lower cardiovascular morbidity and mortality.
- **Cardiac arrhythmias.** Verapamil and diltiazem are both effective in the treatment of a number of cardiac arrhythmias. Nifedipine and all other available 1,4-dihydropyridines are ineffective antiarrhythmic species.

  Verapamil is the agent of choice as a class IV antiarrhythmic drug (see Chapter 28) for the termination of episodes of paroxysmal supraventricular tachycardia (PSVT) that involve regions of the heart, principally the atrioventricular (AV) node, that show calcium channel–dependent responses. Approximately 80% of such patients convert to sinus rhythm after intravenous verapamil. Such arrhythmias have a variety of origins, including AV nodal reentry, accessory pathway reentry (Wolff-Parkinson-White syndrome), and atrial fibrillation and flutter. Verapamil may also be effective against digitalis-induced arrhythmias and ventricular tachycardia and fibrillation due to coronary artery spasm, but ventricular arrhythmias of other origin are not sensitive to verapamil or calcium antagonists in general (see Chapter 28).

Pharmacokinetics

Verapamil, diltiazem, and nifedipine show a broadly similar pattern in their pharmacokinetic behavior. They are all well absorbed following oral administration, all are extensively protein-bound, all are subject to significant first-pass metabolism, and all have durations of action, in the nonsustained release formulations, of 3 to 5 hours.

Hepatic metabolism is the dominant inactivation pathway for all three compounds. The metabolites of nifedipine, pyridine carboxylic acids, are pharmacologically inert. However, major metabolites of diltiazem, desacetyl- and monomethyldiltiazem, are active, as is norverapamil (*N*-desmethylverapamil). However, these activities are significantly less than those of the parent compounds.

The elimination of calcium antagonists is slowed by hepatic disease and by aging.

Side Effects

Adverse effects associated with the calcium antagonists are generally related to their fundamental pharmacological properties and have a low incidence. All of the agents produce a peripheral edema that is not related to salt and water accumulation but rather reflects an unbalance in capillary blood flow. The order of incidence of side effects is nifedipine > verapamil > diltiazem.

- For verapamil, the side effects are, in order of reported frequency of occurrence, constipation, dizziness, headache, peripheral edema, and bradycardia.

- For diltiazem, the side effects are edema, dizziness, headache, and facial flushing.
- For nifedipine, the side effects are facial flushing, headaches, edema, and dizziness (see also long list in Chapter 30).

Contraindications

The calcium antagonists are generally well-tolerated agents. Specific contraindications exist, however, for a number of diseases that may coexist with the primary targets for the calcium antagonists.

Verapamil and diltiazem both have significant cardiac depressant effects on both contractility and conduction. They should be used with caution in any clinical state associated with conduction or contractile failure including cardiac block or AV conduction defect, sinus bradycardia, and sick sinus syndrome. Additionally, calcium antagonists are contraindicated in cardiac failure and following infarct where there is clinical evidence of congestive heart failure. These latter limitations may not apply to the newer and more vascular-selective, 1,4-dihydropyridines.

The calcium antagonists, particularly nifedipine and other 1,4-dihydropyridines, should be avoided in patients with hypotension.

Drug Interactions

A number of drug interactions exist with the calcium antagonists and may be broadly classed as those related to changes in metabolism (predominantly inhibition of cytochrome P-450); those related to changes in altered drug absorption, clearance, or secretion; and those that reflect pharmacological interactions.

- The histamine H_2 antagonist cimetidine, but not ranitidine, increases serum levels of the calcium antagonists. In turn, verapamil, diltiazem, and possibly nifedipine increase serum levels of a number of agents including the anticonvulsant carbamazepine, the receptor antagonists prazosin, propranolol, and metoprolol, and the immune suppressant cyclosporin.
- Nifedipine enhances the gastrointestinal absorption of amoxicillin and propranolol, and all three calcium antagonists inhibit the renal tubular secretion of digoxin.
- A number of pharmacological interactions exist. In particular, verapamil and diltiazem can produce undesired levels of cardiac depression and even AV block when combined with β blockers. Similarly, inhalational anesthetics and these calcium antagonists may produce together undesirable levels of cardiac depression.
- Verapamil and diltiazem appear to potentiate the neurotoxic effects of lithium when the latter is used for mania.
- All calcium antagonists appear to potentiate the actions of a number of cytotoxic anticancer drugs including the anthracyclines, vinca alkaloids, and epipodophyllotoxins. This interaction is related to the ability of the calcium antagonists to block the action of the glycoprotein multiple drug transporter that is overexpressed in drug-resistant tumor cells. This action is unrelated to their calcium channel antagonist properties.

New Agents

New agents have been introduced with pharmacological and pharmacokinetic properties different from those calcium antagonists already available. These agents of the 1,4-dihydropyridine class include amlodipine, felodipine, isradipine, nicardipine, and nimodipine.

The distinctive properties of these agents include 24-hour duration of action with amlodipine as a result of its nonpolar characteristics and slower metabolic rate. Felodipine and amlodipine have enhanced vascular selectivity, a property that may underline a superior antihypertensive profile and a role for these agents in the treatment of congestive heart failure. Nimodipine enjoys a marked regional selectivity for the cerebral vasculature. This defines its use in the treatment of vasospasm associated with cerebral hemorrhage.

Dosage Forms

All calcium antagonists are available in both conventional multidose and extended- and sustained-release formulations. These are summarized in Table 32 – 7.

TABLE 32 – 7. Dosage Forms of Calcium Antagonists

Formulation	Form (mg)		Initial Dose (mg/day)	Maximal Dose/day	Frequency
Conventional					
Verapamil	40, 80, 120		240	480	b.i.d./t.i.d.
Nifedipine	10, 20		30	120 – 180	t.i.d.
Diltiazem	30, 60, 90, 120		90	240 – 360	t.i.d.
Nicardipine	20, 30		60	120	t.i.d.
Isradipine	2 – 5, 5		50	120	b.i.d.
Slow Release					
PLENDIL (felodipine)	5, 10	ER	5	20	q.d.
VERELAN (verapamil)	120, 240	SR	120 – 140	480	q.d.
CALAN SR (verapamil)	180, 240	SR	120 – 180	480	q.d./b.i.d.
ISOPTIN SR (verapamil)	180, 240	SR	120 – 180	480	q.d./b.i.d.
PROCARDIA XL (nifedipine)	30, 60, 90	ER	30 – 60	90 – 120	q.d.
CARDIZEM CD (diltiazem)	180, 240, 300	SR	180 – 240	360	q.d.

b.i.d. = twice a day; ER = extended release; q.d. = every day; SR = sustained release; t.i.d. = three times a day.

REFERENCES

Baker PF (ed): Calcium and Drug Action. New York and Heidelberg: Springer-Verlag, 1987.

Minghetti PP, Norman AW: 1,25 (OH)2-Vitamin D_3 receptors: Gene regulation and genetic circuitry. FASEB J 2:3043–3053, 1988.

Morad M, Nayler WG (eds): The Calcium Channel: Structure, Function and Implications. Berlin: Springer-Verlag, 1989.

Opie LH: Calcium channel antagonists. Part I: Fundamental properties: Mechanisms of classification, sites of action. Cardiovasc Drugs Ther 1:411–430, 1987.

Opie LH: Calcium channel antagonists. Part II: Use and comparative properties of the three prototypical calcium antagonists in ischemic heart disease, including recommendations based on an analysis of 41 trials. Cardiovasc Drugs Ther 1:461–491, 1988.

Tietze KJ, Schwartz ML, Vlasses PH: Calcium antagonists in cerebral/peripheral vascular disorders. Current status. Drugs 32:531–538, 1987.

Triggle, DJ: Calcium antagonists. *In* Antonaccio M (ed): Cardiovasular Pharmacology, 3rd ed. New York: Raven Press, 1990.

Triggle DJ: Calcium-channel antagonists: Mechanisms of action, vascular selectivities, and clinical relevance. Cleveland Clin J Med 59:617–627, 1992.

Triggle DJ: Calcium channel drugs: Antagonists and activators. ISI Atlas Pharmacol 1:319–324, 1987.

Triggle DJ, Janis RA: Calcium channel ligands. Annu Rev Pharmacol Toxicol 27:347–369, 1987.

Young EW, Bukoski RD, McCarron DA: Calcium metabolism in experimental hypertension. Proc Soc Exp Biol Med 187:123–141, 1988.

PART VII

ORGAN SYSTEM PHARMACOLOGY

Drug Therapy for Gastrointestinal Diseases 33

Ravi Vemulapalli and M. Peter Lance

This chapter will address the drugs used in the treatment of a number of different gastrointestinal (GI) disease conditions. It will focus on the drugs and their mechanisms of action in the context of treatment strategies, starting with disorders of the stomach.

TREATMENT OF PEPTIC ULCER DISEASE

Our understanding of the etiology and pathophysiology of peptic ulcer disease has rapidly evolved over the past decade with the discovery of *Helicobacter pylori* in the stomach.

Helicobacter Pylori

Helicobacter pylori is a "comma-shaped" Gram-negative bacterium that has been shown to colonize the stomach. A definite association between *H. pylori* infection and type B gastritis has now been established. A strong correlation with infection and duodenal ulcer also exists, especially in association with gastritis. Association with gastric ulcer and gastric cancer has also been suggested. The mechanisms by which *H. pylori* infection is acquired and the pathophysiology by which it causes peptic ulcer disease are not completely understood at this time. The prevalence of colonization with *H. pylori* increases with age and is higher in lower socioeconomic groups and underdeveloped countries. The prevalence of *H. pylori* increases with age and reaches 60% by 60 years of age.

As *H. pylori* infection has been shown to play a significant role in ulcer pathogenesis and recurrence and possibly plays a role in gastric cancer, it is now felt that all patients with peptic ulcer disease should be checked for the presence of *H. pylori* infection and treated for the infection. This treatment results in a dramatic decrease in the recurrence rate of duodenal ulcers (Fig. 33-1). The impact of eradication of *H. pylori* on the incidence of gastric cancer is still unclear at this time.

It is now the general opinion that eradication of *H. pylori* from the stomach by pharmacological methods should receive first priority in the management of peptic ulcer disease, whereas acid suppression is still used to heal active ulcers.

Peptic ulcers appear to occur when the balance between the "aggressive" mechanisms and the "defensive" mechanisms in the stomach are altered; aggressive mechanisms involved in peptic ulcer disease include

- *Helicobacter pylori*
- Gastric acid
- Gastric pepsin
- Nonsteroidal anti-inflammatory drugs (NSAIDs)

The major endogenous mucosal defense mechanisms, although less well defined, include:

- Bicarbonate
- Mucus
- Mucosal blood flow
- Mucosal growth factors (Soll, 1990; Peterson, 1991)

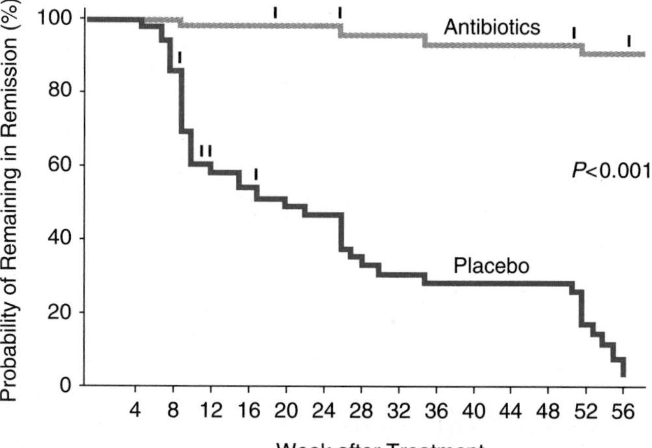

FIGURE 33-1. Probability that a duodenal ulcer would remain in remission during the 1-year follow-up period (Kaplan-Meier plot). The tick marks represent patients who, because of noncompliance, were considered to have withdrawn from the study. The probability of 100% on the vertical axis refers to the proportion of patients whose ulcers were healed at 6 and 10 weeks; the beginning of the follow-up period was defined by the verification of healing at either point. The two patients in the placebo group whose ulcers had not healed by 10 weeks were therefore not included in this life-table estimate. The difference between the groups was significant according to the log-rank test. (Reprinted by permission of *The New England Journal of Medicine*. From Hentschel E, Brandstätter G, Dragosics B, et al: Effect of ranitidine and amoxicillin plus metronidazole on the eradication of *Helicobacter pylori* and the recurrence of duodenal ulcer. N Engl J Med 328:308-312, 1993. ©1993 Massachusetts Medical Society.)

TABLE 33-1. Drug Classes Used to Treat Peptic Ulcers

Inhibit or Neutralize H^+ Secretion
H_2 blockers
  Cimetidine (TAGAMET)
  Ranitidine (ZANTAC)
  Famotidine (PEPCID)
  Nizatidine (AXID)

H^+/K^+ ATPase Inhibitors
Proton pump inhibitors
  Omeprazole (PRILOSEC)
Prostaglandins of E class
  Misoprostol (CYTOTEC)

Antisecretory Agents
Prostaglandins of E class

Coat Mucosa
Sucralfate (CARAFATE)
Bismuth compounds (*eg*, PEPTO-BISMOL)

Act by Other Mechanisms
Sucralfate
Bismuth compounds
Prostaglandins of E class
Antacids—low dose
Antibiotics

Drugs facilitate healing of peptic ulcers and prevent their recurrence by eradication of *H. pylori*, by decreasing the acidity, and by antagonism of the aggressive pathophysiological mechanisms (Table 33-1; Fig. 33-2).

- **Parietal cell secretion is regulated by site-specific agonists and antagonists.** Histamine, gastrin, and acetylcholine all stimulate parietal cell secretion by activation of receptors located on the basolateral membrane of this cell (Fig. 33-2). The $H^+ - K^+$ adenosine triphosphatase (ATPase), located on the apical surface and lining the secretory canaliculi, is the enzyme responsible for secretion of acid. Acid secretion can be inhibited by blocking the histamine, gastrin, or acetylcholine receptors, by activation of the prostaglandin receptor, or by antagonizing the hydrogen-potassium pump. H_2-receptor blockade and H^+/K^+ ATPase inhibition are the only modes of acid inhibition of clinical significance.

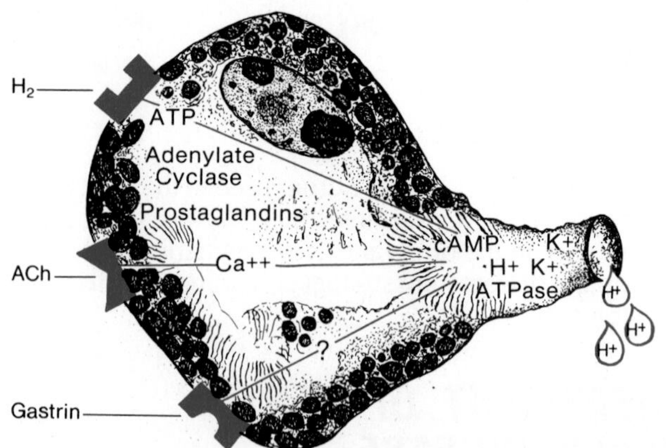

FIGURE 33-2. Diagram of the parietal cell of the gastric mucosa illustrating the three types of membrane receptors and some of the biochemical pathways involved in the secretion of acid into the lumen of the stomach. ACh = acetylcholine receptor; ATPase = adenosine triphosphatase; cAMP = cyclic AMP; H_2 = histamine receptor.

- **Ulcer healing rate is adversely influenced by factors in addition to drugs.**

Impaired healing is associated with:

- Large initial ulcer size
- Smoking
- Continued intake of nonsteroidal anti-inflammatory drugs (NSAIDs)

Accelerated recurrence is associated with:

- *H. pylori* infection
- Smoking
- Gastritis or duodenitis
- Chronic alcohol consumption ± cirrhosis

Regimen for Eradication of *Helicobacter Pylori* Infection

The current regimen for eradication of *H. pylori* infection includes

1. Amoxicillin 500 mg p.o. (orally) three times a day for 14 days (tetracycline in penicillin-allergic patients)
2. Metronidazole 250 mg p.o. three times a day for 14 days
3. Bismuth subsalicylate 300 mg p.o. four times a day for 30 days

All three drugs are given concurrently and attain an eradication rate of over 90%.

Several new regimens are currently being evaluated to increase patient compliance with fewer and less toxic drugs and requiring a shorter course of therapy. The most commonly used alternative regimen at this time is

1. Omeprazole 20 mg p.o. twice a day for 14 days
2. Amoxicillin 500 mg p.o. three times a day for 14 days

This regimen appears to be equally efficacious and better tolerated but is more expensive.

H_2-Receptor Antagonists

ACTIONS. The development of agents that selectively antagonize histamine at the level of its receptor in the parietal cell (H_2 blocker) emphasizes the importance of endogenous histamine in the control of acid secretion. The H_2-receptor blockers produce little interference with any other physiological mechanisms and are a remarkably safe family of drugs. Cimetidine became available in the United States in 1977, and since then more than 10 million patients have been treated with this drug worldwide, making it one of the most widely prescribed drugs in the world.

The chemical structure of H_2-receptor blockers bears some close resemblances to the structure of histamine and H_1 histamine antagonists. Currently there are four H_2-receptor antagonists available on the market for the treatment of peptic ulcer disease: cimetidine, ranitidine, famotidine, and nizatidine. Ranitidine is 10 times more potent than cimetidine, whereas famotidine is 30 times more potent than cimetidine and 8 times more than ranitidine. Nizatidine is similar to ranitidine in potency and dosage. There is no clinically significant difference in efficacy among the H_2 antogonists; they do differ in the frequency of dosing. H_2-antagonists inhibit all aspects of gastric secretion (fasting, nocturnal, postprandial, or pentagastrin).

TIME COURSE OF ACTION. These agents are absorbed rapidly from the GI tract, with peak plasma concentration achieved 45 to 90 minutes after oral administration, with plasma half-lives of approximately 1 to 2 hours. They are eliminated primarily by the kidneys and appear in the urine more than 60% unchanged. Cimetidine, ranitidine, and famotidine are also available in parenteral (IV) formulations.

Although H_2 antagonists suppress all types of acid stimuli, several studies have demonstrated the important role played by nocturnal acid secretion in the pathogenesis of peptic ulcer disease. Figure 33–3 depicts the gastric pH over 24-hour periods in subjects taking placebo or different dosages of cimetidine. These profiles demonstrate that the major deviation from placebo treatment is the acid secretion occurring at night. A single nightly dose of the various H_2 antagonists has been shown to be effective (cimetidine 800 mg; ranitidine 300 mg; famotidine 40 mg). This effectiveness highlights the importance of the suppression of nocturnal acid secretion; moreover, a single nightly dose improves patient compliance over multiple daily doses.

BOX 33–1
THERAPEUTIC USES

Approximately 80% of gastric or duodenal ulcers are healed after 4 to 6 weeks of treatment.

H_2 antagonists are also used in the treatment of hypersecretory syndromes (Zollinger-Ellison syndrome), systemic mastocytosis, basophilic leu-kemia, preoperative prevention of aspiration pneumonia, coadjuvant treatment of pancreatic insufficiency, prevention of stress gastritis, and treatment of reflux esophagitis.

ADVERSE EFFECTS. The H_2 blockers have a good safety record, and the great majority of patients have no side effects. Cimetidine, because it inhibits the drug metabolizing P-450 cytochrome oxidase system of the liver, can induce a prolongation of the action of many drugs that are metabolized by this system. Attention to signs of toxicity and monitoring of serum levels should be obtained when cimetidine is used concomitantly with warfarin, phenytoin, diazepam, chlordiazepoxide, theophylline, and lidocaine. Other H_2 blockers interfere with the P-450 system to varying degrees.

Rare cases of thrombocytopenia, hepatitis, and bone marrow suppression have been described. Cimetidine, but not the others, can cause antiandrogen effects of impotence and gynecomastia. Changes in mental status characterized by confusion, disorientation, and coma have been described in patients using high dosages of the parenteral form of cimetidine, usually in intensive care patients with liver and renal failure or in the elderly. These symptoms usually subside upon discontinuation of drug administration.

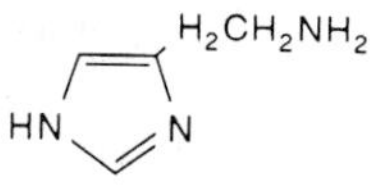

Histamine

Histamine H_2 receptors uniquely blocked by cimetidine and analogs

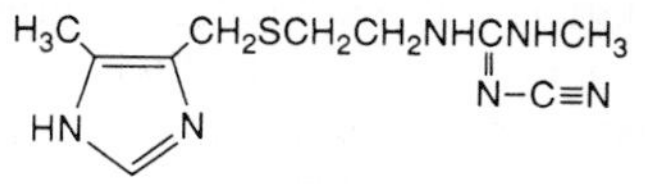

Cimetidine (TAGAMET)

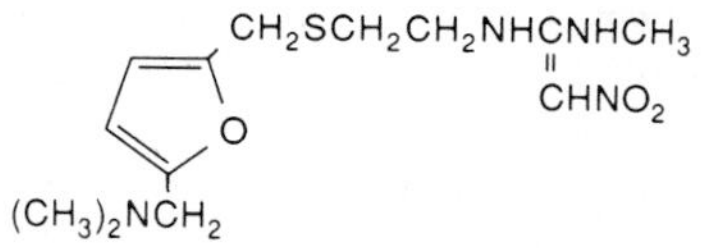

Ranitidine (ZANTAC)

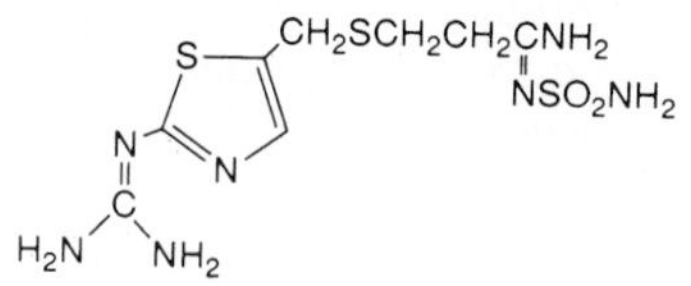

Famotidine (PEPCID)

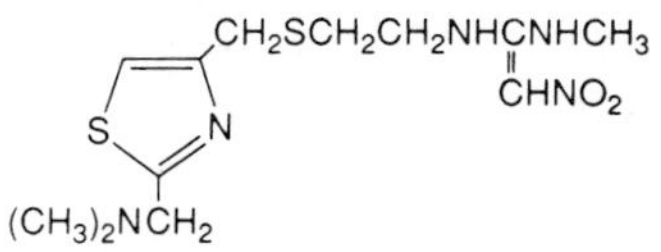

Nizatidine (AXID)

Sucralfate

ACTIONS. Sucralfate (CARAFATE) is a basic aluminum salt of sucrose substituted with eight sulfate groups. In an acid environment some of the $Al_2(OH)_5$ ions dissociate, forming a polymer, sucrose octosulfate. This polymeric viscous substance is thought to adhere to denatured proteins in the base of the ulcer. A barrier is thus formed protecting the ulcer from further aggression by pepsin and HCl. Sucralfate has six to seven times greater affinity for the ulcerated mucosa than for normal mucosa. In addition to this barrier coating of the ulcer base, sucralfate appears to protect cells from damage, that is, has "cytoprotective" properties.

The use of sucralfate is associated also with increased production in the gastric mucosa of prostaglandins, bicarbonate, and increased thickening of the mucus covering the gastric epithelium.

> **BOX 33-2**
> **THERAPEUTIC USES**
>
> Numerous studies have demonstrated that sucralfate is superior to placebo and is as effective as H_2 antagonists in the treatment of peptic ulcer disease.

TIME COURSE AND ADVERSE EFFECTS. Sucralfate is not absorbed by the GI tract, and side effects such as constipation occur in less than 5% of the patients treated. As might be expected, it decreases absorption of some drugs, namely phenytoin and ciprofloxacin. The large size of the pills and the dosage frequency of four times a day make it less appealing to patients and increase noncompliance.

Inhibitors of H^+/K^+ ATPase (Omeprazole)

ACTIONS. Omeprazole (PRILOSEC), a substituted benzimidazole, represents a new approach for the control of

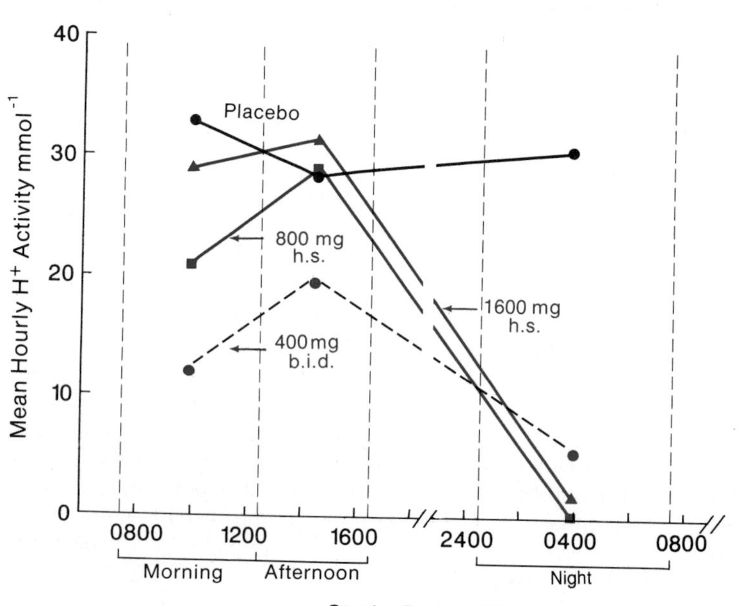

FIGURE 33-3. Temporal pattern of the acid secretion as modified by different regimens and dosages of the histamine receptor (H_2) blocker, cimetidine. Ordinate is the mean hydrogen ion secretion per hour. The abscissa is time plotted as a 24-hour clock divided into the periods over which the acid secretion was measured: morning from 0730 to 1230; afternoon from 1230 to 1630; night from 0030 to 1730. In the placebo condition (*black circles*), acid secretion was high during all three periods. Cimetidine given twice a day (400 mg b.i.d. [*colored circles*]) reduced acid production at all three time periods. Administration of single daily doses of cimetidine at bedtime (800 mg and 1600 mg h.s. [*colored squares and colored triangles, respectively*]) was effective in reducing nocturnal acid secretion to almost zero. Total acid secretion over 24 hours was approximately the same for all three of the cimetidine dosage regimens.

gastric acid secretion. This compound irreversibly inactivates the enzyme H^+/K^+ ATPase (the proton pump) in the secretory membrane of the parietal cell, which represents the final step in the secretion of hydrogen ion (Fig. 33-1).

ADVERSE EFFECTS. Omeprazole is not approved by the FDA for long-term treatment of peptic ulcers, although it has few adverse effects. It has been reported to inhibit some hepatic P-450 enzymes, to decrease the absorption of digoxin, to increase disulfiram toxicity, and to be associated with painful nocturnal erections and gynecomastia. In rats at doses of 100 times those given to humans, gastrinomas have been reported with prolonged use. This has not been found to happen in humans despite some patients being on therapeutic doses of omeprazole for over a decade.

> BOX 33-3
> **THERAPEUTIC USE**
>
> A single dose of omeprazole (the first substituted benzimidazole to undergo clinical trials) can suppress the production of gastric HCl for 24 to 48 hours. It has the greatest efficacy in suppressing acid secretions of all available medications. Already this drug has found extensive use in the treatment of hypersecretory states and gastroesophageal reflux disease.

Prostaglandins of the E Class (Misoprostol)

> BOX 33-4
> **THERAPEUTIC USES**
>
> Prostaglandin derivatives have been found to be especially useful in the treatment of small erosions in the upper GI tract produced by aspirin and other NSAIDs inasmuch as prostaglandin deficiency appears to be an important pathophysiological factor in their development. Their clinical efficacy for treatment of large, symptomatic ulcers is yet to be established.

ACTIONS. Several derivatives of naturally occurring prostaglandins have been developed for the treatment of peptic ulcer disease (misoprostol [CYTOTEC]). Prostaglandins are derived from the metabolism of arachidonic acid catalyzed by the enzyme cyclooxygenase (see Chapter 15). In addition to effects on many organs, they act on gastric mucosa to inhibit production of acid and also possess a cytoprotective action. For example, PGE_2 has been shown to be as effective as the H_2 antagonists in the treatment of ulcer disease.

Antacids

ADVERSE EFFECTS. Abdominal cramping and diarrhea are fairly common at therapeutic doses.

Antacids are only of historical importance in the treatment of peptic ulcer disease. They are currently not used for the treatment of ulcer disease because of the high frequency of dosing that is required to neutralize acid (Fig. 33-4). They also have only limited use in neutralizing nocturnal acid because of their dosing requirements. Calcium-containing antacids may be associated with rebound gastric hypersecretion, resulting in the stimulation of gastrin-producing cells.

Antacids are still the most commonly used medication for dyspepsia, as most of them are available over the counter. Current indications for use of antacids include the use of aluminium-containing antacids in renal failure to bind calcium and as adjuvants to pancreatic supplements in treatment of pancreatic insufficiency.

Aluminum-containing antacids cause constipation, whereas magnesium-containing antacids cause diarrhea at higher doses.

Anticholinergics

Anticholinergics have been used in the past for the treatment of gastric and duodenal ulcers (acid suppression by competitive antagonism of acetylcholine receptors), but their side effect profile has made them obsolete in the treatment of peptic ulcer disease.

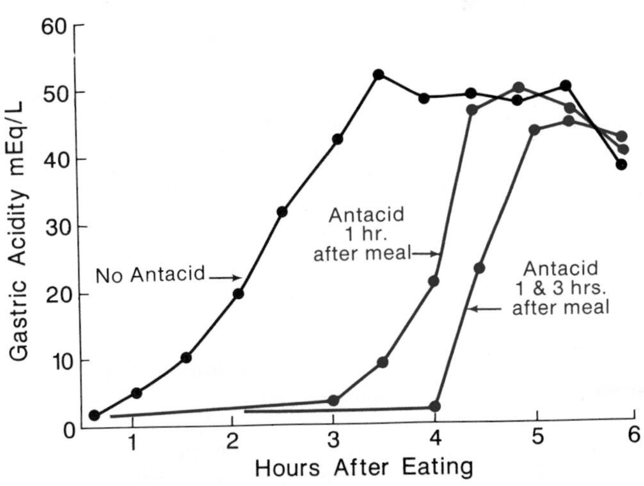

FIGURE 33-4. Effect of timing in relation to a meal of antacid administration on gastric acidity. Ordinate is gastric acidity expressed as milliequivalents per liter. The abscissa is hours after eating a meal. The *curve in black* on the left shows results that were obtained with no antacid, showing a maximal acid secretion within 3 hours following eating. Administration of antacid 1 hour after eating results (*curve in color, on left*) in a delay in the appearance of acid for more than 2 hours, with a peak after 4 hours. Administration of antacid at both 1 and 3 hours (*curve in color, on right*) further delays and reduces acid secretion.

GASTROESOPHAGEAL REFLUX DISEASE (GERD)

The drugs used in the treatment of reflux esophagitis, and which are the most effective clinically, are those that decrease acid secretion or increase gastric emptying, that is, agents that decrease the exposure of the esophagus to the acid gastric contents (bottom two lines in Table 33–2). Practically speaking, the drugs most likely to be used, in order, are the H_2 antagonists, omeprazole, and metoclopramide (discussed below). Omeprazole is the drug of choice because of its superior efficacy, clinical response, and long-term safety profile.

Like ulcer disease, cigarette smoking is a serious risk factor; smoking is associated with functional decrease in the tone of lower esophageal sphincter, thus allowing reflux of gastric contents. Esophageal sphincter tone is also decreased by alcohol, caffeine, chocolate, and mint.

THERAPY FOR CHRONIC PANCREATITIS (PANCREATIC ENZYME SUPPLEMENTS)

Patients with chronic pancreatitis seek medical attention because of abdominal pain or maldigestion (diarrhea, steatorrhea, weight loss). Steatorrhea occurs when the output of pancreatic lipase drops to less than 10% of normal.

The pain of chronic pancreatitis can be at least decreased by pancreatic supplements (however, they are less effective in alcohol-related chronic pancreatitis); the pain reduction appears to be a function of the serine proteases (trypsin, chymotrypsin, elastase) that are released in the duodenum.

Steatorrhea is treated by oral administration of a pancreatic supplement. The critical factor in such treatment is the lipase activity of the pancreatic supplement. Pancreatic lipase is irreversibly inactivated at (gastric) pH < 4.

TABLE 33–2. Strategies for the Treatment of Reflux Esophagitis (GERD)

Mechanisms	Examples
↑ Esophageal acid clearance	Metoclopramide
Mucosal protection	Sucralfate
Neutralize acid	Antacids
↑ Lower esophageal sphincter (LES) tone	Bethanechol, metoclopramide
↓ Acid secretion	H_2 antagonists, omeprazole
↑ Gastric emptying	Metoclopramide, cisapride

BOX 33–5
TREATMENT OF CHRONIC PANCREATITIS

A pancreatic supplement is administered before meals or with meals and at bedtime if nocturnal pain is present. Patients have to be educated about the need for probable lifelong therapy and the necessity of taking a large number of pills, sometimes as many as 16 to 20 a day. 30,000 IU of lipase is required to prevent steatorrhea, and the goal of therapy should be prevention of steatorrhea and weight gain. All pancreatic supplements contain different proportions of lipase, protease, and amylase but are dosed for the lipase content.

- Viokase: eight capsules each time
- Cotazym: six capsules
- Pancrease: three capsules
- Creon: three capsules

If the response is inadequate, sodium bicarbonate or H_2 blocker can be added to increase gastric pH. The dose of sodium bicarbonate is 650 mg before and after meals (± 1300 mg at bedtime).

THERAPY FOR INFLAMMATORY BOWEL DISEASE

A variety of drugs are used to treat patients with inflammatory bowel disease (IBD) (Table 33–3).

The inflammatory cascade of arachidonic acid metabolism begins with the phospholipase-mediated production of

TABLE 33–3. Drug Therapies for Inflammatory Bowel Disease

Symptomatic Therapy
Antidiarrheal
Antispasmodic
Cholestyramine
5-ASA Compounds
Sulfasalazine
Olsalazine
Oral 5-ASA (mesalamine)
Topical 5-ASA and 4-ASA
Corticoids
Oral corticosteroids
Parenteral corticosteroids
Parenteral ACTH
Topical steroids
Immunosuppressives
Azathioprine
6-Mercaptopurine
Cyclosporine
Antibiotics
Metronidazole

ACTH = adrenocorticotropic hormone; ASA = aminosalicylic acid.

arachidonic acid from the phospholipids present in cell membranes. Arachidonic acid is further metabolized to prostaglandins by cyclooxygenase and to leukotrienes by 5-lipoxygenase. Although prostaglandins do not seem to be mediators of tissue injury in IBD (and may even conceivably be protective to the mucosa), the leukotrienes, especially LTB4, probably are mediators of tissue injury. Steroids act to inhibit phospholipase-mediated arachidonic acid release. On the other hand, NSAIDs may exacerbate IBD by shifting arachidonic acid metabolism from prostaglandins to leukotrienes.

Sulfasalazine

ACTIONS. The sulfasalazine molecule is composed of 5-aminosalicylic acid (5-ASA) linked by an azo bond to sulfapyridine. The mechanism of action of sulfasalazine is not clear but inhibition of lipoxygenase is thought to be important.

BOX 33–6
THERAPEUTIC USES

- Ulcerative proctocolitis
  Mild to moderate disease
  For maintenance of remission
- Crohn's disease
  Mild to moderate active disease (colitis > ileitis)
  Maintenance of remission or prevention of postoperative recurrence (unproven)

ADVERSE EFFECTS. Most side effects are due to the sulfapyridine moiety.

- Common side effects: dyspepsia, nausea, anorexia, headache
- Allergic reactions: rash, fever, arthralgia
- Hematological effects:
  Mild: hemolysis, neutropenia, folate deficiency
  Severe: hemolysis, agranulocytosis
- Male infertility (reversible)
- Severe toxic reactions: lung, liver, pancreas, skin, nerve

Sulfasalazine Analogs

Circulating sulfapyridine is responsible for most of the toxicity of sulfasalazine. The development of new sulfasalazine analogs is based upon efforts to deliver 5-ASA to the lower GI tract without using the toxic moiety. Suspensions and suppositories of 5-ASA and 4-ASA have been prepared for direct rectal instillation. Oral preparations include enteric-coated delayed release forms of 5-ASA (mesalamine), or a dimer of 5-ASA (olsalazine) that is split by intestinal bacterial azoreductases into two presumably therapeutic molecules of 5-ASA.

Systemic Corticoids

Oral

These agents are indicated in moderate to severe ulcerative colitis or Crohn's disease; the preparations used are prednisone and prednisolone (see Chapter 55).

Parenteral

Parenteral administration is indicated in severe or toxic ulcerative colitis or Crohn's disease; the preparations used are hydrocortisone and adrenocorticotropic hormone (ACTH) (see Chapter 55). Newer corticoids that have more local effects and fewer systemic actions are under evaluation.

Immunosuppressives—Azathioprine and 6-Mercaptopurine

ACTIONS. The use of immunosuppressive drugs is limited to severe forms of IBD where they can help to avoid the use of steroids (see Chapter 45). The rationale involves decreasing T-cell activity.

In Crohn's disease they are used for steroid sparing, and for fistulae, perineal disease, refractory disease, and maintenance of remission.

Azathioprine and 6-mercaptopurine have been used for refractory Crohn's disease and rarely in ulcerative colitis. Cyclosporine is currently being used for acute exacerbations of ulcerative colitis that are not responsive to steroids in a parenteral form; how it is best used in Crohn's disease is unclear at this time. In view of the potential for severe adverse effects, these agents should be used only by experienced gastroenterologists.

Adverse effects are many and include fever, rash, hepatitis, pancreatitis, bone marrow suppression, and possible teratogenic and carcinogenic effects.

ANTIEMETICS

Nausea and vomiting consist of a complex pattern of sensory and motor events coordinated by the central nervous system involving GI smooth muscle and skeletal muscle, as well as respiratory, cardiovascular, GI secretory, and other systems. Antiemetic drugs act at multiple sites to inhibit vomiting.

Antimuscarinic Drugs

Scopolamine, and histamine H_1 antagonists with prominent antimuscarinic properties, such as diphenhydramine, can be effective antiemetics, especially in postoperative patients. Scopolamine is often used in the prevention of motion sickness. The muscarinic receptor antagonists may produce their antiemetic effects primarily by actions in the vestibular system, including effects on cholinergic (and possibly histaminergic) fibers projecting to the vomiting center (see Chapter 8).

Cannabis

Cannabinoids, including delta[9]-tetrahydrocannabinol (dronabinol; MARINOL) and synthetic congeners, appear to act on the cerebral cortex, the chemoreceptor trigger zone (CTZ), and the vomiting center to reduce emesis. Cannabinoids are particularly useful for the control of chemotherapy-induced emesis.

Dopamine and Serotonin Antagonists

Dopamine receptor antagonists, including phenothiazines such as prochlorperazine and benzamides such as metoclopramide, block proemetic dopamine receptors in the CTZ and in the vomiting center to inhibit emesis.

5-Hydroxytryptamine (5-HT_3) antagonists, including *ondansetron* (ZOFRAN) and *granisetron* (KYTRIL) possess striking antiemetic activity. These drugs are thought to act primarily at the peripheral terminals of vagal afferent neurons to block 5-HT_3 receptors that are involved in afferent signaling of emetic stimuli (see Chapter 13). Certain proemetic drugs, such as cisplatin, may release 5-HT in the vicinity of vagal afferent peripheral terminals. 5-HT_4 agonists, including *cisapride*, may produce their modest antiemetic effects by enhancing gastric emptying due to their gastric prokinetic properties.

Prokinetic Drugs

Prokinetic drugs can improve GI propulsion and increase gastric emptying. The improved GI propulsion results from increased esophageal clearance, gastric emptying, rate of transit in the proximal intestine, rate of transit in distal small intestine, and the rate of transit in colon. The agents can, in some instances, relieve nausea and vomiting.

The increased gastric emptying results from improved antroduodenal coordination and peristalsis. *Motilin* and the motilin agonist, *erythromycin*, act in the proximal portions of motor pathways to initiate a preprogrammed pattern of coordinated propulsive contractions. *Cisapride* stimulates coordinating neurons in the excitatory motor pathway. The dopamine antagonists *metoclopramide* and *domperidone* block inhibitory dopamine receptors on cholinergic motor neurons and consequently increase the amount of acetylcholine released from the nerve terminals. The various prokinetic drugs are compared in Table 33–4.

TREATMENT OF DIARRHEA

(Tables 33–5 and 33–6)

Therapeutic Options

The intestine is an efficient organ for absorption of water and electrolytes in that 98% or more of that ingested is absorbed. The usual net balance is such that approximately 1.8 L per day is absorbed. If the efficiency of absorption is compromised in any way, the result is a stool output that exceeds 200 mL, and diarrhea will occur.

Specific: eliminate cause

- Cure underlying disease (*eg*, enteric infection)
- Correct pathophysiology (*eg*, oral replacement with glucose/saline in cholera)

Nonspecific: decrease net fluid secretion

- Effect on epithelial transport
  Decrease secretion (*eg*, somatostatin)
  Increase absorption (*eg*, short chain fatty acids)
- Effect on motility
  Decrease propulsive contractions (*eg*, opioids)
  Increase mixing contractions (*eg*, opioids)

Most of the acute infectious diarrheas do not require specific therapy because they are usually self-limited. The general approach should be prevention and treatment of dehydration (patients should be on a low-fiber diet, avoiding salads, fruits, and milk products); nonspecific and antimicrobial treatment may be occasionally necessary because of the severe symptoms.

Bismuth Subsalicylate

Bismuth compounds are frequently used (*eg*, PEPTO-BISMOL) for the prevention and treatment of traveler's diarrhea sec-

TABLE 33–4. Comparison of Prokinetic Drugs

Activity	Metoclopramide	Domperidone	Cisapride	Erythromycin
5-HT_3 antagonist	Yes	Yes	Weak	No
5-HT_4 agonist	No	No	Yes	No
Motilin receptor agonist	No	No	No	Yes
Blocked by muscarinic antagonists	Yes	Yes	Yes	Partial
Cross blood-brain barrier	Yes	No	No	No
Antiemetic effect	+++	++	±	±
Prokinetic effect				
Proximal gut	+++	+++	+++	+++
Distal gut	±	±	++	+++
Side effects	Many	Some	Few	Few

Adapted from Burks TF, Goyal RK: Gastrointestinal Pharmacology, AGA-UTPUNIT #24. In The Undergraduate Teaching Project in Gastroenterology and Liver Disease. Distributed by Milner-Fenwick, Inc., 1991.

TABLE 33–5. Antidiarrheal Drug Mechanisms

Drugs	Inhibit Propulsive Contractions	Stimulate Nonpropulsive Contractions	Decrease Fluid Secretion	Enhance Fluid Absorption	Bind Luminal Secretagogues
Opioids	+++	+++	+++	probably	
Alpha$_2$-adrenergic agonists			+++		
Anticholinergics	+++		++		
Somatostatin	+		+++	+	
Bismuth subsalicylate					+++
Cholestyramine					+++

Plus signs indicate presence and relative prominence of the effect.

ondary to *Escherichia coli*. Bismuth subsalicylate (the active ingredient in PEPTO-BISMOL) appears to inhibit the effects of the *E. coli* toxin in the gut in addition to a possible direct antibacterial effect.

Inert Compounds

Kaolin (hydrated aluminum silicate) is claimed to absorb water and toxins and decrease the amount of free water in the GI tract and, therefore, reduce the number of stools in a diarrheal state. Other aluminum salts such as aluminum hydroxide (AMPHOJEL) are known to have a constipating effect directly related to the aluminum component. Other products derived from plants and their fruits include polygalacturonic acid and pectins. These products are not absorbed in the small bowel but are degraded by the colonic bacteria, producing short-chain fatty acids. These short-chain fatty acids (propionate, acetic, and butyrate) facilitate the absorption of sodium and water from the colon. KAOPECTATE (kaolin plus pectin) is a common over-the-counter preparation used in diarrheal illnesses; however, studies definitively documenting its efficacy are lacking.

Opioids

ACTIONS. Opioid drugs act at secretomotor neurons of the submucosal plexus to inhibit secretion into the lumen of the intestine. The overall result of opioid action is to increase net absorption of fluid and electrolytes from the lumen by decreasing secretory stimuli directed at crypt cells. Opioids also induce segmenting contractions that retard propulsion. Opioids act both in the central nervous system and in the enteric nervous system to produce antidiarrheal effects (Tables 33–5 and 33–6).

TABLE 33–6. Opioids Act on CNS and Enteric Nerves

Drug	CNS	Enteric Nerves
Morphine	+++	+++
Codeine	+++	+++
Diphenoxylate	+	+++
Loperamide	0 (does not cross blood-brain barrier)	+++

CNS = central nervous system.

Clonidine

ACTIONS. Clonidine acts at α_2-adrenergic receptors to cause a decrease in GI secretion and to increase absorption. In diabetic autonomic neuropathy, adrenergic nerves may be damaged or absent; these nerves ordinarily release norepinephrine, resulting in an inhibition of the release of vasoactive intestinal peptide (VIP) and acetylcholine by actions at presynaptic α_2 receptors. Clonidine can be especially effective in altering diarrhea in this condition.

Somatostatin

ACTIONS. Somatostatin has several sites of antidiarrheal action. Structural analogs of native somatostatin (*eg*, OCTREOTIDE) have been found that are more potent and metabolically stable.

TABLE 33–7. Laxatives

	Action	Time
1. BULKING AGENTS	Softening/ bulking	1–3 days
Bran		
Methylcellulose		
Psyllium—METAMUCIL		
Wheat husk		
2. OSMOTIC AGENTS	Watery evacuation	1–3 hours
Lactulose		
Magnesium sulphate—EPSOM SALT		
Magnesium citrate		
Magnesium hydroxide/ carbonate—MAALOX		
Phosphates—FLEET'S PHOSPHASODA		
Polyethylene glycol solutions—COLYTE or GOLYTELY		
3. IRRITANTS	Soft/semifluid	6–8 hours
Anthraquinoid derivatives		
Senna		
Diphenylmethane derivatives		
Phenolphthalein		
Bisacodyl		
Miscellaneous		
Glycerol		
Castor oil		
Bile salts		
4. STOOL SOFTENERS	Softening	
Docusate sodium—COLACE		

LAXATIVES

Rarely in medicine is there an absolute indication for the use of laxatives. A high-fiber, well-balanced diet rich in fruits and vegetables supplemented by bran should be enough to normalize bowel function in otherwise healthy individuals. The fear of autointoxication and the constant concern of many patients regarding the frequency and quality of bowel movements make laxatives one of the most popular over-the-counter drugs on the market; this excessive use presents a serious potential for user abuse.

Accepted indications for laxatives and stool softeners include preparation for diagnostic colonic examination (barium enema, colonoscopy); treatment of anorectal disorders (anal fissures, hemorrhoids); and prevention of hepatic encephalopathy. Laxatives can be divided into bulk, osmotic, and irritant (or stimulant) classes (Table 33–7).

Bulk Laxatives

Bulk laxatives, such as the derivatives of psyllium seeds (*eg*, METAMUCIL, KONSYL), natural bran, semisynthetic cellulose, or gum, are substances poorly absorbed through the GI tract, thus causing a retention of water in the lumen, increasing the volume and decreasing the consistency of the fecal bolus. If clinically required, these are the drugs of choice for the treatment of chronic constipation.

Irritant Laxatives

The mechanism of action of the so-called "irritant" laxatives' action involves an interference with normal function of the small bowel and colon, usually reversing the primary absorptive function into a secretory function.

TABLE 33–8. Principal Alterations of Hepatic Morphology Produced by Some Commonly Used Drugs and Chemicals*

Principal Morphologic Change	Class of Agent	Example
Cholestasis	Anabolic steroid	Methyl testosterone†
	Antithyroid	Methimazole
	Antibiotic	Erythromycin estolate, nitrofurantoin
	Oral contraceptive	Norethynodrel with mestranol
	Oral hypoglycemic	Chlorpropamide
	Tranquilizer	Chlorpromazine†
	Oncotherapeutic	Anabolic steroids, busulfan, tamoxifen
	Immunosuppressive	Cyclosporine
	Anticonvulsant	Carbamazepine
	Calcium-channel blocker	Nifedipine, verapamil
Fatty liver	Antibiotic	Tetracycline
	Anticonvulsant	Sodium valproate
	Antiarrhythmic	Amiodarone
	Oncotherapeutic	Asparaginase, methotrexate
Hepatitis	Anesthetic	Halothane‡
	Anticonvulsant	Phenytoin, carbamazepine
	Antihypertensive	Methyldopa,‡ captopril, enalapril
	Antibiotic	Isoniazid,‡ rifampicin, nitrofurantoin
	Diuretic	Chlorothiazide
	Laxative	Oxyphenisatin‡
	Antidepressant	Iproniazid, amitriptyline, imipramine
	Anti-inflammatory	Ibuprofen, indomethacin
	Antifungal	Ketoconazole, fluconazole
	Antiviral	Zidovudine, dideoxyinosine
	Calcium-channel blocker	Nifedipine, verapamil, diltiazem
Mixed hepatitis/cholestatic	Immunosuppressive	Azathioprine
	Lipid-lowering	Nicotinic acid, lovastatin
Toxic (necrosis)	Hydrocarbon	Carbon tetrachloride
	Metal	Yellow phosphorus
	Mushroom	*Amanita phalloides*
	Analgesic	Acetaminophen
	Solvent	Dimethylformamide
Granulomas	Anti-inflammatory	Phenylbutazone
	Antibiotic	Sulfonamides
	Xanthine oxidase inhibitor	Allopurinol
	Antiarrhythmic	Quinidine
	Anticonvulsant	Carbamazepine

Adapted from Zakim D, Boyer TD (eds): Hepatology: A Textbook of Liver Disease. Philadelphia: WB Saunders Co, 1990.
*Several agents cause more than one type of liver lesion and appear under more than one category.
†Rarely associated with primary biliary cirrhosislike lesion.
‡Occasionally associated with chronic active hepatitis or bridging hepatic necrosis or cirrhosis.

Castor Oil

Castor oil's active moiety is ricinoleic acid (a hydroxy fatty acid) that evokes the secretion of water and electrolytes in the colon and small bowel. It also increases small bowel peristaltic activity. Castor oil is commonly used for preparation of patients to undergo diagnostic colonic examination such as barium enema and colonoscopy.

Bile Salts

Bile salts in general have laxative properties, although they are not commercially available as such. One of the major side effects of the use of chenodeoxycholic acid used for the dissolution of cholesterol gallstones is diarrhea. The diarrhea is due to the following mechanisms. Unconjugated bile salts:

- Induce active electrolyte secretion, stimulating adenylate cyclase activities, and increase intestinal cyclic AMP
- Increase intestinal motility
- Increase intestinal permeability

In the colon, unconjugated bile acid reduces absorptive capacity and induces water and electrolyte secretion.

Bisacodyl

Bisacodyl, the active ingredient of DULCOLAX, is an effective laxative. It has a unique mode of action that includes decreased water and glucose absorption in the colon and small bowel, and a stimulatory effect on small bowel peristalsis.

Phenolphthalein

Structurally similar to bisacodyl, phenolphthalein is present in a variety of commonly available laxatives. Its mode of action also involves the interference with absorption at different levels of the GI tract. It also increases intestinal motility.

As indicated earlier, none of the irritant laxatives has absolute indications in medicine. Moreover, chronic use may be responsible for colonic atonia and inability to have spontaneous bowel movements ("cathartic colon").

Cathartic Solutions (Osmotic Laxatives)

The mode of action of these agents is based on the increase in stool osmolarity; water trapped in the stool results in reduced consistency. A combination of polyethylene glycol and electrolytes (COLYTE OR GOLYTELY) is used now for the preparation for diagnostic procedures of the colon (barium enema or endoscopy). The advantage of colonic lavage is that instead of 2 days of clear liquids and administration of castor oil or bisacodyl, patients ingest 1 gallon of the solution a few hours before the procedure.

Mineral Oil

Mineral oil, a mixture of aliphatic hydrocarbons derived from petroleum, has been used extensively as an over-the-counter preparation, most commonly in children. After 2–3 days, the stools soften, and colonic absorption of water is decreased. It also interferes with the absorption of fat-soluble vitamins, and its administration presents the risk of aspiration.

TABLE 33–9. Drugs Associated with Acute Pancreatitis

Azathioprine	Estrogens
Thiazide diuretics	Valproic acid
Furosemide	Chlorthalidone
Ethacrynic acid	Phenphormin
Pentamidine	Methyldopa
Sulfonamides	L-Asparaginase
Tetracycline	Furadantin
Procainamide	6-Mercaptopurine
Calcium	

Stool Softeners

DOCUSATE SODIUM. This is not a true laxative but is a surface-active agent that keeps stool soft. It is useful in constipation secondary to hard stools or in painful anorectal conditions. Glycerol is also used as a stool softener.

GASTROINTESTINAL SIDE EFFECTS OF MEDICATIONS

Gastrointestinal manifestations are among the most common side effects of all medications used, with nausea, vomiting, and diarrhea being the most common of these. Drug-induced hepatotoxicity and pancreatitis warrant brief mention, although an in-depth discussion of these is beyond the scope of this chapter (see also Chapter 50).

Drug-induced hepatoxicity most commonly presents as a hepatitislike picture or a cholestatic picture. A short list of drugs causing various types of hepatotoxicities is listed in Table 33–8. Whenever hepatotoxicity is suspected, the medication must be promptly discontinued. Liver function abnormalities may take weeks to months to resolve and need close monitoring.

A list of medications commonly associated with pancreatitis as a side effect appears in Table 33–9. The exact pathophysiology of medication-induced pancreatitis is unclear at this time.

REFERENCES

Ciaran PK, Charalabos P, LaMont JT: *Clostridium difficile* colitis [Review]. N Engl J Med 330:257–262, 1994.

Fennerty MB: *Helicobacter pylori* [Review]. Arch Intern Med 154:721–727, 1994.

Hixson LJ, Kelley CL, Jones WN, Tuohy CD: Current trends in the pharmacotherapy for peptic ulcer disease. Arch Intern Med 152:726–732, 1992.

Holt S: Chronic pancreatitis [Review]. South Med J 86:201–207, 1993.

Lee WM: Drug-induced hepatoxicity [Review]. Aliment Pharmacol Ther 7:477–485, 1993.

Marshall JB: Chronic constipation in adults. How far should evaluation and treatment go? Postgrad Med 88:49–51, 1991.

Peterson WL: *Helicobacter pylori* and peptic ulcer disease. N Engl J Med 324:1043–1048, 1991.

Podolsky DK: Inflammatory bowel disease [Review]. N Engl J Med 325:1008–1016, 1991.

Soll AH: Pathogenesis of peptic ulcer and implications for therapy. N Engl J Med 322:909–916, 1990.

Yamada T, Alpers DH, Owyang C, et al (eds): Textbook of Gastroenterology. Philadelphia: JB Lippincott Co, 1995. [The single best reference source.]

34 Drug Acting on the Blood and Blood-Forming Organs

Richard E. Bettigole

MEDICATIONS USED TO TREAT ANEMIA

Anemia is defined as a hemoglobin level or hematocrit (packed red cell volume) more than two standard deviations below the mean for healthy individuals the same age and sex as the patient. By this definition, assuming a normal distribution, 2.5% of healthy individuals are anemic (and 2.5% are polycythemic).

Mechanisms of Anemia

Anemia almost always results from blood loss, decreased red cell production, decreased red cell survival, or some combination of these. Expansion of the blood volume (intravascular volume) can cause the hemoglobin to fall. This occurs normally in pregnant women, without any change in red cell mass. Rarely, it may be seen in young children with sickle cell anemia whose spleens enlarge rapidly in what is called a sequestration crisis. Average red cell survival is about 120 days in healthy people.

Red cells are produced in bone marrow. An otherwise healthy person's response to chronic tissue hypoxia is to increase the production of erythropoietin by the kidneys. This glycoprotein stimulates stem cells in the bone marrow to differentiate into red cell precursors, which as they divide and mature eventually extrude their nuclei, leave the bone marrow, and enter the blood circulation.

There also is a stimulus to red cell production simply as a result of increased red cell destruction or even chronic blood loss without anemia or oxygen lack in the tissues of the body. The physiological mechanism for this is unknown. For example, a nonhypoxemic person with a compensated hemolytic anemia (normal hemoglobin and hematocrit, increased red cell production, and increased red cell destruction) clearly has increased erythropoiesis but no tissue hypoxia. Similarly, a healthy person who donates blood frequently but whose iron stores are maintained will have reticulocytosis without anemia.

Iron

Iron has been used for the treatment of anemia for over 2000 years. It is an essential component not only of hemoglobin but also of myoglobin and of several essential enzymes. However, even severe iron deficiency does not seem to show itself clinically except as anemia.

Total body iron in adults is 3 – 5 g, of which 0.5 g or less is in myoglobin and iron-containing enzymes. Depending on the blood volume and the hematocrit, about 1.5 – 3 g of iron exist as hemoglobin in red cells. Iron stores average about 0.5 – 1.5 g. Iron deficiency causes a hypochromic, microcytic anemia with a mean red cell volume (MCV) usually well below normal, and increased variation in the size of red cells.

Humans have no known excretory system for iron. Healthy people average about 0.5 mg iron/mL blood. Blood loss is the main cause of iron deficiency in older children and adults. Menstruating women lose, and therefore require an average of about 1 – 2 mg iron daily, whereas men and nonmenstruating women need only half that amount. The amount of menstrual blood loss varies widely, however, even in women who consider their menstrual cycles entirely normal. Absent iron stores and anemia due to iron deficiency are rather frequent among menstruating women. A full-term infant has about 1g of iron, obtained from its mother during gestation.

In infancy and childhood when body growth is rapid, the need to fill the expanding blood volume can easily lead to iron deficiency despite the absence of blood loss unless foods other than milk are started in a timely fashion. In adults, nutritional iron deficiency is virtually never seen. It cannot be stressed too often that in adults iron deficiency anemia is not a disease; it is a sign of blood loss.

Iron-containing compounds are useful in the treatment of anemia due to iron deficiency and as a dietary supplement for pregnant women.

ABSORPTION. Adults with normal iron stores absorb over one third of ingested heme iron, compared with only about one twentieth or less of nonheme iron. Vitamin C and meat increase the absorption of nonheme iron. Thus, diets vary in the bioavailability of iron. With increasing iron stores, the absorption of dietary iron is increasingly inhibited.

IRON TRANSPORT. Absorbed ferrous iron is bound to transferrin, a plasma protein produced by the liver. Transferrin is measured by its ability to bind iron and is reported as total iron-binding capacity (TIBC). Iron deficiency in otherwise healthy individuals leads to a fall in serum iron and a rise in transferrin (TIBC), so that the percent of plasma iron saturation, which normally is about 30–35%, falls to less than 13% in iron deficiency. (In acute and chronic illnesses, because both serum iron *and* TIBC fall, despite the low serum iron the percent iron saturation usually exceeds 13%.)

Iron from transferrin is used either in heme synthesis (one atom of iron in each heme group, four of which, combined with four globin chains, form a tetramer that is the hemoglobin molecule) or is stored in the reticuloendothelial system, hepatocytes, or elsewhere as single molecules of the protein ferritin or as microscopically visible aggregates of ferritin called hemosiderin.

Over 80% of the iron used for red cell formation normally comes from heme iron derived from the roughly 1% of those red cells that, having lived out their life span, are destroyed daily. Much of the rest comes from transferrin-bound, newly absorbed dietary iron. Iron stores normally lie relatively undisturbed unless there is iron deficiency. The rate of clearance of iron from plasma is increased in iron deficiency and decreased when iron stores are ample.

In iron deficiency, serum ferritin levels are low; in iron overload, levels are quite high. However, serum ferritin is a reactive protein (like fibrinogen, haptoglobin, and Factor VIII) and tends to rise with acute or chronic illness; therefore, although a low serum level of ferritin is good evidence of iron deficiency, a normal level does not rule it out.

Iron deficiency is present in millions of people all over the world. Even in prosperous nations with good nutrition and medical care, many infants and many women in the years between menarche and menopause are iron-deficient. Iron deficiency always should be suspected when there is microcytosis (small red cells), even without overt anemia. The other common causes of microcytosis are the thalassemia syndromes. Even with an obvious possible cause of iron deficiency such as excessive menstrual blood loss, gastrointestinal blood loss may also be a factor. One possible cause of iron deficiency does not relieve one of the responsibility to search for other causes.

Iron Preparations

ORAL. Ferrous salts are better absorbed than ferric salts. Ferrous sulfate has about the same bioavailability as other ferrous compounds when calculated as milligrams of iron. The usual therapeutic dose is 2–3 mg/kg of iron. For ferrous sulfate ($FeSO_4 \cdot 7H_2O$), iron is about 20% by weight, so for a 50-kg woman the $FeSO_4$ dose would be $50 \times 5 \times 2$ to $50 \times 5 \times 3 = 500$ to 750 mg/day. In actual practice 300 mg three times a day (900 mg) is a widely used dose regardless of the adult patient's size. Dosage probably should be adjusted more often for the weight of adult patients, as of course it always must be for children. As the dose of iron is increased, the percent absorbed decreases. At the usual adult dose of about 180 mg/day of iron (300 mg three times a day of $FeSO_4$), about 15–20% is absorbed (27–36 mg). At a dose of 60 mg (one 300 mg $FeSO_4$ tablet), probably 25–30% is absorbed (15–18 mg). Thus, cutting the dose to one third only cuts the absorbed amount by about one half.

Duration of Treatment With Oral Iron. Correction of anemia caused by iron deficiency by the use of oral iron in an otherwise healthy adult can take up to 2 months, assuming iron absorption is normal and there is no continuing loss of blood. If blood loss continues or if there are additional illnesses, return to a normal hemoglobin level may take longer or may not take place at all. Assuming that blood loss is not continuing, oral therapy is continued from 3 to 6 months after the hemoglobin has returned to normal in order to replenish iron stores. Because the rate of iron absorption decreases as iron stores increase, this kind of prolonged therapy is needed in order to replace iron stores.

Side Effects of Oral Preparations of Iron. Intolerance to oral preparations of iron is mainly a function of the iron content of the particular medication. Some studies have shown relatively few side effects of oral iron compared to placebo. Side effects relate mainly to the abdomen and gastrointestinal (GI) tract and include abdominal distress, constipation, diarrhea, and nausea. If there has been a history of intolerance to oral iron, or if the anemia is not severe, therapy can be started with a small dose, gradually increasing to the desired level. Symptoms are reported by about one fourth of treated individuals compared with about one seventh of controls receiving a placebo. However, this is at a dose delivering approximately 200 mg of iron per day (300 mg of ferrous sulfate taken three times a day delivers approximately 180 mg of iron per day).

Iatrogenic Iron Overload. Long-term toxicity may result from continued administration of oral iron in therapeutic amounts to patients who are not iron-deficient, with the gradual production of an overload of iron. This has resulted, in general, either from the careless notion that all anemia should be treated with iron, or that all microcytic anemia should be treated with iron. Thalassemia minor affects millions of people on every continent. Although it is seen most often in the United States in blacks and Italian Americans, it is widespread in people from Greece, India, Southeast Asia, and China and occurs also in many other populations. These people with alpha or beta thalassemia syndromes have microcytic (small) red cells and usually have little or no anemia. Unless they are iron-deficient, oral iron therapy is inappropriate and can lead over a period of years to iron overload. This form of iron toxicity can never be justified.

It is vital to establish whether an anemia is due to iron deficiency because a diagnosis of iron deficiency means an obligation to seek the source of the blood loss, except in growing infants who are known to lack the usual dietary sources of iron.

Iron Poisoning

Iron poisoning due to the ingestion of large amounts of ferrous salts of iron is a common cause of childhood poisoning in infants in some parts of the world, although not particularly common in the United States. Iron pills are often dispensed in bottles of 100. The availability of oral iron preparations in many households, whether for the treatment of iron deficiency or as an iron supplement during pregnancy, makes the problem a difficult one. The use of childproof containers has helped greatly in preventing this form of poisoning.

Ferrous salts are directly toxic to the upper GI tract, and signs of a toxic overdose often occur within an hour or less, although they may be delayed for several hours longer. Nausea and vomiting (often of grayish black or bloody stomach contents) may occur, with abdominal pain and diarrhea. In patients who die, there is hepatocellular damage with a diffuse hemorrhagic lesion of the GI tract. Iron pills are opaque to x-rays and may be seen in radiographs of the abdomen.

BOX 34–1
TREATMENT OF IRON POISONING

If the level of serum iron is less than 500 μg/dL, there should be no immediate danger. However, emergency measurement of serum iron is not often available.

The iron-chelating agent deferoxamine is available as 500-mg vials of deferoxamine mesylate. It can be given intravenously (IV) if the patient is hypotensive but usually is given intramuscularly (IM) at an initial dose of 1 g followed by 500 mg 4 hours and 8 hours after the initial dose. Depending on the clinical response, injections may be continued, but it has been recommended that the dose not exceed 6 g/day. The IV route is used only for patients in shock with an infusion rate that does not exceed 15 mg/kg/hour, with return to the IM route as soon as hypotension is no longer a problem.

Deferoxamine is also used in subcutaneous infusions with a battery-powered pump worn on the forearm of the patient. This has been useful in preventing and treating iron accumulation in patients such as those with thalassemia major who receive transfusions throughout their lives. Remembering that each blood transfusion contains about 250 mg of iron, it is easy to see that an adult getting 40 or 50 units a year is getting around 10–12 g of iron per year. Because the maximal excretion of iron, even in the iron-loaded adult, is only about 10 mg a day, maximal iron excretion is less than 4 g per year. In patients requiring continuing transfusions, phlebotomy obviously is not an available means of decreasing body iron. Subcutaneous infusion of deferoxamine is currently extending the lives and preserving the health of many patients with thalassemia major, but its chronic use is not without problems, including allergic reactions, abdominal pain, and cataracts.

Parenteral Iron Therapy

Iron dextran injection has been available in the United States for many years. During most of this time, it was available only in a preparation for IM use. Despite this, the IM preparation was used IV, particularly in the "Third World," as a means of rapid replacement of the total iron deficit in iron-deficient individuals. It is available now both as an IM preparation containing 0.5% phenol and in 2-mL ampules containing 50 mg/mL of iron for IM or IV administration. The iron from iron dextran must be processed by the body before it becomes available for hematopoiesis. The compound is taken in by reticuloendothelial cells where the sugar portion of the complex is removed and the iron becomes available. The iron gradually leaves the reticuloendothelial cells, becoming bound to transferrin, but the availability of the administered iron dextran takes weeks to months to become complete. IM injection is usually in the buttock, using a Z-track injection to prevent leakage of the material to the skin where it can discolor the skin surface. At 2 mL per injection, which is the usual dose, it takes 20 injections to give the patient 2 g of iron if that is the goal in replacing iron stores.

Severe reactions to parenteral iron dextran have been recorded, including a few fatal anaphylactic reactions. Other reported reactions include joint pain, hives, headache, and fever. Thus there must be specific indications for the parenteral administration of iron.

INTRAVENOUS IRON DEXTRAN. When the physician believes an iron-deficient patient is likely neither to take oral iron nor to return for follow-up, IV iron dextran may be a suitable option despite its small but real risks. The same is true when continuing blood loss requires an amount of iron replacement with which only IV iron dextran can keep up, as in some patients with hereditary hemorrhagic telangiectasia. To try to avoid anaphylactic reactions, one usually starts the injection of IV iron dextran with 0.1 or 0.2 mL over a period of 5 minutes and then gives the remaining amount over 5–10 minutes if there is no sign of a reaction. The total dose may be calculated in a simple fashion by estimating what proportion of the roughly 2 g of iron in hemoglobin in an average-sized adult is missing and adding to that an additional 1–2 g of iron for replenishment of iron stores. For larger or smaller adults, and especially for children, obviously the dose has to be adjusted in proportion to size. It is better to figure out this total dose using common sense rather than to apply a formula blindly, because if it is known that the maximum for any iron-deficient adult is about 3 g of iron replacement, it can be estimated how the results should come out in smaller adults and children, and arithmetic errors cannot be made without recognizing them.

FAILURE TO RESPOND TO IRON THERAPY. The only common causes for an iron-deficient patient not to respond to oral iron (if the patient is not otherwise ill) are not taking the medication or continued bleeding. Good rapport with the patient should enable one to deal with this. Starting therapy with lower doses makes it more likely that the patient will comply with the physician's recommendation. It cannot be stressed too much that because there is really no life-threatening toxicity from the use of oral iron in the usually prescribed doses, the small risk of a fatal anaphylactic reaction to parenteral iron cannot be justified if a little bit more time and attention can achieve the same objective using oral therapy. Parenteral iron should be used when only parenteral iron would be useful.

Vitamin B_{12}

Humans obtain vitamin B_{12} largely from animal protein, including dairy products and eggs. Total body stores are about 1-10 mg. The daily requirement for an average adult is probably no more than 1 μg. About 3 μg daily are secreted in the bile and reabsorbed in the ileum. This secretion and reabsorption accelerates the development of vitamin B_{12} deficiency when intestinal vitamin B_{12} absorption is defective.

Normal individuals have plasma vitamin B_{12} concentrations between 200 and 900 pg/mL. Values of less than 100 pg/mL are definitely abnormal; those between 100 and 200 pg/mL raise a suspicion of vitamin B_{12} deficiency. Cobalamin deficiency, including neuropsychiatric manifestations, can exist, albeit infrequently, in the face of normal serum cobalamin levels and in the absence of anemia. Vitamin B_{12} is mainly bound in the plasma to a globulin called transcobalamin II, by which it is transported to the tissues. Vitamin B_{12} bound to transcobalamin II is rapidly cleared from the plasma, being taken up by hepatic parenchymal cells. Urine or serum levels or methylmalonic acid have been used as a sign of the metabolic effects of vitamin B_{12} deficiency.

Function of Vitamin B_{12}

The active vitamin B_{12} coenzymes are thought to be methylcobalamin and 5-deoxyadenosylcobalamin. These are essential for the growth of cells and for mitosis. Methylcobalamin is necessary for the formation of methionine from homocysteine. Also, folic acid cannot be used properly in the presence of vitamin B_{12} deficiency, so there is a functional deficiency of folic acid metabolites in vitamin B_{12} deficiency. Changes analogous to those in bone marrow occur also in the GI mucosa, both in vitamin B_{12} deficiency and in folic acid deficiency. These changes in the GI mucosa may lead to decreased absorption of vitamin B_{12}. Thus, folic acid deficiency can lead to decreased absorption of vitamin B_{12}, which becomes normal after folic acid repletion. Even with vitamin B_{12} deficiency that is not due to lack of intrinsic factor (see "Absorption," below) but instead is a result of some cause such as a blind-loop syndrome, vitamin B_{12} absorption may in part be decreased because of the mucosal changes caused by the deficiency.

Five-deoxyadenosylcobalamin is used for the conversion of L-methylmalonyl CoA to succinyl CoA and therefore is the mechanism for the methylmalonic acidemia and methylmalonic aciduria seen in vitamin B_{12} deficiency.

ABSORPTION. Vitamin B_{12} is absorbed in the terminal ileum but only if it is bound by a material known as intrinsic factor (IF), which is synthesized by gastric parietal cells. Addisonian pernicious anemia is an autoimmune disorder in which there is atrophic gastritis and decreased-to-absent synthesis of IF with consequent decreased-to-absent absorption of vitamin B_{12}-IF complex. Pancreatic enzymes help release vitamin B_{12} from proteins so that it can be bound by IF, and this explains the vitamin B_{12} malabsorption that may be seen in some forms of pancreatic disease. Vitamin B_{12} absorption obviously may be decreased by ileal disease and certainly is prevented by surgical removal of the stomach or of the terminal ileum. Bacterial overgrowth in blind-loop syndromes prevents an adequate supply of vitamin B_{12} from reaching the ileum. The fish tapeworm *Diphyllobothrium latum* is thought to use vitamin B_{12} as it passes through the upper small intestine, preventing vitamin B_{12} from reaching the terminal ileum. Congenital absence of vitamin B_{12}-binding protein results in megaloblastic anemia, which responds to large dosages of parenteral vitamin B_{12}, apparently by permitting unbound vitamin B_{12} in the plasma to gain access to the cells where it is needed. A functional deficiency of vitamin B_{12} has been reported also in individuals with large increases in transcobalamin I and III as a result of hepatic disease or myeloproliferative disorders.

VITAMIN B_{12} DEFICIENCY. Vitamin B_{12} deficiency causes ineffective red cell production with megaloblastic changes in the bone marrow. The peripheral blood shows macrocytosis, hypersegmented neutrophils, and often thrombocytopenia and leukopenia. Red cell survival tends to be decreased. Usually the MCV is increased and the hemoglobin level is decreased. It is vital to remember that the neurological and psychiatric results of vitamin B_{12} deficiency can occur without anemia, without macrocytosis, or without both. In contrast to the neurological changes, the hematological changes due to vitamin B_{12} deficiency are all reversible. Neurological damage due to vitamin B_{12} deficiency is not always completely reversible. The classic neurological disorder of vitamin B_{12} deficiency is subacute combined degeneration. It is associated with degeneration of axons in the posterior and lateral columns of the spinal cord. Vitamin B_{12} deficiency causes demyelination and cell death both in the spinal column and the cerebral cortex. Paresthesis of the hands, feet, and tongue occur in 5-10% of patients, along with the more common decreases in vibratory and position senses and motor disturbances. Psychological changes can occur in the presence or absence of anemia; these include hallucinations, emotional lability, and dementia. There may also be more subtle personality changes. In general, the changes reversible with treatment are milder and recent, whereas those most likely to be incompletely reversible are more severe and of longer duration (see Chapter 57).

BOX 34-2
THERAPY

Vitamin B_{12} is given IM, usually in 100-μg doses. Initially, it usually is given daily for a few days, then weekly three or four times, and then monthly.

Even though therapy for vitamin B_{12} deficiency is given only once a month after repletion of stores, it is an injection once a month for the remainder of the life of the patient. For this reason, it is important that the physician be sure that the treatment is justified, and that the patient understands the importance of continued treatment. It is important to suspect, diagnose, and treat vitamin B_{12} deficiency. Without adequate sustained treatment the patient can be damaged permanently by a condition that is completely treatable once the need is known.

Vitamin B_{12} deficiency due to a lack of B_{12} in the diet occurs only in strict vegetarians (vegans) who avoid all animal-derived food including eggs and dairy products; vitamin B_{12}-deficient babies may be born to women who are vegans.

Vitamin B_{12} has no known toxicity. (How many other medications come to mind about which this can be said?)

Uses of Vitamin B_{12}

The only proven indication for the use of parenteral vitamin B_{12} is vitamin B_{12} deficiency. The standard work-up for dementia, especially in the elderly, includes a search for hypothyroidism, intracranial abnormalities and vitamin B_{12} deficiency, possibly including a therapeutic trial of vitamin B_{12} for suspected deficiency because, in rare instances, laboratory levels can be normal in the presence of actual vitamin B_{12} deficiency.

Vitamin B_{12} has been widely used also for an assortment of neurological and psychiatric disorders and as a tonic for a wide variety of patients, some of whom are certain the injections help them. None of these uses has been shown to be effective.

Folic Acid

Folic acid or pteroylglutamic acid is the usual pharmaceutical form of this vitamin. The daily requirement in a normal adult is approximately 25–50 μg. During pregnancy or when nursing their babies, women may require 100–200 μg or more daily. Folic acid is used up in the synthesis of hemoglobin. Therefore, patients with high rates of red cell turnover also require increased amounts of folic acid. The standard American diet provides between 50 and 500 μg or more daily, the main sources being fresh green vegetables. Cooking can destroy up to 90% of the folic acid content of food if the cooking is prolonged. In addition to fresh green vegetables, most foods contain some folates. Folate in food occurs mainly in the form of polyglutamates. Most dietary folate is absorbed in the upper portion of the jejunum and in the duodenum. Small intestinal disease in these areas may result in decreased absorption of folate and therefore in its deficiency. Various forms of the coenzyme have different functions: conversion of serine to glycine, synthesis of thymidylate, conversion of homocysteine to methionine, and synthesis of purines. The folates present in food are transported as methyltetrahydrofolate to tissues, where they are stored as polyglutamates.

Folate deficiency is most common where small intestinal disease is most common. Because sprue is widespread in tropical areas, folate deficiency is widespread there too. In temperate climates, folate deficiency is commonly seen in alcoholics, who can become deficient in folic acid in 2 or 3 weeks if, as often is the case, their diet lacks folic acid and they are drinking heavily. It is seen also in people with small intestinal disease such as regional enteritis (Crohn's disease). Folic acid deficiency due to an increased need for folic acid may occur in hemolytic anemias. The cause of the rapid onset of folate deficiency in acute and chronic alcoholism probably is interference with the enterohepatic cycle of the vitamin due to damage to hepatic cells by alcoholism. Some anticonvulsants and, occasionally, oral contraceptives, may interfere with the absorption and storage of folates. Methotrexate, which inhibits dihydrofolate reductase, was designed to have antifolate activity. Folate deficiency, like deficiency of vitamin B_{12}, causes a macrocytic, megaloblastic anemia. The hematological findings in folate deficiency and in vitamin B_{12} deficiency are indistinguishable, although leukopenia and thrombocytopenia may be less common in uncomplicated folic acid deficiency. Folic acid cures the hematological abnormalities, but not the neurological abnormalities seen in vitamin B_{12} deficiency. Vitamin B_{12} does not cure the hematological abnormalities seen in folic acid deficiency. Because administration of therapeutic dosages of folic acid can cure the hematological manifestations of vitamin B_{12} deficiency, it can obscure the presence of vitamin B_{12} deficiency and lead to neurological damage that can be severe and, at least in part, irreversible. For this reason, folic acid was removed some years ago from most multivitamin preparations. It is present in the multivitamin preparations prescribed for pregnant women; therefore, those preparations should not be used except during pregnancy.

SIDE EFFECTS. Unlike vitamin B_{12}, there are rare reports of systemic reaction to parenteral injections of folic acid or its relative, folinic acid (leucovorin). Oral folic acid is not toxic. However, large doses of oral folic acid may decrease the effect of antiepileptic medications.

> BOX 34–3
> **THERAPEUTIC USE**
>
> Folate deficiency in adults usually is treated with oral folic acid: 1 mg, given up to two or three times daily. When folic acid is given prophylactically (as for patients with chronic hemolytic anemias), 1 mg daily is the usual adult dose. Patients receiving pharmacological doses of folic acid should be examined periodically for any sign of the neurological manifestations of vitamin B_{12} deficiency; although there is no known association of vitamin B_{12} deficiency with the usual causes of folate deficiency, there is also no reason to think that individuals with disorders leading to folate deficiency are immune to deficiency of vitamin B_{12}.

Other Agents for Treating Anemia

Recombinant *erythropoietin* was released by the Food and Drug Administration (FDA) in 1989. It is a glycoprotein normally produced by the kidney that stimulates marrow erythroid progenitors to produce red cells. Its therapeutic indications include the anemia of renal failure and the anemia of acquired immunodeficiency syndrome (AIDS). Response requires adequate iron, folic acid, and vitamin B_{12}. The rise in hematocrit in patients with renal failure may be complicated by hypertension, seizures, and clotting of the vascular access or of the dialysis apparatus. Headache, arthralgia, vomiting, and diarrhea also occur more often in treated patients than controls. Erythropoietin is given IV or subcutaneously with a target hematocrit of 30–33%. Other uses of erythropoietin that have been reported include its use to ameliorate the anemia of chronic disease (as in chronic rheumatoid arthritis, metastatic cancer, and others) and to enable such patients to raise their hematocrits so that they can donate blood for their own use in elective surgery. It should be remembered that treatment with erythropoietin is costly.

Anemia resulting from *copper* deficiency has been reported after surgical therapy for obesity (intestinal bypass) and also in people receiving total parenteral nutrition. Daily doses (0.1 mg/kg) of copper sulfate have been given by mouth in such patients and have resulted in clinical responses. A portion of this amount may be added to the material given for total parenteral nutrition. *Cobalt* has been used in the treatment of anemia. It is thought that it tends to raise the hemoglobin level by increasing erythropoietin production as a response to cobalt-induced tissue hypoxia. It has never been shown that anemic patients are clinically benefited by cobalt.

Pyridoxine (vitamin B_6) has produced clinical improvement in up to half of patients both with hereditary and acquired sideroblastic anemias. In these patients, pyridoxine is given orally, 100–200 mg daily. These are amounts far above the usual requirement (pharmacological rather than physiological doses). Hence, these are called pyridoxine-responsive (not pyridoxine deficiency) anemias. These are anemias characterized by a mixed red cell population in the peripheral blood, some of which are hypochromic, and by marrow iron stains showing a ring of intramitochondrial iron surrounding the nuclei of red cell precursors. Pyridoxine, administered in order to prevent the occurrence of isoniazid-induced peripheral neuropathy, has also corrected the sideroblastic anemia associated occasionally with the use of isoniazid.

ANTICOAGULANT, ANTITHROMBOTIC, AND THROMBOLYTIC AGENTS

Thrombosis is merely the obverse of normal hemostasis. We need our circulating blood to stay liquid so that it can perform its numerous vital functions. But we need a mechanism by which bleeding can be stopped, so that a hole in the plumbing does not result in excessive loss of fluid. The same mechanism that seals a leaking small blood vessel can cause a thrombus at the site of an area of abnormal endothelium, such as an atherosclerotic plaque.

When a vessel is injured or the endothelium is damaged, platelets adhere to the exposed basement membrane or collagen. These platelets then normally release a number of substances including serotonin and adenosine diphosphate (ADP). The released ADP causes other passing platelets to agglutinate and stick to the area of damage. This is the mechanism called primary hemostasis, and at the same time it is a mechanism by which an atherosclerotic plaque in a coronary artery can lead to a coronary artery occlusion. This is the origin of the so-called white thrombus seen in the arterial system when there is an abnormal surface to which the circulating blood is being exposed.

Agglutination of platelets has been studied by examining the reactivity of platelets in citrated plasma when ADP, collagen, and other materials are added, using light transmission through a cuvette containing stirred platelet-rich plasma as the method of measurement.

In normal hemostasis, if flow from a cut vessel is stopped by a platelet plug, the platelets also serve as the nidus for the formation of fibrin strands when fibrinogen is clotted by thrombin. On the venous side, thromboses in this low-flow, low-pressure system are usually clots rather than platelet thrombi; these are the red thrombi of the venous system as opposed to the white thrombi of the arterial system. Platelet plugs tend to be unstable and to disaggregate unless they are reinforced by fibrin formation within and around the platelet plug.

Because both platelet plug formation and clot formation are normal adaptive activities leading to protection of the organism, interference with platelet plug formation, interference with blood clot formation, and the use of agents to accelerate the disappearance of clots all affect both normal and pathological platelet plugs and clots. A "magic bullet" has not been found that affects only unwanted clots or platelet agglutinates, while leaving intact those that are useful.

Heparin

Heparin was discovered accidentally in 1916 by a medical student who was investigating ether-soluble materials that accelerated blood clotting. Heparin was purified further in the 1920s and used *in vitro* to prevent the clotting of blood. It seemed logical that such an agent might also be used to treat venous thrombosis. Clinical trials with large doses took place in the late 1930s. However, studies of the efficacy of low doses of heparin did not begin until the 1960s and 1970s.

CHEMISTRY. Heparin is not a single substance. It is a group of straight-chain, anionic mucopolysaccharides or glycosaminoglycans. Heparin has a low pH because of its covalently linked carboxylic acid groups and sulfate groups. Commercially available heparins are polymers of two disaccharides, prepared from the intestinal mucosa of pigs or the lungs of cattle. The incidence of heparin-induced thrombocytopenia is said to be lower with the porcine product. Semisynthetic heparins have been prepared also from sulfated polymers of the disaccharides d-glucosamine and d-glucuronic acid. The physiological function of the heparin normally present in mammalian mast cells is unknown. Low-molecular-weight heparins have been studied in recent years, and now are starting to become available for clinical use; it is claimed that low-molecular-weight heparin can produce an adequate antithrombotic effect with less risk of bleeding than with standard heparin.

ACTIONS OF HEPARIN. Heparin itself is not an anticoagulant. Its anticoagulant effect requires the presence of a plasma factor known as antithrombin III. Heparin vastly potentiates the activity of antithrombin III in neutralizing activated Factors II, IX, X, XI, XII, and XIII. Activated Factor II, of course, is thrombin, the proteolytic enzyme that acts on fibrinogen resulting in the formation of a fibrin clot. Even low concentrations of heparin considerably increase the activity of antithrombin III, especially against activated Factor X and thrombin, which is the rationale for the experimental administration of low doses of heparin that has proved to be therapeutically useful.

Injection of heparin causes the disappearance of turbidity from lipemic plasma due to the release of lipid-hydrolyzing enzymes, especially lipoprotein lipase. Lipoprotein lipase acts on chylomicrons and low-density lipoproteins bound to capillary endothelial cells.

ABSORPTION. Heparin is a polar molecule with an average weight of 15,000 daltons. Probably for this reason it is not absorbed through the GI tract or the skin, nor does it pass the placenta. It is given subcutaneously or IV, but IM heparin is not used because of reports of large IM hematomas at the sites of injection. IV use can be either intermittent or continuous. The higher the dose, the longer the half-life. Liver cells metabolize heparin by means of the enzyme heparinase. Its inactive by-products are excreted in the urine. Both renal and hepatic insufficiency cause prolongation of the half-life of heparin. The larger heparin doses recommended for patients with pulmonary embolism are thought to be required because of rapid heparin clearance in such patients.

SIDE EFFECTS. Allergy to heparin is unusual, with fever, urticaria, or anaphylactic shock. For this reason, a trial dose of 1000 units is given before the usual therapeutic dose. The most common long-term side effect of heparin is osteoporosis, in patients treated for over 3 months with over 15,000 units per day.

Hemorrhage is the most common and most dangerous complication of the use of heparin. All aspirin-containing medications should be avoided. Any bleeding in a patient receiving heparin or any other anticoagulant should be viewed as a sign of a possibly significant lesion. There are many reports of GI hemorrhage while on anticoagulants as the first sign of a GI malignancy.

Thrombocytopenia of a mild and transient nature occurs in a significant minority of people receiving heparin. This is of no clinical significance. On the other hand, severe thrombocytopenia may occur, usually in the second week of heparin therapy. This is characterized by marked thrombocytopenia and multiple episodes of thromboembolism. An IgG antibody directed against a heparin antigen has been detected in the plasma of some patients with this reaction. This is a life-threatening complication, both because of the severe thrombocytopenia and because of the possibility of disease and death from thrombotic complications. If this form of heparin-induced thrombocytopenia is present, heparin must be stopped immediately. If another agent to inhibit thrombosis is needed, oral anticoagulants, antiplatelet agents, or both should be used. This form of severe heparin-induced thrombocytopenia with thromboembolism also has been seen in patients on low-dose heparin. Tests of serum antiheparin antibodies are being developed and may be able to provide a definitive diagnosis of heparin-induced thrombocytopenia. Perhaps this will provide a means of monitoring patients so that heparin can be stopped before severe thrombocytopenia and thrombosis occur.

CONTRAINDICATIONS. Because patients who are actively bleeding can only do so via gaps in the walls of blood vessels, it is obvious that heparin is contraindicated in such patients unless the bleeding can be controlled by other means, such as pressure. Heparin is generally also contraindicated in patients with thrombocytopenic purpura, congenital or acquired coagulation disorders, intracranial hemorrhage, and bacterial endocarditis. It should be avoided after surgery on the eye, central nervous system, or other critical areas.

THERAPY OF HEPARIN-ASSOCIATED BLEEDING. If time is not of the essence, the heparin therapy should be decreased or stopped. If the bleeding is more severe, protamine sulfate may be used. This is available as a solution for IV use containing 10 mg/mL. One milligram of protamine sulfate blocks the anticoagulant effect of 100 units of heparin. Protamine sulfate should not be given at a rate of more than 20 mg/minute nor more than 50 mg in a 10-minute period. Rapid injection of protamine has been reported to cause flushing, hypertension, and other symptoms, possibly as a result of histamine release.

BOX 34-4
THERAPEUTIC USE

Heparin has been standardized at various times both as units and as milligrams. However, because of considerable variation in activity per milligram, only units now are used. A unit of heparin is the amount that prevents 1 mL of recalcified citrated plasma from clotting. Low-dose heparin is given by deep subcutaneous injection for prophylaxis of venous thrombosis. If done in connection with surgery, it is usually started several hours before surgery with a dose of 5000 units in an average-sized adult patient, repeated two or three times daily for a week. Therapy is stopped sooner if the patient is ambulatory earlier, and continued longer if not. *One should obtain a baseline blood count (including platelets), prothrombin time (PT), and partial thromboplastin time (PTT), before beginning to give heparin to any patient.*

Patients receiving heparin usually should not receive medications that interfere with platelet function. Interfering with two hemostatic systems at the same time is more likely to produce bleeding. Heparin used for therapy rather than prophylaxis (standard-dose heparin) is usually given by continuous IV infusion. For IV therapy, start with a "loading dose" of 80 to 100 units/kg. Follow this immediately with an IV infusion of about 20 units/kg/hour. Obtain PTT every 6 to 8 hours adjusting units/hour until the PTT is within the therapeutic range (1.5–2 × control) for 24 hours on the same dose. Thereafter, check PTT daily and adjust dose as needed. Some use intermittent IV therapy through heparin locks, giving 5000–10,000 units initially, followed by 5000–10,000 units every 4 to 6 hours, adjusting the dosage so that the PTT shortly before the next dose is 1.5 to 2 times the patient's control value. Heparin also can be given by deep subcutaneous injection at a dose in adults of 5000–10,000 units every 6 hours, adjusting the dose according to the PTT as with intermittent IV therapy.

When intravenous heparin is given for pulmonary embolism, the loading dose should be at least 100 μ/kg.

Oral Anticoagulants: Warfarin

Warfarin sodium is the only commonly used oral anticoagulant in the United States at this time, although several other agents are available. Its anticoagulant properties were discovered in 1924 as a result of the observation of cattle with a hemorrhagic disorder traced to eating spoiled sweet clover. The effect of warfarin is to cause the synthesis of inactive forms of the vitamin K–requiring Factors II, VII, IX, X, protein C, and protein S. Note that whereas lack of Factors II, VII, IX, and X would be expected to have an anticoagulant effect, lack of protein C or S leads to a thrombotic tendency. Warfarin is the active agent in commonly used rat poisons that cause the animals to bleed to death internally. Warfarin can be used as an example of the many ways one medication may affect the biological activity of another. Some medications, such as phenobarbital, increase the rate of disappearance of warfarin by enzyme induction and decrease its anticoagulant effect. Other agents, such as aspirin, potentiate the effect of warfarin. As a general rule, it is not safe to add or withdraw any medication in a patient on warfarin without checking to see whether there is an effect on the amount of warfarin needed to maintain therapeutic anticoagulation. Warfarin, like heparin, is not itself an anticoagulant. However, its action is different from that of heparin, which immediately becomes an anticoagulant when linked to antithrombin III.

FACTORS THAT AFFECT THE ACTIVITY OF WARFARIN. There are a few reports of congenital resistance to warfarin. Factors that increase the effect of warfarin include any conditions that might lead to vitamin K deficiency, including the use of antimicrobial agents that produce vitamin K deficiency in as little as 10 days to 2 weeks without the use of oral anticoagulants. This effect of antibiotics on the vitamin K synthesized by intestinal bacteria is sometimes overlooked as a possible cause of prolonged coagulation tests and postoperative bleeding. Patients with damaged livers and already impaired hepatic synthesis of coagulation factors are likely also to have a greater effect from warfarin. (All the clotting factors except Factor VIII are thought to be synthesized by hepatocytes.) Older people in general are more sensitive to warfarin, as are those with fever or hyperthyroidism. Aspirin should ordinarily not be used with oral anticoagulants because it interferes with platelet function, leads to increased blood loss from the GI mucosa even without anticoagulation, and potentiates the effect of the oral anticoagulants.

ABSORPTION AND DOSAGE. Warfarin is rapidly and uniformly absorbed after oral administration. It is given once daily. Peak plasma concentrations are reached within 1 hour. Ingestion of food with warfarin decreases the rate but not the extent of absorption. Because warfarin is essentially totally bound to plasma albumin, it does not enter breast milk. However, it is *teratogenic.* Because small amounts cross the placenta, warfarin should not be given to pregnant women. Warfarin usually is started at a dose of 5–7.5 mg daily, adjusting the dose after 3–5 days and thereafter so as to maintain the PT at 1.2 to 1.5 times control. As noted below, ordinarily patients who need anticoagulation are first started on heparin, which is discontinued when they are stable on the oral agent.

ADMINISTRATION AND SIDE EFFECTS. Hemorrhage is by far the greatest and most frequent complication due to oral anticoagulants. It may occur even when the prothrombin time is within the expected therapeutic range. In Europe, less hemorrhage has seemed to occur with warfarin than has been the American experience. Apparently this is due to the different thromboplastin used in the monitoring of oral anticoagulant therapy in the United States as opposed to Western Europe. It is now recommended that the patient/control ratio of the prothrombin time, using the standard United States commercial rabbit brain thromboplastin, should be in the range of 1.2–1.5, going up to a ratio of 1.5–2.0 only for the prophylaxis of thrombosis in patients with recurrent systemic embolism on lower dosages and those with prosthetic heart valves. Prothrombin times now are sometimes reported not in seconds but as an INR (International Normalized Ratio). The INR is calculated as follows: INR = patient's PT/control PT × ISI. The ISI (International Sensitivity Index) is specific both to the reagent and to the instrument used to perform the PT. By using the INR, a patient's prothrombin time measured in any laboratory and with any reagent can be used to adjust the patient's dose, making travel and moving safer for patients. Use of the INR is recommended particularly for patients on long-term oral anticoagulation whose prothrombin time is stable.

Treatment of hemorrhage caused by oral anticoagulants depends on the severity of the hemorrhage. One can simply stop the drug and wait for the coagulation abnormality to disappear. If bleeding is an active problem, 10–20 mg of vitamin K_1 (phytonadione) can be given orally, which should return the prothrombin time to normal within 24 hours. For serious or life-threatening bleeding, IV vitamin K_1 should be used with doses usually of 5–10 mg, although up to 50 mg can be used. The effect of vitamin K is not a coagulant one, however, and correction of the hemorrhagic tendency must await hepatic synthesis of normal Factors II, VII, IX, and X. For this reason, the only rapidly effective means to correct the hemorrhagic tendency due to warfarin is by the use of plasma. This can be either fresh-frozen plasma or cryoprecipitate-depleted plasma (which has less fibrinogen and Factor VIII than normal plasma, but should have normal amounts of Factors II, VI, IX, and X).

Rarely, patients may have a complication known as skin necrosis, or other thrombotic tendencies. It is thought that the reason for this is that protein C (an inhibitor of activated Factors V and VIII) falls to low levels more rapidly than Factor IX at the beginning of a course of warfarin. *For this reason, it is recommended that when a patient is anticoagulated for venous thrombosis, heparin should be started first* and then warfarin is added on the first or second day, usually at a dose of 5 mg/day in adults. The dose is then adjusted as needed. Using this more gradual approach to oral anticoagulation allows heparin to protect the individual if the protein C gets particularly low before Factor IX falls, and skin necrosis should not occur. In the event of what is thought to be warfarin skin necrosis, heparin should be reinstituted (or instituted if not given before) and consideration should be given to the administration of thawed frozen plasma as a source of protein C.

The warfarin-related purple toes syndrome is another rare complication of oral anticoagulant therapy. It presents several weeks after the start of oral anticoagulation and gradually improves after oral anticoagulants are stopped. This syndrome appears to be due to cholesterol microembolization.

Thrombolytic Drugs

Thrombolytic agents are enzymes that cause the dissolution of clots. *Streptokinase* is a protein derived from Group C hemolytic streptococci. It binds to plasminogen, and the streptokinase-plasminogen complex activates uncomplexed plasminogen to the proteolytic enzyme plasmin. Streptokinase is an effective fibrinolytic agent for reasonably fresh clots even up to 4 days old. It also induces bleeding from surgical wounds, sites of arterial puncture, and so forth. Fever is a common side effect. Because it is derived from streptococci, allergic reactions are not uncommon. *Urokinase* probably is at least as effective as streptokinase, is not antigenic, but costs several times as much. It directly converts plasminogen to plasmin. The incidence of bleeding complications is probably about the same with urokinase as with streptokinase.

BOX 34-5
REGIMENS FOR FIBRINOLYTIC THERAPY

The usual loading dose of streptokinase is 250,000 International Units (IU) given over a 30-minute period. Thereafter, 100,000 units/hour is a common dosage, with therapy continued for 1–3 days. Therapy can be monitored by any coagulation test which shows that there is a therapeutic effect of the lytic agent. Because PTs and PTTs are influenced by low levels of fibrinogen, these tests are adequate. The most sensitive test is a thrombin time, but it is not available at all times of the day in many hospitals. PT is a perfectly adequate way of telling whether the desired effect has been achieved. For urokinase the usual loading dose is 4400 IU/kg given IV over 10 minutes followed by a continuous IV infusion at 4400 IU/kg/hour for 12 hours. Because urokinase does not bind to plasminogen, it is not possible (as it is with streptokinase) to give a dose such that all of the plasminogen is bound and none is available for conversion to plasmin. Therefore, it is not necessary to monitor the lytic effect of urokinase. Urokinase should work unless there is a grossly low level of plasminogen.

Regimens for tissue plasminogen activators are still evolving. Bleeding complications are the main untoward effects—especially GI and intracranial bleeding. Reperfusion arrhythmias often occur when fibrinolytic agents are used in patients with recent myocardial infarction. Arterial and venous punctures should be minimized. Check for current regimens and precautions.

Tissue plasminogen activators (TPA) are much-heralded agents about which a great deal of enthusiastic expectation had been generated. This enthusiasm was based on the idea that these agents would have a greater effect on clots but cause less bleeding than streptokinase because they are not fibrinogenolytic but only fibrinolytic. However, in reports of their clinical use, bleeding complications seem to be about as common. It appears that these agents may be slightly superior to streptokinase. It would be expected that urokinase, if it becomes more inexpensive, will replace streptokinase as a therapeutic agent because it is not antigenic.

Antiplatelet-Aggregation Agents

Use of these agents is aimed at the arterial system. There is scanty evidence that antiplatelet agents have any effect on venous thrombosis.

Platelet aggregation seems to be involved not only in thromboembolic disorders but also in the formation of atherosclerotic plaques. Clearly, this is an area of great clinical and research interest.

Different prostaglandins have opposing effects on platelet function. Thromboxane, a platelet product, potentiates platelet aggregation. Prostacyclin (PGI_2) is synthesized by vascular endothelium and inhibits aggregation of platelets. Aspirin inhibits synthesis both of prostacyclin and of thromboxane. Its effects on platelets last for the 8- to 9-day life span of the platelets affected. Low doses of aspirin (60–75 mg/day) have been shown to inhibit thromboxane synthesis more than prostacyclin synthesis. Platelet aggregation is inhibited but there is no significant decrease in the antiaggregatory effect of the prostacyclin at the vessel wall. Essentially, all the studies of the antithrombotic effects of aspirin, however, have used larger doses (usually at least 300 mg/day), which effectively inhibit both thromboxane and prostacyclin synthesis. For this reason, it is not now possible to know what dose of aspirin is best.

Aspirin probably is useful in preventing transient ischemic attacks (TIAs) and strokes. It reduces the risk of myocardial infarction and of reinfarction after myocardial infarction. In a widely publicized study of middle-aged male American physicians, aspirin reduced acute cardiac deaths but had no effect on overall mortality. Aspirin also reduces mortality in acute myocardial infarction.

Sulfinpyrazone has been used as a uricosuric agent in the past to reduce elevated serum levels of uric acid but has largely been supplanted for this indication by allopurinol. Sulfinpyrazone inhibits the platelet-release reaction as well as inhibiting the adherence of platelets to subendothelial structures; it also inhibits the synthesis of prostaglandins. Reports have indicated a reduction in the incidence of sudden death after myocardial infarction, but there has been criticism of the methodology of the studies and sulfinpyrazone is not approved by the FDA as an antithrombotic agent.

Dipyridamole has been in use for some years as a vasodilator. It probably interferes with platelet function by inhibiting phosphodiesterase. The only present official recommended use of dipyridamole as an antithrombotic agent is in conjunction with warfarin for the prevention of thromboemboli in patients who have had prosthetic heart valves implanted.

Use of Drugs to Reduce Surgical Blood Loss

Blood transfusion is well-known to carry a risk of disease transmission. It is the risk of human immunodeficiency virus (HIV) transmission that has created truly widespread concern (some would say hysteria), although the current risk of contracting HIV from one transfusion is believed to be less than 1 in 200,000.

The intuitive response to the problem of limiting surgical blood loss is to tie off or cauterize more bleeders. However, normal hemostatic mechanisms clearly are required to limit surgical blood loss from capillaries, venules, and arterioles.

- *Prostacyclin* (PGI_2) inhibits platelet aggregation. Given IV just before cardiopulmonary bypass in patients having coronary artery bypass grafting procedures, it results in higher intraoperative and postoperative platelet counts but has no significant effect on total blood loss.
- *DDAVP* (desmopressin, a synthetic analog of arginine vasopressin) shortens the bleeding time and the partial thromboplastin time in normal people and people with uremia, platelet function defects, von Willebrand's disease, and hemophilia A (Factor VIII deficiency). It increases plasma levels of high-molecular-weight multimeters of von Willebrand factor. DDAVP has been shown in several studies to decrease blood loss in cardiac and noncardiac surgery.
- *Aprotinin* inhibits trypsin, plasmin, and kallikrein. Its use has been reported to produce impressive decreases in blood loss in both cardiac and noncardiac surgery.

Adverse effects of these drugs include hypotension with prostacyclin and DDAVP, and water retention and hyponatremia with DDAVP. The obvious possibility of increasing the risk of thromboembolism with DDAVP and aprotinin is also a major concern.

The appropriate use and proper dosage (if any) of these agents remains to be established. Use of autologous (autogenic) blood donation in people having elective surgery and/or intraoperative and postoperative salvage and reinfusion of shed blood often can reduce or eliminate the need for transfusion of patients having surgery.

Reflections on the Future

The appropriate use of anticoagulant, antithrombotic, and thrombolytic drugs remains an area of active research. The risk of severe thrombocytopenia and thromboembolism with heparin was totally unsuspected in the mid-1970s. The risk to patients of the presence of lupus inhibitors and what should be done about them in each patient is not well-defined. The risk of bleeding is probably greatest with thrombolytic drugs, intermediate with anticoagulants, and least with antiplatelet agents. If these agents are given in combination, risks as well as benefits can be expected to increase. Low-molecular-weight heparins may give equivalent antithrombotic efficacy with less risk of bleeding.

Platelet aggregation and fibrin clot formation are involved not only in thromboembolism but also in arteriosclerosis and the spread of cancer. Fish oils as well as some ingredients of traditional Chinese cooking have inhibitory effects on laboratory tests of platelet function. Therapeutic effects are less well established, but Eskimos' diet does seem to give them a mild bleeding disorder. Cancer cells grow better in a fibrin mesh than without one; anticoagulation in experimental animals slows the growth of experimental metastases and decreases their numbers. Anticoagulation inhibits formation of a positive tuberculin test in tuberculin-sensitized animals, although other aspects of cellular immunity can be demonstrated in these animals. Clearly these are areas for further study.

REFERENCES

Clouse LH, Comp PC: The regulation of hemostasis: The protein C system. N Engl J Med 314:1298-1304, 1986.

Hirsh J: Drug therapy: Heparin. N Engl J Med 324:1565-1574, 1991.

Hirsh J: Is the dose of warfarin prescribed by American physicians unnecessarily high? Arch Intern Med 147:769-771, 1987.

Hirsh J: Oral anticoagulant drugs. N Engl J Med 324:1865-1875, 1991.

National Conference on Antithrombotic Therapy. Chest 89:1S-106S, 1986.

Samama MM: Thrombolytic agents and treatments. Semin Thromb Hemost 13:131-227, 1987.

35 Renal Pharmacology

Margaret A. Acara

PREREQUISITE RENAL PHYSIOLOGY

Pharmacological agents that alter renal function can be useful in disease states where composition and volume of body fluids are abnormal; the most frequently prescribed of these drugs are diuretics. The goal of diuretic therapy is to achieve a more normal composition of body fluids and thereby maintain normal physiological cellular function. Understanding renal function and fluid balance is required for the understanding of the mechanism of action of these agents.

The three major fluid compartments of the body—plasma, interstitial fluid, and intracellular fluid—are in continual turnover. Although circulating plasma is most immediately subject to influxes and effluxes of water and electrolytes, intracellular and interstitial spaces respond quickly to changes in volume and composition of plasma. Imbalances are generally reflected in the plasma or extracellular fluid compartment, which is continually monitored and adjusted by the kidney. The causes of fluid and electrolyte disorders vary, but the therapeutic approaches must involve the kidney because it controls electrolyte and water excretion.

Salt and Water Balance

In one day one kidney of a normal adult receives over 1700 L of blood (about 1200 mL/minute or 660 mL/minute plasma flow). It filters through the glomeruli 180 L/day or 125 mL/minute (20% of the entering plasma volume) containing 25,200 mEq sodium/day. An ultrafiltrate containing electrolytes and other small-molecular weight solutes is formed through this process. As fluid is forced through the glomerular endothelium, the plasma proteins remain in the vasculature, maintaining oncotic pressure (the sum of the protein osmotic pressure and the osmotic pressure of obligated cations). The hydrostatic pressure from the heart is the major force for the filtration and the difference in pressure between the afferent and efferent arterioles along with the permeability of the filtering membranes contribute to the regulation of the filtered load. The glomerular filtration rate (GFR) is the unit volume of fluid passing through the glomerulus per unit time (generally in mL/minute).

After the fluid is filtered at the glomerulus, it is processed by the tubules, which normally reabsorb greater than 99% of the filtrate; the composition of the reabsorbed filtrate approximates the composition of the extracellular fluid. Sodium is the major electrolyte of the extracellular compartment, and the mechanisms for its reabsorption are associated with the recapturing of filtrate (Fig. 35-1).

Glomerular tubular balance describes the concept that changes in GFR are compensated for by parallel changes in tubular reabsorption of sodium (an increase in GFR is accompanied by an increase in the absolute amount of sodium reabsorbed, while the fraction of sodium reabsorbed by the tubule remains the same). This is also true for excretion; when GFR increases, the amount of sodium excreted also increases but fractional excretion remains the same. One can regulate water and electrolyte excretion by changing ei-

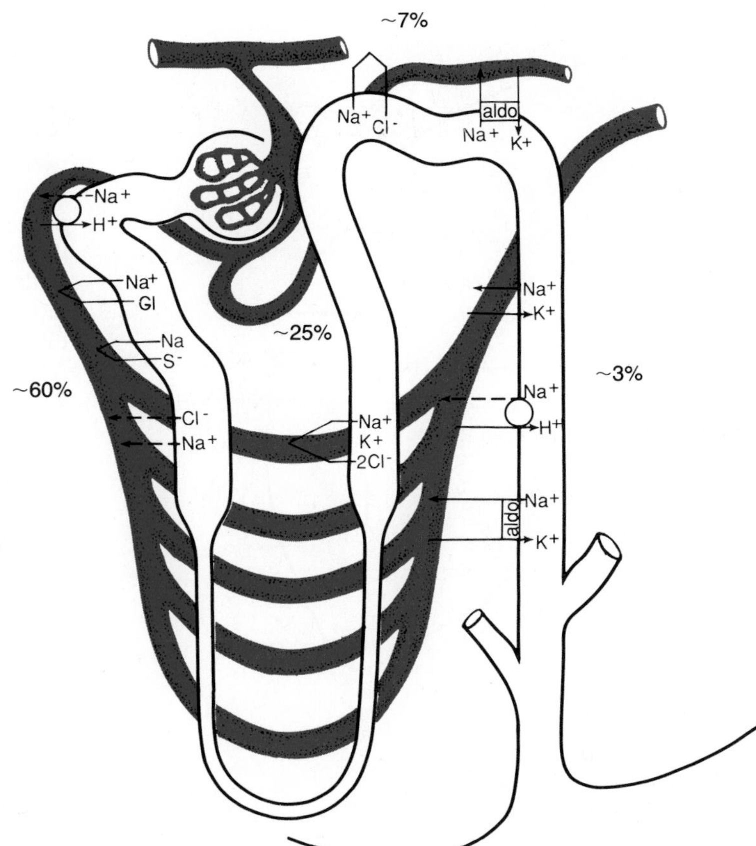

FIGURE 35–1. Diagram of a nephron indicating tubular sites for sodium reabsorption, the capacity of the different segments, and the mechanisms for sodium entry into the cell at each site. Sodium is actively transported out of the cell across the basolateral membrane into the blood by the sodium/potassium pump. In the proximal tubule, approximately 65% of filtered sodium is reabsorbed through (1) countertransport with hydrogen, (2) cotransport with glucose or neutral organic solutes, (3) cotransport with nonchloride anions, or (4) diffusion following a chloride gradient. In the thick ascending limb, approximately 25% of filtered sodium is reabsorbed through the electroneutral cotransport of one K^+, one Na^+, and two Cl^-. In the distal convoluted tubule, approximately 7% of filtered sodium is reabsorbed against an electrochemical gradient through a sodium chloride cotransport. In the late distal tubule, approximately 3% of filtered sodium is reabsorbed mainly through sodium/potassium exchange, some of which is under aldosterone control. The sodium/hydrogen exchange in the distal tubule is associated primarily with urine acidification.

ther tubular reabsorption or GFR. In general, clinically useful diuretic agents have tubular actions that inhibit reabsorption, although secondary effects may alter GFR.

As the filtrate proceeds along the tubule, reabsorption takes place because tubular cells move certain solutes and water back into the postglomerular peritubular capillaries. Cells in particular segments of the nephron are associated with mechanisms for the movement of particular ions. These mechanisms differ with respect to which other electrolytes are involved in the reabsorptive process for sodium and in which segment they are located.

In the reabsorptive process, sodium passively enters the tubule cell across the brush border or luminal membrane, down an electrochemical gradient.

Mechanisms for sodium entry into the cell from tubule fluid are (Fig. 35–1):

1. "*Per se*" entry of sodium;
2. Carrier-mediated cotransport with organic solutes such as sugars and amino acids;
3. Carrier-mediated countertransport with hydrogen;
4. Carrier-mediated electroneutral cotransport of one sodium, one potassium, and two chloride ions; and
5. Carrier-mediated electroneutral cotransport of sodium and chloride.

In addition, sodium also may diffuse back into peritubular capillaries by paracellular pathways. Sodium moves against a concentration gradient from the cell into the blood by active transport through the sodium-potassium exchange pump fueled by adenosine triphosphate (ATP) that moves sodium out of the cell and potassium into it across the basolateral membrane.

Reabsorptive Processes in Particular Nephron Segments

Most diuretics act primarily on sodium movement in one or another segment of the nephron. Nevertheless, the urinary electrolyte excretion profile reflects the combined action on all nephron segments.

The *proximal tubule* reabsorbs approximately 60% of the filtered load, which involves mechanisms 1, 2, and 3 above. *In the early part of the proximal tubule, sodium is reabsorbed preferentially without chloride by:*

1. Sodium and bicarbonate transport linked to hydrogen ion secretion;
2. Cotransport with neutral organic solutes such as glucose and amino acids; and
3. Cotransport with nonchloride anions—acetate, phosphate, citrate, and lactate.

The proximal tubule is freely permeable to water, and reabsorption at this site is isotonic.

In the reabsorption of sodium bicarbonate, a hydrogen ion combines with bicarbonate in the filtrate and forms carbonic acid. Carbonic anhydrase is abundant in the brush border of the proximal tubular cell and in its presence luminal carbonic acid is dehydrated to CO_2 and water. The un-

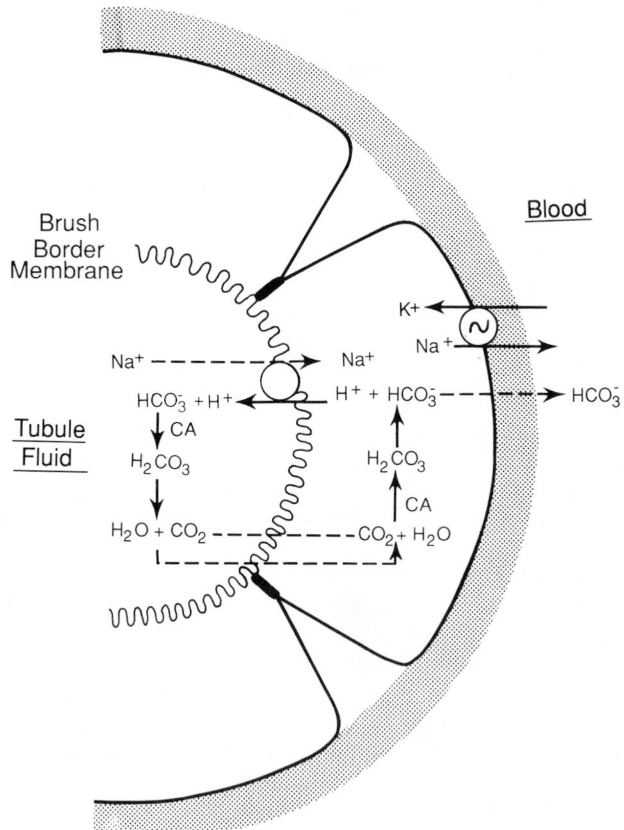

FIGURE 35–2. Sodium/hydrogen exchange and carbonic anhydrase (CA). Sodium enters the tubule cell in exchange for a hydrogen, which has been generated by dissociation of carbonic acid produced from carbon dioxide (CO_2) and water (H_2O) by the hydration action of carbonic anhydrase inside the cell. Carbonic anhydrase, associated with the brush border, also catalyzes the dehydration reaction of carbonic acid to CO_2 and H_2O.

charged CO_2 gas freely diffuses across the luminal membrane into the tubular cell, where it is hydrated to carbonic acid. This acid dissociates to yield a hydrogen ion that may be secreted back into the lumen in exchange for a sodium ion, which may then exit across the peritubular membrane of the cell with a bicarbonate anion. The net effect of this process is the reabsorption of filtered sodium bicarbonate and the secretion of a hydrogen ion. Both the hydration and dehydration reaction are under the control of carbonic anhydrase, whereas the ionic dissociation of H_2CO_3 occurs spontaneously (Fig. 35–2).

The reabsorption of sodium bicarbonate and water early in the proximal tubule results in an increase in the concentration of chloride in the later proximal tubule fluid. Thus, there is a chloride gradient favoring its movement into the peritubular capillary. This nephron segment is highly permeable to chloride and sodium follows chloride to maintain electrical neutrality. Water accompanies the solutes by osmotic obligation.

Although some diuretics directly inhibit sodium reabsorption in the proximal tubule, most act distally. Because the loop of Henle has a high capacity for sodium reabsorption, the sodium that is inhibited from being reabsorbed in the proximal tubule can be almost completely reabsorbed at more distal sites. This process thus negates the effect of proximally active diuretics. Carbonic anhydrase inhibitors have their major site of action in the proximal tubule because that is where the enzyme is mainly localized.

In the thick ascending limb of the loop of Henle, 20–50% of filtered sodium is reabsorbed through the electroneutral cotransport of a sodium ion, a potassium ion, and two chloride ions from the lumen of the tubule into the tubular cell (Fig. 35–3). The Na-K-2Cl cotransporter in the apical or luminal membrane facilitates the entry of these ions from the tubular fluid. Thus, transepithelial NaCl movement is secondary active transport, driven by the inward gradient for sodium across the apical cell membrane. The driving force for this transport is again provided by sodium-potassium ATPase. The existence of potassium conductance in the apical membrane allows potassium to recycle to the cotransporter, whereas the existence of chloride conductance in the basolateral membrane allows chloride to exit from the cell. Net reabsorption of Na^+ and Cl^- ions against their concentration gradients occurs, and the potassium ion is quickly recycled to maintain this activity. One Na^+, 2 Cl^-, and 1 K^+ cotransported across the luminal membrane and K^+ being recycled generate a lumen positive transepithelial potential difference.

An important aspect of reabsorption of filtrate in the ascending limb is that this segment is impermeable to water. Unreabsorbed water remains in the tubule, and fluid leaving the thick ascending limb is hypotonic compared with plasma. Solute movement into the interstitium contributes to osmolality and acts as an osmotic force for water reabsorption in the presence of vasopressin in the concentration of urine through the counter current multiplier action of the

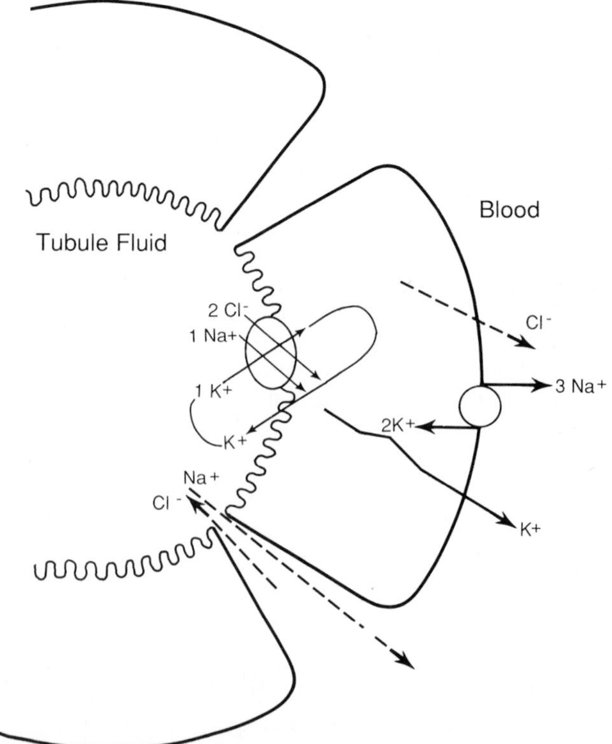

FIGURE 35–3. Mechanism for sodium reabsorption in the thick ascending limb: cotransport of one K^+, one Na^+, and two Cl^-. Sodium and potassium enter the cell along with two chloride ions. Potassium recycles through conductance across the apical membrane to the cotransporter, and chloride conductance occurs across the basolateral membrane.

kidney. Diuretics that act at this site interfere with the development of a concentrated interstitium and may lead to an isotonic urine.

Prostaglandins and Medullary Washout

The concept of "medullary washout" refers to the contribution of the vasa recta in establishing a concentration gradient from cortex to medulla to permit formation of a concentrated urine. The vasa recta act as passive conduits for the equilibration of osmolar solutes in the interstitium. The greater the flow rate through the medullary region, the less time there will be for the blood to equilibrate with the more concentrated interstitium. Osmolar solutes will be picked up and carried away, effectively diluting the medullary interstitium.

The dynamics of blood flow through the medullary region are in part under the control of prostaglandins, particularly prostaglandin E_2, which acts as a medullary vasodilator promoting blood flow to this region. The interactions between the prostaglandin-induced medullary vasodilation and the ability of loop diuretics to increase prostaglandin (PG) concentrations in the medulla provide evidence for a contribution of this system to a diuretic effect. That is, the inability to establish as concentrated an interstitium in the presence of PGE_2 interferes with the formation of negative and positive free water and contributes to the diuresis.

The *thick ascending limb ends and the early distal tubule begins at the macula densa.* In this portion of the nephron, the tubule returns to touch upon the glomerulus from which it originates (juxtamedullary apparatus). The distal tubule extends from the macula densa to a site where other distal tubules come together to form cortical collecting tubules. Sodium is actively reabsorbed against an electrochemical gradient in the distal convoluted tubule (early distal tubule), and provides the driving force for passive potassium entry. Calcium also is reabsorbed here by an active sodium-independent mechanism. In this segment carbonic anhydrase activity is related primarily to the sodium/hydrogen exchange that participates in urine acidification. The flow rate of tubule fluid through this segment and the production of hydrogen ion are major factors for regulating potassium excretion in the urine.

Active reabsorption of sodium and chloride occurs in the *cortical collecting tubule.* Potassium secretion under the control of mineralocorticoids occurs here. Aldosterone stimulates distal tubular sodium reabsorption and potassium secretion. The collecting tubule becomes more permeable to water in response to vasopressin, and in the medullary collecting tubule solute free water is reabsorbed toward a hypertonic interstitium.

Exchange sites for sodium reabsorption and potassium secretion in the distal and collecting tubules regulate the amount of potassium excreted in the urine. Almost all of the filtered potassium is reabsorbed in the proximal tubule; thus variations in urinary potassium reflect the activities of these distal segments. Potassium excretion increases in response to (1) increased amounts of sodium reaching these sites and (2) increased levels of circulating aldosterone. The two major ways for increased amounts of sodium to reach the distal tubule are inhibition of sodium reabsorption at a more proximal site and an increased flow rate through the distal tubule.

Renin-Angiotensin-Aldosterone

The fact that sodium is reabsorbed in the distal tubule with and without aldosterone stimulation is the basis for the existence of two types of potassium-sparing diuretics, one of which is dependent on the presence of aldosterone. Aldosterone stimulates both potassium and hydrogen ion excretion in exchange for sodium. This steroidal hormone enters the distal tubule cell and binds to cytoplasmic receptors; this receptor complex eventually interacts with the nucleus to cause the encoding of new mRNA, directing the synthesis of new aldosterone-induced proteins (AIP), which act to increase sodium reabsorption.

Aldosterone itself is released from the zona glomerulosa in response to stimulation by angiotensin II and/or III. The concentration of angiotensin is in turn regulated by plasma renin levels. The major stimulus for renin release from the granular cells of the juxtamedullary apparatus is a falling renal perfusion pressure. This stimulus is eventually overcome by aldosterone-induced sodium reabsorption and subsequent volume expansion.

Another major action of angiotensin II is systemic, as well as renal, vasoconstriction. Inhibition of the enzyme that produces angiotensin II (known as angiotensin-converting enzyme, ACE, and also as peptidyldipeptidase or kininase II) is an important therapeutic strategy in the treatment of hypertension.

Vasopressin (Antidiuretic Hormone)

The ability to form a concentrated urine is dependent upon circulating levels of vasopressin (antidiuretic hormone, ADH) and the development of an osmotic gradient of increasing concentration from cortex to medulla. This gradient results in part from the cotransport of 1 Na^+, 2 Cl^-, and 1 K^+ in the thick ascending limb (TAL) (Fig. 35–4).

Vasopressin acts on the distal tubule and collecting duct to increase the water permeability of these cell membranes. Under the condition of a concentrated interstitium, water is reabsorbed toward an osmotic driving force. Diuretics that interfere with reabsorption of sodium and chloride in the TAL produce the largest diuretic effect and interfere with the production of both positive and negative free water.

Free water is an operational concept that describes the ability of the diluting segment to dilute and of the concentrating segment to concentrate. Both concentration and dilution result from the cotransport of sodium, potassium, and chloride in the ascending limb. Arithmetically, it is equal to urine flow rate minus osmolar clearance and is expressed in units of mL/minute. *Positive free water* is formed by the removal of sodium and chloride from the tubular fluid without the removal of water, and this results in a hypotonic fluid

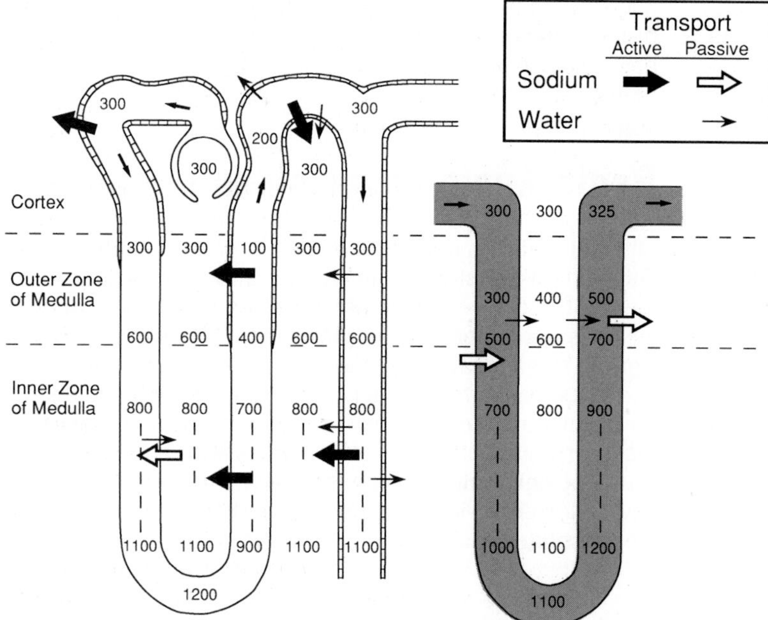

FIGURE 35–4. Concentrating mechanisms in the kidney. As tubule fluid flows through the nephron (*left side* of figure) and blood through the vasa recta (*right side* of figure), the osmolality increases as the inner medulla is reached and then decreases as fluid moves back toward the cortex. Sodium and chloride are moved into the interstitium without water in the thick ascending limb, creating a slightly higher interstitial osmolality. Water from the descending limb moves toward this osmotic force, and sodium chloride moves into the descending limb. Reabsorbed fluid is carried off in the vasa recta, where alteration of flow rate affects the amount reabsorbed. (Modified from Koushanpour E, Kriz W: Renal Physiology—Principles, Structure, and Function. 2nd ed. New York: Springer-Verlag, 1986.)

reaching the early distal tubule. This part of the nephron where salt is reabsorbed without water is designated the *diluting segment.*

Negative free water is water that is reabsorbed primarily in the medullary collecting tubules in the presence of vasopressin and toward an osmotically concentrated interstitium. This portion of the nephron is called the *concentrating segment.*

If the reabsorption of sodium chloride in the cortical diluting segment is inhibited, there will be a decrease in the production of positive free water. If sodium chloride reabsorption in the medullary diluting segment is inhibited, there is not only a decrease in positive free water but also a decrease in the osmotic driving force. Thus, the force drawing water into the interstitium in the presence of vasopressin is decreased and so is negative free water production.

The major stimulus for vasopressin release is an increasing plasma osmolarity and the response of increased water reabsorption decreases plasma osmolarity back toward normal. The increasing plasma osmolarity is sensed by the supraoptic nuclei of the hypothalamus. The message is transmitted through a neurophysin to the posterior pituitary, from which vasopressin is released. The cellular action of vasopressin includes binding of the hormone to an adenyl cyclase-activated membrane receptor on the basolateral membrane. *These tubule receptors have been designated V_2 receptors* (as opposed to the vascular or V_1 receptors for vasopressin). Cyclic AMP activates a protein kinase that phosphorylates membrane proteins, resulting in a more water permeable state on the brush border membrane. Development of V_2 antagonists may provide a new approach to diuretic therapy.

Diabetes insipidus is the disease related to hyposecretion of vasopressin or hyporesponsivity of its target sites, the distal tubules and collecting ducts. An insufficient amount of water is reabsorbed and hypovolemia ensues. The syndrome of inappropriate secretion of antidiuretic hormone (*SIADH*) is related to hypersecretion of vasopressin or hyperresponsivity of the receptors and is characterized by hypervolemia. A paradoxical use of diuretics is involved in the treatment of hypovolemic, nephrogenic diabetes insipidus (negative water balance); the rationale is based on a decreased delivery of filtrate to the diluting segment (discussed below under thiazide diuretics).

Atrial Natriuretic Peptide (Factor, Hormone), Atriopeptin

This hormone is secreted by specific granules in the atria of the heart in response to an increasing vascular volume. In general, the effects of this hormone are hypotension and natriuresis. The latter effect is associated with inhibition of sodium reabsorption and increases in GFR. Atrial natriuretic peptide (ANP) increases vascular permeability, decreases cardiac output and blood volume, and increases hematocrit; it is present in abnormally high levels in congestive heart failure.

Edema

Edema is an excessive accumulation of fluid in the interstitial space. Alteration of cardiac, renal, hepatic, or endocrine function may be of primary importance in its etiology. In this pathological state, widespread swelling of most interstitial spaces occurs. The distribution of edema fluid can be explained by simple physical forces. Changes in Starling forces across the capillary in the direction of increased systemic venous hydrostatic pressure and/or decreased plasma oncotic pressure promote loss of fluid from the vascular system. Distention of vessels contributes to the loss of fluid and proteins from the vascular system to the interstitium through "leaky" capillaries.

The decreased excretion of sodium (or increased retention) is the focus for treatment of disease states characterized by edema. Although accumulation of edema fluid compromises the vascular system through an inadequate circulating volume, the normal renal responses continue to contribute to sodium retention. The decrease in the effective circulating volume sensed by the juxtaglomerular apparatus as a decrease in perfusion pressure results in the release of renin. Increased renin leads to the formation of angiotensin II and an increase in aldosterone release, which causes an increase in sodium reabsorption. This retention of sodium is a vicious cycle, associated with the retention of fluid that is subsequently redistributed as additional edematous fluid. Moreover, decreases in GFR, occurring because of the compromised circulatory system, not accompanied by a decrease in sodium reabsorption, result in glomerular tubular imbalance and contribute further to sodium retention.

RENAL EXCRETION OF DRUGS

Clearance Measurements of Renal Function and Drug Excretion

Clearance is the measurement of the removal of a substance from a fluid such as blood. It is expressed as volume "cleared" per unit time (usually mL/minute). When applied to the kidney, as in renal clearance, it expresses the contribution of this organ to the clearance of a substance from plasma.

In the conventional measurement of renal clearance, timed urine samples are obtained and the excretion rate of the compound under study in amount per minute is divided by its plasma concentration to determine the volume of plasma from which it was derived. The traditional formula for clearance is UV/P; U is the concentration of compound in urine, V is urine flow rate, and P is the concentration of compound in plasma.

Clearance is defined in relation to the compartments observed. Clearance by the whole kidney should include the amount of substance that was lost from the blood to the organ, as well as to the urine and is appropriately designated *renal clearance.* Clearance that describes loss to urine only may be appropriately designated *urinary clearance.*

Renal clearance is calculated as the product of the extraction ratio and renal plasma flow (RPF). It represents the total volume of blood from which a substance, S, has been removed by the kidney in 1 minute. Renal clearance or $R\ Cl_S = E \times RPF$, where the extraction ratio, $E = (A - V)/A$ and A and V represent the concentrations of S in arterial and venous plasma respectively. Renal clearance describes the integrated functions of the whole kidney. It accounts for all pathways of deposition of S in the kidney: what appears in the urine; what is metabolized by the kidney; and what is stored in the kidney.

Urinary clearance, on the other hand, describes the clearance of the substance attributable to the urine only and does not account for the disposition of the substance in other renal compartments. Urinary clearance uses the traditional clearance calculation to express the volume of plasma which contained the amount of S that was excreted in the urine in 1 minute. $U\ Cl_S = UV/P$, where U and P represent the concentrations of S in urine and plasma respectively and V is the urine flow rate. It is only when a substance is neither metabolized nor stored in the kidney that its renal clearance is equal to its urinary clearance; this is true for those substances that measure renal plasma flow, such as p-aminohippuric acid (PAH) and those that measure GFR such as inulin. It also follows that the difference between renal clearance and urinary clearance represents storage and metabolism by the kidney. For pharmacokinetic parameters useful in the measurement of plasma clearances, see Chapter 5.

The fractional excretion (FE) of a substance (S) is the ratio of the urinary clearance of S, calculated as $U\ Cl_S$, to the GFR. A ratio greater than 1.0 reflects tubular addition of S from blood to tubule fluid associated with a secretory component resulting in net excretion. A ratio less than 1.0 is generally interpreted to indicate movement of S from tubule fluid back into blood resulting in apparent net reabsorption. However, the procedure does not account for possible metabolism of the substance; a ratio less than 1.0 simply indicates net disappearance of the substance from tubule fluid.

Renal Handling of Drugs

The majority of drugs are eliminated at least in part by the kidney. The actions of the kidney that affect the amount of drug in the plasma are hemodynamic, metabolic, and transport related. *Factors governing the role of kidney in drug elimination are:*

1. Renal plasma flow
2. Proportion of blood reaching kidney that is filtered—20%
3. GFR—for example, predictable decreases in GFR in the elderly
4. Degree of protein binding, because protein bound is not filtered and only free drug is present in the ultrafiltrate
5. Reabsorption by active or passive processes
6. Amount of passive back diffusion in the distal tubule
7. Metabolism of the drug by the kidney

The amount of drug reaching the kidney is determined by renal plasma flow (RPF). This is calculated as RPF times the concentration of drug in plasma. Approximately 20% of the blood that reaches the kidney is filtered by it. The amount of drug filtered is determined by the GFR and the degree of plasma protein binding of the drug. The protein bound portion of the drug is not filtered, and only the free drug is present in the ultrafiltrate. The portion of drug that is filtered may remain in the tubule to be excreted in the urine, or the drug may be reabsorbed through either passive or active processes.

Many drugs undergo nonionic passive back diffusion in the distal tubule. As filtrate moves along the tubule, water is reabsorbed. This results in the drug becoming more concentrated in the tubule fluid and a gradient is created that favors back diffusion. This process occurs for the most part in the distal tubule since water reabsorption prior to this site has resulted in a large concentration gradient from tubule fluid to blood.

REABSORPTION INVOLVING ACTIVE PROCESSES. Nonfiltered blood carries both free and bound drug into the postglomerular peritubular capillary system. An equilibrium exists between protein-bound and free drug, and free drug binds to receptors or carriers on the tubule cell. Drugs are then moved by active transport systems from the postglomerular peritubular capillary system across the tubule cell into the lumen of the tubule.

Separate excretory transport systems exist for organic acids and organic bases. These systems are saturable and are identified by their ability to be inhibited by prototypical competitors. Probenecid inhibits the organic anion transport system, and quinine inhibits the organic cation system. PAH (p-aminohippurate), an organic acid, is used to measure renal plasma flow because at concentrations less than its transport maximum, all of the compound that reaches the transport system in the proximal tubule is secreted by it. TEA (tetraethylammonium) is the comparable organic cation. Administration of specific inhibitors of these transport systems can result in the prolongation of the half-life of a drug handled by them.

Active reabsorption of organic compounds occurs in the proximal tubule and two of these systems have been well studied: glucose reabsorption and amino acid reabsorption. Certain drugs may be handled in a similar manner. Frequently, these mechanisms for reabsorption are linked to a biotransformation of the substrate being reabsorbed. Glucose, for example, is metabolized to glucose-6-phosphate as it moves across the luminal membrane into the cell. Choline is transformed to its oxidized metabolite, betaine, during its transit from lumen to blood.

The same substances may be actively transported in both directions in the proximal tubule by carrier-mediated mechanisms. For example, the renal handling of uric acid includes filtration and reabsorption as well as secretion. Thus, any drug that occupies the organic acid transport system has the potential to affect plasma uric acid concentration. For example, sulfonamide-type diuretics can inhibit uric acid excretion and contribute to hyperuricemia. On the other hand, probenecid is used as a uricosuric agent to inhibit the reabsorption of uric acid and decrease hyperuricemia. Other drugs also occupy these systems.

PASSIVE PROCESSES OF REABSORPTION. Inasmuch as it is in their nonionized form that drugs cross cell membranes, the pK_a of the drug and the pH of the tubule fluid govern the reabsorption of drugs back into peritubular capillaries. Numerous drugs are either weak acids or weak bases and exist in a mixture of ionic and nonionic forms depending upon their dissociation constant and the pH of their environment. *Weak acids will be nonionized in acid urine and reabsorption favored. Weak bases will be nonionized in alkaline urine and reabsorption favored.* This same principle is taken advantage of when toxic levels of weak acids are reached and rapid elimination is important, such as in salicylate poisoning. The urine is made alkaline (*eg*, by sodium bicarbonate or acetazolamide), favoring ionization of the salicylate and reduction of reabsorption and increased excretion.

The opposite occurs for weak bases. Reabsorption of the nonionized form of weak bases is favored in an alkaline tubular fluid and their excretion as charged molecules is favored in an acid urine.

Increased renal excretion of drugs by interference with nonionic back diffusion is reasonably achievable when the pK_a of the drug falls within an attainable urine pH range. Urine pH may be decreased to 5.0 using acidifying salts and increased to 8.0 as above.

DRUG METABOLISM. The kidney plays a major role in the metabolism of many drugs, and certain renal enzymes can transform a molecule to a more polar and water soluble metabolite. For example, glucuronidation and sulfation act to enhance drug excretion.

In addition to these kidney functions, the kidney is especially vulnerable to damage from various chemical insults. It receives a major percentage of the cardiac output, and through filtration and transport processes renal tubular cells can be exposed to high concentrations and amounts of drugs and chemical substances (see Chapter 50; Abuelo, 1990). Both peritubular membranes (exposed to the blood) and brush border membranes (exposed to tubular fluid) are vulnerable. In addition, because of concentrating mechanisms, drugs and chemicals can become 100–1000 times more concentrated in tubule fluid over that in plasma.

Drug Excretion in Renal Failure

Patients with renal failure may undergo treatment for multiple medical problems and receive various medications. Renal dysfunction leads to abnormal excretion and metabolism of drugs. Decreased renal blood flow (RBF) and GFR, for example in association with advancing age, result in decreases in the amounts of drug reaching the kidney, the amount of drug filtered, and thus the amount of drug excreted; such decreased excretion results in plasma drug concentrations that are higher than desired.

Patients with inadequate renal function have inappropriate responses to ordinary doses of many drugs. This may be the consequence not only of decreased excretion, but an abnormality in absorption, distribution, or metabolism or an altered sensitivity of the target tissue to the drug. The effect of uremia itself to induce alterations in receptor environment may result in untoward effects of drugs. Thus, disturbances in renal function call for judicious drug selection and careful dose modification.

Sometimes in unpredictable fashion, a change in protein binding occurs. In renal failure there is generally a decreased binding of drugs, especially highly bound acidic drugs such as furosemide. Also, in certain conditions, such as the nephrotic syndrome, hypoalbuminemia may be present or the ratio of different globulin fractions changes and a new binding picture emerges. In uremia, an alteration of the binding sites themselves may occur, or certain compounds present in uremia may compete with drugs for binding. Interference with carrier transport systems can occur. *The usual outcome in renal failure is that more free drug is present in plasma than would normally have been predicted.*

The uremic state has differential effects on enzyme systems and may lead to increased or decreased formation of drug metabolites. Some oxidations that occur in hepatic endoplasmic reticulum are accelerated in uremia (*eg*, phenytoin). If the metabolic step leads to an active metabolite, a more intense drug effect could occur.

Drugs Contraindicated in Renal Failure

Two classes of drugs are noteworthy for significant adverse effects in the presence of renal failure. Both nonsteroidal anti-inflammatory drugs (NSAIDs) and angiotensin converting enzyme (ACE) inhibitors further compromise already existing renal failure.

NSAIDs are cyclooxygenase inhibitors and decrease the production of prostaglandins thus preventing prostaglandin-induced maintenance of blood flow in renal failure. However, this effect does not appear to be important so long as kidney function is normal.

Glomerular filtration is maintained in part by the pressure difference across the glomerulus, and angiotensin II apparently has a greater effect to constrict the efferent arteriole than the afferent arteriole; in doing so it enhances the GFR. Administration of ACE inhibitors prevents this efferent vasoconstriction thus decreasing GFR and tubule flow rate.

DIURETICS

A diuretic is any substance that results in increased urine volume. Ingestion of large volumes of fluid increases urine output through an increase in volume in the vascular compartment, which causes an increase in RBF and GFR. Glomerular tubular balance demands that increases in GFR result in increases in urine volume and sodium excretion. Currently useful diuretic drugs act on certain sites along the nephron to interfere with particular sodium reabsorptive pathway(s). The resulting natriuresis and diuresis is a tubular effect, and a decrease in the amount of sodium reabsorbed generally obligates a decrease in the amount of tubule fluid reabsorbed. The loss of fluid decreases plasma volume and hydrostatic pressure and increases plasma oncotic pressure so that fluid returns from the interstitium to the vascular system and is excreted. The overall result is the loss of fluid and weight and the establishment of a new steady state.

Most clinically used diuretics are organic anions with particular pharmacokinetic characteristics. They are tightly bound to plasma proteins and not filtered at the glomerulus in significant amounts but are moved across the tubule cell from the postglomerular peritubular capillary blood into the lumen by the active organic acid transport system in the straight segment of the proximal tubule. They travel in the lumen to their tubular site of action, and their concentration in the lumen determines the diuretic response. Therefore, in order for the diuretic to reach its site of action, sufficient renal function must exist.

Attempting to classify diuretic agents by their chemical structure is of limited value in understanding their renal action. Classifying them according to their major site of action is the traditional and more useful procedure (Fig. 35–5). Because inhibition of sodium reabsorption in a given nephron segment affects electrolyte excretion in a specific manner, the nephron site at which a particular class of diuretic acts confers the relative potency to other classes of diuretics. *Clinically used diuretics are classified by their actions on specific sites:*

- Site 1 is the proximal tubule.
- Site 2 is the thick ascending limb of Henle's loop.
- Site 3 is the early distal tubule or cortical portion of the diluting segment.
- Site 4 is the late distal and early collecting tubule.

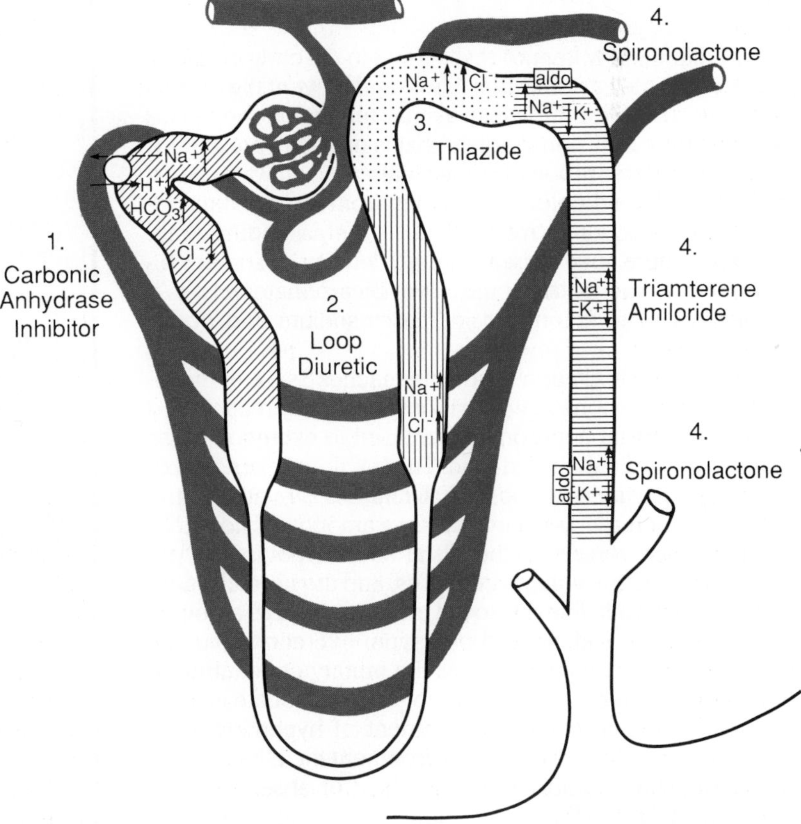

FIGURE 35–5. Sites at which different classes of diuretics act and the effect on particular electrolytes at that site. (1) Carbonic anhydrase inhibition results in a decrease in hydrogen and chloride ions and an increase in sodium and bicarbonate ions in the proximal tubule. (2) Loop diuretics result in an increase in sodium and chloride ions in the thick ascending limb. (3) Thiazides interfere with the reabsorption of sodium in the early (convoluted) distal tubule. (4) Spironolactone, triamterene, and amiloride result in increased sodium and decreased potassium concentrations in the late distal tubule.

Proximal Tubule Diuretics (Carbonic Anhydrase Inhibitors) — Site 1

The only diuretics with their major site of action on the proximal tubule are those that inhibit carbonic anhydrase; carbonic anhydrase exists both in the tubule lumen and in the cytoplasm of the cell. Although other classes of diuretics may have some proximal tubule action, their major activity lies in other nephron segments.

Acetazolamide

ACTIONS. Acetazolamide (DIAMOX) is the prototypical carbonic anhydrase inhibitor. Its mechanism of action as a diuretic can be completely accounted for by noncompetitive inhibition of renal carbonic anhydrase. When this enzyme is inhibited, there is a decreased generation of hydrogen ion to exchange for sodium and less sodium enters the tubule cell. A decrease in hydrogen ion in the lumen results in a decrease in the hydration of bicarbonate to carbonic acid and its subsequent dissociation to carbon dioxide and water. It is as carbon dioxide and water that diffusion back into the cell occurs. The bicarbonate ion itself does not readily diffuse back across the cell. It remains in the lumen and is excreted along with sodium.

CH_3CONH — S — SO_2NH_2 (thiadiazole ring, N—N)

Acetazolamide

Sodium and water not reabsorbed in the early proximal tubule reach the late proximal tubule and prevent the normal differential increase in late proximal tubule chloride. This decreases the diffusion gradient that is normally present for the passive reabsorption of sodium chloride and water. Most of the sodium and chloride escaping from the proximal tubule are subsequently reabsorbed in the ascending limb. However, there is an increase in the delivery of sodium bicarbonate to the distal tubule. Here bicarbonate acts as a nonreabsorbable anion and increases sodium and potassium excretion.

Fractional excretion of sodium reaches 3–5% of the filtered load. Bicarbonate, which is only minimally reabsorbed in the more distal nephron, is increased in excretion by as much as 30% of the filtered load. The fractional excretion of potassium may increase up to 70% and this is related to the delivery of increased sodium and large amounts of nonreabsorbable bicarbonate to the distal sodium/potassium exchange area. Urine volume increases, and the normally acid urine becomes alkaline due to the presence of large amounts of bicarbonate. Sodium and potassium excretions parallel the loss of bicarbonate, whereas the urinary concentration of chloride decreases. The excretion of bicarbonate instead of chloride leads to the development of hyperchloremic metabolic acidosis. In an acid environment the effect of carbonic anhydrase inhibitors is decreased or absent and refractoriness to the diuretic develops within a few days.

(Although thiazide diuretics also inhibit carbonic anhydrase, this is not considered the principal mechanism of their diuretic activity and their carbonic anhydrase inhibitory potencies differ from their diuretic potencies. Also, the electrolyte excretory profile observed after administration of the thiazide diuretics differs greatly from electrolyte excretion observed after the administration of carbonic anhydrase inhibitors.)

TIME COURSE OF ACTION—PHARMACOKINETICS. Acetazolamide has excellent bioavailability and reaches its peak plasma concentration within 2 hours following oral administration. It has a half-life of 13 hours and is eliminated unchanged in the urine. Because it is an organic acid diuretic, it is tightly bound to plasma proteins, undergoes negligible filtration and is secreted by the organic acid transport system.

BOX 35–1
THERAPEUTIC USES

Acetazolamide (DIAMOX) is never a "first choice" diuretic. It is chosen as a diuretic when the addition of a proximally acting agent to the therapeutic regimen is warranted. It is primarily used in patients with preexisting metabolic alkalosis, such as those with congestive heart failure who previously have been treated with more distally acting diuretics. Its proximal action is taken advantage of when it is given along with a distally acting diuretic to produce a sequential blockade.

These diuretics have been used effectively in disorders unrelated to renal function such as in the treatment of grand and petit mal epilepsy where sodium movement into cerebral spinal fluid is associated with carbonic anhydrase activity of glial and choroid plexus cells. Inhibition of this enzyme decreases sodium entry into the cerebrospinal fluid (CSF) and the rate of CSF formation.

In the eye, inhibition of carbonic anhydrase lowers the rate of aqueous humor formation by 45–60%. The decreased fluid formation decreases intraocular pressure. Acetazolamide, methazolamide, dichlorphenamide, and ethoxzolamide have been used for the treatment of wide angle and chronic glaucoma and to reduce intraocular pressure following cataract surgery. When used for these conditions the agents are given systemically because their limited lipid solubility restricts their transcorneal permeability.

The alkaline diuresis that occurs with the use of carbonic anhydrase inhibitors is taken advantage of in the treatment of overdose and poisoning with agents that are organic acids such as salicylates or phenobarbital. Intravenous administration of acetazolamide may more quickly counteract the toxicity. The production of an increased volume of alkaline urine also facilitates the renal elimination of uric acid and is sometimes useful to treat the hyperuricemia associated with gout.

The oral dose effective in humans is 250–375 mg/day. When used as a diuretic, it is given once a day or every other day. For its metabolic acidosis effects, it is given every 8 hours. For chronic simple glaucoma, 250–1000 mg is given in divided doses.

ADVERSE EFFECTS. Only a few toxic effects have been observed with carbonic anhydrase inhibitors; the most notable of these is the loss of potassium leading to hypokalemia. This occurs through the delivery of increased amounts of sodium to the distal tubule along with the nonreabsorbable anion, bicarbonate. More potassium exchanges for the increased sodium and stays with the bicarbonate anion.

In large doses acetazolamide may produce drowsiness and paresthesias. Hypersensitivity reactions are rare and when they do occur they consist of fever, skin reactions, bone marrow depression, and sulfonamidelike renal lesions. Decreases in urinary citrate may lead to calculus formation and ureteral colic. Because teratogenic effects have been demonstrated in animals, these drugs should not be used in pregnant women.

DRUG INTERACTIONS. Thyroidal iodine uptake may be depressed by acetazolamide and should be considered when a patient on acetazolamide is undergoing treatment for thyroid disorders. Alkalinization of the urine may interfere with the action of the urinary tract antiseptic methenamine. Coadministration of phenytoin has been reported to result in drug-induced osteomalacia.

Loop or High-Ceiling Diuretics—Site 2

Furosemide, Bumetanide, and Ethacrynic Acid

Loop diuretics consist of a group of compounds, dissimilar in chemical structure, but with a similar mechanism and site of action. The most commonly used loop diuretic is furosemide (LASIX and others). Two other loop diuretics about which much is known are ethacrynic acid (EDECRIN) and bumetanide (BUMEX and others). (For these and other diuretics see Table 29-5 for names and usual dosages for treatment of hypertension.)

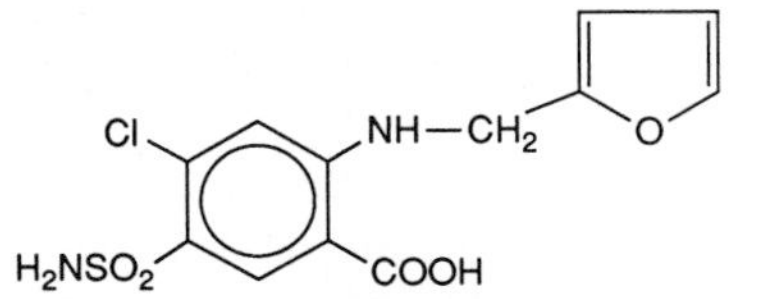

Furosemide

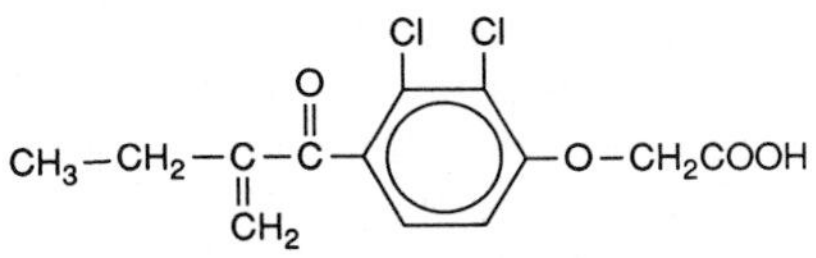

Ethacrynic acid

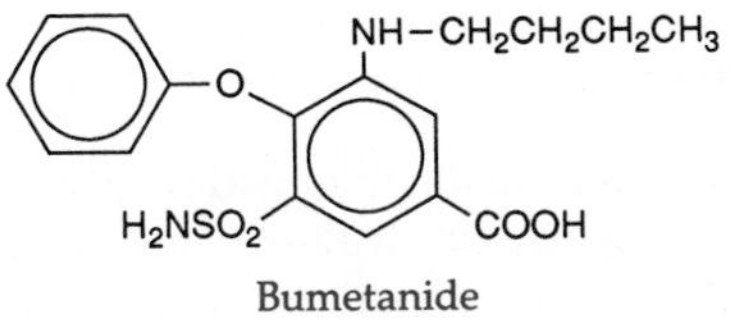

Bumetanide

ACTIONS. Loop diuretics inhibit sodium chloride reabsorption at the high-capacity site in the thick ascending limb of the loop of Henle (site 2). In view of this site of action they have the greatest potential diuretic effect of any of the classes of diuretics; they are capable of producing a diuresis that is 25% of the filtered load. They are called "loop" diuretics because they act at a site immediately distal to the loop of Henle; they are called "high ceiling" because they produce the greatest diuretic effect.

The sodium-potassium pump in the peritubular membrane moves sodium out of the cell and maintains a large electrochemical sodium gradient across the luminal membrane. This gradient provides the driving force for the cotransport of one sodium cation, one potassium cation and two chloride anions in an electroneutral process into the cell from the tubular fluid. A cotransport system implies that the individual flows of the cotransported ions are tightly coupled with each other at a fixed stoichiometry. The system has been shown to be inhibited by furosemide, bumetanide, and the cysteine adduct of ethacrynic acid, and this inhibition is strongly correlated to their diuretic effect.

Loop diuretics decrease both positive and negative free water production by inhibiting the removal of sodium chloride from the lumen, which leaves the lumen less dilute; by the same step (inhibition of the cotransport of one sodium, two chloride, one potassium), they prevent addition of sodium chloride to the interstitium, thus decreasing the osmotic force of the interstitium. The inhibition of sodium chloride reabsorption in the ascending limb delivers more salt to the early distal tubule and decreases the dilution of the urine and thereby positive free water formation. The same action decreases the osmotic gradient in the medullary portion of the kidney, which is the force for water reabsorption under the influence of antidiuretic hormone, so that less water is capable of being reabsorbed (negative free water formation). Thus, positive free water (urine dilution) and negative free water (urine concentration) are affected.

Loop diuretics produce a dose-dependent diuresis characterized by increases in the excretion of water, sodium, chloride, potassium, calcium, and magnesium. There is "washout" of the renal medulla and decreased hypertonicity of the inner zones of the kidney. Increased potassium excretion is mostly due to the increase in volume flow rate through the distal tubule and the increased delivery of sodium to the sodium/potassium exchange site.

Certain hemodynamic effects are characteristic of loop diuretics. One of these is an increase in venous capacitance. The increased renal vasodilation permits an increase in renal blood flow. The increase in renal blood flow is primarily in the inner cortical and medullary blood flows, which is important for the diuresis induced by these agents. Increased medullary flow leads to washout of medullary hypertonicity and decreases water reabsorption in the collecting duct. Evidence indicates that this is a prostaglandin-induced process. Loop diuretics can lead to increased amounts of the vasodilator PGE_2 by inhibiting the enzyme prostaglandin dehydrogenase. PGE_2 also acts directly on the medullary thick ascending limb to inhibit chloride transport.

Loop diuretics appear to interfere with tubuloglomerular feedback so that the decrease in GFR associated with increased distal delivery of fluid generally does not occur. They inhibit chloride flux into the macula densa cells and prevent the expected decrease in GFR secondary to enhanced tubular flow rate.

> **BOX 35–2**
> ## THERAPEUTIC USES
>
> Loop diuretics are commonly used in the treatment of edema of cardiac, hepatic, or renal origin. Because of their efficacy and potency, initial doses are recommended to be relatively low. Also because of their efficacy, they are sometimes useful in the early stages of renal failure, probably because of their ability to increase renal prostaglandin levels. Although these drugs are effective in renal impairment, when GFR can be as low as 2 mL/minute, higher than normal doses may be needed to achieve diuresis. In order to be effective, loop diuretics must be secreted by the proximal tubule and travel to their luminal site of action so that some degree of renal function must exist.
>
> Their rapid action and their effectiveness have made them the *drugs of choice in treatment of pulmonary edema resulting from left heart failure*. Even before the onset of diuretic action, furosemide decreases left ventricular filling pressure and increases venous capacitance. Hemodynamics seem to improve even before significant diuresis has occurred. Diuresis then contributes to a further reduction in filling pressure. Pulmonary edema is an acute situation and furosemide can be effective within 10 minutes after intravenous administration. In such treatment furosemide is given at frequent intervals so that the urine flow rate can be titrated to the desired level while avoiding excessively rapid volume depletion.
>
> The ability of these drugs to inhibit calcium reabsorption by the thick ascending limb makes them *useful in hypercalcemic crisis*. When used for this, it is necessary to replace the large urinary losses of other electrolytes, particularly sodium and chloride, during the diuresis.

ADVERSE EFFECTS. The major toxic effect of the loop diuretics is fluid and electrolyte imbalances due to excessive diuresis. The loss of electrolytes and volume contraction can lead to secondary events such as hypovolemia, hyponatremia, hypokalemia, hyperuricemia, and hyperglycemia.

Ototoxicity may occur as a result of the alteration of electrolyte composition in the inner ear. The potential for ototoxicity for the major drugs is in the order of ethacrynic acid > furosemide > bumetanide. In general, this is a reversible effect that disappears upon withdrawal of the drug. Nevertheless, permanent hearing loss has been reported with ethacrynic acid.

Hyperuricemia may be associated with contraction of plasma volume but is also attributed to the ability of loop diuretics to interfere with the excretion of uric acid by the organic acid excretory transport system. This may be a problem in patients with a predisposition to gout.

A decrease in glucose tolerance has been reported occasionally. The rationale for its occurrence is unclear but it may be associated with diuretic-induced hypokalemia or insulin activity.

DRUG INTERACTIONS. Because of the potential for ototoxicity, drugs with similar potential, such as aminoglycoside antibiotics, should not be coadministered with loop diuretics.

These organic acid drugs are significantly bound to plasma albumin and may compete for protein binding with similarly bound drugs such as warfarin and clofibrate.

Increased cephaloridine nephrotoxicity has been noted with furosemide, and careful use of cephalosporin is recommended.

PREPARATIONS AND PHARMACOKINETICS. In general, loop diuretics have a wide dosage range and maintain their efficacy in impaired renal function. They have a steep dose-response curve and a rapid onset of action. These diuretics are absorbed quickly, with peak concentrations attained within 0.5 to 2 hours. Their half-lives are approximately 1–2 hours and their onset of action is 30–90 minutes. While they are extensively bound to plasma proteins, they have strong affinity for the organic acid excretory transporter, and this accounts for their relatively short half-lives.

Furosemide is excreted unchanged in the urine by secretion in the proximal tubule, mostly within 4 hours of an oral dose. One third of ethacrynic acid is excreted in the bile and the remainder by the kidney. The urinary products of ethacrynic acid are equally divided into three fractions: unchanged drug, a cysteine conjugate, and an undetermined metabolite. It appears that the major diuretic action of ethacrynic acid is mediated through its cysteine conjugate.

Clinically, furosemide has two advantages over ethacrynic acid. It has a broader dose-response curve, which allows greater accuracy in titrating a dose to a particular patient, and there are fewer gastrointestinal side effects. Bumetanide is structurally related to furosemide and is comparable in its activity and maximal effect but is considerably more potent on a weight basis.

Other loop diuretics that have more recently reached the market and have a more prolonged action than those previously mentioned are piretanide, muzolimine, and xipamide. They differ from each other mainly in their pharmacokinetics. The potency of piretanide is intermediate to furosemide and bumetanide. Muzolimine and xipamide also have longer durations of action. Muzolimine has a half-life of approximately 13 hours, and only negligible amounts are excreted in the urine.

Indapamide (LOZOL) is similar in structure to furosemide and bumetanide but different in that it has a prolonged diuretic action. It provokes natriuresis despite renal impairment. In addition, indapamide has a vasodilator antihypertensive effect that is independent of any induced natriuresis. It is extensively metabolized, and only 5% of the unchanged drug is excreted in the urine. Indapamide is 80% bound to plasma proteins and concentrated in red blood cells.

Thiazides—Site 3

Hydrochlorothiazide and Chlorthalidone

Many compounds are available: widely used compounds include hydrochlorothiazide (SIDRIX and others) and chlorthalidone (HYGROTON and others).

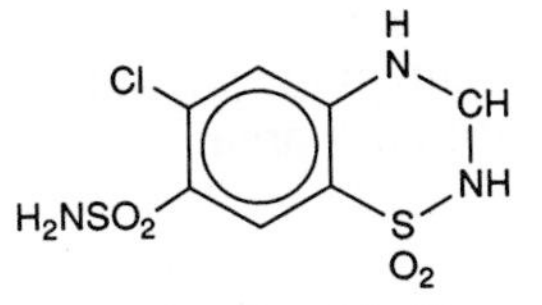

Hydrochlorothiazide

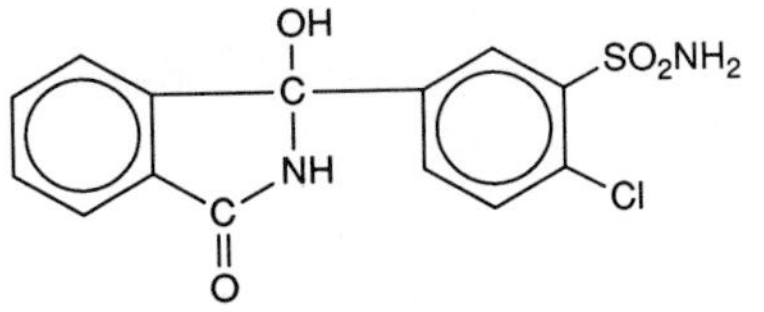

Chlorthalidone

ACTIONS. Thiazides (benzothiadiazines) inhibit the electroneutral sodium chloride cotransport in the distal convoluted tubule, which they reach after secretion in the proximal tubule. Because thiazides inhibit sodium and chloride reabsorption at this cortical diluting segment (site 3), they have a relatively moderate efficacy ("potency") and can lead to excretion of 5–8% of the filtered load.

Action at the cortical diluting site decreases the production of positive free water because sodium is prevented from being reabsorbed and remains in the tubule fluid. Thiazides do not interfere with negative free water production because they have little effect on medullary sodium reabsorption and the osmolar gradient for water reabsorption.

Their potency as diuretics is inversely related to their potency as carbonic anhydrase inhibitors, and no thiazide is equal to acetazolamide in its ability to inhibit the enzyme. The diuresis occurring with thiazide diuretics is associated with increased water, sodium, potassium, chloride, bicarbonate, and phosphate excretion.

Resistance to thiazides may develop and is associated with compensatory sodium reabsorption at a site either more distal or more proximal to that inhibited by the thiazides. Delivery of more sodium to the distal sodium/potassium exchange site stimulates sodium reabsorption there. Contraction of plasma volume as a result of continued diuresis may decrease the filtered load, and a larger proportion of filtrate will be reabsorbed in the proximal tubule and thick ascending limb.

The disadvantages of thiazide therapy include relatively low potency (*ie*, efficacy) and resistance to its effects in the presence of renal impairment. They have no diuretic value in patients with a GFR less than 25–30 mL/minute.

BOX 35-3
THERAPEUTIC USES

Congestive heart failure—thiazide diuretics are used in the management of chronic cardiac decompensation in mild to moderate congestive heart failure (in general, right heart failure). They are also effective in the treatment of edema caused by chronic hepatic or renal disease.

Hypertension—thiazide diuretics have been the mainstay of initial therapy for hypertension. Their beneficial hypotensive effects are present after the edema fluid has been removed. Administration of thiazides results in increased excretion of salt and water accompanied by weight loss and a slightly negative state of sodium balance. As treatment continues, the antihypertensive effect persists even though a return toward sodium balance occurs. With little decrease in cardiac output, there is a decrease in total peripheral resistance. Along with salt restriction, these drugs are frequently sufficient to control mild to moderate hypertension. Because this is generally long-term therapy, periodic assessment of laboratory measurements, particularly serum potassium levels, is required (see Chapter 29).

Diabetes insipidus—therapy with thiazide diuretics results in a fall in urine volume and a rise in urine osmolarity. The diuretic-induced contraction of blood volume is associated with a decrease in filtration rate and increased proximal reabsorption of filtered load. This results in a decrease in the delivery of fluid to the distal nephron. More of the filtrate is absorbed than would occur without the thiazide. The patient is not cured but a better water balance is achieved.

Hypercalcemia—thiazides are the only diuretics that increase the reabsorption of calcium. Because of this, their chronic administration has been found effective in the treatment of hypercalciuric renal stones. Thiazides increase calcium reabsorption from the lumen and prevent the build-up of calcium deposits in the tubule. Their action at the luminal side of the early distal tubule dissociates the reabsorption of sodium and calcium, decreasing sodium and increasing calcium reabsorption by a mechanism that remains unclear. Long-term treatment may lead to hypercalcemia, and serum calcium should be monitored.

Hypertensive emergencies—diazoxide (HYPERSTAT) is related chemically to thiazides and is employed in hypertensive emergencies. It is administered intravenously and rapidly lowers blood pressure. It has no carbonic anhydrase inhibitory or diuretic effect. On the contrary, its use frequently leads to fluid retention (see Chapter 29).

ADVERSE EFFECTS. *As with all diuretics that act proximal to the distal tubule site for sodium/potassium exchange, the development of hypokalemia is a major risk.* An increase in sodium reaching this segment is the main cause of potassium loss in the urine. Carbonic anhydrase activity is associated with the thiazides, which contributes to the kaluresis through the presence of increased bicarbonate in the distal tubule acting as a nonreabsorbable anion. However, inhibition of carbonic anhydrase is variable and not the main mechanism for potassium loss. A clearly dangerous situation occurs when therapy includes cardiac glycosides; diuretic-induced hypokalemia can sensitize the heart to digitalis-induced arrhythmias. Kaluresis may also result in metabolic alkalosis.

Chronic administration of thiazide diuretics can result in hyperuricemia. Like uric acid, thiazides occupy the organic acid transport system, and competition may result in hyperuricemia. In addition, contraction of plasma volume may also serve to increase uric acid reabsorption in the proximal tubule.

The decrease in calcium excretion, although beneficial in one regard, requires guarding against the development of hypercalcemia and its attendant serious side effects. In this regard, thiazides are unlike most of the other diuretics, which cause an increase in calcium excretion.

Although hyperlipidemia and hyperglycemia have been reported during thiazide therapy, such increases are relatively small and their clinical significance controversial.

PREPARATIONS AND PHARMACOKINETICS. Although many structural variations in thiazide diuretics exist, they are all capable of producing the same maximal effect and thus have the same intrinsic activity. If one thiazide is not effective, it is unlikely another one will be.

Hydrochlorothiazide (ESIDRIX, HYDRODIURIL, ORETIC) is the prototypical short-acting *thiazide, and chlorthalidone* is the prototypical long-acting agent. Thiazides begin to act in 1–2 hours. They vary widely in their duration of action and in their plasma half-lives. Differences appear to be proportional to plasma protein binding and the degree of reabsorption in the renal tubule. The half-lives of bendrofluazide, hydrochlorothiazide, hydroflumethiazide, and polythiazide are 3, 10, 17, and 26 hours, respectively. Most compounds are rapidly excreted by the kidneys within 3–6 hours after oral administration.

The various thiazides differ in their degree of metabolism. Hydrochlorothiazide is excreted unchanged, whereas polythiazide is metabolized extensively.

Thiazidelike Agents

Quinazolinones (quinethazone, metolazone, chlorthalidone) act in the same segment of the nephron as the thiazides although they are structurally different. Their activity as diuretics and their electrolyte excretion profile are similar to the thiazides. Quinethazone is orally active within 2 hours with an 18–24-hour duration of action.

Chlorthalidone is similar to thiazide diuretics except for its prolonged half-life. Peak plasma concentrations occur in 2–4 hours. Its prolonged half-life of several days has been attributed to its strong binding to red blood cells. It is about 70 times more potent than hydrochlorothiazide in inhibiting carbonic anhydrase, and in higher doses it increases renal excretion of bicarbonate. It is excreted mainly unchanged by the kidney.

The nonthiazide agent **metolazone** (DIULO, ZAROXOLYN, MYKROX) acts at the same site as the thiazides in the distal nephron. Metolazone is long-acting and retains its effect in renal impairment (as does indapamide). It also has a minor proximal tubule effect on phosphate-linked sodium reabsorption that may be useful in sequential blockade. Metolazone has an onset of action of 1 hour and a duration of action similar to quinethazone. It has been classified as both a loop diuretic and a thiazide diuretic.

Potassium-Sparing Diuretics—Site 4

Spironolactone, Triamterene, and Amiloride

ACTIONS. Their mechanism of action is to inhibit the distal sodium/potassium exchange (site 4), resulting in an increase in the excretion of up to 2–3% of filtered sodium and chloride inasmuch as only a small amount of water and solutes is delivered to this area.

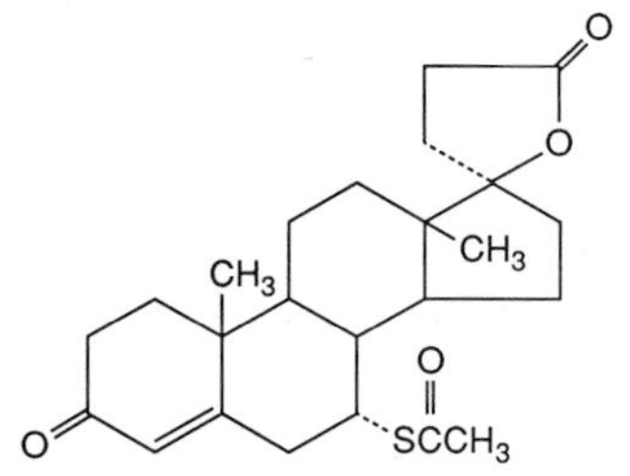

Spironolactone

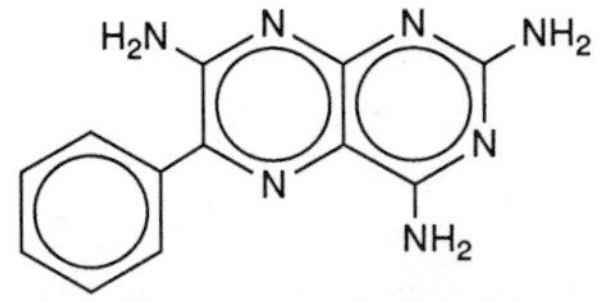

Triamterene

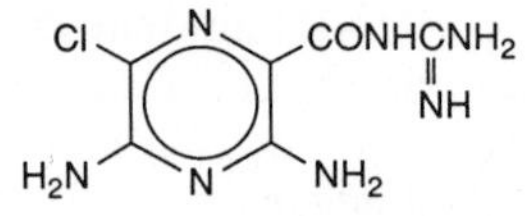

Amiloride

This class is divided into two categories, depending on their effectiveness in the presence of aldosterone. A portion of the sodium/potassium exchange in the distal tubule is aldosterone-controlled; competitive antagonism of aldosterone results in inhibition of the exchange. The major drug acting as an antagonist of aldosterone is spironolactone (ALDACTONE). The aldosterone-independent sodium/potassium exchange is interfered with by agents that directly block uptake of sodium into the distal tubule cell; the two major drugs in this category are triamterene (DYRENIUM) and amiloride (MIDAMOR).

Spironolactone is a competitive antagonist for the aldosterone receptor, a soluble cytoplasmic protein in the cortical collecting tubules. Binding of spironolactone to the receptor prevents it from assuming its active conformation. The subsequent biochemical chain of events leading to the synthesis of physiologically active transport proteins is arrested. Its metabolite, canrinone, is also an active antagonist of aldosterone. Spironolactone is effective when mineralocorticoid activity is high but has little activity in the absence of aldosterone. Because it is a competitive inhibitor, its action is overcome by higher concentrations of aldosterone. It is not effective in adrenalectomized patients or in individuals on a high-sodium diet. Calcium excretion is increased through a direct effect of aldosterone on tubular transport.

Both amiloride and triamterene act on the distal tubule at an aldosterone-independent site to inhibit sodium/potassium exchange that occurs in response to a voltage-dependent process. Triamterene is effective from the peritubular side and irreversibly inhibits the transbasolateral potential difference in the collecting duct. Amiloride acts at the luminal surface of the tubule cell and reversibly inhibits transluminal potential difference in the distal tubule and collecting duct resulting in a decrease in sodium permeability and a natriuresis without potassium loss. There is little if any loss of potassium.

A slight alkalinization of the urine caused by the inhibition of hydrogen ion secretion in the distal tubule occurs with the use of these diuretics. The mechanism for this inhibition is unknown although it is known that these compounds do not inhibit carbonic anhydrase.

> **BOX 35–4**
> **THERAPEUTIC USES**
>
> Although potassium-sparing diuretics may be used alone, their ability to protect against potassium loss has made them beneficial as adjunct therapy with other, more effective, diuretics. These agents conserve both hydrogen and potassium and so tend to counteract the metabolic alkalosis obtained when sodium and potassium are excreted with chloride (as with the loop diuretics).
>
> Spironolactone has been found to be effective in the treatment of primary aldosteronism. It may be useful in the treatment of heart failure because hyperaldosteronism is commonly seen in this condition.

ADVERSE EFFECTS. Chronic use of this class of diuretic has the potential to produce *hyper*kalemia; however, it is not a common occurrence.

Although spironolactone was once used widely for the treatment of hypertension, it has lost popularity because of its side effects, including hyperkalemia and gynecomastia; breast cancer and fibroadenomas have been reported in a few male patients during and after spironolactone therapy, but a cause-effect relationship has not been established (Stierer et al, 1990). Spironolactone, triamterene, and amiloride have the potential to induce hyperchloremic acidosis.

PREPARATIONS AND PHARMACOKINETICS. Spironolactone, which begins to act in 8 hours, is almost wholly metabolized to canrenone and/or canrenoate, which are active, and its overall effect extends over several days. The metabolites have a plasma half-life of 17–22 hours, and any change in dosage will not reach a peak effect for 3–4 days.

Both triamterene and amiloride have considerably shorter half-lives than spironolactone. Triamterene has an onset of action within 2 hours and a half-life of 2–4 hours. Thus, there is a need for multiple daily doses. Although the p-hydroxy metabolite of triamterene is pharmacologically active, the sulfate ester of the metabolite accounts for most of the diuretic activity. Most of the dose excreted is the active metabolite.

Amiloride is pharmacologically similar to triamterene but is a stronger base and more water soluble than triamterene. It is secreted into the proximal tubule fluid by the organic base pathway, and drugs that are organic bases may interfere with its excretion. After oral administration, only 20% of amiloride is absorbed and ultimately excreted unchanged by the kidney. Its half-life and peak are both at approximately 6 hours, with a duration of less than 24 hours. Its use is associated with a moderate increase in urinary pH.

DRUG INTERACTIONS. None of these agents (amiloride, triamterene, and spironolactone) should be prescribed together because this combination therapy has been observed to produce an unexpectedly high degree of hyperkalemia.

Osmotic Diuretics

Mannitol

The mechanism of action of osmotic diuretics is to contribute nonabsorbable osmolar particles to the tubular fluid and obligate water to remain with the extra solute. Thus, substances that act as diuretics by contributing to the osmotic force of the tubule fluid have no specific cellular receptor. The presence of additional solute and the resulting increase in tubular fluid flow rate interfere with reabsorption of filtrate and with normal urinary concentration, resulting in the excretion of large amounts of solute and water.

> **BOX 35–5**
> **THERAPEUTIC USES**
>
> The main use of osmotic diuresis is related to increased tubule flow rate and not mobilization of generalized edema fluid. These diuretics are used to prevent acute renal failure, and this is a clear and important indication. When the GFR falls, there is a more complete reabsorption of tubular fluid, which may lead to anuria. During surgical procedures where a large loss of blood is anticipated, patients may be primed with intravenous fluids and mannitol to maintain a diuresis throughout the surgery and during the immediate postoperative period. Maintenance of tubule flow also prevents precipitation of toxins in the kidney. Toxins can reach very high concentrations in the tubules. A decreased tubular fluid volume favors the precipitation of compounds with low solubility and this may cause physical damage. In drug overdosage, in which the kidney is the major route of elimination, increasing urine flow rate will increase excretion of the drug.
>
> Osmotic agents are not used therapeutically for the mobilization of edema fluid associated with congestive heart failure. Addition of osmolar particles to the plasma may contribute to the edema rather than alleviate it, and expansion of the extracellular fluid is an undesirable hazard.
>
> The contribution of mannitol to the extracellular fluid compartment makes it useful in conditions which require dehydration of cells. Intraocular and intracranial pressure are alleviated by the use of mannitol. Water is drawn toward the osmotically active solute in the plasma.

Osmotic diuretics are given intravenously and contribute to the osmolality of the plasma. Because they are freely filterable at the glomerulus and undergo limited reabsorption, they also contribute to the osmolality of the tubular fluid and interfere with reabsorption throughout the nephron. While sodium and water reabsorption is inhibited in the proximal tubule, there is also a major effect in the thick ascending limb. In part this latter action may be attributed to a decrease in the osmolar solute concentration of the medulla with a concomitant decrease in water reabsorption from the thin ascending limb of Henle's loop.

Mannitol (OSMITROL) is the most commonly used osmotic diuretic. It is a metabolically inert hexose sugar that is poorly permeant into cells. Administration of isotonic or hypertonic solutions of mannitol result in increased total renal plasma flow as well as medullary and papillary plasma flow. Urine flow increases as do excretions of sodium, potassium, chloride, bicarbonate, calcium, and magnesium.

ADVERSE EFFECTS. Administration of osmolar solutes may contribute to extracellular osmolality and will be accompanied by expansion of the extracellular fluid volume. In a patient with congestive heart failure, this is hazardous and contraindicated. Mannitol infusion should be terminated if a patient develops signs of progressive renal failure, heart failure, or pulmonary congestion. Otherwise, headache, nausea, and vomiting are relatively common complaints.

PREPARATIONS AND PHARMACOKINETICS. Mannitol is available for intravenous administration in concentrations of 5–25%. The adult dose for diuresis ranges from 50–200 g over a 24-hour infusion period. When used for the prevention of acute renal failure during surgery or for the treatment of oliguria, the total adult dose is 50–100g.

Other Diuretics

Xanthines

Xanthines (theobromine, caffeine, and theophylline) are the most common over-the-counter diuretics and are weak compared with the thiazides. Their major mechanism of action is unclear. It has been demonstrated that they have both a hemodynamic and tubular effect. Xanthines have a cardiac stimulatory effect and produce renal arteriolar vasodilation leading to increases in RBF and GFR. They also decrease sodium and chloride reabsorption at the level of the tubule, although the exact site is not known. Theophylline is commonly used as a bronchodilator, and the coexistence of its diuretic action should be kept in mind.

Aquaretics

Aquaretics represent a class of diuretics infrequently discussed but that may have a use in diseases associated with abnormal vasopressin activity. They are antagonists of the vasopressin (V_2) receptor and interfere with water reabsorption. *Decinine*, an alkaloid extracted from the *Lythraceae* plant family and the antibiotic *demeclocycline* are examples.

Combination Therapy

The ability of different classes of diuretics to produce a diuresis through actions at different nephron segments provides the rationale for effective and appropriate combination therapy. Therapy based on the principle of sequential blockade is frequently useful when a patient develops resistance to one diuretic or when it is desirable to counteract potassium loss by adding a site 4–acting drug.

A common combination of diuretic agents is that of site 2– or 3–acting agents with a site 4–acting agent. In this way the common side effect of loop and thiazide diuretics, potassium loss, may be avoided. The combination of diuretics that act at sites 2 and 3 also produces additive diuretic effects.

The site 1–acting diuretic, acetazolamide, is given in combination with loop diuretics in patients refractory to the latter. It is thought that refractoriness to loop diuresis is due to avid proximal tubule reabsorption of solute. This compensatory reabsorption of filtered solute results in the delivery of only small amounts of sodium chloride to the more distal segments and thus little diuresis. The addition of acetazolamide to inhibit proximal reabsorption is thought to "flush" the solute load to the loop of Henle, where its reabsorption can be blocked by the loop diuretic with a resulting significant natriuresis.

Particular Ions Affected by Diuretic Therapy—Potential Drug Interactions

Sodium

Diuretic-induced hyponatremia, although usually mild and clinically innocuous, is occasionally severe. Impaired renal conservation of sodium can be associated with chronic administration of diuretics. Reduced delivery of filtrate to the diluting sites is caused by volume depletion–induced reductions in GFR and stimulation of isotonic proximal tubule reabsorption.

Hyponatremia is a serious situation in the presence of diuretics. *Drugs with the potential to induce hyponatremia include drugs that:*

- Stimulate thirst, such as antihistamines, anticholinergics, phenothiazines, butyrophenones, thioxanthene derivatives, tricyclic antidepressants
- Stimulate antidiuretic hormone release, such as acetylcholine, barbiturates, carbamazepine, clofibrate, isoprenaline, morphine, nicotine, and vincristine
- Enhance antidiuretic hormonelike actions—chlorpropamide, tolbutamide, phenformin, oxytocin, nonsteroidal anti-inflammatory drugs, and paracetamol
- Impair renal dilution—acting by unknown mechanisms, such as cyclophosphamide, amitriptyline, thiothixene, fluphenazine, monoamine oxidase inhibitors, and adrenocorticotropic hormone

Potassium

Potassium loss in the urine is an inevitable consequence of effective action by loop and thiazide diuretics that increase flow rate and deliver more sodium to the distal nephron. In addition, contraction of extracellular fluid volume may cause secondary hyperaldosteronism. Potassium depletion can interfere with renal tubular function, impair glucose tolerance and, in severe cases, depress force of skeletal muscle contraction. Considerable controversy exists as to whether treatment is indicated for the typically mild hypokalemia (serum K = 3.0 - 3.5 mEq/L) that occurs with diuretic therapy. Extracellular hypokalemia can exist with little change in intracellular potassium concentrations. When hypokalemia requires treatment, dietary potassium, potassium supplements, or a potassium-sparing agent is added. Most table salt substitutes contain potassium.

Certain patients are at particular risk if not treated for hypokalemia, including those:

- With high circulating aldosterone levels (already excreting too much potassium)
- On digoxin (low potassium potentiates the arrhythmogenic action of the cardiac glycosides)
- On high doses of long-acting diuretics (already potassium depleted)
- Receiving coincidental therapy with corticosteroids, carbenoxolone, or potent purgatives (drugs that further contribute to the hypokalemia)
- Who are diabetic (hypokalemia impairs glucose tolerance)
- Who are elderly or chronically sick (particularly susceptible to the effects of low potassium)

Magnesium

The thiazides and loop diuretics also enhance the excretion of magnesium, whereas the potassium-sparing agents conserve this ion. Magnesium depletion is common during long-term diuretic therapy, especially when loop diuretics are used.

Calcium

Significant amounts of calcium are ordinarily reabsorbed in the ascending limb of the loop of Henle, and loop diuretics inhibit this. Thiazides retain calcium and have been used to prevent the formation of recurrent renal calculi and to prevent osteoporosis. Spironolactone and amiloride have been shown to increase urinary calcium.

Uric Acid

Up to 65 - 70% of patients treated with diuretics develop hyperuricemia. However, clinical gout rarely occurs and then only in susceptible individuals.

Diuretic Resistance

Resistance to a particular diuretic therapy may develop because of an impaired delivery to its site of action or because of a decreased delivery of sodium to the site of action. Decreased sodium delivery may be associated with a decreased GFR and/or increased proximal sodium reabsorption. Increased reabsorption of solute at sites distal to the site of action of the diuretic may occur. Impaired secretion of diuretics into the renal tubular lumen from blood may also result in reduced diuretic effect.

Salt Restriction

Salt ingestion may impede therapy. During diuretic therapy patients not unusually develop salt hunger and increase salt intake, blunting the diuretic or antihypertensive effect of the drug. If sodium intake is too high, diuretics may achieve their pharmacological effect, increased excretion of salt and water, without affecting a weight loss. Thus it is necessary to control salt intake. A salt-restricted diet should be prescribed for patients on diuretics. A recommended diet is 100 mEq/day, which amounts to about 6 g/day. A normal salt diet is about 9 g/day.

REFERENCES

Abuelo JG: Renal failure caused by chemicals, foods, plants, animal venoms, and misuse of drugs: An overview. Arch Intern Med 150: 505-510, 1990.

Eknoyan G, Martinez-Maldonado M (eds): The Physiological Basis of Diuretic Therapy in Clinical Medicine. San Diego: Grune & Stratton, 1986.

Koushanpour E, Kriz W: Renal Physiology—Principles, Structure, and Function, 2nd ed. New York: Springer-Verlag, 1986.

Puschett JB, Greenberg A: Diuretics IV: Chemistry, Pharmacology and Clinical Applications. Proceedings of Fourth International Conference on Diuretics. The Netherlands: Elsevier Science Publications, 1993.

Puschett JB, Winaver J: Effects of diuretics on renal function. *In* Windhager EE (ed): Handbook of Physiology, Section 8, Vol II. Renal Physiology. London: Oxford University Press, 1992.

Stierer M, Spoula H, Rosen HR: Mammakarzinom beim Mann—Eine retrospektive Analyse von 15 Fallen. Ourologie 13:128-131, 1990.

Suki WN, Eknoyan G: Physiology of diuretic action. *In* Seldin DW, Giebisch G (eds): The Kidney. Physiology and Pathophysiology. New York: Raven Press, 1992.

Weiner IM: Diuretics and other agents employed in the mobilization of edema fluid. *In* Gilman AG, Rall TW, Nies AS, Taylor P (eds): Goodman and Gilman's The Pharmacological Basis of Therapeutics, 743-748. New York: Pergamon Press, 1990.

PART VIII

CHEMOTHERAPY

36 Principles of Anti-infective Chemotherapy

Thomas R. Beam, Jr., deceased

USE OF ANTIMICROBIAL DRUGS

Anti-infective drug products may be used for the prevention of infections, the empirical treatment of suspected infections, or the treatment of a known pathogen recovered from a specific body site. Although it is preferable to have a target micro-organism and laboratory-defined susceptibility determinations, the majority of prescriptions for antimicrobials are written in the absence of such information. Therefore, it is important to know the composition of the normal body microbial flora and the likely organisms that colonize and infect hospitalized patients.

Prophylaxis

The first use of antimicrobials is to prevent infections, or prophylaxis. Prophylaxis may be divided into four categories:

1. Surgical
2. Medical
3. Primary
4. Secondary

Surgical

The rationale for surgical prophylaxis was established by Burke using a guinea pig model of wound infection. Results of these studies are summarized in Figure 36 – 1. In an experimental model, multiple surgical incisions were made on the abdomens of guinea pigs. Wounds were contaminated with staphylococci, washed, and then sutured closed. Positive (heat-killed bacteria) and negative (sterile saline) controls were included. An antibiotic was administered before, during, or after surgery. The greatest efficacy was obtained when antibiotics were given shortly before surgery. No benefit was conferred when antibiotics were given 4 or more hours after the incision was created. These results have been confirmed in clinical (human) trials.

However, appropriate prophylactic antibiotics are only one component of many factors that determine wound infection rates. Other factors include:

Patient circumstances
- Age over 60 years
- Nutritional status
- Diabetes mellitus
- Malignancy
- Immunosuppressive chemotherapy or radiotherapy
- Corticosteroids
- Underlying medical conditions

Operative circumstances
- Duration of preoperative hospitalization
- Use of antibacterial soaps
- Elective versus emergency surgery
- Timing of hair removal
- Use of drains
- Implantation of foreign bodies
- Reoperation
- Duration of surgical procedure

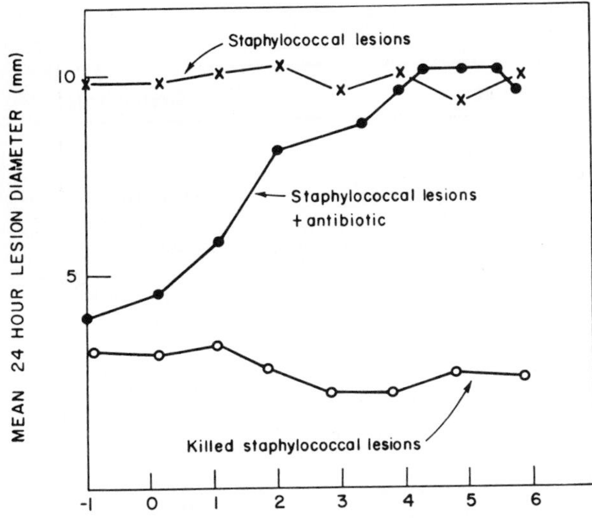

FIGURE 36–1. Active control (infected) lesions showed about 10 mm of induration in the absence of antibiotic. Negative control (killed staphylococci) showed about 3 mm of induration. The effect of antibiotic is progressively reduced after surgery begins, reaching control values at 4 hours. The most effective time of administration is 1 hour before surgery begins. (From Burke JF: The effective period of preventive antibiotic action in experimental incisions and dermal lesions. Surgery 50:162, 1961.)

Wound classification
- Clean
- Clean with prosthesis
- Clean-contaminated
- Contaminated
- Dirty

The most important of these factors in determining the potential for infectious complications of surgery is the wound classification. Prophylactic antibiotics cannot be provided to patients with contaminated or dirty wounds because bacterial contamination has occurred prior to the surgical procedure. Prophylactic antibiotics can be given to patients undergoing clean or clean-contaminated surgical procedures because the drug employed can achieve concentrations in excess of the amount needed to inhibit bacterial growth before any contamination occurs. Specific recommendations for common surgical procedures are provided in Table 36–1.

Medical

Medical prophylaxis is provided to prevent infections in clinical situations that are perceived to be high-risk. Both childhood and adult infections may be targeted. Medical conditions warranting prophylactic use of antibiotics are listed in Table 36–2.

Primary and Secondary

Primary prophylaxis for medical conditions prevents the original infection from occurring. This use of antibiotics can either prevent the organism from colonizing the host or prevent a colonizing organism from invading deeper tissues. All surgical prophylaxis is primary prophylaxis.

Secondary prophylaxis is directed against an organism that has invaded the host but has not yet caused clinically apparent disease. The best example of this use of antibiotics is prevention of active tuberculosis after an individual is known to be infected, as demonstrated by a positive purified protein derivative (tuberculin) skin test.

Presumptive Therapy

Many patients show clinical manifestations of infection. Symptoms may include fever, chills, sweats, loss of appetite, and a sense of malaise. Signs may include erythema, edema, pain, and warmth at a specific body site such as the skin. Supporting laboratory evidence may include leukocytosis, elevated gamma globulin titers, positive C-reactive protein, and increased erythrocyte sedimentation rate. Cultures of the site suspected to be infected may identify no pathogen or normal body flora. An antibiotic prescription should be written to treat the suspected infection (empiric therapy). Several questions help the physician choose a drug that is likely to be successful.

- Where was the infection acquired?
- What is the organ system involved in the infection?
- What is the normal body flora at the presumed site of infection?
- If infection is caused by organisms other than those that are part of the normal flora, what are these organisms likely to be?
- What is the expected susceptibility pattern for the presumed pathogen?
- What is the usual course of therapy for an infection at the body site?
- How sick is the patient?

Determining the place of acquisition of infection is critically important. The first distinction that must be made is community-acquired versus hospital-acquired infection. If community-acquired infection is suspected, questions should be asked about travel history, exposure to pathogens at the work site, and illness among family members or other close contacts. Resistance to antimicrobials is more likely to occur among organisms acquired in the hospital setting.

The organ system involved is defined by the constellation of signs and symptoms. If no localizing features to the complaints are present, then the blood stream is presumed to be infected.

If the site of infection is normally sterile (*eg*, urine), then a priority list of likely pathogens must be conceptualized. In the urinary tract, *Escherichia coli* is by far the most likely causative organism. If the site of infection has a normal flora (*eg*, the respiratory tract), then the most likely pathogens are those of the normal flora (*Streptococcus pneumoniae, Haemophilus influenzae, Moraxella catarrhalis*). Acquisition of an exogenous organism is less likely, but the likelihood can be influenced by time of year, prevalence of the pathogen in the community, and illness among family members. For example, influenza virus infection usually appears between December and March, is detected by public health officials, and affects school-age children before adults.

The susceptibility patterns of micro-organisms should be known by physicians or other health care providers

TABLE 36–1. Common Surgical Procedures and Recommended Prophylactic Antibiotics

Type of Surgery	Documented Need	Drug of Choice	Alternative(s)
Clean Surgery			
CARDIAC			
Prosthetic valve	No	Cefazolin or vancomycin	Nafcillin
Coronary artery bypass	Equivocal	Cefazolin	Vancomycin
Pacemaker implantation	No	None	None
ORTHOPEDIC			
With prosthesis	No	Cefazolin	Vancomycin
Without prosthesis	No	None	None
VASCULAR			
Involving groin	Yes	Cefazolin	Cefuroxime
Abdominal aorta	Equivocal	Cefazolin	Cefuroxime
Other vascular	No	None	None
UROLOGICAL			
Orchiectomy	No	None	None
Anterior cystourethropexy	No	None	None
Varicocelectomy	No	None	None
Insertion of prosthesis	Equivocal	Cefazolin	TMP/SMZ
Clean-Contaminated Surgery			
HEAD AND NECK WITH TRANSECTION OF OROPHARYNX	Yes	Cefazolin	Cefotaxime or cefoperazone
THORACIC (NONCARDIAC)	Equivocal	Cefazolin	
GASTROINTESTINAL			
Gastric, small intestine	Yes	Cefazolin	Cefoxitin or cefotetan
Biliary tract	High risk†	Cefazolin	Cefoxitin or cefotetan
Appendix	Equivocal	Cefoxitin or cefotetan	Clindamycin and gentamicin
Colorectal	Yes	Oral erythromycin and neomycin	Cefoxitin or cefotetan
GYNECOLOGICAL			
Vaginal hysterectomy	Yes	Cefazolin	Cefoxitin or cefotetan
Abdominal hysterectomy	Yes	Cefazolin	Cefoxitin or cefotetan
Cesarean section	Yes	Cefazolin	Cefoxitin or cefotetan
UROLOGICAL			
Ureterolithotomy	High risk‡	Cefazolin	TMP/SMZ
Pyelolithotomy	High risk	Cefazolin	TMP/SMZ
Nephrectomy	High risk	Cefazolin	TMP/SMZ
Partial cystectomy	High risk	Cefazolin	TMP/SMZ
Cystotomy	High risk	Cefazolin	TMP/SMZ

†High risk (biliary tract)—age over 70, past or present jaundice, previous biliary surgery, sepsis within 1 week, common bile duct pathology, diabetes, obesity.
‡High risk (urological)—elderly, malnourished, debilitated, diabetic, immunosuppressed, prosthetic device.
TMP/SMZ—trimethoprim/sulfamethoxazole.

writing prescriptions for antimicrobials. For community-acquired infections, the patterns of resistance are relatively stable over time. For hospital-acquired pathogens, continual change occurs. Resistance to antimicrobials is monitored by the microbiology laboratory, reported on a quarterly basis to the physician staff, and made available on laboratory report forms, computer networks, or pocket-sized cards.

The definition of an appropriate course of antimicrobial therapy is usually arbitrary. Few studies have been performed to determine specifically how long antibiotics should be given to assure a successful outcome. In general, antibiotics are continued until fever has abated for at least 48 hours and the signs and symptoms of infection have improved but not necessarily resolved. Laboratory values should be tending toward the normal range. The patient essentially should be returned to his or her pre-existing status. The degree or severity of illness generates two concerns. The first is choice of drugs. The second is dosing (see Pharmacokinetics and Dosing of Antimicrobials). So far as choice of drugs is concerned, the sicker the patient, the broader the spectrum of antimicrobial therapy. In essence, the aim is to provide activity against most possible pathogens

BOX 36–1

SELECTED GUIDELINES FOR DURATION OF TREATMENT BY SITE OF INFECTION

Urinary Tract	
Uncomplicated (healthy women)	3 days
Complicated (men, kidney infection)	14 days
Respiratory Tract	
Pharyngitis, sinusitis, otitis	7–10 days
Bronchitis	7–10 days
Pneumonia	10–14 days
Skin, Skin Structure	
Uncomplicated (cellulitis)	7–10 days
Complicated (pressure sore)	10–14 days
Bone and Joint	
Arthritis, bursitis	21 days
Osteomyelitis	4–6 weeks

TABLE 36–2. Prophylaxis Against Infection for Medical Diseases

Condition	Proven Efficacy	Agent of Choice	Alternative(s)
Childhood Illnesses			
Ophthalmia neonatorum—standard	Yes	Erythromycin or tetracycline ointment	Silver nitrate
Ophthalmia neonatorum—high risk	Yes	Penicillin G	Cefotaxime
Pertussis	Equivocal	Erythromycin	TMP/SMZ*
Recurrent otitis media	Equivocal	Sulfisoxazole	Amoxicillin, TMP/SMZ
Haemophilus influenzae	Equivocal	Rifampin*	None
Splenectomy; pneumococcal infection	Equivocal	Penicillin V	Amoxicillin*
Rheumatic fever	Yes	Benzathine penicillin G	Sulfadiazine, penicillin V
Children and Adults			
Meningococcal disease	Yes	Rifampin	Sulfadiazine, minocycline
Recurrent urinary tract infections in females	Yes	TMP/SMZ	Nitrofurantoin, trimethoprim
Influenza A	Yes	Amantadine*	None
Bacterial endocarditis	No	Amoxicillin, ampicillin plus gentamicin, or vancomycin with or without gentamicin†	Erythromycin, clindamycin
Adults			
Traveler's diarrhea	Equivocal	TMP/SMZ	Ciprofloxacin, doxycycline, PEPTO-BISMOL
Malaria	Yes	Chloroquine or mefloquine	Primaquine, FANSIDAR
Contact of person with STD	Equivocal	Variable—depends on STD	Variable

*Vaccination recommended when clinically appropriate.
†Drug depends on type of procedure to be performed.
STD = sexually transmitted disease; TMP/SMZ = trimethoprim/sulfamethoxazole.

until culture results become available. If cultures do not identify a causative organism, then therapy is continued based on clinical response. If the patient has not had a favorable response within 48–72 hours, additional antimicrobial drugs are usually provided.

Defined Therapy

For defined therapy, the pathogen is identified, the antimicrobial susceptibility pattern is known, and the site of infection is established. Antimicrobial therapy should be targeted to the organism using the most active, least toxic drug available. Cost also should be considered in making the choice because often several drugs from which to choose are available. The duration of therapy should usually follow the general guidelines previously listed. However, specific courses of therapy are defined for certain organisms. For example, the treatment of pneumonia caused by *Legionella pneumophila* is 21 days.

Another quality of the drug chosen should be a relatively narrow spectrum of activity. Those antimicrobial drugs with the broadest range of activity are also associated with the greatest risk of superinfection. *Superinfection* means acquisition of an organism resistant to the current or previously prescribed antimicrobial, which results in a clinical worsening of the patient. The new infection may develop at the same site as the original infection or at a new site. The new organism may be of the same type (bacterial superinfection) or a new type (*eg*, fungal superinfection).

A third quality of the drug chosen should be its capability to kill (cidal) rather than to suppress (static) the pathogen. Cidal activity is important in treating infections located in body sites with compromised host defenses. Such sites include heart valves (endocarditis), the central nervous system (meningitis, encephalitis), and bone (osteomyelitis). The distinction between static and cidal activity is concentration-dependent and organism-specific. For example, chloramphenicol is bacteriostatic against Gram-negative bacilli such as *E. coli* but bactericidal against Gram-positive cocci such as *S. pneumoniae.*

The final consideration should be the need for more than one drug to kill the pathogen. Drugs are combined to gain greater antibacterial effect than that provided by a single drug (*ie*, synergy). Examples are ampicillin plus gentamicin to treat enterococcal infections or piperacillin plus tobramycin to treat pseudomonas infections. Alternatively, drugs are combined to minimize the risk of resistance developing while the patient is receiving treatment. Isoniazid plus rifampin (with or without pyrazinamide and ethambutol) is used to avoid resistance when treating tuberculosis.

PHARMACOKINETICS AND DOSING OF ANTIMICROBIALS

Severity of Infection

Early dosing schemes endorsed one principle: more is better. Drugs that have a high therapeutic index, such as penicillin, could be given in large amounts, at more frequent intervals, or both without producing significant adverse effects. Cephalosporins share a similar safety profile.

However, the discovery of aminoglycoside antimicrobials such as gentamicin and glycopeptide antibiotics, including vancomycin, taught physicians that pharmacokinetic principles are clinically relevant. In particular, functional status of the organ that excretes the drug is critically important in determining the dose and dosing interval.

Pharmacokinetic Principles

Clinical pharmacokinetics is the study of drug absorption, distribution, metabolism, and excretion over time in an individual patient. All recently marketed anti-infective drugs and all antimicrobials in development have had or will have their pharmacokinetic properties determined before marketing approval is granted by the Food and Drug Administration. New drugs are also studied in clinical settings that reflect the patient population likely to be treated with the product. These requirements were not in place more than 15 years ago. Therefore, less pharmacokinetic information is available about older antimicrobials unless clinical problems developed. The current objectives of clinical trials are to establish a dose and a dosing regimen that maximize efficacy, minimize toxicity, and are appropriate to the patients likely to be treated with the drug.

Pharmacodynamics is the study of drug concentration at the receptor site and the pharmacologic response it produces. For anti-infective drugs, the pathogen is the receptor, and the objective is either to inhibit growth or to kill the microbe while exerting minimal effect on the host.

Different antimicrobials inhibit or kill bacteria by different mechanisms. For β-lactam antimicrobials (penicillins, cephalosporins), the critical variable of effectiveness is the time above the minimum inhibitory concentration (MIC) or minimum bactericidal concentration. These drugs may best be delivered by continuous infusion, targeting a serum or tissue concentration in excess of the MIC of the pathogen for each patient. However, no practical way exists to accomplish this at the present time.

Aminoglycoside antibacterial activity is dose-dependent, and the drugs exert a postantibiotic effect. That is, although the concentration of aminoglycoside drops below the amount necessary to inhibit bacterial growth, no growth occurs. In contrast to β-lactam antibiotics, time above the MIC is not important. β-Lactam antibiotics are usually administered two to four times each day, but for an aminoglycoside, once-a-day dosing produces similar efficacy and less toxicity.

Irrespective of the dosing schedule, drugs with a low therapeutic index should be monitored by determining the concentration in serum at defined points in time. These are the serum *peak* and *trough concentrations*. The peak is defined as the serum concentration 30 minutes after intravenous or 60 minutes after intramuscular administration. The trough is the serum concentration measured within the 30 minutes prior to administering the next dose of drug. The mechanism for determining aminoglycoside dosing is summarized in Table 36–3. An initial loading dose is followed by maintenance doses given at intervals based on age, sex, and renal function. Further refinements are guided by the peak and trough serum concentrations, which should be obtained at least every 3 days.

TABLE 36–3. Aminoglycoside Dosing

Determination of Loading Dose

Aminoglycoside	*Loading Dose**	*Expected Serum Peak*
Gentamicin	1.5–2.0 mg/kg	4.0–10.0 μg/mL
Tobramycin	1.5–2.0 mg/kg	4.0–10.0 μg/mL
Amikacin	5.0–7.5 mg/kg	15.0–30.0 μg/mL
Kanamycin	5.0–7.5 mg/kg	15.0–30.0 μg/mL
Netilmicin	1.3–3.3 mg/kg	4.0–12.0 μg/mL

Determination of Interval Dose

Administer 50% of loading dose at estimated serum half-life or calculate creatinine clearance

$$C_{cr}\text{ male} = \frac{140 - \text{age}}{\text{serum creatinine}}$$

$$C_{cr}\text{ female} = 0.85 \times C_{cr}\text{ male}$$

Choose the preferred dosing interval and percentage at loading dose interval

C_{cr} (mL/mm)	*Half-Life (hours)*	*8 Hours (%)*	*12 Hours (%)*	*24 Hours (%)*
90	3.1	84	—	—
60	4.5	71	84	—
30	8.4	48	63	86
20	11.9	37	50	75
10	20.14	24	34	56

Adapted from Cockcroft DW, Gault MH: Prediction of creatinine clearance from serum creatinine. Nephron 16:31, 1976. By permission of S. Karger AG, Basel.

*Based on ideal body weight: male—50 kg + 2.3 kg for every inch over 5 feet; female—45.5 kg + 2.3 kg for every inch over 5 feet.

ANTIMICROBIAL RESISTANCE

Despite appropriate and judicious use of antimicrobials, the threat of resistance to available drugs always exists. The amount of resistance among bacteria often correlates with the frequency of clinical use, the total quantity of drug dispensed, the location of the patient when receiving treatment, and the immune status of the patient.

Resistance may develop through one or more of the following mechanisms:

- Intrinsic
- Mutation
- Plasmid-mediated

Each class of antimicrobials has its own rate of vulnerability for the development of resistance. Most understanding of resistance patterns has been gained from the evaluation of outbreaks of infection among hospitalized patients. Although these events are dramatic, they often are not valid predictors of widespread resistance problems.

Intrinsic

Intrinsic resistance is a form of resistance that antedates introduction of new antimicrobial drugs into the marketplace. It is a survival mechanism possessed by one or more species of bacteria to ensure reproduction and successful growth of progeny. One form of intrinsic resistance is inducible β-lactamase. This is an enzyme whose expression is repressed until exposure to certain drugs occurs. In the presence of drug, enzyme production is derepressed, the resultant enzyme molecules catalyze the splitting of the β-lactam ring, the antibiotic is rendered inactive, and bacterial proliferation (infection) continues to occur.

A second form of intrinsic resistance is bacterial modification of surface structure. The normal channel through the cell membrane is made of a substance known as OmpF. In the presence of antimicrobials, bacteria can change to OmpC production, a smaller, more restrictive channel that can preclude entry of antimicrobials through the cell envelope.

Mutational

Mutational events can yield resistance to a variety of antimicrobial drugs. Examples are provided below.

- Altered penicillin-binding protein (PBP) — β-lactams
- Altered PBP binding capability — β-lactams
- Altered amino acids in ribosome — aminoglycosides
- Altered DNA gyrase — fluoroquinolones
- Altered protein of ribosome — macrolides, lincosamides
- Altered pathway to synthesize folate — trimethoprim/sulfamethoxazole

Plasmid-Mediated

Plasmids are extrachromosomal pieces of DNA that may confer resistance to antimicrobial drugs. Because they are extrachromosomal, this genetic information is readily shared among bacteria of the same species and sometimes among bacteria of other species as well. Plasmids may confer resistance by

- Reduced affinity of the drug for the target
- Production of new synthesis pathways to bypass a metabolic block
- Reduced uptake of the drug
- Enhanced efflux of drug from the bacteria

Combinations of Resistance Mechanisms

Finally, bacteria may combine these resistance mechanisms and become difficult or impossible to treat. Two examples of such species are methicillin-resistant *Staphylococcus aureus* and multiple drug-resistant tuberculosis. Both of these pathogens

- Are becoming more prevalent among hospitalized patients
- Can be spread to vulnerable hosts in the health care setting
- Are associated with high mortality rates (40 – 90%)

Both pathogens have been associated with indiscriminate use of antimicrobial drugs. Thus, every antibiotic prescription must be written carefully. Factors favoring resistance include excessive dose and duration of therapy, use in unwarranted circumstances, and broad-spectrum coverage when organism-targeted therapy would suffice. The responsibility for maintaining therapeutic viability of antimicrobial drugs rests with every practitioner.

Acknowledgment

This work was supported by the Department of Veterans Affairs.

REFERENCES

PROPHYLAXIS

Altemeier WA, Burke JP, Pruitt BA Jr, Sandersky WR: Definitions and classifications of surgical infections. *In* Altemeier WA (ed): Manual on Control of Infection in Surgical Patients, 2nd ed, 1. Philadelphia: JB Lippincott Co, 1984.

Beam TR Jr: First-generation cephalosporins in surgical prophylaxis. Infect Med 10:275, 1988.

Burke JF: The effective period of preventive antibiotic action in experimental incisions and dermal lesions. Surgery 50:161, 1961.

Conte JE Jr, Jacob LS, Polk HC Jr: Antibiotic Prophylaxis in Surgery. Philadelphia: JB Lippincott Co, 1984.

DOSING AND DOSE MODIFICATION

Barza M: Principles of tissue penetration antibiotics. J Antimicrob Chemother 8(Suppl C):7, 1981.

Bundzten RW, Gerber AU, Cohn DL, et al: Postantibiotic suppression of bacterial growth. Rev Infect Dis 3:28, 1981.

Cockcroft DW, Gault MH: Prediction of creatinine clearance from serum creatinine. Nephron 16:31, 1976.

Moore RD, Smith CR, Leitman PS: The association of aminoglycoside plasma levels with mortality in patients with gram-negative sepsis. J Infect Dis 149:443, 1984.

RESISTANCE

Bryan LE: General mechanisms of resistance to antibiotics. J Antimicrob Chemother 22(Suppl A):1, 1988.

Levy SB: Microbial resistance to antibiotics. An evolving and persistent problem. Lancet 2:83, 1982.

O'Brien TF, Members of Task Force 2: Resistance of bacteria to antibacterial agents: Report of task force 2. Rev Infect Dis 9(Suppl 3):S244, 1987.

37 Penicillins and Other Cell Wall Active Agents

Alan J. Lesse

PENICILLINS

Penicillin and its derivatives form one of the most studied and useful groups of antimicrobial agents. Discovered in 1929 by Alexander Fleming, penicillin has altered both our understanding and treatment of bacterial infections.

Chemistry

Fleming originally discovered the antibacterial properties of a *Pencillium* mold when he noticed that a contaminating mold lysed bacteria that he was studying on a culture dish. Purification of the compound resulted in the eventual discovery of penicillin and ushered in the modern antibiotic era.

The penicillins are a class of bicyclic compounds, consisting of a four-membered, β-lactam ring and a five-membered, sulfur-containing thiazolidine ring, as shown in Figure 37–1.

The four-membered β-lactam ring is inherently unstable, allowing the β-lactam ring to interact with and acylate its bacterial targets. When the β-lactam ring reacts with water, hydrolysis ensues, converting the carbonyl (C = O) into a carboxyl group (COOH) and opening the ring. The lack of ring structure obviates the reactivity of the penicillin molecule. The side chains (represented by an *R* in Figure 37–1) confer unique properties on the penicillins in terms of antibacterial activity, half-life, and stability to acid hydrolysis (and hence usefulness as an oral agent). Penicillin G (benzyl penicillin) and penicillin V (phenoxymethyl penicillin) are both products of fermentation and are referred to as natural penicillins. All other penicillins are formed from synthetic chemical modifications of the naturally occurring compounds and are referred to as semisynthetic penicillins. Derivatives of penicillin can be divided into four major categories, both chemically and functionally. These are natural, antistaphylococcal, amino, and extended-spectrum penicillins. The frequently used term, penicillinase-stable penicillins, is avoided, as seen in the following categorization:

Natural	Antistaphylococcal	Amino	Extended-Spectrum
Penicillin G	Methicillin	Ampicillin	Carbenicillin
Penicillin V	Nafcillin	Amoxicillin	Ticarcillin
	Oxacillin		Azlocillin
	Cloxacillin		Mezlocillin
	Dicloxacillin		Piperacillin

Mechanism of Action

Although much has been learned since Fleming's discovery over 60 years ago, the absolute mechanism of action of penicillin is still under intense investigation. What is clear, however, is that the basic antibacterial action of penicillin is to inhibit bacterial cell wall synthesis in one of the terminal steps of cell wall biosynthesis, a complicated enzymatic process governed by over 20 separate enzymes.

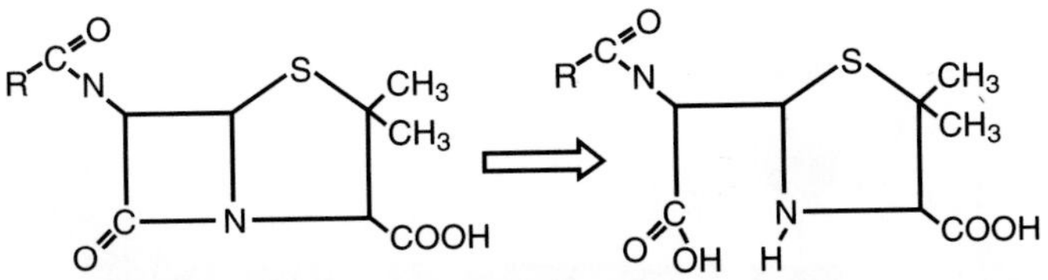

FIGURE 37–1. Hydrolysis of the penicillin molecule results in opening of the *β*-lactam ring. The resultant molecule loses the ability to acylate bacterial targets.

Bacteria, both Gram-positive and Gram-negative, are composed of a rigid cell wall that protects the organisms from osmotic pressures. This rigid cell wall also provides a fixed structure for the more fluid cytoplasm and confers a recognizable shape to the bacteria (eg, cocci, bacilli, coccobacilli).

The rigid nature of these cell walls is imparted by peptidoglycan layers in both Gram-positive and Gram-negative bacteria. In Gram-positive bacteria, the cell wall is composed of a peptidoglycan layer, 50 to 100 molecules thick, adjacent to the plasma membrane. Other molecules such as proteins, teichoic acid, and polysaccharides also populate the cell wall.

Gram-negative bacteria, however, have an alternative membrane structure composed of a plasma membrane and an outer membrane separated by a periplasmic space (Fig. 37–2). The peptidoglycan structure, composed of only 1 or 2 molecules of peptidoglycan, is a rigid structure at the base of the trilaminar outer membrane. The outer membrane contains porins (transmembrane proteins that regulate the entry of substances into the periplasmic space), lipopolysaccharides, and other proteins arranged in a phospholipid bilayer.

Despite the different topographic structure of Gram-positive and Gram-negative bacteria, peptidoglycan biosynthesis occurs in a defined manner in both groups. Peptidoglycan is composed of complex alternating carbohydrates, *N*-acetylglucosamine and *N*-acetylmuramic acid (Figs. 37–3 and 37–4). This alternating *N*-acetylglucosamine–*N*-acetylmuramic acid complex is further associated with short peptides covalently attached to the lactic acids of the *N*-acetylmuramic acid moieties. Figure 37–3 shows the construction of the Gram-positive bacteria *Staphylococcus aureus*, with a pentaglycine attached to the L-lysine of the peptide side chain. Figure 37–4 shows the structure of the Gram-negative *Escherichia coli*, with no secondary peptide chain attached to the lysine. The composition of the peptide chain and degree of branching are different for each species of bacteria, but the chain always contains a terminal D-alanine–D-alanine dipeptide, a unique dipeptide restricted to this bacterial structure. (Please see mechanism of resistance for vancomycin for an exception to this process.) These long polymers of alternating structures are called peptidoglycans.

Strength is added to the cell wall by cross-links between the peptide side chains of adjacent peptidoglycan molecules. Cross-linking, or transpeptidation, is facilitated by an enzyme, transpeptidase (see Figs. 37–3 and 37–4), which catalyzes the covalent linking of the penultimate D-alanine to a specific amino acid on the adjacent strain. In Figure 37–3, the penultimate D-alanine is covalently linked to the terminal glycine of the branched peptide side chain attached to the *N*-acetylmuramic acid. Figure 37–4 shows the covalent linkage seen in *E. coli*, with the penultimate D-alanine covalently bonding with the L-lysine of the adjoining muramyl peptide. The degree of cross-linking is variable but is much more pronounced in Gram-positive bacteria such as *S. aureus* (≈90%) compared with Gram-negative bacteria such as *E. coli* (≈20%).

The transpeptidases appear to be a member of the group of enzymes responsible for peptidoglycan synthesis. Penicillin binding studies of both Gram-positive and Gram-negative bacteria have shown that these proteins bind peni-

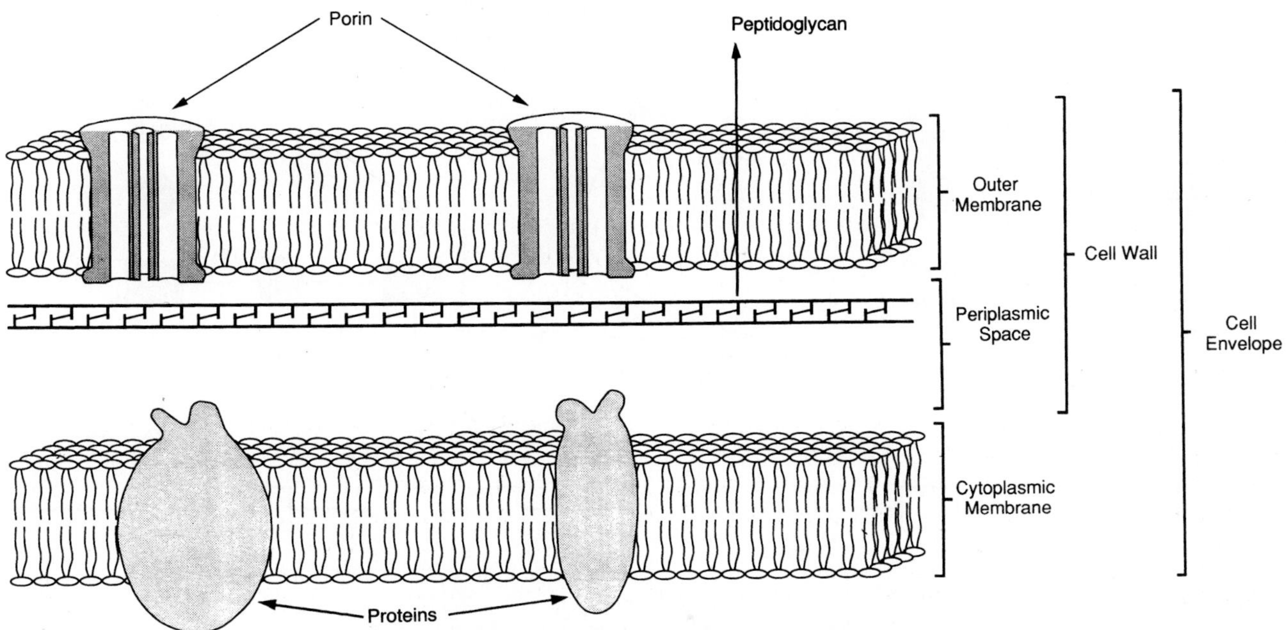

FIGURE 37–2. The Gram-negative cell envelope.

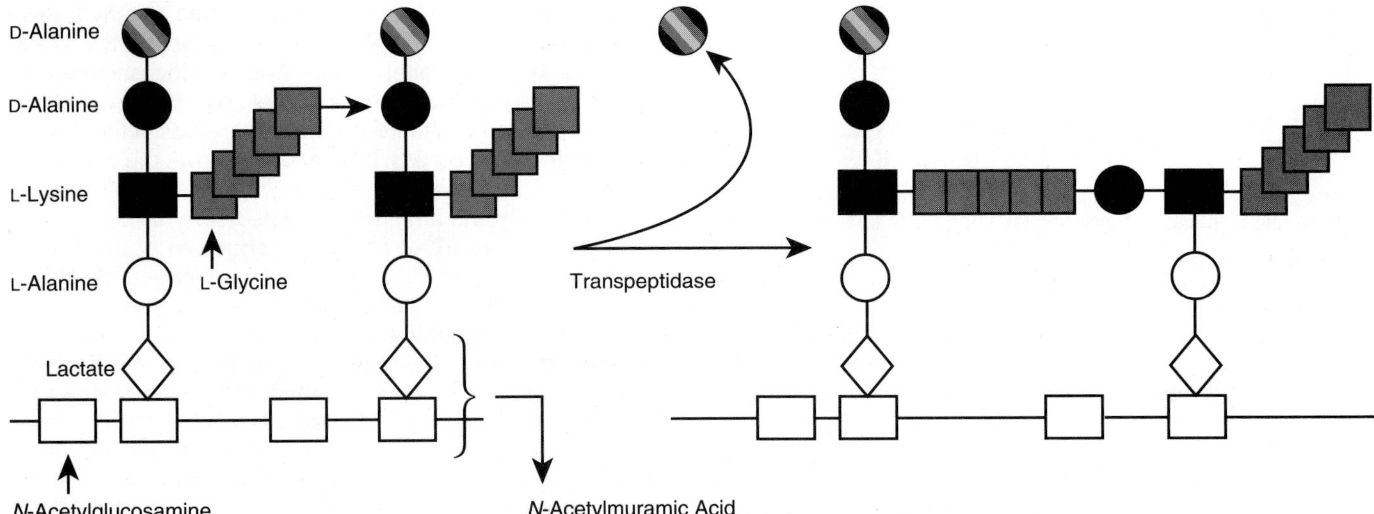

FIGURE 37–3. The transpeptidation reaction in *Staphylococcus aureus*. The penultimate D-alanine is covalently linked to an adjacent terminal L-glycine of a nearby branched peptide chain. The terminal D-alanine is removed from the side chain, as shown here.

cillins. These proteins, referred to as penicillin-binding proteins (PBPs), most likely represent many of the enzymes involved in these terminal assembly steps. A variety of PBPs are expressed on bacteria. Although they do not occur at a specific molecular weight in all bacteria, the relative molecular mass of a PBP can suggest its mechanism of action. High-molecular-weight PBPs such as 1a and 1b are involved in cell elongation and probably represent a major class of transpeptidases. PBP 2 is an interesting class responsible for maintenance of cell integrity; and β-lactam binding to PBP 2 causes rapid cell death. Other PBPs have other binding specificities and mechanisms of actions that span a wide range of functions.

One mechanism by which penicillins inhibit the transpeptidation reaction has recently been elucidated. The three-dimensional structure of the penicillins approximates the structure of the D-alanine–D-alanine side chain recognized by the transpeptidase enzyme. Binding of the penicillin to the transpeptidase results in acylation of the transpeptidase, causing irreversible inhibition of the enzyme.

Because the peptidoglycan layer is responsible for the rigid structure that protects the bacteria from osmotic stress, inhibition of this crucial synthetic, replicative, and reparative system has a lethal outcome on bacterial populations subjected to penicillin. Inhibition of cell wall synthesis therefore results in cell death and is termed bactericidal.

It should be noted that the mechanism of action involves the assembly, maintenance, and repair of bacterial cell wall components, which is why penicillins are only active on actively replicating organisms. Static or stationary-phase bacteria are not killed by penicillins.

Disruption of the cell membrane may ultimately reside in bacterial membrane proteins called autolysins, which are necessary for peptidoglycan disruption, presumably as part of the normal growth and division cycle. Activation of the autolysins results in cell disruption and death, and autolysin-

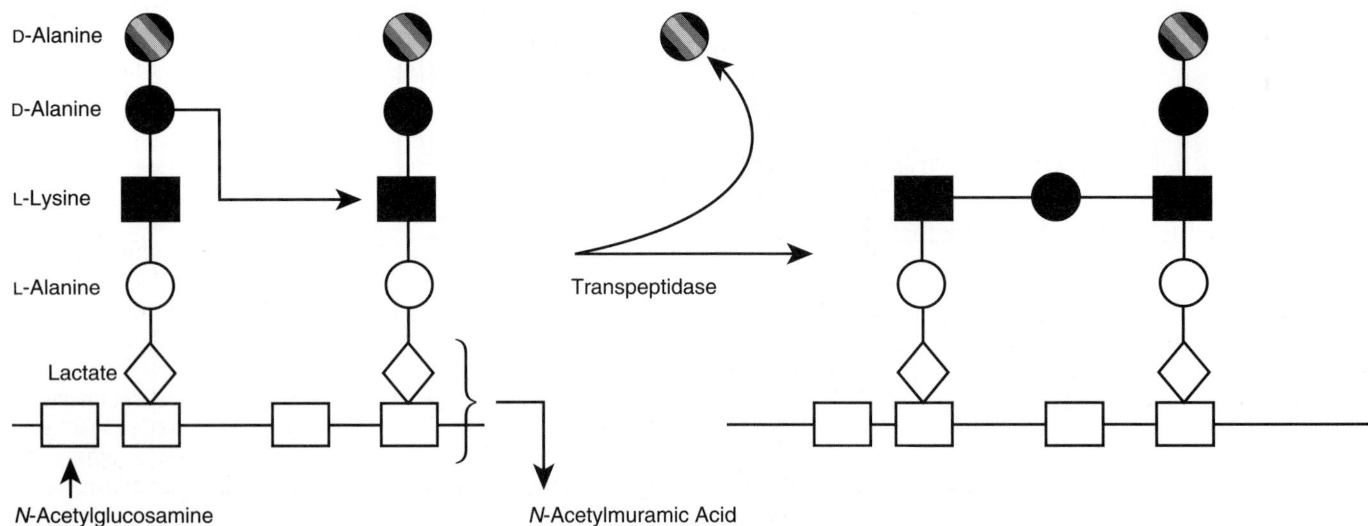

FIGURE 37–4. The transpeptidation reaction in *Escherichia coli*. The penultimate D-alanine is covalently linked to an adjacent L-lysine of a nearby peptide chain. The terminal D-alanine is removed from the side chain, as shown here.

deficient bacteria may be resistant to the bactericidal activity of the penicillins.

Bacterial Resistance

The most frequent cause of bacterial resistance to penicillins is the secretion of enzymes by the bacteria that hydrolyze the β-lactam ring and prevent the penicillins from acylating the transpeptidase. The enzymes, called penicillinases, or more generically, β-lactamases, are most commonly encoded on plasmids that can transfer this resistance from bacteria to bacteria. Gram-positive bacteria secrete these β-lactamases into the extracellular environment, whereas Gram-negative organisms secrete the enzyme into the periplasmic space, resulting in high concentrations of β-lactamase within the small space adjacent to the PBPs. Penicillins that maintain their activity against bacteria that secrete β-lactamases are not hydrolyzed by those β-lactamases.

Resistance to penicillin has existed since its initial clinical introduction. Prior to the introduction of penicillin, almost all staphylococcal isolates were susceptible to penicillin. Over time, *S. aureus* acquired plasmids that conferred β-lactamase, and penicillin resistance became the dominant phenotype. Although it was initially a hospital phenomenon of the 1960s, penicillinase activity is seen in over 90–95% of hospital strains and in probably more than 85–90% of community-acquired strains of *S. aureus*, making penicillin G routinely inactive for staphylococcal infections. Some penicillins, referred to in this chapter as antistaphylococcal penicillins, are highly stable against the specific β-lactamases secreted by *S. aureus*. Many authors refer to these agents as β-lactamase–resistant penicillins because of this property. However, this classification is confusing. Gram-negative bacteria also secrete β-lactamase, but the same hydrophobic side chains that allow for stability against the β-lactamase of *S. aureus* in an extracellular environment markedly increase the hydrophobicity of the drug. This decreased hydrophilicity restricts the passage of the antistaphylococcal penicillin through the Gram-negative outer membrane and prevents these penicillins from binding to the PBPs of Gram-negative bacteria. Students frequently infer that the term β-lactamase–stable penicillins indicates that these penicillins are active against all β-lactamases, when in fact their enhanced spectrum is significantly limited to *S. aureus*.

Because penicillins must bind to PBP to function, alterations in PBPs can decrease susceptibility to many penicillins. This is best seen in *S. aureus* and other staphylococcal species where altered PBPs confer resistance to even the antistaphylococcal penicillins. These strains are commonly referred to as methicillin-resistant *S. aureus* (MRSA). This resistance to penicillin applies to all currently available β-lactam antibiotics, including cephalosporins. This intrinsic, chromosomally mediated resistance is frequently accompanied by multiple-drug resistance. Unfortunately, although MRSA started initially as isolated outbreaks, incidence figures in some hospitals have shown that more than 40% of strains are resistant to methicillin.

Because penicillins must be able to reach the inner membrane of Gram-negative bacteria to bind to their targeted PBPs, their ability to bind to these targets is a function of their concentration, affinity for the PBPs, and affinity for enzymatic degradation by the periplasmic β-lactamases. Factors that decrease antibiotic entry into the periplasma (regulation of porin structure or membrane permeability of the antibiotic) or increased rate of hydrolysis of the penicillin relative to the binding of the penicillin to the PBP decrease the activity of the penicillin in question.

Absorption, Distribution, Metabolism, and Excretion

Only acid-stable compounds have a place in oral therapy. Clinicians should be aware that several acid-labile forms of penicillin, such as penicillin G, are available in pill form. Great caution should be exercised in use of these agents orally. Only penicillin V, ampicillin, amoxicillin, cloxacillin, dicloxacillin, and possibly oxacillin should be given orally.

Penicillins are widely distributed but because of their acidic nature may be markedly decreased in concentration in basic environment, such as prostatic fluid. Because penicillins are administered as salts and have a net negative charge, they cannot passively cross cell membranes. Distribution of penicillins into the spinal fluid is restricted by the blood-brain barrier and blood–cerebrospinal fluid (CSF) barrier to approximately 10% of serum concentrations in normal subjects. In the presence of meningeal inflammation during meningitis, almost 40% of serum levels can be achieved. Because of the large therapeutic index with the penicillins, serum concentrations can be significantly raised and can increase the diffusion of these compounds into the CSF to well above the concentration needed to kill bacteria.

The majority of penicillins are handled by the kidneys as organic acids and excreted by tubular excretion. Probenecid, an inhibitor of tubular organic acid secretion, increases the half-life and raises the serum level of all penicillins that are secreted by the kidney. Students and clinicians must remember that nafcillin and the isoxazolyl penicillins (oxacillin, cloxacillin, and dicloxacillin) are lipophilic and are excreted by biliary means. No dosage adjustment for renal dysfunction is necessary for those four penicillins. The relative dosage adjustment for hepatic dysfunction for those penicillins cleared via biliary excretion is difficult to calculate and should be individually tailored.

Table 37–1 shows selected pharmacokinetic parameters for many of the agents.

Adverse Effects

Penicillins are a remarkably safe class of antibiotics. The major adverse reaction to the penicillins is allergy. Significant allergic reaction, anaphylaxis, and death still occur despite the widespread knowledge of the potentially fatal adverse effects.

Penicillins are perhaps some of the most immunogenic compounds known. The penicillin structure is of insufficient size to act as an immunogen on its own; however, when covalently linked to serum proteins, penicillins function as potent haptens.

The immunology of penicillin allergy is complex. Penicillin undergoes hydrolysis in physiologic conditions, result-

TABLE 37–1. Selected Pharmacokinetic Parameters for Penicillins and Other Cell Wall Active Agents

		Half-Life		Dosing Interval	
Name	**Route**	*CrCl > 80 (hours)*	*CrCl < 10 (hours)*	*CrCl > 80 (hours)*	*CrCl < 10 (hours)*
Natural Penicillins					
Penicillin G	Intravenous	0.4–0.9	7–20	4–6	12
Penicillin V	Oral	0.5	4	6	12
Procaine penicillin	Intramuscular	*	*	*	*
Benzathine penicillin	Intramuscular	*	*	*	*
Aminopenicillins					
Ampicillin	Oral	0.5–1.5	8–20	6	12
	Intravenous	0.5–1.5	8–20	4–6	12
Amoxicillin	Oral	0.9–2.3	5–20	8	12–24
Antistaphylococcal Penicillins					
Methicillin	Intravenous	0.5–1.0	4	4	12
Nafcillin	Intravenous	0.5	1.2	4	4
Oxacillin	Intravenous	0.4–0.5	1–2	4	4
Cloxacillin	Oral	0.5	0.8	6	6
Dicloxacillin	Oral	0.7	1–2	6	6
Extended-Spectrum Penicillin					
Carbenicillin	Intravenous	0.5–1	10–20	4	12
Ticarcillin	Intravenous	1–1.5	13–16	4	12
Azlocillin	Intravenous	0.8–1.5	5–6	4	12
Mezlocillin	Intravenous	0.6–1.1	1.6–5.4	4	8–12
Piperacillin	Intravenous	0.8–1.5	2.1–5.1	4	12
Monobactams					
Aztreonam	Intravenous	1.3–2.9	6–9	8	12–36
Carbepenems					
Imipenem	Intravenous	1	2.7–4	6	12–24
Meropenem	Intravenous	0.8–2.2	4–10	6	24
β-Lactamase Inhibitors					
Clavulanic acid	Oral	0.7–1.5	3–4.3	8	12–24
	Intravenous	0.7–1.5	3–4.3	4–6	12
Sulbactam	Intravenous	1	14–20	6	12–24
Tazobactam	Intravenous	1.1–1.7		6	
Glycopeptide					
Vancomycin	Intravenous	6–8	200–250	12	96–168

*Procaine penicillin and benzathine penicillin have prolonged absorption because of their administration by intramuscular injection and poor solubility. Therefore, despite their having the same half-life as the native penicillin, the apparent serum half-lives of these agents are greatly increased because of prolonged absorption of hours to weeks. These compounds produce serum levels for hours to days, depending on the compound. See individual agent for specific pharmacokinetics.

ing in pencilloyl groups. These penicilloyl groups form complexes with serum proteins and form the majority of the covalently complexed degradation products of penicillins (major determinant). Other minor degradation products also form complexes with serum proteins and although they are stoichiometrically less common (minor determinant), account for a significant proportion of immunoglobulin E–sensitizing haptens.

Accelerated or severe reactions can occur in patients with negative histories but are far more common in patients with positive histories for penicillin allergy.

Skin testing has proved to be a reliable predictor in patients with a positive history of penicillin allergy. *When properly administered*, a negative skin test reliably indicates that penicillin can be given without producing an anaphylactic reaction. Unfortunately, proper administration of penicillin skin testing is nearly impossible outside the research setting because both major and minor determinants, in addition to penicillin, must be evaluated. The only commercially available product for skin testing that evaluates the potentially anaphylactic degradation products of penicillin evaluates only major determinants. Multiple penicilloyl determinants covalently coupled to a poorly immunogenic polylysine carrier are synthesized to produce penicilloyl-polylysine (PPL). This compound only predicts allergic reactions to the major determinant. No commercial product is available for evaluation of reactions to minor determinants. The most accurate preparation of minor determinants includes benzylpenicillin and its alkaline (benzylpenicilloate) and acid (benzylpenilloate) hydrolysis products and is known as *minor determinant mixture* (MDM). The highly predictive MDM is not a stable mixture and cannot currently be synthesized for commercial production.

In the absence of MDM, if PPL were to be used as the

sole testing agent, 10–25% of all truly allergic patients who would have reacted to MDM would be missed. Many clinicians substitute a diluted benzylpenicillin as the minor determinant, but this substitution does not give positive skin test reactions in 5–10% of patients who react to properly synthesized MDM and who represent a group still at risk for a serious or anaphylactic reaction. Therefore, in the absence of being able to generate MDM, skin testing achieves only 90–95% accuracy for a potentially life-threatening complication. Because skin testing itself may precipitate an anaphylactic reaction, this procedure should only be performed at facilities capable of initiating cardiopulmonary resuscitation and monitoring. Skin testing should be performed by an experienced physician skilled in the procedure and prepared for possible anaphylactic reactions to the testing.

Luckily, patients with either positive skin tests or significant prior allergic reactions can still receive penicillin, if it is the drug of choice, after either parenteral or oral desensitization. The more classic approach of parenteral desensitization has given way to a safer, rapid oral desensitization schedule that many investigators find easier to administer (Wendel et al).

Penicillins not only cause Type I (immediate hypersensitivity reactions) but also can cause Type Ii (cytotoxic antibody), Type III (immune complex), Type IV (cell-mediated hypersensitivity), and Type V (idiopathic) reactions. Skin rashes appear to follow ampicillin more often than other forms of penicillin. More than 95% of patients with acute mononucleosis from Epstein-Barr virus have a macular skin eruption if treated with ampicillin.

Other adverse reactions to penicillin are generally less severe than anaphylaxis. Historically, methicillin has a high incidence of allergic interstitial nephritis that has resulted in an almost total discontinuation of the clinical use of the agent. Other penicillins can still cause allergic interstitial nephritis, and this diagnosis should be considered in patients with a rising creatinine level and eosinophilia or eosinophiluria. Electrolyte disturbances can be seen with high doses of penicillins — especially the older preparations such as carbenicillin and ticarcillin — because these agents are

BOX 37–1

INDICATIONS AND CONTRAINDICATIONS OF NATURAL PENICILLINS

Penicillin G. Penicillin G should always be given by the intravenous route. Its primary indications have been reduced over the years because of the development of resistance; however, it still remains the drug of choice for serious streptococcal infections, especially skin and soft tissue infections and endocarditis. The treatment of many streptococcal species causing endocarditis also requires the addition of an aminoglycoside, such as gentamicin, to improve the bactericidal activity. Pneumococcal infections, once exquisitely sensitive to penicillin, have become more resistant over the years. The number of strains of *Streptococcus pneumoniae* that are tolerant to penicillin have increased to the point that serious consideration must be given in some areas for empiric therapy of known or suspected pneumococcal infections with alternative agents (ceftriaxone or vancomycin). Resistance to penicillin has also recently removed penicillin G from recommended empiric therapy of *Neisseria gonorrhoeae* and *Neisseria meningitidis* infections until penicillin sensitivity is confirmed. Most staphylococci are currently resistant to penicillin G. Infections with anaerobes of oral origin, such as infection of the oral cavity, lung abscess, and others are still effectively treated with penicillin G, although some studies of anaerobic lung infections report a higher success rate with clindamycin. Finally, the therapy of the central nervous system (CNS) phase of two spirochetal diseases, syphilis and Lyme disease, utilizes high-dose intravenous penicillin. Current recommendations for neurosyphilis suggest 10 days of high-dose intravenous penicillin G, whereas therapy for Lyme disease includes either penicillin or ceftriaxone for the neurologic, cardiac, or severe rheumatic stages of the disease. Despite the decreasing number of recommendations for the empiric or routine use of penicillin, it is still safe to say that it is generally the drug of choice for treating an organism that is sensitive to penicillin.

Penicillin V. Phenoxymethyl penicillin (PEN-V) is acid-stable and is frequently used for mild or moderate streptococcal infections. Penicillin V is still recommended as therapy for group A streptococcal pharyngitis because resistance to penicillin in group A streptococcal species has not occurred to date. Prior recommendations promoting penicillin V for prophylaxis of bacterial endocarditis have been updated recently, and penicillin V is no longer recommended for this indication.

Procaine Penicillin. This form of penicillin is the procaine salt of penicillin G. The drug is dissolved *in vivo* to produce penicillin G over time and significantly increases the apparent serum half-life. The drug is administered only as an intramuscular injection. Clinical indications for this form of therapy are more limited to the era of frequent intravenous administrations and the availability of broader spectrum agents via intramuscular injection.

Benzathine Penicillin. Benzathine penicillin is the benzathine salt of penicillin G. This product has a low solubility and provides an intramuscular reservoir for low levels of penicillin over a long period of time. Serum levels of the drug can be detected up to 12 weeks after injection, and useful levels can be seen for some micro-organisms up to 4 weeks. The major clinical uses of this form of penicillin include the therapy of syphilis and the prevention of rheumatic fever. Many of the stages of syphilis, excluding the late phases of neurosyphilis, can be effectively treated with one or more injections of benzathine penicillin. Because treatment recommendations are reviewed frequently by the Centers for Disease Control and Prevention, clinicians should confirm current dosing recommendations prior to treatment. In general, syphilis with a duration of less than 1 year requires a single intramuscular injection of 2.4 million units of benzathine penicillin. Syphilis with a duration of more than 1 year without evidence of CNS involvement may be treated by weekly injections of 2.4 million units of benzathine penicillin intramuscularly for 3 weeks (total of 7.2 million units). Prevention of rheumatic fever is generally accomplished with monthly injections of benzathine penicillin.

BOX 37–2
INDICATIONS AND CONTRAINDICATIONS OF ANTISTAPHYLOCOCCAL PENICILLINS

This group is composed of methicillin, nafcillin, cloxacillin, and dicloxacillin, respectively. Although many sources refer to this group as the penicillinase-resistant penicillins, these drugs are clearly inactive against many bacteria secreting β-lactamases, especially Gram-negative bacteria (see Bacterial Resistance). Because these agents are not hydrolyzed by staphylococcal β-lactamases and staphylococci are their primary clinical indications, the more appropriate term should be *antistaphylococcal penicillins.*

Methicillin. Methicillin is not frequently used in the clinical arena because of the incidence of interstitial nephritis and the availability of equally efficacious alternatives (nafcillin and oxacillin). Susceptibility testing with this agent does identify a group of staphylococcal strains with chromosomally mediated alteration in PBPs of staphylococcus. *MRSA* (*m*ethicillin-*r*esistant *Staphylococcus aureus*) is the common term used to describe these strains. Students should note that resistance to methicillin, nafcillin, or oxacillin implies resistance to ***any*** of these agents. The term *methicillin-resistant* therefore implies resistance to all antistaphylococcal penicillins, as well as to other penicillins and cephalosporins.

Nafcillin and Oxacillin. These intravenous preparations are used in the treatment of serious staphylococcal and streptococcal infections. Their activity against enterococcal species is poor, and these agents are inactive against Gram-negative bacteria. Oxacillin may be associated with a lower incidence of phlebitis after intravenous administration.

Cloxacillin and Dicloxacillin. These agents are orally available compounds with a spectrum of activity similar to that of nafcillin and oxacillin. Both agents have decreased absorption with food and should not be taken with meals. Their primary use is to treat mild to moderate infections caused by staphylococci and streptococci. Skin and soft tissue infections account for the majority of their use.

BOX 37–3
INDICATIONS AND CONTRAINDICATIONS OF AMINOPENICILLINS

This group of agents is characterized by the amino substitution of penicillin G with an increase in the activity of these agents against some Gram-negative bacteria and increased activity against enterococci. The two drugs, ampicillin and amoxicillin, are widely used for a variety of indications. The major difference in the drugs is the higher oral absorption, higher serum levels, and longer half-life for amoxicillin compared with ampicillin. Other factors being equal, amoxicillin is the preferred oral drug, whereas ampicillin is the only available intravenous aminopenicillin. Drug susceptibility testing for ampicillin can be used to predict susceptibility to amoxicillin.

When first introduced, ampicillin significantly increased the spectrum of penicillin into the Gram-negative realm with activity against *E. coli*, *Proteus mirabilis*, and some enteric pathogens. However, at the current time, ampicillin is only active against *E. coli* and *P. mirabilis* and a few other Gram-negative pathogens from non–hospital-acquired infections. Most nosocomial Gram-negative rods are now resistant to ampicillin.

Ampicillin provides good activity against streptococcal species and has significantly increased activity against enterococcal species compared to penicillin G. Activity against *Listeria* is also significantly increased with ampicillin and amoxicillin.

Ampicillin and amoxicillin are actively degraded by staphylococcal β-lactamase secreted by the vast majority of *S. aureus* and therefore are not considered good antistaphylococcal agents.

Ampicillin and amoxicillin are active against 70–80% of *Haemophilus influenzae*; however 20–30% of strains carry a β-lactamase plasmid. Use of these agents should therefore be confirmed by susceptibility testing. For life-threatening or serious disease caused by *H. influenzae*, empiric therapy should not rely on ampicillin or amoxicillin alone. Instead, a second- or third-generation cephalosporin or some other agent that is stable in the presence of the *Haemophilus* β-lactamase should be chosen. Combination of ampicillin with chloramphenicol also achieves this antimicrobial spectrum and was used extensively prior to the development of the later-generation cephalosporins. *Neisseria* species also encode a similar plasmid and prohibit the use of ampicillin and amoxicillin for the empiric treatment of gonorrhea.

Recent recommendations have made use of the excellent pharmacokinetic profile and streptococcal activity of amoxicillin for the prophylaxis of bacterial endocarditis. One 3-g dose of amoxicillin prior to dental procedures in endocarditis-prone patients followed by 1.5 g 6 hours after the procedure is currently recommended by several authorities and panels for routine prophylaxis. Complete prophylactic recommendations must be consulted for individual patients because different procedures and patients have different risks and treatment recommendations.

BOX 37–4
INDICATIONS AND CONTRAINDICATIONS OF EXTENDED-SPECTRUM PENICILLINS

The original members of this class, the carboxypenicillins (carbenicillin and ticarcillin), have given way to the newer ureidopenicillins (azlocillin, mezlocillin, and piperacillin). In large part this was due to the decreased activity of carboxypenicillins and their narrower spectrum when compared with the ureidopenicillins. Because the carboxypenicillins were less active, much higher doses were required for clinical effectiveness, and because these agents are administered as the sodium or potassium salts, electrolyte

Continued

BOX 37–4

INDICATIONS AND CONTRAINDICATIONS OF EXTENDED-SPECTRUM PENICILLINS (*Continued*)

disturbances were more common. Additionally, the carboxypenicillins were mainly active against *Pseudomonas aeruginosa* and not members of the family Enterobacteriaceae

The ureidopenicillins, on the other hand, are active against a broad range of Gram-negative pathogens including *P. aeruginosa*. Azlocillin has excellent activity against *P. aeruginosa* but of the group has the poorest activity against other Gram-negative rods and should be considered predominantly as an agent for the treatment of infection with *P. aeruginosa*. Although they are inactive against *S. aureus*, mezlocillin and piperacillin are active against enterococci. Both mezlocillin and piperacillin have good activity against a broad array of Gram-negative pathogens and *P. aeruginosa*. Use of these agents singly against *P aeruginosa* rapidly develops resistance to single-agent therapy with any β-lactam antibiotic. Therapy for *P. aeruginosa* infection should always include both an extended-spectrum penicillin or β–lactam with antipseudomonal activity **and** an aminoglycoside. Many authorities also discourage the use of the extended-spectrum penicillins as single agents to treat other infections to avoid exposing colonizing strains of *P. aeruginosa* to the drug as a single agent, thereby promoting resistance.

administered in high dosages as the sodium or potassium salts. Leukopenia is a well-reported side effect of high-dose penicillin therapy, especially with nafcillin. Thrombocytopenia and a Coombs'-positive hemolytic anemia occur rarely. Platelet dysfunction is seen more frequently with carbenicillin and ticarcillin but still can be seen with high doses of the other extended-spectrum penicillins. Seizures may also be seen with large intravenous dosages of penicillin, especially in the presence of renal failure. Finally, as with most other antimicrobial agents, selection of *Clostridium difficile* with subsequent pseudomembranous colitis can result from any form of penicillin therapy.

AZTREONAM

Chemistry

Aztreonam is a cell wall active antibiotic that contains a *β*-lactam ring like the penicillins and cephalosporins, but does not possess either a five- or six-membered ring seen with the cephalosporins or carbepenems. Aztreonam is a member of the class of antimicrobials referred to as monobactams, indicating their single-ring structure (see structure). Aztreonam is currently the only member of this class to be used clinically.

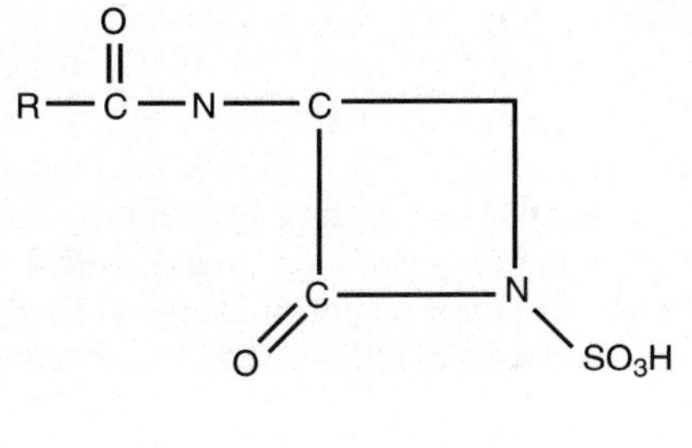

R—C(=O)—N—C (four-membered ring: C—C(=O)—N—SO_3H)

Monobactams

Mechanism of Action and Mechanism of Resistance

The mechanism of action of aztreonam is inhibition of cell wall synthesis through binding to penicillin binding proteins. Unlike penicillins, however, this agent has **no** activity against aerobic Gram-positive bacteria or anaerobic bacteria (either Gram-positive or Gram-negative) because this monocyclic structure does not bind to PBPs of these species. Most Enterobacteriaceae are readily inhibited by clinically achievable concentrations of aztreonam, as are most strains of *P. aeruginosa*. Non-aeruginosa strains of *Pseudomonas* are frequently resistant to aztreonam. Aztreonam is resistant to many of the plasmid-associated *β*-lactamases that inactivate penicillins and first-generation cephalosporins may be susceptible to chromosomally mediated inducible *β*-lactamases, such as those seen in *Enterobacter* species. The compound is not a potent inducer of *β*-lactamases.

Absorption, Distribution, Metabolism, and Excretion

Aztreonam is only available in intravenous and intramuscular forms. The drug is distributed in a manner similar to that for penicillins, but its CSF penetration and use in meningitis have not been studied well enough to recommend it for the treatment of infections of the CNS. Aztreonam is excreted almost exclusively via renal mechanisms, and dosages must be adjusted in patients with renal failure.

Adverse Effects

Few adverse effects of aztreonam have been reported, and despite the structural similarities, aztreonam has little, if any, immunologic cross-reaction with the penicillins and cephalosporins. Patients with documented anaphylactic reactions to penicillin and strongly positive skin test reactions to penicillins can be treated with aztreonam safety. Although it is true that the side-chain structure of aztreonam is the same as that seen in ceftazidime, allergic reaction directed against the side chain is a rare event clinically, presumably related to the strong immunogenic potential of the *β*-lactam ring.

No significant drug interactions have been reported with aztreonam.

BOX 37–5

INDICATIONS AND CONTRAINDICATIONS

The major use of aztreonam is for the treatment of serious Gram-negative infections requiring a parenteral antibiotic. Aztreonam has a spectrum similar to that of the aminoglycosides and thus is frequently thought of as an aminoglycoside substitute. Although this is

Continued

> **BOX 37-5**
> **INDICATIONS AND CONTRAINDICATIONS (*Continued*)**
>
> correct for a majority of indications, one must bear in mind the marked differences between the aminoglycosides and aztreonam. The combination of an aminoglycoside and a penicillin is frequently synergistic (*eg*, penicillin and gentamicin for enterococci, or piperacillin and gentamicin for *Pseudomonas*). No reliable synergy can be predicted if aztreonam were to be used in place of an aminoglycoside in those combinations. Aztreonam also has no Gram-positive or anaerobic activity. Finally, aztreonam does not have the dose-dependent killing seen with the aminoglycosides. Therefore, aztreonam should be used to treat documented or suspected Gram-negative infections that do **not** rely on the synergy of a β-lactam–aminoglycoside combination for cure, and should be used empirically as a single agent if the spectrum of activity does not have to cover anaerobic or Gram-positive bacteria. Aztreonam can be very useful as an alternative to an aminoglycoside, given those caveats, with significantly less toxicity than aminoglycoside antibiotics. Aztreonam can also be given safely to patients with documented penicillin allergies without risk of allergic reactions.

IMIPENEM

Chemistry

Imipenem is a very active antibiotic with a remarkable spectrum of action. Imipenem is the first of a class of carbapenems. The structure, shown here, places the sulfur outside the ring structure and has specific stereochemical bonding unique to this class.

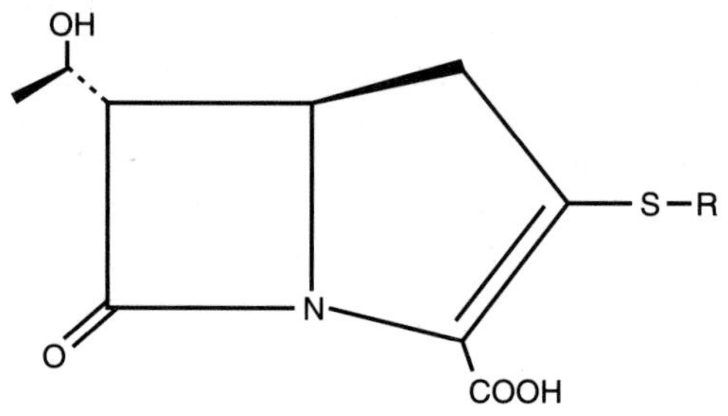

OH

S—R

N

O

COOH

Mechanism of Action

Imipenem has a mechanism of action similar to that of the penicillins in that it inhibits cell wall formation, but unlike most other *β*-lactam antibiotics, it also binds to PBP 2 in addition to PBPs 1 and 3. The combination of binding to PBP 1 and PBP 2 results in rapid cellular lysis. Additionally, imipenem demonstrates a significant postantibiotic effect (PAE) *in vitro* that is unique among *β*-lactam antibiotics. (The PAE is a laboratory observation of bacterial inhibition or bacterial killing after removal of the antimicrobial agent. Most penicillins have no PAE, and rapid regrowth of bacteria occurs upon removal of the agent from the media. Aminoglycosides, quinolones, and imipenem cause a significant PAE. The clinical relevance of this observation is uncertain.) The antibiotic is active against most Gram-positive and Gram-negative bacteria, both aerobic and anaerobic. Like penicillins, imipenem inhibits the growth of enterococci. Imipenem has excellent activity against *Bacteroides fragilis* and other anaerobic bacteria (with the exception of *C. difficile*) and is active against most Gram-negative rods, with the exception of *Pseudomonas cepacia* and *Xanthomonas (Pseudomonas) maltophilia.*

Mechanism of Resistance

The major mechanism of resistance is secretion of specific metallo-*β*-lactamase that hydrolyze imipenem. These enzymes have excellent activity for carbapenems but generally do not hydrolyze penicillin, monobactam, or cephalosporin targets. Therefore, resistance to imipenem does not confer resistance to other *β*-lactam antibiotics. Additionally, chromosomally mediated, inducible *β*-lactamases, such as those seen in *Enterobacter*, are generally inactive against imipenem, although a few recent reports discuss inducible *β*-lactamases that hydrolyze imipenem.

Administration, Absorption, Distribution, Metabolism, and Excretion

Imipenem is acid-labile and must be given parenterally. The drug is well distributed, but only small amounts enter the CNS. Even during meningitis, imipenem levels are not predictable enough to recommend as standard therapy of infections within the CNS. Despite the broad spectrum of activity, imipenem is rapidly metabolized in the renal tubules by the enzyme dehydropeptidase-1, found on the renal tubule brush border. To achieve adequate urinary levels of imipenem, the drug is always administered in combination with cilastatin, a drug that inhibits dehydropeptidase and allows imipenem to enter the urine in an active form. All commercially available imipenem is administered as a combination of imipenem and cilastatin. A newer carbapenem, meropenem, which is inherently stable to dehydropeptidase, may be introduced shortly into the American market and may offer different pharmacokinetic and side-effect profiles from the combination drug without the need for cilastatin. Imipenem is excreted exclusively via renal mechanisms, and dosage adjustments in renal failure are extremely important.

Adverse Effects

This class of agents has significant cross-reactivity with the penicillins, and patients considered at high risk for allergic reaction with penicillins should not receive imipenem. Nausea and vomiting are seen in some patients treated with imipenem. The other major adverse reaction seen with the combination of imipenem and cilastatin is seizures. Patients with a prior history of seizures are at higher risk, but this complication has also been seen in patients with no underlying seizure disorder. Most cases have been seen either with high doses of imipenem or with renal insufficiency and resulting increased serum levels due to impaired renal excretion. Whether this side effect is caused by the imipenem or cilastatin is unclear at this time.

BOX 37–6

INDICATIONS AND CONTRAINDICATIONS

Because of the extremely broad antimicrobial spectrum, imipenem could be considered one of the antibiotic choices in most clinical situations except for infections of the CNS. Many authorities recommend its use in selected situations in which an extremely broad spectrum agent is required, generally a mixed aerobic-anaerobic infection, or when a highly resistant bacteria is confirmed or suspected. Mixed infections with aerobes and anaerobes, such as perforated abdominal viscus, diabetic foot ulcers, decubitus ulcers, gynecological infections, infections in the immunocompromised host, and necrotizing infections, would be appropriate indications for imipenem therapy, as would infections with bacteria already resistant to β-lactam or other antibiotics. The drug must be administered cautiously in patients with renal dysfunction and in those with seizure disorders.

Clinicians should always be encouraged to tailor the spectrum of antimicrobial agents as narrowly as possible to avoid possible superinfection. Therapy with agents with a spectrum as broad as imipenem cannot achieve this goal; therefore, many authorities would not view this highly effective antibiotic as appropriate routine therapy for uncomplicated infections.

β-LACTAMASE INHIBITORS

Chemistry and Mechanism of Action

Most resistance to β-lactam antibiotics is mediated through bacterial production of β-lactamases. Most of these are encoded on plasmids and confer resistance to either single or multiple antimicrobial agents. These β-lactamases hydrolyze the β-lactam antibiotic before it can bind to its PBP. Inhibition of the β-lactamase, therefore, would allow the penicillin to bind to its PBP and result in restoration of the antibacterial activity of the penicillin in question. This mechanism is exploited by the β-lactamase inhibitors clavulanic acid, sulbactam, and tazobactam. Each of these agents binds irreversibly to certain classes of β-lactamases and allows the coadministered penicillins to reach their target site. This "suicidal inhibition" has no antibacterial activity itself but does effectively "tie up" any susceptible β-lactamase, preventing the accompanying penicillin from destruction. All of these agents are combined in fixed ratios with specific penicillins (amoxicillin–clavulanic acid [oral], ticarcillin–clavulanic acid [intravenous], ampicillin-sulbactam [intravenous], and piperacillin-tazobactam [intravenous]). β-Lactamases of *S. aureus*, *Haemophilus*, *Neisseria*, *Branhamella*, *Klebsiella*, and *Bacteroides* are generally inhibited by the agents and expand the spectrum of activity against these bacteria. Chromosomally mediated β-lactamases for the genera *Enterobacter*, *Citrobacter*, *Serratia*, and *Pseudomonas* are not inhibited by these agents, and no increased activity against these bacteria can be expected.

Administration, Absorption, Distribution, Metabolism, and Excretion

Clavulanic acid is the only oral β-lactamase inhibitor currently available in the United States. Sulbactam and tazobactam are only available for parenteral administration. The β-lactamase inhibitors have a similar (but distinct) distribution and excretion as the penicillin they are combined with. All of the compounds are excreted via renal mechanisms.

Adverse Effects

The major adverse reactions to these compounds are nausea and vomiting, especially with clavulanic acid. Because these agents are both immunologically cross-reactive with penicillins and always administered in fixed combinations with a penicillin, these drugs are obviously contraindicated in penicillin-allergic patients.

BOX 37–7

INDICATIONS AND CONTRAINDICATIONS

Increased activity against β-lactamase–producing strains of *S. aureus*, *Haemophilus*, *Neisseria*, and *Branhamella* organisms is seen with these combinations. Expanded Gram-negative coverage against many strains of *E. coli*, *Klebsiella*, and *Proteus* is also seen. Excellent anaerobic activity is also produced by these combination agents.

Amoxicillin-clavulanic acid is a useful agent for most bacteria causing otitis media, sinusitis, bronchitis, and skin and soft tissue infections. The additional anaerobic and Gram-negative activity of this combination also makes it useful for treatment of infections such as chronic sinusitis and diabetic foot ulcers in which anaerobes and Gram-negative rods are seen with greater frequency. Some authorities consider amoxicillin-clavulanic acid to be the drug of choice for treating animal bites when the physician needs to have an active agent against streptococci, staphylococci, and *Pasteurella multocida*, a normal flora of cats and dogs. First-generation cephalosporins and antistaphylococcal penicillins are not active against *Pasteurella*, which is effectively treated by amoxicillin.

The addition of clavulanic acid to ticarcillin increases the Gram-negative spectrum of ticarcillin to include many members of the family Enterobac-

Continued

BOX 37–7

INDICATIONS AND CONTRAINDICATIONS (*Continued*)

teriaceae, anaerobes, and β-lactamase–producing staphylococci. No increase in activity is seen with respect to pseudomonads because resistance to the extended-spectrum penicillins in pseudomonads is not mediated by β-lactamases susceptible to the β-lactamase inhibitors. Reports of staphylococcal bacteremia after use of ticarcillin-clavulanic acid have appeared; use of any of the β-lactamase inhibitor combinations for serious staphylococcal disease or bacteremia should be avoided.

Ampicillin-sulbactam has excellent activity against most anaerobic bacteria and is used in the treatment of infections caused by mixed aerobic and anaerobic bacteria, such as intra-abdominal infections, diabetic foot ulcers, and decubitus ulcers. Addition of the sulbactam to ampicillin also increases the activity against β-lactamase–producing strains of *S. aureus*, *Haemophilus*, *Neisseria*, and *Branhamella* organisms. Ampicillin-sulbactam is therefore useful as an empirical therapy for most cases of community-acquired sinusitis, otitis, bronchitis, and pneumonia (except where *Mycoplasma* or *Legionella* are suspected). The drug should also be useful in the treatment of aspiration pneumonia and anaerobic lung infections.

Piperacillin-tazobactam has recently been released for use in the United States. Increased Gram-negative activity, anaerobic activity, and staphylococcal activity are seen with this combination when compared with piperacillin. No increased activity is seen against pseudomonads. The drug should be useful for mixed aerobic-anaerobic infections as outlined previously.

VANCOMYCIN

Chemistry

Vancomycin is a complex glycopeptide antibiotic. Although its primary mechanism of action is inhibition of cell wall synthesis, the drug is structurally dissimilar to the *β*-lactam antibiotics.

Mechanism of Action

The major mechanism of action is believed to be rapid, irreversible binding of vancomycin via hydrogen bonding to the acyl-D-alanyl-D-alanine terminus of the membrane-bound peptidoglycan precursor. This results in rapid inhibition of cross-linking and causes direct membrane permeability defects. Additional data suggest that vancomycin may also impair RNA synthesis.

Mechanism of Resistance

Resistance to vancomycin had remained low since the time of its introduction more than 30 years ago. However, resistance has increased recently, especially among enterococci. Because this resistance is predominantly plasmid-mediated, great concern exists that the spread of this plasmid into strains of methicillin-resistant staphylococci will effectively eliminate the only useful antibiotic for the treatment of these infections. The consequences of this resistance could be analogous to a return to the preantibiotic era for the treatment of resistant staphylococcal disease.

Elegant studies have recently identified one mechanism of vancomycin resistance. Binding of vancomycin to the bacteria requires direct hydrogen bonding at the site of the acyl-D-alanyl-D-alanine subunit. Some vancomycin-resistant bacteria have substituted a terminal D-lactate for the D-alanine normally seen in peptidoglycan synthesis. This chemical modification results in an ester link instead of the normal amide linkage of acyl-D-alanyl-D-alanine. It is believed that the absence of this amide group inhibits binding of vancomycin to the complex and allows transpeptidation to proceed. The D-alanyl-D-lactate linkage is still an acceptable substrate for the transpeptidase, and peptidoglycan cross-linking is unaffected by the D-lactate moiety.

Administration, Absorption, Distribution, and Metabolism

Systemic levels of vancomycin are only achieved after parenteral administration via intravenous injection. Oral administration of vancomycin results in excellent concentrations of the agent in the gut lumen with little or no absorption of the drug from the gastrointestinal tract. (Minimal serum levels have been seen in patients with colitis, especially in the face of renal dysfunction.) Vancomycin is widely distributed in the body and reaches therapeutic levels in the CSF only in the presence of inflammation of the meninges.

Excretion

Vancomycin excretion is predominantly renal, and the drug has a serum half-life of 4–6 hours in patients with normal renal function. Serum half-life increases markedly in patients with renal insufficiency, with an average half-life of ≈150 hours in patients with creatinine clearances less than 10 mL/minute. Because the drug is only minimally removed by dialysis, single administration of vancomycin may provide useful serum concentrations for 7 days or longer in dialysis patients, and dosage adjustment with renal insufficiency is mandatory with this agent.

Adverse Effects

Early literature concerning vancomycin reported significant renal toxicity. Initial commercial production of vancomycin was difficult, and many authorities now believe that a substantial proportion of the early nephrotoxicity of this agent was related to impurities in the original formulations. Nephrotoxicity is difficult to demonstrate with currently available preparations of vancomycin; however, vancomycin may potentiate the nephrotoxicity of other coadministered agents.

Ototoxicity has been seen with vancomycin and may be more common with higher serum levels, generally in excess of 80 μg/mL. Clear correlation between serum levels of vancomycin and either ototoxicity or nephrotoxicity has not been proved, and the interpretation of "toxic" levels of vancomycin is difficult.

A particular reaction seen with vancomycin is a hypotensive reaction accompanied by flushing and erythema of the face, chest, neck, and upper extremities. This reaction, coined the "red man's syndrome" or the "red-neck syndrome," is exclusively related to the rapidity of administration of vancomycin. The hypotension and erythema of this syndrome are related to the production of histamine, and are the result of the rapid infusion of the agent, and do not represent a true allergic reaction. Decreasing the rate of administration or pretreating the patient with an antihistamine prevents the syndrome. Vancomycin should never be administered rapidly and should be given over a 1-hour period. Rapid administration prior to surgery is thought to be responsible for the labile hemodynamics seen in some patients given vancomycin prior to general anesthesia.

Vancomycin may cause thrombophlebitis at the injection site and may be a cause of drug fever. Other adverse effects include allergy, hypersensitivity reactions, nausea, vomiting, and bitter taste after oral administration.

BOX 37-8

INDICATIONS AND CONTRAINDICATIONS

The use of vancomycin should be divided into two treatment categories: oral and parenteral. Clinicians must remember that oral administration is totally ineffective for systemic infections and should be reserved exclusively for the treatment of specific forms of colitis.

The major use of intravenous vancomycin is the treatment of serious Gram-positive infections, most commonly staphylococcal and streptococcal, in patients with an allergic reaction to the penicillins. The choice of vancomycin over other alternatives such as erythromycin or clindamycin is generally based on the severity of the infectious process, when the clinician desires the bactericidal activity of vancomycin over the bacteriostatic activity of the former agents.

Vancomycin is the drug of choice for the treatment of methicillin-resistant staphylococci, both *S. aureus* and coagulase-negative staphylococci. Institutions vary widely in their incidence of methicillin-resistant staphylococci; empirical therapy at some institutions requires vancomycin for nosocomial infections. The increasing use of artificial devices in medicine (*eg*, indwelling catheters, prosthetic valves, prosthetic joints) has increased the frequency of infections with coagulase-negative *Staphylococcus* and has resulted in a greater role for vancomycin.

Vancomycin is indicated for the treatment of enterococcal infections, generally in combination with an aminoglycoside. Development of resistance to vancomycin in enterococci has recently increased. This may become a major problem because β-lactamase production and high-level resistance to the aminoglycosides has occurred in conjunction with vancomycin resistance, resulting in an inability to provide bactericidal therapy for these organisms.

Endocarditis prophylaxis for prosthetic heart valves in penicillin-allergic patients requiring parenteral therapy is another indication for vancomycin, again in combination with an aminoglycoside.

Vancomycin is generally active against most Gram-positive bacteria except *Leuconostoc* and *Erysipelothrix*. Vancomycin has no activity against Gram-negative bacteria.

Because of the long duration of action in patients on hemodialysis, vancomycin is frequently administered for suspected Gram-positive infections in dialysis patients. A single dose of vancomycin may provide adequate serum levels for over a week.

Vancomycin is quite active against a major etiologic agent of antibiotic associated colitis, *C. difficile*. Infection with toxin-producing strains of *C. difficile* produces pseudomembranous colitis (PMC), which ranges from a mild to fatal disease. Oral vancomycin is highly effective in the treatment of PMC. Resistance to vancomycin has not been seen to date in *C. difficile*.

Just as oral vancomycin is ineffective in the treatment of systemic disease, intravenous vancomycin is ineffective in the treatment of PMC. Luminal levels of vancomycin are subtherapeutic after intravenous vancomycin, and PMC has been reported in patients receiving intravenous vancomycin. Treatment of PMC can be accomplished with 125 mg vancomycin four times daily.

REFERENCES

Donowitz GR, Mandell GL: Drug therapy. Beta-lactam antibiotics (1). N Engl J Med 318:419–426, 1988.

Donowitz GR, Mandell GL: Drug therapy. Beta-lactam antibiotics (2). N Engl J Med 318:490–500, 1988.

Penicillins: *In* AHFS Drug Information, 207–228. Bethesda: American Society of Hospital Pharmacists, 1993.

Neu HC: Penicillins. *In* Mandell GL, Douglas RG Jr, Bennett JE (eds): Principles and Practice of Infectious Diseases, 3rd ed, 230–246. New York: Churchill Livingstone, 1990.

Neu HC: Other β-lactam antibiotics. *In* Mandell GL, Douglas RG Jr, Bennett JE (eds): Principles and Practice of Infectious Diseases, 3rd ed, 257–263. New York: Churchill Livingstone, 1990.

Brewer NS, Hellinger WC: The monobactams. Mayo Clin Proc 66:1152–1157, 1991.

Wilhelm MP: Vancomycin. Mayo Clin Proc 66:1165–1170, 1991.

Wendel GD Jr, Stark BJ, Jamison RB, et al: Penicillin allergy and desensitization in serious infections during pregnancy. N Engl J Med 312:1229–1232, 1985.

38 Cephalosporins

Thomas R. Beam, Jr., deceased

The cephalosporins bind to penicillin-binding proteins (PBPs) with varying affinity, inhibit protein synthesis, and prevent formation of an autolysin. In the absence of autolysin, bacterial cells rupture and die. However, in cells that lack a natural autolysin, cephalosporins still may inhibit bacterial growth and exert a bacteriostatic effect.

Cephalosporins have been divided into generations to characterize the spectrum of antimicrobial activity, describe the time of introduction to the marketplace, and simplify the characteristics of a multitude of compounds. In general, first-generation cephalosporins are short-acting and possess excellent activity against Gram-positive cocci, limited activity against Enterobacteriaceae, and no activity against Pseudomonaceae. Second-generation cephalosporins have slightly longer serum half-lives, less Gram-positive and more Gram-negative activity, and no activity against *Pseudomonas.* Third-generation cephalosporins have longer half-lives, weak activity (particularly against staphylococci), and very potent activity against Gram-negative bacilli. Some are effective in the treatment of infections with *Pseudomonas* species.

CHEMISTRY

Cephalosporin C provides the molecular structure from which other cephalosporins have been derived. It contains a β-lactam ring and an adjacent dihydrothiazine ring. Acid treatment of cephalosporin C hydrolyzes the compound to 7-aminocephalosporanic acid (7-ACA). Substitutions at position 7 of the 7-ACA nucleus alter antibacterial activity. Insertion of a 7-methoxy group yields compounds called cephamycins; cefoxitin is an example. Substitutions at position 3 of the dihydrothiazine ring are associated with altered pharmacokinetics of the drug. The cephalosporin nucleus is shown in Figure 38 – 1.

MECHANISM OF ACTION

Cephalosporins bind to and inactivate PBPs located on the inner bacterial cell membrane. PBPs are enzymes that facilitate synthesis of the peptidoglycan component of the cell wall. The effect on bacterial growth depends on the PBPs to which the cephalosporin binds. Certain PBPs (1,2,3) are important to bacterial survival; binding by a cephalosporin to these PBPs results in a lethal effect. Other PBPs (4,5,6) are not essential to bacterial survival. Binding may produce elongated forms, but the bacteria are not killed. However, host defenses such as polymorphonuclear leukocytes and macrophages, with assistance from immunoglobulin, can eliminate these damaged bacterial cells.

RESISTANCE

The main vulnerability of cephalosporins is to enzymatic degradation through cephalosporinases or β-lactamases. These enzymes may be specified by plasmids that are transferred readily from species to species or by chromosomes and limited to a single bacterial species. Bacteria also may become resistant or may possess native resistance through the development of a permeability barrier at the cell wall. A few types of bacteria combine these mechanisms of resistance.

The type of resistance has also been described as *constitutive* (present all the time) or *inducible* (present only after exposure to the antibiotic). The latter type is of greatest concern clinically because an isolated pathogen initially tests susceptible in the microbiology laboratory. Treatment with a cephalosporin of the patient infected with these strains does not result in clinical improvement. Reisolation and repeated testing of the organism from the infected site show the bacteria to be cephalosporin-resistant.

For first- and second-generation cephalosporins, no clinically relevant activity is demonstrable against pathogens such as *Pseudomonas aeruginosa.* This is attributable to a failure to penetrate through the porin found in the outer membrane of these Gram-negative bacteria.

For all cephalosporins, methicillin-resistant staphylococci are also cephalosporin-resistant. These organisms develop new PBPs to which the penicillins and cephalosporins cannot attach. The normal PBPs are suppressed by the bacteria.

Most second- and third-generation cephalosporins were developed to be β-lactamase stable, particularly to β-

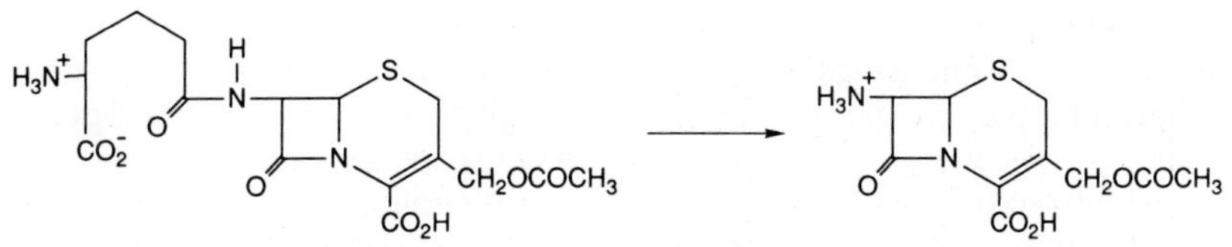

cephalosporin C → 7-ACA

FIGURE 38-1. The basic cephalosporin structure.

lactamases produced by Gram-negative bacilli. These drugs have been extensively used in the hospital setting with great therapeutic success. However, the high usage patterns also have promoted development of resistance. A broad-spectrum β-lactamase specified by a plasmid and capable of producing resistance to all cephalosporins has been identified in *Klebsiella* and *Enterobacter* species. The organisms have disseminated rapidly in certain hospitals, causing epidemics of disease.

A β-lactamase found in the chromosomes of *Enterobacter*, *Serratia*, *Citrobacter*, and *Pseudomonas* species also has been described. Production of this enzyme is derepressed upon exposure to the drug. Rather than catalyze the hydrolysis of the cephalosporin, it has been proposed that this enzyme simply binds to the antibiotic molecule and prevents it from reaching its target site (a spongelike effect).

Most recently, penicillin-resistant pneumococci have become prevalent in certain areas of the United States. Some of these strains have resistance to other classes of antimicrobials (chloramphenicol, macrolides, tetracyclines). A few have also been resistant to all generations of cephalosporins. Clearly, resistance to cephalosporins must be carefully considered before prescribing these drugs in the mid- to late 1990s.

ABSORPTION, DISTRIBUTION, METABOLISM, AND EXCRETION

Cephalosporins may be administered by the oral or parenteral routes. Most cephalosporins are tolerated poorly when given by intramuscular injection because of pain at the injection site. Drugs that can be administered intramuscularly include cefazolin and ceftriaxone (Table 38-1).

TABLE 38-1. Pharmacokinetic Parameters of Cephalosporin Antibiotics

Name	Route of Administration	Protein Binding (%)	Serum Half-Life (Hours)	Metabolized (%)	Secreted	Urine Recovery (%)
First-Generation						
Cephalothin	IV	70	0.5-0.9	20-30	Yes	50-80
Cephapirin	IV	45-50	0.6-0.8	40	Yes	50-90
Cefazolin	IV/IM	85	1.5-1.8	None	Yes	95
Cephalexin	PO	10-15	0.9-1.3	None	Yes	90
Cephradine	IV/PO	10-20	0.8-1.3	None	Yes	90
Cefadroxil	PO	15-20	1.4-1.5	None	Yes	90
Second-Generation						
Cefamandole	IV/IM	70-80	0.6-1.0	None	Yes	80-95
Cefoxitin	IV/IM	70-80	0.75-1.0	<2	Yes	80-95
Ceforanide	IV/IM	80	2.7-3.0	None	Yes	80-95
Cefuroxime	IV/IM	33	1.3-1.7	None	Yes	90-95
Cefuroxime axetil	PO	50	1.2	None	Yes	90-95
Cefaclor	PO	25	0.6-0.9	None	No	60-85
Cefonicid	IV/IM	95-98	3.5-4.5	None	Yes	90
Cefotetan	IV/IM	88	3.5	7	Yes	80
Cefprozil	PO	36	1.3	None	Yes	60
Cefmetazole	IV	65	1.2	None	Yes	85
Loracarbef	PO	25	1.0	None	Yes	90
Third-Generation						
Cefotaxime	IV/IM	38	1.0-1.1	30-50	Yes	85
Moxalactam	IV/IM	50	2.0-2.3	None	No	70-95
Ceftizoxime	IV/IM	30	1.4-1.8	None	Yes	80-90
Ceftriaxone	IV/IM	83-96	6.0-9.0	None	No	40-65
Cefoperazone	IV/IM	87-93	1.9-2.1	None	No	25
Ceftazidime	IV/IM	17	1.6-1.9	None	No	75-90
Cefixime	PO	65	3-4	None	Yes	50
Cefpodoxime proxetil	PO	28	2.5	Minimal	Yes	33

IM = intramuscular; IV = intravenous; PO = oral.

The chemical formulation differs for the oral and parenteral routes of delivery. Furthermore, some drugs available as oral medications do not have comparable parenteral formulations (and vice versa).

Cephalosporins distribute into extravascular sites (interstitial fluid) relatively well. Only third-generation cephalosporins and cefuroxime penetrate reliably into the central nervous system and may be used to treat bacterial meningitis. No cephalosporin penetrates intracellularly; thus, these drugs are not effective in the treatment of intracellular pathogens (*eg*, *Legionella*, *Chlamydia*, and *Rickettsia* species).

ADVERSE EFFECTS

Gastrointestinal side effects of the cephalosporins include nausea, vomiting, diarrhea, anorexia, and pseudomembranous colitis. Hepatic enzyme levels may be transiently and reversibly elevated during therapy, but true hepatotoxicity is rare. Cephalosporins are not generally nephrotoxic, although cephalothin has been reported to cause tubular necrosis. Cephalosporins may interact with nephrotoxic drugs (particularly aminoglycosides) to increase the amount of toxicity.

Cephalosporins may cause a positive Coombs' reaction, but this is rarely associated with hemolysis. When used in high doses for an extended period of time, cephalosporins may cause neutropenia.

Bleeding diathesis and a disulfiram (ANTABUSE)-like effect have been associated with cephalosporins containing a methylthiotetrazole ring. Cephalosporins with this structure include cefamandole, cefotetan, cefmetazole, moxalactam, and cefoperazone. Moxalactam also induces platelet aggregation abnormalities and is the most likely of these agents to cause bleeding. It therefore is the least used among these compounds.

INDICATIONS AND CONTRAINDICATIONS

Cephalosporins may be used for the prophylaxis or treatment of a wide variety of infectious diseases. The drug of choice to prevent postoperative wound infections for many clean and clean-contaminated procedures is cefazolin. Second-generation cephalosporins including cefoxitin and cefotetan are advocated for prophylaxis in gynecologic and

TABLE 38–2. Indications for Use of Cephalosporin Antibiotics*

	Respiratory Tract		Urinary Tract		Skin/Skin Structure		STD					
Name	*CA*	*HA*	*Uncomp*	*Comp*	*Uncomp*	*Comp*	*GC*	*Bacteremia*	Bone or Joint	Intraabdominal	Meningitis	Surgical Prophylaxis
First-Generation												
Cephalothin	x	—	x	—	x	—	—	x	x	—	—	—
Cephapirin	x	—	x	—	x	—	—	x	x	—	—	—
Cefazolin	x	—	x	—	x	—	—	x	x	—	—	x
Cephalexin	x	—	x	—	x	—	—	—	x	—	—	—
Cephradine	x	—	x	—	x	—	—	—	x	—	—	—
Cefadroxil	x	—	x	—	x	—	—	—	—	—	—	—
Second-Generation												
Cefamandole	x	—	x	—	x	—	—	—	x	—	—	x
Cefoxitin	x	—	x	—	x	x	x	x	x	x	—	x
Ceforanide	x	—	x	—	x	—	—	x	x	—	—	x
Cefuroxime	x	—	x	—	x	—	x	x	x	—	x	x
Cefuroxime axetil	x	—	x	—	x	—	x	—	—	—	—	—
Cefaclor	x	—	x	—	x	—	—	—	—	—	—	—
Cefonicid	x	—	x	—	x	—	—	—	x	—	—	x
Cefotetan	x	—	x	—	x	—	—	—	x	x	—	x
Cefprozil	x	—	—	—	x	—	—	—	—	—	—	—
Cefmetazole	x	—	x	x	x	x	—	—	—	x	—	x
Loracarbef	x	—	x	—	x	—	—	—	—	—	—	—
Third-Generation												
Cefotaxime	x	x	x	x	x	x	x	x	x	x	x	x
Moxalactam	x	x	x	x	x	x	—	x	x	x	x	—
Ceftizoxime	x	x	x	x	x	x	x	x	x	x	x	—
Ceftriaxone	x	x	x	x	x	x	x	x	x	x	x	x
Cefoperazone	x	x	x	x	x	x	x	x	—	x	—	—
Ceftazidime	x	x	x	x	x	x	—	x	x	x	x	—
Cefixime	x	—	x	—	—	—	x	—	—	—	—	—
Cefpodoxime proxetil	x	—	x	—	x	—	x	—	—	—	—	—

*x = yes; — = no.
CA = community-acquired; Comp = complicated; GC = *Neisseria gonorrheae*; HA = hospital-acquired;
STD = sexually transmitted diseases; Uncomp = uncomplicated.

colon surgery because of their activity against two major pathogens associated with surgical procedures, *Escherichia coli* and *Bacteroides fragilis*.

The cephalosporins are indicated for treatment of a wide variety of infectious diseases, depending on the individual drug's spectrum of activity. In general, first-generation cephalosporins should be targeted toward streptococcal and staphylococcal infections or toward those caused by a limited number of susceptible Gram-negative strains (*E. coli*).

Second-generation cephalosporins add activity against *Haemophilus influenzae* or *B. fragilis*. Cefuroxime is approved for the treatment of meningitis caused by susceptible strains of *H. influenzae*, *Streptococcus pneumoniae*, and *Neisseria meningitidis*. Other cephalosporins possessing this type of activity are limited to treatment of infections outside the central nervous system. Cefoxitin, cefotetan, and cefmetazole are indicated for treatment of intra-abdominal and pelvic infections. Cefoxitin has also been used to treat serious foot infections in patients with diabetes mellitus.

Third-generation cephalosporins are divided into those with anti-*Pseudomonas* activity (cefoperazone, ceftazidime) and the rest. These drugs have been most useful for treatment of meningitis and hospital-acquired Gram-negative infections in a wide variety of body sites. Included are pneumonia, bacteremia, urinary tract infections, intra-abdominal infections, and skin and skin-structure infections. Ceftriaxone has been commonly employed for single-dose treatment of gonococcal infections and for treatment of late manifestations of Lyme disease.

Indications for use of individual drugs are presented in Table 38-2. In general, community-acquired infections are caused by organisms less resistant to antimicrobials than hospital-acquired infections. Uncomplicated infections occur in individuals without anatomic compromise at the infected site. Indications are for treatment of infections caused by susceptible organisms. Finally, respiratory tract infections may include one or more of the following: tonsillitis/pharyngitis, otitis media, sinusitis, bacterial complications of acute bronchitis, acute exacerbations of chronic bronchitis, and community or hospital-acquired pneumonia. The only contraindication to the use of cephalosporins is previous hypersensitivity to the drugs.

Acknowledgment

This work was supported by the Department of Veterans Affairs.

REFERENCES

Chow JW, Fine MJ, Shlaes DM, Quinn JP, Hooper DC, Johnson MP, Ramphal R, Wagener MM, Miyashiro DK, Yu VL: Enterobacter bacteremia: Clinical features and emergence of antibiotic resistance during therapy. Ann Intern Med 115:585-590, 1991.

Donowitz GR, Mandell GL: Beta-lactam antibiotics. New Engl J Med 318:490, 1988.

Griffith RS, Black HR: Cephalothin—A new antibiotic. JAMA 189:823, 1964.

Meyer KS, Urban C, Eagan JA, Berger BJ, Rahal JJ: Nosocomial outbreak of klebsiella infection resistant to late-generation cephalosporins. Am Coll Phys 119:353-358, 1993.

Quintiliani R, Nightingale CH: Cefazolin. Ann Intern Med 89(Part I):650, 1978.

Tartaglione TA, Polk RF: Review of the new second-generation cephalosporins. Cefonicid, ceforanide and cefuroxime. Drug Intell Clin Pharm 19:188, 1985.

39 Drugs That Act on the Bacterial Ribosome: Aminoglycosides, Tetracyclines, Chloramphenicol, and Erythromycin

Alan M. Reynard

All the drugs covered in this chapter have a relatively broad spectrum of action. In particular, the tetracyclines and chloramphenicol became known as the broad-spectrum antibiotics because of their activity against some nonbacterial species as well as the Gram-positive and Gram-negative bacteria. All these drugs inhibit bacterial protein synthesis by virtue of their actions on the ribosome.

THE AMINOGLYCOSIDES

The currently available aminoglycosides are streptomycin, kanamycin, gentamicin, amikacin, neomycin, netilmicin, paromomycin, and tobramycin.

Although the aminoglycosides have a number of similarities, differences have led to a decrease in use of some of the aminoglycosides and an increase in use of others. Most of the aminoglycosides are still used at least in some circumstances. Over the years since the discovery of streptomycin, kanamycin replaced streptomycin for general use because of a slightly lower toxicity and better activity against Gram-negative bacilli; gentamicin replaced kanamycin because of a broader spectrum of action and lower susceptibility to bacterial resistance; and amikacin replaced gentamicin when resistance to gentamicin rose to unacceptable levels.

Chemistry

The aminoglycosides have several structural features in common; they each contain one or more sugar moieties and a streptidine ring. They each have one or more amino or guanidino groups. The aminoglycosides are very soluble in water, are stable in solution, and are more active in alkaline than in acid media. This last property is of importance in treatment of a variety of infections, because the relatively low pH at the site of infection (urinary tract, respiratory tract, secretions, abscess, *etc*) compromises the activity of these drugs. The structures of streptomycin, gentamicin, and amikacin are shown in Figure 39 – 1.

Mechanism of Action

The aminoglycosides all act by the same mechanism. They bind to proteins on the 30S ribosome of bacteria, thereby in-

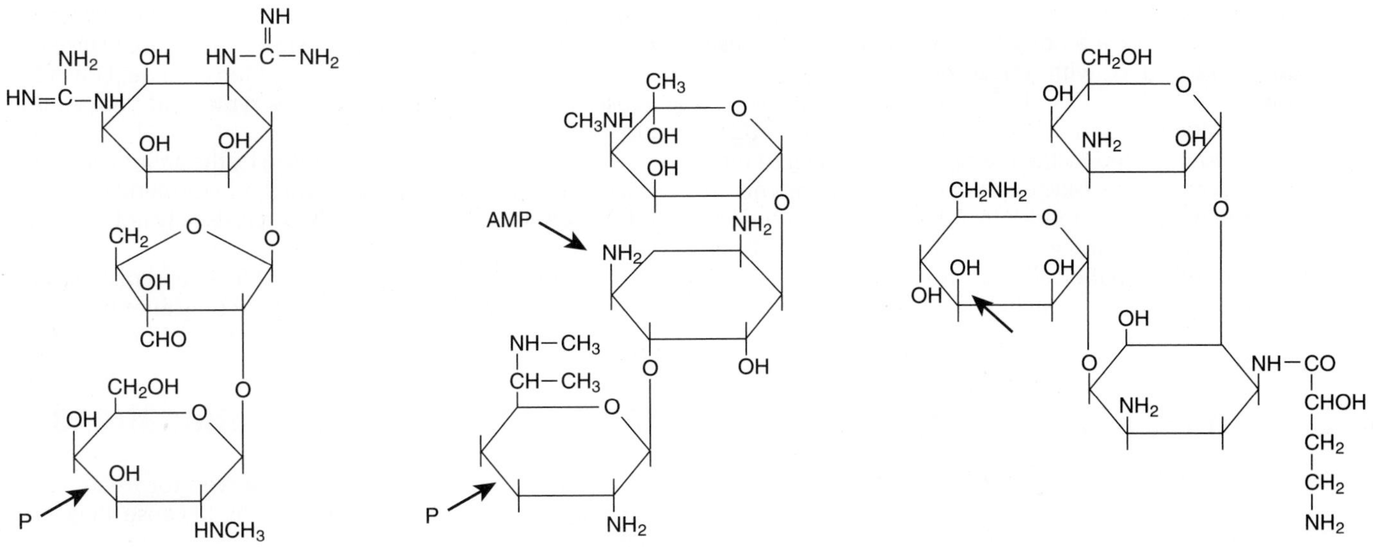

Streptomycin Gentamycin C_1 Amikacin

FIGURE 39–1. Structures of streptomycin, gentamicin, and amikacin. The arrow labeled P shows the site of phosphorylation of streptomycin and the site on gentamicin where the lack of a hydroxyl group protects gentamicin from phosphorylation. The arrow labeled AMP shows where the AMP portion of ATP is attached to gentamicin. The sites for attachment of both the phosphate and the AMP moieties are blocked by the alpha-aminobutyryl group on amikacin.

hibiting protein synthesis, particularly the initiation step. Inhibition of protein synthesis is not a lethal event in bacteria in the same sense as destruction of the cell envelope. Nevertheless, the aminoglycosides bind so strongly to their receptors that the binding is essentially irreversible and the end result is death of the bacterial cell. Thus, the aminoglycosides are considered to be bactericidal. This is in contrast to other inhibitors of protein synthesis such as chloramphenicol and the tetracyclines, in which binding to the ribosome is weaker and the drugs are bacteriostatic.

The aminoglycosides also cause misreading of the genetic code, so that incorrect amino acids are incorporated into proteins of the bacterial cell, but this mechanism is probably less important than inhibition of protein synthesis in killing cells.

At high concentrations, aminoglycosides cause disruption of membranes of both bacterial and mammalian cells. The concentration required for this is higher than that usually achieved in the blood during therapy. However, aminoglycosides accumulate in the fluids of the ear and the kidney in high concentration, and this high concentration is probably responsible for the adverse effects seen in these two organs.

Resistance

Bacteria can become resistant to the aminoglycosides in several ways. The most important, clinically, is the plasmid-mediated production of drug-inactivating enzymes by resistant cells. Three different enzymes have been identified. They catalyze the reactions below:

$$\text{AcCoA} + \text{AG} \longrightarrow \text{Ac-AG} + \text{CoA}$$

$$\text{ATP} + \text{AG} \longrightarrow \text{P-AG} + \text{ADP}$$

$$\text{ATP} + \text{AG} \longrightarrow \text{AMP-AG} + \text{PP}_i$$

In the first reaction, an amino group on the aminoglycoside (AG) is acetylated (AcCoA = acetylcoenzyme A). In the second, a hydroxyl group on the aminoglycoside is phosphorylated (ATP = adenosine triphosphate; ADP = adenosine diphosphate). In the third, a hydroxyl group on the aminoglycoside receives the adenosine monophosphate (AMP) portion of ATP (the aminoglycoside is adenylylated) (PP_i = inorganic pyrophosphate). In all cases the conjugated aminoglycoside is inactivated.

The phosphorylation reaction was discovered soon after the discovery of plasmid-mediated resistance. Phosphorylation causes inactivation of the first two aminoglycosides, streptomycin and kanamycin. Gentamicin, lacking the hydroxyl group (see the two arrows labeled P in Figure 39–1) that is the target of that reaction, was free of inactivation for a number of years. Eventually, a plasmid appeared that specified the enzyme that catalyzes adenylylation, a reaction to which gentamicin is susceptible. In this reaction the AMP portion of ATP is attached to an amino group on the gentamicin (see arrow labeled AMP in Fig. 39–1). At about the same time, a derivative of kanamycin, amikacin, was produced that was not susceptible to either phosphorylation or adenylylation. Amikacin is essentially kanamycin B with an α-amino-γ-hydroxybutaryl moiety attached. This group protects the molecule from the inactivating enzymes by steric hindrance.

In general, plasmid-mediated resistance results in low-level resistance where minimal inhibitory concentrations range from 25 to 200 μg/mL.

Another mechanism of resistance is a mutation that results in the production of a 30S ribosomal subunit that contains an altered protein. The ribosome still functions in protein synthesis but no longer binds an aminoglycoside. This mechanism results in an organism with very high levels of resistance (1000–3000 μg/mL). This mechanism has less clinical significance than enzyme-mediated resistance in the

Gram-negative rods, but has become an increasingly common form of resistance among enterococci and can cause infections associated with these organisms to be untreatable.

A third mechanism derives from the fact that aminoglycosides are transported to the interior of a cell, where they bind to ribosomes by an oxygen-dependent transport mechanism. Some organisms flourish in anaerobic conditions. In this circumstance, aminoglycosides are not transported into the bacterial cells, and the cells survive despite the presence of high concentrations of aminoglycoside in the environment.

Absorption, Distribution, Metabolism, and Excretion

The most common route of administration of the aminoglycosides is intravenous. Intramuscular injection is used for streptomycin with good absorption; peak plasma levels are achieved in 30 – 90 minutes. Administration is rarely oral except for neomycin. Aminoglycosides are not absorbed from the gastrointestinal tract. Neomycin, when administered orally, affects only the microbes in the gastrointestinal tract and is used in combination with erythromycin for elective colon surgery. Neomycin is also present in some topical antimicrobial creams.

Less than 20% of absorbed drug is bound to plasma protein. The aminoglycosides are highly charged and do not enter mammalian cells readily. There is little metabolism of the drugs. Excretion is largely by glomerular filtration and is reduced in renal damage. In patients with reduced kidney function, the dose of an aminoglycoside must be reduced. A number of nomograms are available to calculate dose on the basis of creatinine clearance, ideal body weight, and sex of a patient.

Adverse Effects

The principal dangers associated with the use of aminoglycosides are ototoxicity and nephrotoxicity. In both types of toxicity the high concentration of drug that accumulates in the fluids of these tissues probably plays a role.

The ototoxicity is associated with either hearing loss (cochlear damage), vertigo (vestibular damage), or both. An early sign is tinnitus accompanied by loss of high-frequency hearing. The hearing loss, if detected early, can be reversed, but it becomes permanent after prolonged treatment. Patients receiving aminoglycosides such as streptomycin should have periodic hearing tests. The various aminoglycosides differ in the relative proportion of hearing loss and vertigo that they produce. The high amount of hearing loss produced by neomycin precludes its systemic use. Ototoxicity is not a problem with the other aminoglycosides as long as serum concentrations are monitored.

The nephrotoxicity caused by the aminoglycosides is dose-related and reversible if not too severe. Among the commonly prescribed aminoglycosides, gentamicin is the most nephrotoxic, followed by tobramycin and amikacin.

The concomitant administration of other drugs that cause similar adverse effects will potentiate the adverse effects caused by the aminoglycosides. Drugs that cause ototoxicity include ethacrynic acid and furosemide. Drugs that cause nephrotoxicity include ethacrynic acid, furosemide, cisplatin, and polymyxin.

A third adverse reaction caused by the aminoglycosides is a curare-like neuromuscular blockade resulting in respiratory paralysis. This occurs rarely and is usually not of clinical concern.

Allergic reactions in the form of fever and rash may occasionally occur. These usually appear only after prolonged contact with the drug, as in the treatment of tuberculosis.

Indications and Contraindications

The aminoglycosides are usually reserved for treatment of the more serious microbial infections because they have very severe adverse effects.

There is a narrow window of plasma concentration of gentamicin between the minimum needed to produce a therapeutic effect (8 μg/mL) and a toxic effect (12 μg/mL). In addition, there is considerable variability in achievable plasma levels between individuals. Therefore, the plasma concentration of gentamicin is often monitored.

Because amikacin has a broader spectrum of activity against Gram-negative bacilli than does gentamicin, it has replaced gentamicin for general use in some hospitals because of the increased resistance to gentamicin.

Tobramycin and netilmicin have essentially the same spectrum of action as gentamicin. Netilmicin, because of its structure, is protected from inactivation by the phosphorylating enzyme and, therefore, exhibits less resistance than gentamicin. Tobramycin has greater *in vivo* activity against *Pseudomonas aeruginosa*. Paromomycin is rarely used.

BOX 39-1
THERAPEUTIC USES

Streptomycin is currently used mainly in the treatment of tuberculosis, usually in conjunction with other agents such as isoniazid, rifampin, and pyrazinamide or ethambutol. Streptomycin is also used in the therapy of plague and tularemia.

Gentamicin may be used for treatment of many aerobic Gram-negative infections such as those caused by *Escherichia coli*, Klebsiella, Enterobacter, Proteus, and Serratia. Another use for gentamicin is in treatment of certain infections caused by methicillin-resistant staphylococci. Gentamicin and piperacillin act synergistically in the treatment of *Pseudomonas aeruginosa*.

Neomycin, because of its high toxicity, is never administered parenterally, but it is available in a variety of over-the-counter preparations for topical administration. Neomycin is administered orally for preparation of the lower bowel for surgery. It is not absorbed from the gastrointestinal tract, except in patients with renal dysfunction. It is excreted in the feces.

TETRACYCLINES

The tetracyclines are a group of drugs with a common 4-ring structure, hence the name.

Chemistry

The tetracyclines are bright-yellow compounds, poorly soluble in water as the free base but soluble as the hydrochloride. The hydrochloride is the form available for clinical use. With the exception of chlortetracycline, tetracyclines are moderately stable in solution. However, breakdown products form over a period of several years even in solid form, and these products can be toxic. The tetracyclines chelate divalent and trivalent metal ions. This chelation is responsible for their incorporation into tooth and bone material and for poor absorption from the gastrointestinal tract, particularly in the presence of milk and other milk products. The structure of tetracycline illustrates the 4-ring system from which the name is derived.

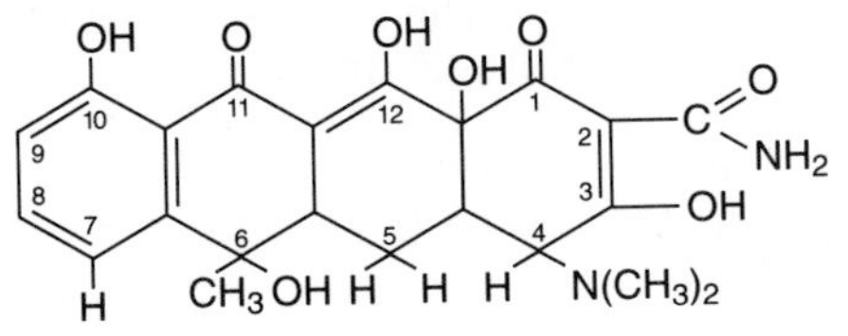

Mechanism of Action

The tetracyclines bind to the 30S subunit of microbial ribosomes, which results in inhibition of protein synthesis by interference with attachment of aminoacyl-tRNA. Tetracyclines are actively transported into microbial cells but not into mammalian cells; this is the basis for their selective toxicity. Tetracyclines are bacteriostatic drugs.

Resistance

Plasmid-mediated resistance to the tetracyclines is extremely common among the Gram-negative rods. It results from an increased efflux of drug from the resistant cells, thereby reducing intracellular concentration. There is no known chromosomally mediated resistance to the tetracyclines.

Absorption, Distribution, Metabolism, and Excretion

Absorption of the tetracyclines following oral administration is somewhat variable. In general, chlortetracycline is least well absorbed, and doxycycline and minocycline are almost completely absorbed. Because absorption is poor in the presence of food, the drugs should be taken at least 1 hour before or 2 hours after a meal.

The tetracyclines are bound in various amounts to plasma proteins and are distributed to most tissues. Unlike chloramphenicol, the tetracyclines do not reach useful concentrations in cerebrospinal fluid.

A considerable portion of an oral dose of a tetracycline is excreted in the feces. This varies among the tetracyclines. Tetracyclines are relatively lipophilic and therefore appear in the enterohepatic circulation, which also contributes to fecal excretion. Absorbed tetracyclines are excreted largely by glomerular filtration, making their plasma levels very dependent on kidney function. Exceptions are minocycline and doxycycline; for these drugs glomerular filtration appears to have little role in excretion.

Adverse Effects

The tetracyclines produce a variety of dose-related gastrointestinal effects, including nausea, vomiting, and epigastric distress. Diarrhea may also result and should be distinguished from the pseudomembranous colitis associated with growth of *Clostridium difficile*.

Tetracyclines, like other broad-spectrum antibiotics, have a relatively high potential to produce superinfection. This is caused by the suppression of certain body flora with subsequent appearance of other organisms, particularly staphylococci, clostridia, and candida. Drugs with a narrow spectrum of action, such as penicillin, produce superinfection much less frequently. When there is evidence of superinfection, administration of the causative drug, in this case tetracycline, should be stopped if the original infection has been adequately treated. New antimicrobial therapy should be provided for the superinfection.

Hepatic toxicity can occur with administration of large doses (usually 2 g/day or more) of drug. The symptoms include jaundice, azotemia, acidosis, and possibly shock. Biopsy of the liver reveals a diffuse, fatty infiltrate.

Nephrotoxicity in the form of azotemia has been observed in some patients, especially in the presence of preexisting kidney failure. The shelf life of tetracycline is limited, and ingestion of outdated tetracycline has been the cause of a clinical picture similar to that of the Fanconi syndrome, presumably due to the effects of degradation products. The symptoms include nausea, vomiting, and kidney failure.

Treatment with tetracyclines, especially demeclocycline and doxycycline, may cause sensitivity to sunlight (phototoxicity), leading to mild to severe skin reactions.

Tetracycline, because it chelates divalent metals, binds strongly to bone and tooth material. The binding can cause depression of bone growth. Tetracycline is a bright-yellow compound and can cause discoloration of teeth that changes from yellow to grayish brown over time. Because of these effects, tetracyclines are contraindicated in children of tooth-formation age and also in pregnant women from mid-pregnancy onward.

Administration of minocycline has been associated with vestibular reactions such as dizziness and nausea.

Intravenous (IV) administration of a tetracycline can lead to thrombophlebitis at the IV site.

Various hypersensitivity reactions to the tetracyclines have been described including rash, fever, glossitis, angioedema, and anaphylaxis. However, these reactions, especially the more serious ones, are quite rare.

Great benefit has been derived from the use of tetracyclines. However, the enormous amounts of tetracycline used have contributed to greatly increased numbers of resistant organisms.

Indications and Contraindications

Tetracyclines are contraindicated in children up to about 8 years of age, in whom long bones or tooth enamel is being formed, and are contraindicated in pregnant women.

BOX 39–2

THERAPEUTIC USES

The tetracyclines are the drugs of choice for treatment of rickettsial infections such as Rocky Mountain spotted fever, rickettsialpox, Q fever, Brill's disease, murine typhus, and scrub typhus; chlamydial infections such as pneumonia, psittacosis, inclusion conjunctivitis, and trachoma; and mycoplasma infections such as pneumonia.

Rickettsial and mycoplasma infections are usually treated with tetracycline, whereas chlamydial infections are often treated with doxycycline.

Neisseria gonorrhoeae is susceptible to the tetracyclines, and treatment of gonorrhea in areas in which there is a high prevalence of penicillinase-producing *N. gonorrhoeae* can be accomplished with tetracycline or doxycycline. However, resistance to the tetracyclines has also increased, reducing effectiveness of these drugs, and ceftriaxone (see Chapter 38) has become the treatment of choice. Tetracyclines are effective against chlamydia, which often accompanies gonorrhea. They should be administered along with ceftriaxone for treatment of cervicitis, urethritis, and inflammatory pelvic disease.

The tetracyclines can be useful in cases of syphilis when it is not possible to use a penicillin or a cephalosporin because of allergy.

Minocycline has been used to eradicate the meningococcal carrier state, but its serious toxicity (vertigo) limits its usefulness.

Tetracycline is often used in treatment of acne when it occurs in young people and in adults as acne rosacea. It is thought that inhibition of propionibacteria results in a decrease in the amount of fatty acids occurring in sebaceous follicles. The low dose of tetracycline used seems to produce few adverse effects, but there is the possibility, because of the long term of treatment, of developing tetracycline-resistant organisms.

Tetracyclines may be used for a number of infections for which they are no longer the drug of choice. This is particularly true when the drug of choice is not useful because of hypersensitivity, resistance, or some other reason. These infections include cholera, brucellosis, tularemia, urinary tract infection by some Gram-negative strains, actinomycosis, Lyme disease, yaws, relapsing fever, tetanus, and plague.

CHLORAMPHENICOL

Chemistry

Chloramphenicol has a relatively simple structure. It is produced by chemical synthesis, in contrast to most other antibacterial agents, which are produced as a byproduct of mold growth. It is a colorless compound, relatively insoluble in water.

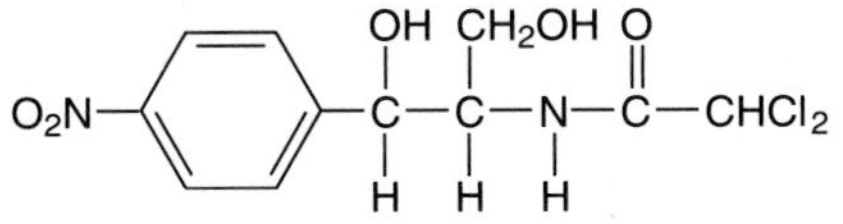

$$O_2N-C_6H_4-\underset{H}{\overset{OH}{C}}-\underset{H}{\overset{CH_2OH}{C}}-\underset{H}{N}-\overset{O}{\overset{\|}{C}}-CHCl_2$$

Mechanism of Action

Chloramphenicol binds to the 50S ribosomal subunit of susceptible species and inhibits the peptidyl transferase enzyme that is part of the subunit. The result is inhibition of protein synthesis. It is a bacteriostatic drug.

Resistance

As with the tetracyclines, plasmid-mediated resistance is very common in Gram-negative rods. This resistance is especially troublesome with *Haemophilus influenzae* because chloramphenicol and ampicillin were the drugs of choice before the prevalence of resistant strains became too high. One mechanism of resistance is production by the resistant bacterium of an intracellular enzyme that catalyzes the acetylation of chloramphenicol, thereby inactivating it. Another mechanism is reduced permeability to the drug by the bacterial membrane.

Absorption, Distribution, Metabolism, and Excretion

Chloramphenicol is administered orally either as chloramphenicol or as chloramphenicol palmitate. The palmitate ester is hydrolyzed to free drug in the intestine and absorbed. Chloramphenicol is not very soluble in water and is marketed for injection as the succinate ester. The inactive ester is hydrolyzed to free drug in various tissues in the body.

The drug is distributed well to most tissues of the body, including the cerebrospinal fluid, whether or not there is inflammation. It can be found in bile and in maternal milk, and it crosses the placenta. It is bound to plasma proteins.

Chloramphenicol is inactivated in the liver by glucuronide formation. Therefore its concentration in plasma is dependent on liver function. Patients with liver disease may have abnormally high concentrations of the drug if the dose is not adjusted. Similarly, infants with immature liver development are subject to abnormally high concentrations of the drug, leading to toxicity.

Excretion of chloramphenicol and the glucuronide is mainly in the urine, but the dose does not have to be altered in the presence of renal failure.

> **BOX 39–3**
> **THERAPEUTIC USES**
>
> Chloramphenicol is sometimes used for treatment of typhoid fever due to *Salmonella typhi*, but ampicillin is also highly effective. Resistance may occur to one or both of these drugs. In such cases trimethoprim-sulfamethoxazole and several of the cephalosporins may be used. Meningitis due to *H. influenzae* or *N. meningitidis* usually responds well to chloramphenicol. Again, ampicillin is also effective, but resistance to ampicillin has increased to over 25% of *H. influenzae*. Meningitis due to *N. meningitidis* or *S. pneumoniae* is usually treated with penicillin, but when the patient is allergic to ampicillin, chloramphenicol is an alternative. It is often stated that a static drug should not be used in combination with a penicillin antibiotic. Nevertheless, chloramphenicol has been used, with good results, in conjunction with ampicillin for treatment of meningitis, especially in children between 3 months and 10 years of age, in which *H. influenzae* is the most likely causative organism.
>
> Chloramphenicol is effective in treatment of infection by several anaerobic organisms, particularly *Bacteroides fragilis*, and is sometimes used for treatment of brain abscess. Metronidazole is also effective against bacteroides and is often combined with penicillin for these infections. Clindamycin has activity against bacteroides but, unlike chloramphenicol and metronidazole, does not reliably penetrate the blood-brain barrier sufficiently to provide therapeutic concentrations.
>
> Chloramphenicol is an alternative drug for treatment of infection due to rickettsiae and brucella when tetracycline cannot be used.

Adverse Effects

The most important adverse effect of chloramphenicol is a rare (about 1 in 30,000 to 60,000 courses) but often fatal aplasia of the bone marrow, leading to pancytopenia. The mechanism is not yet understood. In patients who survive there is an abnormally high incidence of leukemia. There seems to be no correlation between outcome following aplastic anemia and dose, but the incidence of the malady increases with increased length of treatment with chloramphenicol.

Chloramphenicol also causes a dose-related anemia characterized by a defect in red cell maturation. This probably results from an inhibition by chloramphenicol of mitochondrial protein synthesis. This may be fatal but usually reverses after the drug is discontinued.

Administration of chloramphenicol has produced fatal results in infants. Infants under approximately 4 weeks of age have immature liver function and are not able to inactivate chloramphenicol by glucuronidation. In addition, such infants have immature kidneys and cannot excrete the drug at the same rate as older children or adults. In this circumstance chloramphenicol can accumulate and cause vomiting, hypothermia, and shock. When the infants die, they are a cyanotic gray color; from which the name, the gray syndrome, is derived.

Chloramphenicol, like the tetracyclines, has a propensity to predispose to superinfection.

Hypersensitivity reactions are relatively rare.

Indications and Contraindications

Chloramphenicol is effective against a large number of microorganisms but is used for only a limited number of infections because of its adverse effects. The infections for which it is used tend to be the more serious types such as meningitis.

Drug Interactions

Chloramphenicol has been reported to increase the toxicity of phenytoin and to decrease the effects of iron salts and vitamin B_{12}.

ERYTHROMYCIN

Erythromycin is the principal drug in a class of drugs known as macrolides. Others include clarithromycin, azithromycin, and oleandomycin.

Chemistry

Erythromycin base is a bitter-tasting crystalline substance that is poorly water-soluble. It is a weak base (with a pK of 8.8), and susceptible to inactivation by acid. *In vitro* activity of the drug progressively increases from pH 5.5 to 8.5. It is a stable compound in isotonic saline and 5% dextrose in water, with preservation of activity for 21 days at 25°C.

The term macrolide comes from the large ring structure, as seen in the figure below.

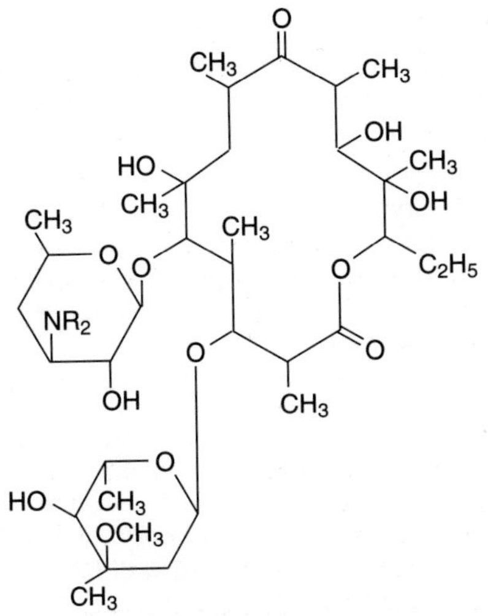

O
CH_3 CH_3
OH
HO CH_3
CH_3 OH
CH_3 CH_3
O O O C_2H_5
NR_2
O O
OH CH_3
O
HO CH_3
OCH_3
CH_3

Because of its vulnerability to acid inactivation, two mechanisms have been employed to avoid acid degradation in the stomach. The first is to apply an enteric coating; unfortunately, this also tends to diminish absorption. The second is to alter the chemical structure specifically to lessen acid inactivation. This has been accomplished by formation of a salt (stearate), ester (ethyl succinate or propionate), or lauryl sulfate salt of an ester (estolate).

Mechanism of Action

Erythromycin is a bacteriostatic antibiotic against most susceptible strains. It binds to the 50S subunit of 70S ribosomes, resulting in inhibition of protein synthesis. Erythromycin antagonizes chloramphenicol action by binding to the 50S subunit. But erythromycin differs by inhibiting a translocation reaction, whereas chloramphenicol inhibits a peptidyl transferase reaction.

Erythromycin has a broad spectrum of activity against Gram-positive and Gram-negative aerobic and anaerobic bacteria, plus mycobacteria, mycoplasma species, and chlamydia. It may be bacteriostatic or bactericidal, depending on the concentration achieved at tissue sites of infection. It possesses bactericidal activity against *Enterobacteriaceae* and *Pseudomonadaceae* in strongly alkaline conditions that can be achieved only by systemic alkalization.

Resistance

Resistance in some species develops because an altered ribosomal RNA reduces ribosomal binding of the erythromycin.

Absorption, Distribution, Metabolism, and Excretion

Erythromycin base or stearate is absorbed from the upper small intestine. Food reduces absorption of these preparations. Peak serum concentrations are reached approximately 4 hours after ingestion of enteric-coated tablets. The estolate is less susceptible to acid degradation, and absorption is minimally inhibited by food. Peak serum concentrations are reached in 2 hours. However, the estolate must be hydrolyzed to the base, and only the base interacts with bacterial ribosomes. Actual concentrations of base are similar to those achieved by giving the base preparation of drug, as noted earlier. Erythromycin ethylsuccinate is less acid-vulnerable, and absorption is less inhibited by food. However, serum concentrations also approximate those of the base. Thus, none of the preparations has unique pharmacokinetic advantage.

Erythromycin gluceptate and lactobionate are IV formulations of the drug.

Protein binding of different erythromycin formulations varies from 40 to 90%. The drug persists in tissues longer than blood, therefore allowing some accumulation over time. Erythromycin distributes throughout the total body water. It achieves therapeutic concentrations for susceptible organisms in most body sites, including aqueous humor, ascitic fluid, bile, middle ear fluid, pleural fluid, prostatic fluid, sinus fluid, and tonsils—all in the presence of inflammation.

BOX 39-4
THERAPEUTIC USES

Erythromycin is the drug of choice for treatment, prophylaxis, or reduction of risk of dissemination of pathogens by eliminating the carrier state of several infectious diseases. These include:

- *Mycoplasma pneumoniae* respiratory tract infections
- *Legionella pneumophila* pneumonia
- *Chlamydia trachomatis* pneumonia or conjunctivitis in newborns
- Chlamydia pelvic infection during pregnancy (even though safety is not fully established)
- *Campylobacter jejuni* gastroenteritis

It has been used in combination with neomycin as oral prophylaxis for elective colorectal surgery, oral prophylaxis against dissemination of pertussis, and topical prophylaxis to prevent neonatal ophthalmia caused by chlamydia. It is also used to eradicate the carrier state of *Corynebacterium diphtheriae*. Many infectious disease specialists consider it the drug of choice for these conditions.

Erythromycin is an important alternative, particularly in the penicillin-allergic patient, for treatment of Group A, B, C, or G streptococcal infection, pneumococcal infections, and disseminated gonococcal disease. Nongonococcal urethritis, usually treated with tetracycline, may be treated successfully with erythromycin as an alternative. Erythromycin is also recommended as an alternative therapy for early and late syphilis, although its efficacy is unproven. It is recommended for treatment of syphilis in pregnancy for the penicillin-allergic patient. Erythromycin has been employed in the treatment of anaerobic bronchopulmonary infections with success, Q fever pneumonitis among patients unable to tolerate tetracycline, and pneumonitis caused by nocardia or *Actinomyces israelii*. Acne vulgaris may be treated with oral or topical erythromycin. Lymphogranuloma venereum, granuloma inguinale, and chancroid may be treated with this drug also. It should be considered as a therapeutic alternative for these conditions.

As a prophylactic agent, erythromycin represents a valuable alternative to penicillin for the prevention of rheumatic fever. It may also be used for prophylaxis against bacteremia among patients undergoing dental procedures who are at risk for endocarditis.

Erythromycin also penetrates through host and bacterial cell membranes. Therefore, it has proved useful in the treatment of intraphagocytic infections such as Legionella and infections caused by organisms lacking a true cell wall, such as chlamydia and mycoplasma. Three mechanisms may contribute to intracellular concentration of erythromycin:

- Engulfment of surrounding fluid by phagocytic vacuoles
- pH gradients
- Active transport using an energy-dependent process

Erythromycin enters the enterohepatic circulation and most drug is excreted in the feces. A small percentage is excreted in urine. Dose adjustment is not required in renal failure.

Adverse Effects

The most common adverse effect associated with oral administration of erythromycin is gastrointestinal (GI) distress including epigastric pain or discomfort, nausea, vomiting, and diarrhea. The effect is often dose-related. Relief may sometimes be obtained by switching from one preparation to another, or by administering the drug with food. However, it should be remembered that food inhibits the absorption of certain preparations.

Hypersensitivity reactions are unusual. The most serious side effect is cholestatic hepatitis, which is most commonly associated with the estolate preparation. All cases reported have occurred in patients older than 12 years. The reaction characteristically begins 10 or more days after initiation of therapy and progresses rapidly. Rare adverse effects include sensorineural hearing loss and pseudomembranous colitis. Safety in pregnancy has not been established; the estolate ester should probably be avoided in the pregnant woman.

Indications and Contraindications

Erythromycin is contraindicated only in patients with a known hypersensitivity to the drug.

Drug Interactions

IV erythromycin is incompatible with a variety of other medications that might be administered through the same infusion. These include vitamins B and C; antibiotics—cephalothin, tetracycline, chloramphenicol, and colistin; and other drugs—heparin, and diphenylhydantoin. Simultaneous administration of oral erythromycin and theophylline results in elevated theophylline concentrations and potential toxicity. A similar phenomenon has been observed with cyclosporine, carbamazepine, warfarin, and methylprednisolone. All are assumed to be due to erythromycin-induced inhibition of hepatic metabolism of these drugs.

CLARITHROMYCIN AND AZITHROMYCIN

These two newer members of the macrolide family have characteristics similar to erythromycin. Clarithromycin is more stable to acid than is erythromycin and is absorbed better in the presence of food. Clarithromycin has activity against *Toxoplasma gondii* and *Mycobacterium intracellulare.* Azithromycin has activity against chlamydia and gonococci in the treatment of pelvic infections, urethritis, and cervicitis.

REFERENCES

Gump DW: Chloramphenicol: A 1981 view [Editorial]. Arch Intern Med 141:573, 1981.

Kucers A, Bennett N: Chloramphenicol and thiamphenicol. The Uses of Antibiotics, 4th ed, 757-807. Philadelphia: JB Lippincott Co, 1987.

Meyer RD: Drugs five years later. Ann Intern Med 95:328, 1981.

Neu HC: New antibiotics: Areas of appropriate use. J Infect Dis 134 (Suppl):S3, 1987.

Neu HC: A symposium on tetracyclines: A major appraisal. Introduction. Bull NY Acad Med 54:141-155, 1978.

Phillips I: Aminoglycosides. Lancet 2:311, 1982.

Standiford HC: Tetracyclines and chloramphenicol. *In* Mandell GL, Douglas RG Jr, Bennett JE (eds): Principles and Practice of Infectious Diseases, 3rd ed, 284-295. New York: John Wiley & Sons, 1990.

Tedesco FJ: Pseudomembranous colitis. Pathogenesis and therapy. Med Clin North Am 66:655, 1982.

Washington JA, Wilson WR: Erythromycin: A microbial and clinical perspective after 30 years of clinical use. Mayo Clin Proc 60:189, 271, 1985.

40 Miscellaneous Agents: Quinolones, Sulfonamides and Trimethoprim, Urinary Tract Agents, Metronidazole, Spectinomycin, Bacitracin, and Antimycobacterial Drugs

Alan J. Lesse

FLUOROQUINOLONES

This class of antimicrobial drugs has witnessed an explosion in both clinical use and in continued development of new agents. The group has broad activity against many Gram-negative pathogens, including *Pseudomonas aeruginosa.* The availability of both oral and intravenous formulations with such potent antibacterial activity has significantly altered prescribing patterns by physicians. Unfortunately, this has also led to an overuse of these agents and the development of resistant bacteria.

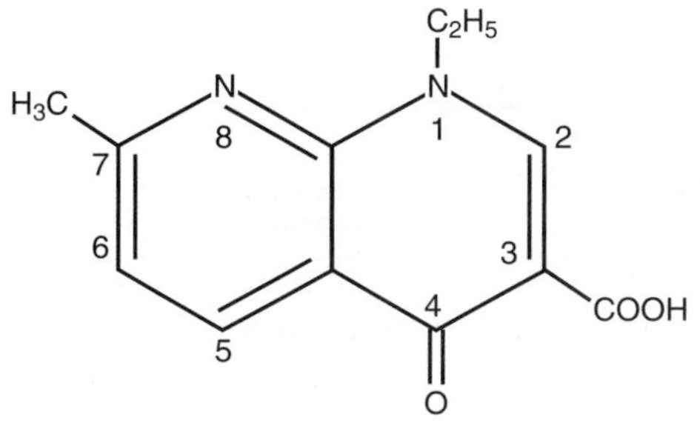

Nalidixic Acid

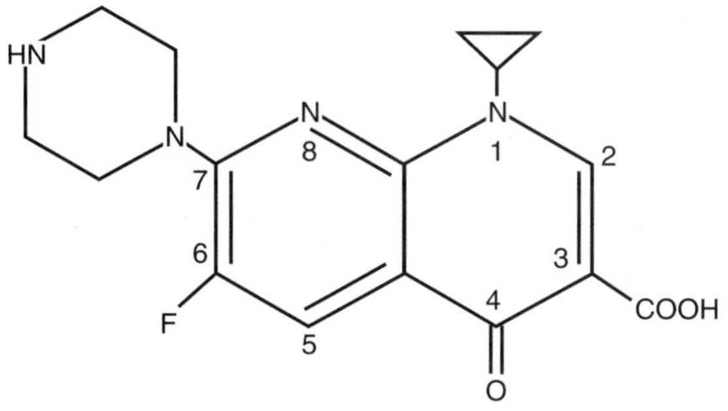

Ciprofloxacin

FIGURE 40–1. Structures of nalidixic acid and ciprofloxacin.

Chemistry

The fluoroquinolones are fluorinated derivatives of nalidixic acid. The currently available fluoroquinolones have a fluorine atom at the 6 position of the quinolone nucleus and have a piperazine nucleus at the 7 position of the quinolone ring (Fig. 40–1), which increases the activity against *P. aeruginosa.* These chemical modifications have resulted in a marked increase in the antimicrobial spectrum of the agents. Unlike nalidixic acid, bacteria do not rapidly develop resistance while on therapy. Chemical modifications of the quinolones have also altered the pharmacological profiles; therefore, many of the agents now in use or in development have adequate serum and tissue levels for the treatment of systemic infections. However, some of the quinolones, such as norfloxacin, only have sufficient distribution for the treatment of urinary and gastrointestinal infections.

Mechanisms of Action

The fluoroquinolones inhibit a crucial bacterial enzyme, DNA topoisomerase (adenosine triphosphate-hydrolyzing), a type II DNA topoisomerase responsible for the negative supercoiling of bacterial DNA. The enzyme, also referred to as DNA gyrase, is composed of four subunits, two A monomers and two B monomers. The enzyme transiently nicks the DNA during supercoiling, then repairs the nicks after completion of the supercoiling. Nalidixic acid appears to interfere with the A subunit, whereas the quinolones may interact with both the A and B subunits, although the greater affinity appears to be to the A subunit. The exact mechanism of inhibition is unclear, as some studies suggest that the quinolones bind to the DNA gyrase, whereas others show binding to the DNA template. Mammalian topoisomerase is unaffected by clinical concentrations of the quinolones and unlike bacterial DNA gyrases, does not supercoil the DNA target.

Mechanisms of Resistance

Resistance to the quinolones falls into two categories: one specific mechanism—altered binding to DNA gyrase—and one less specific mechanism—altered bacterial permeability to the agent. Specific resistance to the agents generally results from mutations in the A subunit of the DNA topoisomerase of the bacteria, which alters quinolone binding and confers resistance. Spontaneous mutation in Gram-negative bacteria occurs at a low frequency *in vitro* compared with nalidixic acid and is not encountered during therapy of most Gram-negative infections. Resistance to the quinolones in Gram-positive infections occurs more rapidly.

Although development of resistance during therapy of Gram-negative bacteria is uncommon with the quinolones, selective pressure in the hospital environment in the face of widespread use of the quinolones has led to relatively rapid selection of resistant bacteria at some institutions. Resistance among Gram-positive bacteria, particularly methicillin-resistant *Staphylococcus aureus,* occurs rapidly, and many institutions have seen staphylococcal isolates go from 100% susceptible to less than 20% susceptible in as little as 1 year. For that reason and because of the decreased activity of the currently available quinolones, the use of these agents for Gram-positive bacterial infections is limited and discouraged.

Alteration of DNA gyrase binding of the quinolones is chromosomally mediated and is not transmitted on plasmids, although laboratory data have suggested that plasmid-mediated resistance is possible.

The second mechanism of resistance to the quinolones is decreased membrane permeability, which is relatively nonspecific in nature. Although this mechanism is generally mediated through altered porins, such porin alterations may also affect the permeability of other antimicrobial agents.

Route of Administration, Absorption, Distribution, Metabolism, and Excretion

The currently available quinolones can be divided into two groups based on their pharmacological properties (Table 40–1). One group, represented by norfloxacin, has serum and tissue levels that are not sufficient for the treatment of systemic infections and are only effective in the treatment of infections in the urinary and the gastrointestinal tracts. The second group—ciprofloxacin, ofloxacin, enoxacin, and lomefloxacin—all attain excellent serum and tissue levels and can be used for infections outside the urinary and the gastrointestinal tracts. At the current time, enoxacin is only approved for use in treating urinary tract infections.

Norfloxacin is 50% absorbed after oral administration and is distributed widely. Norfloxacin, however, does not achieve adequate tissue or serum levels for the therapy of

TABLE 40–1. Selected Pharmacokinetic Parameters of the Quinolones

Quinolone	Formulation	Half-Life/ Routine Administration	Useful for Systemic Infections	Theophylline Interaction	Clearance
Norfloxacin	Oral	3–4 hours/b.i.d.	No	Yes	Renal/hepatic
Enoxacin	Oral	6 hours/b.i.d.	Yes	Highly significant	Renal/hepatic
Ofloxacin	Oral, intravenous	6–8 hours/b.i.d.	Yes	Minimal	Renal
Ciprofloxacin	Oral, intravenous	3–4 hours/b.i.d.	Yes	Significant	Renal/hepatic
Lomefloxacin	Oral	8 hours/daily	Yes	Minimal	Renal

Gram-negative infections outside the urinary or the gastrointestinal tract. The drug is metabolized and cleared in both the urine and bile, and approximately 30% is delivered to the colon, providing excellent drug concentrations for the treatment of pathogens in the gastrointestinal tract. Urinary concentrations of the drug are high and provide excellent concentrations for the treatment of most urinary pathogens. The drug has a half-life of 3–4 hours with normal renal function. Dosages do not need to be altered until creatinine clearance falls below 30 mL/minute.

Ciprofloxacin, ofloxacin, enoxacin, and lomefloxacin are also well absorbed after oral administration. All of these drugs achieve serum concentrations that are above the minimal inhibitory concentrations (MICs) of most Gram-negative pathogens, and they are useful in the treatment of systemic infections as well as urinary tract infections. The drugs are widely distributed, with a large apparent volume of distribution and excellent concentrations in many body fluids. Excretion of the agents is dependent on the compound. Renal clearance is the major route of excretion for ofloxacin and lomefloxacin, whereas renal and hepatic clearance is used for ciprofloxacin and enoxacin. Pefloxacin, a quinolone that is yet to be introduced, is excreted predominantly by hepatic routes. Only ciprofloxacin and ofloxacin are available for intravenous administration at the current time, but intravenous preparations of several newer quinolones are currently under investigation. Treatment of central nervous system (CNS) infections with quinolones is possible, but insufficient data exist to recommend them for primary therapy. Because of their penetration into the prostate and the prostatic fluid, the quinolones are highly effective in the treatment of prostatitis.

Adverse Effects

Quinolones have an excellent side-effect profile with a low overall incidence of adverse reactions (2–4%). Nausea and vomiting account for most of the adverse reactions.

Central nervous system effects can also be seen with the quinolones. Insomnia, confusion, headaches, dizziness, and anxiety have all been reported. Because nalidixic acid was associated with an increased frequency of seizures, it is currently advisable to assess the risk-benefit ratio of quinolone administration in seizure-prone patients, although the association with seizures in patients treated with quinolones is not convincing.

Photosensitivity has been reported with all quinolones, and patients should be warned about this potential side effect.

Toxicological studies in animals revealed cartilage damage in developing animals; therefore, the quinolones are not indicated for the treatment of children. Further studies are ongoing to assess this risk in humans.

Students and clinicians should also be aware that another quinolone, temafloxacin, was approved for use by the Food and Drug Administration (FDA) on February 24, 1992. On June 5, 1992, the drug was voluntarily removed from the market by the manufacturer after nine initial reports of hypoglycemia were followed shortly thereafter by reports of anaphylaxis, hepatic failure, hemolytic anemia, renal failure, and even death. Analysis of this potentially fatal reaction indicated an incidence of approximately 1 in 3500. Premarketing trials enlisting 4000 patients for FDA approval could not identify this reaction prior to marketing. Although several theories have been advanced to explain this reaction, none have been proved, and subsequent release of intravenous antibiotics and other drugs may be impacted by the experience with temafloxacin. Clinicians and students should realize that low-frequency adverse reactions may not be discovered within the FDA-mandated clinical trials and may only appear during postmarketing surveillance.

Drug Interactions

This class of compounds has significant drug-drug interactions. Magnesium, calcium, and aluminum antacids significantly decrease the bioavailability of the oral quinolones. Sucralfate also reduces the oral absorption of the quinolones, and iron salts may decrease their oral bioavailability. Such interactions may result in therapeutic failures secondary to inadequate drug absorption.

Ranitidine and cimetidine may also affect quinolone pharmacokinetics, although the literature is not in complete agreement on this interaction. Ranitidine appears to be less likely than cimetidine to decrease clearance of the quinolones.

Interaction with theophylline can be serious or life-threatening (Table 40–1). Enoxacin can significantly decrease theophylline clearance (43–75%) and cause significant elevations of theophylline levels. Because the therapeutic index of theophylline is low, these drug-drug interactions can theoretically increase a therapeutic serum concentration into the toxic range. Ciprofloxacin and norfloxacin also produce significant but smaller increases in serum theophylline concentrations. However, individual variations in metabolic interactions may result in significant increases of theophylline concentrations with ciprofloxacin and norfloxacin in many patients. Ofloxacin and lomefloxacin have little effect on theophylline concentration to date,

BOX 40–1
CLINICAL USE (INDICATIONS AND CONTRAINDICATIONS)

The quinolones as a group are very active against most gram-negative rods, including the majority of enterobacteriaceae, and fastidious gram-negatives such as *Neisseria*, *Haemophilus*, and *Moraxella (Branhamella) catarrhalis*. In general, all of the agents have the same MICs, with the exception of ciprofloxacin, which is generally twice as active as other agents. This advantage is balanced by the lower achievable serum concentrations of ciprofloxacin compared with the other quinolones (except for norfloxacin).

Although all of the quinolones are generally active against *P. aeruginosa*, the level of activity of ciprofloxacin is higher than that of the others. Most strains are inhibited at less than 1 μg/mL, whereas the other quinolones range from 2–8 μg/mL for inhibition, with most strains requiring 4 μg/mL for inhibition. Nonaeruginosa strains of *Pseudomonas* are generally less susceptible to quinolones with correspondingly higher MICs.

Although therapy of Gram-negative bacteria is a strength of the quinolones, the activity of the agents against Gram-positive bacteria is generally unacceptable for routine clinical use. When the quinolones were first introduced, most strains of methicillin-resistant *S. aureus* were susceptible to the agents. Use of these agents for methicillin-resistant *S. aureus* brought an astonishingly rapid development of resistance at many centers, and none of the currently available quinolones can be recommended for the treatment of staphylococcal or other Gram-positive infections. In fact, patients have developed pneumococcal bacteremia and meningitis while receiving ciprofloxacin for the treatment of community-acquired pneumonias.

Anaerobic bacteria have MICs generally above the clinical achievable concentrations, and quinolones should not be relied on for anaerobic activity.

The quinolones do have specific activity against many bacterial and nonbacterial pathogens. Laboratory evidence suggests that these agents should be active against both *Mycoplasma* and *Legionella*, although clinical experience with these agents is lacking. *Chlamydia* are also susceptible, especially to ofloxacin. Both *Mycobacterium tuberculosis* and atypical mycobacteria are inhibited by the quinolones, and these agents have a role in multidrug combinations for the therapy of both multidrug-resistant tuberculosis and atypical mycobacteria, especially *Mycobacterium avium-intracellulare*.

Quinolones are bactericidal and, unlike β-lactams, can kill stationary-phase organisms. The bactericidal concentrations are generally only two to four times the MIC. The quinolones also exhibit a significant postantibiotic effect, the clinical significance of which is not known. These features may make quinolones more active in the clinical settings of slower bacteria replication, such as osteomyelitis.

Norfloxacin is indicated in the treatment of complicated and uncomplicated urinary tract infections and most bacterial causes of diarrhea, including infection with *Salmonella*, *Shigella*, *Yersinia*, and *Campylobacter*. Because serum concentrations are not sufficient to treat systemic infections, this agent cannot be recommended for infections outside the urinary or gastrointestinal tract. Some studies have shown a use for selective decontamination of the gut by norfloxacin in neutropenic patients and in patients at risk for spontaneous bacterial peritonitis. This agent can be used for the treatment of urethral gonococcal infections but has no advantages over ciprofloxacin or ofloxacin, which are the primary quinolones recommended for the therapy of gonorrhea.

Enoxacin, despite its excellent serum levels, is approved only for use in urinary tract infections, although it should be as broadly active as other quinolones. The marked interactions with theophylline should limit its use in patients requiring theophylline.

Ciprofloxacin has the lowest MIC of the available quinolones against most Gram-negative pathogens. Serum levels, however, are generally lower than those of other agents, balancing its enhanced antimicrobial activity against enterobacteriaceae. Ciprofloxacin is, however, generally more active than the other quinolones against *Pseudomonas* species, generally at a serum concentration-MIC ratio that favors ciprofloxacin, despite its lower serum concentrations. Gram-negative infections at most clinical sites, including the urinary tract, skin and soft tissue, bones, and joints, as well as systemic and pulmonary infections are treated effectively with ciprofloxacin and other quinolones. Sexually transmitted diseases such as gonorrhea and chancroid can be treated with ciprofloxacin and other quinolones. Bacterial diarrhea, including traveler's diarrhea, is also effectively treated.

Ofloxacin obtains higher serum concentrations than does ciprofloxacin but is less active against *Pseudomonas* species. Ofloxacin is active against *Chlamydia trachomatis* and is recommended for the treatment of both cervicitis and urethritis caused by either *Chlamydia* or *Neisseria gonorrhoeae*. Single-dose therapy for the latter is sufficient, and 7 days of therapy is required for adequate cure rates with *Chlamydia*. Ofloxacin may also be particularly active against multidrug-resistant *M. tuberculosis*. Recent outbreaks of a highly resistant strain have prompted the use of ofloxacin in both treatment and prophylaxis regimens.

Lomefloxacin has a pharmacokinetic profile that allows once-daily dosing. The antibacterial spectrum of the agent is similar to that of ofloxacin; its use has been limited in the United States.

but the possibility of altered theophylline kinetics with the quinolone class should raise the clinical awareness of the clinician, even with the use of ofloxacin and lomefloxacin.

Quinolones may inhibit caffeine metabolism, and patients should be alerted to this interaction. Additionally, warfarin and ciprofloxacin interactions have been reported, and patients taking a quinolone and warfarin should be closely monitored.

NALIDIXIC ACID

Nalidixic acid is a naphthyridine derivative, first introduced in the early 1960s. As described in the quinolone section, nalidixic acid is only effective in the treatment of urinary tract infections. Resistance may develop during therapy, and adverse reactions, such as seizures, have been described. Most of the clinical use of nalidixic acid has therefore been replaced with the fluorinated derivatives of nalidixic acid, the fluoroquinolones.

SULFONAMIDES

Sulfonamides represent a useful but older class of antimicrobial agents. Although the development of newer classes of antimicrobial agents has limited the therapeutic usefulness of sulfonamides, they are still indicated in specific circumstances.

Chemistry and Mechanism of Action

Sulfonamides are structurally similar to para-aminobenzoic acid (PABA) (Fig. 40-2). In many bacteria, PABA is a substrate for the synthesis of tetrahydrofolic acid, the reduced form of folic acid. Sulfonamides competitively inhibit the enzyme dihydropteroate synthetase, which converts PABA to dihydropteroic acid, a precursor of tetrahydrofolic acid, by binding to the enzyme with a greater affinity than PABA. Because these cofactors are required in the synthesis of cellular components of DNA (thymidine and purines), sulfonamides effectively inhibit cellular growth in these bacteria. Sulfonamides, therefore, are predominantly bacteriostatic agents.

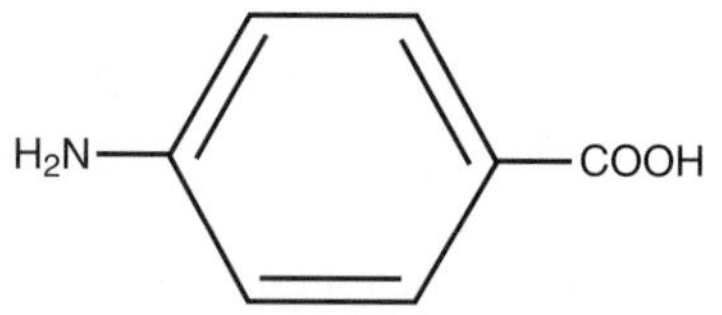

H_2N—[benzene ring]—COOH

Para-aminobenzoic Acid

H_2N—[benzene ring]—SO_2NHR

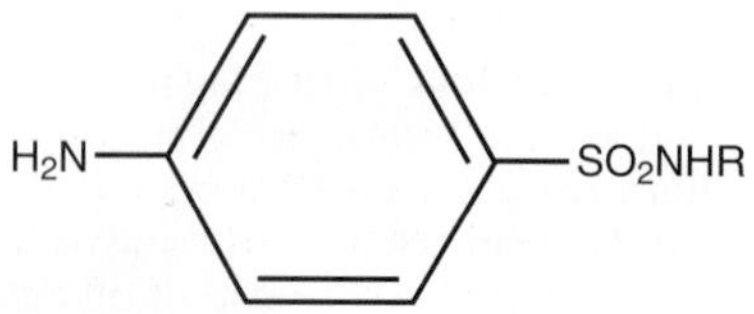

Sulfonamide Nucleus

FIGURE 40-2. Structures of a sulfonamide and para-aminobenzoic acid.

Mammalian cells cannot synthesize tetrahydrofolic acid and require preformed folic acid. Therefore, sulfonamides do not inhibit mammalian folic acid metabolism and, via an analogous mechanism, are inactive against bacteria that can utilize preformed folic acid or folic acid precursors.

Absorption, Distribution, Metabolism, and Excretion

Historically, many sulfonamides have been developed. Today only two major groups remain in clinical practice. The first group is rapidly absorbed and excreted (sulfisoxazole, sulfamethoxazole, and sulfadiazine). The second group (sulfasalazine) is poorly absorbed and is recommended only for the treatment of ulcerative colitis.

Sulfisoxazole, sulfamethoxazole, and sulfadiazine are all well absorbed orally and achieve excellent serum levels. These drugs are distributed widely throughout the body, including in cerebrospinal fluid (CSF) and in serosal fluids such as pleural, peritoneal, synovial, and prostatic fluid.

Most sulfonamides are acetylated in the liver prior to excretion in the kidneys via glomerular filtration. Dosage adjustment in renal failure is indicated, but accurate predictions of clearance are not easily calculated.

Adverse Effects

The major toxicity of this class of agents is the allergic reaction. The predominant manifestations are dermatological and range from a minor rash to life-threatening exfoliative dermatitis, toxic epidermal necrolysis, and Stevens-Johnson syndrome. Many of the more serious adverse reactions are preceded by a rash; therapy with sulfonamides should be discontinued after the appearance of this rash. (A possible exception to this rule may be seen with acquired immunodeficiency syndrome [AIDS] patients, in whom dosage reduction and continued treatment in the face of simple skin rashes have been advanced by some authorities.) Despite the extreme usefulness of this class of drugs in AIDS patients with *Pneumocystis carinii*, over one third of AIDS patients treated with sulfonamides may develop a skin rash caused by sulfonamides at some point in their disease.

Hematological effects can be seen with sulfonamides and include leukopenia, granulocytopenia, thrombocytopenia, and aplastic anemia. Patients with glucose-6-phosphate dehydrogenase (G6PD) deficiency may suffer acute hemolytic crisis after therapy with these oxidizing agents, although hemolytic anemia may be seen in the absence of G6PD.

Nephrotoxicity was seen with older less-soluble sulfonamides but is rarely seen today. The most damaging form of renal disease, crystalluria from precipitation of the sulfonamide or its metabolite, was frequently irreversible but is not commonly seen with the currently available agents. Alkalinization of the urine with hydration increases sulfonamide solubility in the urine. Acute tubular necrosis has also been seen less commonly, and the use of sulfa drugs in patients with renal impairment is controversial.

Other potential adverse reactions include hepatotoxicity, nausea and vomiting, anorexia, and neurological dysfunction, such as headache, confusion, neuropathy, insomnia, seizures, and other neurological abnormalities.

Sulfonamides can displace bilirubin from albumin binding sites, and their use in infants has led to kernicterus. These drugs are therefore contraindicated in pregnant women and infants.

Sulfonamides may also displace oral hypoglycemics and coumarin anticoagulants from albumin binding sites and increase serum levels of these drugs. Sulfonamides may also decrease warfarin clearance and increase prothrombin times. Sulfonamides may decrease phenytoin metabolism and result in increased phenytoin levels.

BOX 40–2
CLINICAL USE (INDICATIONS AND CONTRAINDICATIONS)

Clinical indications for sulfonamide therapy for routine bacterial infections have been decreasing over the last two decades with the development of bacterial resistance to these agents and the concomitant increase in therapeutic alternatives to the sulfonamides. However, the impact of AIDS on medicine has resulted in an increased use of these agents, particularly in combination with other agents.

Outpatient urinary tract infection is the major indication for single-agent sulfonamide therapy. Although most authorities no longer utilize these agents as front-line therapy, they still serve a useful role as therapeutic options for these infections.

Historically, sulfonamides were recommended both for eradication of the carriage of *Neisseria meningitidis* and for rheumatic fever prophylaxis for group A streptococcus. Currently, resistance among both of these pathogens is too high to routinely recommend these agents any longer.

Therapy of *Nocardia* infections is still based on single-agent treatment with a sulfonamide.

The onslaught of AIDS has markedly increased the use of sulfonamides, in combination with pyrimethamine, for the therapy of toxoplasmosis. Most clinicians currently recommend sulfadiazine with pyrimethamine for both initial and maintenance therapy of brain abscess from *Toxoplasma gondii*. Sulfamethoxazole, in fixed combination with trimethoprim (see Trimethoprim), is first-line therapy for non–sulfa allergic patients with *P. carinii* pneumonia (PCP) and other infections.

Finally, the long-acting sulfonamide, sulfadiazine, is recommended for the therapy of chloroquine-resistant *Plasmodium falciparum* infection by some authorities. Prophylactic use of this fixed combination was associated, however, with an unacceptable risk of Stevens-Johnson syndrome, and its use as a preventive agent is no longer sanctioned by the Centers for Disease Control and Prevention.

TRIMETHOPRIM

Trimethoprim is an inhibitor of the enzyme dihydrofolate reductase, which catalyzes the conversion of dihydrofolic acid to tetrahydrofolic acid. Unlike sulfonamides, the enzymatic target for trimethoprim is present in mammalian systems. However, binding to the bacterial dihydrofolate reductase occurs at concentrations several thousand times lower than it does in its mammalian counterpart and allows trimethoprim to be used as an antibacterial agent without significant host toxicity. Trimethoprim is reported to be bactericidal in its action.

Absorption, Distribution, Metabolism, and Excretion

Trimethoprim absorption approaches 100% after oral administration. Distribution of trimethoprim is extensive. Very high concentrations are found in many tissues and body fluid, and the agent appears readily in prostatic secretions.

Trimethoprim is excreted predominantly in the kidneys after metabolism in the liver and peripheral tissues. Dosage adjustments need to be made for patients with renal dysfunction.

Adverse Effects

The most common adverse reactions to trimethoprim are rash and gastrointestinal intolerance. Thrombocytopenia, leukopenia, and megaloblastic anemia may be seen as a result of effects on the mammalian dihydrofolate reductase, as high serum concentrations of trimethoprim may inhibit the mammalian enzyme. Folinic acid may correct the enzyme inhibition in humans with no effect on its antibacterial activity because sensitive bacteria cannot utilize the compound.

Trimethoprim inhibits the hepatic metabolism of phenytoin and can cause significant increases in serum phenytoin levels. Because of its antifolate properties, the drug should be used with caution in patients with folate deficiency.

BOX 40–3
CLINICAL USE (INDICATIONS AND CONTRAINDICATIONS)

The primary indication for single-agent trimethoprim is acute, uncomplicated, urinary tract infections caused by susceptible pathogens. The drug may also be useful in the prophylaxis of recurrent urinary tract infections. The major indication for the agent is in combination with sulfamethoxazole, as outlined in Trimethoprim-Sulfamethoxazole Combinations.

PYRIMETHAMINE

Pyrimethamine is another dihydrofolate reductase inhibitor with a mechanism of action similar to that of trimethoprim. The drug is well absorbed from the gastrointestinal tract and is widely distributed throughout the body. Pyrimethamine has an exceptionally long serum half-life of 111 hours. The drug is excreted unchanged in the urine.

The major adverse reactions to pyrimethamine are hypersensitivity and hematological reactions. The drug causes an array of dermatological effects similar to those caused by the sulfonamides, ranging from rashes to life-threatening manifestations of erythema multiforme and Stevens-Johnson syndrome. The hematological toxicity of pyrimethamine appears to be greater than that of trimethoprim, resulting in megaloblastic anemia, leukopenia, thrombocytopenia, or pancytopenia. Supplemental folinic acid administration is more routine with pyrimethamine than with other folic acid antagonists. Other less-common reactions may be seen and are difficult to attribute to pyrimethamine alone because it is frequently given as a component of a combination therapy.

The two major uses of pyrimethamine are in combination with other drugs for the treatment of toxoplasmosis and malaria. The combination of pyrimethamine with sulfadiazine represents first-line therapy for toxoplasmosis in patients with AIDS. Drug-induced leukopenia and pancytopenias may be seen more frequently in this setting, given the hematological compromise of these patients from their underlying human immunodeficiency virus (HIV) infection and their concomitant antiretroviral therapy. Patients are initially treated with high doses of pyrimethamine for several weeks; the doses are reduced to life-long, suppressive doses in AIDS patients because of the recurrence of disease when therapy is discontinued. Combination of pyrimethamine with clindamycin or dapsone also has been reported in patients with allergic reactions to the sulfonamides. Pyrimethamine and sulfadiazine also have been effective in the treatment of chloroquine-resistant malaria.

TRIMETREXATE

Trimetrexate is a potent inhibitor of dihydrofolate reductase. It is currently indicated as salvage therapy in patients with severe *P. carinii* infections who fail to respond to treatment with trimethoprim with sulfamethoxasole (see next section) or pentamidine (see Chapter 43). The drug has considerable antifolate properties in humans and must be used with folinic acid. The human antifolate properties of this compound are so potent that the drug is also used in experimental chemotherapy protocols in cancer chemotherapy.

TRIMETHOPRIM-SULFAMETHOXAZOLE COMBINATIONS

Trimethoprim with sulfamethoxazole (abbreviated TMP-SMZ or co-trimoxazole) is marketed in a fixed ratio of 1:5 trimethoprim-sulfamethoxazole for both parenteral and oral administration. The combination represents a good example of antibacterial synergy, in which the combination of the agents is more active than either agent administered singly. Theoretically, this is the result of a two-site inhibition of folic acid synthesis by these agents acting on the same biosynthetic pathway. The same logic also suggests that resistance to this two-step inhibition is less likely. The combination is frequently bactericidal.

Adverse Effects

Adverse reactions are predominantly the sum of the adverse reactions of the individual agents. Overall, the most significant reactions are hypersensitivity and hematological effects. Skin rash is the most common and is usually attributed to hypersensitivity to the sulfa component. Although generally mild and reversible on discontinuation of treatment, toxic epidermal necrolysis, erythema multiforme, exfoliative dermatitis, and the Stevens-Johnson syndrome may occur. Allergic or toxic suppression of bone marrow cells also has been reported. Chills, fever, allergic vasculitis, and a systemic lupus erythematosus syndrome may be seen. AIDS patients, as stated previously, appear to have a very high rate of dermatological toxicity to the drug combination. Skin rashes have been reported in up to 30% of HIV-infected patients treated with TMP-SMZ. Because of the extreme utility of the drug combination in this patient population and the generally mild dermatological manifestations seen in HIV-infected individuals, some authorities have recommended continuing therapy if the only dermatological manifestation is a macular rash. This approach should only be attempted by health care workers who are intimately familiar with the multiple adverse reactions seen in this patient group. Those unfamiliar with these complications should either discontinue therapy or consult experienced physicians before continuing therapy in the face of a rash with TMP-SMZ in HIV-infected patients.

Other toxicities are similar to those with the individual agents, especially the hematological reactions.

BOX 40–4

CLINICAL USE (INDICATIONS AND CONTRAINDICATIONS)

Although the indications for the use of either sulfonamides or trimethoprim alone are rather meager, this cannot be said for the combination drug. Clinical use of this combination is widespread and continues to be effective, despite the availability of newer agents.

TMP-SMZ is a drug of first choice for the therapy of many urinary tract infections. Acute uncomplicated urinary tract infection may be treated by single-dose, 3-day, or 7- to 10-day regimens with approximately equal efficacy. Recurrent infections and complicated urinary tract infections may need alternative therapy. Prophylaxis for frequent recurrent disease also may be given with TMP-SMZ. Additionally, prostatitis can be effectively treated with this combination.

TMP-SMZ is a drug of choice for acute otitis me-

BOX 40-4

CLINICAL USE (INDICATIONS AND CONTRAINDICATIONS) (*Continued*)

dia, sinusitis, and bronchitis. The most likely etiologies for these infections, *Streptococcus pneumoniae*, *Haemophilus influenzae*, and *Branhamella catarrhalis*, are all effectively treated by trimethoprim-sulfamethoxasole. The agent may also be an acceptable alternative to erythromycin for the eradication of *Bordetella pertussis*.

Enteric infections with known susceptible strains of *Salmonella* or *Shigella* may be treated with TMP-SMX; however, worldwide resistance is increasing. Empirical therapy of these infections and of traveler's diarrhea from enterotoxigenic *Escherichia coli* may be more effective with a quinolone.

Over the last 10 years, TMP-SMX has emerged as the first-line therapy for the prevention and treatment of PCP in AIDS patients. Treatment regimens utilizing either oral or intravenous TMP-SMX are effective and are first-line therapy in nonallergic patients with suspected PCP. Prevention of the primary episode (primary prevention) in patients with CD_4 counts under 200 cells per microliter, and prevention of recurrent disease (secondary prophylaxis) are highly effective with TMP-SMX. Prophylaxis with TMP-SMX is more effective than that with aerosolized pentamidine and carries the advantage of prophylaxis against extrapulmonary disease that is not prevented with pentamidine. TMP-SMX is also highly effective in the prevention of PCP in the non-AIDS population at high risk (such as patients with acute lymphocytic leukemia).

Although some evidence may exist for the decreased incidence of toxoplasmosis in patients receiving TMP-SMX prophylaxis, this drug is not effective in treating TMP-SMZ.

Other infections such as brucellosis, *Listeria* meningitis in the penicillin-allergic patient, meilioidosis, and chlamydial infection may be treated with TMP-SMZ.

URINARY TRACT ANTISEPTICS

Two compounds, methenamine and nitrofurantoin, are used clinically to treat infections of the urinary bladder. These agents, referred to as urinary tract antiseptics, are so labeled because they are effective agents in sterilizing the urine but carry no significant antibacterial effect for treatment of infections outside of the urinary tract.

Methenamine

Methenamine (hexamethylenetetramine) has an interesting ring structure, as is shown in Figure 40-3. In an acidic environment, the compound is hydrolyzed to form ammonia and formaldehyde. Because the antibacterial activity is imparted by the formaldehyde, the drug is only antibacterial at an acidic pH.

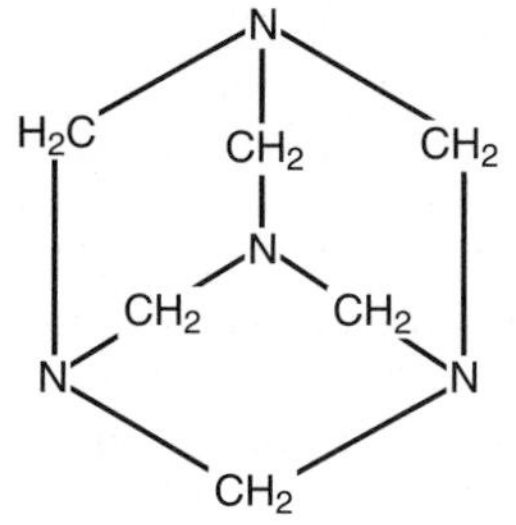

N, H_2C, CH_2, CH_2, N, CH_2, CH_2, N, N, CH_2

Methenamine

FIGURE 40-3. Structure of methenamine.

Mechanisms of Action and Resistance

Formaldehyde is toxic to most micro-organisms at concentrations of about 20 μg/mL. Bacteria do not develop resistance to formaldehyde, which is nonspecific in this mechanism of action.

Route of Administration, Absorption, Distribution, Metabolism, and Excretion

Methenamine is well absorbed orally in the stomach and in the small bowel when administered as either the free drug or the hippurate or mandelate salt. In the absence of an enteric coating, 10-30% of the drug is converted to formaldehyde in the stomach. The drug is widely distributed throughout the body but is neither toxic nor antibacterial at physiologic pH, because formaldehyde generation via hydrolysis is negligible at this pH. The drug is exclusively excreted in the urine, where it is converted in the acidic environment to formaldehyde and ammonia. If urine pH is above 6, no antibacterial activity is seen. Currently available preparations of methenamine include methenamine and its acid salts (hippurate and mandelate) to decrease urine pH and to promote urinary hydrolysis. In acidic urine, formaldehyde generation occurs slowly, and sufficient concentrations of formaldehyde require 1 hour or longer to accumulate. Additional urinary acidification agents, such as ascorbic acid and the hippurate and mandelate salts of methenamine, are of questionable benefit in acidification of the urine. Normal urine, in the absence of diuresis, however, is generally sufficiently acidic to hydrolyze methenamine.

Adverse Effects

Methenamine is generally well tolerated. The major adverse reactions are nausea and vomiting. Prolonged administration of high doses can produce dysuria, hematuria, and bladder irritation, presumably from prolonged increased formaldehyde concentrations.

Use of the mandelate and hippurate salts should be avoided in patients with renal failure, as acid excretion is generally inhibited by these agents. Mandelate salts have crystallized in patients with renal insufficiency and are contraindicated. Both mandelate and hippurate salts may precipitate urate crystals in the urine and should be avoided in patients with gout.

The presence of urea-splitting organisms in the urine, such as *Proteus* species, may result in an inability to acidify the urine, preventing an antibacterial effect from being generated.

Drug Interactions

Methenamine complexes with sulfonamides in the urine, resulting in antagonism of both agents, and their use is mutually exclusive.

> BOX 40-5
>
> **CLINICAL USE (INDICATIONS AND CONTRAINDICATIONS)**
>
> The major use of methenamine is the treatment of cystitis, both bacterial and fungal. Because urine flow above the bladder is too rapid to allow sufficient formaldehyde generation, the drug is ineffective in upper urinary tract disease. Methenamine is used in patients with indwelling urinary catheters and chronic recurrent lower urinary tract infections; however, the more rapid elimination of urine from a catheterized bladder may actually decrease formaldehyde concentrations in the bladder and decrease the effectiveness.

Nitrofurantoin

Chemistry and Mechanisms of Action and Resistance

Nitrofurantoin is a nitrofuran analog with effective antibacterial activity. The drug appears to inhibit bacterial replication by damaging bacterial DNA, although the exact mechanism is unknown. Resistance mechanisms are unclear.

Route of Administration, Absorption, Distribution, Metabolism, and Excretion

The drug is given by oral administration. A macrocrystalline form is more commonly prescribed because of decreased gastrointestinal side effects. The drug is rapidly absorbed and excreted into the urine and has a half-life of 20 minutes with normal renal function. The drug is distributed widely throughout the body, including the CNS and placenta. The drug is rapidly metabolized in many tissues, and only 33% of the administered dose is excreted into the urine by glomerular filtration and tubular excretion. Urinary concentrations are related to renal function in that urinary levels decrease and serum levels increase as renal function declines.

Adverse Effects

The most common side effect of nitrofurantoin is gastrointestinal irritation. Anorexia, nausea, and vomiting occur and may be decreased by administering the drug with food, which does not decrease its absorption.

Hypersensitivity reactions are a particularly disturbing side effect of nitrofurantoin. Dermatological reactions including rashes, urticaria, pruritus, and angioedema may be seen and are generally reversed on discontinuance of the drug.

Pulmonary toxicity is of particular concern and ranges from mild to severe. Exacerbation of underlying asthma may be seen in patients treated with nitrofurantoin. Acute pneumonitis with eosinophilia, fever, chills, cough, and infiltrates on chest radiograph can be seen, especially in elderly patients. Subacute pulmonary syndromes are less severe, are seen with long-term administration, and may be reversible with discontinuance of the drug. The most feared complication of nitrofurantoin is chronic interstitial lung disease with fibrosis. Permanent lung disease can be seen and may be related to the duration of drug administration after the onset of clinical symptoms. Discontinuance of the drug at this stage will not reverse the fibrosis, and the condition may progress to permanent lung dysfunction.

Peripheral neuropathy is seen in patients treated with nitrofurantoin, especially in those with renal insufficiency and higher serum levels. Headache, myalgia, vertigo, and other CNS effects may also be seen, as well as hematological and hepatic effects.

> BOX 40-6
>
> **CLINICAL USE (INDICATIONS AND CONTRAINDICATIONS)**
>
> Nitrofurantoin is effective in the treatment of lower urinary tract infection. Its use in upper tract disease is debatable, and a systemic antibiotic would provide more reliable renal parenchymal concentrations. Although some physicians prescribe this agent for the chronic suppressive therapy of recurrent urinary tract infections, its use should be balanced against the potentially severe pulmonary toxicity. Given the potential for toxicity, most physicians would avoid chronic suppressive therapy with this agent. The drug should be avoided in patients with renal insufficiency because urine levels are decreased and serum levels (and, therefore, side effects) are increased.

OTHER AGENTS

Metronidazole

Although originally used for its activity against parasitic agents (*Trichomonas* and *Entamoeba*), metronidazole has become an extremely useful agent in the treatment of anaerobic bacteria. (See Chapter 43, Antiparasitic Agents, for a description of the pharmacology of the agent.)

BOX 40-7
CLINICAL USE (INDICATIONS AND CONTRAINDICATIONS)

Metronidazole is one of the most effective drugs for the therapy of infection with Gram-negative anaerobic bacteria. The drug is bactericidal against most anaerobic Gram-negative rods found in the digestive tract, including *Bacteroides*. The drug is highly effective against many Gram-positive anaerobic bacteria such as clostridia, including *Clostridium difficile*, but is not as active against some other Gram-positive anaerobic bacteria such as *Peptococcus*, *Peptostreptococcus*, and microaerophilic streptococci. For this reason, metronidazole is not the drug of first choice in the therapy of anaerobic infections from Gram-positive anaerobic bacteria of the upper gastrointestinal and respiratory tracts. Oral infections and anaerobic lung abscesses, frequently caused by mixed infections, which include infection with Gram-positive anaerobic bacteria, may respond better to agents such as penicillin G, clindamycin, or combinations of a penicillin and a β-lactamase inhibitor.

Metronidazole has become a drug of first choice in the treatment of mild to moderate pseudomembranous colitis caused by *C. difficile*. Authorities who recommend metronidazole over vancomycin frequently cite the cost difference between metronidazole and vancomycin as the primary reason for this choice. Metronidazole has an additional advantage over vancomycin in that the parenteral form of metronidazole achieves acceptable colonic concentrations for the treatment of *C. difficile*, whereas parenteral vancomycin produces unsatisfactory drug levels in the colon. Rare strains of *C. difficile* have been found to be resistant to metronidazole.

Spectinomycin

Spectinomycin is an aminocyclitol antibiotic available only for intramuscular injection. The drug is related to the aminoglycosides but devoid of oto- or nephrotoxicity. Spectinomycin is only given for the therapy of urogenital gonorrhea in penicillin-allergic patients who are intolerant to cephalosporins and quinolones. The use of this agent has decreased significantly with the introduction of ceftriaxone, ofloxacin, and ciprofloxacin. Spectinomycin has no activity against *Chlamydia*, and additional therapy for this sexually transmitted pathogen must be included in the treatment regimen.

Bacitracin

Bacitracin is a polypeptide antibiotic that inhibits cell wall synthesis and causes direct damage to cell wall structure. The agent has significant toxicity that is manifested by renal tubular damage and glomerular injury. Renal failure can result from use of bacitracin. Other adverse reactions include gastrointestinal intolerance, rash, and potentiation of neuromuscular blockade.

Because of the toxicity of this agent and the availability of other agents, parenteral bacitracin is not currently used in clinical medicine. Topical formulations still contain bacitracin as an active antibacterial agent; however, because of lack of absorption, systemic toxicity is not seen.

TREATMENT OF TUBERCULOSIS

Over the past 10 years, no area of antimicrobial therapy has undergone such a radical change in emphasis as the drug therapy of tuberculosis. The explosion of tuberculosis coinciding with the AIDS epidemic has resulted in an increase in the number of cases of tuberculosis and a large increase in the number of drug-resistant isolates of *M. tuberculosis*. What were once called "second-line" agents are now recommended for routine therapy. (This author's classification is based on 1993–1994 recommendations and significantly reclassifies the antimycobacterial agents.)

Students are strongly cautioned that therapy of tuberculosis must be properly prescribed, and treatment regimens must be followed strictly. Failure to follow the basic tenets of tuberculosis therapy not only results in treatment failures for the affected individual but also poses a public health problem when inappropriately treated patients infect others with resistant strains of tuberculosis. Studies have clearly shown that treatment of tuberculosis in the presence of resistance to either of the two major antitubercular agents, isoniazid or rifampin, has a substantially higher mortality. Knowledge of the pharmacological principles and toxicities of the various agents is imperative.

Pathophysiology

Knowledge of the pathophysiology of tuberculosis is essential to being able to provide proper therapy. No other area of antimicrobial therapy relies so heavily on combination therapy as does the treatment of mycobacterial disease. For this reason, the clinical use section of this chapter discusses these agents in groups rather than discussing the use of single agents (with the exception of the single-agent use of isoniazid).

Review of the pathogenesis of tuberculosis is essential to the understanding of the therapy for the disease. Infection is initiated with the inhalation of airborne droplet nuclei of correct size to reach the terminal air space. Mycobacteria are ingested by alveolar macrophages, replicate within the phagocyte, and destroy the macrophage. Other macrophages enter the area with lymphocytes, and an area of pneumonitis develops. Infected macrophages spread to regional lymph nodes and may spread throughout the body. This is thought to precede the development of tuberculin reactivity. Depending on the balance between cellular immunity and local antigen concentration, the immune system works to control infection. In the vast majority of cases (90% in the absence of immunocompromised states), bacterial destruction is rapid, and the only indication of infection is a positive skin test for tuberculosis. Some patients have antigen concentrations in the parenchyma and hilar nodes sufficient to cause necrosis and visible calcification on chest radiograph (Ghon complex). Some may go on to develop active disease, especially when the patient has an immunodeficiency such as AIDS. An important consequence of infection is seeding of the apical posterior lobe, where infection may progress immediately or may be delayed for several years. During the stages before active disease (visible on chest radiograph), the number of tuberculous bacilli is relatively small ($\approx 10^3 - 10^4$) and far below the number seen in active cavitary disease (10^9).

The presence of a reaction to a purified protein derivative (PPD) skin test for tuberculosis therefore indicates that the patient has, or had, live-replicating tuberculous bacilli within his or her body. If a patient has no evidence of clinical disease (as evidenced by a negative chest radiograph and no clinical symptoms) and a positive PPD test, he or she either has eradicated all of the mycobacteria and is cured, or has live mycobacteria and has not progressed to clinical disease. A patient whose only manifestation of exposure to tuberculosis is a positive PPD either may have subclinical disease, which can go on to develop clinical tuberculosis, or may have successfully eradicated the mycobacteria via immune mechanisms. The terminology frequently used for the treatment of patients with positive PPD skin tests and no active disease ("prophylaxis") is, therefore, a misnomer. Discussion of the treatment of positive skin tests should revolve around the *therapy* of subclinical disease, or less correctly, the prophylaxis of progression from subclinical to clinical disease.

Several populations of tuberculous bacilli are thought to be present in active infection, depending on the environmental conditions presented to the bacteria. These are: (1) rapidly growing bacilli in the hyperoxic, neutral-pH, and extracellular environment of the cavity; (2) slowly metabolizing bacilli in the somewhat hypoxic, acidic environment of caseous material; and (3) slowly metabolizing bacilli in the acidic intracellular environment of the macrophage. A fourth population of dormant bacilli is also thought to exist. These populations are differentially susceptible to the various antimycobacterial agents and can influence treatment options.

Antimycobacterial Agents

Isoniazid

CHEMISTRY. Isoniazid (isonicotinic acid hydrazide) is a synthetic antitubercular agent that was discovered in the early 1950s.

MECHANISMS OF ACTION. Although the exact mechanism of action is not fully defined, isoniazid inhibits mycolic acid synthesis. Because mycolic acid is an integral, structural component of *myco*bacteria, inhibition of mycolic acid synthesis results in antimycobacterial activity. Isoniazid is bactericidal against the rapidly growing extracellular mycobacteria that are present in cavitary lesions; against intracellular mycobacteria in the acid, intracellular environment; and against slowly replicating organisms within caseous material. Therefore, isoniazid is bactericidal against all major populations of mycobacteria that are seen in tuberculosis. Dormant mycobacteria are an exceptionally resistant population to treat, with only rifampin and possibly the quinolones having any effect.

MECHANISMS OF RESISTANCE. It has been appreciated for some time that *M. tuberculosis* organisms that lack catalase activity have a high incidence of resistance to isoniazid. The molecular mechanism of this resistance was recently elucidated and was shown to be, in part, related to the catalase/peroxidase enzyme product of the myocobacterial gene *katG.* Strains that fail to metabolize isoniazid because of defective catalase/peroxidase are resistant to isoniazid, suggesting that a bacterial metabolite of isoniazid is the biologically active moiety.

Resistance to isoniazid occurs in untreated populations of mycobacteria at a frequency of 1 in 10^6 bacilli. This resistance is an independent event with respect to other antibacterial resistance. Single-drug therapy with isoniazid of large concentrations of *M. tuberculosis* ($> 10^6 - 10^7$) may therefore select for drug-resistant populations. Bacterial densities of 10^9 or 10^{10} bacteria can frequently be seen in cavitary pulmonary tuberculosis; contrasted with a total body burden of 10^3 to 10^4 bacteria in asymptomatic infection without clinical disease (as manifested by a positive PPD test). Although single-agent isoniazid therapy for the treatment of preclinical disease (so-called isoniazid prophylaxis) would not be expected to result in isoniazid resistance; single-agent isoniazid therapy in the presence of clinical disease can reliably be shown to result in the development of isoniazid resistance. Physicians are strongly cautioned that development of resistance to isoniazid is associated with a significantly increased morbidity and mortality.

ROUTE OF ADMINISTRATION, ABSORPTION, DISTRIBUTION, METABOLISM, AND EXCRETION. Isoniazid is generally given in the oral form, although intramuscular and intravenous administration are possible. The drug is well absorbed after oral administration and is widely distributed. Concentrations in spinal fluid are quite high even in the absence of meningeal inflammation. In addition, isoniazid concentration in caseous material is high and results in therapeutic levels of the drug within the caseation.

Isoniazid is metabolized in the liver, predominantly by acetylation. Genetic factors determine the rate of acetylation, with so-called slow and fast acetylators being identified. Although they are clearly identifiable, rates of acetylation have little impact on the clinical use of the agent. The metabolite is excreted through the kidneys. Dosage adjustment may be necessary in the presence of severe hepatic or renal failure.

ADVERSE EFFECTS. Many adverse effects can be seen with isoniazid. In many clinical situations, however, the *fear* of toxicity is greater than the *risk* of toxicity and many patients have appropriate therapy withheld because of the fear of toxicity.

Nausea, vomiting, and other gastrointestinal side effects are common adverse reactions seen with isoniazid.

Hepatotoxicity is a major adverse reaction to isoniazid. Hepatocellular inflammation with elevated transaminases is seen with isoniazid and may progress to fatal hepatitis. Recent reports have identified several cases of isoniazid-induced hepatic failure requiring liver transplantation. Hepatic injury is age-related, with an increased incidence in older populations. The majority of cases of hepatitis occur within the first 4 – 8 weeks of therapy. Increased rates of hepatotoxicity are seen with prior liver injury, alcohol consumption, and coadministration of hepatotoxic agents.

Isoniazid is frequently used in asymptomatic patients for the therapy of subclinical disease and for the prevention of the development of clinical tuberculosis. However, because over 90% of normal patients with tuberculous infection do not go on to develop clinical disease (see Pathophysiology), the risk of development of tuberculosis versus isoniazid-associated hepatitis must be weighed. Patients should be alerted to the symptoms of hepatitis and instructed to call their physician should symptoms develop. The risk of hepatotoxicity versus the ability of the drug to prevent clinical tuberculosis markedly influences the indications for isoniazid prophylaxis. The paradigm is to balance the risk of toxicity with the risk of development of clinical tuberculosis. As patients' risk factors change, the decision as to which action is less toxic will also change.

Isoniazid administration causes increased excretion of pyridoxine (vitamin B_6), which can result in a peripheral neuropathy. Therefore, pyridoxine is always coadministered with isoniazid to prevent this complication. Other nervous system complications of isoniazid include ataxia, seizures, psychosis, encephalopathy, and other CNS abnormalities. Although it is very rare, optic neuritis also has been seen with isoniazid.

Hypersensitivity reactions to isoniazid, such as fever, rash, vasculitis, and other immune-mediated reactions, can occur in patients receiving isoniazid. A difficult diagnostic dilemma may be encountered in patients receiving isoniazid for tuberculosis who develop drug fever from the isoniazid, because discontinuation of the drug during tuberculosis therapy is difficult to manage clinically.

A lupus-like reaction to isoniazid with positive serological findings for antinuclear antibodies can be seen. Additionally, hematological toxicity in the form of leukopenia, eosinophilia, and thrombocytopenia has been seen with isoniazid.

Overdose with isoniazid can produce an anion gap metabolic acidosis; supportive therapy including pyridoxine should be initiated rapidly.

Some reports suggest that rates of acetylation may influence toxicity, causing patients with slow acetylation to have a higher incidence of adverse reactions related to higher drug concentrations (*eg*, peripheral neuropathy) and patients with fast acetylation to have a higher incidence of hepatotoxicity.

DRUG INTERACTIONS. Isoniazid administration can interfere with the hepatic metabolism of carbamazepine and phenytoin, resulting in increased serum concentrations of both agents. Serum levels of both medications must be monitored in patients receiving either drug concomitantly with isoniazid.

Coadministration of isoniazid and ketoconazole may result in subtherapeutic concentrations of ketoconazole.

Reports of coordination difficulties and psychosis resulting from concomitant administration of disulfiram and isoniazid suggest that this combination should be avoided.

Rifampin

CHEMISTRY. Rifampin is a semisynthetic derivative of the rifamycin complex. The drug has a complex chemical structure and is noted for its deep orange color. The drug is called rifampicin in the United Kingdom, Europe, Australia, and other areas of the world.

MECHANISM OF ACTION. Rifampin inhibits the enzyme DNA-dependent RNA-polymerase. The drug is very specific for the bacterial form of the enzyme and has little effect on the mammalian version of this essential enzyme. The resulting interference with bacterial protein synthesis is frequently bactericidal and mycobactericidal.

The major indication for rifampin is in the treatment of tuberculosis and other mycobacterial diseases. Rifampin is bactericidal for all populations of tuberculous bacilli, including intracellular mycobacteria in the acidic environment of the cell or caseous material, and is bactericidal for intracavitary bacilli in the hyperoxic alkaline environment of the cavity. Even dormant tuberculous bacilli may be killed by rifampin.

MECHANISMS OF RESISTANCE. One-step resistance to rifampin occurs in populations of *M. tuberculosis* at a frequency of ≈ 1 in 10^8 organisms, even in the absence of selective pressure of rifampin. Students and clinicians are cautioned that administration of rifampin to large concentrations of tuberculous bacilli results in the selection of rifampin-resistant strains.

ROUTE OF ADMINISTRATION, ABSORPTION, DISTRIBUTION, METABOLISM, AND EXCRETION. Rifampin is well absorbed orally and reaches adequate serum levels easily after oral administration. A recent parenteral formulation was introduced for intravenous administration but is reserved for patients who are unable to use their gastrointestinal tract. Rifampin is well distributed throughout the body, as confirmed by the orange color imparted after administration to most bodily fluids, including tears, saliva, urine, and serum. Penetration into the CSF in the absence of meningeal inflammation is variable but obtains approximately 50% of serum concentrations in the presence of meningitis. Rifampin is highly lipophilic and enters cells readily. The intracellular distribution of this agent enhances the drug's activity against its primary intracellular target, *M. tuberculosis.* Rifampin is metabolized by deacetylation in the liver, and the active metabolite undergoes intrahepatic circulation. Metabolism of rifampin induces cytochrome P-450 systems; this accelerates the metabolism of rifampin and the metabolism of several other agents (see Drug Interactions). The serum half-life of rifampin is 2–5 hours and is not significantly affected by renal disease but is prolonged in hepatic dysfunction.

ADVERSE EFFECTS. The major adverse reaction to rifampin is hepatotoxicity. While on rifampin, many patients have minimally abnormal liver enzyme levels that do not require discontinuation of the drug. The reaction is classically more cholestatic than that seen with isoniazid, as reflected by increased alkaline phosphatase and bilirubin concentrations. However, a necroinflammatory reaction with elevated transaminases can be seen with rifampin, and significant alterations of liver enzymes must be carefully evaluated before treatment continues. Administration of rifampin in the presence of liver disease should proceed cautiously. Fatal hepatitis and a shocklike state have been reported in patients treated with rifampin, especially in the presence of preexisting liver pathology.

Gastrointestinal effects of rifampin may reflect underlying hepatic dysfunction but also may be seen without hepatic abnormalities. Symptoms such as nausea, vomiting, diarrhea, and abdominal pain may be seen with rifampin.

Significant discoloration of most bodily fluids occurs as a consequence of rifampin therapy. Patients who wear soft contact lenses must be warned of the possibility of permanent discoloration of their lenses while taking rifampin. Patients must also be warned of a significant red-orange discoloration of the urine while taking rifampin.

An unusual flulike illness may be seen with rifampin administration. Fever, chills, and myalgias accompanied by headache, dizziness, and bone pain have been described. Dermatological reactions including pruritus, urticaria, rash, exfoliative dermatitis, eosinophilia, and anaphylaxis can also occur. The reaction is said to occur at a higher frequency with intermittent administration. Changing to a lower dosage or to daily administration frequently corrects these abnormalities.

Rare renal toxicity, including interstitial nephritis, acute tubular necrosis, and cortical necrosis, has been seen.

Intravenous rifampin formulations may contain sodium formaldehyde sulfoxylate and cause severe bronchospasm in atopic, sulfite-sensitive individuals. Just as with isoniazid, the parenteral formulation should be reserved for those patients who are absolutely unable to take oral medications.

Other adverse effects, including neurological effects (*eg*, headache, nervousness, behavioral changes, confusion), have been seen rarely with rifampin. Leukopenia, thrombocytopenia, and hemolytic anemia have also occurred and occur at an increased frequency with intermittent administration.

DRUG INTERACTIONS. Drug interactions with rifampin are extremely important because of the significant induction of the cytochrome P-450 system. It is a good habit to review all medications in patients who are about to receive rifampin and determine whether an interaction might be expected. Although this practice would be prudent for many medications, the severity and frequency of drug-drug interactions with rifampin warrants this cautious approach. Rifampin may decrease serum levels of verapamil, oral anticoagulants, cyclosporine, oral hypoglycemic agents, oral contraceptives, corticosteroids, methadone, quinidine, digitalis, β blockers, narcotics, diazepam, mexiletine, theophylline, and analgesics. Such adverse reactions as unexpected pregnancy in patients taking birth control pills, organ rejection in patients taking cyclosporine, hyperglycemia in patients taking oral hypoglycemics, and adrenal insufficiency during corticosteroid replacement therapy are but a few examples of the significant drug-drug interactions that can occur with rifampin and other therapeutic agents.

Significant (>90%) reductions in verapamil serum levels can be seen when oral verapamil is used in combination with rifampin. Failure to recognize this drug-drug interaction can render verapamil clinically inactive and can result in possible severe clinical outcomes. Significant reduction in serum ketoconazole levels have also been seen with administration of rifampin, and concomitant use of these agents is difficult.

ANTIBACTERIAL ACTIVITY. The primary use of rifampin is for the therapy of tuberculosis. A discussion of its therapeutic use in tuberculosis follows. Rifampin is unique among other agents used in the therapy of tuberculosis because of its usefulness as an antibacterial agent. Because of its impressive distribution, rifampin is an excellent drug to eradicate the nasal carriage of many bacterial pathogens, including *Meningococcus*, *H. influenzae*, and *Staphylococcus* (generally in combination with an antistaphylococcal penicillin or trimethoprim-sulfamethoxasole). Rifampin is also useful in combination with other agents in the treatment of less common diseases in the United States, such as Q fever and brucellosis. However, because of its extreme usefulness as an antitubercular agent, physicians should avoid the temptation to routinely prescribe rifampin. The indiscriminate use of rifampin could lead to an increased likelihood of patients who are silently harboring tuberculosis being exposed to rifampin as a single agent, which would increase the potential for rifampin resistance within the population.

Pyrazinamide

CHEMISTRY. Pyrazinamide, an analog of nicotinamide, is an older antitubercular drug that has recently been recognized as an important first-line agent in the therapy of tuberculosis, especially in regimens of short duration.

MECHANISM OF ACTION. Although the exact mechanism of action is unknown, pyrazinamide is bactericidal against intracellular organisms at an acidic pH. Pyrazinamide exerts its action only on metabolically active organisms. Despite the long-held belief that pyrazinamide is bactericidal in acidic vesicles of macrophages, this hypothesis cannot be fully substantiated by experimental observations. Although the exact mechanism of action remains to be clarified, pyrazinamide is clinically quite active in combination with other agents and forms a cornerstone of short-course, multidrug regimens.

ROUTE OF ADMINISTRATION, ABSORPTION, DISTRIBUTION, METABOLISM, AND EXCRETION. Pyrazinamide is well absorbed orally and distributed widely, including the CNS. No parenteral forms of pyrazinamide exist. The drug has a long half-life of 12–24 hours and can be administered as a single daily dose. Pyrazinamide is metabolized in the liver, and the metabolites are excreted via renal mechanisms. Renal failure can therefore result in significant accumulation of pyrazinamide metabolites and can represent a major problem in administration of the agent.

The drug is generally administered at 20–35 mg/kg/day in divided doses but can be given as a single administration if tolerated by the patient. Twice-weekly and weekly dosing schedules can also be adopted for observed therapy or for increased compliance.

ADVERSE EFFECTS. The major adverse reaction to pyrazinamide is hepatotoxicity. Original reports of parenchymal liver disease suggested that this agent was associated with a marked risk of liver damage. Lower drug dosages and shorter duration of therapy have resulted in a significantly lower toxicity profile than was originally described. Pyrazinamide is now one of the initial drugs used in most antitubercular regimens. The hepatotoxicity is necroinflammatory, resulting in elevated transaminase levels. The toxicity is generally seen early in the course of administration, is dose-related, and is usually reversible on discontinuation of the drug.

Hyperuricemia is commonly seen in patients who are treated with pyrazinamide. Marked elevations of serum uric acid concentrations may be seen, but development of clinical gout is unusual unless the patient has a history of gout.

Arthralgia, arthritis, nausea, vomiting, fever, and malaise are also seen with the use of pyrazinamide.

Ethambutol

CHEMISTRY. Ethambutol was discovered during the screening of compounds for antimycobacterial activity. The drug is synthetic and is not a product of microbiological origin.

MECHANISM OF ACTION. Ethambutol is active only against mycobacterial species. By an ill-defined interaction with mycolic acid, ethambutol is tuberculostatic. Resistance to ethambutol, like that to all other antituberculous agents, develops when the agent is used as a single drug to treat clinical disease.

ROUTE OF ADMINISTRATION, ABSORPTION, DISTRIBUTION, METABOLISM, AND EXCRETION. Ethambutol is available only as an oral agent. The drug is well absorbed orally and distributed widely. CSF concentrations are low in the presence of normal meninges but increase significantly with meningeal inflammation. The drug is minimally metabolized (15%), and the majority of the drug is excreted unchanged by the kidneys. Dosage adjustment is necessary with renal dysfunction.

ADVERSE EFFECTS. The primary toxicity of ethambutol is neuropathy. The major form of this is retrobulbar neuritis, which results in alteration of color vision, potentially leading to decreased visual fields and blindness. The neuropathy is frequently reversible on discontinuance of the medication. The toxicity is dose-related and is seen more commonly at the higher dosing range. The patient should be warned to report any alterations in vision while on ethambutol; the physician may wish to use the lower dosing range when it is clinically indicated. In addition to retrobulbar neuritis, peripheral neuropathies may occur.

Hyperuricemia may occur with ethambutol, and patients on ethambutol plus pyrazinamide may experience significant increases in serum uric acid concentrations.

Streptomycin

CHEMISTRY. Streptomycin is an aminoglycoside antibiotic. Pharmacological details of the drug are covered in Chapter 39.

MECHANISMS OF ACTIONS. Streptomycin is bactericidal against rapidly growing tuberculous bacilli in the hyperoxic environment of cavitary tuberculosis. The drug is inactive against intracellular or dormant organisms.

MECHANISMS OF RESISTANCE. Like other antitubercular medications, resistance develops rapidly to streptomycin when the drug is used as a single agent. Approximately 1 in 10^6 tuberculous bacilli are resistant to streptomycin in the absence of selective pressure.

ROUTE OF ADMINISTRATION, ABSORPTION, DISTRIBUTION, METABOLISM, AND EXCRETION. The drug is available only as an intramuscular injection.

Clinical Use of Antitubercular Medication

Isoniazid "Prophylaxis"

Although this text is not intended as a therapeutic guide, significant confusion exists over the use of isoniazid for the prevention of clinical tuberculosis, and this confusion is addressed here. A better understanding of the use of isoniazid and the interaction of epidemiological and pharmacological principles should lead to a better understanding of the use of isoniazid and therefore is briefly reviewed in this section.

As outlined previously, the term *isoniazid prophylaxis* is a misnomer. The term, however, has become ingrained in the medical jargon and is used for this discussion. It should be strongly stated that single-agent isoniazid is used to treat subclinical disease and to prevent the development of clinical tuberculosis. Guidelines from the Centers for Disease Control and Prevention are summarized in this section and in the algorithm shown in Figure 40–4. Modifications of the original recommendations, as suggested by Barnes and Barrows (1993), are also incorporated in the discussion. Please note that recommendations may change rapidly in the future. A static text reference should never be considered as the final determination in any area undergoing as rapid a change as the therapy of tuberculosis. Readers are cautioned that these recommendations represent a synopsis, and they are encouraged to familiarize themselves with the references and the current literature before instituting therapy.

It cannot be overemphasized that *isoniazid prophylaxis must never be given before the diagnosis of active tuberculosis is excluded. The use of single-drug therapy in the presence of clinical disease leads to the development of drug-resistant strains and causes treatment failures.* If the patient has a normal chest radiograph and no other symptoms of tuberculosis, it is necessary to determine whether he or she has been previously treated for tuberculosis. If the patient had received appropriate therapy in the past for either clinical disease (multidrug regimen) or subclinical disease (isoniazid alone) and shows no evidence of reactivation, then no therapy is indicated.

Patients at the highest risk of tuberculosis should be treated, even if they have a negative PPD. These populations include HIV-infected individuals with close contact with tuberculosis, HIV-infected individuals with a prior positive PPD with no treatment history, or HIV-infected individuals with radiographical evidence of old tuberculosis. Children 5 years of age and younger who have close contact with known infectious patients should be tested and begun on therapy regardless of the PPD result. If initial testing and repeat testing at 3 months show negative results, then therapy can be discontinued.

A 5-mm PPD is indication for isoniazid prophylaxis in HIV-positive patients, patients in close contact with infectious tuberculosis, and in patients with chest radiographic evidence of previously untreated tuberculosis.

Any person whose PPD increases by more than 15 mm within a 2-year period should receive isoniazid prophylaxis, *regardless of the age of the patient.* Increases in PPD diameter of 10 mm are considered significant in persons younger

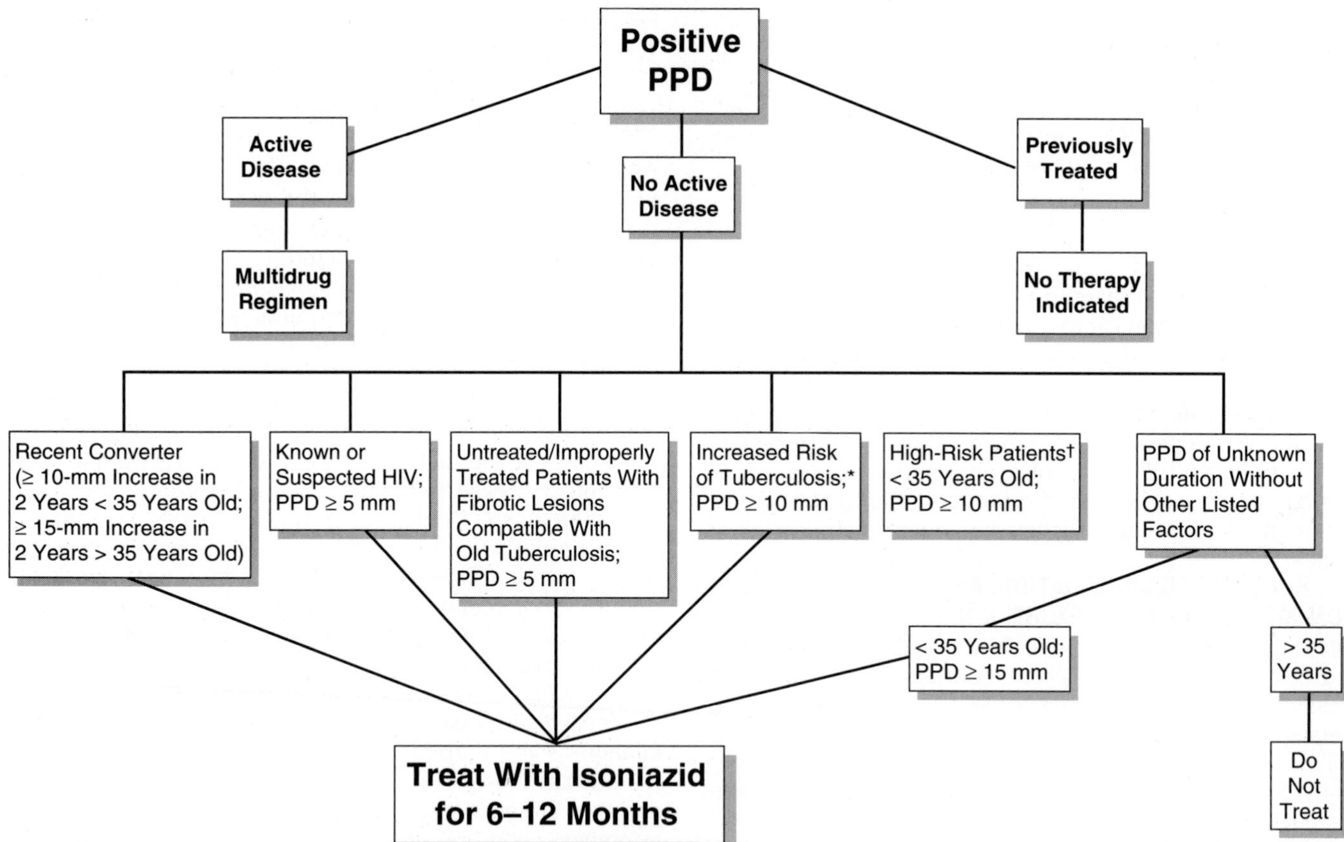

FIGURE 40–4. Algorithm for therapy following a positive skin test for tuberculosis (purified protein derivative [tuberculin; PPD]). Note that several indications for isoniazid therapy exist in the absence of a positive PPD (see text for explanation). *Asterisk* indicates conditions at high risk for development of tuberculosis, which include but are not limited to intravenous drug use, diabetes, end-stage renal disease, silicosis, malnutrition, gastrectomy, immunosuppressive therapy, and malignancy. *Dagger* indicates persons at high risk for developing tuberculosis, who include foreign-born residents from countries with high rates of tuberculosis, people of lower socioeconomic status, and residents of long-term care facilities, such as nursing homes and prisons.

than 35 years of age. (The difference in PPD size for determination of significance is related to the age incidence for isoniazid hepatotoxicity. Because the older population may have a higher exposure to nontuberculous mycobacteria and is at higher risk of isoniazid hepatotoxicity, a higher cutoff for PPD positivity is less sensitive but more specific for tuberculosis.)

Any person with a PPD diameter of 10 mm or greater and a coexistent condition such as intravenous drug use, diabetes, end-stage renal disease, silicosis, malnutrition (greater than 10% reduction from ideal body weight), gastrectomy, immunosuppressive therapy, malignancies, and other conditions should receive isoniazid prophylaxis.

Persons who were born in countries with high rates of tuberculosis, those of lower socioeconomic status, and residents of long-term care facilities or prisons who have a PPD diameter of 10 mm or more should receive isoniazid.

At the current time, patients older than 35 years of age with a positive tuberculin skin test (> 15 mm) of *unknown duration, with a negative chest radiograph and none of the above risk factors* are thought to have a greater risk of suffering adverse reaction to isoniazid therapy than they are at risk for developing active tuberculosis. Please note that despite several age criteria within the recommendations, *recently exposed individuals*, as identified by the conversion of a negative PPD to a positive PPD, are candidates for isoniazid therapy *regardless of age* because of the higher rate of active tuberculosis within the first 2 years of exposure. Despite the prevailing concept that the first determination of isoniazid use is age, the previous discussion should highlight the fact that the age of the patient is only a cofactor in the decision to treat. Age is generally considered only after other determinations have been established. In the algorithm (Fig. 40–4), age as the single defining criteria for isoniazid prophylaxis is not reached until after at least six other factors (activity of disease, recent exposure, recent conversion of PPD, HIV status, chest radiographic evidence of old tuberculosis, and risk status for tuberculosis) have been considered.

If a question ever exists as to whether a chest radiograph represents active disease, a multidrug regimen must be chosen to avoid treating clinical disease with a single agent. If cultures of tuberculosis are negative at 3 months, then the other agents may be discontinued and isoniazid continued for the remainder of the prophylaxis regimen.

Duration of therapy ranges from 6–12 months and can be given either daily or twice weekly. The 12-month treatment regimen is preferred for patients with chest radiographic evidence of old tuberculosis and for patients with significant immunosuppression, such as infection with HIV.

Therapy of Active Tuberculosis

Therapy of tuberculosis is initially started with four of the five first-line agents, isoniazid, rifampin, pyrazinamide, and either streptomycin or ethambutol. The use of four agents is recommended because of several considerations. First, the background rate of resistance to either isoniazid or rifampin is now clinically significant in many areas of the United States. Prior recommendation of only isoniazid and rifampin may therefore be unacceptable. Second, the use of intensive therapy "up front" allows for shorter treatment courses (sometimes as short as 6 months). Third, the use of four drugs initially can result in better cure rates if patients stop taking medications before completing their full treatment regimen; aggressive treatment at the outset allows the cure rates with abbreviated courses to be better with the four-drug regimens than with the two- or three-drug regimens, although the rates are lower than with full-course regimens. Fourth, the addition of pyrazinamide has been extremely useful in the shortened courses; failure to include pyrazinamide in short-duration chemotherapy results in significantly poorer cure rates. Fifth, the addition of streptomycin, which is bactericidal against extracellular organisms, and pyrazinamide, which is bactericidal against intracellular organisms, results in bactericidal activity against all of the major populations of tuberculous bacilli.

The four-drug regimen usually includes daily streptomycin via intramuscular injection for 1 month, 2 months of pyrazinamide, along with a 6–9 month regimen of isoniazid and rifampin. All isolates of tuberculous bacilli should be routinely tested against the five first-line agents and therapy adjusted in the face of resistance.

Drug-Resistant Tuberculosis

The incidence of resistance to antituberculosus agents is increasing. Prior therapy for tuberculosis, acquisition of tuberculosis outside of the United States, HIV infection, and the infection of prison and homeless populations all have caused an increased risk of drug-resistant tuberculosis. Previously treated patients represent a particular problem in the choice of therapy prior to obtaining sensitivity testing. Because of the increased likelihood of resistance to drugs used to treat prior disease, *at least two antitubercular drugs should be added to any failing (or failed) tuberculosis treatment regimen.* This strategy avoids inadvertent single-drug therapy, should the patient's isolate be resistant to all of his or her prior medications. In addition, because many treatment failures are from noncompliance rather than primary drug resistance, many experts recommend that drugs be added to prior regimens instead of just using new regimens.

Recent reports have detailed highly resistant strains of tuberculosis in prisoners and in AIDS patients. These isolates are resistant to isoniazid, rifampin, ethambutol, streptomycin, and other agents. Mortality associated with infection from these strains is high, and treatment options are limited. Poor compliance with prescribed regimens and inappropriate treatment regimens are felt to be responsible for the development of these strains. The rapid spread of these isolates has been accelerated by the AIDS epidemic, as AIDS patients frequently have a high bacillary burden of mycobacteria and are highly susceptible to the development of active tuberculosis. Treatment and prophylaxis regimens for these strains include pyrazinamide and ofloxacin, along with standard first-line agents for treatment until sensitivities are available. These highly resistant tuberculous bacilli should serve as a reminder of the importance of appropriate therapy for all patients with tuberculosis and of the consequences of inappropriate therapy of this disease. Many recommendations for the treatment of infection with tuberculosis strains that are resistant to both isoniazid and rifampin include surgical excision, highlighting the high failure rate of chemotherapy for resistant tuberculous bacilli.

In the event of infection with multi-drug resistant strains or the development of adverse reactions to the primary agents, secondary agents need to be added to the regimen. In general, the use of the so called second-line drugs should be reserved for atypical patients or presentations. It has clearly been shown that resistance to either isoniazid or rifampin increases tuberculosis mortality, and resistance to both significantly increases the risk of death. For this reason, physicians prescribing second-line agents should be intimately familiar with tuberculosis and the drug therapy of the disease.

Second-Line Agents

ETHIONAMIDE. Ethionamide, a congener of isonicotinic acid, is a tuberculostatic oral agent. The drug is well absorbed orally and is distributed well throughout the body, including in the CSF. The drug is primarily a second-line agent by virtue of its bacteriostatic nature and the high frequency of gastrointestinal tract intolerance. Most patients on ethionamide develop nausea and vomiting. Other side effects include neuropathies, orthostatic hypotension, and a metallic taste.

PARA-AMINOSALICYLIC ACID. Para-aminosalicylic acid is a structural derivative of para-aminobenzoic acid and inhibits mycobacterial growth by altering folate metabolism. The drug is poorly absorbed after oral administration and causes significant nausea and vomiting. Hypersensitivity reactions and a lupus-like syndrome are also seen after administration of this agent. Because of its toxicity and the availability of other agents, para-aminosalicylic acid is seldom prescribed in the United States, but because of its low cost, it is still used in the developing world.

CYCLOSERINE. Cycloserine is a well absorbed antibacterial and antimycobacterial agent that inhibits cell wall synthesis. The drug is widely distributed and is excreted by the kidneys. Toxicity of cycloserine significantly restricts its use, however. Psychosis, seizures, and behavioral changes are frequent with cycloserine. These toxicities relegate cycloserine to a largely unused agent.

KANAMYCIN, CAPREOMYCIN, VIOMYCIN, AND AMIKACIN. These aminoglycoside antibiotics have activity against tuberculosis. Kanamycin is rarely if ever used because of marked ototoxicity. Capreomycin and viomycin are similar agents and must be given via intramuscular injection. Cross-resistance between capreomycin and viomycin occurs commonly. Amikacin is available by intravenous and intramuscular injection. Amikacin is probably the most active aminoglycoside against mycobacterial species. Expense and the risk of renal toxicity and ototoxicity have limited the use of this agent compared with streptomycin. However, accurate assays exist for amikacin serum concentrations and allow for careful monitoring.

CIPROFLOXACIN AND OFLOXACIN. The quinolones, ciprofloxacin and ofloxacin, are highly active against *M. tuberculosis*. Currently, the quinolones are used as an adjunct to therapy and are primary drugs in the presence of resistance to both rifampin and isoniazid. Resistance may be a problem in the future, as the use of the quinolones in the community is massive and the chances of exposing undiagnosed tuberculosis to single-agent quinolones in the community must be higher than with other agents.

DRUG THERAPY FOR OTHER MYCOBACTERIA (INCLUDING LEPROSY)

The AIDS epidemic has markedly increased the number of cases of infection with atypical mycobacteria. *Mycobacterium avium* complex (MAC) (also called *M. avium-intracellulare*) is a frequent infection in AIDS patients who have CD_4 counts below 100 cells per square millimeter. Because therapy of this infection is difficult, prevention of the disease is attempted with a rifampin analog, rifabutin.

Rifabutin

Rifabutin is a structural analog of rifamycin S and is highly active against MAC and *M. tuberculosis in vitro*. The drug has similar pharmacokinetics to rifampin and is available as an oral formulation. Adverse reactions in clinical trials for MAC infection include rash, gastrointestinal intolerance, and neutropenia. Other adverse reactions include a flulike syndrome, hepatitis, hemolysis, arthralgia, myositis, and skin discoloration.

Rifabutin is currently indicated as prophylaxis of MAC infection in AIDS patients with CD_4 counts below 100 cells per cubic millimeter. Many physicians also include rifabutin in treatment regimens for the therapy of infections caused by MAC. Current therapeutic recommendations for infections caused by MAC include rifabutin, ciprofloxacin, and either azithromycin or clarithromycin. Some experts recommend a five- or six-drug regimen that includes rifabutin, ethambutol, ciprofloxacin, clofazamine, amikacin, and azithromycin.

Dapsone

Dapsone is a sulfone antibiotic. The mechanism of action is felt to be bacteriostatic, as the effects of dapsone are inhibited by para-aminobenzoic acid in the laboratory. The mechanism of action is therefore felt to involve folate biosynthesis, but this is not proved.

The drug is well absorbed orally and is distributed widely. Clearance of the agent varies widely among individuals. The drug is metabolized in the liver and is excreted by the kidneys.

Adverse reactions to dapsone may be significant. Dapsone may cause hemolytic anemia and methemoglobinemia. Hemolytic anemia may occur with or without G6PD deficiency but is severe in patients with the disorder. Cutaneous reactions to the drug are common. Peripheral neuropathy, anorexia, hepatitis, cholestatic jaundice, and a drug-induced lupus-like reaction have been reported in addition to other side effects. Patients receiving the drug for leprosy may also experience erythema nodosum leprosum or lepromatous lepra reactions in conjunction with therapy.

Drug interaction can occur in patients receiving dapsone. Some reports suggest that coadministration of dapsone with didanosine may decrease dapsone absorption by buffering gastric acidity. Rifampin may decrease dapsone concentrations, and trimethoprim may increase serum concentrations of dapsone.

The major use worldwide for dapsone is for the therapy of leprosy, either alone or in combination with rifampin. Recently, the drug has been shown to be useful in the prophylaxis of *Pneumocystis carinii* pneumonia (PCP) infections in AIDS patients. Use of dapsone may be considered to prevent PCP infection in patients who are unable to take cotrimoxazole or pentamidine.

Clofazimine

Clofazimine is a phenazine dye with antimycobacterial activity. The drug is available in an oral preparation and is poorly absorbed from the gastrointestinal tract. Administration with food may increase absorption. The drug is lipophilic and is distributed to fatty tissue, resulting in excellent intracellular concentrations, which may explain its activity against intracellular organisms. The drug has a long apparent tissue half-life, probably related to its wide lipophilic distributions, and may be recovered weeks, months, or years after discontinuing therapy.

Adverse reactions to clofazimine include a marked bronze discoloration of the skin in 75–100% of patients taking the drug. Patients should be cautioned about this before taking the medication. Abdominal pain, nausea, vomiting, and gastrointestinal intolerance are common side effects of clofazimine and may be dose-limiting. Other adverse reactions include anxiety, dizziness, headaches, and eosinophilia in addition to other less-common effects.

The major use of clofazamine is the therapy of leprosy, generally in combination with rifampin. In the United States, the major use of the agent has been in multiple-drug regimens for the treatment of MAC infections.

Acknowledgment

This chapter was supported by the Department of Veterans Affairs.

REFERENCES

Alford RH: Antimycobacterial agents. *In* Mandell GL, Douglas RG Jr, Bennett JE (eds): Principles and Practice of Infectious Diseases, 3rd ed, 350–360. New York: Churchill Livingstone, 1990.

Barnes PF, Barrows SA: Tuberculosis in the 1990s. Ann Intern Med 119:400–410, 1993.

Centers for Disease Control and Prevention: Recommendations of the Advisory Committee for Elimination of Tuberculosis. MMWR 39:9-12, 1990.

Cockerill FR III, Edson RS: Trimethoprim-sulfamethoxazole. Mayo Clin Proc 66:1260-1269, 1991.

Des Prez RM, Heim CR: *Mycobacterium tuberculosis*. *In* Mandell GL, Douglas RG, Bennett JE (eds): Principles and Practice of Infectious Diseases, 3rd ed, 1877-1906. New York: Churchill Livingstone, 1990.

Frieden TR, Sterling T, Pablos-Mendez A, et al: The emergence of drug-resistant tuberculosis in New York City. N Engl J Med 328:521-526, 1993.

Goble M, Iseman MD, Madsen LA, et al: Treatment of 171 patients with pulmonary tuberculosis resistant to isoniazid and rifampin. N Engl J Med 328:527-532, 1993.

Initial therapy for tuberculosis in the era of multidrug resistance. Recommendations of the Advisory Council for the Elimination of Tuberculosis. MMWR 42(RR-7):1-8, 1993.

Iseman MD: Treatment of multidrug-resistant tuberculosis. N Engl J Med 329:784-791, 1993.

Neu HC: Quinolone antimicrobial agents. Ann Rev Med 43:465-486, 1992.

Peloquin CA: Pharmacology of the antimycobacterial drugs. Med Clin North Am 77:1253-1262, 1993.

Severe isoniazid-associated hepatitis—New York, 1991-1993. MMWR 42:545-547, 1993.

Smilack JD, Wilson WR, Cockerill FR III: Tetracyclines, chloramphenicol, erythromycin, clindamycin, and metronidazole. Mayo Clin Proc 66:1270-1280, 1991.

Stratton C: Fluoroquinolone antibiotics: Properties of the class and individual agents [Review]. Clin Ther 14:348-375, 1992.

Sulfonamides. *In* AHFS Drug Information 93, 472-482. American Society of Hospital Pharmacists, 1993.

Sulfones. *In* AHFS Drug Information 93, 482-486. American Society of Hospital Pharmacists, 1993.

Transformation with *katG* restores isoniazid-sensitivity in *Mycobacterium tuberculosis* isolates resistant to a range of drug concentrations. Mol Microbiol 8:521-524, 1993.

Transmission of multidrug-resistant tuberculosis among immunocompromised persons in a correctional system—New York, 1991. MMWR 41:507-509, 1992.

Urinary anti-infectives. *In* AHFS Drug Information 93, 486-493. American Society of Hospital Pharmacists, 1993.

The use of preventive therapy for tuberculous infection in the United States: Recommendations of the Advisory Committee for Elimination of Tuberculosis. MMWR 39:9-12, 1990.

Walker RC, Wright AJ: The fluoroquinolones. Mayo Clin Proc 66:1249-1259, 1991.

Zinner SH, Mayer KH: Sulfonamides and trimethoprim. *In* Mandell GL, Douglas RG Jr, Bennett JE (eds): Principles and Practice of Infectious Diseases, 3rd ed, 325-334. New York: Churchill Livingstone, 1990.

41 Antifungal Agents

Alan J. Lesse

Antifungal therapy is undergoing rapid change. Fear of toxicity from standard therapy with amphotericin B has evolved to therapy with newer agents that have broad antifungal activity. Comparative trials of these agents are still ongoing, but the pressure to avoid toxicity has pushed many clinicians to choose the less toxic agents. However, a less toxic, less efficacious regimen is not an appropriate therapeutic substitute for an efficacious but more toxic therapy. Only when the results of comparative trials establish the efficacy of the newer agents can the increased toxicity of the older regimens be replaced by the new treatment modalities.

SYSTEMIC ANTIFUNGAL AGENTS

Polyene Antifungal Agents

Amphotericin B

CHEMISTRY. Amphotericin B is a polyene macrolide with a complicated ring structure. Because amphotericin is amphoteric, its salts are soluble in both acidic and basic media. However, amphotericin B is insoluble at physiologic pH and requires sodium desoxycholate as a solubilizing agent. The colloid of amphotericin-sodium desoxycholate is the intravenous formulation currently licensed by the Food and Drug Administration (FDA). Some authors believe that a significant portion of the toxicity of amphotericin B may be related to administration of the sodium desoxycholate.

MECHANISMS OF ACTION. Amphotericin B binds to membrane sterols in fungal cell membranes. This interaction appears to form pores or channels and results in increased cell permeability, cell leakage, and death. At low concentrations, amphotericin appears to be fungistatic, whereas at higher concentrations, the drug appears to be fungicidal, presumably because of the increased cell permeability that results from higher concentrations of amphotericin B–induced pores.

MECHANISMS OF RESISTANCE. Many fungal species that affect man, including the dimorphic fungi, are susceptible to amphotericin B. Fungi such as *Pseudoallescheria boydii, Cladosporium carrioni, Fonsecaea pedrosoi, Fusarium* species, and dematiaceous fungi frequently are resistant to amphotericin B.

ROUTE OF ADMINISTRATION, ABSORPTION, DISTRIBUTION, METABOLISM, AND EXCRETION. Amphotericin B is administered only via intravenous injection for the therapy of systemic fungal diseases. Oral absorption of the agent is poor. Intravenous administration of 50 mg of amphotericin B yields serum concentrations of about 2 μg/mL. The drug has limited distribution, with cerebrospinal fluid (CSF) concentrations of the agent only 3% of serum levels. Despite the failure to recover amphotericin from spinal fluid in therapeutic concentrations, the drug is still effective in the therapy of many forms of fungal meningitis. Intrathecal administration of amphotericin B, once more common than it is today, is now indicated for the therapy only of coccidioidal meningitis.

Metabolism and excretion of amphotericin are difficult to quantify. The route of clearance is unknown and the drug can be detected for weeks in the serum after discontinuance of therapy. The drug is presumed to enter an equilibrium with tissue membranes (cholesterol) and to be slowly released over time.

Comparisons of selected pharmacokinetic parameters of the commonly used antifungal agents are found in Table 41–1.

ADVERSE EFFECTS. Although amphotericin B is regarded as the gold standard of antifungal therapy in most fungal infections, the drug is primarily known for its extreme toxicities. Immediate reactions to amphotericin B can occur and include hypotension, arrhythmia, anaphylactoid reactions, and even death. Physicians frequently administer a 1-mg test dose of amphotericin B slowly over one-half hour in order to test the patient's response; this is done because toxicity to the agent appears to be dose-related.

Many patients who receive amphotericin B develop fever, chills, and rigors upon administration of the drug. Accompanying symptoms include headache, arthralgias, myalgias, nausea, vomiting, and hypotension. The time course is rather distinctive, with many reactions occurring 30 to 90 minutes after the start of the infusion; frequently, reactions begin with a rigor. Many pretreatment modalities have been tried in order to prevent these reactions, including acetaminophen, aspirin, diphenhydramine, and meperidine. None of these measures has been shown to be efficacious. Some studies, however, have

TABLE 41–1. Selected Pharmacokinetic Parameters of Systemic Antifungal Medications

Parameter	Amphotericin B	Ketoconazole	Fluconazole	Itraconazole
Mechanism of action	Binds to cell membrane sterols	Inhibition of ergosterol synthesis	Inhibition of ergosterol synthesis	Inhibition of ergosterol synthesis
Route of administration	Intravenous	Oral	Oral Intravenous	Oral
Protein binding	Low	High	Low	High
Urine concentration	Low	Low	High	Low
Cerebrospinal fluid concentration	Low	Low	High	Low
Requires gastric acidity for absorption	—	Yes	No	Yes

shown that 25 to 50 mg of hydrocortisone administered intravenously before or with amphotericin B can decrease the severity of the reaction. Some authorities caution against concomitant administration, because *in vitro* studies have shown a decrease in amphotericin B antifungal activity in the presence of hydrocortisone. In some patients, acetaminophen may be used for mild febrile reaction instead of hydrocortisone. Because not all patients develop these reactions, premedication is not indicated in all patients. It is suggested that the patient's reaction to therapy be monitored in the absence of premedication before committing the patient to additional medications.

Renal toxicity and azotemia are thought to be unavoidable consequences of full-dose therapy with amphotericin B. Possible mechanisms include renal vasoconstriction and membrane damage to the cholesterol-laden renal tubular cells. Several studies have shown that sodium repletion and salt loading may decrease amphotericin B nephrotoxicity. Patients given amphotericin B should be well hydrated and not sodium restricted or sodium depleted. Although much of the loss of renal function returns on discontinuation of therapy, partial permanent loss of function is a common sequela.

Because the route of clearance is unknown, dosage adjustment in renal failure is generally unnecessary. However, it is common practice to go to alternate-day therapy when the creatinine level increases above 3 mg/dL.

Thrombophlebitis is a common complication of therapy. Heparin has been recommended by some authorities; however, studies have not shown the efficacy of heparin. Administration via central veins avoids this complication.

Electrolyte disturbances are common, with hypokalemia and hypomagnesemia being the most common. A renal tubular acidosis secondary to amphotericin B appears to accentuate the hypokalemia.

Normocytic normochromic anemia is common with amphotericin B. Other toxicities include hypertension, cardiac arrhythmia, thrombocytopenia, leukopenia, agranulocytosis, allergic reaction, visual impairment, hepatitis, and liver failure; these are but a sampling of the potential toxicities of the agent.

In short, amphotericin B may represent the most toxic noncancer chemotherapeutic agent in clinical use.

DRUG INTERACTIONS. Amphotericin B may potentiate the nephrotoxicity of other agents such as aminoglycosides and cyclosporin. Concomitant administration of glucocorticoids may exacerbate electrolyte disturbances, especially hypokalemia. Synergistic and antagonistic action have been described with other antifungal agents and amphotericin B. Mechlorethamine and other anticancer agents may potentiate the nephrotoxic, bronchospastic, and hypotensive effects of amphotericin B.

BOX 41–1
CLINICAL USE (INDICATIONS AND CONTRAINDICATIONS)

Amphotericin B is indicated in a wide variety of systemic fungal infections. These include infections with *Candida, Cryptococcus, Histoplasmosis, Blastomycoses, Coccidioidomycosis, Paracoccidioidomycosis, Aspergillosis, Mucormycosis,* disseminated *Sporotrichosis,* and other fungal infections.

Many authorities still recommend amphotericin B as the drug of choice for the initial therapy of cryptococcal meningitis in acquired immunodeficiency syndrome (AIDS) patients, despite the excellent activity of fluconazole for maintenance therapy and prevention of relapse. This is in part because of the good track record with amphotericin B in initial therapy and an advantage in some studies of amphotericin B over fluconazole in patients with more than mild disease.

Administration of amphotericin B usually involves a test dose of amphotericin. Many authorities recommend a slow increase in dosage, up to 0.6 to 0.7 mg/kg/day. However, this gradual approach does not decrease toxicity and delays achieving therapeutic drug concentrations for several days. In patients who tolerate the test dose, it is advisable to proceed to the full dose. Administration is frequently given over 4 hours, despite studies showing an equal incidence of adverse reactions in either 1- or 4- hour administrations.

Intra-articular administration is still recommended for some patients with sporotrichosis or coccidioidomycosis, but these indications are rare. Intrathecal administration of amphotericin B was the

Continued

BOX 41–1

CLINICAL USE (INDICATIONS AND CONTRAINDICATIONS) (*Continued*)

mainstay of therapy for coccidioidal meningitis and is still recommended; however, recent studies with the newer triazole, fluconazole (see below), may significantly reduce the need for this difficult form of therapy.

Despite its significant toxicity, amphotericin B is frequently given to febrile, neutropenic patients who fail to become afebrile after 7 days of broad-spectrum antibacterial treatment. Studies have shown that a significant percentage of those patients have undiagnosed fungal infections and respond to therapy with amphotericin B. Administration of amphotericin B under these circumstances should not wait for the culture identification of a fungus prior to starting therapy.

Because of the marked toxicity, several attempts have been made to reduce the toxicity of amphotericin B. Liposomal administration of the agent appears to be promising, and significantly higher dosages of liposomal amphotericin B can be administered with decreased toxicity. Formulations of the standard desoxycholate-amphotericin B combined with intravenous lipid preparations have recently been associated with decreased toxicity, but without significant efficacy data. Studies of these and other formulations of amphotericin B are ongoing.

Azole Antifungal Agents

Two groups of azole antifungal agents are currently available for systemic use in the United States. The first group, the imidazoles, includes ketoconazole and miconazole; and the second group, the triazoles, includes fluconazole and itraconazole. Other members of each group are available for topical therapy, but the drugs listed here are the only ones currently in use for systemic disease.

Ketoconazole

CHEMISTRY. Ketoconazole is an imidazole antifungal by virtue of the two nitrogen atoms in the five-member imidazole ring. Triazoles, by contrast, have three nitrogen atoms in their imidazole ring structure.

MECHANISMS OF ACTION. The azole antifungal agents act by inhibition of cytochrome P-450 enzymes that are involved in cell membrane synthesis in fungi. The principal target for these drugs is 14α-demethylase, which converts lanosterol to ergosterol in the fungal cell membrane. Although the activity is highly selective, clinically achievable concentrations of ketoconazole may inhibit mammalian cytochrome P-450 systems. These interactions are responsible for many of the adverse effects seen with the agent. The drug is fungistatic at clinically achievable concentrations.

MECHANISMS OF RESISTANCE. Resistance mechanisms to the azoles are poorly understood. Specific mechanisms are not yet known; however, resistant isolates have clearly been described. Although most strains of *Candida albicans* are inhibited by ketoconazole, *Candida tropicalis* frequently is resistant.

ROUTE OF ADMINISTRATION, ABSORPTION, DISTRIBUTION, METABOLISM, AND EXCRETION. Ketoconazole is administered via the oral route only. The drug requires acid pH in the stomach for conversion of the drug to the hydrochloride salt and its subsequent absorption. Achlorhydria or medications that interfere with gastric acidity significantly alter ketoconazole drug levels. In addition, significant interpatient variability exists in the absorption of ketoconazole.

After absorption, the drug is distributed widely, is highly protein-bound, and is present in low concentrations in urine and CSF. Less than 3% of the drug is excreted in the urine, and CSF concentrations are insufficient for the treatment of fungal infections in the central nervous system (CNS). The drug is metabolized in the liver and excreted into the stool. See Table 41–1 for comparisons to other agents.

ADVERSE EFFECTS. The most common adverse reaction to ketoconazole is nausea and vomiting. This effect appears to be dose-related, with a higher incidence seen with increasing dosages. Some authors report that this side effect can be diminished by administration of the drug with meals.

Hepatotoxicity and fatal hepatic necrosis occur infrequently on administration of ketoconazole. Transient transaminase elevations may be seen in as many as 10% of patients during the first 2 weeks of ketoconazole administration. Clinical hepatitis has been reported at a much lower rate of 1 : 10,000 to 1 : 50,000 patients. Although discontinuation of the drug usually results in normalization of liver function tests, continued administration of ketoconazole in the presence of drug-induced hepatitis has resulted in fatal hepatic necrosis. Patients must be warned to alert their physician should constitutional symptoms develop while taking ketoconazole. Immediate discontinuation of the drug is indicated in the presence of significantly elevated transaminase levels.

Despite the fact that ketoconazole inhibits fungal enzymes 100-fold more than mammalian enzymes, the selectivity is not absolute and ketoconazole can decrease conversion of mammalian lanesterol to cholesterol. Because cholesterol is necessary for steroid hormone precursor synthesis, potential endocrine abnormalities may occur in patients who are treated with ketoconazole. Additionally, ketoconazole can inhibit several key enzymes in hormone biosynthesis, such as 14α-demethylase and 11β-hydroxylase, thereby further decreasing key hormones and their precursors. Decreased testosterone concentrations have been reported in men on ketoconazole, especially when higher doses of ketoconazole are employed. Resultant gynecomastia, hair loss, and decreased libido and potency have been reported. Decreased response to corticotropin has also been described, and there are rare reports of adrenal insufficiency.

Other adverse reactions, such as pruritus, headache, CNS dysfunction, arthralgias, and hematologic toxicity, are rarely seen with the drug. Transient decreases in serum cholesterol have also been described in up to 20% of patients treated with ketoconazole.

Patients with decreased gastric acidity may not absorb ketoconazole. Dissolution of the drug in 0.2 N HCl increases ketoconazole absorption in patients with defective acid production. Achlorhydria, especially when it occurs as a consequence of an human immunodeficiency virus (HIV)-related gastropathy, results in profound malabsorption of ketoconazole and therapeutic failure due to poor drug levels.

DRUG INTERACTIONS. Many drug interactions are seen with ketoconazole. Although some are mild, others may have life-threatening consequences. Physicians must carefully review medication profiles of patients being started on ketoconazole.

A life-threatening drug interaction of ketoconazole with the nonsedating antihistamines terfenadine and astemizole has recently been described. Ketoconazole and a new triazole antifungal, itraconazole, can decrease the hepatic metabolism of both terfenadine and astemizole (presumably through inhibition of cytochrome P-450 enzymes). Increased levels of these antihistamines and their metabolites can cause prolongation of the QT and QT_c intervals, resulting in arrhythmia, tachycardia, *torsades de pointes*, and even death. Patients receiving either antihistamine should not be given ketoconazole. Structurally related compounds such as fluconazole, miconazole, and metronidazole should not be administered with either terfenadine or astemizole.

Another life-threatening drug interaction may occur between ketoconazole and cyclosporine. Ketoconazole reduces the hepatic clearance of cyclosporine and results in marked increases in serum concentrations of cyclosporine. Failure to adjust cyclosporine dosage while receiving ketoconazole can result in massively elevated cyclosporine concentrations and accompanying profound immunosuppression and renal dysfunction.

Because ketoconazole requires gastric acidity for conversion to the hydrochloride salt and for absorption, agents that interfere with gastric acidity can significantly decrease absorption of ketoconazole. Antacids and H_2-blockers such as cimetidine and ranitidine can cause decreased absorption of ketoconazole, as can sucralfate.

Administration of rifampin and ketoconazole concomitantly may result in decreased ketoconazole concentrations due to increased ketoconazole metabolism induced by rifampin. Isoniazid coadministration may also decrease ketoconazole concentrations by a similar mechanism.

Ketoconazole has been noted to decrease serum concentrations of theophylline and to increase the concentrations of warfarin, methylprednisolone, prednisone, and possibly sulfonylurea hypoglycemic agents. Interactions with phenytoin are difficult to predict and may affect either or both agents. Serum levels of phenytoin must be followed during ketoconazole therapy.

BOX 41-2
CLINICAL USE (INDICATIONS AND CONTRAINDICATIONS)

Ketoconazole has been used in serious dermatophyte infections; cutaneous, oral, esophageal, and vaginal *Candida* infections; and an uncommon condition known as chronic mucocutaneous candidiasis. Large-scale, national trials have shown good results in the treatment of nonmeningeal histoplasmosis and blastomycosis in patients with normal immune function, with the possible exception of osseous involvement with these fungi. Ketoconazole therapy for paracoccidioidomycosis and nonmeningeal coccidioidomycosis has also been successful.

AIDS patients have a higher failure rate with ketoconazole therapy secondary to the decreased absorption of ketoconazole (see above). Therapy of histoplasmosis in HIV-infected patients has been particularly disappointing; although this drug may be given to prevent relapse after amphotericin B therapy, itraconazole (see below) is now the preferred agent.

Despite its activity against esophageal and mucocutaneous candidiasis, ketoconazole plays no role in the therapy of candidemia or deep-seated candidal infections.

Because of its poor aqueous solubility, ketoconazole does not distribute effectively into the CSF or urine. Ketoconazole therefore should not be used in the therapy of fungal infections in the CNS or urinary tract.

Fluconazole

CHEMISTRY. Fluconazole is the first triazole marketed for the therapy of fungal disease. The drug is pharmacologically quite different from either of the two commonly prescribed azoles, ketoconazole and itraconazole. Fluconazole is freely soluble in water, and this property differentiates fluconazole in terms of distribution, absorption, and therapeutic efficacy. Additionally, the agent is unique at this point in time in having both an oral and intravenous formulation.

MECHANISMS OF ACTION. The drug is similar in action to ketoconazole; however, fluconazole is reported to be 10-100 times more specific for the fungal rather than mammalian cytochrome P-450 enzymes than ketoconazole. This enhanced specificity is probably responsible for the lower number of drug interactions and toxicity when compared to ketoconazole.

MECHANISMS OF RESISTANCE. Although the mechanism of resistance to the azoles is not clearly defined, it should be noted that many non-albicans strains of *Candida* are resistant to fluconazole. *Candida krusei* and *Torulopsis glabrata* frequently are resistant to fluconazole, and this drug should not be thought of as a primary drug for fungemia prior to organism identification. Use of fluconazole in routine prophylaxis in bone marrow transplant patients and neutropenic patients resulted in an increased incidence of *C. krusei* infection.

In vitro testing of fluconazole and other azoles frequently does not parallel clinical and experimental models in animals and may not be reliable for prediction of therapeutic efficacy. This may explain the efficacy of fluconazole in animal models and humans against such pathogens as *Histoplasma* and *Blastomyces*, despite high *in vitro* minimal inhibitory concentrations.

ROUTE OF ADMINISTRATION, ABSORPTION, DISTRIBUTION, METABOLISM, AND EXCRETION. Fluconazole may be given either intravenously or orally. Oral administration results in almost complete absorption from the gastrointestinal tract, regardless of gastric acidity. The drug is widely distributed throughout the body, including the CSF and urine. The drug is cleared through the kidneys and has a long half-life of 25 hours, allowing once-daily administration. Dosages are adjusted in renal failure. See Table 41 – 1 for comparisons to other agents.

ADVERSE EFFECTS. Fluconazole appears to be well tolerated. Because the drug was initially introduced for the therapy of cryptococcal meningitis in patients with AIDS, many of the toxicities are difficult to firmly attribute to the drug, because this population has an increased incidence of adverse reactions to all medications. Additionally, the underlying disease, AIDS, may be responsible for many of the reported drug effects.

Transient, mild increases in serum transaminase concentrations have been reported with fluconazole. Reports of fulminant hepatitis are not seen with fluconazole as compared to ketoconazole. Nausea, vomiting, and abdominal pain occasionally also occur. Rashes, including exfoliative dermatitis, and eosinophilia have been seen in up to 5% of patients treated with fluconazole. Other side effects, including fever, arthralgias, myalgias, anaphylaxis, and hypokalemia, have all been reported.

DRUG INTERACTIONS. Although fluconazole has less activity on mammalian cytochrome P-450 enzymes than does ketoconazole and although the drug interactions are fewer, fluconazole nevertheless has significant interactions with several medications.

Despite a paucity of reports of interactions with terfenadine and astemizole, the structural analogy of fluconazole and ketoconazole indicates that neither nonsedating antihistamine should be administered with fluconazole.

Fluconazole may decrease the hepatic metabolism of several agents. Decreased clearance of cyclosporine may result in significant immunosuppression, leukopenia, and renal dysfunction in patients who receive both agents. A similar drug interaction with phenytoin can produce toxic phenytoin serum concentrations in patients who are taking fluconazole and phenytoin. Fluconazole-induced increases in concentrations of warfarin and sulfonylurea hypoglycemics can result in prolonged prothrombin times and hypoglycemia, respectively.

Fluconazole concentrations can be decreased on coadministration of rifampin, whereas thiazide diuretics have been shown to increase fluconazole levels, presumably mediated through inhibition of renal clearance of fluconazole by the thiazides.

Gastric acidity is not important in the absorption of fluconazole, and a 15% decrease in fluconazole serum concentrations with cimetidine administration is not considered clinically significant.

BOX 41 – 3
CLINICAL USE (INDICATIONS AND CONTRAINDICATIONS)

Fluconazole is an excellent agent for the therapy of infections caused by *Cryptococcus*. Although most authorities prefer amphotericin B for the initial therapy of cryptococcal meningitis in AIDS patients (amphotericin B therapy results in a more rapid sterilization of the spinal fluid), fluconazole is an excellent agent to complete the initial course of therapy. Fluconazole is, however, the drug of choice for the lifelong preventive therapy of cryptococcal disease after primary therapy in patients with AIDS.

Fluconazole also has excellent activity in the treatment of esophageal candidiasis in patients with AIDS and cancer. The drug is more effective than topical nystatin or clotrimazole.

Therapy of systemic candidal infections is debatable. Large, multicenter studies are underway to assess the efficacy of high doses of fluconazole compared to amphotericin B. Given the decreased activity of fluconazole against some non-albicans *Candida* and the fungistatic nature of fluconazole, the drug should not be considered as a substitute for amphotericin B in the therapy of candidemia or systemic candidal disease until further studies are completed.

Fluconazole is active against other systemic fungal infections such as histoplasmosis, blastomycosis, and coccidioidomycosis. A few reports also show utility in the therapy of paracoccidioidomycosis and sporotrichosis. Histoplasmosis and blastomycosis may be more effectively treated with either ketoconazole or, more likely, itraconazole.

Recent data suggest that high-dose fluconazole may provide a therapeutic alternative to intrathecal amphotericin B for the treatment of CNS involvement with coccidioidomycosis. High-dose fluconazole was nearly as efficacious as intrathecal amphotericin B for coccidioidal meningitis and was not associated with the significant morbidity associated with placement of the CSF shunt.

Because fluconazole is soluble in aqueous media and excreted in the urine, it may be appropriate therapy for fungal urinary tract infections. Other azoles—miconazole, ketoconazole, and itraconazole—do not achieve adequate urinary concentrations for the therapy of urinary infections and cannot be used for this indication.

Itraconazole

CHEMISTRY. Itraconazole is a highly lipophilic triazole that is poorly soluble in water.

MECHANISMS OF ACTION. The mechanism of action is similar to the other azoles: inhibition of fungal cytochrome P-450 enzymes. Itraconazole is significantly more selective for fungal cytochrome P-450 enzymes than for mammalian enzymes. Itraconazole has approximately the same cytochrome P-450 specificity as fluconazole (10- to 100-fold more selective than ketoconazole). Unlike other triazoles, itraconazole has clinically useful activity against *Aspergillus*.

MECHANISMS OF RESISTANCE. As with other azoles, the mechanism of resistance of itraconazole is poorly understood. Many strains of *Candida glabrata* are resistant to itraconazole.

ROUTE OF ADMINISTRATION, ABSORPTION, DISTRIBUTION, METABOLISM, AND EXCRETION. The current formulation of itraconazole is for oral administration. The drug is 50% absorbed after oral administration. This can be increased by administration with food, and the manufacturer recommends taking the medication with a fatty meal. As with ketoconazole, decreased gastric acidity may inhibit drug absorption. The drug is highly protein-bound and is not well distributed into CSF or urine. Despite the poor concentration in CSF, itraconazole has been shown to be effective in fungal meningitis, presumably related to the excellent tissue levels. Tissue concentrations of itraconazole are higher than serum concentration, particularly in adipose tissue. The drug is metabolized in the liver and is excreted in the feces. Metabolites of itraconazole may appear in the urine, but only one metabolite has antifungal activity. The drug has a long half-life of 15–25 hours, which lengthens on chronic administration, presumably related to the increased tissue stores. Concentrations of the drug in skin, nails, and keratin are excellent and provide sustained concentrations at these tissue sites. See Table 41–1 for comparisons to other agents.

ADVERSE EFFECTS. Itraconazole was released for clinical use in November, 1992. Clinical data regarding adverse reactions, therefore, are limited. Nausea and vomiting are noted on administration, but drug discontinuance for this side effect is not common. Edema has also been reported as an adverse effect of the drug. Hepatic enzyme elevations are seen, but fatal hepatic necrosis has not been strongly associated with itraconazole.

DRUG INTERACTIONS. Drug interactions with itraconazole occur but appear to be fewer than those seen with ketoconazole. Cyclosporine clearance is decreased by itraconazole, and serum concentrations must be monitored to prevent potentially life-threatening complications. Interaction with terfenadine has been documented, and the use of itraconazole with either terfenadine or astemizole should be avoided. Decreased itraconazole serum concentrations can result either from decreased absorption or from increased metabolism. Agents that inhibit gastric acidity, such as antacid and H_2-blockers, decrease itraconazole absorption, whereas rifampin reduces serum concentrations of itraconazole through increased metabolism of the drug. Itraconazole has been reported to decrease digoxin clearance, and serum digoxin concentrations should be measured while itraconazole therapy continues.

BOX 41–4

CLINICAL USE (INDICATIONS AND CONTRAINDICATIONS)

No comparative trials have demonstrated the therapeutic efficacy of itraconazole for systemic candidal disease. However, the agent is highly effective for nonsystemic forms of *Candida* infections.

Activity of itraconazole against the routine dimorphic fungi of humans is excellent. Itraconazole is effective in the therapy of nonmeningeal blastomycosis, histoplasmosis, and coccidioidomycosis. In fact, itraconazole is the only effective azole for the therapy of histoplasmosis in AIDS patients, both for initial and chronic maintenance therapy.

Despite poor CSF concentrations of itraconazole, the drug has been used successfully in the treatment of coccidioidal meningitis.

Itraconazole is unique among the currently available azole antifungal agents in its activity against *Aspergillus*. Although comparative trials are ongoing, noncomparative trials of itraconazole have shown considerable efficacy against infections caused by *Aspergillus*. Several trials are evaluating the use of itraconazole for therapy and prophylaxis of *Aspergillus* infections in the neutropenic host.

Itraconazole has shown excellent activity against dermatophyte infections. This may be due in part to the excellent tissue concentrations of the agent. The agent may become the oral azole of choice for severe dermatophyte infections. In comparison to ketoconazole for most indications, itraconazole is more potent and less toxic. However, at the current time, itraconazole is a more costly agent.

OTHER SYSTEMIC ANTIFUNGAL AGENTS

Flucytosine

Flucytosine is a water-soluble, fluorinated pyrimidine. Susceptible fungi contain the enzyme cytosine deaminase, which can convert flucytosine to 5-fluorouracil. Fluorouracil metabolites inhibit both DNA synthesis and RNA-directed protein synthesis. Mammalian cells cannot convert flucytosine to fluorouracil, thereby allowing the mechanism of action to be selective for fungi. Flucytosine is well absorbed orally and distributed widely, including in urine and CSF. The drug is cleared by renal mechanisms.

The most common toxicities include nausea, vomiting, and diarrhea. Severe toxicity is related to bone marrow suppression and is seen more commonly when serum concentrations are elevated above 100 μg/mL. Leukopenia and thrombocytopenia are common toxicities. Conversion of flucytosine to 5-fluorouracil by intestinal microbes has been postulated as the mechanism of action of this toxicity. Renal dysfunction strongly predisposes to this toxicity, because of the renal clearance of flucytosine and its metabolites.

The use of flucytosine has been decreasing after introduction of the azoles. The primary indication for this agent is combination therapy of cryptococcal meningitis with amphotericin B. Because the vast majority of patients with cryptococcal disease currently have AIDS, many patients cannot tolerate the additional hematopoietic toxicity of flucytosine. Several authorities still recommend this combination as the best therapy for cryptococcal meningitis, but lack of ready access to flucytosine levels limits this form of therapy. Early therapeutic conversion of fluconazole has also limited the use of flucytosine.

Prior to the development of fluconazole, flucytosine was used for urinary candidal infections because of its renal excretion. Fluconazole has largely replaced flucytosine in this indication.

Miconazole

Miconazole was the first imidazole agent available for systemic fungal infections. The agent has poor aqueous solubility and requires polyethoxylated castor oil for intravenous administration. Significant toxicity, possibly related to the vehicle, was seen with the preparation. With the advent of both oral and intravenous azoles with increased activity and significantly less toxicity, parenteral miconazole is seldom prescribed.

Griseofulvin

Griseofulvin is an orally administered antifungal agent that is restricted predominantly to the therapy of dermatophyte infections of the skin and nails. Griseofulvin inhibits microtubules of the mitotic spindle and cytoplasm and disrupts mitosis in actively growing fungi. The drug is administered only by the oral route.

Griseofulvin is widely distributed, especially to skin, hair, and nails. The most common side effect is headache, with serious adverse reactions being rare. Other adverse reactions include gastrointestinal complaints, hepatotoxicity, hematologic toxicities, and rashes, including erythema multiforme.

TABLE 41–2. Topical Antifungal Agents

Agent	Class	Mechanism of Action	Over the Counter	Formulations
Amphotericin B	Polyene macrolide	Binds to sterols in fungal cell membrane	No	Cream Lotion Ointment
Butaconazole	Imidazole	Inhibition of ergosterol synthesis	No	Vaginal cream
Ciclopirox olamine	Hydroxypyridinone	Decreases intracellular concentrations of essential nutrients	No	Cream Lotion
Clioquinol	Hydroxyquinolone	Unknown	No	Cream Lotion Ointment
Clotrimazole	Imidazole	Inhibition of ergosterol synthesis	Yes	Lozenges Topical cream Topical lotion Topical solution Vaginal cream Vaginal tablets
Econazole	Imidazole	Inhibition of ergosterol synthesis	No	Cream
Haloprogin	Polychlorinated phenyl ester	Unknown	No	Cream Solution
Ketoconazole	Imidazole	Inhibition of ergosterol synthesis	No	Cream Shampoo
Miconazole	Imidazole	Inhibition of ergosterol synthesis	Yes	Aerosol spray Cream Powder Vaginal cream Vaginal suppository
Naftifine	Allylamine	Inhibition of sterol synthesis by squalene monooxygenase	No	Cream Gel
Nystatin	Polyene macrolide	Binds to sterols in fungal cell membrane	No	Oral suspension Lozenges Cream Ointment Powder Vaginal tablets
Oxiconazole	Imidazole	Inhibition of ergosterol synthesis	No	Cream
Terconazole	Triazole	Inhibition of ergosterol synthesis	No	Vaginal cream Vaginal suppository
Tolnaftate	Synthetic antifungal	Unknown	Yes	Aerosol Powder Cream Gel

Griseofulvin is indicated for dermatophytic infections, except tinea versicolor. Therapeutic efficacy of the more costly itraconazole is generally higher, and cost-benefit analysis may be necessary in the treatment decision for significant dermatophytic infections.

TOPICAL ANTIFUNGAL AGENTS

Many topical antifungal agents are available for the treatment of superficial fungal infections. Some of the most effective agents (clotrimazole and miconazole) now are available without a prescription. Table 41-2 summarizes selected properties of some of these agents. Several agents have unique mechanisms of action. Selection criteria for individual agents are not presented here. The reader should, however, take note of the troche formulation of clotrimazole for oral and esophageal candidiasis. Although less effective than fluconazole, clotrimazole troches provide a nonsystemic alternative for this common problem.

Acknowledgment

This chapter was supported by the Department of Veterans Affairs.

REFERENCES

Antifungal antibiotics. *In* AHFS Drug Information 93, 68-92. American Society of Hospital Pharmacists, 1993.

Antifungals. *In* AHFS Drug Information 93, 2172-2199. American Society of Hospital Pharmacists, 1993.

Berestein GL: Liposomal amphotericin B in the treatment of fungal infections. Ann Intern Med 105:130, 1986.

Bodey GP: Azole antifungal agents. Clin Infect Dis 14(Suppl 1):S161-169, 1992.

Como JA, Dismukes WE: Oral azole drugs as systemic antifungal therapy. N Engl J Med 330:263-272, 1994.

Hoeprich PD: Clinical use of amphotericin B and derivatives: Lore, mystique, and fact. Clin Infect Dis 14(Suppl 1):S114-119, 1992.

Terrell CL, Hughes CR: Antifungal agents used for deep-seated mycotic infections. Mayo Clin Proc 67:69-91, 1992.

42 Antiviral Drugs

Ann M. Arvin and Alan M. Reynard

The replication of both RNA and DNA viruses is an intracellular process that is difficult to inhibit without disrupting the metabolism of the host cell. The analysis of the biochemistry of viral synthesis has led to the development of effective antiviral therapy for infections caused by some herpesviruses, some respiratory viruses, and human immunodeficiency virus (HIV).

VIDARABINE

The chemical structure of vidarabine, 9-d-arabinofuranosyladenine monohydrate, is identical to that of adenosine except for the substitution of arabinose for ribose (Fig. 42 – 1).

Mechanism of Action

The drug is taken up by mammalian cells in its intact form and as arabinosylhypoxanthine, an inactive metabolite produced by deamination. The intact form of the drug is phosphorylated intracellularly by cellular enzymes. The triphosphate form, ara-adenosine triphosphate (Ara-A), inhibits the DNA polymerase of herpes simplex virus (HSV) and other herpesviruses and also acts as chain terminator when incorporated into HSV DNA. The drug binds to cellular DNA polymerases but its specificity is several-fold greater for the viral DNA polymerases. Vidarabine inhibits many DNA viruses *in vitro* but not most RNA viruses.

Organ System Pharmacology

Vidarabine is distributed into all tissues but undergoes rapid deamination into arabinosylhypoxanthine extracellularly as well as after its uptake by cells. Cerebrospinal fluid concentrations are proportional to plasma concentrations, with a ratio of approximately 1:3. Both the native and the metabolized forms of the drug are eliminated primarily by renal excretion.

Adverse Effects

Common side effects of vidarabine that do not require the interruption of therapy include nausea, vomiting, and diarrhea. Its most serious adverse effect is encephalopathy associated with headache, dizziness, confusion, hallucinations, ataxia, and tremors, which can progress to coma. Patients with impaired renal function are at particular risk of this adverse effect. At dosages above 20 mg/kg/day, hematological suppression can occur, causing a decrease in hemoglobin and in granulocyte and platelet counts. Liver function tests such as serum glutamic-oxaloacetic transaminase (SGOT) may become elevated. Vidarabine administration occasionally causes rash and pruritus or malaise. The clinical use of the drug is complicated by its relative insolubility, requiring its administration in large volumes of intravenous (IV) fluid.

BOX 42-1

INDICATIONS AND CONTRAINDICATIONS

Vidarabine has been replaced by acyclovir as the drug of choice for the treatment of HSV encephalitis. Preliminary data indicate that the efficacy of vidarabine is comparable to acyclovir in neonatal HSV infections, but acyclovir therapy avoids the problem of IV fluid volume required for vidarabine administration. Acyclovir was more effective for the treatment of herpes zoster in bone marrow transplant recipients than vidarabine.

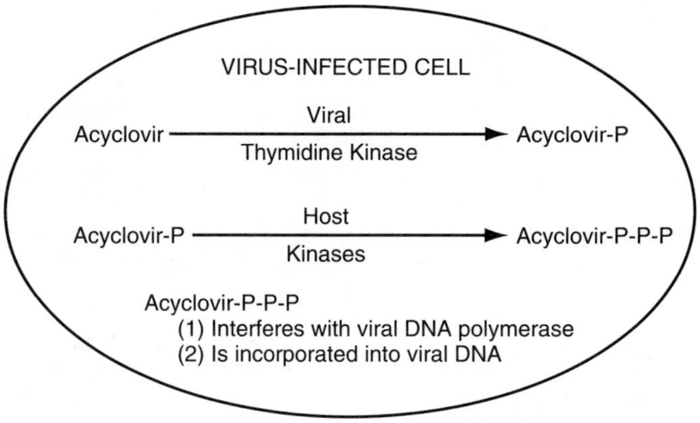

VIRUS-INFECTED CELL

Acyclovir —Viral Thymidine Kinase→ Acyclovir-P

Acyclovir-P —Host Kinases→ Acyclovir-P-P-P

Acyclovir-P-P-P
(1) Interferes with viral DNA polymerase
(2) Is incorporated into viral DNA

FIGURE 42-2. Acyclovir inhibits viral DNA synthesis in virus-infected cells.

ACYCLOVIR

Acyclovir is a synthetic acyclic purine nucleoside, 9-[(2-hydroxyethoxy)methyl] guanine (Fig. 42-1).

Mechanism of Action

Acyclovir is taken up selectively by cells infected with herpesviruses. Like vidarabine, its activity depends upon conversion to the triphosphate form. However, the antiviral specificity of acyclovir for HSV and varicella zoster virus (VZV) is enhanced relative to vidarabine because its phosphorylation is mediated selectively by the thymidine kinase of these viruses (Fig. 42-2). The consequence of this is that phosphorylation of acyclovir occurs mainly in virus-infected cells, thereby sparing cells not infected with the virus. The triphosphate form of acyclovir interferes with HSV DNA polymerase; incorporation of the compound into viral DNA results in chain termination. The initial conversion of acyclovir to the monophosphate form does not occur in uninfected cells, so that drug toxicity for host cells is minimal. The triphosphate form does have some inhibitory effect on the cellular a-DNA polymerase. Natural resistance of HSV and VZV strains to acyclovir is rare but can occur if the strain is a thymidine kinase-deficient mutant. Other viruses, including herpesviruses such as cytomegalovirus (CMV) and Epstein-Barr virus (EBV), do not require viral thymidine kinase for replication, so that their inhibition by acyclovir is limited. EBV replication is reduced by the drug because the viral DNA polymerase of EBV is highly sensitive to acyclovir triphosphate.

Organ System Pharmacology

The pharmacokinetics of acyclovir is consistent with a two-compartment model with the distribution at steady state being approximately equal to the body fluid volume. The plasma half-life of acyclovir given orally to adults is 3-4 hours. Drug levels are measurable in saliva, lesion fluid, and vaginal secretions; cerebrospinal fluid levels are approximately half the plasma concentration. More than 80% of a drug dose is eliminated by renal excretion through glomerular filtration and, to a lesser extent, by tubular secretion. Renal tissue levels are substantially higher than plasma concentrations.

Adverse Effects

Clinical symptoms reported by some patients include nausea, vomiting, and headache, but these side effects rarely interfere with drug treatment. The drug can precipitate in the renal tubules with excessive dosages or when the therapeutic dosage is given by rapid infusion or to patients who are dehydrated. Impaired renal function, as reflected by an increase in serum creatinine, and decreased creatinine clearance may result. A few cases of encephalopathy, with signs including lethargy, tremors, hallucinations, seizures, and

FIGURE 42-1. The structures of vidarabine, acyclovir, and amantadine.

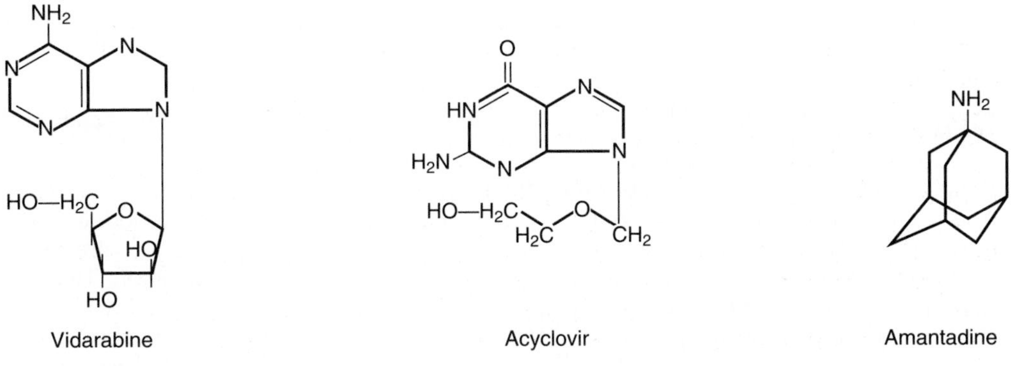

Vidarabine

Acyclovir

Amantadine

coma, have been reported in patients with deficient renal clearance. Extravasation of the drug into soft tissues can produce severe cutaneous lesions. Theoretically, the selection of drug-resistant mutants of HSV and VZV could occur during acyclovir therapy, but the emergence of resistance has been quite unusual in clinical experience with the drug. Prolonged, low-dose therapy in immunocompromised patients, especially those with acquired immunodeficiency syndrome (AIDS), is associated with a high risk of emergence of resistance and should be avoided.

BOX 42–2

INDICATIONS AND CONTRAINDICATIONS

Acyclovir is most active against HSV-1 and HSV-2; HSV-2 is only slightly less sensitive than HSV-1. IV acyclovir is indicated for HSV encephalitis, neonatal HSV, and life-threatening HSV and VZV infections in immunocompromised patients. Oral acyclovir is indicated for the treatment of primary and recurrent genital herpes. Topical acyclovir reduces the duration of primary genital herpes but is not effective for recurrences. Treatment of primary HSV infections with acyclovir does not prevent recurrent disease, indicating that the drug does not prevent the establishment of latent neural cell infection. Acyclovir ophthalmic ointment is effective for herpes simplex keratitis. Acyclovir is not effective for CMV infection. The safety of acyclovir administration during pregnancy has not been established. Acyclovir, given orally as 800 mg per dose five times a day, is effective for the treatment of herpes zoster in nonimmunocompromised patients in clinical trials.

New acyclovir derivatives that provide much higher plasma concentrations after oral administration are being developed. The experience to date with acyclovir for treatment of infectious mononucleosis caused by EBV does not suggest significant clinical efficacy. Oral acyclovir prophylaxis has been useful for the suppression of recurrent HSV infections in organ and bone marrow transplant recipients.

Acyclovir is the drug of choice for HSV infections and has proven clinical value for the treatment of VZV infections in immunocompromised patients. The possible emergence of drug resistance in clinical strains of HSV and VZV has not yet created a major therapeutic problem but will require careful monitoring as the drug is used widely. Drug resistance has been encountered in severely immunocompromised patients given prolonged acyclovir therapy.

Drug Interactions

Concurrent administration of other drugs that reduce renal clearance, such as amphotericin, would be expected to raise the plasma and renal concentrations of acyclovir. Some patients given acyclovir and interferon or intrathecal methotrexate have had severe neurological complications, but these reactions were not clearly related to acyclovir. Probenecid reduces its renal excretion.

Preparations

Acyclovir capsules contain 200 mg of drug. The bioavailability of the oral dose is 15–20%. The oral regimens for HSV infections are (1) a 200-mg capsule five times a day for 10 days for initial episodes or for 5 days for recurrences, and (2) a 200-mg capsule three times a day for up to 6 months for suppression of recurrent genital herpes. Topical acyclovir ointment (5%) is prescribed for initial genital herpes in otherwise healthy patients and for recurrent mucocutaneous herpes in immunocompromised patients. The ointment is used to cover the lesions every 3 hours, six times a day for 7 days. IV acyclovir (500 mg/vial) is given as 750 mg/sq m/day divided into three dosages and given every 8 hours for HSV infections in immunocompromised patients and as 1500 mg/sq m or 30 mg/kg/day (500 mg/sq m or 10 mg/kg every 8 hours) for VZV infections in high-risk patients. The dosage for neonatal HSV and HSV encephalitis is 30 mg/kg/day (10 mg/kg every 8 hours). The IV drug must be given as a 1-hour infusion. The dosage is adjusted for impaired clearance if the creatinine clearance is less than 50 mL/minute/1.73 sq m.

GANCICLOVIR

Ganciclovir is 9-(1,3 dihydroxy-2-propoxymethyl) guanine; the drug is sometimes referred to as DHPG.

Mechanism of Action

Like acyclovir, ganciclovir is phosphorylated by the viral thymidine kinase of HSV-1 or HSV-2 to its monophosphate form within infected cells; the triphosphate form, which is generated by the activity of cellular enzymes, interferes with viral replication by insertion into the viral DNA. DNA replication is inhibited by chain termination and competitive inhibition of viral DNA polymerase. Ganciclovir also inhibits VZV replication *in vitro*, probably by the same pathway. The drug has antiviral effects on CMV and EBV as well. However, because these viruses do not have viral thymidine kinases, the mechanism by which ganciclovir inhibits CMV and EBV replication is less certain. The initial phosphorylation of ganciclovir is presumed to occur by the action of viral or cellular deoxyguanosine kinases, allowing its incorporation into replicating CMV or EBV DNA. The triphosphate form of the drug is known to accumulate in significantly higher concentrations in CMV- or EBV-infected cells, compared with uninfected cells. Viral infection is then restricted by the phosphorylated drug because of chain termination and inhibition of the viral polymerase.

Organ System Pharmacology

Animal studies have demonstrated that ganciclovir is excreted by the kidneys without undergoing any metabolic change, in concentrations equaling 90% of the dose given by IV administration. The drug is widely distributed in tissues, including brain, and concentrations can be maintained in plasma that are above the mean inhibitory concentration for CMV isolates, which is 0.02–3.0 μg/mL.

Adverse Effects

Ganciclovir has bone marrow suppressive effects in animals and also reduces spermatogenesis. The drug has been shown to have tumorigenic potential in mice. Therefore, the use of ganciclovir has been restricted to life-threatening or sight-threatening infections in immunocompromised patients. The severity of the underlying illnesses in these patient populations has complicated assessments of ganciclovir toxicity in clinical use. However, patients can develop neutropenia, thrombocytopenia or anemia, gastrointestinal symptoms, rashes, and abnormal hepatic and renal function; neurological syndromes including altered mental status, seizures, hallucinations, and psychosis have also been described during ganciclovir therapy. Suppression of the bone marrow is dose-related and occurred within 10 days after initiating ganciclovir treatment of CMV infection in transplant recipients. Approximately 40% of patients given the drug can be expected to have neutrophil counts less than 1000 cells/cu mm. Adverse effects on reproductive function and carcinogenicity are also possible, based on observations in animals. Phlebitis is common with ganciclovir administration.

BOX 42-3

INDICATIONS AND CONTRAINDICATIONS

Because of its potential for causing serious adverse effects, ganciclovir is indicated only for life-threatening or sight-threatening infections caused by CMV. The patients who are most likely to experience such infections include bone marrow and organ transplant recipients and patients with AIDS caused by HIV. The licensed indication for ganciclovir is limited to CMV retinitis. Ganciclovir has antiviral activity in severely immunocompromised patients with CMV pneumonia, when measured as a reduction in the quantity of infectious virus in urine, blood, and respiratory secretions. However, the impact of drug treatment on the survival rate of severely immunosuppressed patients with CMV pneumonitis has been variable in clinical trials. Although it has the capacity to inhibit HSV and VZV, its potential toxicity is a contraindication to the clinical use of ganciclovir for HSV and VZV infections, even in severely immunocompromised patients.

CMV isolates that are resistant to ganciclovir have been recovered from AIDS patients following ganciclovir treatment.

Ganciclovir is the only antiviral agent that is currently licensed for the treatment of CMV infection in high-risk patients.

Drug Interactions

Because of the potential of both ganciclovir and azidothymidine to cause severe bone marrow suppression, the concomitant administration of these drugs is not recommended. Theoretically, other drugs, such as chemotherapeutic agents, that inhibit rapidly dividing cells may have additive toxicity in patients receiving ganciclovir. As in the case of acyclovir, probenecid is likely to reduce the renal clearance of ganciclovir. Seizures have been reported in some patients who were receiving ganciclovir and imipenem-cilastin.

Preparations

Ganciclovir is available as an IV preparation. The use of ganciclovir for CMV retinitis is based on an induction phase, in which the drug is given at a dose of 5 mg/kg, as a 1-hour IV infusion, administered every 12 hours for 14–21 days. Maintenance therapy consists of 5 mg/kg/day for 5–7 days per week. Excretion of the drug by the kidneys requires adequate hydration; dosage reductions are essential if renal function is impaired.

AZIDOTHYMIDINE

Azidothymidine (zidovudine, 3-azido-3-deoxythymidine) was originally synthesized as a compound with potential antitumor activity. Its specific therapeutic value remained undefined until its substantial *in vitro* activity against HIV was demonstrated in the search for agents to treat AIDS. Clinical trials are in progress to determine the value of combinations of azidothymidine with other drugs or lymphokines, such as interferons, in symptomatic HIV infection.

Mechanism of Action

The conversion of azidothymidine to its triphosphate form by cellular enzymes produces a compound that is very active as a competitive inhibitor of the reverse transcriptase of HIV and other retroviruses. This effect is manifest at low intracellular concentrations of the drug (<1 μg/mL) whereas the cellular a-DNA polymerase is much less sensitive to the agent, so that host cell toxicity is minimal. Incorporation of the drug also acts to terminate DNA synthesis.

Organ System Pharmacology

Azidothymidine is absorbed at more than 50% of the oral dose, and the plasma and body fluid concentrations produced are well above the 1–5 μm required to inhibit HIV *in vitro.* The drug is detected in cerebrospinal fluid after oral or IV administration.

Adverse Effects

Patients treated with azidothymidine for 4–6 weeks can be expected to develop anemia severe enough to require intermittent blood transfusions. Most patients also have granulocytopenia. Patients receiving the drug should have a complete blood count every 1–2 weeks. Clinical data are lacking, but like vidarabine and acyclovir, the toxicity of azidothymidine is probably increased in patients with impaired renal or hepatic function.

> BOX 42-4
> **INDICATIONS AND CONTRAINDICATIONS**
>
> Azidothymidine is indicated for the treatment of HIV infection in patients who have symptomatic HIV infection with past *Pneumocystis carinii* pneumonia or an absolute CD4 T lymphocyte count less than 200/cu mm. It also has value for the treatment of HIV infection, which is asymptomatic, by prolonging the interval until the development of symptomatic disease. Azidothymidine is the first drug with proven efficacy against HIV infection, but the initial clinical experience does not indicate that HIV infection can be eradicated by the drug.

Drug Interactions

Any drugs that have adverse effects upon bone marrow or renal function may enhance the toxicity of azidothymidine, for example, dapsone, pentamidine, amphotericin B, flucytosine, interferon, and cancer chemotherapeutic agents. Probenecid reduces the renal excretion of the drug and may inhibit glucuronidation; it has been recommended that patients receiving azidothymidine should not be given acetaminophen, aspirin, or indomethacin. Neurological symptoms have been described in a few patients given azidothymidine and acyclovir.

RIBAVIRIN

Ribavirin is 1-D-ribofuranosyl-11-1,2-triazole-3-carboxamide and is most closely related to guanosine by x-ray crystallography studies.

Mechanism of Action

Ribavirin is phosphorylated intracellularly by cellular enzymes with the triphosphate form being the most active antiviral form. In contrast to vidarabine and acyclovir, ribavirin has broad activity against both RNA and DNA viruses. Its mode of action is best understood for respiratory viruses. *In vitro* studies of activity against influenza A infection of mammalian cells demonstrated a decrease in the intracellular nucleoside pool, inhibition of 5-cap formation of cellular mRNAs, and viral RNA polymerase inhibition. RNA viruses are generally more susceptible to ribavirin, but the replication of HSV, CMV, and many other viruses is inhibited by this agent.

Organ System Pharmacology

Information about the tissue distribution of ribavirin in human subjects is limited. Ribavirin is actively taken up by erythrocytes when given orally or IV with the half-life in these cells being 40 days. Penetration of the drug into cerebrospinal fluid has been documented. Most of the drug is excreted by the kidneys without undergoing metabolism. The drug is detected in plasma after 3 or more days of aerosol administration at concentrations of 3-6 μm; these concentrations are 1000-fold lower than concentrations in respiratory secretions.

Adverse Effects

Oral ribavirin administration causes a transient, dose-related anemia. Its administration by aerosol has produced serious mechanical interference with assisted ventilation because of drug precipitation in mechanical ventilators. Deterioration of respiratory function has been documented in some infants and adults treated with aerosolized ribavirin, but the role of the drug in causing such clinical events is not certain.

> BOX 42-5
> **INDICATIONS AND CONTRAINDICATIONS**
>
> Ribavirin given by aerosol into an infant oxygen hood has been effective for the treatment of respiratory syncytial virus (RSV) pneumonia. It is not approved for use in infants with RSV pneumonia who require assisted ventilation. Ribavirin, given systemically, is highly effective for the treatment of Lassa fever, a rare arenavirus infection. The oral drug is not useful for the treatment of respiratory viral infections.
>
> Despite its activity *in vitro*, ribavirin is not effective clinically in patients with HIV infection. Further experience with its aerosol administration to infants who require mechanical ventilation for RSV pneumonia is needed to determine the safety and efficacy of the drug in these patients. Although oral ribavirin has been used for hepatitis A and measles infections elsewhere, these indications for the drug have not been established definitely.
>
> Ribavirin is the first antiviral agent licensed for the treatment of RSV, which is the most common cause of severe pneumonia in infants and has been lifesaving for patients with Lassa fever. Its efficacy for respiratory and other viral infections in adults remains to be established, although initial studies indicate some benefit from aerosol therapy of influenza A and B infections.

Preparations

Ribavirin is prepared as both oral and IV formulations. Only the aerosol formulation is available in the United States. The drug is aerosolized by putting 20 mg/mL of drug in the reservoir of a small particle Collison generator and administering it along with humidified air and oxygen for 12-18 hours/24 hours. The usual duration of treatment is 3-7 days.

INTERFERONS

The interferons (IFNs) constitute a family of glycoproteins that are made by mammalian cells exposed to viruses, double-stranded RNAs and other compounds. The IFNs are classified as alpha-, beta-, and gamma-IFN. Alpha-IFN and beta-IFN exhibit a significant degree of homology in amino acid sequences, whereas gamma-IFN differs substantially. Alpha-IFN is produced primarily by leukocytes, beta-IFN by fibroblasts and epithelial cells, and gamma-IFN by T lymphocytes. Genetic engineering methods have been used to prepare recombinant IFNs of each class.

Mechanism of Action

IFNs have diverse effects upon viral replication, including interference with viral uncoating, viral RNA transcription, viral protein synthesis, and the assembly of whole virions. The antiviral efficacy of IFNs is probably enhanced by their natural activities as immunomodulating lymphokines *in vivo.*

Organ System Pharmacology

The tissue distribution and metabolism of IFNs is incompletely understood. IFN activity is detected in serum after intramuscular administration but diminishes rapidly, probably because of the catabolism of IFN protein by the liver. Topical and intralesional administration does not produce detectable serum concentrations of IFN.

> **BOX 42-6**
> **INDICATIONS AND CONTRAINDICATIONS**
>
> IFNs have been effective against several viral infections in clinical trials, but licensure for a specific indication is in treatment of hepatitis C. Clinical benefit has been demonstrated with alpha-IFN used in placebo-controlled trials for treatment of primary and recurrent VZV infections in immunocompromised patients, prophylaxis of recurrent HSV-1 infections, CMV prophylaxis in renal transplant recipients, prophylaxis and treatment of respiratory viral infections, and systemic and intralesional therapy for papillomavirus infections.
>
> The evaluation of the antiviral efficacy of IFNs against human viral infections has been limited by the difficulty of producing sufficient quantities of the protein. The preparation of IFNs using recombinant DNA technology will allow much broader investigation of their value as antiviral agents alone and in combination with other compounds.
>
> Although IFNs and IFN inducers were considered promising early in the effort to identify antiviral agents of clinical value, widespread use has been limited by short supply and by the concomitant development of other drugs, such as acyclovir, that have met the need for treatment of some herpesviral infections. However, better understanding of these natural antiviral substances is likely to generate new approaches to their clinical application.

Adverse Effects

IFN therapy has been associated with fever, malaise, and fatigue; prolonged administration produces hair loss. A dose-related leukopenia occurs with natural and recombinant IFNs. The topical intranasal application of alpha-IFN was associated with punctate hemorrhages of the nasal mucosa in some patients.

Drug Interactions

Concurrent therapy using alpha-IFN and vidarabine or acyclovir can cause neurological toxicity.

Preparations

Most clinical trials have been carried out with human leukocyte alpha-IFN in dosages of $1-3 \times 106$ U per dose given once or twice daily by intramuscular injection.

AMANTADINE

Amantadine (1-adamantanamine hydrochloride) has a unique chemical structure (Fig. 42-1). It is a tricyclic amine derived from a 10-carbon alicyclic compound, adamantane.

Mechanism of Action

The mechanism of the antiviral activity of amantadine is not fully defined. Its action appears to occur early in the course of viral infection of the mammalian cell with effects upon uncoating and fusion as well as assembly of progeny virions.

Organ System Pharmacology

Amantadine hydrochloride is not metabolized, and more than 90% of the dose is excreted by the kidneys. Plasma and tissue fluid concentrations of 0.5-1 μg/mL are observed with the usual dosage, whereas concentrations in respiratory secretions are about two thirds of the plasma levels. Higher plasma concentrations occur in patients with impaired glomerular filtration.

Adverse Effects

Amantadine causes mild adverse effects including dizziness, anxiety, and insomnia; some patients have had ataxia and confusion. In some controlled clinical trials of amantadine as an antiviral agent, such symptoms were reported as commonly by participants receiving aspirin or acetaminophen only. Urinary retention is another potential side effect. Serious adverse effects in patients treated for Parkinson's disease have included hypotension, congestive failure, altered mental status including psychosis and depression, seizures, and leukopenia.

> **BOX 42-7**
> ## INDICATIONS AND CONTRAINDICATIONS
>
> Amantadine is indicated for the prophylaxis and treatment of influenza A virus infections. Low concentrations of the drug, achievable after its oral administration, inhibit clinical isolates of all types of influenza A, that is, H1N1, H2N2, and H3N2 strains. Amantadine is considered an adjunct to the primary management of patients who are at risk for severe influenza A infection, which consists of annual influenza immunization. Those who may develop severe influenza A infection include the elderly, patients with chronic pulmonary or cardiac disease, and immunocompromised patients. Those who have not received vaccine prophylaxis can benefit from amantadine prophylaxis given for at least 10 days after a known exposure to influenza A or up to 90 days during a community epidemic. The early treatment of influenza A pneumonia with amantadine, continuing for 24–48 hours after the resolution of symptoms, also reduces the severity of the illness in high-risk patients. Amantadine is contraindicated during pregnancy.
>
> Rimantadine is a compound that is closely related to amantadine but that produces higher concentrations in respiratory secretions. Rimantadine appears to cause fewer side effects and is now being evaluated for the therapy of influenza A infections. This compound has been used extensively in the Soviet Union and was comparable to amantadine in initial clinical trials in the United States.
>
> Amantadine is an antiviral agent that is underutilized currently in clinical practice, given its demonstrated efficacy for the prophylaxis and treatment of influenza A infections. This circumstance is due to the difficulty of making a specific diagnosis of influenza A and should be alleviated as rapid viral diagnostic methods become available for this purpose.

Drug Interactions

Amantadine hydrochloride interacts with anticholinergic drugs to produce atropine-like effects unless the dosage of the anticholinergic drug is reduced. Alterations of mental status may occur if patients are receiving central nervous system stimulants. Decreased excretion of the drug has been reported after concomitant administration with hydrochlorthiazide and triamterene. Amantadine prophylaxis or treatment does not interfere with the immune response to influenza vaccination given concurrently.

Preparations

Amantadine is available as a capsule (100 mg) and as a pediatric suspension (50 mg/5 mL).

REFERENCES

Couch RB, Six HR: The antiviral spectrum and mechanism of action of amantadine and rimantadine. *In* Mills J, Corey L (eds): Antiviral Chemotherapy: New Directions for Clinical Application and Research, 50–57. New York: Elsevier, 1986.

Elion GB: History, mechanism of action, spectrum and selectivity of nucleoside analogs. *In* Mills J, Corey L (eds): Antiviral Chemotherapy: New Directions for Clinical Application and Research, 118–137. New York: Elsevier, 1986.

Fischl FA, Richman DD, Grieco MH, et al: The efficacy of azidothymidine (AZT) in the treatment of patients with AIDS and AIDS-related complex. A double-blind placebo-controlled trial. N Engl J Med 317:185–191, 1987.

Hirsch MS, Kaplan JC: Treatment of human immunodeficiency virus infections. Antimicrob Agents Chemother 31:839–843, 1987.

Laskin OL, Stahl-Bayliss CM, Kalman CM, Rosecan LR: Use of ganciclovir to treat serious cytomegalovirus infections in patients with AIDS. J Infect Dis 155:323–327, 1987.

Merigan TC, Rand KH, Pollard RB, et al: Human leukocyte interferon for the treatment of herpes zoster in patients with cancer. N Engl J Med 298:891–897, 1978.

Whitley RJ, Alford CA, Hirsch MS, et al: Vidarabine versus acyclovir therapy in herpes simplex encephalitis. N Engl J Med 314:144–149, 1986.

Antiparasitic Agents

43

Elizabeth A. Vande Waa

Parasitic diseases present major health problems throughout the world, particularly in developing countries. Although the mortality associated with these diseases impacts on populations, the morbidity associated with them also has a tremendous impact on the economic development of regions where these diseases are endemic. Health professionals around the world are becoming increasingly familiar with the parasitic diseases as a group due to increased travel and immigration from endemic regions. Granted, the major parasitic diseases, such as malaria and schistosomiasis, are associated with tropical climates; however, parasites are cosmopolitan in distribution. In the United States alone, it is estimated that over 60 million individuals harbor a helminth parasite, and the prevalence of infection with the protozoan *Entamoeba histolytica* is 2–4% of the general population. Finally, many otherwise innocuous parasites are becoming common health problems for individuals who are immunocompromised.

COUNSELING TRAVELERS

Although the health professional in the United States may have little contact with life-threatening parasitic diseases *per se*, he or she may encounter individuals who travel to regions where tropical diseases are endemic. In these cases, it is the physician's role to counsel travelers with respect to health risks, as well as to prescribe prophylactic medications. Awareness of drug-resistant strains of parasites in endemic areas is key information for both the traveler and his or her physician. Furthermore, patient education regarding the course of certain diseases is important, because many parasitic diseases do not manifest themselves immediately. Careful follow-up examination of the patient upon return from an endemic area is essential.

There are four ways to approach the treatment and spread of parasitic diseases: (1) vector control, (2) improved sanitation and hygiene, (3) vaccines, and (4) chemotherapy. Vector control has had limited success in controlling the spread of these diseases. There are many problems inherent in this approach, including toxicity of the chemicals used to eradicate the vector, resistance of the vector, and the need for frequent application of the chemicals in areas where this may not be possible either geographically or financially. Economic barriers also must be crossed in order to improve hygiene and sanitation in areas where many tropical diseases are inherent. Vaccines would be an attractive means of preventing disease spread, particularly because a highly efficacious vaccine would provide long-lasting immunity. This in turn would reduce the frequency of treatment and, eventually, as individuals became immunized, the incidence of disease would decline. Unfortunately, although this is a growing area of research interest, no vaccine exists for any of the parasitic diseases. Chemotherapy, then, becomes the major means whereby to prevent and control diseases caused by parasites. Although many drugs exist with which to treat these invading organisms, chemotherapy has limitations, particularly in developing countries, where drug storage, availability, and distribution to individuals in outlying areas provide challenges. These factors, combined with emerging drug resistance, make the study of antiparasitic

TABLE 43–1. Drugs Used to Treat Parasitic Infections

Parasitic Infection	Drug of Choice	Alternative Drugs	Comments
Helminth Infections			
INTESTINAL NEMATODE INFECTIONS			
Ascariasis			
Ascaris lumbricoides	Mebendazole	Albendazole,*† pyrantel, Piperazine, ivermectin*	
Hookworm infection			
Necator americanus	Mebendazole	Albendazole,*† pyrantel	
Ancylostoma duodenale	Mebendazole	Albendazole,*† pyrantel	
A. braziliense (cutaneous larval migrans)	Thiabendazole	Albendazole*†	
Trichuriasis			
Trichuris trichiura	Mebendazole	Albendazole,*† Oxantel	
Enterobiasis			
Enterobius vermicularis	Mebendazole	Albendazole,*† pyrantel, ivermectin*‡	
Strongyloides stercoralis	Thiabendazole	Albendazole,*† ivermectin*	
Trichinosis			
Trichinella spiralis	Albendazole*†	Thiabendazole	Thiabendazole efficacy limited to intestinal phase
BLOOD AND TISSUE NEMATODES			
Filariasis			
Wuchereria bancrofti	Diethylcarbamazine‡	Ivermectin*	
Brugia malayi	Diethylcarbamazine†	Ivermectin*	
Onchocerca volvulus	Ivermectin	Diethylcarbamazine‡	
TREMATODES			
Schistosomiasis			
Schistosoma mansoni	Praziquantel	Oxamniquine	
S. hematobium	Praziquantel	Metrifonate‡	
S. japonicum	Praziquantel	—	
S. mekongi	Praziquantel	—	
Liver and lung flukes			
Clonorchis sinensis, *Opisthorchis* spp.			
Paragonimus spp.	Praziquantel*		
Fasciola hepatica	—	—	
CESTODES			
Taeniasis			
Taenia saginata	Praziquantel*	Niclosamide	
T. solium	Praziquantel*	—	Use of niclosamide not recommended owing to risk of cysticercosis
Neurocysticercosis due to *T. solium*	Albendazole*		
Diphyllobothriasis			
Diphyllobothrium latum	Praziquantel*	Niclosamide	
Hymenolepiasis			
Hymenolepis nana	Praziquantel*	Niclosamide	
Echinococcosis			
Echinococcus granulosus	Albendazole*†	Mebendazole*	Mebendazole may be only partially effective
Protozoan Infections			
Trichomoniasis			
Trichomonas vaginalis	Metronidazole	—	
Amebiasis			
Entamoeba histolytica			
Asymptomatic cyst passers	Diloxanide furoate†	—	
Noninvasive intestinal form	Diloxanide furoate†	Paramomycin	
Invasive forms; amebic abscess	Metronidazole	Chloroquine, dehydroemetine	Alternative drugs are generally not recommended
Giardiasis			
Giardia lamblia	Metronidazole*	Quinacrine	
Leishmaniasis			
Leishmania tropica	Sodium stibogluconate†		
L. mexicana, *L. braziliensis*	Sodium stibogluconate†	Amphotericin B	
L. donovani	Sodium stibogluconate†	Pentamidine	
Trypanosomiasis			
Trypanosoma brucei rhodesiense	Suramin	Eflornithine, pentamidine	Acute infection
T. brucei gambiense	Eflornithine	Suramin, pentamidine	No central nervous system involvement
T. brucei gambiense	Eflornithine	Suramin, then melarsoprol	Chronic infection, with central nervous system involvement
T. cruzi	Nifurtimox†		

TABLE 43–1. Drugs Used to Treat Parasitic Infections *Continued.*

Parasitic Infection	Drug of Choice	Alternative Drugs	Comments
Protozoan Infections (Continued)			
Malaria			
Plasmodium vivax, P. ovale, P. malariae	Chloroquine	—	For chemoprophylaxis and treatment of clinical attack
P. vivax, P. ovale	Primaquine	—	Radical cure agent
P. falciparum			
Chloroquine-sensitive	Chloroquine	—	For chemoprophylaxis and treatment of clinical attack
Chloroquine-resistant or multidrug-resistant			
Chemoprophylaxis	Chloroquine, proguanil, or pyrimethamine-sulfadoxine	Mefloquine	Dependent on geographical location
Treatment	Mefloquine	Quinine with or without pyrimethamine-sulfadoxine	

*Accepted therapy in some countries. Use is either not approved or is considered investigational in the United States.
†Contact the Parasitic Disease Drug Service, Centers for Disease Control, for availability.
‡Recommendation based on limited clinical trials.

drugs dynamic. Drugs currently used for the treatment of parasitic diseases may be found in Table 43–1.

In the United States, many of the drugs discussed below are not routinely available and must be obtained from the Parasitic Disease Drug Service, Center for Infectious Disease, Centers for Disease Control, Atlanta, GA, 30333. Telephone (404) 329–3670 (days) or (404) 329–2888 (evenings and weekends).

ANTHELMINTIC DRUGS

Helminth parasites infect over 2 billion people worldwide. These parasitic worms can be divided into three groups: nematodes (roundworms), trematodes (flukes), and cestodes (flatworms and tapeworms). The lifecycles of many of the parasitic helminths are quite complex, offering a formidable challenge to disease eradication and even drug treatment. However, many agents do exist with anthelmintic activity. These are discussed in detail.

Intestinal Nematode Infections

Ascariasis

Infection with *Ascaris lumbricoides* is one of the top 20 causes of morbidity in Africa, South America, and much of Asia. In the United States, cases of ascariasis are most often seen in humid regions of the South. Embryonated Ascaris eggs are found in the soil, and infection is usually due to ingestion of feces-contaminated raw vegetables. Adult ascarids live in the lumen of the small intestine, where the female may lay up to 200,000 unembryonated eggs per day. The eggs embryonate in soil, and their ingestion by a human host perpetuates the lifecycle.

TREATMENT. Mebendazole, a 5-substituted benzimidazole, is the drug of choice for the treatment of ascariasis (Cook, 1990). Mebendazole is given orally and is well-tolerated. Absorption of mebendazole is poor (5–10%), and the drug has a plasma half-life of approximately 1 hour. The absorbed drug is metabolized in the liver via a first-pass effect to a number of metabolites, about 48% of which appear in the urine. Much of the drug is excreted via the bile into the feces. Because mebendazole is so poorly absorbed, it is highly efficacious in the intestinal tract, where the adult ascarids reside. The mechanism of action of mebendazole is thought to involve inhibition of the assembly of tubulin dimers into tubulin polymers. This causes a lack of formation of microtubules and may ultimately cause them to break down. Microtubules are important to parasites in a number of capacities, such as larval development, transport of carbohydrates, and enzyme function. They are also needed in order to maintain the parasite tegument and digestive apparatus (Lacey, 1990; Roos, 1990). Mebendazole also has affinity for mammalian tubulin; as a result, it is embryotoxic—it thus is contraindicated in pregnancy.

SIDE EFFECTS AND OTHER CONSIDERATIONS. Because mebendazole is so poorly absorbed, side effects associated with its use are few. Abdominal pain and diarrhea are occasionally seen, but systemic effects are rare. Mebendazole is teratogenic, but flubendazole, another benzimidazole not yet approved for use, has been shown to be safe in pregnancy. As will be discussed below, mebendazole is efficacious against a variety of intestinal nematodes, and thus it is considered a broad-spectrum agent for treatment of these parasites.

Hookworm Infection

Hookworm infection is due to either *Necator americanus* (in the Americas) or *Ancylostoma duodenale* (in other parts of the world). Adults of both species inhabit the lumen of the small intestine, where they feed on villous tissue and suck blood. Thus, the main goals of therapy for treatment of this infection involve both the eradication of the parasite as well as correction of the anemic state of the host. The antiparasitic drug of choice for hookworm is mebendazole, which was discussed previously. Oral iron therapy added to this corrects anemia.

Trichuriasis

Infection with *Trichuris trichuria* (whipworm) is the result of ingestion of embryonated eggs. Eggs can be found in moist, warm soil that is contaminated with human feces. Adult parasites become imbedded in the epithelium of the large intestine; the posterior end of the worm protrudes into the lumen of the large bowel. Treatment for this parasite is oral mebendazole.

Enterobiasis

Infection with *Enterobius vermicularis* (pinworm) is the most common helminth infection in the United States, although its distribution is cosmopolitan. Adult parasites inhabit the colon, where they mate. Gravid female worms, in response to lowered oxygen tension or reduced body temperature, migrate to the perianal region — usually while the infected host is asleep. Here, they deposit their eggs. The presence of the parasite in the perianal area causes an intense itching, and autoinfection may result if the host has oral contact with contaminated fingers. Ingestion of embryonated eggs continues the cycle and, because the eggs may survive for a few days outside the host, clearing an infection relies on both excellent hygiene as well as chemotherapy. The drug of choice for treatment of pinworms is mebendazole. Because the infection is easily spread, it is recommended that all individuals who live with the infected host undergo treatment.

Strongyloidiasis

Strongyloides stercoralis is commonly found in the tropics and subtropics, but may also be encountered in warm, humid areas of the United States. The lifecycle of this parasite is complex, with a large component of it taking place with the parasite as a free-living organism in warm, moist soil. In addition, dogs and monkeys may serve as reservoir hosts for Strongyloides. The infection begins when third-stage larvae are ingested or penetrate the skin of the host. Ultimately, parasites end up in the small intestine, where they develop into adults. These larvae develop only as hermaphroditic females, because male worms exist only in the free-living state. Eggs produced by the female parasite develop to second-stage larvae, then are passed out into the environment. If deposited in warm soil, the larvae can develop into free-living males and females that can reproduce. These third-stage larvae may then penetrate another host and continue the lifecycle. Another interesting consideration of Stronglyoides infection may occur in the immunocompromised individual. Here, the second-stage larvae may actually develop into third-stage worms in the large intestine. These parasites may then penetrate the large intestine, enter the bloodstream and, after migrating through the lung, be swallowed. Development to adult females then occurs in the small intestine.

TREATMENT. The drug of choice for the treatment of strongyloides is thiabendazole. This drug, like mebendazole, is a benzimidazole that is effective against a wide spectrum of intestinal nematodes, acting to disrupt tubulin polymerization. The drug is metabolized to 5-hydroxythiabendazole, and the glucuronide or sulfate conjugates of this are almost completely eliminated within 24 hours via the kidneys. Generally, a 2-day course of thiabendazole produces a cure in about 90% of patients infected with *S. stercoralis.* A longer course of treatment may be necessary in the immunocompromised patient with disseminated disease.

SIDE EFFECTS AND OTHER CONSIDERATIONS. Unlike mebendazole, thiabendazole is readily absorbed from the gastrointestinal tract, reaching peak plasma concentrations within 1 hour. The bioavailability of the drug is responsible for a number of systemic side effects associated with its use. These include nausea, vomiting, headache, and abdominal pain, as well as dizziness. While thiabendazole has not been found to be teratogenic, its use in pregnancy is limited due to its side effects.

Trichinosis

Trichinosis is caused by infection with the parasite *Trichinella spiralis*, the larvae of which may be ingested when eating raw or undercooked meat. These parasites have a complex lifecycle; the treatment of disease caused by these organisms is challenging. Upon ingestion, the larvae become male or female adults within 28 hours. Within 30 hours, mating begins and, within 5 – 6 days, newborn larvae are shed. The larvae penetrate into blood vessels and eventually become distributed throughout the body. Larvae remain only in striated skeletal muscle cells. Here, the larva induces a unique process whereby it rearranges the host cell cytoplasm so that it serves as a "nurse cell" to the larva. The larva – nurse cell unit can thereby efficiently extract nutrients and dispose of wastes. By 20 days after infection, the larva – nurse cell complex is fully grown and infective. In the United States, infected pigs most often serve as reservoir hosts for this disease, and the ingestion of infected undercooked pork initiates trichinosis.

TREATMENT. The treatment of trichinosis is complicated by the fact that the disease often goes unnoticed until the parenteral, or muscle, phase. In the enteral phase, adult worms are highly susceptible to the benzimidazoles and thiabendazole is the drug of choice for trichinosis. Larvae that have embedded in skeletal muscle have shown some response to thiabendazole in certain studies, although steroids coadministered with the drug are recommended to reduce inflammation.

Other Drugs Used for the Treatment of Intestinal Nematodes

Albendazole

Albendazole is another benzimidazole derivative with a broad spectrum of activity against nematodes residing in the gut. Specifically, this drug has shown activity against *A. lumbricoides*, *N. americanus*, *A. duodenale*, and *E. vermicularis*. In contrast to mebendazole, however, this drug also has some efficacy against Strongyloides and trichinosis. Albendazole is rapidly absorbed from the gastrointestinal tract, but its systemic side effects are few. These include minor epigastric pain and diarrhea. As of yet, albendazole is not approved for use in the United States.

Pyrantel

Pyrantel pamoate is considered a broad-spectrum anthelmintic; it is the drug of second choice for the treatment of hookworm, ascariasis, and pinworm infections. The mechanism of action of pyrantel involves the binding of the drug to the nicotinic receptor, causing depolarization and a spastic paralysis of the parasite. Paralyzed worms are then expelled from the intestines of the infected individual. The drug is poorly absorbed from the gastrointestinal tract, so side effects associated with its use are few. An analog of pyrantel, oxantel, is effective against whipworm. Pyrantel and oxantel may be given in combination when the patient is infected with mixed species of soil-transmitted nematodes.

Tissue-Dwelling Nematode Infections

Bancroftian and Brugian Filariases

Disease caused by infection with *Wuchereria bancrofti* or *Brugia malayi* is extremely debilitating. Adult parasites of these species live in the lymph nodes of the infected host. Here, they cause lymphadenopathy and swelling of the extremities, and the term *elephantiasis* has been coined to describe this pathology. These filarial worms are transmitted via infected mosquitoes. When the insect bites, the third-stage larvae crawl onto the skin and through the bite wound left by the mosquito. Worms are transmitted via the lymph to lymph nodes, where they develop to adults. Adult parasites excrete microfilariae, which circulate in the blood. These may then be ingested when a mosquito bites the host, and the lifecycle is continued.

TREATMENT. The drug of choice for both bancroftian and brugian filariases is diethylcarbamazine. This drug causes a rapid disappearance of the microfilariae from the blood, although its effects on these worms is thought to be indirect. Presumably, diethylcarbamazine sensitizes the microfilariae so that they become targets of the host's reticuloendothelial system. Adult worms are also affected by the drug, although this effect is slow in onset. The molecular mechanism of action of diethylcarbamazine remains unknown. Diethylcarbamazine is administered as the citrate salt. It is rapidly absorbed, reaching peak plasma concentrations within 1 to 3 hours after administration. Most of the drug ($> 50\%$) is excreted unchanged in the urine; a minor amount is excreted as the *N*-oxide, and small amounts may also be found in the feces. Excretion of the drug via the urine is highly pH-dependent, greatly increasing with acidification of the urine. Plasma half-life is prolonged severalfold when urine is alkalinized to pH 8.

SIDE EFFECTS AND OTHER CONSIDERATIONS. In general, the side effects associated with the use of diethylcarbamazine are not severe, but they are common. These include headache, malaise, joint pain, nausea, vomiting, and anorexia. The drug is not recommended in pregnancy due to these effects. Currently, diethylcarbamazine is the only agent available for the treatment and suppression of infection with either *W. bancrofti* or *B. malayi.*

Onchocerciasis

Filariasis caused by infection with *Onchocerca volvulus* is a problem in parts of Africa and in Central and South America. This parasite is transmitted by the blackfly *Simulium damnosum*, which breeds in rapidly flowing water. Individuals living close to these bodies of water are more likely to become infected. In the host, the adult parasite lives in subcutaneous nodules, where it may live for 8 to 10 years. During this time, the female worms produce hundreds of thousands of microfilariae that migrate through the skin, from where they may be transferred back to a biting fly. Microfilariae may also migrate to the eye, however, where they cause a great deal of pathology and, ultimately, blindness. Thus, onchocerciasis is called *river blindness.*

TREATMENT. Although the microfilariae are responsible for the pathology associated with onchocerciasis, eradication of the adult worm from the infected host would prevent further pathology. However, as of yet, no drug has been found to be effective against adult *O. volvulus.* A surgical procedure known as a nodulectomy is the only treatment for the adult worm. To clear the microfilariae, diethylcarbamazine has some efficacy. It is thought that this drug sensitizes the microfilariae to the host's immune system, as discussed previously. This effect, however, leads to a severe side effect called the Mazzoti reaction, which is described below. Due to this reaction, another drug, ivermectin, is being used with greater frequency for the treatment of onchocerciasis and is considered the drug of choice for the disease (Campbell, 1989).

Ivermectin is a macrocyclic lactone produced by the actinomycete *Streptomyces avermitilis.* This drug is a broad-spectrum agent with efficacy against a variety of ecto- and endoparasites. Its first use was in veterinary medicine, but it is now approved for use against nematodes in humans. The drug is ineffective against trematodes and cestodes.

The mechanism of action of ivermectin is not entirely known; however, it has been shown to potentiate the release and binding of γ-aminobutyric acid (GABA) at postsynaptic sites in the neuromuscular junction. A dose-dependent increase in chloride ion permeability at these sites is also seen. The result of this is a paralysis of the parasite. *O. volvulus* microfilariae are sensitive to the effects of ivermectin, whereas adult worms are not. There is evidence, however, the ivermectin inhibits the release of microfilariae from the female worm.

Upon oral administration, peak plasma concentrations of ivermectin are reached within 4 hours. The half-life of the drug is approximately 12 hours, and most of it appears in the feces. The potency and selectivity of ivermectin are remarkable. A single dose of 150 μg/kg significantly reduces skin and eye microfilariae in the infected patient. This effect may last up to 1 year, so an annual dosing regimen is recommended.

SIDE EFFECTS AND OTHER CONSIDERATIONS. Ivermectin has few serious side effects. Those recorded include dizziness, pruritis, and swelling of the face and lower limbs. Ivermectin does not penetrate the blood-brain barrier, so no effects on mammalian GABA-mediated neurotransmission are seen.

> **BOX 43–1**
> **THE MAZZOTI REACTION**
>
> In some patients, a mild Mazzoti reaction may be seen after treatment with the drug. This reaction describes an immune response to antigens that are released from dead or dying microfilariae. Specifically, this involves a papular rash, severe itching, tachycardia, and headache. This side effect is directly related to the microfilarial load in the patient; when this is high, exacerbation of ocular pathology may also be seen. In patients treated with diethylcarbamazine, the Mazzoti reaction is a very common side effect and may be fatal. Because ivermectin is less likely to cause this reaction, it is the drug of choice for onchocerciasis.

Ivermectin is also effective against bancroftian filariasis, ascariasis, and trichuriasis. Its efficacy against Strongyloides infection offers it as an alternative to thiabendazole.

Trematode Infections

Of the trematodes or flukes that affect humans, the schistosomes cause the most significant pathology. There are three species of schistosome that infect humans: *Schistosoma mansoni*, *S. japonicum*, and *S. haematobium*. These parasites cause significant mortality and morbidity in over 73 countries worldwide. Infection with the parasite begins after contact with water that harbors a snail (Fig. 43–1), the intermediate host for the infection.

Eggs that remain in the host may become trapped in the liver, where they induce an immune response with resultant granuloma formation. This ultimately leads to hepatomegaly and splenomegaly, and esophageal varices — characteristic pathology associated with schistosomiasis.

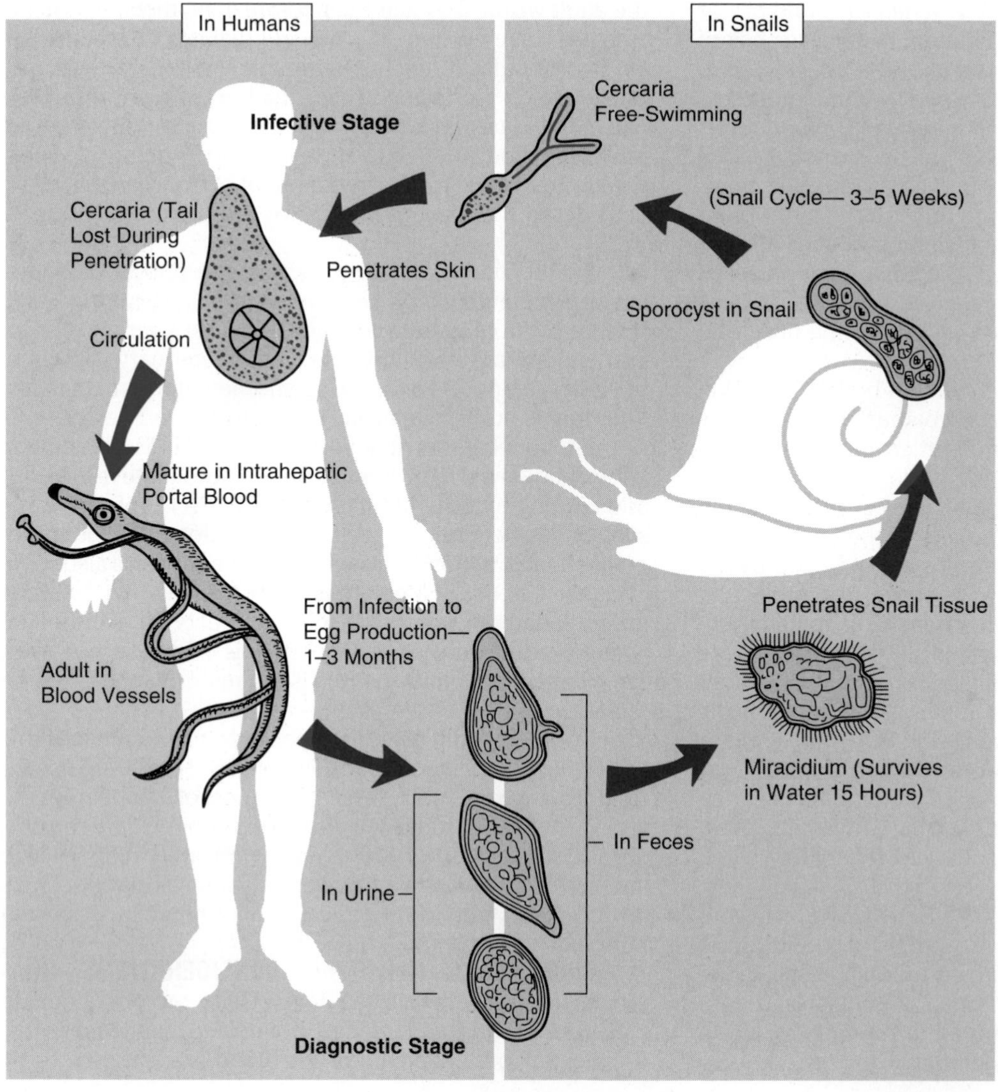

FIGURE 43–1. The life cycle of *Schistosoma* species.

BOX 43-2
LIFE CYCLE OF SCHISTOSOMA SPECIES

The infected snail sheds cercariae, which penetrate the skin of the host. The parasites then migrate through the lungs to the liver, where they mature into adult males or females and begin to mate. In the case of *S. mansoni* and *S. japonicum*, adult worms remain *in copula* in the blood vessels of the mesentery. *S. haematobium* adults migrate to the venous plexus surrounding the bladder, where the female begins producing eggs. Many of the eggs are passed out into the environment via the urine or feces. These hatch and infect a snail, thereby perpetuating the life cycle.

Treatment

For the treatment of all infections caused by *Schistosoma* spp., praziquantel is the drug of choice. Praziquantel is considered to be a broad-spectrum agent, with efficacy against a variety of both trematodes and cestodes. The mechanism of action of this agent is thought to involve an increased permeability of the parasite to divalent cations, particularly calcium, in the presence of the drug. As a result, spastic paralysis of the parasite is seen, as well as blebbing of the parasite's protective tegument. This vacuolization of the tegument is thought to make the parasite more susceptible to host immune attack, and once antibody is bound to these sites, subsequent complement fixation or the binding of white blood cells to the area results in complete tegumental disruption. Praziquantel is usually effective in a single oral dose. The drug is subject to a first-pass effect in the liver, and over 90% of it can be detected as hydroxylated or conjugated metabolites in the urine.

Side Effects and Other Considerations

Praziquantel is a very safe drug to use; its single oral dosing regimen and limited side effects add to its attractiveness as an anthelmintic. Side effects associated with praziquantel use include headache and dizziness, abdominal pain, and skin rashes. All of these side effects are self-limiting and short in duration. Skin eruptions are rare, but are thought to result from antigens being released from the dying parasites, thereby inducing an immune response. Praziquantel has not been found to be teratogenic in any trials. As stated above, praziquantel is effective against a variety of other trematodes, including the lung fluke *Paragonimus*, and the liver flukes *Opisthorchis* spp. and *Clonorchis sinensis*.

Other Drugs for the Treatment of Schistosomiasis

METRIFONATE. This organophosphorous compound has efficacy against *S. haematobium* infections only. In the host, metrifonate is metabolized to dichlorvos, which has antiparasitic activity. Like other organophosphates, this compound is a potent inhibitor of acetylcholinesterase; however, the basis for the specific antiparasitic activity in this infection is unknown. Metrifonate is a drug of second choice against *S. haematobium*.

OXAMNIQUINE. Oxamniquine is effective only against *S. mansoni* infections. It is a tetrahydroquinoline derivative that is given orally. Within the host, it is speculated that oxamniquine is metabolized to an unstable intermediate, which subsequently forms a reactive carbonium ion. This species is thought to then alkylate parasite macromolecules. Metabolism of the drug occurs largely in the intestine, and metabolites are seen in the urine, which they color orange to dark red. The use of oxamniquine is limited, and drug resistance has been detected in Brazil.

Cestode Infections

A variety of species of cestodes, or tapeworms, infect humans. These include *Taenia saginata*, the beef tapeworm; *T. solium*, the pork tapeworm; *Hymenolepis nana*, the dwarf tapeworm; and *Diphyllobothrium latum*, the fish tapeworm. Adult tapeworms live in the intestines; generally, infection with these organisms is asymptomatic. Infection begins when the host ingests either eggs or the cysticercus, which lodges in the connective tissue of pigs, cows, or fish. The cysticercus then forms a scolex, which lodges in the mucosa of the small intestine. As the parasites mature, they form proglottids or segments that are excreted into the feces. Either these proglottids, which are loaded with eggs, or the embryonated eggs from these segments may then be ingested by an animal and the lifecycle is perpetuated. The most serious consideration of tapeworm infection involves that with *T. solium*. In certain cases, infectious cysticerci may pass into the host tissue. Most specifically, cysts may pass into the central nervous system (CNS), where the resulting cysticercosis may be fatal.

Treatment

The treatment of tapeworm infection relies on two drugs, praziquantel and niclosamide. Niclosamide is well-tolerated orally, and in the gut it is readily taken up by cestodes. Once in the parasite, niclosamide acts to uncouple oxidative phosphorylation. As a result, the parasite cannot synthesize adenosine triphosphate (ATP) from adenosine diphosphate (ADP); eventually, this leads to paralysis, and the parasite is passed out of the intestine in the feces. Side effects resulting from niclosamide use are mild and are limited to nausea and transient gastrointestinal pain. Niclosamide may be used safely in pregnancy. This drug is effective against all species of adult cestodes; however, it is ineffective against the cysticerci of *T. solium*. If infection with *T. solium* is suspected, the patient must be treated with praziquantel (described above), so that the individual is not put at risk for cysticercosis.

ANTIPROTOZOAL DRUGS

The parasitic protozoa have a tremendous impact on world health. Over half the world population is at risk for malaria alone, a disease that kills over 1 million children in Africa each year. Protozoa with a more cosmopolitan distribution, such as trichomonads and amebae, are increasing in prevalence, particularly in immunocompromised individuals, such as those with the human immunodeficiency virus (HIV). Strategies for chemotherapeutic attack of these parasites is complicated both by the immune state of the host, as well as by emerging drug resistance.

Malaria

Malaria is the most prevalent of all parasitic diseases. It is caused by infection with one of the four species of Plasmodium: *P. falciparum*, *P. vivax*, *P. ovale*, and *P. malariae*. The species that causes the highest morbidity and mortality in humans is *P. falciparum*.

> **BOX 43-3**
> **LIFE CYCLE OF PLASMODIUM SPECIES**
>
> The lifecycle of the malaria parasite is complex and relies on a mosquito vector. The infected mosquito, upon taking a blood meal on the host, releases infective sporozoites. This form of the parasite leaves the circulation and resides in the liver, where it multiplies, forming schizonts. This stage of the lifecycle is known as the exoerythrocytic stage and is largely asymptomatic. After several days, the schizonts break out of the liver parenchyma and enter the circulation. The parasite, now known as a merozoite, invades red blood cells, where it multiplies to the point where the red blood cell cannot accommodate the protozoa. The blood cell bursts, and the merozoites are freed—at which time they invade other red blood cells. This stage of malaria is called the erythrocytic stage, and results in the pathology associated with malaria infection. During this stage, the patient develops fever cycles that correspond to the bursting of erythrocytes. After several of these asexual multiplications, the organism can form gametes within the red blood cell. These may be taken up by a mosquito vector in a subsequent blood meal. In the mosquito, the gametes form sporozoites, the infective stage for man. The duration of an acute attack of malaria may be only about 2 weeks; however, the febrile episodes associated with the disase may be very severe, particularly in the case of *P. falciparum*. In contrast, infection with either *P. ovale* or *P. vivax* results in mild manifestations of the disease; however, the schizonts of these species can form hypnozoites in the liver that may remain dormant for years. The hypnozoites can once again become active schizonts at any time, putting the patient at risk for relapse of the disease.

Treatment

The treatment of malaria is highly dependent on the species of the invading organism, as well as on the life stage of the parasite. The lifecycle of the parasite is shown in Figure 43-2. Drugs effective at each stage in the lifecycle are as shown; they are discussed in detail below.

CHLOROQUINE. Chloroquine is an aminoquinoline that has been the mainstay against malaria infection. Its mechanism of action is not completely understood; however, it is known that the drug binds to ferriprotoporphyrin IX, a heme breakdown product. This product is highly lytic to red blood cells and, normally, the malaria parasite complexes it so that the blood cell does not lyse. In the presence of chloroquine, however, the ferriprotoporphyrin IX is bound to the drug and, as such, maintains its lytic activity. As a second possible mechanism, it is also known that chloroquine accumulates into acidic compartments of the parasite, such as lysosomes. As a weak base, the drug neutralizes these compartments, so that the parasite is unable to utilize proteases involved in hemoglobin breakdown, a process essential for parasite survival (Krogstad et al, 1987).

Chloroquine is tolerated well orally and is usually given as the diphosphate. It is concentrated in tissues, particularly the liver, spleen, and kidneys. Chloroquine and its major metabolite (desethylchloroquine) are excreted in the urine.

Side Effects and Other Considerations. Use of chloroquine is associated with relatively mild side effects. These may include headache, nausea, and visual disturbances. The drug is concentrated in the liver and kidneys, so care should be used when it is administered to a patient with compromised hepatic or renal function. Chloroquine is safe to use in pregnancy. The drug is effective against the asexual blood stages of all species of Plasmodium, but it is not effective against the tissue forms of malaria. Therefore, it will not cure malaria caused by *P. vivax* or *P. ovale*. After administration, chloroquine lowers the fever associated with an acute attack of malaria within 24 to 48 hours; parasites are cleared from the bloodstream within 48 to 72 hours postdosing.

> **BOX 43-4**
> **CHLOROQUINE PROPHYLAXIS**
>
> To the individual living in or travelling to an area endemic for malaria, chloroquine is given prior to exposure to the disease. In this sense, the drug is thought of as having a prophylactic effect. Actually, chloroquine is not a true prophylactic agent—that is, it does not prevent malaria infection. Rather, it rapidly and completely suppresses the clinical aspects of malaria once the individual is exposed to the parasite, resulting in a suppressive cure. Chloroquine is the drug of choice for the treatment of all chloroquine-sensitive strains of malaria.

QUININE. Quinine is the oldest antimalarial agent. It is an alkaloid derived from the bark of the cinchona tree, and has been used to treat malarial fevers since 1633. Quinine is given orally and is well-absorbed, reaching peak plasma concentrations within 3 hours. The drug is extensively metabolized in the liver, but it does not bind to this or other tissues to the same extent as chloroquine. The antimalarial mechanism of action of quinine is not understood—it is thought to be similar to that of chloroquine.

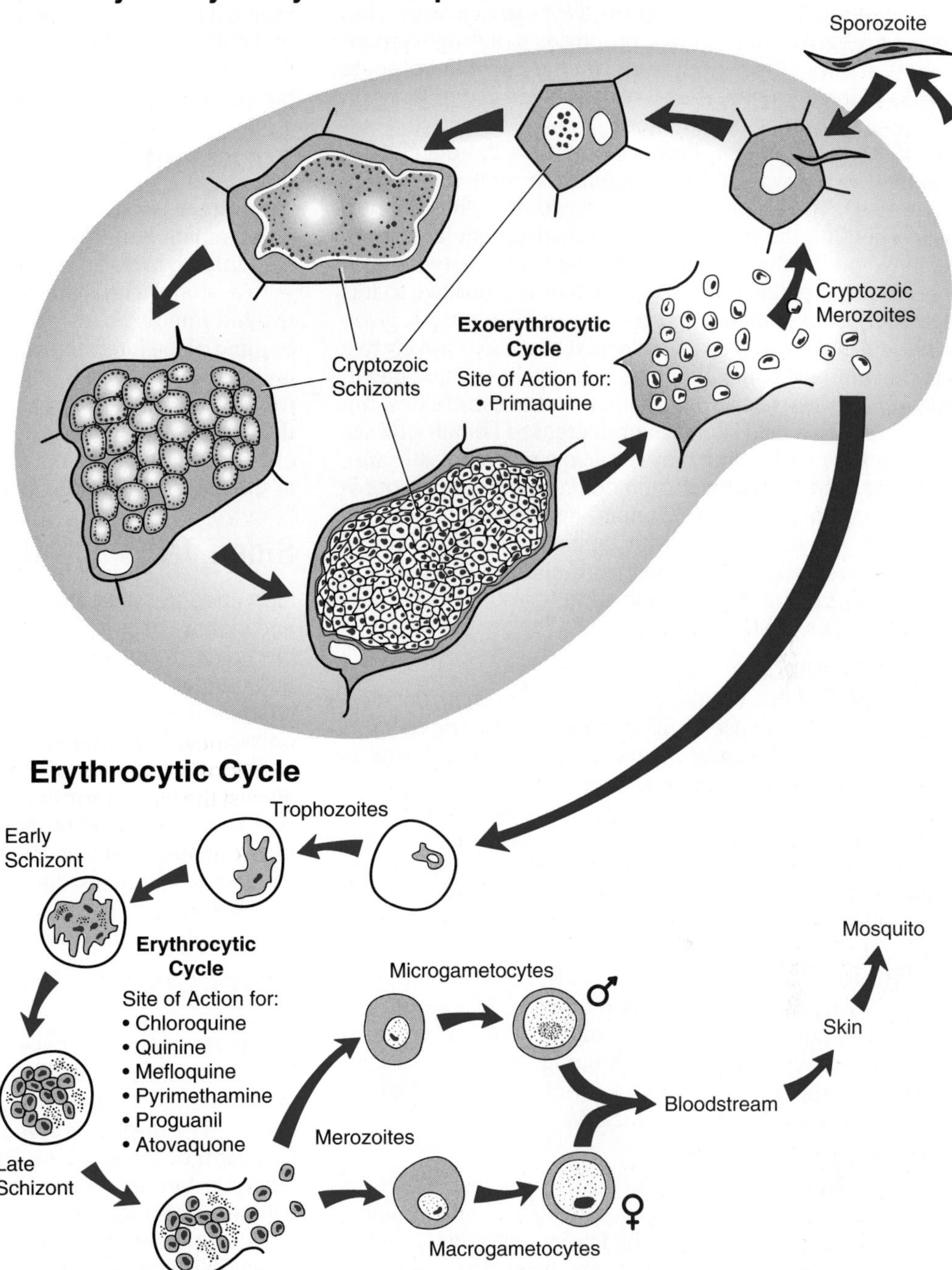

FIGURE 43–2. The lifecycle of malaria. Drugs effective at either the erythrocytic or exoerythrocytic stages of the parasite's development are noted.

Side Effects and Other Considerations. Quinine has a unique group of neurotoxic side effects associated with its use. These are referred to as *cinchonism* and include tinnitus, headache, vertigo, and blurred vision. Visual disturbances may be severe enough to include photophobia, diplopia, altered color perception and, in rare instances, blindness. High doses of the drug can affect the cardiovascular system and can be lethal. Quinine is effective against blood stages of malaria parasites. It has no effect on tissue stages, but it is gametocytocidal for *P. vivax* and *P. malariae.* Because of the toxicity associated with its use, quinine is reserved only for cases of chloroquine-resistant malaria or for cases of cerebral malaria. It is usually given in combination with an antibiotic such as tetracycline or pyrimethamine-sulfadoxine (discussed below).

MEFLOQUINE. Mefloquine is a structural derivative of quinine. It is the newest antimalarial agent, and is used only for the treatment of chloroquine-resistant *P. falciparum.* Because resistance to this agent is already emerging, limitations on its use are prudent. The mechanism of action of mefloquine is unknown, although it is concentrated within the parasite, as is chloroquine. Mefloquine is given orally and is much less toxic than quinine. It has a half-life of 17 days, probably due to the fact that it undergoes extensive enterohepatic and enterogastric circulation. Side effects associated with mefloquine's use are minor and include nausea, vomiting, and dizziness; however, due to a lack of clinical data, mefloquine is not yet approved for use in infants, children, or pregnant women. For prophylaxis of drug-resistant malaria, mefloquine is given alone; for the treatment of acute attacks of infection, the drug is usually given in combination with pyrimethamine-sulfadoxine.

PYRIMETHAMINE. Pyrimethamine, a 2,4-diaminopyrimidine, is always used in combination with sulfadoxine (FANSIDAR). The combination of the two drugs has a synergistic effect on the biosynthesis of dihydropteric acid. Specifically, pyrimethamine inhibits dihydrofolate reductase, and the plasmodium enzyme is much more sensitive to this drug than is its mammalian counterpart. The drug is given orally and is metabolized in the liver. It binds extensively to a number of tissues, including the kidneys, liver, and spleen. Side effects associated with pyrimethamine use are few, but can present as a mild skin rash or decreased hematopoiesis. Extended use of the drug may result in a megaloblastic anemia. Uses of pyrimethamine-sulfadoxine include chemoprophylaxis (even in pregnant women) against falciparum malaria and, in combination with quinine, the treatment of acute malarial attacks resulting from chloroquine-resistant *P. falciparum*. This drug combination is also used for chemoprophylaxis of vivax malaria.

OTHER DRUGS

PRIMAQUINE. Primaquine is a tissue schizonticide that brings about a cure from infections with *P. vivax* or *P. ovale*. The mechanism of action of this aminoquinoline is unknown. An interesting side effect of primaquine is hemolysis, which is seen in patients with a glucose-6-phosphate dehydrogenase deficiency. This inherited disorder is seen in some blacks and certain ethnic groups of Eastern Mediterranean origin, and it is recommended that patients receiving primaquine be screened for this deficiency prior to drug treatment.

PROGUANIL. Proguanil is a blood schizonticide that inhibits plasmodial dihydrofolate reductase. As a result, the synthesis of purines, pyrimidines, and certain amino acids within the parasite is blocked. Although rarely used anymore, proguanil is recommended for chemoprophylaxis in areas of chloroquine-resistant malaria.

NEW DRUGS

ATOVAQUONE. Among the new drugs with which to treat malaria, atovaquone appears to hold some promise (Hudson, 1993). This agent is a hydroxynaphthoquinone derivative, and it inhibits plasmodial dihydro-orotate dehydrogenase, an enzyme essential to parasite pyrimidine synthesis. Its unique mechanism of action has rendered atovaquone efficacious even against multidrug-resistant strains of malaria. In trials, atovaquone combined with proguanil or tetracycline produced radical cures in patients infected with drug-resistant *P. falciparum*. This drug is also efficacious for the treatment of *Pneumocystis carinii* and *Toxoplasma gondii* (discussed later), both of which are particularly problematic in the acquired immunodeficiency syndrome (AIDS) patient.

Trichomoniasis

Trichomoniasis is caused by a flagellated protozoan, *Trichomonas vaginalis*. This is a sexually transmitted disease, resulting in vaginitis in females and urethritis and prostatovesiculitis in males. Infected males often remain asymptomatic, thereby acting as reservoirs for the organism. Thus, it is important that both an infected female and her sexual partner be treated for trichomoniasis once it is diagnosed.

Treatment

The drug of choice for treating trichomoniasis in both males and females is metronidazole. The mechanism of action of this drug involves its enzymatic reduction of the nitro group —this occurs within the parasite. Once metabolized to reactive intermediates, cytotoxicity results, probably due to the binding of the intermediates to parasite DNA. Metronidazole is well-tolerated orally, and is rapidly absorbed. It is then distributed to tissues and reaches therapeutic concentrations in the semen, vaginal secretions, and breast milk. The drug is cleared by oxidative metabolism in the liver and is excreted in the urine, which may become reddish-brown.

Side Effects and Other Considerations

Side effects associated with metronidazole are usually mild and include nausea, anorexia, diarrhea, epigastric pain, and cramping. More serious side effects include neurotoxicity and numbness in the extremities, but these are rare. Metronidazole causes a disulfiram-like reaction when alcohol is consumed, so the patient must be warned to avoid alcohol while using the drug. Additionally, the drug should not be given to pregnant women in the first trimester.

Metronidazole has a broad spectrum of activity against invading organisms. It is effective against trichomoniasis, amebiasis, giardiasis, and certain strains of obligate anaerobic bacteria.

Amebiasis

By far the most clinically important species of ameba in humans is *Entamoeba histolytica*. This organism is distributed throughout the world, and affects 2–4% of the U.S. population. The disease is spread via fecal-oral contact with the cyst form of the amebae. One may come into contact with the cysts through water, fruits or vegetables contaminated with infective feces, or through direct contact with an infective cyst-passer. The pathological course that the disease may take is illustrated in Figure 43–3. Many individuals who pass infective cysts are asymptomatic or only mildly symptomatic. In these patients (known as carriers), liver abscesses eventually form, but this often results in little or no clinical distress. In other individuals, however, amebiasis may progress to severe dysentery which, left untreated, could be fatal. In these cases, hepatic amebiasis, including amebic hepatitis and abscesses of the liver, is common.

BOX 43–5

TREATMENT OF AMEBIASIS

Once the infective cyst is ingested by the host, it migrates to the lower small bowel, where its wall dissolves, releasing eight trophozoites. These move to

BOX 43-5
TREATMENT OF AMEBIASIS (*Continued*)

the large intestine, where they replicate and may form cysts that pass out in the feces. In some cases, the trophozoites may become invasive, penetrating the intestine and forming ulcerative lesions. Abscesses may form in the liver or in other organs. The treatment of infection caused by *E. histolytica* depends on the lifecycle stage of the parasite.

Luminal amebicides are active against trophozoites and are used to treat mild or asymptomatic forms of the disease. Systemic amebicides are used to treat invasive forms of amebiasis, particularly in cases of amebic dysentery or hepatic abscesses. Mixed amebicides are active against both the invasive and noninvasive forms of the disease. Examples of each of these drugs include luminal amebicides, diloxanide furoate and paromomycin; systemic amebicides, chloroquine and dehydroemetine; and the mixed amebicide, metronidazole.

Treatment

DILOXANIDE FUROATE. Diloxanide furoate is orally effective for the treatment of amebiasis, although its mechanism of action is unknown. It is a drug of choice for asymptomatic cyst-passers, but it can be combined with metronidazole in cases of systemic amebiasis. Diloxanide is well-tolerated and is metabolized to the glucuronide in the liver. Side effects associated with its use are generally mild and may include vomiting, diarrhea, and flatulence. In the United States, the drug is available only from the Parasitic Disease Drug Service, Centers for Disease Control.

CHLOROQUINE. Although ineffective against luminal amebiasis, chloroquine is highly efficacious against hepatic abscesses that result from infection. The drug is concentrated in the liver, but can be used with a luminal amebicide to treat both invasive and noninvasive forms of the disease. Chloroquine was discussed in greater detail under antimalarial drugs in this chapter.

DEHYDROEMETINE. This drug is rarely used as a systemic amebicide; its use is limited to cases where metronidazole is contraindicated.

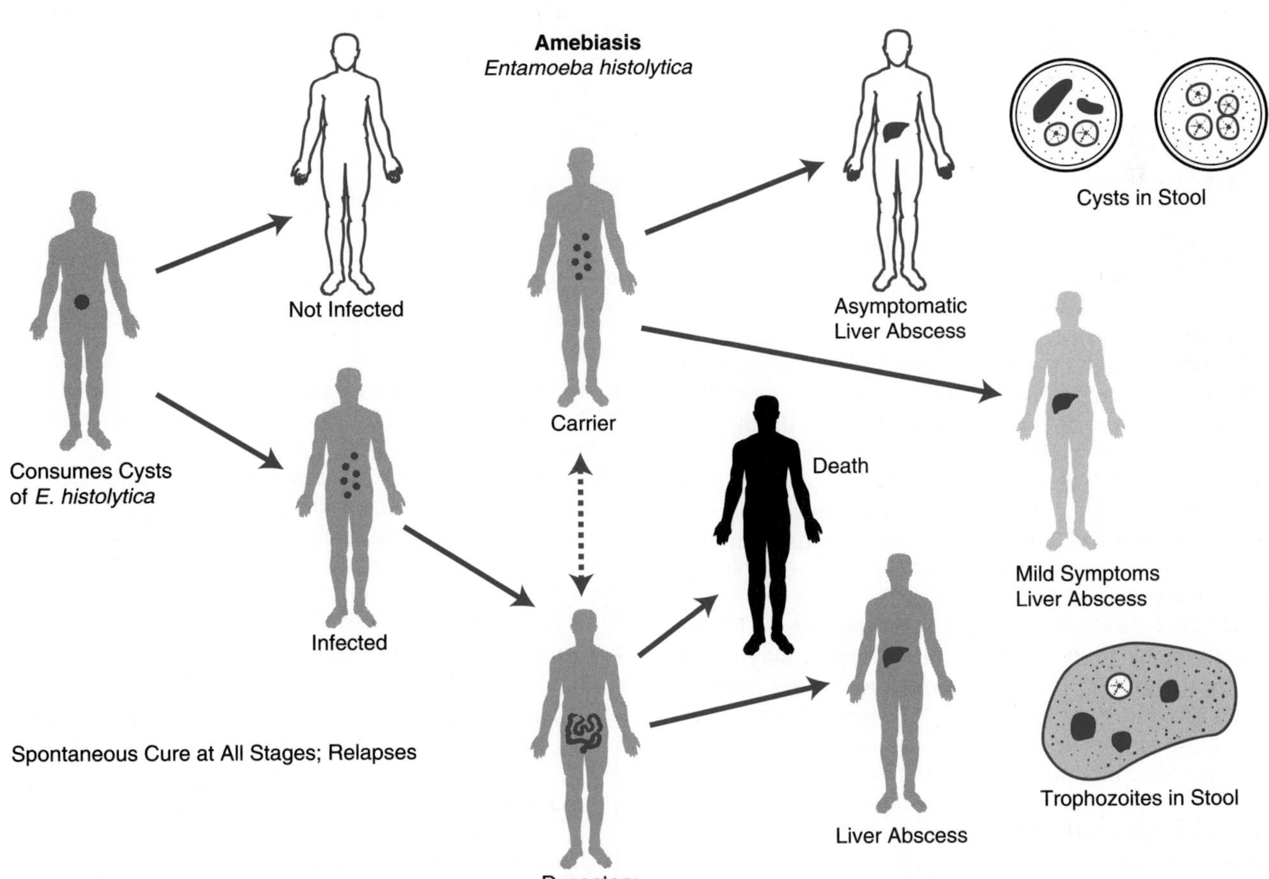

FIGURE 43-3. Possible pathological courses of infection with *Entamoeba histolytica*.

METRONIDAZOLE. Metronidazole is the drug of choice for all cases of symptomatic amebiasis; it is not used for asymptomatic cyst passers. Uses and side effects associated with the use of metronidazole were discussed under trichomoniasis in this chapter.

PAROMOMYCIN. This drug is an aminoglycoside antibiotic. It is poorly absorbed from the gastrointestinal tract and, as such, it reaches high concentrations in the lumen of the intestine. Thus, it is an effective luminal amebicide.

Giardiasis

Giardiasis is caused by the flagellated protozoan *Giardia lamblia.* This disease is the most common intestinal protozoan infection in the United States and is spread by the oral-fecal route. Typically, feces-contaminated water or fresh vegetation are carriers for the infective cysts. Once ingested, the cysts form trophozoites that may cause severe diarrhea, malabsorption, and significant weight loss. Children and the immunocompromised are especially prone to the acute or chronic gastrointestinal symptoms. In immunocompetent adults, the asymptomatic cyst-passer is usually seen.

Treatment

A drug that is highly effective against giardiasis is quinacrine. This agent was developed as an antimalarial, but is highly efficacious against *G. lamblia.* It is well-absorbed after oral administration, but it is not well-tolerated. Side effects associated with the use of this drug include vomiting, headaches, exfoliative dermatitis, urticaria, and dizziness.

Metronidazole is increasingly used for the treatment of giardiasis, primarily because this broad-spectrum antiprotozoal is well-tolerated.

Leishmaniasis

Leishmaniasis in humans is caused by three species of Leishmania: *L. donovani*, *L. tropica*, and *L. braziliensis.* The disease is spread by a sandfly vector, which passes the infective stage to humans during a blood meal. Once in the host, these organisms multiply within mononuclear and polymorphonuclear macrophages, as well as in cells of the reticuloenothelial system. The three species of parasite cause distinct pathology and differ in their geographic distribution and species of vector. The three forms of leishmaniasis and their causitive agents are *L. donovani*, which causes visceral leishmaniasis (kala-azar); *L. tropica*, which causes cutaneous leishmaniasis (oriental sore); and *L. braziliensis*, which causes mucocutaneous leishmaniasis.

Of the three species, *L. donovani* is responsible for the most significant pathology. All internal organs may be affected, but the liver, spleen, and bone marrow are severely compromised. If left untreated, kala-azar is always fatal. Disease resulting from infection with *L. tropica* or *L. braziliensis* is usually self-limiting, but often lesions are located on the face or head and can be terribly disfiguring. Treatment of leishmaniasis is difficult because the available drugs are quite toxic and not very effective; however, recovery from kala-azar and oriental sore gives a lasting immunity.

Treatment

HEAVY METALS. Therapy for leishmaniasis has relied on the heavy metals, particularly sodium stibogluconate. The mechanism of action of this agent is unknown, but it may act by inhibiting parasite enzymes with essential sulfhydryl groups. Sodium stibogluconate is given only by intravenous or intramuscular injection. After intravenous injection, about 80% of the drug is excreted by the kidneys within 6 hours. In the United States, the drug is available from the Parasitic Disease Drug Service, Centers for Disease Control.

Side Effects and Other Considerations. Sodium stibogluconate, being a heavy metal poison, is a fairly toxic drug. Its main side effects include pain at the injection site, joint pain, and gastrointestinal distress. In some cases, renal and hepatic failure may result. Currently, stibogluconate encapsulated into liposomes is being tested for efficacy against leishmaniasis. Because the liposomes would be selectively taken up by infected mononuclear cells, systemic side effects should be greatly reduced.

AMPHOTERICIN B. This antifungal agent has some efficacy against leishmaniasis. However, its use is also associated with a number of severe side effects, including renal failure.

NEW AGENTS FOR THE TREATMENT OF LEISHMANIASIS. Currently, a number of drugs are undergoing clinical trials to determine their efficacy against this disease. Among these are allopurinol, which is used to treat gout; imipramine and 3-chloroimipramine, antidepressants that are being tested in a liposome-encapsulated form; and primaquine, an antimalarial. For the treatment of cutaneous leishmaniasis, topical ointments are being developed. One of these, which contains paromomycin and methyl benzithonium chloride, has been shown to be effective in over 95% of patients in certain clinical trials (Croft, 1988).

Trypanosomiasis

Two forms of trypanosomiasis affect humans; namely, African trypanosomiasis and American trypanosomiasis (Chagas' disease). African trypanosomiasis is characterized by

- Transmission is via the tsetse fly.
- The disease is caused by two subspecies of *Trypanosoma brucei.*
- *T. brucei rhodesiense* causes a rapidly progressing and usually fatal form of the disease.
- *T. brucei gambiense* causes a chronic form of the disease called sleeping sickness.

American trypanosomiasis is characterized by

- Transmission is via blood-feeding reduviid bugs.
- The disease is caused by *T. cruzi.*
- Chagas' disease results in destruction of myocardial cells and neurons of the myenteric plexus.

Treatment

The majority of drugs available for the treatment of trypanosomiasis are effective only against the African forms of the disease. As a rule, all of the drugs used are highly toxic and cause significant side effects in the patient.

MELARSOPROL. This agent is a heavy metal poison effective against African trypanosomiasis. Its mechanism of action is unknown, but it is thought to inhibit enzymes with essential sulfhydryl groups. The drug is administered only to hospitalized patients by intravenous infusion. A small amount of the drug crosses the blood-brain barrier, and thus it is effective in treating the disease even after it has reached the CNS. Side effects associated with the use of melarsoprol are many and may be severe. They include fever, encephalopathy, and hypersensitivity reactions. Hemolytic anemia may be seen in patients with a glucose-6-phosphate dehydrogenase deficiency.

PENTAMIDINE. For the treatment of African trypanosomiasis, pentamidine is given by intramuscular or intravenous injection. It can be used as a prophylactic agent for African trypanosomiasis, with doses repeated every 6 months. Pentamidine does not cross the blood-brain barrier; as a result, it is virtually ineffective for the treatment of *T. brucei rhodesiense*, which progresses to the CNS rapidly, but it is effective against *T. brucei gambiense* only in the early stages of the disease, before CNS involvement is apparent. The mechanism of action of the drug in the parasite is unknown, but may involve binding of pentamidine to parasite DNA. The drug has many side effects, including tachycardia, dizziness, vomiting, rash, fatal hypoglycemia, and renal dysfunction.

SURAMIN. Suramin is most effective as a prophylactic agent against African trypanosomiasis. It does not penetrate the CNS, so it is not used for the treatment of *T. brucei rhodesiense* or for late stages of infection due to *T. brucei gambiense.* Side effects associated with the use of this drug are many; thus it is not recommended for prophylaxis in the infrequent or short-term traveler to regions where the disease is endemic. Serious effects include nausea, vomiting, shock, and unconsciousness. Other common adverse effects are fever, skin rashes, and neurotoxicity.

EFLORNITHINE. The most recent advance in the treatment of African trypanosomiasis is the drug eflornithine. This drug is a selective, irreversible inhibitor of parasite ornithine decarboxylase, an enzyme necessary for the synthesis of polyamines. In the trypanosome, polyamines are needed for the formation of trypanothione, a cellular nucleophile that protects the organism from reactive oxygen species. Polyamines are also needed for the synthesis of DNA, RNA, and proteins. Eflornithine is selectively toxic to the trypanosome because the turnover rate of ornithine decarboxylase is very slow in the parasite (several days) compared to that in mammalian cells (20 – 30 minutes). Rapid enzyme synthesis in the host cells allows for a rescue from the drug effect. The drug is administered intravenously in four divided doses over a 2-week period. It is effective against both *T. brucei gambiense* and *T. brucei rhodesiense.* Interestingly, it has been found to be particularly effective in arousing comatose sleeping sickness patients — it has thus been called the resurrection drug (WHO Report, 1990).

NIFURTIMOX. The only available agent with limited efficacy against *T. cruzi* is nifurtimox. This nitroheterocyclic drug exerts its effect by forming free radicals such as superoxide and hydrogen peroxide within the parasite. Because *T. cruzi* lacks catalase and peroxidase, it is extremely sensitive to these reactive compounds. Nifurtimox is given orally and is well-absorbed from the gastrointestinal tract. In the treatment of acute Chagas' disease, daily drug therapy must be continued for 75 days; chronic disease is less responsive to the drug and requires a 120-day course. Unfortunately, nifurtimox use is associated with many side effects, and these may be serious enough to consider withdrawal of the drug. Among these are nausea, vomiting, and malaise. With long-term use, peripheral neuropathy, weight loss, and hypersensitivity reactions may occur. Nifurtimox is also immunosuppressive. If left untreated, however, the cardiac pathology associated with Chagas' disease is usually fatal, so nifurtimox use is generally warranted.

Other Protozoal Infections

A variety of other parasitic protozoa can infect humans. Typically, the infections caused by these organisms are mild and self-limiting, so the diseases are not clinically as relevant. However, as more is learned about the immune response to parasitic diseases, it is increasingly recognized that diseases that may be innocuous in the immunocompetent individual may be devastating to the immunocompromised patient. Among these are infections caused by *Pneumocystis carinii*, *Toxoplasma gondii*, Cryptosporidium spp., and *Isospora belli.*

Patients with HIV are particularly at risk for chronic manifestations of otherwise self-limiting diseases caused by these organisms. An acute flare-up of these diseases is easily treated, but in the HIV patient, treatment for any one of these protozoa will mean maintenance doses of antiprotozoal drugs for the lifetime of the individual.

Pneumocystis carinii

Pneumocystis carinii causes a highly fatal pneumonia. This organism is an opportunist and is seen primarily in patients with underlying disease such as leukemia, Hodgkin's lymphoma, or HIV. It may also be seen in transplant patients or others receiving corticosteroids as immunosuppressive therapy. The treatment of pneumocystis pneumonia relies on sulfa antibiotics, intravenous pentamidine, or atovaquone.

Toxoplasma gondii

Toxoplasma gondii grows in any mammalian or avian organ. The disease may be contracted from raw or undercooked meat, or from contact with infected cat feces. Typically, disease manifestations are rare, but transplacental transmission of the infection can occur. In neonates, the disease may be fatal, with cerebral lesions, spasticity, and pathology of the retina. In the patient with HIV, CNS lesions, pneumonia, or hepatitis may be indicators of toxoplasmosis. Treatment for this disease is a combination of sulfadiazine and pyrimethamine or sulfadiazine plus clindamycin.

Cryptosporidium

Cryptosporidium spp. usually cause a mild diarrheal disease in humans. The organism is carried by a wide variety of hosts, and may be transmitted to man via water or improperly prepared food products. In the immunocompromised individual, cryptosporidiosis can cause a protracted diarrhea. There is no known treatment for this organism, although paromomycin has had some efficacy in patients with HIV.

Isospora belli

Isospora belli has a worldwide distribution. The organism inhabits the small intestine where it causes slight pathology, usually seen as diarrheal disease. Again, the immunocompromised individual is at risk for developing chronic diarrhea due to infection. In these cases, sulfa antibiotics have been efficacious in treating the disease.

REFERENCES

Campbell WC (ed): Ivermectin and Abamectin. New York: Springer-Verlag, 1989.

Cook GC: Use of benzimidazole chemotherapy in human helminthiases: Indications and efficacy. Parasitol Today 6:133-136, 1990.

Croft SL: Recent development in the chemotherapy of leishmaniasis. Trends Pharmacol Sci 9:376-381, 1988.

Hudson AT: Atovaquone—a novel broad spectrum anti-infective drug. Parasitol Today 9:66-68, 1993.

Krogstad DJ, Gluzman IY, Kyle DE, et al: Efflux of chloroquine from Plasmodium falciparum: Mechanism of chloroquine resistance. Science 238: 1283-1285, 1987.

Lacey E: Mode of action of the benzimidazoles. Parasitol Today 6:112-115, 1990.

Medical Letter: Drugs for parasitic infections. Med Lett Drugs Ther 30:78, 1988.

Roos MH: The molecular nature of benzimidazole resistance in helminths. Parasitol Today 6:125-127, 1990.

World Health Organization: "Resurrection" drug approved. TDR News 34: 1-2, 1990.

Cancer Chemotherapy: Antineoplastic Drugs 44

Joseph R. Bertino

The modern era of cancer chemotherapy began after World War II with the introduction of nitrogen mustard, an alkylating agent developed for clinical use as a consequence of the hematopoietic toxicity encountered with sulfur mustard (a war gas) and aminopterin, a folate antagonist. These compounds produced dramatic remissions in patients with lymphoma and in children with acute lymphocytic leukemia. Unfortunately, cures were not obtained, due to the rapid development of drug resistance, a problem that has been noted with single-agent treatment using each new drug introduced into the clinic.

These encouraging results were followed by a vigorous anticancer drug development program, especially in the United States, and were fostered by support and screening facilities provided by the National Cancer Institute for academic and industrial researchers. Since this time over 30 drugs have been approved for use in treating patients with malignancies. Based on principles derived mainly from treatment of rodent tumors, combination regimens have been devised that cure a majority of patients with choriocarcinoma, testicular cancer, acute lymphocytic leukemia, certain childhood solid tumors, and several types of lymphoma, including Hodgkin's disease, large cell lymphoma, and Burkitt's lymphoma.

Cure is also obtained with combination treatment in patients with other tumors such as ovarian cancer and acute myelocytic leukemia, but these cure rates are only in the range of 10–20%. Other diseases are less susceptible to treatment with chemotherapeutic drugs, although effective palliation and prolongation of survival may be obtained in some.

Another important use of chemotherapy that has evolved over the past 20 years is in the adjuvant situation. In this circumstance drugs are administered either before (neo-adjuvant) definitive treatment (surgery and or X-ray treatment), or following definitive treatment. Encouraging results have been obtained in patients with breast cancer and recently in patients with colon cancer treated in this manner.

PRINCIPLES OF CHEMOTHERAPY

Doses and schedules are important for successful chemotherapy. Studies in experimental tumors have clearly established that optimal antitumor effect occurs when doses used are the highest achievable, consistent with host tolerance. In recent years the term "dose intensity" has been employed to define the amount of drug delivered per unit time, usually in milligrams per square meter per week. For certain drugs, such as alkylating agents that are not very schedule dependent, dose intensity delivered directly relates to treatment outcome. In most tumors in which cure is possible, this issue becomes a critical one, and less than optimal dosing may result in treatment failure.

In most human tumors that are curable by combination chemotherapy, a certain subset of patients, usually with advanced, bulky tumors, are not effectively treated by these programs. The possibility of curing even this subset of patients by increasing dose intensity using autologous marrow rescue and or hematopoietic growth factors (G-CSF, GM-CSF, IL3, and so forth) is under active investigation in many centers. Preliminary results in chemotherapy-sensitive tumors (lymphoma, acute leukemia, testicular cancer) are encouraging. This approach is also being attempted for patients with other malignancies not usually cured by chemotherapy (*eg*, breast cancer, low-grade lymphoma). It is too early to tell if this aggressive treatment policy will benefit these patients.

In most cases, combination chemotherapy is necessary for optimal results. As mentioned earlier, drug resistance occurs rapidly when treatment with a single drug is used. The introduction of combination chemotherapy for acute lymphocytic leukemia (ALL) and Hodgkin's disease in the 1960s was an outgrowth of experimental studies that showed that combination of effective drugs gave additive cell kill, and delayed or prevented drug resistance. Drugs are used in combination when the dose-limiting toxicity of one drug is nonoverlapping with the other, and if evidence has been obtained in experimental tumors that the combination gives additive or synergistic antitumor effects. When two drugs are combined that both have bone marrow suppression as the limiting toxicity, it is usually possible to use each drug at two thirds of the optimum dose without increasing toxicity. If both drugs are equally effective, the combination increases dose intensity by 1.5×. There may also be important reasons to sequence the use of drugs in combination, especially if one drug is used to modulate or increase the activity of a second drug. An example is the methotrexate-5-fluorouracil sequence used to treat colorectal carcinoma. An increase in the response rate was noted when methotrexate administration preceded fluorouracil treatment by 24 hours, as compared with the results obtained when both drugs were administered together.

The disadvantage of combination chemotherapy is that the assumption is that both (or more than two) drugs are equally effective. If not, less tumor cell kill may result, because the dose of the most effective drug is decreased. When toxicity occurs, it may be difficult to adjust subsequent drug doses, because the major offending agent may not be known.

During more recent years, the idea of using alternating cycles of chemotherapy of two or more drug combinations has been tested in the clinic. This concept derived from theoretical modeling that showed that drug-resistant cells were less likely to survive alternating drug combinations as compared with repeated dosing with a fixed drug combination. Another approach now under investigation is the sequential use of combinations: the first combination is used until a maximal response is obtained (usually several months) followed by treatment with several courses of the second combination. The second combination is used at the time when there are theoretically only few resistance cells remaining. If there is no cross-resistance to the drugs of the first combination, the second combination treatment may eradicate cells surviving the treatment with the first combination.

DRUG RESISTANCE

The major obstacle to cure with chemotherapeutic agents is survival and proliferation of cells that are resistant to further treatment. A great deal has been learned in the past 15 years of the genetic mechanisms that cause cells to become resistant to various drugs (Table 44–1). There is often more than one resistance mechanism that may allow a cell to survive increasing concentrations of a drug. Resistance occurring after a tumor population has been initially susceptible is called acquiring resistance. Some tumors may not be initially responsive to a drug, that is, they are intrinsically resistant. Presumably, this difference reflects the number of cells in the population that are resistant. When there is good tumor regression (*eg*, complete responses) to treatment, the frequency of mutant cells that have a resistant phenotype may be low (1 in 10^6). In tumor populations naturally resistant to a drug (*ie*, no or minimal tumor regression), a substantial number of tumor cells may have a resistant phenotype (*ie*, greater than 10%).

An important new development in the understanding of drug resistance has been the elucidation of a type of resistance called multidrug resistance (MDR).

MDR resistance may be acquired or intrinsic in tumors —its importance derives from the finding that resistance to any one of several drugs (usually alkaloids: vinca alkaloids, anthracyclines, etoposide, actinomycin D) results in cross-resistance to all of the other drugs that share this phenotype. The basis of this form of resistance is the presence of a protein (P-glycoprotein) that is capable of rapidly effluxing MDR-type drugs, thus protecting the cells from damage by preventing these drugs from reaching their intracellular targets.

CYCLE-ACTIVE AND NON-CYCLE-ACTIVE AGENTS

Cycle-active agents are drugs that require a cell to be "in cycle," *ie*, actively going through the cell cycle preparatory to cell division in order to be cytotoxic. Some of these drugs are effective primarily against cells in one of the phases of the cell cycle (*ie*, G_1, S, G_2, or M). The importance of this des-

TABLE 44–1. Mechanisms of Drug Resistance to Anticancer Agents

Mechanism	Examples
Insufficient drug uptake	Methotrexate, nitrogen mustard
Increased drug efflux	MDR drugs: vinca alkaloids, anthracyclines, etoposide
Insufficient drug activation	5-Fluorouracil, 6-mercaptopurine
Increased inactivation	Cytosine arabinoside
Increased target enzyme	Methotrexate
Altered target enzyme	Methotrexate (dihydrofolate reductase)
	Etoposide (topoisomerase II)
Increased repair of DNA damage	Cisplatin

MDR = multidrug resistance.

TABLE 44-2. Phases of the Cell Cycle and Drug Effects

Phase	Description	Drug Sensitivity
G_0	Resting stage (not in cycle)	X-rays Alkylating agents
G_1	RNA synthesis	Alkylating agents Actinomycin D
S	DNA, RNA, protein synthesis	Antimetabolites
G_2	RNA, protein synthesis	Bleomycin
M	Mitosis	Vinca alkaloids Taxol

ignation is that "cell cycle-active agents" are usually schedule-dependent, and that duration of exposure is as important and usually more important than dose. In contrast, non-cell cycle-active agents are usually not schedule-dependent, and effects depend on the total dose administered, regardless of the schedule. Alkylating agents are generally considered to be non-cycle-active, whereas antimetabolites are prototypes of cycle-active compounds (Table 44-2).

THE FUTURE OF CHEMOTHERAPY

Optimal use of these agents requires a thorough knowledge of chemotherapy principles, the mechanism of action, and pharmacology (pharmacokinetics and risk/benefit). Many of these drugs have both acute and long-term toxicities. Efforts to reduce these toxicities have followed two major avenues—developing analogs that have fewer of these toxicities, or decreasing toxicity by the use of other agents. Progress has been made in both directions, and less toxic analogs of cisplatin (carboplatin) and doxorubicin (mitoxantrone) are examples of the first approach, whereas development of antinausea medication (*eg*, metoclopramide) and protective agents (*eg*, mesna for ifosfamide toxicity) are examples of the second approach.

Our knowledge of the role of oncogenes (growth factors) in normal and abnormal growth, as well as the role of the immune system in controlling abnormal cell growth, has markedly increased, and the latter half of the 1990s will see the introduction into the clinic of new types of treatment that may be more selective and possibly less toxic. Because this field is investigational and no products other than interferon have been approved for use yet, we will not discuss them further in this chapter.

ANTIMETABOLITES

Methotrexate

The folate antagonist aminopterin was the first antimetabolite shown to induce complete remissions in children with ALL. Unfortunately it was soon appreciated by Farber and his associates that these remissions were short-lived, and the patients' leukemia became resistant to subsequent courses of this drug. In the 1950s, methotrexate (amethopterin, MTX) supplanted aminopterin in the clinic, based on experimental studies showing that it has an improved therapeutic index as compared to aminopterin. The structure of folic acid, aminopterin, and methotrexate is shown in Figure 44-1.

MECHANISM OF ACTION. Methotrexate and aminopterin are analogs of the vitamin folic acid. The major mechanism of action of MTX is to powerfully inhibit the enzyme dihydrofolate reductase (DHFR). As a consequence of this inhibition, intracellular folate coenzymes are rapidly depleted (by blocking uptake of reduced folates, restoration of folate stores is also impaired). Because folate coenzymes are required for thymidylate biosynthesis as well as purine biosynthesis, DNA synthesis is blocked and cell replication stops.

More recent work has shown that MTX is retained in certain cells for long periods of time, as a consequence of an enzymatic process that adds additional glutamates (up to five) to the antifolate. This may be an important determinant of MTX selectivity because cells capable of this conversion (*eg*, lymphoblasts) may be expected to be more susceptible to cell kill by this drug.

Acquired resistance to MTX in patients with leukemia has been shown to be due to increased levels of dihydrofolate reductase as a consequence of gene amplification, defective polyglutamylation, and impaired uptake of this drug. Alterations of DHFR enzyme leading to decreased binding of MTX have not yet been reported.

CLINICAL USES. MTX continues to be a key drug in the treatment of acute lymphocytic leukemia, choriocarcinoma, and in combination therapy of intermediate-grade and high-grade lymphomas, breast cancer, head and neck cancer, and bladder cancer.

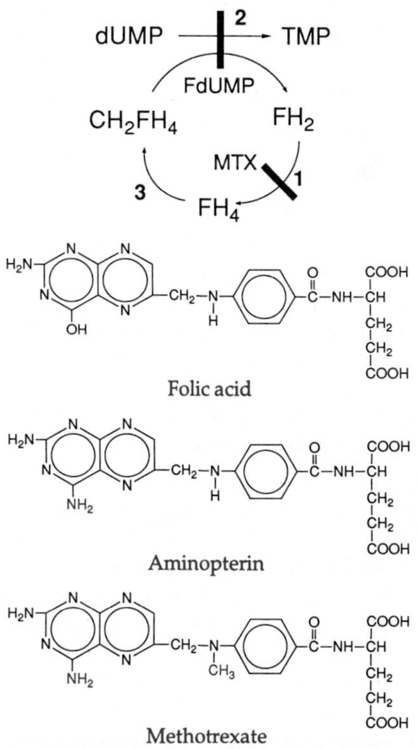

FIGURE 44-1. Sites of action of methotrexate (MTX) and the fluoropyrimidine antimetabolite, fluorodeoxyuridylate (FdUMP); (1) DHFR, dihydrofolate reductase; (2) TS, thymidylate synthase; (3) SHM, serine hydroxymethylate; FH_2, dihydrofolate; FH_4, tetrahydrofolate; CH_2FH_4, N^5,N^{10}-methylenetetrahydrofolate. Also shown are the structures of folic acid, aminopterin, and methotrexate. (TMP = thymidine 5′-monophosphate.)

TABLE 44–3. Antimetabolites

Drug	Route Administered	Pharmacokinetics	Indications	Toxicity: *Acute*	Toxicity: *Long-term*
FOLIC ACID ANTAGONISTS					
Methotrexate	PO, IV, SC, IM, Intrathecally May be used in high dose with folinic acid (leucovorin) "rescue"	$t_{1/2}\beta = 3-4$ hours Excreted mainly unchanged in urine; metabolized to 7-hydroxy-methotrexate	Acute lymphocytic leukemia Breast cancer Choriocarcinoma Head and neck cancer	Myelosuppression Mucositis Skin rash (10%)	Rare: liver fibrosis
PYRIMIDINE ANTAGONISTS					
5-Fluorouracil	IV, bolus weekly, daily by continuous infusion	$t_{1/2}\beta = 10-15$ minutes rapidly metabolized by liver	Breast cancer Colon cancer Head and neck cancer	Myelosuppression Mucositis, diarrhea Cerebellar toxicity (high doses)	
5-Fluorodeoxyuridine	Intra-arterially (hepatic artery)	Rapidly metabolized by liver	Colon cancer metastatic to liver	Liver toxicity	Biliary sclerosis (5–10%)
Cytosine arabinoside	IV, intrathecal, rapidly metabolized ($t_{1/2}\beta = 7-20$ min) to ara-uracil	Rapidly metabolized by deamination	Acute leukemia Lymphoma	Marrow suppression Nausea and vomiting CNS toxicity (high doses)	
PURINE ANTAGONISTS					
6-Mercaptopurine	PO	Metabolized by xanthine oxidase to 6-thiouric acid (inhibited by allopurinol)	Acute leukemia	Marrow suppression Occasional nausea and vomiting	Rare: cirrhosis
6-Thioguanine	PO, IV	Metabolized by initial methylation	Acute leukemia	Marrow suppression	
2′-Deoxycoformycin (pentostatin)	IV	$t_{1/2}\beta = 2.6-9.4$ hours; excreted unchanged in urine	T-cell lymphoma Hairy cell leukemia	Dose related: Acute renal failure CNS effects	
Fludarabine	IV		Chronic lymphocytic leukemia	Marrow suppression	
2-chlorodeoxyadenosine	IV	$t_{1/2}\beta = 7$ hours	Hairy cell leukemia Low-grade lymphoma	Marrow suppression T-cell depletion	
Hydroxyurea (hydroxycarbamide)	PO	Excreted mainly by kidney, unchanged	Chronic myelocytic leukemia	Leukopenia Nausea and vomiting (large doses)	

CNS = central nervous system; IM = intramuscularly; IV = intravenously; PO = orally; SC = subcutaneously.

CLINICAL PHARMACOLOGY. MTX is reasonably well absorbed by mouth when administered in low doses (5–10 mg), but when doses exceed 30 mg, progressively less of the drug is absorbed, with significant interpatient variation. Therefore, doses of MTX of 30 mg or greater should be administered intravenously (IV), intramuscularly (IM), or subcutaneously. The pharmacology and toxic effects of this drug are given in Table 44–3.

Fluoropyrimidines (5-fluorouracil and 5-fluorodeoxyuridine)

5-Fluorouracil (5-FU) was developed by Heidelberger and others as a consequence of the observation that uracil was salvaged more efficiently by certain malignant cells than by normal tissues.

MECHANISM OF ACTION. 5-Fluorouracil exerts its cytotoxic effects by inhibition of DNA synthesis, and/or by incorporation into RNA, thus inhibiting RNA processing and function. The active metabolite of 5-FU that inhibits DNA synthesis via potent inhibition of thymidylate synthetase is 5-fluorodeoxyuridylate (5-FdUMP). Conversion of 5-FU to 5-FdUMP occurs in cancer cells, a fact that contributes to its selective toxicity.

In rapidly growing tumors, inhibition of thymidylate synthase appears to be the key mechanism of cell death caused by 5-FU; however, in other tumors, cell death is better correlated with incorporation of 5-FU into RNA. Incorporation of 5FU into DNA can also occur, and may contribute to 5FU cytotoxicity. Recent studies indicate that the dose schedule of 5-FU may change its mechanism of action; that is, "pulse" 5-FU may kill cells via incorporation into RNA, whereas continuous-infusion 5FU may kill cells by inhibition of thymidylate synthesis.

CLINICAL USE. The principal use of 5-FU is for gastrointestinal (GI) tumors (colon, stomach) and breast cancer.

The ternary complex formed by FdUMP and the folate coenzyme, N^5, N^{10}-methylenetetrahydrofolate with thymidylate synthase has been noted to dissociate slowly, with a half-life of several hours. The presence of excess folate coenzyme ensures maximal ternary complex formation, and in addition retards the dissociation of FdUMP from the complex. Based on this understanding, recent clinical trials have employed high doses of leucovorin, a stable reduced folate precursor of N^5, N^{10}-methylenetetrahydrofolate, followed by 5-FU treatment, in the hope of maximizing ternary complex formation in malignant cells, and subsequent cell death. MTX pretreatment may also increase 5-FU cytotoxicity by inhibiting purine synthesis and thus increasing 5-phosphoribosyl-1-pyrophosphate (PRPP) levels in cells, thus increasing 5-FU nucleotide formation. In addition, inhibition of dihydrofolate reductase by MTX leads to an increase in dihydrofolate polyglutamates in cells, a folate that also enhances FdUMP binding to thymidylate synthase. Sequential MTX–5-FU treatment has led to an increase in response rate in certain solid tumors, notably colon cancer.

Other strategies to modulate 5-FU cytotoxicity are also being tested in the clinic; these include pretreatment with the *de novo* pyrimidine synthesis inhibitor phosphonacetyl-L-aspartate (PALA); the use of dipyridamole, an inhibitor of nucleoside salvage; and uridine "rescue."

CLINICAL PHARMACOLOGY. 5-FU is absorbed erratically after oral administration and therefore is administered intravenously. The clinical pharmacology of this drug is given in Table 44–3. Various dosage schedules of 5-FU have been investigated, including bolus treatment daily for 5 days once a month, weekly bolus treatment, and infusions lasting 24, 48, or 120 hours or longer.

Cytosine Arabinoside

Cytosine arabinoside (ara-C) is an antimetabolite analog of deoxycytidine.

MECHANISM OF ACTION. Cytosine arabinoside is converted intracellularly to the nucleotide triphosphate (ara CTP); this latter compound is an inhibitor of DNA polymerase and is also incorporated into DNA. The latter event is considered to cause the lethal action of ara-C because incorporation results in a defect in ligation of newly synthesized fragments of DNA.

Cytosine arabinoside and its mononucleotide are inactivated by two intracellular enzymes, cytidine deaminase and deoxycytidylate deaminase.

RESISTANCE MECHANISMS. Although several mechanisms for acquired resistance to ara-C have been elucidated in experimental tumor systems, an explanation for acquired resistance in leukemia cells of patients is still not clear. Deletion of deoxycytidine kinase, an increased pool size of dCTP, and increased activity of cytidine deaminase have been described to occur in ara-C–resistant cell lines. The level of intracellular ara-CTP formation in tumor cells has been reported to be useful in monitoring drug efficacy.

CLINICAL USE. Cytosine arabinoside is used in the treatment of acute leukemia (in combination with an anthracycline) and in the treatment of intermediate-grade or high-grade non-Hodgkin's lymphoma (in combination therapy).

There is some evidence that high doses (1–3 g/sq m) of cytosine arabinoside given at 12-hour intervals for 6 to 12 doses may be more effective alone or in a combination with anthracyclines than conventional doses (100–300 mg/sq m) in the treatment of acute myelocytic leukemia (AML).

CLINICAL PHARMACOLOGY. Cytosine arabinoside is administered IV as a pulse dose or a continuous infusion (Table 44–3). Ara-C is not active orally because of degradation by cytidine deaminase present in gastrointestinal epithelium and in the liver. The drug distributes rapidly into body water, and unlike many drugs, a high concentration (50% of the plasma level) may be reached in the cerebrospinal fluid (CSF) 2 hours after IV administration. As in the case of MTX, single-bolus infusions (over 0.5–1 hour) of doses as high as 5 g/sq m produce little marrow toxicity because of its rapid clearance whereas doses of 1 g/sq m over 48 hours produce severe marrow toxicity.

6-Mercaptopurine and 6-Thioguanine

The purine analogs 6-mercaptopurine (6-MP) and 6-thioguanine (6-TG), introduced into the clinic soon after methotrexate, are also key drugs in the curability of ALL.

Other important purine analogs have found a use in the clinic, including azathioprine, a 6-mercaptopurine "pro drug" that is a potent immunosuppressive agent; allopurinol, an inhibitor of xanthine oxidase, useful in the prevention of uric acid nephropathy; and antiviral compounds such as ara-adenine.

2-deoxycoformycin (pentostatin), a potent inhibitor of adenosine deaminase, has also been found to be a useful agent in the treatment of T cell malignancies. This compound, as well as 2-chloro-2′-deoxyadenosine have impressive activity in the treatment of a rare type of chronic leukemia (hairy cell leukemia). Fludarabine has been recently approved for use in the treatment of chronic lymphocytic leukemia (CLL). The structure of these compounds is shown in Figure 44–2.

MECHANISM OF ACTION. Both 6-MP and 6-TG have a thiol group substitution for the 6-oxo or 6-hydroxyl group found in hypoxanthine or guanine, respectively. Both compounds are converted to nucleotides by the enzyme hypoxanthine-guanine phosphoribosyl transferase (HPRT). *De novo* purine synthesis is blocked by the 6-thiopurine nucleotide (phosphoribosyl transferase), as well as the conversion of purine analogs. The nucleotides of both these drugs are also incorporated into DNA after conversion to the triphosphates. This incorporation may also contribute to the cytotoxic effects of the thiopurines.

RESISTANCE MECHANISMS. In experimental tumor cells, resistance is most commonly found to be a consequence of markedly decreased activity of the activating enzyme HPRT. In human ALL, resistance was found to be asso-

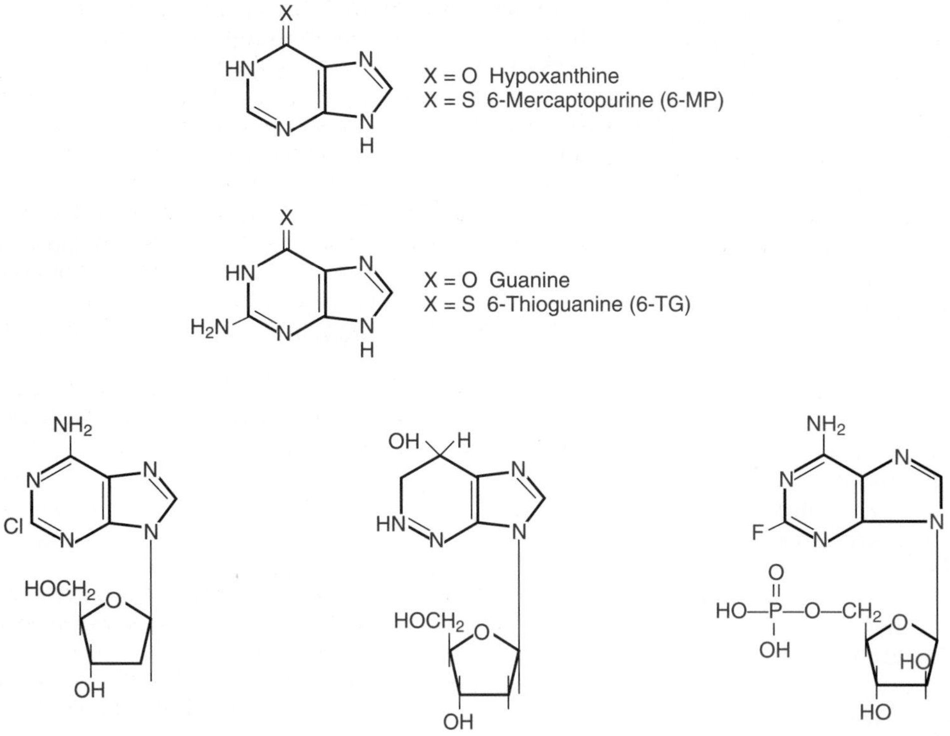

X = O Hypoxanthine
X = S 6-Mercaptopurine (6-MP)

X = O Guanine
X = S 6-Thioguanine (6-TG)

2-Chloro-2'-deoxyadenosine (CdA)

Pentostatin (2'-Deoxycoformycin [2'-DCF])

2-Fluoro-ara-AMP (Fludarabine)

FIGURE 44–2. Structure of purine analogs.

ciated with an increase in activity of alkaline phosphatase, found in membranes and capable of degrading on the nucleotides of the 6-thiopurines. Absence of HPRT activity was a rare cause of resistance in AML, and an alteration of this enzyme leading to decreased thiopurine binding to the enzyme was found in the blast cells of some patients.

CLINICAL PHARMACOLOGY. Both 6-TG and 6-MP are administered orally, although absorption may be erratic. These drugs differ in their catabolism, and as a consequence, metabolism of 6-MP but not 6-TG is inhibited by allopurinol.

6-Mercaptopurine is metabolized primarily by xanthine oxidase to 6-thiouric acid, which is inhibited by allopurinol, whereas 6-TG is principally methylated, followed eventually by oxidation and elimination of the sulfur moiety. *Therefore, a dosage reduction in 6-MP of 75% is recommended when allopurinol is used with 6-MP*; no dosage reduction is necessary when 6-TG and allopurinol are administered together.

Another difference between these two drugs is gastrointestinal toxicity; 6-TG causes less nausea and vomiting than 6-MP, presumably because of metabolism of this latter drug by the GI mucosa.

Hydroxyurea

MECHANISM OF ACTION. Hydroxyurea is an inhibitor of ribonucleotide reductase, the enzyme that converts ribonucleotides at the diphosphate level to deoxyribonucleotides. While not an antimetabolite in the true sense, that is, it is not a substrate analog, it is a cell cycle agent that acts in S-phase.

RESISTANCE MECHANISMS. Resistance to hydroxyurea occurs in experimental tumors as a consequence of an increase in ribonucleotide reductase activity and/or an alteration of this activity leading to decreased binding to the active site of the enzyme.

CLINICAL USE. Hydroxyurea has resurfaced as an excellent drug for the treatment of chronic myelogenous leukemia, and appears to be equally effective as busulfan, with potentially less toxicity. Hydroxyurea has also been used to lower the blast count rapidly during the blast crisis of chronic myelocytic leukemia (CML) and in patients with ALL.

CLINICAL PHARMACOLOGY. The clinical pharmacology and toxicity of this drug are shown in Table 44–3.

TUBULIN INHIBITORS

The structures of the tubulin inhibitors are shown in Figure 44–3. These compounds are all plant alkaloids.

The Vinca Alkaloids

Of the three vinca alkaloids tested extensively in the 1970s and 1980s—vinblastine, vincristine, and vindesine—only the former two are now available for use in the United States.

MECHANISM OF ACTION. The vinca alkaloids exert their cytotoxic action through binding to tubulin, a dimeric protein found in the cytoplasm of cells. Microtubules are essential for forming the spindle along which the chromosomes migrate during mitosis, and for maintaining cell struc-

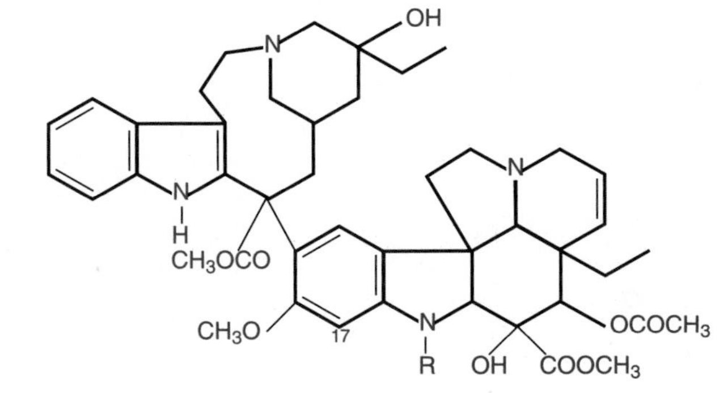

Vinblastine R = CH_3
Vincristine R = CHO

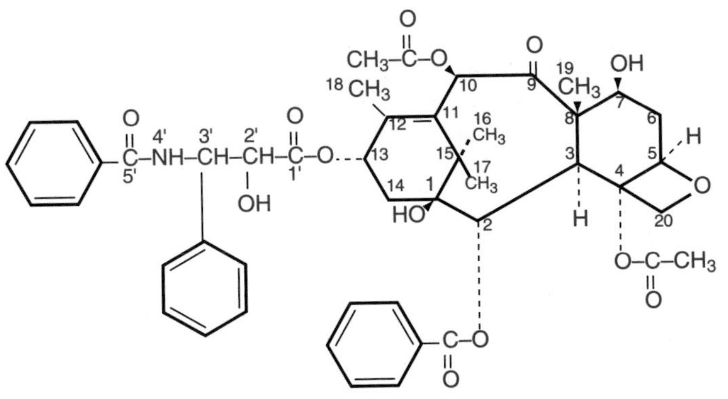

Paclitaxel (TAXOL)

FIGURE 44–3. Structure of tubulin inhibitors.

ture. Binding of the vinca alkaloids to tubulin leads to inhibition of the process of assembly and dissolution of the mitotic spindle. As a consequence, cells are arrested in metaphase, although some studies indicate that cell kill also occurs in late S phase.

RESISTANCE MECHANISMS. Resistance to the vinca alkaloids has been shown in experimental cells to be associated with other drugs sharing the MDR phenotype and related to increased efflux of these drugs. Resistance has also been reported to be a consequence of mutations in tubulin, leading to decreased binding of the vinca alkaloids to this protein.

CLINICAL USE. These drugs are used widely in the treatment of hematological neoplasms: vinblastine because of its excellent activity in the treatment of Hodgkin's disease, and vincristine for its broad spectrum of activity in non-Hodgkin's as well as Hodgkin's disease, and in acute lymphocytic leukemia.

CLINICAL PHARMACOLOGY. Both vincristine and vinblastine are administered IV. Toxicity and indications for use of these drugs are given in Table 44–4.

Taxol

Taxol, recently approved for treatment of ovarian cancer, inhibits tubulin depolymerization. This drug also has significant activity in breast cancer and in lung cancer, and its use in these and other neoplasms is under study. The clinical pharmacology of this drug is given in Table 44–4.

TOPOISOMERASE INHIBITORS

Anthracyclines

The next four agents are all anthracyclines. Their structures are presented in Figure 44–4.

Daunorubicin

Daunorubicin, like the other anthracyclines discussed below, can intercalate into DNA, produce superoxide free radicals, and also bind to cell membranes. More recently, inhibition of topoisomerase II, important for DNA replication,

TABLE 44–4. Tubulin Inhibitors

Drug	Route Administered	Pharmacokinetics	Indications	Toxicity	
				Acute	*Long-term*
VINCA ALKALOIDS					
Vinblastine (VELBAN)	IV	$t_{1/2}\beta = 53$ minutes Metabolized by liver	Hodgkin's disease	Bone marrow suppression, chiefly leukopenia Mucositis at high doses Local toxicity if extravasation occurs	
Vincristine (ONCOVIN)	IV	$t_{1/2}\beta = 164$ minutes Metabolized by liver	Hodgkin's disease Lymphomas	Neurologic toxicity (peripheral neuropathy) Local toxicity if extravasation occurs	
TAXOL	IV	$t_{1/2}\beta = 5–17$ hours; extreme metabolism	Ovarian cancer Breast cancer	Neutropenia Neurologic toxicity	

IV = intravenously.

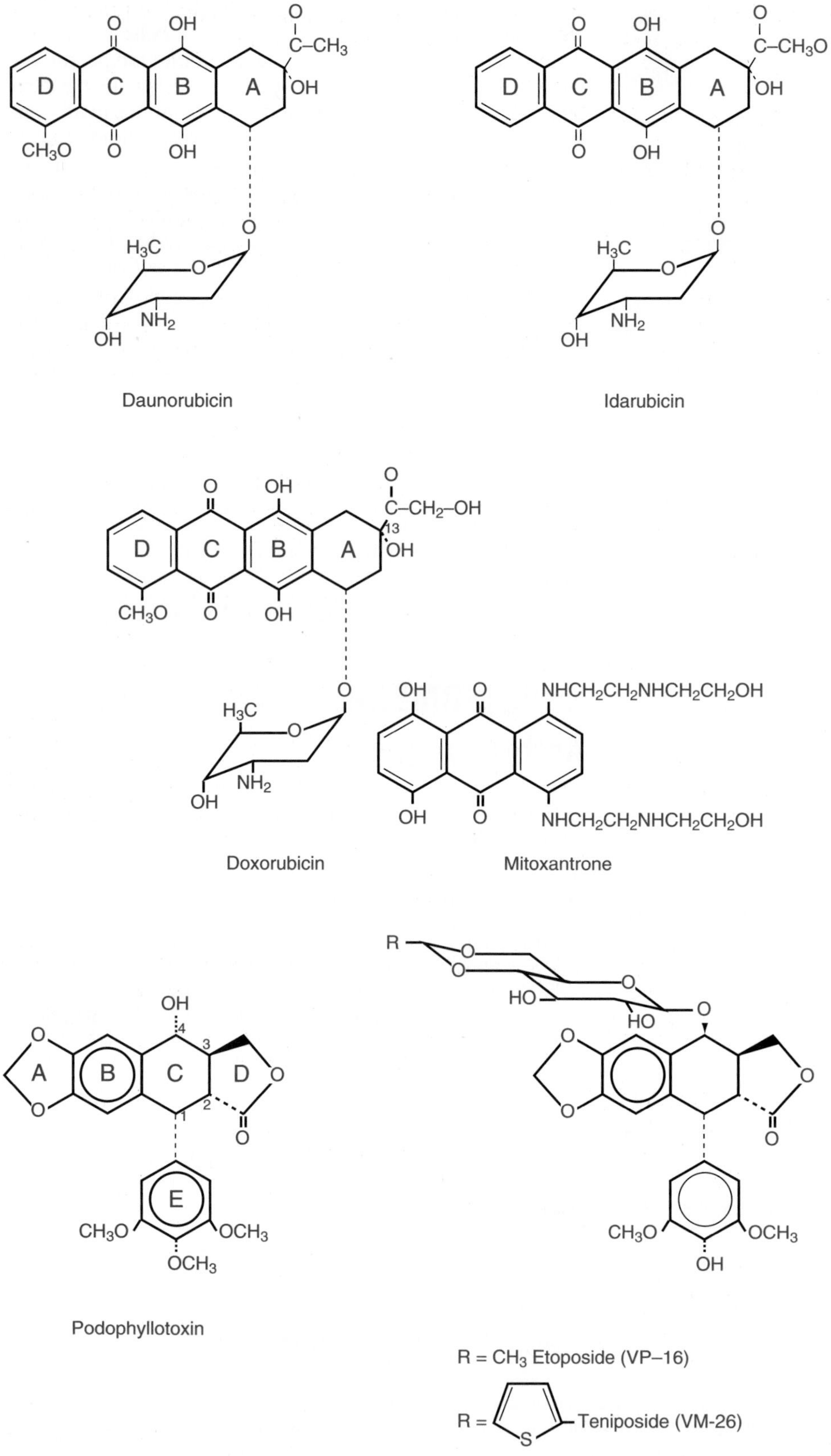

Daunorubicin

Idarubicin

Doxorubicin

Mitoxantrone

Podophyllotoxin

R = CH_3 Etoposide (VP–16)

R = (thienyl) Teniposide (VM-26)

FIGURE 44–4. Structure of topoisomerase II inhibitors.

has been implicated as its major mechanism of action. Generation of free radicals as a result of formation of a semiquinone intermediate may be the cause of the cardiotoxicity of this class of drugs.

The major use of daunorubicin is to treat acute leukemia, usually in combination with cytosine arabinoside.

The toxicities and clinical pharmacology of this drug are given in Table 44-5.

Doxorubicin

The mechanism of action and toxicities of doxorubicin are similar to daunorubicin (Table 44-5). Doxorubicin has a wide spectrum of antitumor activity, and is used to treat acute leukemia, lymphoma, small cell lung cancer, breast cancer, and sarcoma.

Idarubicin

Compared to daunorubicin, idarubicin is more lipophilic, and is taken up more rapidly into cells. It is also slightly more effective than daunorubicin or doxorubicin as an inhibitor of topoisomerase II. Idarubicin has recently been approved for use in the treatment of patients with AML.

Mitoxantrone

This synthetic anthracycline lacks the daunosamine sugar of the previously discussed compounds (Fig. 44-4). Its toxicity profile is less than doxorubicin in that alopecia and cardiac toxicity is less commonly observed. In comparative studies it appears to have equal efficacy in combination treatment of acute leukemia and lymphoma, but probably is less efficacious in the treatment of breast cancer.

Epipodophyllotoxins

Two glycosidic semisynthetic derivatives of podophyllotoxin have received extensive clinical trials. Etoposide (VP-16) and tenoposide (VM.26) are now available in the pharmacy. These structures are given in Figure 44-4. Both drugs inhibit activity of topoisomerase II.

Etoposide has significant clinical activity in Hodgkin's disease, diffuse aggressive lymphomas, leukemias and in small cell lung cancer. Tenoposide has been used primarily in combination with cytotosine arabinoside to treat children with ALL.

Etoposide may be administered either orally or IV. When administered orally, about 50% of the dose is absorbed; therefore, the dose should be increased twofold over the IV dosage. The clinical pharmacology of this drug is given in Table 44-5.

DRUGS THAT DAMAGE DNA

All the classes of drugs that are discussed in this section damage DNA by various mechanisms. Although the major mechanism of cytotoxicity is believed to occur as a consequence of this interaction, these agents usually have other sites of action and often react with other cellular targets, such as membranes. The classes of drugs that are discussed are alkylating agents, nitrosoureas, platinum compounds,

TABLE 44-5. Inhibitors of Topoisomerase II

				Toxicity	
Drug	**Route Administered**	**Pharmacokinetics**	**Indications**	***Acute***	***Long-term***
ANTHRACYCLINES					
Doxorubicin	IV	β elimination phase 30 hours; metabolized externally; elimination primarily biliary	Acute leukemia Lymphoma Breast cancer	Myelosuppression Alopecia Mucositis	Cardiac toxicity
Daunorubicin	IV	β phase 48 hours; metabolized to daunorubicinol	Acute leukemia	Myelosuppression Alopecia	Cardiac toxicity
Idarubicin	IV	$t_{1/2}\beta = 3-27$ hours, metabolized to IDR-ol; an alcohol that is also cytotoxic	Acute leukemia	Myelosuppression Alopecia	Cardiac toxicity
Mitoxantrone	IV	Metabolized extensively long-term β $t_{1/2}$	Acute leukemia Lymphoma Breast cancer	Myelosuppression	
EPIPODOPHYLLOTOXINS					
Etoposide (VP-16)	IV PO (50% absorbed)	50% metabolized, rest excreted unchanged in urine	Lung cancer Lymphoma Acute leukemia	Hypotension if administered too rapidly Bone marrow suppression Alopecia	2° acute leukemia

PO = orally; IV = intravenously.

and natural products, which include bleomycin, and actinomycin D.

The DNA-damaging agents are all capable of producing long-term toxicities because of their mutagenic properties, namely an increased risk of malignancy (usually acute leukemia 3 – 7 years after treatment) and gonadal damage that leads to infertility.

They are all potent inhibitors of bone marrow cell proliferation, and this is usually their dose-limiting toxicity.

The Alkylating Agents

These drugs are important in the treatment of malignancies, either as single agents or as components of effective combination regimens. In combination they may eradicate noncycling cells not killed by the cycle-active components of the treatment.

There appears to be little or no cross-resistance of alkylating agents with other classes of drugs. It is of importance that a cell resistant to one alkylating agent may not be resistant to other alkylating agents. This has led to renewed interest in combinations of alkylating agents, especially in preparative regimens for autologous bone marrow transplantation.

The major cytotoxic and mutagenic effects of these agents are believed to result from their interactions with DNA. Alkylating agents are able to form positively charged carbonium ions, which react with nucleophilic groups, such as SH, PO_4, and NH_3, on nucleic acids, proteins, and smaller molecules. The N7 atom of guanine is particularly susceptible to alkylation and is believed to be the major lesion in DNA. As a consequence of alkylation of DNA, cell damage may occur from single-strand breakage and cross-linking of DNA, thus interfering with cell division.

There are several drugs now on the market that are derivatives of the parent compound mechlorethamine.

Mechlorethamine (MUSTARGEN)

This nitrogen mustard is the most rapidly acting of this group of compounds and must be freshly prepared and administered into a rapidly flowing IV. *If extravasated, it can cause severe local tissue damage.*

MECHANISM OF ACTION. This agent enters cells through a transport system in place for choline, and resistance to this drug has been attributed to a decrease in its uptake.

CLINICAL USES. Mechlorethamine is used in treatment of Hodgkin's disease, for which it is a component of MOPP (mechlorethamine, ONCOVIN [vincristine], procarbazine, prednisone) chemotherapy.

Mechlorethamine is used topically to treat patients with mycosis fungoides, a T-cell lymphoma of skin.

ADVERSE EFFECTS. Like other alkylating agents, the dose-limiting toxicity to mechlorethamine is myelosuppression that may cause leukopenia and thrombocytopenia, sometimes of several weeks' duration.

Local tissue reactions due to extravasation should be treated immediately with administration of sodium thiosulfate and application of ice. Mechlorethamine also causes severe nausea and vomiting that occurs within the first hour or two after drug administration.

The major long-term toxicities of this drug, as with all alkylating agents, are gonadal damage, often leading to infertility, and an increased risk of secondary malignancies, in particular acute leukemia.

CLINICAL PHARMACOLOGY. This compound is administered IV, but may also be used intrapleurally for the control of effusions. It disappears rapidly from plasma (Table 44 – 6).

Cyclophosphamide

This nitrogen mustard was synthesized based on the rationale that it would be specifically cleaved and activated by tumor cells that contained an enzyme capable of cleaving the N-P bond in the molecule. This drug is relatively inert until activated by bond cleavage and may be administered orally. However, it is activated by the P-450 system in liver as well as in tumors; therefore, the basis of its selectivity is not clear.

CLINICAL USES. Cyclophosphamide, unlike nitrogen mustard, has a wide spectrum of antitumor and immunosuppressive activity. It is used as part of combination therapy regimens to treat lymphoma, breast cancer, bladder cancer, small cell lung cancer, ovarian cancer, and various childhood malignancies. It is used widely in high-dose regimens with autologous marrow replacement to treat refractory lymphoma.

ADVERSE EFFECTS. Cyclophosphamide differs in certain ways from other nitrogen mustards. It is relatively "platelet sparing," that is, there is less thrombocytopenia observed with this drug compared with other alkylating agents; there is more alopecia (hair loss); and sterile hemorrhagic cystitis is seen in 5 – 10% of patients treated with high doses unless vigorous hydration and bladder emptying are employed.

Long-term toxicity that includes sterility and carcinogenesis is also noted with this agent.

CLINICAL PHARMACOLOGY. The half-life after IV administration is 6 – 7 hours (Table 44 – 6). With time, the toxic metabolites phosphoramide mustard and acrolein are generated; the former compound is believed to be important in antitumor effects, and the latter compound responsible for bladder toxicity. After oral administration, peak levels are achieved in 1 hour.

Ifosfamide

Activation of ifosfamide, like cyclophosphamide, also occurs predominantly in liver by the P-450 mixed-function oxidase system. Ifosforamide mustard, the active compound, is generated. Acrolein and chloroacetic acid are the principal toxic metabolites.

CLINICAL USE. Ifosfamide, like cyclophosphamide, has a broad spectrum of activity. Antitumor effects are seen in patients with lymphomas, ovarian cancer, testicular cancer, and in various solid tumors. Its role in combination therapy is still under investigation.

There appears to be a lack of cross-resistance with cyclophosphamide in the treatment of some tumors (lymphoma, sarcoma).

TABLE 44–6. **DNA Damaging Agents**

Drug	Route of Administration	Pharmacokinetics	Indications	Toxicity	
				Acute	*Long-Term*
Mechlorethamine (HN_2, Mustargen)	IV (freshly prepared) Intrapleural Topical	Disappears rapidly from plasma	Hodgkin's disease (in combination). Sclerosing agent for malignant pleural effusion. Topical—mycosis fungoides.	Severe nausea and vomiting Bone marrow depression.	Sterility Secondary neoplasms
Cyclophosphamide	PO, IV	Converted to active species by P-450 system in liver (phosphoramide mustard and acrolein [$t_{½}$ = 6–7 hours])	Lymphoma Breast cancer Bladder cancer Lung cancer Ovarian cancer Solid tumors of children	Nausea and vomiting (high doses) Bone marrow suppression (relatively "platelet sparing") Alopecia (hair loss) Hemorrhagic cystitis (5%)	Sterility Secondary neoplasms
Ifosfamide	IV with hydration and mesna to protect bladder	Activation occurs predominantly in liver by P-450 mixed-function oxidase system ($t_{½}$ = 7–8 hour)	Lymphoma Ovarian cancer Testicular cancer Sarcomas	Nausea and vomiting Bone marrow suppression CNS toxicity with high doses Bladder toxicity (decreased by hydration, mesna)	Sterility Secondary neoplasms
Phenylalanine mustard	PO	$t_{½}$ (PO) = 90 min; 10–15% excreted unchanged in urine	Multiple myeloma	Nausea and vomiting Alopecia Marrow suppression	Sterility Secondary neoplasms
Chlorambucil	PO	Absorbed well. Little or no free drug found in urine	Chronic lymphocytic leukemia Low-grade lymphoma	Bone marrow depression	Sterility Secondary neoplasms
Triethylenemelamine (TEM)			Retinoblastoma	Bone marrow depression	Sterility Secondary neoplasms
Thiotepa	PO, IV, intrathecal, intravesical	Penetrates CNS	High-dose regimen with autologous marrow transplant	Bone marrow depression	Sterility Secondary neoplasms
Hexamethylmelamine	PO	Well absorbed, intensely metabolized Urinary recovery low	Ovarian cancer	Occasional nausea and vomiting Occasional neurologic toxicity	Sterility Secondary neoplasms(?)
ALKYL SULFONATES					
Busulfan	PO	Almost 100% excreted in urine as methane sulfonic acid	Chronic myelocytic leukemia	Bone marrow depression	Skin pigmentation Pulmonary fibrosis Gynecomastia Secondary neoplasms Sterility
NITROSOUREAS					
Carmustine (BCNU, bischloroethyl-nitrosourea)	IV	Rapidly metabolized (6 min)	Lymphoma Brain tumors	Delayed bone marrow depression Nausea and vomiting	Sterility Secondary neoplasms Nephrotoxicity
Lomustine (CCNU, 1-[2-chloroethyl])-3-cyclohexyl-1-nitrosourea)	PO	Rapidly absorbed and metabolized	Lymphoma Brain tumors	Delayed bone marrow depression Nausea and vomiting	Sterility Secondary neoplasms Nephrotoxicity
PLATINUM COMPOUNDS					
Cisplatin	IV with forced hydration	Extensively plasma bound Only 25% excreted in urine 1st 24 hr	Ovarian cancer Testicular cancer Lung cancer Head and neck cancer Bladder cancer	Nephrotoxicity Severe nausea and vomiting Anemia	Neurotoxicity
Carboplatin	IV (does not require forced hydration)	$t_{½}\beta$ = 1–3 hr 90% excreted in urine in 24 hr	Ovarian cancer	Bone marrow suppression Less nausea and vomiting than cisplatin	

Continued

TABLE 44–6. DNA Damaging Agents *Continued.*

Drug	Route of Administration	Pharmacokinetics	Indications	Toxicity: Acute	Toxicity: Long-Term
TRIAZENES					
Dacarbazine (DTIC, dimethyltriazeno-imidazole-carboxamide)	IV	Metabolized by hepatic P-450 system ($t_{1/2}$ = 5 hr), 50% excreted unchanged	Hodgkin's disease (in combination) Sarcoma Melanoma	Nausea and vomiting Flu-like syndrome Pain and tissue necrosis if extravasation occurs	Sterility Secondary neoplasms
ANTITUMOR ANTIBIOTICS					
Bleomycin	IV or IM	$t_{1/2}\beta = 2–4$ hr Excreted in urine	Lymphoma Epidermoid carcinoma Testicular cancer	Mucositis Pigmentation	Pulmonary fibrosis
Actinomycin D	IV	$t_{1/2}\beta = 36$ hr	Choriocarcinoma Wilms' tumor	Nausea and vomiting Marrow suppression Vesicant	
MISCELLANEOUS AGENTS					
Procarbazine	PO	?	Hodgkin's disease	Marrow suppression Nausea and vomiting	Secondary neoplasms
Hexamethylmelamine	PO	$t_{1/2}\beta = 5$ hr	Ovarian cancer	Neurologic toxicity	

CNS = central nervous system; IV = intravenously; PO = orally.

ADVERSE REACTIONS. The dose-limiting toxicity of this drug is bladder toxicity, presumably due to accumulation of acrolein and chloroacetic acid in the bladder. Dose fractionation and vigorous hydration with diuretics will decrease this toxic effect. Mesna, a thiol that is excreted in the urine, is now used routinely in ifosfamide-containing regimens because of its ability to inactivate the toxic metabolites of ifosfamide in the bladder. Mesna is generally well tolerated but may cause some nausea and vomiting.

The nausea and vomiting produced by ifosfamide are less than that observed with large doses of cyclophosphamide, as is the degree of myelosuppression. Central nervous system (CNS) toxicity is occasionally seen in patients treated with high doses of ifosfamide/mesna and is manifested by changes in mental status, cerebellar dysfunction, and even seizures.

Phenylalanine Mustard

The rationale for synthesis of phenylalanine mustard (melphalan) was based on the premise that certain tumors, in particular myeloma and melanoma, might preferentially accumulate compounds that were analogs of phenylalanine or tyrosine.

CLINICAL USES. The major use of this agent has been in the treatment of multiple myeloma, usually in combination with prednisone. It has also been used to treat breast cancer and melanoma, but it has been supplanted by other drugs in the treatment of these diseases.

CLINICAL PHARMACOLOGY. Phenylalanine mustard is well absorbed orally (Table 44–6) and, unlike mechlorethamine, reacts slowly with nucleophiles. It enters cells through the l-amino acid active transport system.

ADVERSE EFFECTS. Nausea and vomiting are infrequent with this agent, as is hair loss. The major toxicities are similar to those of other alkylating agents: marrow suppression and similar late effects.

Chlorambucil

Chlorambucil, like melphalan, is a slow-acting nitrogen mustard. It was synthesized with the hope that it would penetrate tumor tissue readily and slowly react with DNA. Chlorambucil is used primarily to treat patients with chronic lymphocytic leukemia and low-grade lymphomas, in particular, follicular lymphomas and Waldenstrom's lymphoma. Chlorambucil is well-tolerated, and usually does not cause nausea or vomiting. Its cytotoxicity is similar to that of phenylalanine mustard.

This drug is administered orally, and it is absorbed well (Table 44–6). It is metabolized completely, and little or no free drug is found in the urine.

Miscellaneous Drugs that Damage DNA

Triethylenemelanine (TEM)

This compound was first synthesized by chemists for use in industry. Because of the ethylenimine group in its structure and the recognition that it was an alkylating agent, it was studied as an anticancer drug. Currently it is not used in the clinic except for the treatment of retinoblastoma.

Thiotepa

This compound was introduced into the clinic in 1953. There has been a resurgence of interest in this compound for use in autologous marrow transplant regimens because its limiting toxicity is bone marrow suppression.

Busulfan

Busulfan, an alkyl sulphonate type of alklating agent, causes predominantly myelosuppression, with little other pharmacological action. It is used exclusively to treat CML. The drug has some unusual side effects in addition to its myelosuppressive activity. It may cause generalized skin pigmentation, gynecomastia, and pulmonary fibrosis.

Carmustine and Lomustine

Carmustine (bischloroethylnitrosourea, BCNU) was the first of the nitrosourea compounds in clinical trial to receive extensive clinical evaluation. *An unusual feature of these highly reactive compounds is their lipid solubility and, thus, their ability to cross the blood-brain barrier.* Lomustine (CCNU, 1-[2-chlorethyl]-3-cyclohexyl-1-nitrosourea) is similar to carmustine in its mechanism of action and clinical activity. It is administered orally and is rapidly absorbed and biotransformed.

The nitrosoureas, in particular carmustine and lomustine, have been extensively studied in animal tumor models and in the clinic. The nitrosoureas show some degree of cross-resistance with other alkylating agents, and more recent studies indicate that these compounds are primarily alkylating agents. A base-catalyzed decomposition of these compounds generates the alkylating chlorethyldiazonium hydroxide entity.

The nitrosoureas, like other alkylating agents, are potent bone marrow toxins. However, the hematopoietic depression produced by the nitrosoureas occurs later than that seen with other alkylating agents. Leukocyte and platelet nadirs occur 4 – 5 weeks after drug administration. Thus, the nitrosoureas appear to damage a primitive stem cell. The late marrow depression and cumulative toxicity make these drugs difficult to use clinically.

Nausea and vomiting occur frequently with the nitrosoureas. Nephrotoxicity may also result from nitrosourea treatment. Both drugs may produce hepatotoxicity; this side effect is less common with lomustine. A large adjuvant study of lomustine with 5-FU by the GI cancer group has shown that treatment with this combination was associated with *an increased incidence of acute leukemia,* presumably attributable to the nitrosourea.

Streptozocin

Like the other nitrosoureas, this drug functions as an alkylating agent. The plasma half-life is short (35 minutes), and the drug is excreted in the urine as metabolites (Table 44 – 6). This drug selectively destroys islet cells of the pancreas and causes diabetes in animals.

The major use for streptozocin is in the treatment of carcinoid and islet cell tumors. It has also been used in combinations to treat Hodgkin's disease and colon cancer, but its contribution to the antitumor effects seen is not well defined.

Unlike carmustine and lomustine, the dose-limiting side effect of streptozocin is nephrotoxicity. *Little or no bone marrow depression is seen with this drug,* thus allowing it to be used in combinations.

Diabetes is not seen in humans, but mild glucose intolerance may occur as a result of its use. Similar to the other nitrosoureas, nausea and vomiting may be severe.

Dacarbazine

Dacarbazine (DTIC, dimethyltriazenoimidazolecarboxamide) is believed to act by alkylating DNA after metabolism by the P-450 system. Dacarbazine is used in combination with doxorubicin, bleomycin, and vinblastine to treat Hodgkin's disease (ABVD), and is also used to treat soft tissue sarcoma and malignant melanoma.

Severe nausea and vomiting occur with therapeutic dosages of this drug. Myelosuppression is uncommon with the usual dosages but occasionally can be severe. Other toxic effects are a flu-like syndrome and facial flushing. Hepatoxicity has occasionally been noted. Dacarabazine may cause severe pain and tissue necrosis if infiltration occurs.

Cisplatin

Cisplatin (diammine-dichloro-platinum, DDP) is a platinum coordination complex that has broad-spectrum antitumor activity in humans. The story of its discovery is one of serendipity and the prepared scientific mind.

MECHANISM OF ACTION. Cisplatin is a reactive molecule and is able to form inter- and intrastrand links with DNA to cross-link proteins with DNA.

CLINICAL USES. Cisplatin has significant antitumor effects in ovarian, testicular, lung, and head and neck carcinomas. Of great importance is the ability of cisplatin, when used in combination, to give additive or synergistic activity. The use of cisplatin with vinblastine and bleomycin, or more recently with etoposide, has led to a cure rate (77%) in patients with advanced testicular cancer.

In combination with cyclophosphamide, it is the treatment of choice in the treatment of ovarian cancer, leading to a high response rate (70%), and some cures (about 10%).

Cisplatin and 5-FU infusions also are highly effective in causing tumor regressions in patients with squamous cell carcinoma of the head and neck, although the remissions produced are only temporary.

DRUG RESISTANCE. Drug-resistant cell lines have been produced, and resistance has been attributed to various mechanisms, including decreased uptake, an increase in repair of DNA lesions, and an increase of the metal-binding protein metallothionine.

CLINICAL PHARMACOLOGY. Cisplatin is administered IV with forced hydration. Following drug administration, the drug is rapidly bound to protein and persists in serum for long periods of time, with only 20 – 40% excreted in the urine within the first few days following drug administration. High concentrations of platinum, as measured by atomic absorption, persist in liver, intestines, and kidney.

ADVERSE EFFECTS. The dose-limiting toxicity of cisplatin is nephrotoxicity due to tubular injury. This complication may be largely, but not completely, avoided by vigorous hydration before and after cisplatin administration. The use of 3% sodium chloride may allow for even higher doses to be safely administered, because the chloride ion may decrease activation of this compound and renal injury. Hypomagnesemia may also result from tubular damage.

Severe nausea and vomiting are noted with this drug; recently, antiemetic therapy has been shown to control this problem. Myelosuppression is not a major problem, although anemia has been noted frequently in patients receiving multiple courses of this drug. Neurotoxicity is a problem with patients receiving multiple courses; this includes peripheral neuropathy and ototoxicity, especially high-frequency hearing loss. Rarely, Ig-mediated hypersensitivity reactions have occurred.

TABLE 44–7. L-Asparaginase

Route of administration	IV, IM (preferred)
Pharmacokinetics	Elimination half-life up to 48 hours
Indications	Acute leukemia (pre-B, T-cell ALL)
Toxicity	Hypersensitivity reactions (less with IM use than with IV use) Hemorrhagic pancreatitis (high doses) Azotemia Reversible liver dysfunction Depletion of clotting factors Neurologic dysfunction (somnolence, confusion)

ALL = acute lymphocytic leukemia; IM = intramuscularly; IV = intravenously.

Carboplatin

This platinum complex has been approved by the Food and Drug Administration (FDA) for the treatment of ovarian cancer. It has the same mechanism of action as cisplatin, and there is some cross-resistance between it and cisplatin. A major advantage of carboplatin over cisplatin is its lack of nephrotoxicity; it may be administered without the need for hydration. Limiting toxicity is bone marrow depression, especially thrombocytopenia.

Bleomycin

This antitumor antibiotic was isolated by Umezawa and colleagues in Japan from *Streptomyces verticillis.* It is mainly used in combination regimens to treat lymphoma, testicular cancer, and squamous cell carcinomas.

Bleomycin is a mixture of peptides, containing several unusual amino acids. The mechanism of action of this drug has been shown to be due to its binding to DNA and subsequent strand scission.

Unlike many anticancer drugs, a useful feature of this drug is its relative lack of marrow toxicity. However, a major toxicity of large cumulative doses is pulmonary fibrosis. The clinical pharmacology of this agent is given in Table 44–6.

Actinomycin D

Actinomycin D (dactinomycin) is also isolated from a *Streptomyces* species. Dactinomycin is believed to kill cells by intercalating between adjacent guanosine-cytosine pairs in DNA. The drug is used to treat Wilms' tumor, choriocarcinoma, and rhabdomyosarcoma. Clinical pharmacology and toxicity of this agent are given in Table 44–6.

Procarbazine

Procarbazine is a methylhydrazine derivative, and its use in the clinic is restricted primarily to the treatment of Hodgkin's disease, as part of the MOPP regimen.

This drug has many side effects. It is a weak monoamine oxidase inhibitor, and ingestion of foods with high tyramine content (cheese) can lead to serious reactions. Significant drug interactions with tricyclic antidepressants and sympathomimetic amines have also been reported. The toxicities and clinical pharmacology of this compound are given in Table 44–6.

Hexamethylmelamine

This compound has recently been approved for combination therapy or second-line treatment of patients with ovarian cancer. It is believed to act via alkylation of DNA. It causes only mild myelosuppression in therapeutic doses (Table 44–6).

ANTITUMOR ENZYMES

L-Asparaginase

L-asparaginase is an enzyme used to treat patients with pre-B- or T-cell acute leukemia. These types of leukemia are auxotrophic for L-asparaginase, and the depletion of this amino acid in the serum of these patients can cause marked tumor regression.

Effects of this enzyme are limited by the development of drug resistance, shown to be due to the emergence of cells able to synthesize L-asparaginase.

Allergic reactions including anaphylaxis can occur to the enzyme from E. coli; fortunately another preparation from *Erwinia carotovora* may be substituted with safety. Other toxicities and clinical pharmacology are given in Table 44–7.

L-asparaginase is usually given in combination with other antileukemic agents; a particularly effective combination is L-asparaginase followed 24 hours later by methotrexate; larger doses of methotrexate can be tolerated with this schedule with enhanced leukemic effects.

REFERENCES

Black DJ, Livingstone RB: Antineoplastic drugs in 1990. Drugs 39:652–673, 1990.

Chabner BA, Collins JM (eds): Cancer Chemotherapy: Principles and Practice, 1–15. Philadelphia, JB Lippincott Co, 1990.

Goldie JH, Coldman AJ: Genetic instability in the development of drug resistance. Natl Cancer Inst 81:116–124, 1989.

Holland JF, Frei E III, Bast RC, et al: Cancer Medicine, Vol 1, 3rd ed. Philadelphia, Lea and Febiger, 1993.

Mihich E: Drug Resistance: Mechanism and Reversal. New York, John Libbey & Co, 1990.

Rothenberg MI, Ling V: Multidrug resistance: Molecular biology and clinical relevance. Natl Cancer Inst 81:907–910, 1989.

Immunopharmacology 45

Alan Winkelstein

Pharmacological agents capable of suppressing immune responses have assumed increasing importance in clinical medicine. These drugs are essential for inhibiting histoincompatible organ transplant rejection reactions and are clinically important in the treatment of diseases thought to be caused by aberrant immune responses. These disorders are believed to result from abnormalities in immune regulation; the immune system loses its ability to discriminate between self and foreign antigens. As a consequence, immune responses can be directed at self antigens. Immunosuppressive drugs reduce the magnitude of these autodirected reactions and thus are potentially able to limit tissue injury.

The ideal immunosuppressant selectively inhibits a single immune response without impairing other reactions. In addition, it is not toxic to other organ systems. With the possible exception of Rh_0(D)immune globulin (RHOGAM), an antibody to the D antigen of the Rh system on red blood cells that is used to prevent immune sensitization after exposure, none of the immunosuppressants available at present fulfill these criteria. Specifically, none selectively inhibit a single response; rather they induce a state of generalized immunosuppression. Although this may be beneficial to the target aberrant immune response, it also renders treated patients more susceptible to infections and may increase their risk of developing selected malignancies.

The major compounds used to suppress immune responses can be subdivided into several categories. Corticosteroids are the drugs most widely used to suppress manifestations of potentially harmful immune responses. Certain cytotoxic drugs, originally developed for their antineoplastic activities, exert profound immune inhibitory effects. More recently, a series of new immunosuppressants has been developed; these drugs, which include both cyclosporine and FK-506, interfere with selected functions of immunologically competent lymphocytes. The last group of immunosuppressants includes monoclonal antibodies that either kill the subsets of lymphocytes mediating the unwanted responses or interfere with the functions of these cells through binding and inactivating essential receptors.

CORTICOSTEROIDS

Drugs derived from the adrenal cortical glucocorticoid hormones are extensively used to suppress manifestations of pathological immune responses. Their effectiveness was first reported in 1949 when hydrocortisone (cortisol), the major corticosteroid secreted by the adrenal gland, was discovered to inhibit manifestations of rheumatoid arthritis, a presumed autoimmune disease. This was rapidly followed by successful clinical trials that investigated both other connective tissue diseases and systemic autoimmune disorders.

Because of hydrocortisone's beneficial activities as an inhibitor of inflammatory and immunological reactions, numerous synthetic steroid compounds have been developed. These have advantages over cortisol; they possess greater anti-inflammatory properties while displaying reduced salt-retaining activities. The synthetic compounds also differ from cortisol in their biological half-lives; their anti-inflammatory effects persist for longer durations. Despite these differences, all corticosteroid compounds exert their anti-inflammatory and immune-modulating activities by similar mechanisms.

Clinically, the most widely used synthetic steroid is prednisone. Because of its popularity, it is generally used as the standard for comparing the activities of other corticosteroids. The major preparations used clinically and a comparison of their relative potencies are listed in Table 45–1.

Pharmacological quantities of corticosteroids can effectively inhibit a spectrum of clinical manifestations associated with immune-mediated diseases. In numerous circumstances, these effects are life-saving. Their beneficial effects result from a combination of two separate activities, immunosuppressive and nonspecific anti-inflammatory properties. The relative contributions of each cannot be accurately quantified; either can produce the desired therapeutic goal—suppression of the underlying clinical disease. In general, statements such as "corticosteroids have broad immunosuppressive activities" usually refer to the drugs'

TABLE 45–1. Clinical Properties of Corticosteroid Preparations

Preparation	Anti-inflammatory Potency	Equivalent Dose (mg)	Sodium-Retaining Potency	Approximate Plasma Half-Life (minutes)
Hydrocortisone (cortisol)	1.0	20.00	2+	90
Cortisone	0.8	25.00	2+	30
Prednisone	4.0	5.00	1+	60
Prednisolone	4.0	5.00	1+	200
Methylprednisolone	5.0	4.00	0	180
Triamcinolone	5.0	4.00	0	300
Betamethasone	20–30	0.60	0	100–300
Dexamethasone	20–30	0.75	0	100–300

Adapted from Claman HN: Glucocorticosteroids II: The clinical response. Hosp Pract 18:144, 1983.

ability to inhibit disease-associated manifestations, not to their effect on specific immune responses.

In clinical trials, corticosteroids alone do not appear to have potent immunosuppressive activities. By contrast, they have considerable activity in combination with other immunosuppressants. Thus, drug combinations containing steroids have proved extremely useful both in suppressing transplant rejection reactions and in inhibiting manifestations of autoimmune diseases.

Steroid therapy appears to exert differential effects on acute and chronic manifestations of immune-associated diseases. These agents are primarily active in suppressing acute inflammatory reactions and in inhibiting the immediate consequences of aberrant immune responses. However, in many disorders, they do not alter the chronic course of the underlying disease. For example, these hormones are potent inhibitors of acute articular inflammatory reactions in patients with rheumatoid arthritis but have little effect on the chronic course of this disease.

The anti-inflammatory and immunosuppressive activities of corticosteroids can be grouped conveniently into three general categories: their effects on leukocyte circulation, their ability to alter functions of immunologically competent cells, and a series of miscellaneous anti-inflammatory properties.

Effects on Cellular Traffic

One of the important activities of corticosteroids is to transiently alter the numbers of circulating leukocytes. Figure 45–1 depicts the quantitative changes in each cell type following a single intravenous injection of a glucocorticoid. A prompt increase in the number of neutrophils and a concomitant decrease in the total number of lymphocytes, monocytes, eosinophils, and basophils results. Maximal effects are observed 4–6 hours after drug administration. In general, the numbers of each cell type return to their baseline values within 24 hours.

The neutrophilia is caused by at least two distinct activities, the release of mature neutrophils from bone marrow reserves and a reduction in the ability of circulating cells to migrate into inflammatory exudates. The latter effect accounts for the increase in the half-life of circulating neutrophils. In

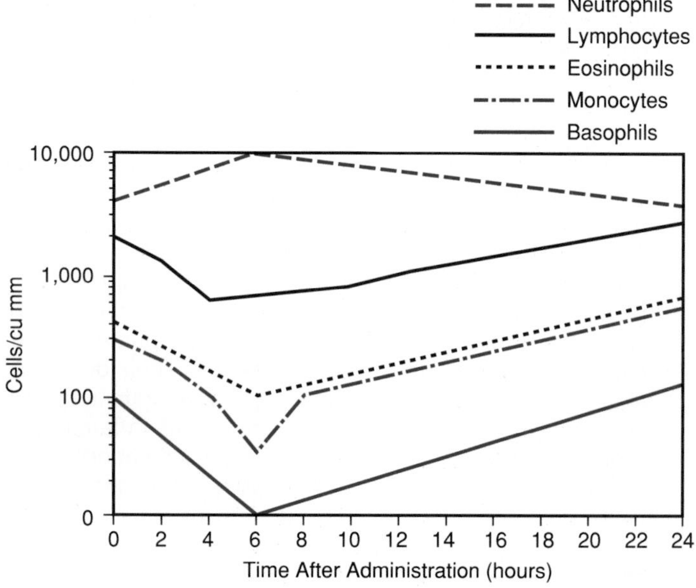

FIGURE 45–1. Quantitative changes in cell type following intravenous glucocorticoid injection. (Reprinted [adapted] with permission. Claman HN: Glucocorticosteroids. I. Anti-inflammatory mechanisms. Hospital Practice Volume 18, issue 7, pages 123–134, 1983.)

this circumstance, the numerical increase in blood neutrophils actually may be detrimental to the patient. Because of this activity, these phagocytes have reduced access to extravascular sites of inflammation or infection.

In contrast to the neutrophilia, steroids induce a reduction in the number of circulating lymphocytes. This effect is not caused by lympholysis, but rather by cell sequestration into lymphoid tissues, including the bone marrow. Lymphocyte subset analysis indicates that the number of T cells is markedly depressed. B cells are only modestly reduced, and the concentrations of natural killer (NK) and other null cells are not significantly altered. T helper/inducer ($CD4^+$) cells are decreased to a greater extent than T suppressor/cytotoxic ($CD8^+$) lymphocytes.

An important steroid effect is to cause a profound monocytopenia. The number of these cells is reduced to a greater extent than any other type of leukocyte; monocyte counts frequently decline to almost undetectable levels. This activity appears to be a result of margination of these cells; they show increased adherence to vascular endothelial cells. The number of eosinophils and basophils is also reduced; these effects also result from cellular redistribution.

Functional Changes

In addition to altering leukocyte distribution, corticosteroids affect important functional activities of both lymphocytes and monocytes. Neutrophil activities, such as chemotaxis, are relatively resistant to steroids. Formerly, it was believed that these agents inhibited the release of lysosomal enzymes; this was theorized to be the basis for limiting tissue damage in immune-induced injuries. However, recent studies suggest that steroids may not significantly affect these neutrophil functions.

Corticosteroids alter the functions of T lymphocytes. A prominent effect is to inhibit *in vitro* lymphoproliferative responses because of a reduction in the synthesis and secretion of interleukin 2 (IL-2), a lymphoid growth factor that is essential for the clonal expansion of activated lymphocytes (Fig. 45–2). The decreased availability of IL-2 is partially due to suppression of another interleukin, IL-1, which is elaborated by monocytes. IL-1 acts in conjunction with the antigen presented on antigen-presenting cells to stimulate $CD4^+$ cells to produce IL-2. Other studies have shown that corticosteroids do not impair the ability of antigen-stimulated T cells to express IL-2 receptors or to respond to exogenous IL-2. Steroids also do not suppress the ability of T cells to elaborate two other inflammatory cytokines, interferon-γ and migration inhibition factor.

Corticosteroids have lesser effects on B lymphocytes. Evidence suggests that patients receiving moderate doses of prednisone respond normally to specific antigens. Nevertheless, a short course of high-dose corticosteroids causes modest reductions in serum concentrations of both immunoglobulin (Ig)G and IgA. Only minimal effects on IgM levels result. Decreased serum concentrations are observed 2–3 weeks after a 5-day treatment course. In asthmatic children, IgE concentration is also reduced. With respect to two other lymphoid effectors, NK cells and killer cells, which are effectors of antibody-dependent cellular cytotoxicity, corticosteroids do not alter their *in vitro* activities.

Paralleling their effects on circulating monocytes, corticosteroids induce striking impairments in monocyte/macrophage functions. One effect is to impair bactericidal activities; this can adversely affect the individual's ability to respond to infectious agents. Steroids also inhibit the antigen-presenting activities of monocytes that are essential for initiating most immune responses. Other activities include decreased capacities of monocytes to undergo directed migration in response to chemotactic factors and impaired responsiveness to the T-cell cytokine migration inhibition factor. Steroids also block monocyte activation and their ability to differentiate into macrophages. As noted previously, an important effect is to inhibit synthesis and secretion of IL-1.

Steroids also impair the *in vivo* ability of reticuloendothelial cells to phagocytize antibody-coated particles. This effect correlates with *in vitro* studies indicating decreased expression of Fc and complement receptors and reduced binding of immune complexes to these receptors. These activities appear to account for the beneficial effects of steroids in diseases such as idiopathic thrombocytopenic purpura (ITP) and autoimmune hemolytic anemia (AIHA).

Delayed hypersensitivity skin tests are suppressed by prolonged treatment with corticosteroids. In general, these hormones must be administered for periods of 10–14 days before skin test reactivity (anergy) is impaired.

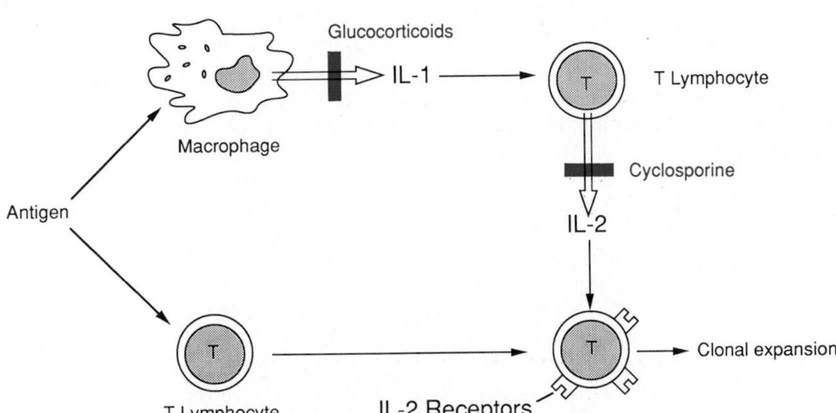

FIGURE 45–2. Clonal expansion of activated T lymphocytes and sites of inhibition by corticosteroids and cyclosporine.

Other Effects

Steroids can also affect the production of soluble mediators that regulate both inflammatory and immune responses. An important activity is to inhibit the synthesis of prostaglandins and leukotrienes, potent mediators of inflammation. This suppression results from the synthesis of a regulatory protein, lipomodulin, an antagonist of the enzyme phospholipase A. The latter catalyzes the release of arachidonic acid from cell membranes. Free arachidonic acid serves as the precursor for both prostaglandins and leukotrienes. Another anti-inflammatory activity is to suppress IgE-mediated histamine release by basophils and mast cells, an important mediator of most allergic disorders.

BOX 45-1
CLINICAL USE

In pharmacological quantities, steroids are effective but nonspecific therapies for many disorders of apparent immune pathogenesis. As noted previously, these compounds are primarily active in suppressing acute inflammatory reactions. They may not alter the clinical course of chronic immunopathological processes.

No defined guidelines for steroid administration exist, but most protocols conform to one of three patterns. The first, often employed when these drugs are administered for extended periods, entails the use of the minimal amount needed to partially suppress disease manifestations (*eg*, the treatment of patients with rheumatoid arthritis). Often patients receive prednisone in doses as low as 7.5–10 mg daily. These amounts are only slightly greater than the comparable amounts of corticosteroids produced by the normal adrenal gland.

The second approach uses higher doses in an attempt to rapidly and completely suppress disease manifestations. In these protocols, a typical dose is prednisone 1–2 mg/kg daily, given either in a single dose or in divided doses. This type of therapy is often used in potentially serious disorders such as AIHA, ITP, systemic lupus erythematosus (SLE), and immunologically induced acute glomerulonephritis.

The third pattern is the pulse intravenous administration of extremely high corticosteroid doses (*eg*, 10–30 mg/kg methylprednisolone). These ultralarge doses are usually reserved for "life-threatening" illnesses. They have also been successfully utilized in reversing acute allograft rejection reactions. Most studies suggest that the immunological effects of these massive-dose steroid protocols do not differ from those resulting from more conventional doses. Although the therapeutic superiority of these regimens has not been proved in controlled trials, they may be more effective than conventional dose therapy.

Prolonged therapy with corticosteroids is not innocuous; these drugs have numerous and potentially serious side effects. A full discussion of toxicities is beyond the scope of this section. However, it is important to recognize that chronic therapy may cause greater morbidity than the underlying disease.

CYTOTOXIC DRUGS

Cytotoxic drugs consist of a group of pharmacological agents that are able to kill cells capable of replication. In the process of responding to an antigen, immunologically competent lymphocytes are transformed from a resting or intermitotic state to an actively proliferating phase (Fig. 45-3). Because of their capacity to replicate, these cells are potentially susceptible to the cytolytic effects of these drugs. Some cytotoxic drugs developed as anticancer agents were subsequently found to possess immunosuppressive activities. This resulted in experimental and clinical trials in which they were successfully used both to treat diseases caused by aberrant immune responses and to inhibit transplant rejection reactions (Table 45-2). At present, four cytotoxic drugs—cyclophosphamide, azathioprine, methotrexate, and chlorambucil—are clinically used for their immunosuppressive properties.

Although the antigen-specific lymphocytes responsible for an unwanted immune response constitute the principal targets for cytotoxic drugs, their inhibitory activities are not restricted to a single lymphocyte subset. In varying degrees, they affect all immunologically competent lymphocytes. Thus, therapy results in generalized immunosuppression, and treated patients are susceptible to opportunistic infections and neoplasms.

Cytotoxic drugs are also used to treat rheumatic disorders (Table 45-3).

Furthermore, these drugs are not selectively toxic for lymphocytes; they can kill nonlymphoid proliferating cells including hematopoietic precursors, gastrointestinal mucosal cells, and germ cells in the gonads. Thus, predictable side effects of all cytotoxic agents include bone marrow suppression, gastrointestinal complications, and reduced fertility.

The lymphocytotoxic activities of cytotoxic drugs can be related to their toxicities for cells in specific phases of the mitotic cycle (Fig. 45-4). One group of drugs, including both azathioprine and methotrexate, are considered phase-specific agents. These drugs are lethal to cells only during a selected phase of the mitotic cycle. Azathioprine and methotrexate kill cells in the S or DNA synthetic phase of the mitotic cycle. Conversely, they are not toxic to cells that are not in this susceptible phase.

TABLE 45-2. Some Immunological Disorders in Which Cytotoxic Drugs Are Either Effective or Probably Effective

Rheumatoid arthritis
Systemic lupus erythematosus
Systemic vasculitis
Wegener's granulomatosis
Polymyositis
Membranous glomerulonephritis
Chronic active hepatitis
Primary biliary cirrhosis
Inflammatory bowel disease
Autoimmune hemolytic anemia
Immune thrombocytopenia
Circulating anticoagulants
Multiple sclerosis
Myasthenia gravis

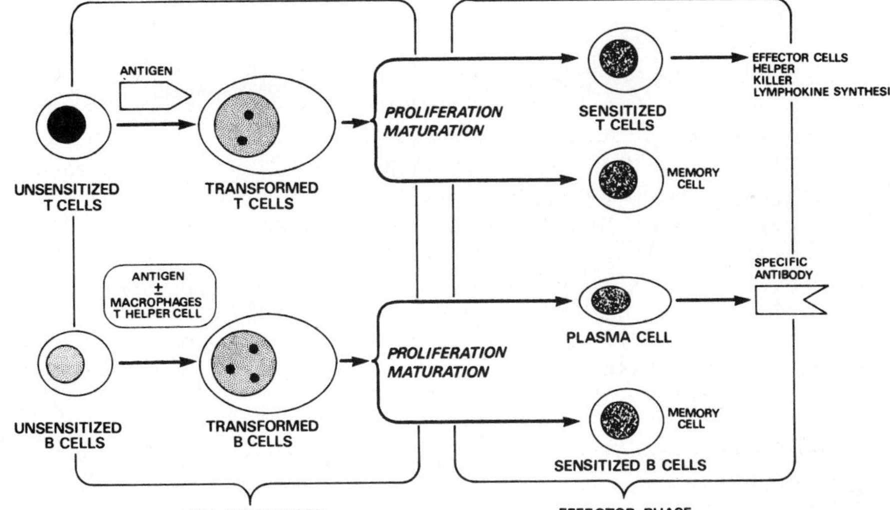

FIGURE 45-3. The development of an immune response. The period from antigenic challenge through the proliferative expansion of transformed lymphocytes is considered the *induction phase*. The period following cellular expansion is defined as the *established (effector) phase*. (From Webb DR Jr, Winkelstein A: Immunosuppression, immunopotentiation, and anti-inflammatory drugs. *In* Stites DP, Stobo JD, Fudenberg HH, Wells JV [eds]: Basic and Clinical Immunology, 5th ed, 271-287. Los Altos, CA: Lange Medical Publications, 1984.)

Cyclophosphamide and chlorambucil are designated as cycle-specific agents. They are toxic for both intermitotic and proliferating cells but are more effective against cells that are in active proliferative cycle. The third group, the cycle-nonspecific compounds, are equally toxic for intermitotic and proliferating cells (Fig. 45-5).

BOX 45-2
CLINICAL USES

Cytotoxic drugs are used to treat a spectrum of autoimmune disorders. Table 45-2 is a partial list of disorders in which cytotoxic drugs have been reported to be effective. One area in which these drugs have been extensively evaluated is in the treatment of connective tissue diseases. Table 45-3 compares the activities of each of the commonly used cytotoxic immunosuppressants in these disorders. Although these agents have been used clinically for more than a decade, it is difficult to ascertain their true effectiveness. This is because of a paucity of controlled studies and the unpredictable courses of autoimmune disorders.

Azathioprine

Azathioprine (IMURAN), a nitromidazole derivative of the purine antagonist 6-mercaptopurine (6-MP), is selectively toxic for proliferating cells. *In vivo*, azathioprine is rapidly converted into 6-MP. Although conflicting data exist, most investigators believe that the addition of the imidazole side chain both enhances its immunosuppressive potency and increases the therapeutic-toxic ratio.

Biochemically, both azathioprine and 6-MP are chemical analogs of physiological purines—adenine, guanine, and hypoxanthine. Both drugs act by competitive inhibition to block synthesis of inosinic acid, the precursor of the purine compounds adenylic acid and guanylic acid. As a result, their major effect is to impair DNA synthesis; this results in the death of replicating cells.

Comparatively, azathioprine appears to preferentially inhibit T-cell responses compared with those resulting from activation of B lymphocytes. Nevertheless, both cell-mediated and humoral responses are inhibited. In addition, azathioprine appears to effectively reduce the number of circulating NK and killer cells.

TABLE 45-3. Clinical Efficacy of Cytotoxic Drugs in Rheumatic Disorders*

	Azathioprine	Chlorambucil	Cyclophosphamide	Methotrexate
Rheumatoid arthritis	++	+	++	++
Rheumatoid vasculitis	0	+	++	0
Systemic lupus erythematosus	+	+	+	0
Polyarteritis nodosa	+	0	++	0
Polymyositis	+	0	0	++
Psoriatic arthritis	0	0	0	+
Wegener's granulomatosis	+	+	++	0
Reiter's syndrome	0	0	0	+

Adapted from Nashel DJ: Mechanisms of action and clinical applications of cytotoxic drugs in rheumatic disorders. Med Clin North Am 69:832, 1985.
*++ = substantial evidence of effectiveness; + = benefit suggested by some studies; 0 = not studied or benefit negligible.

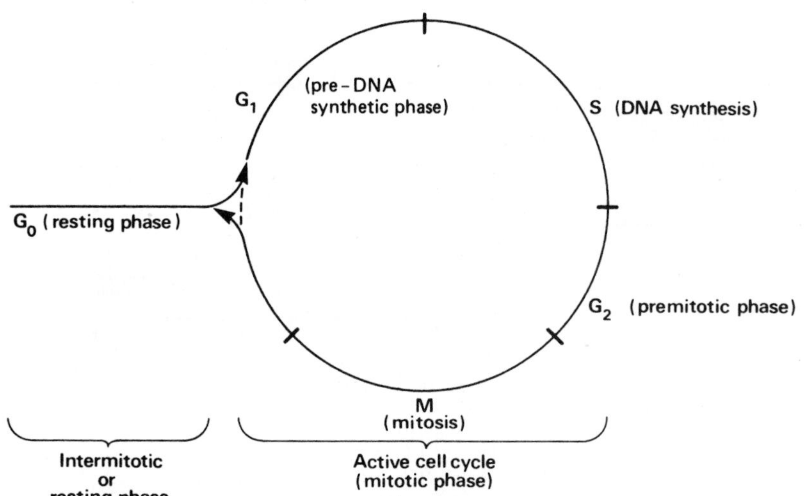

FIGURE 45–4. Mitotic cycle: drugs that are selectively toxic for cells in a discrete phase of their cycle are designated *phase-specific agents.* Most exert their toxicity for cells in the S phase. *Cycle-specific agents* are toxic for both intermitotic and proliferating cells but show greater toxicity for those in active cycle. *Cycle-nonspecific agents* show equal toxicity for all cells regardless of the mitotic activity. (From Webb DR Jr, Winkelstein A: Immunosuppression, immunopotentiation, and anti-inflammatory drugs. *In* Stites DP, Stobo JD, Fudenberg HH, Wells JV [eds]: Basic and Clinical Immunology, 5th ed, 271–287. Los Altos, CA: Lange Medical Publications, 1984.)

Prior to the development of cyclosporine (see Cyclosporine), combinations of azathioprine and corticosteroids were the standard therapy for inhibiting the rejection of organ transplants. These two agents still maintain an important role in this area, particularly in patients who are intolerant to cyclosporine or who require prolonged treatment. In addition, azathioprine is used to treat many connective tissue diseases and other presumed immune-mediated disorders (Table 45–4).

Extensive experience has been gained in patients with severe rheumatoid arthritis. As a therapeutic agent, azathioprine is classified as a "disease-remitting agent," implying that it can alter the course of this disease. Beneficial effects have also been reported in patients with SLE, other connective tissue diseases, autoimmune blood dyscrasias, and immunologically mediated neurological diseases. It is also used as a steroid-sparing agent in the treatment of primary biliary cirrhosis, chronic active hepatitis, and inflammatory bowel disease. Addition of azathioprine permits the use of reduced quantities of corticosteroids. Azathioprine is administered orally, and the maximal beneficial effects generally require continuous daily therapy for several weeks.

The primary lymphocytotoxic effects of azathioprine are directed against actively replicating cells; as such, short therapeutic courses do not alter the numbers of circulating T and B lymphocytes. The drug reduces the numbers of large lymphocytes; these are cells that have been triggered by antigens to enter active proliferative cycle. Immunoglobulin concentrations and titers of specific antibodies are not appreciably reduced by even prolonged azathioprine treatment. In a dose-dependent manner, this drug reduces the number of circulating neutrophils and monocytes. This ef-

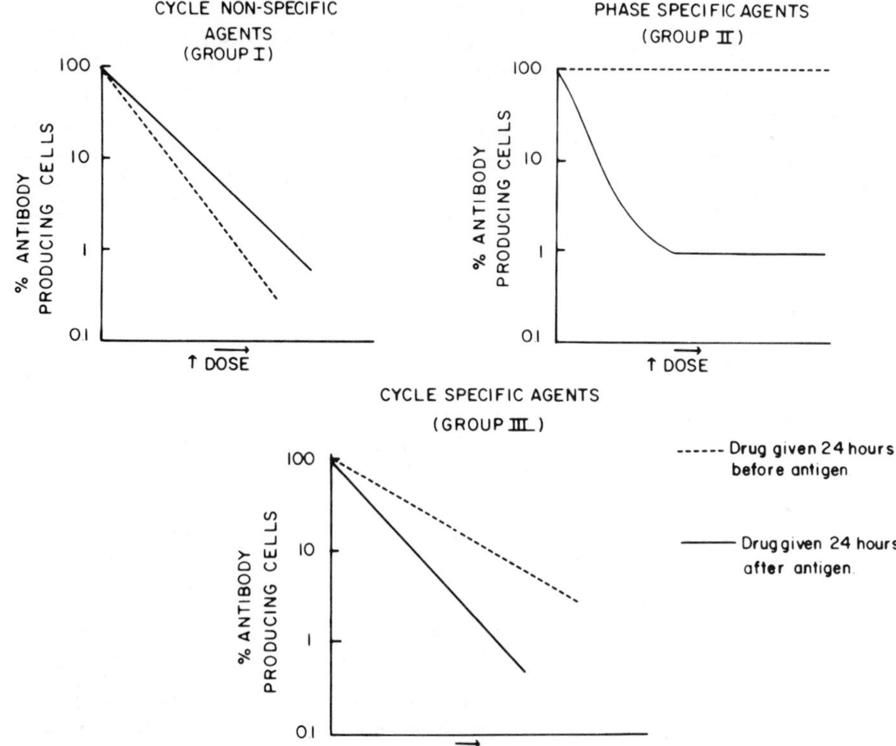

FIGURE 45–5. Schematic representation of the effects of different classes of immunosuppressants on the numbers of antibody-producing cells. The *dotted lines* represent the effects of the drug given 24 hours before the antigen; the *solid lines* represent the effects of the drug given 24 hours after the antigen. (From Winkelstein A: Immune suppression resulting from various cytotoxic agents. Clin Immunol Allergy 4:295–314, 1984.)

TABLE 45–4. Azathioprine

Trade Name	Chemical Structure	Administration	Mechanism of Action	Major Indications	Toxicities
IMURAN	[structure: H_3C–N imidazole with NO_2, S-linked to purine (HN, N)]	Orally, 1.25–2.5 mg/kg/day	S phase toxin (phase-specific agent) Inhibits *de novo* purine synthesis	Transplant rejection reactions Chronic graft-versus-host disease Rheumatoid arthritis ? Systemic lupus erythematosus ? Vasculitis ? Other connective tissue diseases Inflammatory bowel disease Chronic active hepatitis/ primary biliary cirrhosis ? Myasthenia gravis ? Multiple sclerosis	Bone marrow depression Gastrointestinal irritation Hepatotoxicity (rare) Infections Malignancies

fect results from its cytotoxic activities for hematopoietic precursors. Other adverse effects include transient liver dysfunction and skin rashes.

Cyclophosphamide

Both experimentally and clinically, cyclophosphamide (CYTOXAN) is a potent lymphocytotoxic immunosuppressant with a comparatively high therapeutic-toxic ratio (Table 45–5). Studies in both animals and humans indicate that following pulse administration, a dose-related reduction in the numbers of both B and T lymphocytes occurs. Experimental trials with cyclophosphamide indicate that it has diverse effects on different immune responses. Depending upon several factors, including the type of antigen, the dose of the drug, and the timing of the drug relative to the antigenic challenge, targeted immune response may be either inhibited or augmented. Comparatively, this alkylating agent appears to cause more pronounced suppression of humoral responses than those attributed to cellular immunity. This is illustrated by models in which profound inhibition of both IgG and IgM antibody responses occurs without significant changes in T-cell responses.

The effects of this agent on cell-mediated immune responses are particularly variable. Cyclophosphamide can prolong the survival of allogenic skin grafts if administered after grafting. However, if used prior to grafting, it is a potent immune enhancer. In part, this augmentation has been attributed to a preferential toxicity for T suppressor cells.

Cyclophosphamide is probably the most potent immunosuppressant available for the treatment of disorders resulting from aberrant immunity. Beneficial and often lifesaving effects have been documented for Wegener's granulomatosis, other forms of vasculitis, severe rheumatoid arthritis, the nephritis associated with SLE, autoimmune blood dyscrasias such as ITP, AIHA, and pure red cell aplasia, Goodpasture's syndrome, and immune forms of glomerulonephritis.

This alkylating agent can be administered either orally or intravenously. Recent clinical trials suggest that pulse intravenous therapy, particularly when used in combination with corticosteroids, may be more effective than daily low-dose oral treatment. Cyclophosphamide is inactive until it undergoes hepatic transformation to 4-hydroperoxycyclophosphamide. The compound is further metabolized to form phosphoramide mustard and other alkylators. These active metabolites are present in the circulation for only a

TABLE 45–5. Cyclophosphamide

Trade Name	Chemical Structure	Administration	Mechanism of Action	Major Indications	Toxicities
CYTOXAN	[structure: cyclic O–P(=O)–NH ring with $N(CH_2CH_2Cl)_2$]	Orally, 1–3 mg/kg/day Intravenously 10–20 mg/kg/every 1–3 months	Cycle-specific agent Binds and cross-links DNA strands Effects B cells > T cells; T suppressors > T helpers	Rheumatoid arthritis and vasculitis Systemic lupus erythematosus Wegener's granulomatosis Systemic vasculitis Autoimmune blood dyscrasias Immune-mediated glomerulonephritis	Bone marrow depression Gastrointestinal reactions Sterility (may be permanent) Alopecia Hemorrhagic cystitis Opportunistic infections Neoplasms (lymphoma, bladder cancer, acute myelogenous leukemia) Goodpasture's syndrome

few hours. Drug metabolism is not appreciably altered by either hepatic or renal insufficiency.

Cyclophosphamide's cytotoxic effects are primarily caused by its capacity to bind and cross-link DNA chains. It may also react and alter the function of other intracellular macromolecules. The DNA-alkylating activity can result in the immediate death of the target cell, or the cell may incur a lethal injury that is later expressed when the cell is stimulated to divide. In the latter circumstance, the injured cell may function normally in the intermitotic (Go) phase of its cycle. Conversely, if DNA repair can be effected, the cell may survive and be able to successfully undergo subsequent mitotic divisions. DNA aklylation is the prime mechanism acting to decrease the *in vitro* lymphoproliferative responses.

In animal studies, cyclophosphamide causes a depletion of both T and B lymphocytes; its selectivity for B cells appears to result from their delayed recovery. Clinical studies suggest that the effects on different subsets depend upon the dose of the drug; comparatively low doses primarily reduce the number of B cells and $CD8^+$ lymphocytes, whereas higher doses result in comparable depression in both $CD4^+$ and $CD8^+$ lymphocytes. In patients with rheumatoid arthritis treated with long-term oral cyclophosphamide, immunoglobulin levels are gradually reduced. Therapy is also accompanied by decreases in the titers of many autoantibodies.

Despite a comparatively high therapeutic-toxic ratio, cyclophosphamide therapy is associated with serious and potentially lethal adverse reactions. In general, the major dose-limiting toxicity is suppression of hematopoiesis. Other side effects include infertility and gastrointestinal manifestations such as abdominal pain, nausea, vomiting, and diarrhea. Teratogenesis is also a recognized complication.

In addition, this drug induces specific toxic manifestations not observed with other immunosuppressants; these include both hemorrhagic cystitis and alopecia. Cystitis has been reported in 9–17% of rheumatic patients chronically treated with this drug. The delayed toxicities include an increased risk of opportunistic infections and a higher than expected occurrence of cancers, particularly non-Hodgkin's lymphoma, bladder cancer, acute nonlymphoblastic leukemia, and skin cancers. The incidence of malignancies appears to be related to both the total drug dose and the length of treatment. The overall risk for malignancies is difficult to estimate, but two long-term studies (7 and 11 years of follow-up) report that the incidences of neoplastic diseases were 24–25% in the groups receiving this alkylating agent, as compared with 7–13% in the control groups.

Methotrexate

Methotrexate is a reversible inhibitor of dihydrofolate reductase, an enzyme required for the conversion of folic acid to its active form, tetrahydrofolate. The latter compound serves as a donor of one carbon fragment for thymidine synthesis. Thus, methotrexate is a potent inhibitor of DNA synthesis; this effect results in the killing of proliferating cells during the S (DNA synthetic) phase of their mitotic cycle. The blockade in folate utilization imposed by methotrexate cannot be overcome, even with high doses of folic acid, but can be circumvented with folinic acid (leucovorin), the tetrahydrofolate analog.

Methotrexate was one of the first cancer drugs developed. Shortly after its introduction, it was found to be effective in the treatment of the skin disorder psoriasis. However, initial trials had to be terminated because of the high incidence of hepatic fibrosis. Subsequently, it was shown that smaller quantities were effective in controlling this disease and could be administered for extended periods without causing hepatic injury. During these trials, it was noted that psoriatic patients with coexisting arthritis experienced sustained relief of their articular symptoms. These observations led to trials of methotrexate in patients with rheumatoid arthritis; it was reported that 60–70% of patients with severe rheumatoid arthritis achieved either a complete or partial remission. Other studies showed that it is also effective in the treatment of both polymyositis and Reiter's syndrome (Table 45–6).

A typical treatment regimen for rheumatic diseases is 2.5 mg of methotrexate every 12 hours for three doses; this course is repeated weekly. These doses are considerably lower than those employed in cancer patients. The major toxicity of methotrexate is hepatic fibrosis, an apparent dose-related complication. Liver disease is rarely observed

TABLE 45–6. Methotrexate

Chemical Structure	Administration	Mechanism of Action	Major Indications	Toxicities
H_2N, N, N, N, N, NH_2 CH_3 CH_2N–C$_6$H$_4$–CONH $HOOCCH_2CH_2$–C(H)–COOH	Orally, 2.5–5.0 mg every 12 hours for three doses, repeated weekly	S phase toxin (phase-specific) Competitively inhibits dihydrofolate reductase, thereby restricting synthesis of tetrahydrofolate; this is required for one-carbon transfer reactions involved in thymidine synthesis	Rheumatoid arthritis Psoriasis and psoriatic arthritis Polymyositis/ dermatomyositis Reiter's syndrome Prophylaxis for graft-versus-host disease in bone marrow transplants	Gastrointestinal—stomatitis, diarrhea, mucositis Bone marrow—megaloblastic anemia Hepatic fibrosis Pneumonitis Decreased fertility

until the total dose exceeds 1.5 g. It should be noted that fibrosis can develop despite persistently normal liver function tests.

Pulmonary complications are potential side effects of methotrexate therapy. Rarely does this antimetabolite cause a hypersensitivity pneumonitis; this is an idiosyncratic rather than a dose-related complication. The clinical manifestations are often that of an acute fulminant and potentially life-threatening bilateral pneumonia. In other patients, the toxic effects can lead to slowly progressive pulmonary fibrosis. Other toxic manifestations include mucositis (oral ulcerations are common in methotrexate-treated patients) and megaloblastic anemia because of the drug's interference with folate metabolism.

Animal studies indicate that methotrexate, in doses significantly higher than those used to treat patients with connective tissue diseases, is a potent immune inhibitor with a high therapeutic-toxic ratio. It suppresses both humoral and cellular responses. Short courses *in vivo* do not reduce blood lymphocyte counts or alter *in vitro* lymphoproliferative responses. The mechanisms by which methotrexate exerts its beneficial effects in rheumatic diseases are not well understood at present.

Chlorambucil

Chlorambucil is an alkylating agent that has cytotoxic properties similar to those of cyclophosphamide. Comparatively, most studies suggest that it is less toxic than cyclophosphamide but lacks the latter's potency as an immunosuppressant.

Chlorambucil has been extensively used in Europe to treat immunologically mediated diseases. Most reports suggest a therapeutic spectrum similar to that of cyclophosphamide. It is the drug of choice for the treatment of idiopathic cold agglutinin hemolytic anemia and essential cryoglobulinemia.

Chlorambucil has advantages over cyclophosphamide; it does not cause alopecia or hemorrhagic cystitis and may be less toxic for the gastrointestinal system. However, it is a toxic compound; like cyclophosphamide, it causes bone marrow suppression and interferes with gonadal function. It is also a fetal toxin. Studies in chlorambucil-treated patients with myeloproliferative diseases indicate a high incidence of acute leukemia.

Combinations of Cytotoxic Drugs

Recent clinical studies have attempted to enhance suppression of manifestations of immunologically related diseases while minimizing toxicities by using combinations of two or more cytotoxic drugs. Multidrug therapies, which, are derived in part from cancer chemotherapeutic protocols, are based on the concept that lower doses of two or more drugs have additive or even synergistic effects on effector lymphocytes. The reduced quantities of each agent result in a decreased incidence of toxic side effects, particularly those that are dose-related.

CYCLOSPORINE

Cyclosporine is a novel immunosuppressant that is able to selectively impair immune responses without killing target lymphocytes. This agent acts selectively on T helper/inducer ($CD4^+$) lymphocytes; it has minimal effects on T suppressor/cytotoxic ($CD8^+$) cells, B lymphocytes, granulocytes, and macrophages. Because of its potency, it has become the agent of choice in suppressing transplant rejection reactions, and it also effectively prevents graft-versus-host disease in histocompatible matched allogeneic bone marrow transplants. By contrast, it is relatively ineffective in treating established graft-versus-host disease.

Pharmacologically, cyclosporine is a unique nonpolar, cyclical undecapeptide, derived from the fermentation of soil fungi. The drug is not water-soluble but can be administered either orally or parenterally in a lipid vehicle.

Cyclosporine acts as an immunosuppressant by blocking an early phase of a developing immune response. One of its primary mechanisms of action is to suppress the capacity of $CD4^+$ lymphocytes to elaborate IL-2. It appears that this effect is caused by an inhibition in the synthesis of the mRNA's coding for this interleukin. Likewise, the synthesis of other cytokines may be impaired. The blockade in IL-2 synthesis inhibits the generation of cytotoxic T-cell effectors from precursors. Another consequence is to impair the generation of T helper cells, which suppresses the humoral responses to thymic-dependent antigens. By contrast, cyclosporine does not inhibit the lytic activities of preformed cytotoxic T cells or the antibody responses to thymic-independent antigens.

Recent studies have further defined its mechanisms of action. An intracellular cyclosporine-binding protein, cyclophilin, has been identified, purified, and characterized. This protein, present in nearly all mammalian cells, is a peptide-prolyl *cis-trans* isomerase, an enzyme that catalyzes protein folding. This drug-protein interaction is believed to impair the signal transduction required for lymphocyte activation, which limits the synthesis of the mRNA needed for cytokine production. The activity of this cyclosporine-cyclophilin complex may also be a causative factor for many of the toxic side effects of this drug. Of potential importance, cyclosporine can modify genes controlling multidrug resistance to cancer chemotherapeutic agents. Multidrug resistance is commonly associated with the overexpression of the transmembrane transport protein, P glycoprotein, which is responsible for a drug accumulation deficit seen in certain resistant neoplasms. Thus, cyclosporine or its nonimmunosuppressive derivatives may prove useful in restoring the effectiveness of cancer chemotherapeutic agents.

The immunosuppressive potency of cyclosporine may be augmented by the simultaneous administration of moderate doses of corticosteroids. These two agents act synergistically. Cyclosporine directly inhibits IL-2 production; steroids indirectly suppress the synthesis of this growth factor by blocking monocyte-macrophage release of IL-1.

Cyclosporine has a narrow therapeutic-toxic ratio. Because of its unpredictable pharmacokinetics, drug levels must be closely monitored. Cyclosporine absorption from the small intestines is normally incomplete and unpredictable. The drug is metabolized by the liver and excreted in the bile. As a result, blood levels are significantly altered by abnormal liver function, by drugs that induce or inhibit hepatic metabolism, and by low bile flow.

Unlike cytotoxic drugs, cyclosporine is not toxic for bone marrow stem cells; it does not cause cytopenias. Renal failure and hypertension are its major toxicities. This drug causes an increase in renovascular resistance, which in its early stages is reversible; however, longer-term therapy can lead to persistent ischemia and irreversible intestinal fibrosis and tubular atrophy. Hypertension is probably the result of both renal ischemia and sodium retention.

Cyclosporine treatment has additional side effects. These include gingival hyperplasia, hirsutism, and coarsening of facial features. Reversible hepatotoxicity, resulting in elevations of the serum bilirubin and transaminase levels, is another common side effect. Neurological side effects include tremors, paresthesia, and, infrequently, convolutions. Drug therapy can result in elevations in serum cholesterol and uric acid levels; also, the drug is a potential diabetogenic agent. In patients receiving bone marrow transplantation, cyclosporine may cause a potentially fatal capillary leak syndrome or a hemolytic uremic syndrome.

As is the case with other immunosuppressants, patients treated with cyclosporine are more susceptible to opportunistic infections and certain malignancies. The most frequently encountered neoplasms in organ transplant recipients treated with this immunosuppressant are those involving the skin and non-Hodgkin's lymphoma. A disproportionally high percentage of the skin cancers are Kaposi's sarcoma.

FK-506

This compound, a macrolide antibiotic, has been shown to be an extremely potent immunosuppressant with activities similar to those of cyclosporine. It appears to be approximately 100 times more potent in suppressing transplantation rejection reactions. Recent studies suggest that it may also be useful in treating certain immune-mediated diseases. FK-506 has significantly fewer side effects than cyclosporine. At some institutions, it is used as the primary therapy for transplantation trials for liver, heart, lung, intestinal, kidney, and other organs. Preliminary results suggest that with FK-506 it may be possible to perform transplant procedures that were formerly considered either impractical or impossible.

Although biochemically unrelated to cyclosporine, FK-506 acts by similar mechanisms. Both agents exert their immunosuppressive activities by predominantly affecting the functions of $CD4^+$ T cells. A major effect is to inhibit IL-2 synthesis and secretion. Like cyclosporine, FK-506 is not lympholytic, nor is it toxic for bone marrow progenitors. Furthermore, FK-506 does not inhibit target cell killing by preformed cytotoxic lymphocytes. Recent biochemical studies suggest that the mechanisms of action of both drugs depend on the binding to specific cytosolic receptors. Although these are distinct and different receptors, one of the major results of these drug-receptor interactions is interference with the function of the enzyme peptidyl-prolyl isomerase.

Current evidence suggests that FK-506 has a better therapeutic index than cyclosporine. Like cyclosporine, it is moderately diabetogenic. Both drugs are neurotoxic. FK-506 therapy appears to result in significantly less hypertension than cyclosporine, and it is less nephrotoxic.

Other side effects commonly seen with cyclosporine such as gingival hyperplasia, hirsutism, and coarsening of facial features are rare with FK-506. Finally, this compound does not cause metabolic disturbances such as hyperuricemia and hypercholesterolemia. Long-term complications include both an increased incidence of opportunistic infections and those neoplasms associated with chronic immunosuppression.

ANTIBODIES TO LYMPHOCYTES

Heterologous antisera, reactive to lymphocyte membrane antigens, represent another mode of achieving nonspecific immunosuppression. These antibodies can be divided into two general groups: polyclonal antisera that react with multiple-membrane determinants and monoclonal antibodies that are directed at a single-membrane–associated protein.

Polyclonal Antibodies

Polyclonal antibodies are generally prepared by immunizing animals with human lymphocyte suspensions. If thymus cells are used, the preparation is termed ***antithymocyte serum;*** this is often further fractionated to obtain the globulin portion (***antithymocyte globulin***). Other antisera are prepared from thoracic duct lymphocytes, splenic cells, or blood lymphocytes obtained by leukophoresis. These antisera are referred to as either ***antilymphocyte serum*** or ***antilymphocyte globulin.***

In animal studies, polyclonal antisera are effective immunosuppressants; their primary activity is to inhibit cell-mediated responses. This is in accord with their specificity for T lymphocytes. Although these agents can induce lymphopenia *in vivo*, their exact mechanisms of action are not well understood. Clinically, these antisera are used primarily to treat organ graft rejection reactions.

Several problems are associated with the use of polyclonal antisera. First, the preparations are not standardized, and no laboratory tests measure the *in vivo* immunosuppressive activities of a particular preparation. Thus, the amount needed to achieve a specific immunosuppressive activity cannot be predetermined. Second, these reagents are not selective for T lymphocytes. They cross-react with other cells, including platelets, an effect that can lead to severe thrombocytopenia. Third, these reagents are immunologically recognized as foreign proteins, which may result in a severe serum sickness.

Monoclonal Antibodies

In organ transplant studies, monoclonal antibodies have assumed increasing clinical importance. In fact, recent studies suggest that some may be capable of inducing a state of selective immunological unresponsiveness or tolerance, the ultimate goal of therapeutic immunosuppression. A prominent trend in organ transplantation is to use antibodies with increasing specificity for the lymphocyte subsets directly involved in effecting the reaction. This selectivity serves to preserve the function of other immunologically competent lymphocytes and to maintain immune defense mechanisms.

Monoclonal antibodies can be divided into two general groups, those with specificity for a specific subset of T cells and those reactive with activation antigens present on the lymphocyte subset affecting the targeted immune response. The former includes a group of pan-T cell antibodies; the one most widely used clinically is anti-OKT3, an antibody that reacts with the CD3 polypeptide on all immunologically competent T cells. This monoclonal antibody has been successfully used to treat steroid-resistant acute transplant rejection reactions.

Therapy with OKT3 and other monoclonal antibodies is not without significant side effects; the immediate complications include severe fever and chills, headache, meningism, hypotension, diarrhea, vomiting, respiratory distress, and anaphylactic shock. Fatal reactions to OKT3 occasionally have been reported. Long-term toxicities include an increased incidence of opportunistic infections and lymphoproliferative neoplasms.

More recently, antibodies specifically directed against either the CD4 or CD8 antigens have been tested as selective immunosuppressants in organ transplantation. The initial trials have provided insight into organ rejection mechanisms. For example, it has been widely assumed that $CD8^+$ cytotoxic cells are the prime effectors of graft rejection. However, in experimental models, monoclonal antibodies directed at $CD4^+$ antigen-bearing cells appear to be even more potent than comparable anti-CD8 antibodies. $CD4^+$ T lymphocytes have been shown to have multiple functions including the ability to mount cytolytic reactions against allogenic cells expressing human leukocyte antigen Class II antigens.

The second group of immunosuppressive antibodies are those directed at specific T-cell activation antigens. These membrane receptors are not expressed on resting T cells but appear shortly after the cells are induced to respond to an immunological challenge. The best studied of these inhibitors is the anti-Tac monoclonal antibody, which reacts with the p55 KD peptide of the IL-2 receptor. The Tac antigen is expressed on the effector T lymphocytes of patients with certain autoimmune diseases and of those participating in organ allograft rejection reactions. They are also present on neoplastic cells of patients with specific T-cell leukemias/lymphomas, such as human T-cell leukemia/lymphoma virus-I-induced acute T-cell leukemia.

Both unmodified anti-Tac antibodies and those conjugated with either toxins or radioisotopes are currently being tested for their immune inhibitory properties. Initial results indicate that these are potent inhibitors of transplant rejection reactions and are capable of suppressing manifestations of selected autoimmune diseases. Because of their specificity for activated T cells, they may induce specific immunosuppression without impairing the subsequent capacity of the immune system to respond to other antigens.

A third group of immunosuppressive monoclonal antibodies, those with specificity for cell adhesion molecules, also show promise in experimental studies as immunosuppressants. Adhesion molecules have multiple activities, including those involved in transmitting stimuli from antigen-presenting cells to immunologically competent lymphocytes and in effecting the cytolytic responses of antigen-stimulated lymphocytes.

REFERENCES

Ben-Yehuda O, Tomer Y, Shoenfeld Y: Advances in therapy of autoimmune diseases. Semin Arthritis Rheum 17:206-220, 1988.

Briggs JS: A critical review of immunosuppressive therapy. Immunol Lett 29:89-94, 1991.

Mitchell MS, Fahey JL (eds): Immune suppression and modulation. Clin Immunol Allergy 4:197-451, 1984.

CORTICOSTEROIDS

Meuleman J, Katz P: The immunologic effects, kinetics and use of glucocorticosteroids. Med Clin North Am 69:805-816, 1985.

CYTOTOXIC DRUGS

Nashel DJ: Mechanisms of action and clinical applications of cytotoxic drugs in rheumatic disorders. Med Clin North Am 69:817-840, 1985.

CYCLOSPORINE AND FK-506

Foxwell BM, Ruffel B: The mechanisms of action of cyclosporine. Clin Biochem 24:9-14, 1991.

Freeman DJ: Pharmacology and pharmacokinetics of cyclosporine. Clin Biochem 24:9-14, 1991.

Hohman RJ, Hultsch T: Cyclosporine A: New insights for cell biologists and biochemists. New Biologist 2:663-672, 1990.

Thomson AW: The immunosuppressive macrolides FK-506 and rapamycin. Immunol Lett 29:105-111, 1991.

POLYCLONAL AND MONOCLONAL ANTIBODIES

Chatenoud L, Bach JF: Monoclonal antibodies to CD3 as immunosuppressants. Semin Immunology 2:437-447, 1990.

Cobbold SP: Monoclonal antibody therapy for the induction of transplantation tolerance. Immunol Lett 29:117-122, 1991.

PART IX

POISONING AND ADVERSE REACTIONS TO DRUGS

46 Toxicology: Management of Acute Poisoning

Jill G. Dolgin

This chapter is divided into two parts. The first part reviews the epidemiological characteristics and general management of acutely poisoned patients; the second part reviews the clinical management of those toxins involved most frequently in fatalities.

Although several excellent texts contain valuable information on the toxicity and treatment of poisons (Goldfrank, 1994), the most up-to-date information on both human and animal poisonings is provided by Poisindex (MICROMEDEX, Medical Information Systems, Denver, CO). It contains data on the chemical composition, toxicity, and current medical management of over 750,000 drugs, household chemicals, industrial and environmental toxins, and biologicals (including plant and animal toxins). Poisindex also facilitates the identification of manufactured drugs by providing a visual reference of the symbols imprinted on tablets and capsules and of street drugs by indicating their slang terminology, color, and shape. Poisindex is edited and updated every 3 months.

Another valuable source of information is a regional poison control center. Currently there are over 100 regional poison control centers located throughout the United States; 38 have been certified by the American Association of Poison Control Centers (AAPCC). These centers provide around-the-clock information on poisons and patient care, collect and report poisoning data, and help educate both health professionals and the public.

THE POISONED PATIENT

General Characteristics

A poison is a chemical substance that impairs the biochemical and physiological functions of an organism. Exposure to poisons continues to be a growing problem and challenge for the health care practitioner. Poisonings are the third leading cause of accidental death and the second leading cause of suicide (Centers for Disease Control, 1989). The AAPCC estimated 4.4 million poisonings occurred nationwide in 1991 (Litovitz et al, 1992). Of the 1.8 million poisonings reported to the AAPCC, 764 resulted in death. The majority of all poisonings occurred in the home and were managed without the need for emergency room referral. Nonpharmaceuticals were involved in 58% of all poisonings. In contrast, fatal poisonings most frequently involved pharmaceuticals. Ingestion was the most common route of exposure. Accidental poisonings are most common in children under 5 years of age and in the elderly. Intentional exposures (drug abuse and suicide attempts) are most common in adolescents (>14 years of age) and adults and are the most frequent cause of death.

Pediatric Poisoning

The 1991 AAPCC statistics show that 60% of all poisonings occurred in children under the age of 6 years; 46% involved children under the age of 3 years. Although child-resistant bottle caps have reduced pediatric poisoning fatalities by 70% since their institution in 1972, the unintentional ingestion of drugs by children continues to result in significant morbidity, mortality, and consumption of health care resources (Centers for Disease Control, 1987). Most pediatric poisonings result from exposure to a variety of common household substances and medications. The majority of these poisonings were safely managed at home. However, unintentional pediatric fatalities were increased from 25 deaths in 1990 to 44 in 1991. Ingestion of iron supplements accounted for 65% of these fatalities. In addition to iron, children were most commonly victims of exposures to hydrocarbons (18%), fumes (16%), and household cleaning products (11%).

Multiple factors contribute to the risk of accidental exposure of children to medications. These include their inability to recognize potential hazards, their curiosity about their environment, their tendency to put things in their mouths, and their access to easily reached medicinals in the kitchen and bedrooms. Other factors include ineffective and misused child-resistant closures, as well as the failure of these items to function after continuous use. Public education and awareness efforts conducted by local and regional poison control centers are targeted at persons who have frequent contact with small children, including grandparents and those who may not be used to caring for children. Poison prevention advisements are available for distribution to the public at poison control centers nationwide.

Adolescent-Adult Poisoning

Whereas pediatric poisonings make up the majority of calls received by poison control centers, adolescent and adult poisonings more often result in serious morbidity and mortality. A large percentage of these poisonings are due to drug abuse or suicide gestures. Men aged 20–39 years accounted for 70% of all drug abuse emergency room visits and 65% of all drug abuse deaths in 1987. During the period 1980–1986, cocaine and heroin/morphine were involved in more than one third of these deaths (Centers for Disease Control, 1989). Other commonly abused drugs include barbiturates, benzodiazepines, volatile inhalants such as isobutyl and amyl nitrate ("rush," "locker room"), typewriter correction fluid, trichloroethane, glues, over-the-counter (OTC) sedatives, and diet aids (legal stimulants) that contain either phenylpropanolamine or ephedrine. Most suicide gestures involve drugs prescribed as therapy for the victim. Drugs commonly involved in these gestures include antidepressants, nonopioid analgesics, benzodiazepines and other sedative-hypnotics, psychotropics, central nervous system (CNS) stimulants, and cardiovascular/antihypertensive drugs. Polypharmacy in drug abuse and suicide gestures is common; alcohol is the second most commonly ingested substance. Because of the alarming increase in drug abuse, suicidal intentions may be difficult to distinguish from recreational overdose. Many patients take overdoses as risk-taking behavior and have a history of prior treatment for psychiatric illness. These patients should receive psychiatric assessment before discharge.

EVALUATING THE POISONED PATIENT

Stabilization

Symptomatic medical care that supports vital functions is the mainstay of treatment because there is no antidote for the majority of poisons encountered in clinical toxicology. "Treat the patient, not the poison" remains the most basic tenet. Initial management requires establishing the airway, as well as maintaining adequate breathing and circulation. Serial measurements of vital signs (*ie*, blood pressure, heart rate, respiration, and core temperature), important reflexes, and acid-base status help to judge the progression of toxicity, response to therapy, and the need for additional treatment.

Generally, the use of drugs is limited to those required for resuscitation and antidotes. Patients who present with an altered mental status are an exception. These individuals should receive a diagnostic challenge with glucose (adult: 50 mL of 50% dextrose intravenously [IV]; pediatric: 1–2 mL/kg of 25% dextrose IV) to distinguish hypoglycemia from other causes, as well as naloxone (2 mg for both adults and children as a starting dose), an opioid antagonist. Chronic narcotic users and victims of severe opiate overdoses may require at least 10 mg of naloxone, given in 1- to 2-mg increments, before a possible narcotic overdose can be excluded. Naloxone reverses the respiratory and CNS depression due to narcotics and may be useful in some cases of ethanol and sedative-hypnotic toxicity. Patients with a history of alcohol abuse should also receive 100 mg intramuscularly (IM) of thiamine to prevent Wernicke's encephalopathy.

History

Once vital functions have been stabilized, the diagnosis can be aided by a more detailed evaluation. This includes documenting any available history and performing a thorough physical examination. Historical information combined with the clinical findings may be quite accurate in predicting the toxins involved in the overdose patient. Family, friends, and paramedical personnel should be questioned about the environment in which the patient was found. Syringes and bottles of prescription and OTC preparations located in the vicinity of the patient should be brought to the emergency room.

Physical Examination

A toxicologically oriented physical examination emphasizes vital signs, eyes, mouth, skin, abdomen, and nervous system. The findings can suggest which toxin is involved, as well as clinical interventions and laboratory tests that may confirm or quantitate its presence. A limited number of toxins produce no initial signs, symptoms, or routine laboratory abnormalities. The most important of these is acetaminophen. Serum acetaminophen levels should *always* be determined in patients with an unknown ingestion.

Blood Pressure and Heart Rate

Toxins that stimulate the sympathetic nervous system or block the parasympathetic system peripherally may cause hypertension and tachycardia. These findings are consistent with amphetamines, cocaine, and phencyclidine (PCP), as well as both anticholinergic (*eg*, antihistamines, antispasmodics) and cholinergic (*eg*, nicotine, physostigmine) drugs. In some cases, the initial stimulation of vital signs is followed by a generalized depression (*eg*, monoamine oxidase inhibitors, levodopa, bretylium). Hypotension and tachycardia are common with plant toxins (Amanita mushrooms), drugs that produce peripheral arteriolar dilatation with reflex compensation (antipsychotic agents, 2-stimulants, theophylline), and toxin-induced tissue hypoxia (carbon monoxide, cyanide). Hypotension and bradycardia are characteristic features of narcotics, central β_2-agonists (*eg*, clonidine), sedative-hypnotics, nicotine (late finding), β blockers, and calcium channel blockers.

Respiration

Both the rate and the depth of respiration may be increased by sympathomimetics, by drugs that stimulate the medullary respiratory center either directly (*eg*, salicylates) or indirectly by causing cellular hypoxia (*eg*, carbon monoxide, cyanide), and by metabolic acidosis. Respiration is depressed by opioids and sedative-hypnotics.

Core Temperature

Hyperthermia can be elicited by drugs that increase muscle activity or metabolic rate (*eg*, salicylates, thyroid hormones, sympathomimetics, antimuscarinics) or by those that impair thermoregulation (*eg*, anticholinergics, antidepressants, antipsychotics). Hypothermia is frequently caused by the inability of the body to respond to cool ambient temperatures. Alcohol, phenothiazines, narcotics, and sedative-hypnotics are examples of drugs that promote hypothermia by producing vasodilatation and inhibiting the shivering reflex. Sepsis, hypothyroidism, and hypoglycemia should be eliminated as nondrug-related causes of hypothermia.

Eyes

Constriction of the pupils (miosis) may be due to increased muscarinic tone (*eg*, organophosphates, physostigmine), decreased sympathetic tone (*eg*, narcotics, clonidine, phenothiazines, sedative-hypnotics), or brainstem injury. Dilatation of the pupils (mydriasis) may be due to increased sympathetic tone (*eg*, lysergic acid diethylamide [LSD], cocaine amphetamines) or muscarinic blockade (*eg*, atropine, bethanechol). Horizontal nystagmus (*eg*, phenytoin, ethanol, barbiturates) or vertical nystagmus (*eg*, PCP) are also important findings. Ptosis (eyelid drooping) and ophthalmoplegia are features of botulism.

Mouth

The mouth should be inspected to determine whether the patient has a gag reflex and whether corrosives have caused ulceration in the mouth or pharynx. Some toxins result in detectable odors in the mouth, such as wintergreen (salicylates), acetone (isopropyl alcohol), almonds (cyanide), garlic (arsenic, organophosphate), alcohol, and petroleum distillates. Dry mucous membranes may indicate anticholinergic poisoning, whereas hypersalivation may suggest organophosphate poisoning.

Skin

The patient should be checked for needle tracks, burns or bruises, and abnormal skin temperature or color. Diaphoresis (sweating) may suggest an overdose with stimulants, salicylates, organophosphates, or nicotine. Extremely dry, warm skin may suggest an overdose with anticholinergic drugs, whereas dry, cool skin may indicate sedative-hypnotic or barbiturate poisoning. Cutaneous bullae (skin blisters at pressure points) accompany sedative-hypnotic poisoning and are seen also in patients unconscious for prolonged periods of time. A cherry-red skin coloration (usually an autopsy finding) may suggest severe carbon monoxide poisoning.

Abdomen

Decreased or absent bowel sounds are typical findings in anticholinergic, narcotic, and sedative-hypnotic overdoses. Hyperactive bowel sounds, abdominal cramping, and diarrhea are common findings in poisonings with organophosphate and carbamate insecticides, iron and heavy metals, sympathomimetics, *Amanita phalloides* mushrooms, and in drug/alcohol withdrawal syndromes.

Nervous System

Ataxia and incoordination are symptoms of phenytoin, alcohol, barbiturate, and sedative-hypnotic intoxication. Muscle rigidity and hyperactivity suggest intoxication with sympathomimetic drugs, methaqualone, PCP, or haloperidol. Generalized seizures are often the result of severe intoxication from cyclic antidepressants, stimulants, isoniazid, and phenothiazines. Coma with absent reflexes and flaccid muscle activity may be present with narcotic and sedative-hypnotic drugs and may mimic brain death.

Toxicology Screen

Toxicology screens are often used to diagnose, assess prognosis in, and manage acute poisoning, particularly in comatose or uncooperative patients. However, toxicology screens are time-consuming, expensive, and often unreliable. Their reliability depends on (1) communication between the laboratory and the physician about drugs suspected to be involved, (2) correct sampling of appropriate biological fluids, (3) prompt reporting of the results, and (4) the number of substances listed on the drug analysis profile. Most laboratories limit screens to drugs commonly prescribed and to a few drugs of abuse.

Toxicology screens are no substitute for clinical judgment and should be ordered only in those few instances when the results obtained will influence the therapy provided. For example, plasma levels of a few toxins (*eg*, acetaminophen, salicylates, lithium, carbon monoxide, theophylline, iron, ethylene glycol, methanol) may influence the course of therapy, whereas for many drugs (*eg*, cyclic antidepressants) there is a poor correlation between plasma levels and toxicity. Interpretation of toxicological analyses must consider the clinical condition of the patient, the time elapsed since exposure, and the potential for delayed toxic effects. For example, therapeutic levels of acetaminophen (30 μg/mL) 4 – 8 hours postingestion are associated with little risk of hepatotoxicity; the same level obtained more than 16 hours postingestion indicates a high risk of hepatotoxicity unless antidotal therapy is instituted immediately. Other considerations include the fact that toxic reactions may occur at therapeutic levels if the drug exacerbates an underlying pathology, the possibility of false negatives, and the realization that no assay or combination of assays can detect all possible poisons.

TREATING THE POISONED PATIENT

The three goals in treating acute poisoning are to (1) prevent absorption of the toxin, (2) enhance its elimination, and (3) reverse its toxicity by administering antidotes.

Decrease Absorption

Irrigation-Washing

Decontamination of the skin, eyes, and gastrointestinal (GI) tract should be started after the initial diagnostic assessment and laboratory evaluation. Contaminated clothing should be removed once the patient is removed from further exposure. The skin should be cleansed with copious amounts of soap and water to prevent further percutaneous absorption. The eyes should be irrigated with warm tap water or normal saline solution.

Dilution

Although diluting poisons within the GI tract with large volumes of water has been recommended in the past, the use of water may actually increase the acute toxicity of drugs by enhancing their dissolution and stimulating gastric emptying. The AAPCC has recommended that oral dilution with water be used only to minimize the risk of burns from caustic-type substances. Water can be given with ipecac syrup, but is not required for its efficacy. Inhalation of humidified air or oxygen can dilute toxins in the nasal passages.

Emesis

Induction of vomiting with ipecac syrup is the preferred method for removing ingested substances from the stomach of patients with a gag reflex who are conscious and alert. It is most effective when initiated within 30 minutes of toxin ingestion. Recommended dosages and contraindications to emesis are listed in Table 46 – 1. Upon the advice of a physician or poison control center specialist, ipecac syrup can be used safely and effectively in the home. Other emetics, such as lobeline injection, copper sulfate solution, salt water, and

TABLE 46–1. Ipecac Syrup

Administration

1. Carefully supervise all vomiting patients.
2. Administer ipecac syrup.

Age	*Volume*
6–12 months	10 mL–15 mL
1–5 years	15 mL–30 mL
>5 years	30 mL

3. Repeat dose if vomiting has not occurred within 20 minutes.
4. After vomiting has begun, give fluids (about 15–30 mL) until vomitus is clear.
5. Do not give food or drink for 1–2 hours to allow effects from ipecac to stop.
6. Keep patient in upright position or on side/stomach to prevent vomit aspiration.

Contraindications

1. Child younger than 6 months of age unless in an emergency room.
2. Comatose patient or patient with altered level of consciousness.
3. Presence of seizures or expected onset of seizures owing to toxin involved.
4. Loss of gag reflex.
5. Ingestion of sharp solid material.
6. Ingestion of caustics.
7. Nonaromatic and nonhalogenated hydrocarbons that do not contain other toxic agent.

mustard powder, have been abandoned because they are either impractical or ineffective or have a low margin of safety. Apomorphine is no longer used in humans because of its side effects, but is safely used in animals. A soapsuds solution (2–3 tablespoons of liquid dishwashing detergent, not automatic dishwasher detergent, in 6–8 ounces of water) is recommended as an emetic by some poison control centers in situations where ipecac syrup is not available.

Activated Charcoal and Cathartics

Activated charcoal is the most efficacious procedure for preventing the absorption of drugs, even if the patient presents to the emergency room several hours postingestion. Currently the use of activated charcoal alone, without prior ipecac-induced emesis or lavage, is favored, particularly in patients seen more than 1 hour postingestion. Optimal adsorption occurs when the dose of charcoal is at least tenfold greater than the estimated dose of toxin. Charcoal does not adsorb iron salts, hydrocarbons, simple alcohols, boric acid, lithium, cyanide, and caustics. Thickening agents such as bentonite, 70% sorbitol, or 2% carboxymethylcellulose are effective in suspending charcoal without altering its adsorptive capacity. Flavoring agents such as jam, jelly, milk, cocoa powder, ice cream, and sherbet should be avoided because they compromise the efficacy of the charcoal. Administration of a cathartic with the activated charcoal hastens the removal of toxins from the GI tract and thereby reduces their systemic absorption. Sorbitol (40–70%) is the preferred cathartic agent if heart failure is not present. The use of sorbitol in the commercially available, premixed activated charcoal preparations precludes the need for other cathartics. Magnesium or sodium sulfate and magnesium citrate can be used with the activated charcoal powder. Oil-based cathartics are of no value and are potentially harmful because of the potential for lung aspiration. Table 46–2 lists usual dosages of common cathartics.

Gastric Lavage

Gastric lavage is used primarily in patients who are obtunded, comatose, or uncooperative. The most important factor in determining the efficacy of gastric lavage, as well as ipecac-induced emesis, appears to be the time elapsed between ingestion and implementation of the decontamination procedure. When the decontamination procedure is delayed more than 60 minutes postingestion, the amount of toxin recovered by gastric lavage or emesis is small and not significantly different. Gastric lavage performed more than 1 hour postingestion has shown no benefit over the administration of activated charcoal alone (Kulig et al, 1985). Epidemiological studies report that the mean time from ingestion to hospital presentation is 3.3 hours for adults and 68 minutes for children (Kulig et al, 1985; MacLean, 1973). Another important variable in determining the effectiveness of gastric lavage is the size of the tube. Decontamination with small-bore nasogastric tubes is inferior to ipecac-induced emesis. The larger orogastric tubes are more efficacious and can be used to introduce activated charcoal or a specific antidote. Contraindications for lavage are similar to those for emesis. Aspiration pneumonia, secondary to vomiting during the procedure, is the most common complication.

Whole Bowel Irrigation

Whole bowel irrigation is used primarily as a safe, precolonoscopy procedure. It involves the oral administration of large volumes of a polyethylene-glycol iso-osmotic electrolyte (GOLYTELY, COLYTE) solution that traverses the entire GI tract and is generally well-tolerated. Although superior to gastric lavage and induced emesis, it is both labor-intensive

TABLE 46–2. Activated Charcoal and Cathartics

Single-Dose Activated Charcoal

1. Administer 1.0 g/kg of activated charcoal mixed in water or 70% sorbitol.

Multiple-Dose Activated Charcoal

1. Administer one half of initial dose (without cathartic) every 2–6 hours until patient is asymptomatic.
2. Cathartic may be given every 8–12 hours if patient has not stooled.

Cathartics

1. Sorbitol (70%) is preferred (child: 1–2 mL/kg; adult: 100–150 mL).
2. Magnesium or sodium sulfate (10%); magnesium citrate (10%) (child: 4 mL/kg; adult: 150–250 mL).

Contraindications

1. Absence of bowel sounds.
2. Signs of intestinal obstruction, abdominal trauma, or gastrointestinal bleeding.
3. Shock, poor tissue perfusion.
4. Use cautiously in patient with hematemesis.
5. Avoid magnesium cathartics in patient with renal disease.
6. Avoid sodium cathartics in patient with congestive heart failure.

and time-consuming. It should not be used routinely but may be promising for drugs that are not adsorbed by activated charcoal (*eg*, iron, lithium) or for overdoses with delayed-release pharmaceuticals (Tenenbein, 1988).

Enhance Elimination

Knowledge of basic concepts governing the pharmacokinetic or toxicokinetic (kinetics of a drug in overdose) properties of a drug can assist the clinician in deciding which therapies may accelerate the removal of the toxin and thus decrease morbidity and mortality. Procedures such as changing urinary pH (with or without diuresis, hemodialysis, or peritoneal dialysis), charcoal and resin hemoperfusion, exchange transfusion, repeated oral administration of activated charcoal, and plasmapheresis all have been used in attempts to hasten systemic elimination of drugs and poisons.

These therapies enhance the clearance of drugs but do not affect their volume of distribution (Vd). For drugs eliminated by first-order kinetics, both clearance and Vd are related to the half-life of the drug ($t_{1/2}$), the time necessary to eliminate one half the amount of drug in the body, by the following equation:

$$Ct_{1/2} = \frac{0.693\ Vd(L/kg)}{cl}$$

cl represents clearance (mg/minute); C is the plasma drug concentration (mg/L). Thus, for drugs with a large Vd, the $t_{1/2}$ is prolonged at any given clearance. Conversely, as clearance rate increases, the $t_{1/2}$ shortens for any given Vd. Generally, methods to enhance elimination are clinically effective only for toxins with a Vd less than or equal to total body water, 0.6 L/kg. The degree of plasma protein binding also affects the efficacy of the treatment modality. Except for charcoal or resin hemoperfusion, therapies that enhance drug clearance primarily remove the free or unbound drug from the plasma compartment. Therefore, if a drug has a large Vd (*eg*, cyclic antidepressants, digoxin), the removal of drug from plasma has minimal impact on the total amount of drug in the body. Plasma drug levels rebound to pretreatment levels as the drug exits tissue stores and re-equilibrates with plasma. In cases of massive overdose, elimination pathways that involve hepatic enzyme systems can become saturated. In these instances, drug clearance remains constant and is concentration-independent (zero-order kinetics). Drugs that exhibit zero-order kinetics in overdose include theophylline, salicylates, some barbiturates, chloral hydrate, ethchlorvynol, and acetaminophen. In these instances, using methods to enhance drug elimination may contribute to total body clearance and may significantly improve the clinical outcome.

It is important to understand not only the toxicodynamic (injurious effects of toxins on vital functions) and toxicokinetic properties of toxins, but also to be familiar with the risks versus the benefits of each technique. These methods should be considered only in those instances in which it has been shown to impact the clinical outcome or in high-risk patients who do not respond to traditional supportive care.

Forced Diuresis

Fluid loading and forced diuresis with furosemide or mannitol is one of the oldest techniques used to enhance drug elimination. Only drugs that are minimally protein-bound, eliminated primarily by renal excretion, and passively reabsorbed in the renal tubules are affected by diuresis. Forced diuresis has unproven efficacy but has been utilized in overdoses with bromides, PCP, lithium, and amphetamines. Contraindications include renal or cardiac failure. Pulmonary edema and electrolyte imbalances are potential problems with diuresis.

Acid-Alkaline Diuresis

Renal elimination of a few toxins is enhanced by alteration of urinary pH with or without forced diuresis. This technique takes advantage of the ionization properties (expressed as the negative log of their acid dissociation constant or pKa) of drugs that are weak acids and weak bases. Because the ionized forms of these drugs cannot diffuse through the cell membrane, they are trapped in compartments that promote their ionization. Acids (un-ionized when protonated) are trapped in alkaline compartments; bases (ionized when protonated) are trapped in acidic compartments. When the pH of the urine is altered appropriately, it can cause drugs contained within it to become ionized. In this form, the drug is not reabsorbed by the renal tubules, and its excretion is hastened. Alkaline diuresis is a useful technique for weak acids such as salicylate (pKa = 3.0), phenobarbital (pKa = 7.2), and some oral hypoglycemics (*eg*, chlorpropamide). Acid diuresis has been advocated in strychnine (pKa = 8.0), PCP (pKa = 8.5), and amphetamine (pKa = 9.9) overdoses, but is not clinically useful and may be harmful.

Dialysis

Dialysis refers to the diffusion of a toxin across a semipermeable membrane. Although it has been recommended for a variety of poisons, relatively few patients benefit from it. The physical characteristics of the drug are the major factors limiting its efficacy. The drug must have a small Vd, a molecular weight small enough (<500 daltons) to permit it to pass through the dialysis membrane, hydrophilicity, and low protein binding. Hemodialysis is indicated in renal failure secondary to toxin exposure, when the metabolism of a dialyzable drug is limited by saturation of liver enzymes, and in severe overdose with salicylates, lithium, ethylene glycol, or methanol. It is used also in the presence of fluid and electrolyte imbalances. Peritoneal dialysis is a relatively simple technique, yet is only 10–25% as effective as hemodialysis and only slightly more effective than forced diuresis. It can be useful if short-term dialysis is required, as in salicylate or lithium overdoses.

Charcoal-Resin Hemoperfusion

Hemoperfusion is a technique whereby blood is pumped through a cartridge that contains either charcoal or an amberlite resin. The affinity of the toxin for the adsorbent, the rate of blood flow through the cartridge, and the Vd of the toxin are the factors that contribute to the efficacy of hemoperfusion. Unlike dialysis, hemoperfusion is not limited to small, hydrophilic compounds and effectively extracts large, hydrophobic drugs that exhibit extensive protein binding. Charcoal removes both polar and nonpolar drugs, whereas resin clears nonpolar drugs more effectively than does charcoal. It is the modality of choice in severe theophylline, paraquat, digitoxin, ethchlorvynol, phenytoin, and phenobarbital poisonings. It does not correct fluid and electrolyte imbalances or remove all toxic chemicals. Complications such as depletion of platelets and removal of plasma proteins and solutes have been minimized with increasing clinical experience and the advent of more adsorbent and coated cartridges.

Exchange Transfusion

Exchange transfusion is a technique in which blood of a poisoned patient is removed and replaced with fresh whole blood. Potentially, its most effective applications are in patients with severe methemoglobinemia unresponsive to methylene blue and in severe iron poisoning.

Multiple-Dose Activated Charcoal

The oral administration of multiple doses of activated charcoal (MDAC), also called gastrointestinal dialysis, enhances drug elimination by (1) preventing the absorption of drugs from the GI tract, (2) adsorbing drugs that either diffuse or are transported back into the GI tract, and (3) adsorbing drugs that are excreted into the small intestine from the biliary tract (Levy, 1982; Watson, 1987). The ability of MDAC to remove drugs is influenced by the same pharmacokinetic principles that govern the effectiveness of hemodialysis and hemoperfusion. Drugs that undergo extensive enterogastric or enterohepatic recycling (*eg*, digitoxin) may be removed more efficiently by MDAC. The efficacy of MDAC is affected also by the preparation and dose of charcoal, the time interval between drug intoxication and charcoal administration, the time interval between dosages of charcoal, and the severity of intoxication (Watson, 1987). Advantages of MDAC are that it can be initiated immediately in the primary care setting and that it is noninvasive, inexpensive, and generally well-tolerated. Adverse effects include repeated emesis (especially after ipecac syrup), protracted diarrhea (because of cathartic coadministration), aspiration, and GI obstruction. Although the plasma clearance of phenobarbital, theophylline, salicylates, and carbamazepine (Park et al, 1986; Tenebein, 1988) is enhanced by MDAC, changes in morbidity and mortality have been demonstrated only for theophylline overdoses.

Plasmapheresis

Plasma exchange transfusion refers to the therapeutic removal of large volumes of plasma and its replacement with normal plasma or suitable colloid. It is most applicable to toxins that are highly protein-bound, have a small Vd, and have a prolonged $t_{1/2}$ (*eg*, phenytoin, digitoxin). Because hemodialysis and hemoperfusion clear larger plasma volumes at a faster rate, they should be considered first when supportive care is insufficient. As yet, because of the multiple complications and costs involved, plasmapheresis should be considered an unproven and hazardous form of poisoning therapy.

Antidotes

Antidotes antagonize the effects of toxins by inhibiting the binding of a toxin to its receptor (pharmacological antagonist), causing a physiological response that opposed the actions of a toxin (physiological antagonist), changing the chemical nature of a poison to a less toxic form (chemical antagonism), or decreasing the amount of toxin that reaches its site of action by either preventing its absorption or enhancing its elimination or metabolism (biochemical antagonism). Unfortunately, there are only a small number of toxins for which effective antidotes exist. Major antidotes and dosages are listed in Table 46 – 3. These drugs are supplemented by immunological agents such as snake antivenins and bacterial antitoxins. Flumazenil and immunological agents are being evaluated currently as potential antidotes for benzodiazepine and tricyclic antidepressant poisonings, respectively. Strong acids and bases are treated with water or milk. Neutralization of acids and bases with antacids or lemon juice, respectively, is no longer advocated because of the exothermic reaction produced by these combinations.

Acute Poisons

The AAPCC began collecting data on human poisonings in 1983. Since that time, it has been observed that more than 90% of the chemicals associated with fatalities are distributed among 12 generic classes of chemicals. Figure 46 – 1 depicts the rank of these classes according to the number of deaths with which they were associated in 1988. Although small changes in the relative order of these chemical classifications occur yearly, poisonings from chemicals within these classifications continue to be the major challenge to medical practitioners. The following text provides a general discussion of the toxicity and treatment for those chemicals within each category most frequently associated with fatality. More detailed discussions are available elsewhere (see Goldfrank, 1994).

Antidepressants

Antidepressants constitute the class of drugs found to cause most deaths from acute poisoning. Only street drugs and cardiovascular agents approach this degree of lethality. This observation is probably a reflection of their relatively low margin of safety, as well as the fact that individuals taking antidepressants have a higher potential for suicide. Of the 764 poisons associated with fatality in 1991, 188 were antidepressants. The cyclic antidepressants were most frequently involved (153 deaths), followed by lithium salts (12), monoamine oxidase (MAO) inhibitors (5), other antidepressants (9), and trazodone (5).

Cyclic Antidepressants and Trazodone

Amitriptyline and imipramine are prototypical tricyclic antidepressants and account for 81% of the fatalities within this

TABLE 46–3. Poisons and Antidotes

Poison	Antidote	Dosage
Acetaminophen	*N*-acetylcysteine (MUCOMYST)	Load: 140 mg/kg orally ×1 dose Maintenance: 70 mg/kg every 4 hours for 17 doses
Arsenic, mercury	DMSA (succimer)	See doses for lead (investigational use only)
	EDTA calcium	See doses of lead
	Dimercaprol (BAL IN OIL)	See doses for lead
Atropine, anticholinergics	Physostigmine (ANTILIRIUM)	Adult: 0.5–2 mg IV Pediatric: 0.5 mg (0.01 mg/kg) Repeat as needed
Benzodiazepines	Flumazenil (MAZICON)	0.5 mg over 15 seconds, may repeat 0.5 mg doses to a total of 3–5 mg
Cyanide, nitroprusside	Cyanide antidote kit	1 ampule amyl nitrate (inhaled); sodium nitrite 300 mg at 2.5 mL–5 mL/minute IV, then 12.5 g of 25% sodium thiosulfate IV infusion
	Hydroxycobalamine (vitamin B_{12}) Investigational	Load: 50 mg/kg IV Maintenance: 25 mg/hour (investigational use only)
Digoxin	Fab fragments	Dose according to serum level or amount ingested
Ethylene glycol, methanol	Ethanol	Load: 10 mL/kg of 10% of 5% dextrose in water IV or orally Maintenance: 1.5 mL/kg/hour of 10% in 5% dextrose in water Maintain serum ethanol level 100–130 mg%
	4-Methylpyrazole	20 mg/kg/day p.o. or IV (investigational)
Iron	Deferoxamine (DESFERAL)	90 mg/kg IM to a maximum of 1 g every 4–8 hours or 15 mg/kg/hour IV to maximum of 6 g/24 hours
Isoniazid	Pyridoxine (vitamin B_6)	5 g over 30–60 minutes Repeat to maximum 40 g adults; 20 g children
Lead	EDTA calcium (edetate)	50–75 mg/kg/day deep IM or slow IV in three to six doses for 5 days
	Dimercaprol	3–5 mg/kg dose IM every 4 hours for 48 hours, then 3 mg/kg/dose IM every 6 hours for 48 hours, then 3 mg/kg/dose every 12 hours for 7 days
	DSMA (succimer)	10 mg/kg/dose orally every 8 hours for 5 days, then 10 mg/kg every 12 hours for 14 days
Methemoglobinemia	Methylene blue	0.1–0.2 mL/kg of 1% solution IV infusion, repeat as needed
Opioids	Naloxone	0.4–2 mg initially, repeat every 2–3 minutes until desired effect; continuous IV infusion may be necessary
Organophosphates, carbamates	Atropine	Adult: 0.5–2 mg IV Pediatric: 0.05 mg/kg IV Repeat dosage every 10 minutes until "atropinized"
	Pralidoxime (2-PAM), organophospates only	Adult: 1–2 g over 30 minutes Pediatric: 25–50 mg/kg over 30 minutes Repeat 1 hour after initial dose and then every 6–12 hours
Warfarin	Phytonadione (vitamin K_1)	Adult: 10 mg IM Pediatric: 1–5 mg IM/IV Doses of 100–400 mg/day may be required in severe cases

(DMSA = dimercaptosuccinic acid; EDTA = edetate calcium disodium.)

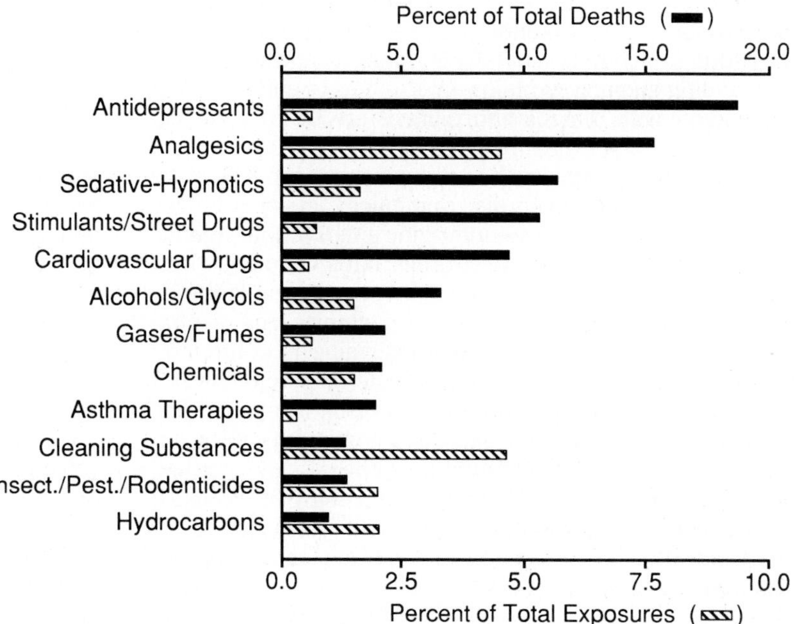

FIGURE 46–1. Distribution of deaths *(solid bars)* and exposures *(open bars)* among 12 categories of poisons. Percentages are based on the total number of poisons known to be involved in human fatalities (741) and exposures (1,437,117). Among the categories of poisons listed by the AAPCC, antidepressants were most frequently associated with fatalities (18.2%), whereas analgesics were most frequently involved in all cases of poisoning (10.0%). (Data from Litovitz, JL, Schmitz BF, Holm KC: 1988 annual report of the American Association of Poison Control Center national data collection system. Am J Emerg Med 7:495–545, 1989.)

category. Amoxapine and maprotiline are representative tetracyclic antidepressants. Trazodone as well as fluoxetine and bupropion are newer (second-generation) antidepressant drugs whose chemical structures differ from those of the cyclic antidepressants.

The cyclic and second-generation antidepressants are pharmacokinetically similar. Most are absorbed incompletely and undergo significant first-pass metabolism. They are eliminated over the course of several days following their oxidation by hepatic microsomal enzymes and eventual conjugation with glucuronic acid. About 15% of the metabolized dose is excreted into the intestines through the bile and may remain biologically active. The half-life of these agents (therapeutic, 8 - 100 hours) may be prolonged in the overdose setting.

Acute intoxication with these drugs usually begins with a brief phase of agitation and restlessness that may include tonic-clonic seizures. This may rapidly lead to coma with depressed tendon reflexes, depressed respiration, hypotension, and hypothermia. Antimuscarinic symptoms such as dry mouth, mydriasis, sinus tachycardia, the absence of bowel sounds, urinary retention, and a flushed, dry skin are also evident. Although sinus tachycardia is most common, a variety of cardiac conduction abnormalities and arrhythmias can also be observed. Amoxapine and maprotiline exhibit fewer cardiovascular effects but have a greater seizure potential than other cyclic antidepressants. Trazodone and fluoxetine exhibit less cardiotoxicity and neurotoxicity than the cyclic antidepressants and have weaker antimuscarinic properties. Overdoses with bupropion, a drug chemically related to amphetamine, commonly result in seizures.

The induction of emesis is contraindicated because it may precipitate seizures; gastric lavage is of limited benefit unless begun within 1 hour of exposure. Activated charcoal adsorbs these compounds and may be particularly efficacious in cases of overdose, because the anticholinergic effects of these drugs prolong their stay in the gut. Although MDAC can be given to interrupt the enterohepatic circulation of these drugs, the risk of bowel obstruction with MDAC outweighs its potential benefit in serious intoxications. The large volumes of distribution (VD, 5 - 60 L/kg) exhibited by these drugs is a function of their lipophilicity and strong protein binding and may explain why attempts to enhance their elimination with dialysis and diuresis are of little clinical value.

The lethality of the cyclic antidepressants is primarily the result of their effect on cardiac rhythmicity. In general, they are more toxic than the phenothiazine antipsychotic agents. There are no antidotes for these drugs. Intoxications are best managed by supporting cardiac function and ventilation by treating the hypotension, seizures, arrhythmias, and respiratory depression. The use of physostigmine is contraindicated due to its potential to exacerbate or precipitate seizures and arrhythmias. Deaths usually result from a cardiac arrhythmia, but respiratory failure and coma also can occur. All patients should be admitted to a critical care unit and be placed on a cardiac monitor for at least 24 hours. If the patient is symptomatic, they should be observed for 24 hours after the resolution of CNS and cardiovascular symptoms.

Monoamine Oxidase Inhibitors

Of this class of drugs, isocarboxazid, phenelzine, and tranylcypromine are the ones used currently in the United States for the treatment of depression. MAO inhibitors are rapidly absorbed from the GI tract. Although little is known of their pharmacokinetics, MAO inhibitors are metabolized in the liver primarily by acetylation. About half the population in the United States and Europe are slow acetylators and are thus more susceptible to MAO toxicity.

Toxic manifestations of drug overdose may be delayed 6 - 24 hours after ingestion and include restlessness, hypertension, hyperreflexia, mydriasis, sinus tachycardia, hyperpyrexia, diaphoresis, muscular rigidity, and coma. Hypertension usually is accompanied by headache, hyperpyrexia, and tachycardia and may lead to cerebral hemorrhage and death. If MAO inhibitors are ingested alone, the late phases of severe intoxications (>4 mg/kg) may be associated with profound hypotension, bradycardia, and cardiac arrest.

Because there is no antidote for MAO intoxication, treatment is supportive care. Particular attention should be given to ensuring adequate ventilation and to controlling blood pressure, hyperthermia, excessive muscle rigidity, and seizures. Because isocarboxazid and phenelzine bind irreversibly with MAO, several weeks may be required to synthesize new enzyme and to restore monoamine metabolism to normal. Intoxications with tranylcypromine are reversed more rapidly, perhaps reflecting the reversible binding between the drug and MAO. Patients should be monitored in the intensive care unit, even if they present asymptomatic initially, for 24 hours.

Lithium Salts

Lithium is well-absorbed from the GI tract, is not bound by plasma proteins, and has a VD (0.8 L/kg) that slightly exceeds total body water (0.6 L/kg). Although lithium quickly diffuses throughout the body's extracellular space, it crosses cell membranes slowly. This is particularly true in the CNS, where equilibrium between plasma and brain takes from 8 to 10 days. This may explain why the toxic symptoms in patients who have not previously received lithium are sometimes limited to nausea and vomiting. Lithium is eliminated almost entirely by urinary excretion. Because there are no specific antidotes for lithium intoxication, treatment is primarily supportive. Emesis or lavage may be of value if initiated shortly after ingestion or when absorption is delayed, as with sustained-release tablets. Sodium polystyrene sulfonate may bind lithium more effectively than activated charcoal, which is of dubious value.

Lithium overdoses accounted for 6% of the fatalities due to antidepressants in 1991. The mechanism responsible for the therapeutic and toxic effects of lithium remains unclear. In patients chronically on lithium therapy, toxicity is common at blood levels of 2 mEq/L; sustained levels of 4 mEq/L are often lethal. Higher levels may be tolerated in naive individuals. Although early signs of lithium overdose include nausea, diarrhea, and polyuria, neurological effects constitute the primary concern. These include mental confusion, drowsiness, dysarthria, blurred vision, tremor, fasciculations, myoclonus, and choreothetosis and may progress to stupor, seizures, and coma. Renal and cardiac conduction abnormalities may be evident in severe cases. It is extremely important to recognize the distinction between lithium and cyclic antidepressant overdoses, because hemodialysis may be beneficial for lithium overdosage but ineffective for enhancing removal of other antidepressants.

Hemodialysis markedly reduces serum lithium levels, although levels rise again after treatment because of the redistribution of lithium from intracellular to extracellular sites. This observation may explain why, even with hemodialysis, recovery remains slow. Approximately 80% of the lithium filtered by the kidney is reabsorbed in the proximal tubule, where it competes with sodium for reabsorption. Thus, maintaining water and sodium balance is a major concern. Forced diuresis with saline solution and osmotic diuretics (mannitol) can result in serious electrolyte imbalances and should not be used unless the glomerular filtration rate is below normal. In those instances of impaired glomerular filtration, volume repletion with IV normal saline for several hours should increase renal lithium clearance. Carbonic anhydrase inhibitors (acetazolamide) and urinary alkalinization have been reported to reduce plasma lithium levels, presumably through their effects on Na^+/H^+ exchange. However, urinary alkalinization is not recommended. Dehydration (vomiting, diarrhea) and hyponatremia (low salt; distal tubule diuretics, thiazides) can potentiate lithium toxicity by increasing its renal reabsorption.

Analgesics

Analgesics made up 190 of the 764 fatal poisons reported to the AAPCC in 1991. Most of the analgesics associated with fatality could be classified as either acetaminophen (82 deaths), a salicylate (60), an opioid (40), or ibuprofen (4).

Acetaminophen

Acetaminophen is rapidly and completely absorbed from the GI tract. Therapeutic dosages are metabolized in the liver by conjugation to glucuronides (60%) and sulfates (35%). A small fraction (4%) is metabolized by the P-450 mixed-function oxidase system to a reactive intermediate, which is detoxified by glutathione to cysteine and mercapturic acid metabolites. At higher dosages, more acetaminophen is converted to the reactive intermediate because the conjugation pathways become saturated. As glutathione stores are depleted, the reactive intermediate binds to other cellular proteins and produces hepatic necrosis. Renal dysfunction has the same etiology. Acetaminophen intoxication is best treated by replenishing glutathione stores with *N*-acetyl-L-cysteine (NAC), a glutathione precursor.

Acetaminophen toxicity results after an acute ingestion of greater than 150 mg/kg or a minimum of 7.5 gm. A dose of greater than 500 mg/kg or 15 gm may be lethal if treatment is not instituted.

Acetaminophen poisoning is divided into four stages. The first (12 – 24 hours postexposure) is characterized by anorexia, nausea, vomiting, and diaphoresis. The second (1 – 2 days) is associated with clinical improvement. The prothrombin time and plasma levels of hepatic transaminases and bilirubin begin to increase. Hepatotoxicity, manifested by centrilobular necrosis, usually reaches its peak during the third stage (3 – 4 days). Mildly poisoned individuals enter stage four (5 – 7 days postexposure) and recover. Severe intoxications lead to hepatic encephalopathy that progresses from confusion to coma to death. Some patients also exhibit acute renal failure.

Emesis or lavage may be useful if initiated early. However, activated charcoal alone should be initiated within 4 hours postexposure. Between 4 to 8 hours postingestion, activated charcoal should be administered if multiple drugs have been coingested. However, in order to prevent hepatotoxicity following exposure, therapy with NAC should not be delayed more than 8 to 10 hours. NAC should be administered orally, starting with a loading dose of 140 mg/kg of 20% solution, diluted to 5%, followed by dose of 70 mg/kg every 4 hours, diluted to 5%, for 17 doses. IV NAC is not yet Food and Drug Administration (FDA) approved. Liver function and renal function tests should be monitored daily.

Salicylates

Salicylates are rapidly and completely absorbed from the GI tract in therapeutic dosages. An acute overdose can result in the formation of drug concretions (bezoars) and delayed gastric emptying. Salicylic acid and methyl salicylate are well-absorbed through the intact skin. Aspirin and methyl salicylate are rapidly hydrolyzed to salicylic acid by esterases in GI mucosa and liver. The plasma half-life of aspirin is 15 – 20 minutes, whereas the half-life of salicylic acid at therapeutic doses is approximately 3 hours. Salicylic acid is metabolized in the liver by conjugation with glycine to form salicyluric acid and with glucuronic acid to form salicylic phenolic and acyl glucuronides. A small portion is hydroxylated to gentisic acid. Because these metabolic pathways are quickly saturated at therapeutic dosages, the half-life of salicylate in cases of overdose can be as long as 36 hours. Salicylates are excreted primarily by the kidney as salicylic acid (10%), salicyluric acid (75%), phenolic (10%) and acyl (5%) glucuronides, as well as gentisic acid (<1%). The salicylic acid content of urine is quite variable because it depends on both dosage and urinary pH.

Common features of acute salicylate poisoning involve the GI tract and the CNS. These include nausea and vomiting, tinnitus and hearing loss, as well as hyperventilation. Hyperventilation is mediated by the stimulatory effect of salicylates on the medullary respiratory center and by the increased plasma CO_2 levels that result from the ability of salicylates to uncouple oxidative phosphorylation. The uncoupling of oxidative phosphorylation also may be responsible for the hyperpyrexia and sweating seen in cases of overdose. Acid-base imbalances are another important clinical manifestation of toxicity. Hyperventilation leads to respiratory alkalosis that is followed by the increased renal excretion of bicarbonate, potassium, and water.

Severe salicylate intoxication is associated with a combination of respiratory alkalosis and metabolic acidosis. High dosages of salicylate depress respiration which, in the presence of low plasma bicarbonate and the enhanced production of CO_2, results in respiratory acidosis. Salicylates produce metabolic acidosis by interfering with the citric acid cycle, which results in the accumulation of organic acids such as lactate, pyruvate, and acetoacetate. Severe intoxication also may lead to pulmonary edema, convulsions, and coma. These effects on the CNS may reflect a reduction in brain glucose levels, as well as the shift of salicylates from the blood to the brain in acidemic patients because of pH-partitioning.

The treatment for salicylate intoxication is primarily symptomatic. Particular attention should be given to correcting hyperpyrexia, dehydration, acid-based imbalances, and hypokalemia. CNS depression should be treated with IV glucose even when serum glucose levels are normal. Absorption from the GI tract can be prevented by emesis or gastric lavage within 2 to 4 hours of exposure or by activated charcoal alone. MDAC may also enhance the elimination of absorbed drug. The elimination of aspirin (pKa = 3.5) and other salicylates can be enhanced by urinary alkalinization (pH = 7–8) with sodium bicarbonate, hemodialysis, and hemoperfusion. Although the latter two treatments are equally effective in removing salicylates, hemodialysis is better able to control acid-base and electrolyte imbalances.

Opioids

Heroin overdosage fatalities contributed to only 17% of the opioid fatalities in 1991. However, poison information center data inadequately represent the true incidence of heroin abuse because the majority of overdose victims die, due to the rapid onset of respiratory failure, before treatment can be initiated in a health care facility. Therefore, these cases are not reported to the poison control centers.

Acute intoxication with opioids is associated with the triad of CNS depression (stupor, coma), respiratory depression, and pinpoint pupils (except meperidine). Opioids (except pentazocine) also produce peripheral vasodilation that, in the presence of hypoxia, may progress to shock. Seizures may be seen following overdoses with meperidine and propoxyphene. Cardiac arrhythmias are not uncommon in propoxyphene overdoses. Pulmonary edema is present in the majority of fatalities.

Treatment of overdose begins with establishing adequate ventilation and circulation and is followed by the administration of naloxone, a pure opioid antagonist. Naloxone does not reverse cardiac arrhythmias seen with propoxyphene. The patient must be monitored carefully because the antagonistic effects of naloxone last for only a few minutes, whereas the toxic effects of long-acting opioids (methadone) may last for several days. Multiple IV doses of naloxone or a continuous infusion may be necessary to maintain adequate ventilation. Induction of emesis is contraindicated; lavage may be effective if initiated early. Activated charcoal alone may be effective any time postexposure because of the decreased GI motility produced by opioids. Forced diuresis and dialysis are of no value because of the large volumes of distribution and high degrees of protein binding exhibited by opioids. Also, forced diuresis may exacerbate pulmonary edema.

Ibuprofen

Next to aspirin, ibuprofen is the most widely used nonsteroidal anti-inflammatory drug (NSAID) in the United States. Because of its greater availability in OTC preparations, ibuprofen overdose has increased over 100-fold since 1984. Although 1991 reported poisoning exposures to all nonsteroidal agents exceeded salicylate exposures by 100%, they result in 80% fewer fatalities.

Acute ibuprofen overdoses may result in mild GI symptoms such as nausea, vomiting, and epigastric pain. A toxic dose-response relationship has not been clearly established in adults. In children, mild to moderate symptoms have been observed in patients ingesting 100–300 mg/kg; severe toxicity is demonstrated by doses of greater than 300 mg/kg. Peptic ulceration and hemorrhage are not common in acute overdoses. Other less commonly observed manifestations of ibuprofen toxicity include metabolic acidosis, hypotension, CNS depression, and renal dysfunction. Renal toxicity is thought to be due to the decreased production of intrarenal prostaglandins, which causes a decrease in both renal blood flow and glomerular filtration rate. In children, aspirin toxicity is associated with hyperventilation, whereas ibuprofen is more commonly associated with apnea (>300–400 mg/kg).

Intoxications are treated with supportive care. Ipecac syrup may be of benefit if administered within 30 minutes of exposure. Activated charcoal alone may be of benefit any time postexposure because it adsorbs many other NSAIDs. Methods to enhance the elimination of ibuprofen are ineffective. There are no antidotes.

Stimulants and Street Drugs

Of the fatalities reported to the AAPCC in 1991, 90 involved stimulants and street drugs. Cocaine was responsible for 60 deaths, followed by amphetamines (11), heroin (10), caffeine (3), and phenylpropanolamine (2). The treatments for heroin (diacetylmorphine, which is rapidly deacetylated to morphine) and nitrite intoxication are presented in this chapter under Opioids and Chemicals, respectively. Caffeine (1, 3, 7-trimethylxanthine) and theophylline (1, 3-dimethylxanthine, discussed later under Asthma Therapies) intoxication are treated similarly.

Cocaine

Cocaine is well-absorbed from nasal, respiratory, and GI mucosa. Following absorption, it is rapidly degraded by plasma and liver cholinesterases; only small amounts (10%) are excreted unchanged in the urine.

The initial CNS effects (euphoria, garrulousness, restlessness) are due to cortical stimulation and are followed by effects (hyperventilation, tachycardia, hypertension, hyperthermia, emesis, tremor, convulsions) caused by the progressive involvement of lower brain centers. The central effects of cocaine on heart rate, blood pressure, and temperature are potentiated by its peripheral effects on the sympathetic nervous system. In high dosages, cocaine depresses the CNS as well as myocardial contractility and conduction. Death results from either respiratory failure or cardiac arrest.

Acute intoxications are best treated with supportive care. Therapeutic measures are aimed at controlling the central effects of cocaine. Particular attention should be given to controlling seizures, cardiac arrhythmias, and hyperthermia. Because cocaine is usually inhaled or injected, decontamination of the gut by lavage or emesis is frequently unwarranted. The short plasma $t_{1/2}$ (1 hour) and relatively large Vd (2 L/kg) of cocaine, as well as the small fraction of cocaine excreted unchanged in the urine, make attempts to enhance its elimination impractical. Diazepam can be used to control hyperactivity, tachycardia, and convulsions. Lidocaine should be reserved for patients with life-threatening cardiac arrhythmias. The use of β blockers for hypertension and tachycardia are no longer advocated and may actually exacerbate hypertension due to the potent α-adrenergic effects demonstrated by cocaine. Hyperthermia, which plays a large role in the mortality associated with cocaine, should be controlled with ice water lavage and external cooling.

Amphetamines and Phenylpropanolamine

Amphetamines refer to a class of drugs with similar pharmacological and toxicological properties. The amphetamines associated most frequently with fatality are amphetamine and two structural analogs, methamphetamine and methylphenidate. Smokable methamphetamine is called ice. The toxic manifestations of amphetamine overdose are similar to those described earlier for cocaine. Phenylpropanolamine (PPA) is an analog of amphetamine that is found in OTC preparations of nasal decongestants and diet aides. PPA is a less-potent CNS stimulant than amphetamine; hypertension is the most serious toxic effect of PPA. High dose (>10 mg/kg) of PPA have an effect on the CNS that is similar to that seen with cocaine.

Intoxication with these drugs is best treated with supportive care, with particular attention given to controlling hyperthermia, hypertension, and seizures. Although all these drugs delay gastric emptying, emesis is not recommended because it may provoke seizures, hypertensive hemorrhage, and cardiac complications. Activated charcoal and a cathartic are recommended. Because amphetamine (pKa = 9.9), methamphetamine (pKa = 10.1), and PPA (pKa = 9.4) are weak bases, their elimination can, theoretically, be enhanced by urinary acidification, although its use is not advocated in the overdose setting. Acidification is contraindicated in the presence of rhabdomyolysis and myoglobinuria because myoglobin may precipitate in the renal tubules and damage the kidneys.

Phencyclidine

Although classified pharmacologically as a dissociative anesthetic, PCP is no longer used in humans because of adverse reactions (delirium, seizures) seen postanesthesia. PCP produces a wide variety of physiological effects. Mild intoxications (5–10 mg) present with altered thought patterns, bizarre behavior, horizontal and vertical nystagmus, normal or pinpoint pupils, hyperthermia, hypertension, and tachycardia. Higher dosages (> 10 mg) result in convulsions, coma, respiratory depression, cardiac arrhythmias, and renal failure secondary to rhabdomyolysis.

Most PCP fatalities are either homicidal or accidental. Intoxications are best treated by isolating the patient from unnecessary external stimuli in order to control self-destructive behavior and by supporting vital functions. Emesis and lavage are of questionable benefit because PCP is usually rapidly absorbed and these procedures may further agitate the patient. PCP is a weak base with a pKa of 8.5. Urinary acidification theoretically enhances PCP elimination, but also increases the risk of renal failure in the presence of myoglobinuria. The large Vd of PCP (5.2 L/kg) may explain why acidification does not always lead to a significant clinical improvement. Activated charcoal may be useful to remove PCP trapped in the acidic environment of the stomach and to interrupt the enterogastric circulation of PCP.

Sedative-Hypnotics

The category of drugs termed sedative-hypnotics ranked third (97 deaths) on the list of substances associated most frequently with fatality in 1991.The benzodiazepines (45), phenothiazines (21), and barbiturates (13) were identified in the majority of fatal overdoses. Other drugs identified less frequently were glutethimide, chloral hydrate, ethchlorvynol, diphenhydramine (present in OTC sleep aids), and meprobamate. Although the spectrum of their effects varies, all these drugs depress the CNS.

The toxic manifestations of these drugs are an increase in the depth of CNS depression (sedation, coma, respiratory depression) and cardiovascular instability (hypotension, decreased contractility, arrhythmias, pulmonary edema). Acute intoxications are best treated with supportive care. This includes establishing a clear airway and maintaining adequate ventilation and cardiovascular function. Emesis or lavage should be initiated within 30 minutes of exposure to be effective. Activated charcoal may be of value at any time after exposure to sedative-hypnotics due to the delay in gastric emptying demonstrated by these agents. Diuresis is generally ineffective because the kidney is not a significant elimination pathway; forced diuresis may exacerbate pulmonary edema. MDAC and urinary alkalinization can increase the excretion of phenobarbital (pKa = 7.2) 5- to 10-fold and may obviate the need for extracorporeal removal. Resin hemoperfusion, when necessary, is generally accepted to be more beneficial than hemodialysis in those patients unresponsive to supportive care.

Diphenhydramine, widely available as an OTC cold medicine and sleeping aid, was responsible for 5 of the 10 fatalities involving antihistamines in 1991. Diphenhydramine is a potent H_1-blocker, noted for its antimuscarinic and sedative properties during both therapeutic use and overdose. Signs of peripheral anticholinergic toxicity include blurred vision, tachycardia, arrhythmias, decreased GI motility, urinary retention, and thickening of bronchial secretions. In children and young adults, CNS toxicity is usually associated with stimulation; in adults, toxicity is associated with CNS depression. The decreased GI motility associated with diphenhydramine overdose may increase the effectiveness of gut decontamination procedures initiated more than 1 hour postexposure. Activated charcoal effectively binds diphenhydramine. Methods to enhance its elimination are ineffective because of its large Vd (6.5 L/kg) and significant protein binding (78%). Physostigmine may be given in life-threatening situations such as supraventricular tachycardia in the presence of coronary artery disease, hypertension, or severe agitation. Cardiac conduction delays contraindicate the use of physostigmine.

Cardiovascular Drugs

In 1991, 87 fatalities were ascribed to cardiovascular drugs. Calcium channel blockers were responsible for 31 deaths, followed by cardiac glycosides (21), β blockers (17), antiarrhythmics (8), antihypertensives (8), and vasodilators (2). They rank second only to the antidepressants as the most lethal category of prescription drugs.

Calcium Channel Blockers

Diltiazem, nifedipine, verapamil, and isradipine were associated with fatalities in 1991. All of these drugs produce vasodilatation. Manifestations of acute toxicity are exacerbations of their therapeutic effects. Bradycardia, conduction block, and hypotension are the major complications seen with verapamil and diltiazem; vasodilatation and tachycardia are the predominant features of intoxication with nifedipine.

Aggressive supportive care is the cornerstone of management. Decontamination of the stomach by the usual measures should be initiated; however, induction of emesis is contraindicated. The ingestion of large quantities of sustained-release preparations may result in a bezoar or bowel obstruction. MDAC or whole bowel irrigation may be warranted in these cases. The pharmacokinetic characteristics of all of these agents indicate that diuresis, hemodialysis, and hemoperfusion are impractical for these lipophilic drugs. Hypotension may be difficult to manage, but usually responds to IV calcium and normal saline solution. Atropine, isoproterenol, glucagon, and external cardiac pacing can be used to treat bradycardia and atrioventricular (A-V) block. 4-Aminopyridine is currently under investigation as an effective calcium channel blocker antagonist.

Cardiac Glycosides

Digoxin was the drug involved in all cardiac glycoside fatalities. Nausea and vomiting are common symptoms of glycoside poisoning. Fatigue, mental confusion, and visual disturbances also may be present. Abnormalities in cardiac rhythm, particularly A-V block and ventricular tachycardia, are the usual cause of death. Acute intoxications are associated also with hyperkalemia, which may exacerbate dysrhythmias. Symptoms of toxicity may begin within 30 minutes; peak effects are noted between 3 and 12 hours. Decontamination of the GI tract with activated charcoal followed by a cathartic is beneficial. Emesis and lavage are not recommended because they may stimulate vagal reflexes and exacerbate bradyarrhythmias. The large Vd of digoxin limits the usefulness of diuresis, dialysis, and hemoperfusion. Hyperkalemia may be present and significantly contributes to the morbidity and mortality. Treatment with IV glucose, insulin, bicarbonate, and oral ion-exchange resins such as sodium polystyrene sulfonate (KAYEXALATE) should be attempted. The electrocardiogram should be monitored closely. The administration of calcium salts is contraindicated due to precipitation of intractable ventricular fibrillation or tachycardia. Atropine is useful in managing A-V block; phenytoin effectively suppresses ventricular arrhythmias and promotes A-V conduction. In severe intoxications, the IV administration of the antidote — Fab fragments of immunoglobulins directed against digoxin (DIGIBIND) — can rapidly reverse cardiac toxicity. Serial monitoring of serum potassium and the electrocardiogram are imperative after Fab fragment administration. The benefits of treatment with Fab fragments must be weighed against the possibility of hypersensitivity reactions and of precipitating congestive heart failure in severely diseased patients.

Beta Blockers

The nonselective (1 and 2) adrenergic-receptor antagonists propranolol and naldolol, and the selective (1) adrenergic-receptor antagonists metoprolol, acebutolol, and atenolol were the blockers identified in fatal overdoses. Because the selectivity of the 1-blockers is lost at high concentrations, the toxic effects of all β blockers are similar. These effects include bradycardia, depressed sinoatrial and A-V conduction, hypotension, and bronchospasm. Lipophilic blockers like propranolol and, to a moderate degree, metoprolol can cause CNS depression, seizures, and sudden apnea.

The mainstay of treatment is to prevent further absorption with either lavage or charcoal, followed by a cathartic. Emesis with ipecac may be contraindicated because of the rapid onset of cardiovascular symptoms. Although hemodialysis and hemoperfusion are of no apparent benefit in overdoses with most blockers, the pharmacokinetic properties of atenolol suggest that these procedures may enhance its elimination. Cardiovascular and CNS toxicity are treated symptomatically. Atropine can be used to reverse bradycardia. Bradycardia and hypotension usually respond to high doses of glucagon (5 – 10 mg initially, followed by IV infusion), which elevates cAMP through β-adrenergic receptor-independent pathway. Because isoproterenol is a nonselective β-adrenergic agonist, it may not correct hypotension. Hypotension is best treated with glucagon or norepinephrine. Aminophylline or isoproterenol can alleviate bronchospasm. Seizures can be controlled with diazepam.

Antiarrhythmics

The drugs in this category associated most commonly with fatality are the class 1A antiarrhythmics disopyramide, procainamide, and quinidine. Acute toxic effects are due to conduction delays (heart block, ventricular arrhythmias) and the depression of myocardial contractility. All three have anticholinergic properties. The negative inotropic and anticholinergic effects are more common with disopyramide. Hypotension may result from the α-adrenergic receptor blockade produced by quinidine. Procainamide and quinidine may produce CNS symptoms (confusion, convulsions, and coma).

The anticholinergic properties of these drugs suggest that decontamination of the stomach (emesis within 30 minutes postexposure, lavage, and charcoal followed by catharsis) will be beneficial. Because disopyramide, procainamide, and quinidine are weak bases, they are concentrated in the acidic environment of the stomach. Repeated doses of activated charcoal (every 3–4 hours) may enhance their elimination. The pharmacokinetic properties of disopyramide indicate that hemoperfusion and hemodialysis should effectively enhance its elimination. Unless renal failure is present, these techniques offer little benefit in intoxications with procainamide and quinidine. Ventricular arrhythmias can be successfully treated with phenytoin, isoproterenol, and overdrive pacing.

Antihypertensives

Drugs in this category associated with fatal poisonings are captopril, clonidine, and methyldopa. Hypotension is the primary manifestation of overdose with all three agents. In severe overdose, clonidine and methyldopa may produce hypertension by stimulating peripheral α-adrenergic receptors. By decreasing sympathetic tone, clonidine and methyldopa can also produce dry mouth, bradycardia, and the impairment of A-V conduction. CNS symptoms of clonidine and methyldopa overdose include coma, hypothermia, miosis, and apnea. The apnea may respond to high doses of naloxone; this should be considered in the initial management. Overdoses are treated by removing these drugs from the stomach by lavage and activated charcoal followed by a cathartic. Primary emphasis should be placed on treating hypotension by fluid infusion and vasopressor amines (dopamine, dobutamine, norepinephrine). Although supportive therapy is usually sufficient, the pharmacokinetic properties of captopril and methyldopa indicate that hemodialysis may be of benefit.

Asthma Therapies

Theophylline

Preparations of theophylline were responsible for 38 of the fatalities reported to the AAPCC in 1991. Caffeine, another methylxanthine-like theophylline, is found in a variety of OTC preparation used as analgesics and diet aids; no deaths were reported in 1991. The pharmacological and toxicological properties of theophylline and caffeine are similar. Nausea and vomiting are the most common symptoms of methylxanthine overdose. Symptoms of CNS toxicity range from agitation to convulsions; symptoms of cardiovascular toxicity include tachycardia and arrhythmias. The hypokalemia that often accompanies acute intoxications may potentiate convulsions and arrhythmias.

Supportive care is the best treatment for methylxanthine intoxication, with emphasis placed on controlling convulsions and cardiovascular complications. Either emesis or lavage can remove methylxanthines from the stomach when initiated within 1 hour of exposure. Activated charcoal is effective at any time postexposure. Because the methylxanthines are weak bases (pKa = 8.75), they concentrate in the stomach because of pH partitioning. Thus, multiple dosages of activated charcoal can reduce the serum $t_{1/2}$ of methylxanthines even when they are administered parenterally. When initiated early, MDAC may obviate the need for extracorporeal removal, yet can be used in conjunction with these methods. The risks of severe morbidity and mortality depend on the patient's age, chronicity of exposure, and concomitant disease states. Serum theophylline levels greater than 40 μg/mL or greater than 80 μg/mL in the chronic or acute-on-chronic intoxication, or acute intoxication, respectively, may require more aggressive treatment with hemodialysis or hemoperfusion. Hemoperfusion is generally more effective than hemodialysis, but in severe intoxications they have been used concomitantly.

Alcohols and Glycols

Chemicals in this category were responsible for 46 fatalities in 1988. The chemicals involved were ethanol (36), methanol (4), ethylene glycol (4), and isopropanol (1).

Ethanol

Ethanol is a short-acting CNS depressant found in a variety of commercial products, including beverages, medicinal liquids (some rubbing alcohols, cold/cough formulations), cosmetics (perfumes, aftershaves, colognes), mouthwashes, and liniments. Severe intoxications produce a general CNS depression that may include hypothermia, coma, and respiratory failure. Hypoglycemia may be present also, especially in children.

Ethanol is well-absorbed from the GI tract. The rapid absorption of ethanol makes GI decontamination procedures of little benefit when they are initiated more than 1 hour postingestion. Activated charcoal does not bind alcohols in significant amounts but should be administered to patients if a multiple drug ingestion is suspected. Most intoxications respond to supportive care that emphasizes maintaining adequate ventilation and body temperature, as well as the IV administration of fluids to correct dehydration, acidosis, and hypoglycemia. Hemodialysis can enhance the elimination of ethanol (Vd of 0.6 L/kg and no protein binding) and is indicated when the patient is comatose, the serum ethanol level exceeds 500 mg/dL, and hepatic function is compromised.

Methanol

Methanol is widely used as a solvent in shellacs, paints, varnishes, and paint removers. It also is contained in windshield washer fluid, gas line antifreeze, and canned fuel (sterno). Initially, methanol produces a mild CNS depression without the euphoria seen with ethanol. This is followed by an asymptomatic period that progresses within 6 to 30 hours to other signs of intoxication. These include GI disturbances (nausea, vomiting, abdominal pain), ocular abnormalities (blurred vision, hyperemia of the optic disk, blindness), and metabolic acidosis. The delayed symptoms are probably due to the accumulation of toxic metabolites, primarily formic acid, resulting from the oxidation of methanol. The pharmacokinetic properties of methanol and ethanol are similar. Methanol is metabolized by alcohol dehydrogenase to formaldehyde, which is oxidized by aldehyde dehydrogenase to formic acid. Formate is subsequently oxidized to carbon dioxide through a folate-dependent pathway. Mortality from methanol intoxication correlates best with serum formate levels.

Treatment strategies emphasize supportive care (ensuring adequate ventilation and circulation, as well as controlling metabolic acidosis) and lowering serum formate levels. The latter is accomplished by decreasing formate formation by emesis or lavage within 1 hour of exposure and the administration of ethanol, and by increasing its elimination via hemodialysis and the administration of folate. The benefits of ethanol are due to its 10-fold greater affinity for alcohol dehydrogenase, which causes it to be oxidized by the enzyme in preference to methanol. 4-Methylpyrazole [4-MP], a potent inhibitor of diphenylchlorarsine (DA), is not a CNS depressant-osmotic diuretic; coincident dehydration associated with it is currently being investigated as a substitute for ethanol, because of its greater affinity for alcohol dehydrogenase and fewer side effects.

Ethylene Glycol

In industry, ethylene glycol is used as a starting material in chemical syntheses; in the home, it is found in radiator antifreeze and cosmetics. Intoxication occurs in three phases. In the first phase (1 - 12 hours), the patient appears inebriated without the odor of ethanol and may experience nausea and vomiting. Other symptoms include acidosis, nystagmus, convulsions, and coma. The second phase (12 - 36 hours) is associated with hyperventilation, which may be indicative of metabolic acidosis or pulmonary edema, and tachycardia. The third phase (48 - 72 hours) is characterized by renal failure, which may be evidenced by lumbar pain, oliguria, and uremia. Calcium oxylate crystals in the urine are also indicative of ethylene glycol intoxication.

Ethylene glycol is well-absorbed from the GI tract. The kidney excretes 20% of the absorbed dose unchanged; the remainder is metabolized in the liver. Alcohol dehydrogenase oxidizes ethylene glycol to glycoaldehyde. Both chemicals are thought to be responsible for the CNS depression seen during the first phase of ethylene glycol intoxication. Glycoaldehyde is oxidized to glycolate, which is primarily responsible for the metabolic acidosis seen in overdose. Glycolate can be oxidized further to oxalate, which chelates calcium. Tissue destruction induced by the deposition of calcium oxalate crystals is thought to result in the toxicity associated with the last two phases of intoxication. Supportive care should emphasize controlling acidemia with bicarbonate and maintaining urinary output. The acidic metabolites of ethylene glycol are more toxic than the parent compound. The accumulation of these metabolites can be inhibited by the administration of ethanol, which has a 100-fold greater affinity for alcohol dehydrogenase than does ethylene glycol. The elimination of these metabolites can be enhanced by hemodialysis and the administration of pyridoxine and thiamine, cofactors in the metabolism of glyoxylate.

Isopropanol

Isopropanol is an industrial solvent that in the home is found primarily in rubbing alcohol, skin lotions, window cleaners, and gasoline antifreeze. Compared with ethanol, isopropanol is about twice as potent a CNS depressant and causes gastric distress (pain, nausea, vomiting) more frequently. Hypotension associated with severe intoxication is a poor prognostic indicator. Death is usually preceded by respiratory arrest in deep coma. Isopropanol is well-absorbed from the GI tract; 20 - 50% of the absorbed dose is excreted unchanged. The remainder is oxidized in the liver, presumably by alcohol dehydrogenase, to acetone. Acetone, also a CNS depressant, is eliminated slowly by the lung and kidney and may be further oxidized to acetate and formate. The fact that isopropanol is metabolized more slowly than ethanol may explain the observation that toxic symptoms of isopropanol overdose last two to four times longer than those seen with ethanol. Treatment consists of gastric lavage or emesis within 1 hour of exposure, followed by supportive care, which includes correcting hypotension and acidosis. Hemodialysis effectively enhances elimination. Ethanol is not useful in the treatment of isopropanol intoxication.

Gases, Fumes, and Vapors

As a category, gases, fumes (submicron particles, usually oxidized, produced during the heating or combustion of a solid), and vapors (gaseous phase of substances that are liquids or solids at room temperature and pressure) were responsible for 49 deaths in 1991. Carbon monoxide (CO, 37 deaths) and hydrogen sulfide (H_2S, 5 deaths) were the gases most frequently involved in fatalities. Other gases associated less frequently with fatality include ammonia (NH_3), methane, and propane. CO, H_2S, and NH_3 are chemical asphyxiants because they produce cellular hypoxia by interferring with oxygen transport and delivery to the tissues. In contrast, methane and propane are termed simple asphyxiants because they produce hypoxia by displacing oxygen from the respiratory environment. Hypoxia from simple asphyxiants is treated by resuscitation in air or with oxygen.

Carbon Monoxide

Carbon monoxide accounts for 35% of the exposures and 76% of the fatalities in this category. It is a colorless and odorless gas that is produced by the incomplete combustion of organic material. In the home, it is a major component of the exhaust gases emanating from automobiles and heating equipment. Following its absorption through the lung, CO binds to hemoglobin with an affinity 250 times greater than oxygen to form carboxyhemoglobin (COHb). Hypoxia ensues because COHb carries less oxygen and has a greater affinity for the oxygen it does carry. Tissues with the greatest metabolic activity (*eg*, brain, heart) are particularly vulnerable to hypoxia. Early symptoms include headache, weakness, irritability, and confusion. Moderate intoxications are associated with nausea and vomiting, as well as increased respirations and tachycardia. Severe intoxications are manifested by coma, convulsions, and cardiopulmonary depression. Death results from respiratory failure. Treatment consists of moving the patient to an area without CO and administering oxygen to enhance its elimination. Pure oxygen (100%) reduces the $t_{1/2}$ of COHb from 5 to 6 hours (in room air) to 40 - 90 minutes; hyperbaric oxygen (3 atmospheric absolute [ATA]) reduces it to less than or equal to 0.5 hour.

Chemicals

Cyanide was involved in 12 of the 37 fatalities caused by chemical toxicity in 1991. Chemicals associated less frequently with fatalities include ethylene glycol, acids and alkali, methylene chloride, as well as nitrates and nitrites. Ethylene glycol (11 fatalities in 1991) was discussed in this chapter under Alcohols and Glycols; acids and alkali and methylene chloride are discussed under Cleaning Substances and Hydrocarbons, respectively.

Cyanide

Hydrogen cyanide (HCN) is an extremely volatile liquid that has the odor of bitter almonds. HCN and its common alkali salts (potassium, sodium, and calcium cyanide) are found in fumigants, metal polishes, electroplating solutions, and ore-extracting processes. Cyanogenic glycosides (*eg*, amygdalin, the active ingredient of LAETRILE) are found naturally in a variety of plants. Enzymes in the plants and the human GI tract hydrolyze the glycosides and release HCN. The toxic effects of cyanide are due to its reversible inhibition of aerobic metabolism. Cyanide blocks cellular respiration by binding to enzymes containing the ferric (3+) ion, particularly cytochrome oxidase, which is involved in the last step of oxidative phosphorylation. Symptoms of cyanide poisoning, which occur rapidly in succession, include headache, dizziness, dyspnea, unconsciousness, convulsions, and respiratory arrest. Although the smell of bitter almonds can aid diagnosis, approximately one third of the population is genetically insensitive to the odor of cyanide.

Cyanides are rapidly absorbed from the skin and mucosal surfaces. Toxic symptoms may appear within seconds following the inhalation of HCN and within a few minutes following the ingestion of cyanide salts. Cyanide has a large Vd (1.5 L/kg) and exhibits significant (60%) binding to plasma proteins. Most of the absorbed cyanide (80%) is metabolized by the enzyme rhodanase which, in the presence of thiosulfate, converts cyanide to the relatively harmless thiocyanate ion that in turn is excreted by the kidney. Although rhodanase is found in a variety of tissues, particularly the liver, rhodanase activity is usually somewhat sluggish because of the body's limited store of thiosulfate. Thus, one treatment in cases of overdose is the IV administration of sodium thiosulfate to enhance cyanide metabolism. To protect cells while this enzymatic transformation is occurring, a portion of the circulating hemoglobin is converted to methemoglobin by the administration of amyl nitrite (inhalation) or sodium nitrite (IV injection; LILLY CYANIDE ANTIDOTE KIT). The ferric ion of methemoglobin, like that of cytochrome oxidase, has a high affinity for cyanide. As the free cyanide concentration is reduced, cyanide is released from the cyanomethemoglobin complex and becomes available for enzymatic detoxification. Oxygen (100%) should be administered in conjunction with nitrite and thiosulfate therapy. High doses (25 mg/hour) of hydroxycobalamine (vitamin B_{12a}) is under investigation to treat cyanide toxicity. It combines with cyanide to form cyanocobalamin (vitamin B_{12}), which is excreted by the kidney. Due to the rapidity with which symptoms appear, gastric lavage should be delayed until the treatments described earlier are initiated. Activated charcoal, hemodialysis, and hemoperfusion are ineffective.

Nitrates and Nitrites

Nitrates ($-NO_3$) and nitrites ($-NO_2$) can be classified as either inorganic or organic. Inorganic nitrates are found in well water contaminated by runoff from various nitrogen sources (*eg*, sewage treatment facilities, decaying matter, fertilizers), as well as certain plants (*eg*, broccoli, cauliflower, spinach) and medicinals (*eg*, diuretics, ammonium nitrate; antidiarrheal agents, bismuth subnitrate; topical burn treatments, silver nitrate). Inorganic nitrites are found also in well water because of the reduction of nitrates to nitrites by bacteria. Organic nitrates and nitrites are used in the treatment of angina and congestive heart failure, as well as in the manufacture of explosives. Organic nitrites ("locker room," "rush") are abused also as adjuncts to sexual intercourse. The toxicity of nitrates and nitrites is due to their ability to dilate smooth muscle and to oxidize hemoglobin to methemoglobin. Methemoglobin produces tissue hypoxia because of its inability to transport and release oxygen. Because the nitrates are weaker oxidizers than nitrites, the nitrates are thus less likely to produce methemoglobinemia. The toxicity of dietary nitrates is primarily a consequence of their conversion to nitrites by bacteria residing in the GI tract. Compared with adults, infants are more susceptible to nitrate poisoning because their GI tracts contain more nitrate-reducing bacteria and because their hemoglobin is more susceptible to oxidation. Toxic symptoms include headache, dizziness, flushed skin, diaphoresis, hypotension, tachycardia and, particularly upon standing, syncope. Cyanosis may be one of the first symptoms, because of the dark brown color of methemoglobin.

Organic nitrates and nitrites are well-absorbed through the GI and respiratory tracts, as well as through the skin. The organic nitrates are hydrolyzed by the liver to inorganic nitrite and both partially and fully denitrated metabolites that may possess some of the vasodilatory activity of the parent compound. The metabolism of organic nitrites is unclear. Treatment of intoxications emphasizes establishing adequate tissue oxygenation (100% oxygen, IV methylene blue) and guarding against hypotension. In the presence of nicotinamide-adenine dinucleotide phosphate (reduced form) (NADPH), methylene blue acts as an exogenous cofactor that enhances the reduction of methemoglobin to hemoglobin by the relatively dormant methemoglobin reductase (diaphorase II) within the erythrocyte. Gastric decontamination may also be of benefit.

Cleaning Substances

There were 26 deaths in 1991 attributable to chemicals used for cleaning. The majority were distributed among acids (10), alkali (8), and detergents (3).

Acids

Acids such as chromic, hydrochloric, nitric, oxalic, phosphoric, and sulfuric are found in a variety of household products, including toilet bowl cleaners, automobile batteries, metal cleaners, and soldering fluxes. These same chemicals, as well as hydrofluoric acid, are used industrially. Most fatalities result from the inhalation of acid vapors and the ingestion of strong acids. The inhalation of acid vapors and the aspiration of ingested acids produces a chemical pneumonitis that may progress to the acute respiratory distress syndrome. The ingestion of a strong acid is usually self-limiting because of the intense pain it produces in the buccal cavity. Once swallowed, however, the acid causes a coagulation necrosis as it moves through the esophagus and along the lesser curvature of the stomach. When the acid reaches the pyloris and antrum, it induces spasms that trap the acid in the distal stomach, where the greatest damage is produced. Death is usually the result of asphyxia because of laryngeal or pulmonary edema, shock or peritonitis because of gastric perforation or, in the more chronic phase of injury, pyloric stenosis. The toxicity of hydrofluoric acid is compounded by the release of fluoride that is itself toxic to the cardiovascular, neuromuscular, and central nervous systems. These effects may be due in part to the ability of fluoride to produce hypocalcemia.

Treatment for the inhalation and ingestion of acids emphasizes maintaining adequate ventilation and circulation. If the ingested acid is not concentrated, it is diluted with water or milk within 30 minutes. Fluids are limited to one or two glasses to avoid the induction of vomiting, which re-exposes the esophagus to the acid. Calcium gluconate is administered in cases of hydrofluoric acid poisoning. The benefits of the removal of concentrated acids or hydrofluoric acid by lavage using a soft rubber catheter may outweigh the risk of perforation. Dilute bases are not administered as a neutralizing agent because they initiate an exothermic reaction that may exacerbate the injury. Bicarbonate is not administered because the release of carbon dioxide may led to gastric distention and perforation.

Alkali

Fatalities in this category result usually from the ingestion of sodium, potassium, or ammonium hydroxide, which are contained in a variety of products, including drain and oven cleaners, clinitest tablets used to test for urinary sugar, alkaline button batteries, and concentrated ammonia (>6%). Alkali elicit a liquefaction necrosis that is more deeply penetrating than the coagulation necrosis seen with acids. The deeper burns produced by alkali result in greater scarring and stricture formation than that seen with acids. Solid alkali that adhere to the oral mucosa usually are associated with oropharyngeal and upper esophageal injuries: liquid alkali produce more distal esophageal injuries that may occur in the absence of oropharyngeal damage. Death may result from asphyxia because of glottic or laryngeal edema, shock, perforation of the esophagus with mediastinitis or, in the more chronic stage of injury, because of progressive dysphagia and anorexia caused by esophageal strictures. Gastric perforation is rare. Household ammonia rarely causes burns, but may produce a chemical pneumonitis if aspirated. Button batteries produce burns by electrical discharge only if they become lodged in the esophagus or GI tract. Alkali and acid poisonings are treated similarly. Gastric lavage is not recommended for alkali ingestions.

Detergents

Detergents are composed of organic and, in many instances, inorganic ingredients. The primary organic ingredient is a synthetic surfactant (surface active agent) obtained from petrochemical precursors. Soaps differ from detergents in that the organic surfactants of soaps are salts of fatty acids obtained from animal and vegetable sources. Surfactants decrease the surface tension of water, which increases the wetting and emulsifying properties of the water-surfactant solution. Surfactants are classified by their electrical charge as either cationic, anionic, nonionic, or amphoteric. Cationic surfactants are the most toxic; fabric softeners are the primary household source. Household detergents usually contain the relatively nontoxic anionic and nonionic surfactants. The other primary ingredient of most detergents is a group of alkaline, inorganic salts called builders. Builders maintain the proper pH of the wash solution and inactivate calcium and other minerals that may interfere with the actions of the surfactant. Builders are contained in heavy-duty laundry detergents and automatic dishwater detergents. High concentrations of cationic surfactants (>7.5%) and builders are capable of causing esophageal and gastric burns, perforations, and peritonitis. Treatment is the same as that for acids and alkali.

Insecticides, Pesticides, and Rodenticides

The majority of the 14 fatalities caused by chemicals in this category were found among the organophosphates (9). Fatalities occurred less frequently in poisonings with carbamates, anticoagulants, and strychnine.

Organophosphates

Diazinon, malathion, and parathion are members of a group of organophosphate insecticides that have achieved great popularity because of their effectiveness as insecticides and their relative lack of persistence in the environment as compared with other insecticides, such as the organochlorines. The organophosphates inactivate acetylcholinesterase (AChE), the enzyme that hydrolyses acetylcholine at cholinergic (muscarinic and nicotinic) synapses in the periphery and CNS. The accumulation of acetylcholine leads to the stimulation and finally the paralysis of these synapses. The effects of organophosphate poisoning are listed in Table 46–4, the symptoms observed clinically are dependent on the balance between the stimulation and the blockade of both muscarinic and nicotinic synapses.

Most organophosphates are well-absorbed through the skin, as well as through the respiratory and GI tracts. They are metabolized by the cytochrome P-450 system in the liver. In some instances, as in the case of the organophosphates listed earlier, the metabolites are more toxic than their parent. Initial treatment of poisonings emphasizes ensuring adequate oxygenation, followed by atropine to noncompetitively antagonize the muscarinic and CNS effects

TABLE 46–4. Clinical Manifestations of Organophosphate Poisoning

Muscarinic Synapses	Physiological Effects
Respiratory system	Wheezing, dyspnea, increased bronchial secretion
Cardiovascular system	Bradycardia, hypotension, ventricular tachycardia
Gastrointestinal system	Cramps, vomiting, diarrhea, tenesmus
Pupils	Miosis
Ciliary body	Blurred vision
Lacrimal glands	Increased lacrimation
Salivary glands	Increased salivation
Sweat glands	Increased perspiration
Bladder	Increased micturition, incontinence
Nicotinic Synapses	
Striated muscle	Cramps, fasciculations, twitching, paralysis
Sympathetic ganglia	Tachycardia, hypertension
Central Nervous System	
	Dizziness, anxiety, restlessness, confusion, insomnia, ataxia, coma, convulsions, absent reflexes, Cheyne-Stokes respiration, respiratory and circulatory depression

of the organophosphates. It usually is recommended that ventilation be established prior to atropinization, because failure to do so may precipitate ventricular fibrillation. However, clinical judgment is required, because the administration of atropine may alleviate respiratory distress by decreasing bronchial secretions and spasms. Pralidoxime (pyridine-2-aldoxime methochloride or 2-PAM) should be used in the presence of muscle fasciculations and muscular weakness in order to antagonize the toxicity of organophosphates on nicotinic synapses. Pralidoxime reactivates AChE if given within 24 to 48 hours of exposure. After that time, the organophosphate irreversibly destroys AChE. Should this occur, supportive care may be required for several weeks until the enzyme is resynthesized. Because organophosphates are absorbed through the skin, contaminated clothing is removed and the skin is washed with soap. Health personnel must avoid direct contact with all contaminated areas.

Gastric decontamination may be of value if initiated within 1 hour of exposure. Because antidotes are available, methods to enhance elimination are not usually required.

Carbamates

Aldicarb (temik) and propoxur (baygon) are the two members of this category that are sometimes associated with fatality. Because the carbamates inactivate AChE, the toxic manifestations of carbamate poisoning mimic those seen with the organophosphates. There are two primary differences in toxicity between the two classes of insecticides. First, the symptoms of carbamate poisoning are less severe and of shorter duration because the carbamate-AChE complex, unlike the organophosphate-AChE complex, readily dissociates. Second, the carbamates produce only minor CNS effects because they poorly penetrate the blood-brain barrier. Like the organophosphates, the carbamates are well-absorbed by all routes. Carbamate and organophosphate poisonings are treated similarly. The only exception is that pralidoxime is not usually indicated in carbamate poisoning because the effects of the carbamates are reversible. Pralidoxime should be considered in severe cases of AChE poisoning when the insecticide is unknown or contains an organophosphate.

Anticoagulants

The coumarin derivatives warfarin and brodifacoum are anticoagulants commonly found in commercial rodenticides. These anticoagulants antagonize the effects of vitamin K_1 (phytonadione), a cofactor in the postribosomal synthesis of clotting Factors II, VII, IX, and X. Brodifacoum is approximately 100 times more potent than warfarin and has a longer half-life (120 days vs 2 days). Hemorrhage is the primary toxic effect of these agents. Gastric decontamination may be of benefit if initiated within 1 hour postexposure. Hemoperfusion and exchange transfusion have theoretical benefits, but are not clinically indicated for these agents. Phytonadione is an effective antidote that restores the prothrombin time and reduces bleeding.

Hydrocarbons

Hydrocarbons were responsible for 36 fatalities in 1991. Half were due to halogenated hydrocarbons; petroleum distillates and aromatic hydrocarbons were associated less frequently with fatality.

Halogenated Hydrocarbons

Chemicals in this classification commonly associated with fatality include carbon tetrachloride (CCl_4), chloroform ($CHCl_3$), trichloroethane (CH_3CCl_3), and methylene chloride (CH_2Cl_2); they are volatile liquids that are used as solvents, aerosol propellants, and in the manufacture of FREON (*ie*, CCl_4). They all depress the CNS, although CCl_4 is the most potent. They are well-absorbed through the respiratory and GI tracts and slightly less so through the skin. The lung excretes most of the absorbed dose of these chemicals unchanged; the remainder presumably is metabolized through the hepatic cytochrome P-450 system.

A small percentage (19%) of deaths were attributed to ingestion and probable lung aspiration by children. Intentional inhalation abuse by teenagers of butane, trichloroethane (found in fabric protectors), and FREON account for the majority of the fatalities. Death due to inhalation is commonly referred to as "sudden sniffers death syndrome" and is thought to be secondary to ventricular fibrillation induced by hypersensitization of the myocardium to endogenous catecholamines. Some of the metabolites are also toxic. CCl_4 is metabolized to free radicals and phosgene, which covalently bind to lipids and proteins and lead to fatty degeneration of the liver and hepatorenal necrosis. The metabolism of $CHCl_3$ is similar to CCl_4, except that $CHCl_3$ does not cause lipid peroxidation. Methylene chloride is metabolized to carbon monoxide, which leads to the formation of carboxyhemoglobin, a result that may prove dangerous to individuals with impaired cardiovascular status. CH_2Cl_2 is a potent irritant; prolonged contact (30 minutes) to high concentrations may cause chemical burns to the skin and mucosal surfaces. Symptoms of intoxication include headache, dizziness, fatigue, and nausea, and may rapidly progress to unconsciousness.

Treatment is supportive and includes removal from exposure (*eg*, physical environment, clothing), administration of supplemental oxygen, and monitoring for dysrhythmias. Gastric decontamination (*eg*, emesis, lavage, and charcoal) should be used following the ingestion of CCl_4 and may benefit ingestions of CH_2Cl_2 greater than a few swallows. The IV administration of NAC (see Acetaminophen earlier in this chapter) may reduce the hepatorenal toxicity because of the depletion of glutathione stores by the reactive metabolites of CCl_4 and $CHCl_3$. There are no methods to enhance elimination.

FREON refers to a group of fluorinated hydrocarbons that are used as aerosol propellants and refrigerants. FREONS are CNS depressants that generally have a lower systemic toxicity than their chlorinated hydrocarbon counterparts. Absorption of FREONS is approximately 40 times greater by inhalation than by ingestion. Concentrations above 5 – 15% may produce lightheadedness and altered consciousness. Higher concentrations of some FREONS, which may be achieved by their accidental or intentional discharge into enclosed spaces (*eg*, plastic bags), can cause sinus bradycardia that terminates in asystole. Like the chlorinated hydrocarbons, FREONS can produce cardiac dysrhythmias. Treatment is symptomatic and supportive.

Petroleum Distillates

Petroleum distillates are crude-oil byproducts than contain varying amounts of saturated and unsaturated aliphatic and aromatic hydrocarbons. Petroleum distillates are responsible for the majority of all hydrocarbon exposures. Although turpentine is a distillate of pine resin, not petroleum, it is usually included in this classification because the presentation and treatment of turpentine and petroleum distillates are similar.

The primary concerns in petroleum distillate exposure are the respiratory, central nervous, and GI systems. Deaths are almost always caused by pulmonary complications that are initiated by aspiration of the distillate. These complications lead to hypoxemia and include the inhibition of pulmonary surfactant, bronchospasm, the displacement of alveolar oxygen by distillate vapors, and direct injury to alveolar parenchyma. In addition to volatility, viscosity is another property of the distillate that determines its aspiration hazard. Chemicals with a low viscosity (below 60 sterile supply units) are more toxic because they are better able to reach distal airways. Distillates with a low viscosity include gasoline, kerosene, turpentine, mineral spirits, mineral seal oil (red furniture polish), various naphthas, as well as both halogenated and aromatic hydrocarbons. Chemicals with a high viscosity (above 100 sterile supply units) have a minimal aspiration risk; they include motor and transmission oils, baby and suntan oils, fuel and diesel oils, grease, tar, petroleum jelly, and paraffin wax. Common symptoms of respiratory distress caused by aspiration include cough, choking, tachypnea, lethargy, and cyanosis.

Central nervous system toxicity, with the exception of volatile aromatic hydrocarbons (*eg*, benzene, toluene, xylene, turpentine), is usually the result of aspiration-induced hypoxemia, because the GI absorption of most petroleum distillates is poor. The major GI concern following ingestion is vomiting, because it increases the risk of aspiration. The treatment for petroleum distillate poisoning is supportive care. Gastric decontamination by the induction of emesis is an area of active controversy and requires that the potential toxicity of ingested petroleum distillates be weighed against their aspiration hazard. The induction of emesis is not recommended for highly viscous or highly volatile (*eg*, mineral seal oil) petroleum distillates with limited GI absorption. Emesis is recommended in the alert patient for large ingestions (several milliliters per kilogram) of other petroleum distillates, the ingestion of chlorinated and aromatic hydrocarbons, as well as the ingestion of distillates that contain highly toxic ingredients. Activated charcoal does not absorb most petroleum distillates but does bind significant amounts of kerosene and turpentine. Cathartics also may be of benefit. Avoid mineral oil cathartics because they increase the risk of aspiration and retard absorption. There are no antidotes or effective methods to enhance elimination.

Aromatic Hydrocarbons

The principal chemicals in this class include benzene (C_6H_6), the prototypical aromatic hydrocarbon, as well as toluene ($C_6H_5CH_3$) and xylene ($C_6H_4[CH_3]_2$). They are used as feedstock in chemical manufacturing, are excellent solvents for paints and glues, and are found in automotive and aviation fuels. In more recent years, household products that contain benzene have been reformulated to contain toluene, a less toxic solvent. The primary effect of acute exposures is CNS depression. Symptoms include headache, drowsiness, nausea, and ataxia at low doses and confusion, respiratory depression, and coma at high doses. Severe inhalations may result in noncardiogenic pulmonary edema. Because they may also cause a feeling of euphoria, aromatic hydrocarbons, like the halogenated hydrocarbons, also are abused by sniffing. Aromatic hydrocarbons can also produce dysrhythmias by sensitizing the heart to circulating catecholamines. Aromatic hydrocarbons are generally well-absorbed through the respiratory and GI tracts and slightly less so through the skin. Approximately 10% of the absorbed dose is exhaled through the lung unchanged. The remainder is biotransformed by the hepatic cytochrome P-450 system; toluene and xylene are also biotransformed by alcohol and aldehyde dehydrogenases. The metabolites of these pathways appear in the urine as conjugates of glucuronic acid, glycine, and sulfate. Treatment is supportive and includes removal from exposure, administration of supplemental oxygen, and monitoring for dysrhythmias. Although emesis may be of value within 30 minutes of ingestion, the potential benefit must be weighed against the risk of aspiration.

REFERENCES

Centers for Disease Control: Unintentional ingestions of prescription drugs in children under five years old. MMWR 36:124, 1987.

Centers for Disease Control: Unintentional poisoning mortality—U.S. 1980-1986. MMWR 38:153, 1989.

Goldfrank LR: Toxicologic Emergencies, 5th ed. New York: Appleton-Century-Crofts, 1994.

Kulig K, Bar-Or D, Cantrill SV, et al: Management of acutely poisoned patients without gastric emptying. Ann Emerg Med 14:562-567, 1985.

Levy G: Gastrointestinal clearance of drugs with activated charcoal. N Engl J Med 307:676, 1982.

Litovitz TL, Schmitz BF, Holm KC: 1991 annual report of the American Association of Poison Control Centers national data collection system. Am J Emerg Med 10:452-505, 1992.

MacLean WC Jr: A comparison of ipecac syrup and apomorphine in the immediate treatment of ingestion of poisons. J Pediatr 82:121, 1973.

Park GD, Spector R, Goldberg MJ, Johnson GF: Expanded role of chemical therapy in the poisoned and overdosed patient. Arch Intern Med 146:969-973, 1986.

Tenenbein M: Whole bowel irrigation as a gastrointestinal decontamination procedure after acute poisoning. Med Tox 3:77, 1988.

Watson WA: Factors influencing the clinical efficacy of activated charcoal. Drug Intell Clin Pharm 21:160, 1987.

47 Environmental and Occupational Toxicology

James R. Olson and Paul J. Kostyniak

The purpose of this chapter is to provide basic information that can be applied to recognizing the role that physical and chemical hazards play in eliciting disease and to understanding how intervention can minimize these hazards. The ultimate goal is the prevention of injuries and adverse health effects that can result from occupational or environmental exposures.

It has long been recognized that in the course of employment, many individuals come in contact with a variety of chemical substances, some of which are recognized as being "toxic." The *toxicity* of a chemical is simply its ability to produce an adverse effect. The toxic effect can be minor (*eg*, involving an upset stomach or headache) and may disappear in a short period of time. The toxic effect may be more severe, and symptoms such as convulsions or coma could be life threatening or could lead to irreversible damage. One chemical may have a wide spectrum of effects, with the more severe effects being elicited as the dose of the chemical is increased.

Toxicity is not equivalent to the term *hazard. Hazard* refers to the degree of risk or danger associated with a specific situation or work practice involving the chemical. One may use *very toxic* compounds under controlled work practices that present *no hazard* to the individual. Similarly, relatively *nontoxic* compounds can be used in situations that do present a *significant hazard.*

IN GENERAL, MINIMIZING EXPOSURE IS KEY TO MINIMIZING THE PROBABILITY OF TOXIC MANIFESTATIONS DEVELOPING FROM CHEMICAL EXPOSURES.

GENERAL PRINCIPLES OF TOXICOLOGY

Exposure

To produce adverse effects in a biological system, a chemical agent or its biotransformation products must reach appropriate target sites in the body at a concentration and for a length of time sufficient to produce the adverse effect. The tissue concentration of a given agent is dependent upon the chemical and physical properties of the agent; the route, dose, duration, and frequency of exposure; the bioavailability of the agent; and the pharmacokinetics of the agent in a given individual. Interindividual differences in pharmacokinetics and susceptibility also play a major role in determining whether an adverse response will occur.

Ingestion is a route of exposure most frequently encountered in accidental poisonings in children and in suicide attempts. However, chronic ingestion of lower levels of chemical toxicants does occur as the result of food contaminants (*eg*, pesticides, heavy metals, chlorinated aromatics) or in an occupational setting from inappropriate decontamination procedures before eating or smoking. For example, cases of chronic lead poisoning have developed in workers because of the contamination of cigarettes with lead glazing compound by hand contact in a china factory when workers were allowed to smoke while performing a glazing operation. Prohibiting smoking during that operation prevented further oral exposure and eliminated the incidence of poisoning.

The *skin* is a relatively effective barrier for most water-soluble toxicants. More lipophilic substances such as chlorinated solvents commonly used in degreasing operations can readily pass through that barrier and result in overexposure. The presence of lipophilic solvents may also enhance the dermal absorption of more hydrophilic drugs and chemicals. Prevention of exposure can be achieved by the use of protective equipment (*ie*, gloves) and barrier creams.

Inhalation exposure is clearly the most important route of exposure for most chemical toxicants in the workplace. This is easily recognized in the exposure standards set by the Occupational Safety and Health Administration (OSHA), in which limits for air concentrations of chemical toxicants are the means by which worker exposures are controlled. Additionally, for processes in which the standard can not be met because of technical limitations, respiratory protective equipment is used to control worker exposure.

In toxicity testing, the duration and frequency of exposure of animals to a chemical are generally classified as acute, subacute, subchronic, or chronic. Acute exposure usually refers to a single administration or continuous exposures within a 24-hour period. Subacute, subchronic, and chronic exposures are repeated exposures to a chemical for 1 month or less, for 1 to 3 months, and for more than 3 months, respectively.

Human exposures to environmental and/or occupational agents are frequently chronic or long-term exposures at low doses. Even at low daily doses, some agents have the ability to accumulate in target tissues to toxicologically relevant doses following several years of exposure. In the case of 2,3,7,8-tetrachlorodibenzo-para-dioxin (TCDD; dioxin), which has a biological half-life of about 11 years in humans, it takes about 4 half-lives or 44 years to approach steady-state levels in target tissues. Therefore, highly persistent agents such as TCDD have a greater potential to accumulate and to elicit adverse effects following chronic exposure.

TABLE 47–1. Approximate Acute LD50s of Some Representative Chemical Agents

Agent	LD50 (mg/kg)*
Ethyl alcohol	10,000
Sodium chloride	4000
Ferrous sulfate	1500
Morphine sulfate	900
Phenobarbital sodium	150
Picrotoxin	5
Strychnine sulfate	2
Nicotine	1
d-Tubocurarine	0.5
Hemicholinium-3	0.2
Tetrodotoxin	0.10
Dioxin (2,3,7,8-tetrachlorodibenzo-para-dioxin; TCDD)	0.001
Botulinum toxin	0.00001

From Klaassen CD, Eaton DL: Principles of toxicology. *In* Amdur MO, Doull J, Klaassen DC (eds): Casarett and Doull's Toxicology: The Basic Science of Poisons, 4th ed. Elmsford, NY: Pergamon Press, 1991. Reproduced with permission of McGraw-Hill, Inc.

*LD50 (median lethal dose) is the dosage (mg/kg body weight) causing death in 50% of the exposed animals.

Dose-Response Relationships

Dose-response relationships are central to establishing the potential that a given agent has to produce a deleterious or toxic response. Paracelsus (1493–1541) clearly recognized this relationship, stating that "All substances are poisonous, there is none which is not a poison. The right dose differentiates a poison and a remedy." This basic principle of toxicology is still accurate, because virtually every chemical has the potential to produce injury or death if present in a sufficient amount. Table 47–1 illustrates the range of doses necessary to produce lethality following acute exposure to a number of agents. Acute toxic potency is expressed as the LD50 (median lethal dose) on a mg/kg body weight basis. The rank order for the toxic potency of toxicants may also be expected to vary depending on the duration and frequency of exposure and the adverse response that is monitored.

RANGE OF ADVERSE EFFECTS

Drugs and other xenobiotics are capable of producing a wide range of biological, therapeutic, and toxicological responses. Adverse or toxic effects are responses that are deleterious to the well-being of humans. The specific toxic effects that a chemical causes may be considered a property of that chemical. Whether an effect develops in an individual following exposure to the chemical is dependent upon how large a chemical dose was received.

Acute Toxicity

Acute toxicity results from a brief exposure to a sufficient dose of a chemical, resulting in specific adverse effects. For example, an acute exposure to ammonia can result in an immediate effect on the membranes of the respiratory tract and the eyes, causing tearing, a choking sensation, irritation, and coughing.

Chronic Toxicity

Chronic toxicity can result from long-term exposures, often lasting months or years. Each dose may not cause any obvious adverse effect. However, depending on the chemical, a potential for accumulation may exist, whereby the chemical is removed from the body at a slower rate than it is taken in. The substance may accumulate to the extent necessary to result in *delayed toxicological effects*, after months or even years of exposure. In other cases, whether or not the chemical is effectively removed from the body, it may cause changes that can result in the manifestation of delayed toxicological effects as long as 20 to 30 years after exposure.

Local Toxicity

Local toxicity refers to adverse effects that occur at the site of first contact between the biological system and the toxicant. Examples of local effects are the direct corrosive effect on the skin or mucosal surfaces that come into contact with a caustic substance, such as a strong base (*eg*, NaOH), during ingestion, and surface irritation leading to bronchoconstriction and coughing caused by the inhalation of an irritant such as ammonia.

Systemic Toxicity

Systemic toxicity requires the absorption and distribution of the toxicant from its entry point to distant sites where deleterious effects are produced. Most substances are capable of producing their primary systemic toxicity at one or two sites or target organs. The target organ may not necessarily represent the site that contains the highest concentration of the chemical. For example, in the case of lead, the brain is a target organ, whereas the majority of the body burden of lead is concentrated in bone.

Reversible Versus Irreversible Toxic Effects

Reversible versus irreversible toxic effects are generally determined by the ability of a tissue to regenerate or repair a given injury. Liver injury in many cases is reversible, because the liver has the potential to regenerate, whereas central nervous system injury is usually irreversible because of the limited ability of highly differentiated nervous tissue to replicate. Teratogenic and carcinogenic responses are also generally considered irreversible effects. Mutagenicity and carcinogenicity are topics that are discussed in greater detail in the later half of this chapter.

Developmental Toxicity

Developmental toxicity refers to adverse effects in developing organisms produced by exposures to chemical, physical, or biological agents. *Embryolethal* lesions are incompatible with survival and result in resorption, spontaneous abortion, or stillbirth. *Teratogenic* responses include irreversible structural or functional abnormalities that are compatible with survival of the offspring. Overall *growth retardation* or delayed growth of specific organ systems is another persistent adverse effect that is also referred to as *embryotoxicity*. Often a given exposure to a developmental toxin results in growth retardation, teratogenicity, and embryolethality in a population. Thalidomide is a teratogen that produced amelia (absence of the limbs) or various degrees of phocomelia (preaxial reductions of the long bones of the limbs) in affected children during the late 1950s and early 1960s. Thalidomide was a sedative-hypnotic used during pregnancy to ameliorate nausea and vomiting. A marked increase in the incidence of these rare malformations resulted in the relatively rapid identification of this teratogenic agent and in its withdrawal from the market. This tragic incident led to much greater emphasis on preclinical testing for drug safety, particularly with regard to assessing potential for developmental toxicity.

Idiosyncratic Reactions

Idiosyncratic reactions to a chemical exposure refer to genetically determined abnormal reactivity to a chemical. Idiosyncratic reactions include extreme sensitivity to low doses of a toxicant or extreme insensitivity to high doses of the chemical. In general, the responses observed are qualitatively similar to those observed in all individuals. An example of an idiosyncratic reaction is the extreme sensitivity of some individuals to nitrites and other chemicals that produce methemoglobinemia. A deficiency in reduced nicotinamide-adenine dinucleotide – methemoglobin reductase has been identified in these sensitive individuals, and the trait has been shown to be inherited in an autosomal recessive manner.

Allergic Reactions

Allergic reactions are immunologically mediated adverse reactions to a chemical resulting from a previous exposure and sensitization to that chemical or to a structurally similar agent. *Hypersensitivity* and *sensitization reaction* are other terms used to describe this response. Table 47 – 2 summarizes the classification scheme for allergic responses based on the mechanisms involved in the responses (Coombs and Gell, 1975). For example, toluene di-isocyanate is a type I agent producing anaphylaxis or immediate hypersensitivity reaction. Both asthma and contact dermatitis have been reported in polyurethane foam makers, plastic foam makers, rubber workers, and others exposed to toluene di-isocyanate. In most cases, removal of the offending agent generally eliminates the allergic response.

Interactions of Chemicals

Interactions of chemicals are of great importance because people are exposed to a complex mixture of xenobiotics in the environment and in the occupational setting. As with therapeutic agents, the adverse effects of xenobiotics exhibit additive, synergistic, potentiating, and antagonistic responses. For example, 2,3,7,8-substituted polychlorinated dibenzo-*p*-dioxins and polychlorinated dibenzofurans are thought to exhibit additive toxicity because they act through a common mechanism, involving binding of the compounds to the Ah (aryl hydrocarbon) receptor. Carbon tetrachloride and ethanol are both hepatotoxic, and the combined effects of these agents result in a *synergistic* or a greater-than-additive hepatotoxic response. Isopropanol is not hepatotoxic but *potentiates* or enhances the hepatotoxic response to carbon tetrachloride following a combined exposure. Conversely, the combined exposure to two or more chemicals may interfere with the actions of the other chemical(s). *Antagonistic* responses can be mediated by functional, chemical, dispositional, or receptor-mediated mechanisms. Therefore, it is important to consider interactive responses that are associated with environmental and occupational exposures.

These potential interactions are recognized in occupational exposure standards, whereby exposure to multiple

TABLE 47–2. Gell and Coombs' Classification Scheme of Allergy

Classification	Symptoms	Mechanism	Chemical Agents
Type I Anaphylaxis or immediate hypersensitivity	Asthma, urticaria, rhinitis, atopic dermatitis	IgE bound to mast cell/basophil triggers release of soluble mediators (*eg*, histamine)	Amino ethanolamine, beryllium, chloramine, copper-ammonia solutions, ethylenediamine, ethylene oxide, formaldehyde, isocyanates (toluene, diphenylmethane, hexamethylene, di-isocyanate), platinum salts, nickel salts, phthalic anhydrides
Type II Cytolytic	Hemolytic anemia, Goodpasture's disease	IgG and/or IgM binds to cells and results in destruction via complement, opsonization, or ADCC	Trimellitic anhydride, mercury
Type III Arthus	Systemic lupus erythematosus, glomerular nephritis, rheumatoid arthritis, serum sickness	Antigen-antibody complexes deposit in various tissues and may then fix complement	Trimellitic anhydride, mercury
Type IV Delayed-type hypersensitivity	Contact dermatitis, tuberculosis	Sensitized T lymphocytes induce a DTH response	Beryllium, chromium, dichlorophene, ethylenediamine, formaldehyde, isocyanates, mercury bichloride, mercaptobenzothiazole, potassium dichromate, paraphenylenediamine, phthalic anhydride

From Coombs RRA, Gell PGH: Classification of allergic reactions responsible for clinical hypersensitivity and disease. *In* Gell PGH, Coombs RRA, Lachman PJ (eds): Clinical Aspects of Immunology. Philadelphia: JB Lippincott, 1975.

ADCC = antibody-dependent cell-mediated cytotoxicity; DTH = delayed-type hypersensitivity; Ig = immunoglobulin.

agents that act by the same mechanism warrants a proportional reduction in the exposure limits for the individual agents, such that the total exposure is kept below levels likely to result in adverse effects.

ASSESSMENT OF RISK FROM CHEMICAL EXPOSURES

Risk

The process of risk assessment is commonly divided into four major steps: hazard identification, dose-response assessment, exposure assessment, and risk characterization (Fig. 47–1). Risk management, which should be distinct from risk assessment, is the process of weighing policy alternatives and selecting the most appropriate regulatory action, integrating the results of risk assessment with engineering data and with social, economic, and political concerns to reach a decision (NAS, 1983).

Risk is defined as the expected frequency of the occurrence of an undesirable effect occurring as a result of exposure to a chemical, physical, or biological agent. Estimation of risk utilizes dose-response data generated in laboratory animals, *in vitro* data, and when available, epidemiological data in humans. The quality and suitability of the biological data are major limiting factors in assessing the risk of an adverse response, such as cancer, associated with a given exposure to a chemical or physical agent. Ultimately, a regulatory agency sets a numerical *limit* for exposure based on this risk assessment. Inherent in that number is a degree of uncertainty that is not stated. This uncertainty is minimized as a function of the quantity and quality of the database upon which the risk assessment is based.

The evaluation of potential adverse effects, assessment of exposures, and extrapolation to predict effects are performed by toxicologists, epidemiologists, and environmental researchers. Results are published in peer-reviewed scientific literature. The assessment of the existence of public health problems and the certainty of that risk, although often speculated upon by individual investigators, usually emanate from expert advisory committees and panels formulated by regulatory agencies. A good example is the current controversy over whether the release of mercury from dental amalgam poses a public health problem that necessitates further regulation of that material. Literally hundreds of papers have been published by toxicologists and epidemiologists in the peer-reviewed literature discussing the toxicity of mercury vapor, the release rates from amalgam, the distribution of that mercury both in animals and in humans, and doses causing specific effects in animals and in humans. Expert committees convened by the Food and Drug Administration have reviewed the available peer-reviewed literature and have advised that no further regulatory action was required. Because risk assessment is based on the data available at a given point in time, as new data become available, it may be necessary to revisit the issue from time to time.

Quantitative Aspects of Risk Assessment

Under ideal conditions, a human risk assessment for a given chemical utilizes dose-response data in humans for the

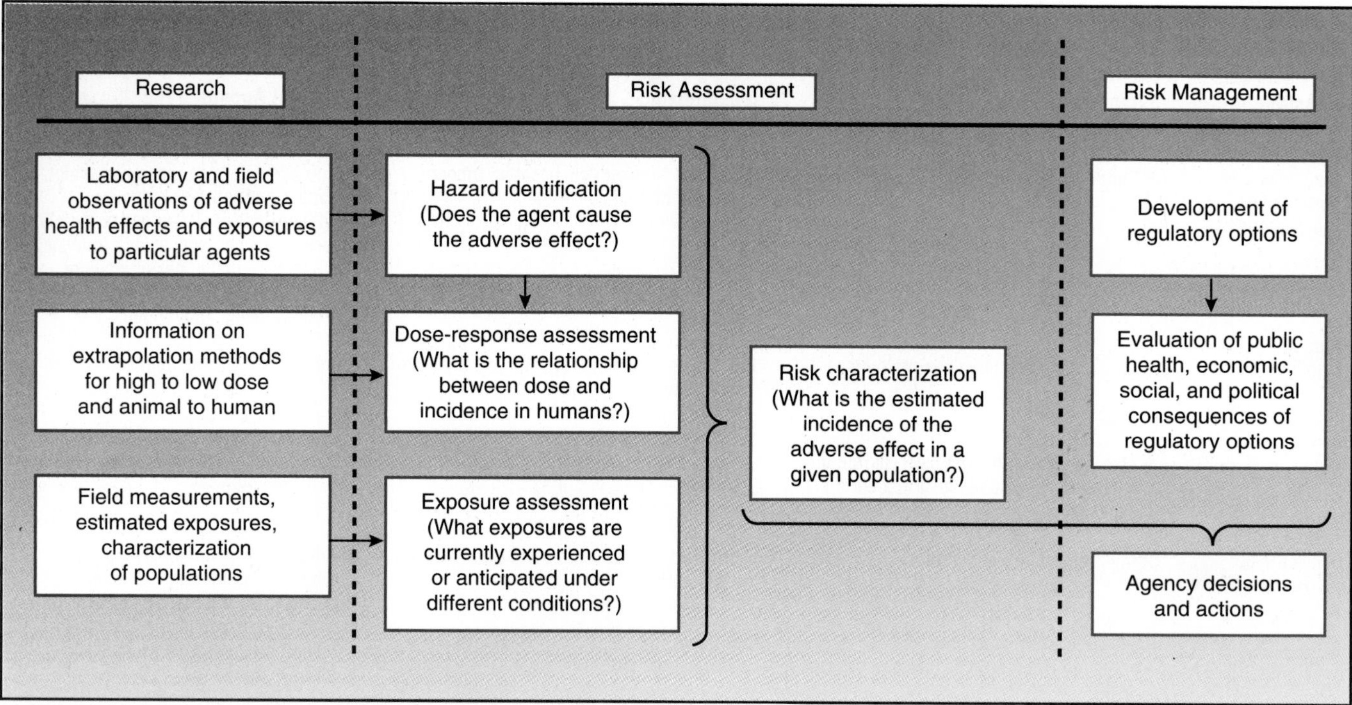

FIGURE 47–1. Elements of risk assessment and risk management. (Reprinted with permission from RISK ASSESSMENT IN THE FEDERAL GOVERNMENT. Copyright 1983 by the National Academy of Sciences. Courtesy of the National Academy Press, Washington DC.)

chemical under relevant exposure conditions. Because such data are generally never available, a need exists to extrapolate high-dosage studies in laboratory animals to cases of low-dose exposure in humans.

Chronic studies in one or more species of laboratory animals are utilized in the risk assessment process. The no-observed-adverse-effect level (NOAEL) is obtained in animals following chronic exposure to several doses of a given chemical. The NOAEL is the highest dose administered that does *not* produce an adverse effect. Establishing an NOAEL for a chemical assumes that the response of interest exhibits a *threshold* or a dose below which the probability of an individual responding is no greater than the background rate of response for the population. For responses that exhibit a threshold, safety or uncertainty factors are utilized with the NOAEL in aminals to establish exposure levels that are protective of human populations. A safety factor of 100 (NOAEL/100) is often used, with the justification of a factor of 10 for interindividual differences in the human population and an additional factor of 10 for interspecies differences. When the reliability of the NOAEL is in question, the original safety factor of 100 is multiplied by 10, resulting in the application of a safety factor of 1000 or NOAEL/1000. This additional factor of 10 is also referred to as a "modifying factor," which is an additional uncertainty factor that allows for "professional judgment" in the estimation of allowable levels. The US Environmental Protection Agency (EPA) utilizes the term *reference dose* to establish exposure levels that are protective of human health. The reference dose value is calculated by dividing the NOAEL determined in animal studies by the product of the uncertainty factors and the modifying factor.

For a response such as cancer that may not exhibit a threshold, a number of models can be used in risk extrapolation. The goal of these models is to provide an estimate of the response at exposure levels that are far below those for which experimental data are available. Extra risk is defined as the lifetime risk of cancer. The US EPA often considers a risk of 1×10^{-6} or one case in a million individuals a maximally acceptable risk. The linearized multistage model is a conservative model that assumes no threshold for carcinogenic and mutagenic effects and assumes a linear dose-response curve at the lowest end of the response scale. This model has been widely used by the US EPA in quantitative risk assessment procedures.

Recently criticism has been raised against the rigid approaches that these agencies have taken in their regulatory process. There has been a trend to incorporate more mechanistic data into the risk assessment process, which takes into account the specifics of toxicant distribution to target sites (physiologically based pharmacokinetic modeling), repair mechanisms, and specific data on the most sensitive population groups. These approaches eliminate some of the uncertainty that is inherent in the risk assessment process.

Risk Perception

Virtually every activity in daily living is associated with a relative health risk. The annual risk of death from various causes is given in Table 47–3. The annual risk of death from a motor vehicle accident is 2.4 deaths per 10,000. The lifetime risk can be estimated by multiplying annual risk by 70 years. Thus, the lifetime risk of death due to a motor vehicle accident is 1.68 deaths per 100 or 168 deaths per 10,000. The risk estimates for motor vehicle accidents, home accidents, electrocution, all cancers, and a few other activities have a relatively small degree of uncertainty because the values are based on actuarial data and represent a best estimate of actual risk. This is in contrast to the high degree of uncertainty associated with the theoretical upper bound estimates of risk from chronic, low-level exposure to chemicals, as seen here for asbestos exposures in schools.

Role of Health Professionals in Managing Risk

In the workplace, where traditionally much of the regulatory effort has been directed, an effective Medical and Industrial Hygiene program strives to promote employee health and to design and monitor workplace practices to minimize on-the-job hazards. The objectives of the industrial hygiene program are to:

1. *Recognize* potential hazards.
2. *Evaluate* the factors in the workplace that can lead to injury, disease, or discomfort.
3. *Control* those factors in the workplace through environmental controls and appropriate work practices.

The occupational physician often works closely with the industrial hygienist and other health professionals and provides baseline medical information through routine physical examinations, specific screening programs, and recordkeeping on the working population. This aids in further identifying unanticipated hazards and in evaluating effectiveness of current industrial hygiene practices.

In recent years, fewer companies are relying on full-time occupational medicine specialists. There is a tendency to interact more closely with individual physicians in addressing medical problems originating in the workplace. It is therefore essential that the practicing physician have some basic understanding of the principles of chemical exposure and its control.

To assist physicians in the recognition of diseases that may in part be related to occupational exposures, Rutstein and colleagues (1983) developed a list of sentinel health events that may be occupationally related (Table 47–4). The prevention of occupational disease depends on reduction of

TABLE 47–3. Some Commonplace Risks (Mean Values With Uncertainty)

Cause	Annual Risk (deaths per million)	Uncertainty
Total asbestos exposure in schools (ages 6–16 years)*	0.3	Factor of 20, downward only
Electrocution	5.3	5%
Sea-level background radiation (except radon)	20	Factor of 3
Home accidents	110	5%
Air pollution, eastern United States	200	Factor of 20, downward only
Motor vehicle accident (total)	240	10%
All cancers	2800	10%
Cigarette smoking, one pack per day	3600	Factor of 3

Reprinted with permission from Wilson R, Crouch EAC: Risk assessment and comparisons: An introduction. Science 236:267–280, 1987. Copyright 1987 American Association for the Advancement of Science.

*Asbestos data from Foster KR, et al (eds): Phantom Risk: Scientific Inference & the Law. Cambridge: MIT Press, 1993.

TABLE 47–4. Occupationally Related Disease

Condition	Industry/Occupation	Agent
Pulmonary tuberculosis	Physicians, medical personnel	*Mycobacterium tuberculosis*
Plague, tularemia, anthrax, rabies, and other infections	Farmers, ranchers, hunters, veterinarians, laboratory workers	Various infectious agents
Rubella	Medical personnel, intensive care personnel	Rubella virus
Hepatitis	Day-care center staff, orphanage staff, medical personnel	Hepatitis A virus, hepatitis B virus
Ornithosis	Bird breeders, pet shop staff, poultry producers, veterinarians, zoo employees	*Chlamydia psittaci*
Malignant neoplasm of nasal cavities	Woodworkers, cabinet and furniture makers Radium chemists and processors Nickel smelting and refining	Hardwood dust Radium Nickel
Malignant neoplasm of larynx	Asbestos industries and utilizers	Asbestos
Malignant neoplasm of trachea, bronchus, and lung	Asbestos industries and utilizers Topside coke oven workers Uranium and fluorspar miners Smelters, processors, users Mustard gas formulators Ion exchange resin makers, chemists	Asbestos Coke oven emissions Radon daughters Chromates, nickel, arsenic Mustard gas Bis(chloromethyl)ether
Mesothelioma	Asbestos industries and utilizers	Asbestos
Malignant neoplasm of bone	Radium chemists and processors	Radium
Malignant neoplasm of scrotum	Automatic lathe operators, metalworkers Coke oven workers, petroleum refiners	Mineral/cutting oils Soots and tars
Malignant neoplasm of bladder	Rubber and dye workers	Benzidine, naphthylamine, auramine, 4-nitrophenyl

Table continued on following page

TABLE 47–4. Occupationally Related Disease *Continued*

Condition	Industry/Occupation	Agent
Malignant neoplasm of kidney	Coke oven workers	Coke oven emissions
Acute lymphoid leukemia	Radiologists, rubber industry	Ionizing radiation
Acute myeloid leukemia	Occupations with exposure to benzene Radiologists	Benzene Ionizing radiation
Erythroleukemia	Occupations with exposure to benzene	Benzene
Non–autoimmune hemolytic anemia	Whitewashing and leather industry Electrolytic processes, smelting Plastics industry	Copper sulfate Arsine Trimellitic anhydride
Aplastic anemia	Explosives manufacture Radiologists, radium chemists	TNT Ionizing radiation
Agranulocytosis or neutropenia	Explosives and pesticide industries Pesticides, pigments, pharmaceuticals	Phosphorus Inorganic arsenic
Toxic encephalitis	Battery, smelter, and foundry workers	Lead
Parkinson's disease (secondary)	Manganese processing, battery makers, welders	Manganese
Inflammatory and toxic neuropathy	Pesticides, pigments, pharmaceuticals	Arsenic and arsenic compounds
	Furniture refinishers, degreasing operations	Hexane
	Plastics, rayon industries	Methyl butyl ketone, copper disulfide, other solvents
	Explosives industry	TNT
	Battery, smelter, and foundry workers	Lead
	Dentists, chloralkali plants, battery makers	Mercury
	Plastics industry, paper manufacturing	Acrylamide
	Microwave and radar technicians	Microwaves
	Radiologists	Ionizing radiation
	Blacksmiths, glass blowers, bakers	Infrared radiation
	Moth repellant formulators, fumigators	Naphthalene
Noise effects on inner ear	Many industries	Excessive noise
Raynaud's phenomenon (secondary)	Lumberjacks, chain sawyers, grinders	Whole body, segmental vibration
	Vinyl chloride polymerization industry	Vinyl chloride monomer
Extrinsic asthma	Jewelry, alloy, and catalyst makers Polyurethane, adhesive, paint workers Plastic, dye, insecticide makers Foam workers, latex makers, biologists Bakers Woodworkers, furniture makers	Platinum Isocyanates Phthalic anhydride Formaldehyde Flour Red cedar and other wood dusts
Pneumoconiosis of coal workers	Coal miners	Coal dust
Asbestosis	Asbestos industries and utilizers	Asbestos
Silicosis	Quarrymen, sandblasters, silica processors, mining, ceramic industries, and foundries	Silica
Talcosis	Talc processors	Talc
Chronic beryllium disease of the lung	Beryllium alloy workers, ceramic and cathode ray tube makers, nuclear reactor workers	Beryllium
Byssinosis	Cotton industry workers	Cotton, flax, hemp, and cotton-synthetic dusts
Acute bronchitis, pneumonitis, and pulmonary edema due to fumes and vapors	Alkali and bleach industries Silo fillers, arc welders Paper, refrigeration, oil industries Plastics industry	Chlorine Nitrogen oxides Sulfur dioxide Trimellitic anhydride
Toxic hepatitis	Solvent utilizers, dry cleaners, plastics industry	Carbon tetrachloride chloroform, trichloroethylene
	Explosives and dye industries Fumigators, fire extinguisher formulators	Phosphorus, TNT Ethylene dibromide
Acute or chronic renal failure	Battery makers, plumbers, solderers Electrolytic processes, smelting Battery makers, jewelers, dentists	Inorganic lead Arsine Inorganic mercury

TABLE 47–4. Occupationally Related Disease *Continued*

Condition	Industry/Occupation	Agent
	Fire extinguisher makers	Carbon tetrachloride
	Antifreeze manufacturers	Ethylene glycol
Male infertility	Formulators and applicators	Dibromochloropropane
Contact and allergic dermatitis	Leather tanning, poultry dressing plants, packing, adhesives and sealant industry, boat building and repair	Irritants (*eg*, cutting fish oil, solvents, acids, alkalis, allergens)

From Rutstein DD, Mullan RJ, Frazier TM, et al: Sentinel health events (occupational): A basis for physician recognition and public health surveillance. Am J Public Health 73:1054–1062, 1983.
TNT = 2,4,6-trinitrotoluene.

hazardous exposure in the workplace and on better education of workers, managers, and physicians.

MUTAGENESIS AND CARCINOGENESIS

Chemical Mutagenesis

A *mutation* is a heritable alteration in cellular DNA, which may lead to changes in cell phenotype. For example, the parent or wild-type *Escherichia coli* has the designation His^+, indicating that the organism can synthesize its own supply of histidine, whereas His^- mutant cells require an exogenous source of histidine in the medium for growth. The ability of micro-organisms to express a mutant phenotype of the nutritional type has become a valuable tool in assessing the mutagenic or genotoxic activity of various chemicals and is commonly known as the Ames Test. A *mutagen* is a physical or chemical agent that causes mutations to occur. X-rays and ultraviolet radiation are examples of physical mutagens. Drugs and chemicals can directly or indirectly affect DNA structure and its function as a template for DNA replication and RNA transcription. Spontaneous mutagenesis occurs at a constant background rate in nature by usually unknown mechanisms; however, induced mutagenesis indicates that some identifiable exogenous agent or agents are involved. The spontaneous mutation rate is in the range of 10^{-7} to 10^{-9} for prokaryotes and 10^{-10} to 10^{-12} for eukaryotes. Thus mistakes in DNA replication occur so rarely that a 1 in 10 million or less chance exists that a gene will mutate when a cell divides. A mutagen may increase the spontaneous rate by a factor of 10 to 1000, depending on its potency.

Several drugs used in cancer chemotherapy, including the nitrogen mustards and certain nitrosourea compounds, can be both mutagenic and carcinogenic in humans. However, most chemically or physically induced DNA lesions or modifications do not result in a heritable mutation or an adverse biological response because of efficient DNA excision repair mechanisms. A mutation and potential adverse response are more likely to occur in repair-enzyme–deficient cells or when the rate of cell division does not allow time for repair to be completed before DNA replication occurs. Xeroderma pigmentosum is an autosomal recessive trait in which individuals have a defective excision repair process and are thus more likely to develop mutation(s) and cancer.

Biological Consequences of Mutation

A mutation to a structural gene can be missense, nonsense, or silent, depending on where an amino acid substitution, addition, or deletion occurs in a protein. A *missense* mutation occurs when an amino acid substitution produces a partially active protein. A *nonsense* mutation results from an alteration that produces a base sequence that no longer codes for an amino acid. A *silent* mutation occurs when a base alteration does not lead to an amino acid change because of redundancy of the genetic code or if the mutation produces an amino acid substitution that does not alter function.

An example of a missense mutation in the hemoglobin molecule is found in patients with sickle cell anemia. In this disease, a single amino acid substitution (a valine instead of a glutamic acid as the sixth amino acid from the amino terminus of the globin β chain) occurs as a result of a single base change in the triplet code word. Hemophilia and various inborn errors of metabolism are other examples of genetically determined diseases resulting from mutations. Mutation during embryonic development may result in congenital malformations or spontaneous abortion when the mutation is incompatible with life. Many cancers also are thought to be the result of a routine mutation or a hereditary trait occurring in cells of the mature organism (non–germ cell). It is also important to note that some mutations are considered beneficial from the evolutionary point of view, resulting in the expression of desirable traits.

Chemical Carcinogenesis

Cancer is a multifactorial disease associated with:

1. Certain chemicals, both natural and synthetic
2. Radiation, ionizing and nonionizing (*eg*, ultraviolet light)
3. Genetic background
4. Biological agents, such as oncogenic viruses

All of these factors can contribute to some degree to the ultimate expression of cancer in a given individual. For example, interindividual variations in the metabolism of a chemical carcinogen can result in enhanced activation of a chemical to its ultimate reactive form or may result in enhanced metabolism via a detoxification pathway. Genetic variability also exists for the relative ability to repair damaged DNA. Although cancer is a complex disease with many causative factors, it is estimated that 80–90% of all human cancers may at least in part be the result of chemicals present in the environment.

Throughout the early history of the field of chemical carcinogenesis, several cases existed in which a compound was first suspected of being carcinogenic in humans and later was found experimentally to be carcinogenic. In 1775, Sir Percivall Pott reported a high incidence of scrotal cancer in the chimney sweeps of London and correctly attributed this to their constant contact with coal tar and soot. However, it was not until 1916 when Yamagiwa and Ichikawa applied coal tar to the ears of rabbits and experimentally produced cancer at the point of application. Ten to fifteen years later, two tons of coal tar were fractionated, isolating the cancer-producing polycyclic aromatic hydrocarbons, benzo[a]pyrene and dibenz[a,h]anthracene. Polycyclic aromatic hydrocarbons (PAHs) are natural products of incomplete combustion. It is estimated that 2000 tons of PAHs are put in the air each year in the United States through various combustion processes, including the burning of wood, coal, petroleum products, and tobacco products.

Since those earlier studies, many diverse agents have been found to be carcinogenic, and several systems for the classification of these agents have been developed based on their mode of action. Chemical carcinogens can be broadly divided into two classes, *genotoxic* and nongenotoxic or *epigenetic*. Genotoxic carcinogens are electrophiles that react covalently with DNA, producing detrimental mutations in specific genes (*eg*, oncogenes and tumor suppressor genes) that are involved in the process of neoplastic conversion. In addition to being DNA-reactive, genotoxic carcinogens are effective after a single exposure, act in a cumulative manner, and may produce responses that are irreversible. The mutagenic, and therefore carcinogenic, potential of these compounds can be detected using a number of short-term *in vitro* and *in vivo* tests, the most common of which is the Ames bacterial mutagenicity test. In contrast, nongenotoxic or epigenetic carcinogens are not mutagenic and do not interact with DNA but may stimulate the process of neoplastic development and progression.

Although the precise mechanisms of action for epigenetic agents are still in doubt, they may interact with protein and/or RNA and alter gene expression. Other possible mechanisms for these agents include cytotoxicity and chronic tissue injury, mitogenesis, altered gap junctions and cell-to-cell communication, intracellular generation of reactive oxygen free radicals, hormonal imbalance, and immunological effects. Carcinogenic effects of nongenotoxic agents generally occur following long-term exposure at relatively high doses of the agents. In contrast to genotoxic carcinogens, the effects of epigenetic agents may be reversible.

Knowledge regarding the biological and chemical properties of chemical carcinogens has assisted in efforts to classify this diverse group of agents. Table 47–5 illustrates a classification of carcinogenic chemicals proposed by Williams and Weisburger (1991).

DNA-reactive or genotoxic carcinogens can be classified according to whether they are active with or without biotransformation by the host to an ultimate carcinogenic product. The non–DNA-reactive or epigenetic carcinogens consist of a wide range of agents, many of which increase DNA synthesis, mitosis, and cell duplication rates. Agents producing effects that might be indirectly considered genotoxic are grouped with epigenetic agents because their activity is thought to be the result of a critical epigenetic biological effect. For example, epigenetic agents such as hormones, peroxisome proliferators, and TCDD can act through receptor-mediated signal transduction pathways, although exactly how the resulting change in gene expression results in cancer is unknown. Therefore, it is important to note that the classification scheme in Table 47–5 is just a practical, working approach that does not preclude the possibility of some genotoxic carcinogens from also having epigenetic effects.

TABLE 47–5. Classification of Carcinogenic Chemicals

Category and Class	Example
A. Genotoxic (DNA-reactive) carcinogens	
1. Activation-independent organic	Alkylating agents
2. Activation-independent inorganic	Nickel, cadmium*
3. Activation-dependent	Polycyclic aromatic hydrocarbon, arylamine, nitrosamine
B. Epigenetic carcinogens	
1. Promoter	Organochlorine pesticides, saccharin
2. Hormone-modifying	Estrogen, amitrole
3. Peroxisome proliferators	Clofibrate, diethylhexylphthalate
4. Cytotoxic	Nitrilotriacetic acid
5. Immunosuppressor	Cyclosporin A, azathioprine
6. Solid state	Plastics, asbestos
C. Unclassified	
1. Miscellaneous	Ethanol, dioxane

From Williams GM, Weisburger JH: Chemical carcinogenesis. *In* Amdur MO, Doull J, Klaassen CD (eds): Casarett and Doull's Toxicology: The Basic Science of Poisons, 4th ed. Elmsford, NY: Pergamon Press, 1991. Reproduced with permission of McGraw-Hill, Inc.

*Some metals have yielded evidence of reaction with DNA; others may operate through epigenetic mechanisms such as alteration of fidelity of DNA polymerases.

Genotoxic (direct-acting, primary) carcinogens are electrophilic chemicals that can interact directly with nucleophilic molecules, including DNA. Bis(2-chloroethyl) sulfide, or mustard gas, is an example of an alkylating agent that is relatively stable in the anhydrous state. However, under aqueous conditions, the chemical undergoes hydrolytic decomposition, liberating an alkylating moiety (carbonium ion) and HCl. As a chemical warfare agent utilized during World War I, severe burning of the skin and fatal lung damage were produced as a result of the local, acute toxicity of the HCl. Delayed toxicity (cancer) could also result from the carbonium ion, which can alkylate DNA at the N-7 of guanine. Bis(chloromethyl) ether, an important chemical intermediate in industry, is another highly reactive alkylating agent that produced cancer of the upper respiratory tract in workers exposed to apparently low levels of the agent. Another group of direct-acting genotoxic alkylating agents includes the cis-platinum(II) coordination complexes, which were developed as antineoplastic drugs. These compounds are a complex chelate of divalent platinum, chlorine, and amino groups.

Most known chemical carcinogens are in the *procar-*

cinogen or activation-dependent class of genotoxic agents. These compounds require metabolic (enzymatic) activation by the host to form a primary- or direct-acting carcinogen. The capacity for biotransformation (activation and detoxification) varies greatly between species and organs, accounting partially for the species differences and organotropism of these agents. PAHs are a group of procarcinogens that are present in complex environmental products such as soot, coal tar, tobacco smoke, petroleum, air pollutants, and cutting oils. Although the PAHs are in part responsible for cases of lung cancer seen in cigarette smokers and tar roofing workers, it is also clear that complex mixtures such as tar and smoke include other chemical promoters that act through epigenetic mechanisms to contribute to the overall carcinogenicity. Figure 47–2 illustrates the multistep metabolic activation of the prototype PAH, benzo[a]pyrene (BP). The first step is a cytochrome P-450–mediated epoxidation, resulting in BP-7,8-epoxide, which in turn is metabolized to BP-7,8-diol by epoxide hydrolase. Cytochrome P-450–mediated metabolism of this product then results in the formation of the primary carcinogenic product, (+)-BP-7,8-diol-9,10-epoxide. The 10 position of this compound is then capable of alkylating DNA at the 2 amino group on guanine. Although this metabolic pathway leads to the metabolic activation of BP to a primary carcinogen, it is also important to note that many other pathways exist for the metabolism of BP that lead to the formation of detoxification products that are readily eliminated.

The tobacco-specific nitrosamines, N-nitrosonornicotine (NNN) and 4-[methylnitroso-amino-1(3-pyridyl)]-1-butanone (NNK), are other procarcinogens found in tobacco and tobacco smoke. They are formed by bacterially mediated nitrosation of nicotine during the curing process. Cigarette smoke represents a major source of carcinogenic nitrosamine exposure in smokers and of involuntary exposure to nonsmokers. Chewing tobacco is another source of human exposure to NNN and NNK, which, in contrast to PAHs, do not depend on combustion for their formation. Increased risk of cancers of the oral cavity is associated with the use of smokeless tobacco products, such as chewing tobacco.

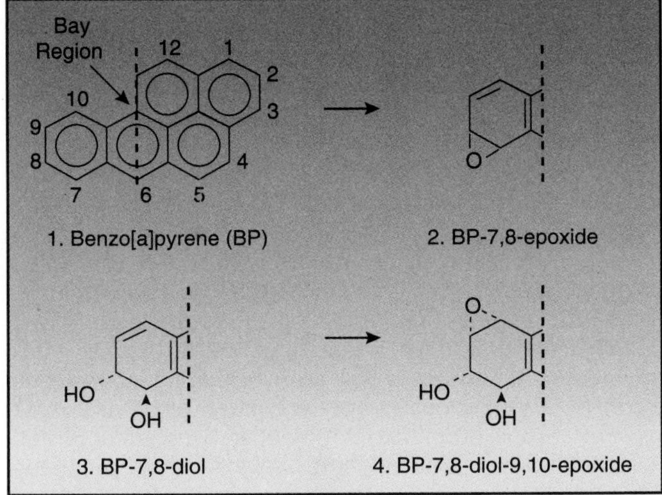

FIGURE 47–2. Bioactivation of benzo[a]pyrene.

Increased risk of cancer of the oral cavity and esophagus is also associated with the combined exposure to cigarette smoke and excessive drinking of alcoholic beverages (more than six drinks per day). This is in contrast to cigarette smokers with low or no alcohol consumption, who have little or no increased risk of cancer at these sites. Alcohol may be producing this response through increasing the metabolism and/or bioavailability of PAHs, NNN, and/or NNK found in smoke in the target tissues of the oral cavity and esophagus. Alcohol under these conditions is acting as a *cocarcinogen* by enhancing the first sequence of the carcinogenic process, neoplastic conversion. Cocarcinogens are defined as agents that enhance the overall carcinogenic process initiated by a genotoxic carcinogen when administered before or together with the genotoxic agent(s) or at a time when carcinogen damage to DNA is still present. A cocarcinogen is an epigenetic agent which may act through (1) increasing the uptake or bioavailability of a carcinogen, (2) enhancing the metabolic activation or decreasing the detoxification of a genotoxic agent, (3) inhibiting the DNA repair process, and/or (4) increasing the proliferation of cells with DNA damage, thereby facilitating mutation.

In contrast to cocarcinogens, *tumor promoters* enhance neoplastic development, the second step in the carcinogenic process. Tumor promoters are not genotoxic carcinogens but enhance the carcinogenic activity of a genotoxic agent when given subsequent to the genotoxic agent. The mechanism for the promoting activity of these chemicals when administered after a primary genotoxic carcinogen is complex and not yet fully understood. A two-stage model for carcinogenesis has been developed experimentally to investigate the process of tumor promotion for various agents. The model consists of tumor initiation, consisting of a single exposure to a genotoxic primary carcinogen, followed by multiple exposures at relatively high doses to a tumor-promoting agent. Phorbol esters, such as 12-O-tetradecanoyl-phorbol-13-acetate, have been extensively investigated for their tumor-promoting activity, which may in part be related to their binding to protein kinase C. Similarly, estrogens and testosterone have tumor-promoting activity that in part is related to their binding to the estrogen and androgen receptors, respectively. The persistent extremely toxic environmental contaminant TCDD (dioxin) is the most potent tumor promoter known. Most, if not all, of the biological and toxicological responses of TCDD are mediated by its binding to a specific high-affinity cytosolic protein referred to as the Ah receptor. Once TCDD is bound to the Ah receptor, the complex undergoes structural transformation, enters the nucleus, binds to specific dioxin-responsive elements on DNA, and transcribes various proteins, including cytochrome P-450 1A1 and 1A2, interleukin 1B, and plasminogen activator-inhibitor 2. Other tumor promoters that do not appear to have a receptor-mediated action include bile acids and fatty acids, which promote colon cancer; saccharin, which promotes bladder cancer; and phenobarbital, dichlorodiphenyltrichloroethane (DDT), and butylated hydroxytoluene, which enhance liver carcinogenesis.

Immunosuppressive drugs are another class of epigenetic agents that through the suppression of the immune system may allow the development of tumors initiated by distinct genetic events. Azathioprine or 6-mercaptopurine has been associated with increased incidence of leukemias or sarcomas but rarely solid tumors. Cyclosporin A use in organ transplant recipients also has been found to be associated with an increase in the incidence of lymphoma.

Solid-state materials such as asbestos are another group of epigenetic carcinogens. Large amounts of asbestos may reach the pleural cavity following chronic inhalation because the fine needle-like fibers are not biotransformed and are poorly excreted. Mining, construction, shipbuilding, and manufacture of asbestos-containing materials have led to high exposures, which have resulted in asbestosis, a progressive pulmonary fibrosis and pleural calcification. An increased incidence of lung cancer is also associated with asbestos exposure. Epidemiological studies have shown that industrial asbestos exposure has resulted in a fivefold greater risk of developing lung cancer. Other behaviors also affect the incidence of lung cancer. Individuals who regularly smoke cigarettes have a 10-fold greater risk of developing lung cancer than nonsmokers. In combining these exposures, individuals having industrial asbestos exposure who were also regular cigarette smokers had a more than additive or 50-fold greater risk of developing lung cancer. Asbestos has also been shown to be a causative agent in the induction of a rare form of cancer not normally seen in unexposed individuals. Mesothelioma is a cancer of the mesothelial membranes in either the pleural or peritoneal cavity. It is this form of cancer that prompted the EPA to regulate exposures of children to asbestos in school under the Asbestos Hazard Emergency Response Act. The reason for this action was primarily because mesothelioma has been reported even for nonoccupational asbestos exposure. For example, mesotheliomas have been reported in the wives of asbestos workers whose only exposure was from laundering the husband's work clothes. Similarly, a study in South Africa indicates that an increase in ambient air levels of asbestos in regions where asbestos was mined and processed was a contributing factor in development of mesothelioma in the local populations. Finally, a long latency period exists from the initial exposure to the actual onset of disease, which approaches approximately 40 years. It is this long latency and the fact that mesothelioma can result from even nonindustrial exposures that led to an initial focusing of asbestos control measures in children during the primary and secondary school years.

Generally, regulations such as the Asbestos Hazard Emergency Response Act are phased in when risk assessment estimates predict more than a one in a million lifetime risk for the particular cancer end-point.

Prevention and Regulation

It is now clear that complex environmental and occupational exposures to chemicals produce cancer through a combination of genotoxic and epigenetic mechanisms. For example, epigenetic agents in cigarette smoke play a major role in the development of lung cancer. This is supported by epidemiological studies of cigarette smokers that found a lower risk of lung cancer with each year following smoking cessation. Epigenetic agents in various diets also are thought to play a major role in the development of cancers of the colon, breast, prostate, and perhaps pancreas. Recommendations of public health programs to stop smoking, lower total dietary fat intake, and increase fiber content in the diet are based on the principle that tumor promotion is a potentially reversible process. Williams and Weisburger (1991) developed a list of risk factors for various cancers and specific preventive approaches that could reduce cancer risk (Table 47 – 6). Many of the preventive measures are simply the increased consumption of fruits and vegetables, which are a source of antioxidants, retinoids, and fiber. Vitamin A or retinoic acid derivatives have been shown to inhibit neoplastic development, possibly through restoring cell-to-cell communication and inhibiting promotion. Vitamin E and synthetic antioxidants such as butylated hydroxytoluene, butylated hydroxyanisole, propyl gallate and ethoxyquin have inhibited tumor induction by chemical carcinogens in several experimental models. Vitamins C and E also prevent the formation of nitrosamines and nitrosamides, which in turn has reduced cancers of the liver, upper gastrointestinal tract, and respiratory tract.

Recently, a number of studies have commenced to study the role of estrogenlike xenobiotics in the development of certain cancer types and the effects on reproduction. A recent review by Davis and colleagues (1993) reviewed both toxicological and epidemiological evidence for chlorinated organic chemicals' involvement in the induction of breast cancer. Table 47 – 7 presents some of the animal and human evidence that they have gathered. Although the commercial use of many of these chemicals is decreasing (*eg*, Atrazine) or has been banned for some years (*eg*, DDT and polychlorinated biphenyls), many are persistent and cycle in the ecosystem for decades. Thus, the potential for further exposure often continues long after a chemical is no longer in commercial use. The long-term effect on the reproductive capacity and general health of the population remains a concern.

Finally, it should be pointed out that the regulation of chemical toxicants is a constantly evolving process. A trend has occurred in the last decade to focus on the more subtle noncarcinogenic effects of chemical exposures. As the toxic end-points become more subtle, the doses necessary to elicit that effect are often considerably lower than those necessary to elicit the more severe effects. This tends to drive exposure standards lower and lower. A good example of this is seen in the recent four- to fivefold reductions in lead exposure standards. There was a time when physicians diagnosed lead poisoning based on rather serious objective findings, including central nervous system effects (lead encephalopathy) and hematological effects (anemia and porphyrin imbalance). Blood lead levels were not viewed as being a particular concern until they exceeded 30 – 50 μg/dL. More recently, lead poisoning has been defined as a child having a blood lead above 10 μg/dL. A child being examined by a physician, in all probability, presents with no objective findings at this blood level. The standard has been set at this level because of findings in epidemiological studies of large populations that children with values in excess of 10 μg/dL had a greater probability of having a reduced intelligence quotient score (2 – 6 points, on average). A concern also exists for exposure *in utero* during development, and a number of studies have shown reduced birth weights, more premature births, and retarded growth in populations having elevated

TABLE 47–6. Factors and Possible Mechanisms in Main Epithelial Cancer Causation and Prevention

Disease	Risk Factors	Mechanism	Protective Elements	Mechanism
Nasopharyngeal cancer	Salted, pickled fish	Contains specific nitrosamine (?)	Vegetables	Micronutrients
	Viral factors	Can increase cell cycling	Vaccination (?)	
	Wood and leather workers	Carcinogens/promoters		
Esophageal cancer	Salted, pickled food (?)	Specific nitrosamine	Yellow-green vegetables	Role of vegetables unknown if risk factor present in food
	Alcohol intake with smoking	Alcohol modifies esophageal metabolism of tobacco-specific carcinogens	Yellow-green vegetables	Carotene, vitamin A protective elements
	Tobacco chewing	Tobacco-specific carcinogens and promoters (?)	Vegetables (?)	β-carotene as antioxidant
Gastric cancer (glandular intestinal)	Salted, pickled food	Nitrosoindoles, phenolic diazotates	Green-yellow vegetables	Role of vegetables unknown if risk factor present in food, but may assist in differentiation
	Geochemical nitrate and salt	Carcinogens formed in stomach	Green-yellow vegetables, fruits, vitamins C and E	Vitamins C and E prevent formation of carcinogen: vitamins increase cellular tissue defenses
Bladder cancer	*Bilharzia*: schistosomiasis	Carcinogens unknown; increased cell proliferation enhances risk	Yellow-green vegetables	Beneficial micronutrients
	Smoking	Unknown	Yellow-green vegetables	Retinoids
	Occupational	Chronic high exposure to some arylamines	Reduce exposure	Reduce exposure
Endocrine-related cancers (prostate, breast, ovary)	Total dietary fat (saturated and ω-6 polyunsaturated lipids)	Complex multieffector elements: hormonal balances, membrane and intracellular effectors	Monounsaturated oil (olive)	Neural action on hormone metabolism
			ω-3 Polyunsaturated oils	Protective effects in hormone metabolism
			Medium-chain triglycerides	Caloric equivalent to carbohydrate
			Cereal fiber and pectin	Affects enterohepatic cycling of hormones
			Yellow-green vegetables	Micronutrients
	Fried/broiled meats	HAAs	Tryptophan and proline	Prevent formation of HAAs
Endometrial cancer	Same as above; excessive body weight	Same as above; fat cells generate high levels of estrogen	Same as above; weight control/loss	Same as above; lowers excessive nonphysiologic estrogen levels
Pancreatic cancers	Same as endocrine cancer (total dietary fat)	High-fat diets increase functional demands, increase cell duplication (?)	Vegetables	Micronutrients
	Cigarette smoking	Tobacco-specific nitrosamines		
	Fried/broiled meats	HAAs	Tryptophan and proline	Prevent formation of HAAs
Colon cancer				
Proximal	?	?	?	?
Distal	Same as endocrine-related cancers	Biosynthesis of cholesterol, thence bile acids, and colon cancer promotion, including higher cell cycling rates	Cereal fiber, especially wheat	Increases stool bulk; dilutes promoters; lowers intestinal pH
Rectal cancer	Alcoholic beverages, especially beer	Increases cell cycling in rectum	Cereal fiber (?)	Dilutes effectors by increasing stool bulk
Liver cancer	Mold-contaminated foods	Mycotoxins	Avoid moldy foods; improve nutrition; more protein, fruits and vegetables	Lower carcinogen intake
	Some plants	Pyrrolizidine alkaloids		
	Pickled foods	Nitrosamines	Avoid pickled foods	
	Chronic virus	Hepatitis B	Vaccination	
	High level of specific alcoholic beverages	Damages liver; risk of cirrhosis potentiates effect of carcinogens	Decrease intake of alcohol	May lower cell duplication rates
	Occupational, iatrogenic	Vinyl chloride, some oral contraceptives (infrequent occurrence)	Lower exposure	
	Cigarette smoking	Tobacco-specific nitrosamines		
	Fried/broiled meats	HAAs	Tryptophan and proline	Prevent formation of HAA

From Williams GM, Weisburger JH: Chemical carcinogenesis. *In* Amdur MO, Doull J, Klaassen CD (eds): Casarett and Doull's Toxicology: The Basic Science of Poisons, 4th ed. Elmsford, NY: Pergamon Press, 1991. Reproduced with permission of McGraw-Hill, Inc.

HAA = heterocyclic aromatic amine.

TABLE 47–7. Experimental Evidence on Mammary Carcinogenesis of Some Chlorinated Organics

Chemical	Animal Studies
Organochlorine Compound	
DDT	Accelerator of mammary tumors in male mice treated with 2-acetamidophenanthrene
Triazines, atrazine	Increased incidence of mammary tumors in male rats
Benzene	Breast cancer after oral and respiratory routes of exposure
Polycyclic Aromatic Hydrocarbons	
Benzo[a]pyrene	Mammary tumors after gastrointestinal route of exposure
Dibenz[a,h]anthracene	Mammary tumors after gastrointestinal route of exposure
Chemical	**Human Case Control Studies**
DDE, PCB	Elevated risk for breast cancer
Hexachlorocyclohexane	Elevated risk for breast cancer; odds ratio = 10.5 (> 0.1 ppm)
DDE	Elevated risk for breast cancer; odds ratio = 4 (10th–90th percentile)

Adapted from Davis DL, et al: Medical hypothesis: Xenoestrogens as preventable causes of breast cancer. Environ Health Perspectives 101:372–377, 1993.

DDE = dichlorodiphenyl dichloroethylene (metabolite of DDT); DDT = dichlorodiphenyltrichloroethane; PCB = polychlorinated biphenyl.

blood lead at birth. Thus, as the toxic end-point upon which a standard is based becomes more subtle, a tendency for the standard to be driven downward will occur to protect the population from that effect.

REFERENCES

Coombs RRA, Gell PGH: Classification of allergic reactions responsible for clinical hypersensitivity and disease. *In* Gell PGH, Coombs RRA, Lachman PJ (eds): Clinical Aspects of Immunology. Philadelphia: JB Lippincott, 1975.

Davis DL, Bradlow HL, Wolff M, et al: Medical hypothesis: Xenoestrogens as preventable causes of breast cancer. Environ Health Perspectives 101:372–377, 1993.

Hayes AW: Principles and Methods of Toxicology, 2nd ed. New York: Raven Press, 1989.

Klaassen CD, Eaton DL: Principles of toxicology. *In* Amdur MO, Doull J, Klaassen CD (eds): Casarett and Doull's Toxicology: The Basic Science of Poisons, 4th ed. Elmsford, NY: Pergamon Press, 1991.

NAS: Risk Assessment in the Federal Government: Managing the Process. Washington, DC: National Academy Press, 1983.

Rutstein DD, Mullan RJ, Frazier TM, et al: Sentinel health events (occupational): A basis for physician recognition and public health surveillance. Am J Public Health 73:1054–1062, 1983.

Williams GM, Weisburger JH: Chemical carcinogenesis. *In* Amdur MO, Doull J, Klaassen CD (eds): Casarett and Doull's Toxicology: The Basic Science of Poisons, 4th ed. Elmsford, NY: Pergamon Press, 1991.

Wilson R, Crouch EAC: Risk assessment and comparisons: An introduction. Science 236:267–280, 1987.

Alcohols 48

Peter K. Gessner

DEFINITIONS

Substances

Alcohols

Alcohol is a term that identifies chemical compounds with aliphatic hydroxy groups. The three simplest alcohols, methanol, ethanol, and ethylene glycol, can be consumed and can be abused.

- ***Methanol*** and ***ethylene glycol*** have slight inebriating properties, but both form toxic metabolites. Accordingly, their consumption, even in small quantities, can precipitate a life-threatening medical emergency.
- ***Ethanol*** is a two-carbon compound bearing one hydroxy group. It is formed when yeast is forced to oxidize sugar in the absence of oxygen. It is imbibed by the majority of the population who enjoy its inebriating effects. A minority do so excessively; the consequences of this constitute a major public health and social problem.

ETHANOL

Drinking Behaviors

The population can be divided into four groups relative to their alcohol consumption. The multiplicity of synonyms used to characterize drinking behaviors reflects, however, a continuing debate regarding how these behaviors should be characterized.

- ***Nondrinking, abstinence, or teetotalism:*** practiced by a significant proportion of the population, particularly in some regions of this country.
- ***Nonproblem, social, or controlled drinking:*** the type

of drinking devoid of negative consequences and practiced by the majority of the population.

- ***Alcohol abuse, problem drinking, or early-stage alcoholism:*** drinking that is excessive in that it brings negative consequences for the imbiber related to health, job, family, or legal system.
- ***Alcohol dependence, alcohol addiction, late-stage or gamma alcoholism:*** drinking that not only brings negative consequences for the subject but also provides evidence of dependence, such as physical dependence and withdrawal, drinking first thing in the morning, or alcoholic blackouts.

Quantification of Consumption

Drinking behavior definitions focus on what is clinically more discernible, which is the *consequences* of the drinking rather than the amount drunk. In the final analysis, however, it is the *absolute amount* of ethanol consumed that determines the consequences of drinking. Beverage type is of little consequence. Realization of this has led to a unitary definition of a unit "drink" that cuts across beverage type:

- A ***drink*** is defined as the quantity of beverage that contains 0.5 oz or 15 mL of absolute alcohol.
- ***Table wine*** is obtained by anaerobic fermentation of grape juice by yeast. Regardless of how much sugar is present in the grape juice, the process stops naturally when the ethanol concentration rises to 12–14%. Hence, a 4-oz glass of wine contains about 0.5 oz of ethanol and constitutes a "drink."
- ***Beer*** is made by fermentation of brews that contain less sugar. Consequently, its ethanol content is lower, usually about 4%; therefore, a 12-oz bottle of beer constitutes a "drink."
- ***Spirits,*** or ***liquor,*** obtained by distilling off the alcohol from fermented brews, are usually marketed as 80 to 100 proof, or 40–50% ethanol (proof = ethanol concentration × 2). Hence a "drink" is a 1-oz shot.

Blood Levels

The acute effects of alcohol on target organs are a function of tissue ethanol levels. These levels are proportional to those in the blood. These have been variously reported:

- ***Scientifically,*** ethanol blood levels are reported in milligrams per deciliter (mg/dL). Earlier, the same units bore the designation mg% (meaning mg of ethanol per 100 mL or 1 dL). Blood ethanol levels can also be reported in units of concentration, namely millimoles (mM), where 1 mM ethanol contains 4.6 mg ethanol per deciliter.
- ***In the courts,*** and thus the media, blood ethanol content is reported in percentages (weight/volume). Thus, the 0.1% blood alcohol level, which in many jurisdictions is considered presumptive evidence of driving while intoxicated, is equivalent to a blood ethanol concentration of 100 mg/dL.

Absorption, Distribution, and Elimination

The following factors determine the speed of onset, the intensity, and the duration of action of ingested ethanol.

• Absorption

Absorption occurs primarily from the small intestine at a rate proportional to concentration. Direct absorption from the stomach does occur but is much slower than that from the intestine. Accordingly, anything that delays gastric emptying (*eg,* food in stomach) also delays absorption and subsequently lowers peak plasma alcohol levels. In concentrations above 50 proof, ethanol inhibits gastric motility and delays gastric emptying.

• Distribution

Ethanol is freely soluble in both water and fat and therefore distributes readily to all tissues at a rate governed by blood flow. If allowed to partition between water and fat, its concentration in the water is 30 times higher than in fat. Accordingly, at equilibrium its distribution *in vivo* is much the same as that of body water.

MEN VERSUS WOMEN. Consumption of a given amount of ethanol leads to higher blood alcohol levels in the average woman than in the average man. First, fat constitutes a higher proportion of the body weight in women than in men, which results in a smaller volume of distribution for ethanol. Second, the body weight of women tends to be lower than that of men.

• Excretion

Alcohol is excreted in breath, urine, and sweat but in amounts that are quantitatively insignificant, although proportional to concentration in blood. Therefore, noninvasive assessment of blood ethanol levels can be performed by measuring alcohol levels in the breath.

• Metabolism

The primary and overwhelming method of elimination of alcohol is metabolic. More than 98% of the process is hepatic, first by oxidation to acetaldehyde, then to acetate, and eventually, to carbon dioxide.

RATE. At all but the lowest blood concentrations, ethanol is eliminated at a constant rate, *ie,* by apparent zero-order kinetics. About two thirds of a "drink" is cleared per hour on average.

ENZYMES. Hepatic alcohol dehydrogenase and aldehyde dehydrogenase are the two enzymes responsible for ethanol metabolism *in vivo.* The alcohol dehydrogenase is a cytosolic enzyme. The aldehyde dehydrogenase involved is a mitochondrial enzyme. In liver homogenates, two other enzymes, namely the microsomal ethanol-oxidizing system, and catalase, oxidize ethanol; however, their *in vivo* role is at best minimal. Nevertheless, ethanol consumption does induce the microsomal ethanol-oxidizing system.

Acute Effects on the Nervous System

Ethanol induces a depression of many central nervous system (CNS) functions. The depression or impairment of function increases progressively with dose.

• Behavioral Effects

The changes after alcohol consumption are caused by a number of mechanisms including both the individual's conscious and unconscious "expectations" and the actions of alcohol on nervous function. For example, many individuals exhibit significantly more aggressive behavior if they believe that they have consumed alcohol, even when they have not.

As another example, ethanol is popularly perceived as generally having stress-relieving properties. Experimentally, it has been found that ethanol ingestion does result in decreased cardiovascular responses in some stressful situations, but the response is very much related to the individual's personality; appreciable differences may also exist in relation to age and gender.

In addition to expectation effects, alcohol consumption clearly alters mood and in most individuals reduces anxiety moderately and promotes a feeling of well-being. Nevertheless, when alcohol is consumed in large amounts, the mood frequently becomes less euphoric and more depressed, with an increase in irritability or dysphoria, especially later in the evening after the alcohol had been consumed.

• Cognitive Function

Cognitive function progressively deteriorates as blood ethanol levels rise. Arithmetic subtraction proficiency, a good test of cognitive function, is shown to be impaired in Figure 48-1; tolerance among moderate and heavy drinkers is evident.

• Judgment

Judgment is impaired progressively as blood ethanol levels increase. For example, in the tests of standing steadiness illustrated in Figure 48-1, subjects with raised blood ethanol levels asserted that their performance had improved even in the face of obvious objective evidence to the contrary, *ie*, even when they were visibly swaying, losing their balance, or falling.

• Cerebellar Function

As blood ethanol levels increase, a progressive monophasic deterioration of standing steadiness is observed. Figure 48-1 shows such impairment in individuals asked to stand steadily with eyes closed and one foot directly in front of the other, a good test of cerebellar function. The effects of any given blood ethanol level are somewhat less in moderate drinkers and markedly less in heavy drinkers than those observed in abstainers, clear-cut evidence of tolerance.

• Driving Ability

All three of the above effects contribute to a decline in performance of complex tasks. Significant impairment of driving ability is observed at blood ethanol levels of 35 mg/dL. An important consequence of such impairment is the increased probability of involvement in a vehicular accident; the probability rises in an exponential manner with blood alcohol levels (Fig. 48-2). More than 50% of fatal automobile accidents involve at least one intoxicated driver. As might be expected, alcoholic intoxication is also found to be a concomitant of a quarter or more of pedestrian highway deaths, serious injuries in the home, and private plane crashes.

• Amnesia

The amnesia associated with an episode of acute intoxication can be of two types. The first and most frequent is a partial, fragmentary loss of memory for some events occurring

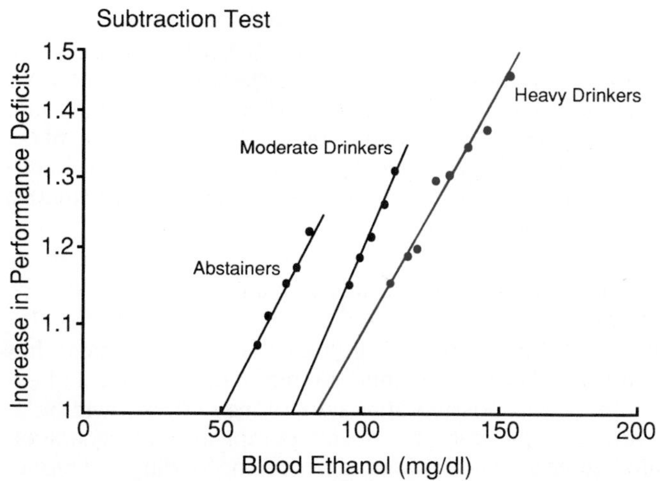

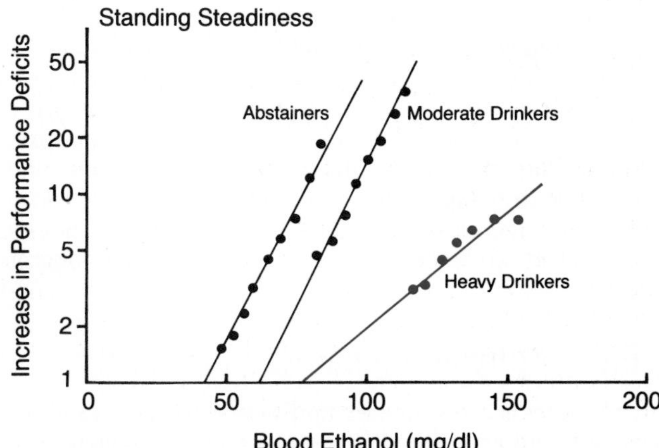

FIGURE 48-1. Effect of blood ethanol levels on cerebellar and cognitive function. (Redrawn from Goldberg L: Quantitative studies on alcohol tolerance in man. Acta Physiol Scand 5:S16, 1943.)

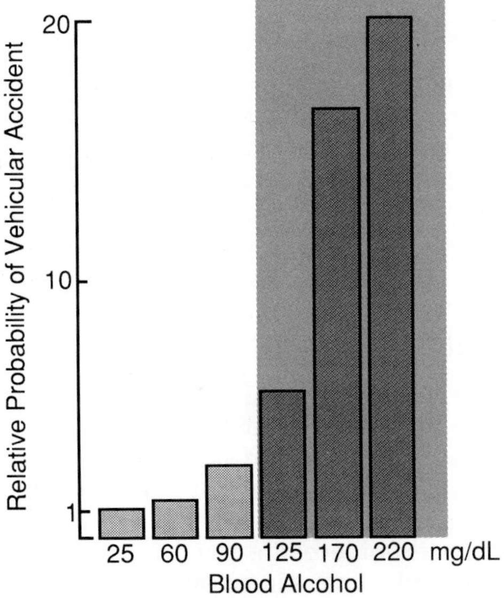

FIGURE 48–2. Relationship between probability of vehicular accident and blood ethanol level.

during intoxication; the individual is usually completely unaware of the memory deficits. The second type of amnesia, usually denoted as a "blackout," consists essentially of a complete loss of memory of events occurring during a period, with a clear-cut time of onset and of recovery of the memory. During such blackouts, the individual characteristically appears to others as behaving and responding in an appropriate but sometimes mildly intoxicated manner. The first type of partial amnesia is nearly universal and is dose/concentration-dependent — the higher the blood level, the greater the degree of memory loss. In contrast, the susceptibility to blackouts appears to vary greatly among different individuals.

• Other Important Actions on Nervous Function

Other actions of alcohol on nervous function include analgesia; sedation with increased likelihood of sleep but a fractured late-night sleep pattern; altered thought processes in the direction of increased fantasies, decreased ability to think abstractly, and decreased ability to focus attention; altered mood and affect, usually including a mild reduction of anxiety, some euphoria, and moderate talkativeness early in an episode of intoxication but with dysphoria and depression after high concentrations of alcohol some hours after the start of drinking; slowing of extraocular muscle movements with increases in lateral gaze nystagmus; slurred speech; and an exaggeration of irritability and aggressiveness.

• Electrophysiological Actions

Ethanol effects are complex and vary with site examined. Some neurons are excited by systemic or local application of alcohol (*eg*, some sensory receptors) in concentration associated with moderate intoxication, some neurons are inhibited or exhibit depression of responsivity, whereas many other neurons are not affected except by very high to lethal concentrations.

• Respiration

In high doses ethanol induces a centrally mediated depression of respiration. At one time this was thought to be the proximal cause of death in acute alcoholic intoxication. Death in such cases is now seen to be the result of cardiovascular collapse secondary to the direct toxic action of ethanol on blood vessels.

Mechanisms of Action

Identification of the mechanism(s) mediating ethanol's pharmacological effects on the CNS has been difficult because of alcohol's many neurochemical and electrophysiological effects. The actions of alcohol exhibit selectivity and specificity in terms of qualitative effects, sites of action, and differential actions on a variety of neuronal systems. Among the probable mechanisms of action are:

• Action at γ-Aminobutyric Acid$_A$ Receptors

γ-Aminobutyric acid (GABA) functions as an inhibitory neurotransmitter in the CNS, where it is the most abundant neurotransmitter. The GABA receptor is an oligomeric one that incorporates a chloride ion channel. GABA increases the chloride ion flux through this channel. This causes hyperpolarization of the neuron and inhibition. Ethanol augments the GABA-induced chloride flux. It does so by acting at a site other than the receptor's GABA recognition site. Increasing evidence suggests that many of the CNS actions of ethanol may be mediated by this mechanism.

• Actions at Other Sites

Actions at other sites may turn out to also involve binding or modification of the binding properties of *N*-methyl D-aspartate, nicotinic and acetylcholine receptors, or effects on adenosine triphosphatases (ATPases), cyclic guanosine monophosphate, and central prostaglandin systems. Ethanol also has been shown to produce vasoconstriction of cerebral vessels, to alter calcium release and neurotransmitter-secretion coupling, and to alter the release of endogenous anxiogenic substances.

• Effects on Membrane Fluidity

In concentrations that would be lethal *in vivo*, ethanol has widespread effects on neuronal membrane fluidity and excitability. It is possible that alcohol may interact with relatively specific macromolecular complexes, *ie*, receptors, analogous to recent evidence of specific binding and recognition sites for a variety of small molecules and even ions such as calcium.

Other Organ System Effects

Ethanol has a large variety of effects on various organ systems. Among the more important are nausea and vomiting; diuresis; catecholamine release with moderate increase in heart rate and blood pressure; complex endocrine effects including decreased testosterone, prolactin, corticotropin, and antidiuretic hormone levels; precipitation of headache; and decreased absorption and increased excretion of thiamine.

Vestibular Effects

Ethanol affects the organs of balance; this is because the density of ethanol is 0.79 times lower than that of the water it displaces and because blood circulates through the inner ear's cupola, but the endolymph in the semicircular canals is secreted and therefore reflects changes in blood ethanol levels more slowly.

• **RISING BLOOD ALCOHOL PHASE.** As blood ethanol levels increase, those in the cupola rise more rapidly than those in the endolymph. Hence, the specific density of the cupola becomes lower than that of the endolymph, and the inner ear, which normally registers only acceleration, becomes sensitive to the effects of gravity. This causes sensations of motion when none is occurring. In the ambulatory individual it can lead to nausea and vomiting.

• **FALLING PHASE.** As blood alcohol levels fall, the process is reversed. Ethanol levels in the cupola fall faster than those in the endolymph, and again the effects of gravity cause spurious sensations of motion.

• **NYSTAGMUS.** Nystagmus accompanies these phenomena. Called the *positional alcohol nystagmus*, it is seen in the supine subject when the head is turned to one side. During the rising phase, the eyes beat to that side; during the falling phase, they beat to the opposite side.

Peripheral Actions

Ethanol induces a number of peripheral effects, most of which are mediated or modulated by its central effects:

- **Cutaneous and mucosal vasodilation** results in a sensation of warmth but also in an overall increase in the rate of heat loss and a lowering of central core temperature; in cold weather this can lead to fatal hypothermia.
- **Gastrin secretion** causes an increase in appetite and enhanced peristalsis; this centrally mediated effect is abolished by vagotomy.
- **Antidiuretic hormone secretion** is inhibited by ethanol; this causes diuresis.

Hepatic Metabolism and Its Effects

The oxidation of ethanol to acetaldehyde occurs in the liver. The process involves the following:

- **Alcohol dehydrogenase,** a zinc-containing cytosolic enzyme that oxidizes ethanol and concurrently transfers reducing equivalents to nicotinamide-adenine dinucleotide (NAD^+).
- $\mathbf{NAD^+}$ is reduced to NADH in the oxidation of ethanol. The regeneration of NAD^+ occurs initially at the expense of other reducible substrates in the cytosol (*eg*, pyruvate); however, the supply of these becomes quickly exhausted, and the regeneration of NAD^+ becomes the rate-controlling step.
- **The respiratory electron transport chain**, which is located in the mitochondria: it regenerates mitochondrial NAD^+ and, less directly, cystosolic NAD^+ (Fig. 48–3). Because NAD^+ cannot cross membranes, the regeneration of the latter is mediated by "shuttles" (*ie*, substrates that

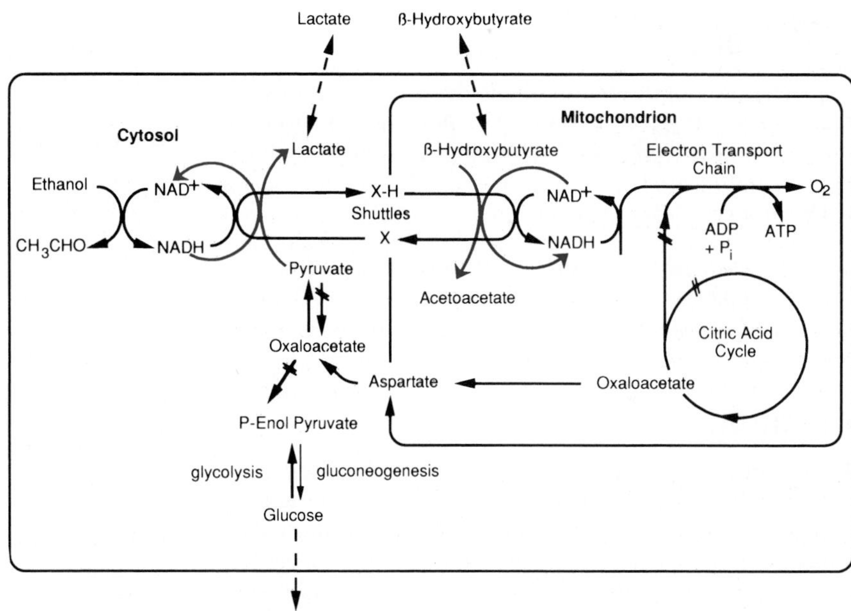

FIGURE 48–3. Metabolic scheme for events related to ethanol metabolism in the hepatocyte. Reactions inhibited or blocked during ethanol metabolism are shown crossed by double lines.

can transport the reducing equivalent across the mitochondrial membrane).

- The rate of operation of the respiratory electron transport chain is determined by the concentration ratio ([ADP] [phosphate]/[ATP]). The utilization of ATP, and hence the ratio, is not acutely affected by ethanol. Therefore, the rate of operation of the electron transport chain, the rate at which NAD^+ is regenerated, and the rate at which ethanol is oxidized all remain constant.
- **Gluconeogenesis** is blocked because it involves formation of enol phosphopyruvate from pyruvate via oxaloacetate, and during ethanol metabolism, the pyruvate is removed by reduction to lactate. The citric acid cycle is also inhibited by the scarcity of NADH.
- **Fatty acid utilization** is inhibited. It involves as a first step β-oxidation, a process that requires reoxidation of cofactors by the electron transport chain. Because β-oxidation is in competition for oxidation with the NADH produced in the oxidation of ethanol, it is also blocked. In heavy drinkers, this inhibition leads to fatty acid infiltration of the liver, a reversible condition.

Chronic Effect of High Doses

• Membrane-Bound Adenosine Triphosphatases

The activity of ATPases, which function as the sodium/potassium pump, increases, leading to higher rates of ATP utilization. These effects may be due to the cell membrane having been rendered more leaky by the action of ethanol.

• Respiratory Electron Transport Chain Activity

This activity increases in response to the higher rate of ATP utilization.

• Ethanol Oxidation

The higher rate of operation of the electron transport chain leads to faster regeneration of NAD^+ and thereby to a more rapid, but still acutely constant, rate of ethanol oxidation.

• Oxygen Utilization

The increased rate of operation of the electron transport chain results in more oxygen being utilized and in the hepatocyte extracting oxygen more efficiently from the blood percolating through the liver.

• Centrolobular Liver Necrosis

Blood percolates through the liver lobule in the direction of the centrolobular vein. Ingestion of ethanol in an amount sufficient to depress respiration and thus oxygenation of the blood, combined with the greater efficiency of hepatocytes in extracting oxygen from the blood, can result in the blood that reaches the centrolobular vein being too low in oxygen to assure viability.

The necrotic area in the liver is invaded by fibroblasts (a healing process), which results in the deposition of fibrous tissue, an action that can impair blood flow. This is a precursor of liver cirrhosis.

Tolerance, Physical Dependence, and Alcoholism

• Tolerance

Acute and chronic tolerance to alcohol's effects develops readily when even moderate amounts of alcohol are consumed. Ethanol induces both functional and metabolic tolerance, although quantitatively, functional tolerance is more important. The degree of tolerance that develops is a function of the amount of alcohol consumed.

• Physical Dependence

Physical dependence is the condition of habituation that results in the occurrence of a withdrawal syndrome upon cessation of alcohol consumption. For physical dependence to develop, the amount of alcohol consumed must be greater than that initially necessary to induce significant pharmacological effects.

• Alcohol Abuse

Alcohol abuse is drinking behavior that results in significant medical, legal, occupational, or economic problems for the imbiber. Abuse usually occurs before the drinker develops physical dependence. The condition responds well to minimal intervention and has a good prognosis. The four types of drinking behaviors (abstinence, social or nonproblem drinking, problem drinking, and ethanol dependence or alcohol addition) represent a behavioral progression. Although the vast majority of individuals who imbibe alcoholic beverages do not become addicted to ethanol, this is the progression followed by those who do.

• Alcohol Dependence

Dependence represents a significantly more morbid condition that usually encompasses physical dependence, requires intense treatment, and has a significantly poorer prognosis than does alcohol abuse.

• Alcoholism

As generally used in this country, *alcoholism* is a term that encompasses both alcohol dependence and problem drinking. It is a term with strong historical roots. How it is defined subsumes beliefs and attitudes regarding the nature of alcohol-related problems. The conceptual formulation of such beliefs has involved four phases:

- Temperance was a strong social movement that developed in the United States in the 18th and 19th centuries and held the belief that ethanol (the "devil rum") imbibed in any quantity possessed a behavioral toxicity that necessarily predestined the drinker to become a hopeless drunkard. These beliefs culminated with the passing of the Prohibition Amendment to the U.S. Constitution in 1919.

- The repeal of the Prohibition Amendment in 1933 marked the culmination of a process whereby the concepts advanced by the temperance movement were rejected. Alcohol came to be viewed as a benign commodity like any other and habitual drunkenness as a personal moral failing of the imbiber. On this basis, individuals with alcohol-engendered health problems were frequently refused medical treatment.
- Alcoholics Anonymous is a fellowship of individuals with serious drinking problems. Those forming it in 1935 adopted the construct that although the majority of the population could drink alcohol safely, they, the alcoholics, formed a subgroup who were in some way biologically different from the rest of the population and consequently was "powerless over alcohol." Accordingly, they viewed life-long abstinence and support of each other in this resolve as their only defense. Taking just one drink, according to this construct, would lead to a loss of control and an inability to stop until drunk. The then-recent discovery of insulin led them to suggest that alcoholism was a disease like diabetes or, alternatively, like an allergy.
- Empirical scientific research, which government financial support has much expanded in the last 30 – 40 years, has frequently failed to affirm previously developed beliefs.

The resulting synthesis leads to the following conclusions:

- **Behavioral toxicity:** in modest quantities, alcohol can be consumed safely and does not cause behavioral toxicity. Consumption of six or more drinks per day is correlated in adult males with a tendency for the consumption to escalate. Chronic consumption of 10 or more drinks per day necessarily leads (in adult males) to the development of ethanol dependence. The generally lower body weight and higher fat content of females suggests they would be susceptible to lower levels of alcohol consumption.
- **Biological differences:** despite extensive research and occasional promising leads, no biochemical, neurological, or other abnormality has been identified that reliably differentiates alcoholics from the rest of the population.
- **Genetic predisposition:** research with twins and adoptees in Scandinavia indicates that a modest degree of genetic predisposition exists for alcoholism among children of alcoholics. It accounts, however, for only one eighth of the overall prevalence of alcoholism. Nonetheless, alcoholism is very much a familial condition, suggesting a strong nurturing influence.
- **Distribution of consumption:** alcoholics do not form a distinct drinking population. Analysis of the distribution of ethanol consumption levels in the population indicates that, like that of other commodities, it is unimodal and continuous. The mean per capita consumption in the population is affected by prices and other socially controlled factors (for instance, the hours during which bars are open). In turn, the per capita consumption determines the fraction of the population drinking in excess of 10 drinks per day.
- **Loss of control:** alcoholics frequently assert that although determined to have no more than one or two drinks, once they have had the first drink, they are unable to stop imbibing. Repeated efforts to elicit alcohol-induced "loss of control" under placebo-controlled conditions have proved unsuccessful. On the other hand, it has been observed that alcoholics led to believe that they are drinking an alcoholic beverage drink more of it than of one that they have come to believe is alcohol-free, regardless of whether the beverage does contain ethanol or not. This suggests that their consumption of alcoholic beverages is driven by something akin to a conditioned response.

The Acute Withdrawal Syndrome

The syndrome is a concomitant of physical dependence. If severe, it can be damaging or even fatal. Because the symptoms of a mild withdrawal and the early phase of a severe one are the same, how the syndrome develops in any given patient should be carefully monitored.

• Etiology

In individuals physically dependent on ethanol, cessation or significant reduction in the consumption of ethanol leads to the development of the alcohol withdrawal syndrome. In individuals with a high degree of functional tolerance to ethanol, the syndrome can develop as a the result of a major drop in blood alcohol levels, although the resulting levels are still high enough so that they would cause a nontolerant subject to be intoxicated. The peak severity of the syndrome is proportional to the level of magnitude of the prewithdrawal alcohol consumption.

• Time Course

The early symptoms of the withdrawal syndrome are observed within hours of the reduction or cessation of alcohol intake. The symptoms and signs peak, as a rule, after 48 hours, and an improvement in the patient's condition ensues. In patients who are dependent on very high levels of ethanol (more than 26 drinks per day) a secondary condition called delirium tremens develops after the withdrawal syndromes have peaked.

• Early Symptoms and Signs

Most prevalent is a characteristic gross tremor. It can become extreme. Severe weakness, effusive perspiration, hyperreflexia, insomnia, anorexia, nausea, retching, vomiting, and diarrhea are other early manifestations.

• Symptoms and Signs of Severe Withdrawal

An elevation of blood pressure, hallucinations (during which the patient tends to retain insight), and grand mal – type seizures are symptoms and signs of severe withdrawal.

• Delirium Tremens

Delirium tremens is not a withdrawal syndrome but rather a consequence of it. It is characterized by overactivity of the autonomic nervous system, with tachycardia, dilated pupils, excessive sweating, and fever of noninfectious origin. The gross delirium that develops is characterized by a loss of insight — an inability to identify people or to interpret properly what is seen, heard, or perceived by other sensory means. Untreated, delirium tremens has a mortality rate as high as 30%. Even among those receiving expert care, a 3–7% mortality rate exists.

Therapy for the Withdrawal Syndrome

Because it is a withdrawal syndrome, the condition responds well to readministration of CNS depressants, although ethanol itself is not used to this end clinically.

• General Supportive Therapy

General supportive therapy is sufficient if the withdrawal is mild. It includes the following:

Reality orientation, including checking on the patient at 30-minute intervals, engaging him or her in conversation with emphasis of where and who he or she is, provision of windows and good lighting, appears to inhibit the development of hallucinations.

Thiamine administration reverses Wernicke's encephalopathy and is thought to prevent the development of Korsakoff's psychosis, an irreversible impairment of the ability to transform short- to long-term memory.

Hydration because patients in withdrawal frequently suffer from dehydration.

• Pharmacotherapy With Central Nervous System Depressants

Administration of increasing amounts of a relatively short-acting depressant should occur until signs of mild CNS depression are evident, *ie*, until tolerance is exceeded. Thereafter, the patient is maintained on the depressant, but its dose is gradually reduced until none is given over a 10-day period. If pharmacotherapy is instituted within the first 2 days of withdrawal, the condition responds well to it. The drugs that have been found most effective in this respect are

Chlordiazepoxide

Oxazepam

Paraldehyde (now obsolete)

• Pharmacotherapy of the Adrenergic Concomitants

Drugs such as phenothiazines, propranolol, and clonidine control the adrenergic concomitants of the withdrawal but do not control its more severe manifestations. Consequently, monitoring of the development of withdrawal becomes more problematic. Phenothiazines also lower the threshold for seizures and therefore are contraindicated.

• Anticonvulsant Pharmacotherapy

Phenytoin and other anticonvulsants are not effective in controlling the seizures of alcohol withdrawal and should not be used in the absence of a history or other evidence of epilepsy.

• Delirium Tremens

Appropriate treatment of the withdrawal syndrome within the first 2 days of its emergence prevents the later appearance of delirium tremens. Once delirium tremens emerges, however, it tends to be resistant to treatment.

Hangover

In the majority of, but not all, individuals, acute ingestion of five or more alcoholic drinks is followed some hours later by a discomforting set of postintoxication symptoms collectively referred to as a hangover.

• Time Course

The symptoms start soon after blood alcohol levels begin to decline and peak before ethanol is completely cleared from the blood.

• Intensity

The intensity of the symptoms is related to the quantity of alcoholic beverage consumed. The symptoms are worse following consumption of beverages with a high congener content, such as bourbon, than ones free of them, such as vodka.

• Symptoms

Thirst, the most common hangover symptom, is likely the result of the diuresis induced by ethanol.

Headache, the next most common symptom has an etiology that is not known.

Giddiness, nausea, and vomiting form a cluster of symptoms probably caused by the vestibular effects of ethanol.

Withdrawal syndrome–related symptoms include tremor, disturbances of thermoregulation (*eg*, sweating, hot flashes, cold chills), and nervousness.

Toxicity

Ethanol consumed in large quantities acutely or chronically (the amount imbibed by alcoholics can be 150–600 g, or 10 to 40 drinks per day) is a systemic poison. Among imbibers the incidence of medical conditions is quantitatively correlated with the amount they consume (Fig. 48–4). The toxic sequelae involve so many organ systems that it has been said that to know ethanol toxicity is to know medicine. The most important among the sequelae of high-level chronic consumption are those on the CNS, the induction of liver cirrhosis and pancreatitis, the hypertensive and teratogenic ef-

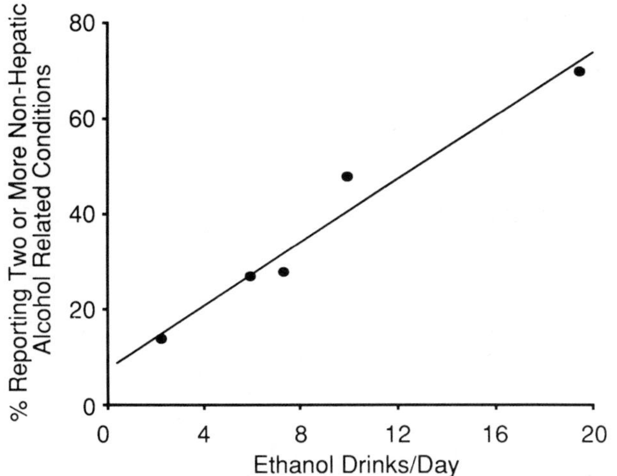

FIGURE 48–4. Percentage of alcoholics reporting two or more medical conditions (anemia, weakness in limbs, numbness of legs, dizziness, loss of balance, or fractures) in the previous 6 months as a function of their mean daily alcohol consumption. (Data from Polich JM, Armor DJ, Braiker HB: The Course of Alcoholism: Four Years After Treatment. Santa Monica, CA: Rand Corp, 1980.)

fects, and the ability to cause damage to skeletal and cardiac muscle.

Acute Poisoning

Rapid consumption of large amounts of ethanol can result in life-threatening effects:

- **Cardiovascular shock** secondary to severe hypotension that is unresponsive to norepinephrine and is the result of a direct toxic action of ethanol on peripheral blood vessels
- **Renal failure** secondary to the severe hypotension: to preserve adequate blood circulation to the brain, severe hypotension causes the normally high blood flow to the kidneys to be reduced to the point that renal ischemia results
- **Aspiration pneumonia** due to the combination of emesis with unconsciousness and the resulting aspiration of vomitus
- **Respiratory arrest** can occur if the ingestion of ethanol is combined with that of other CNS depressants; the respiratory depression caused by the action of ethanol on the brainstem respiratory center, however, usually is not sufficiently severe for ethanol alone to cause the arrest

Chronic Central Nervous System Toxicity

• **INTELLECTUAL AND MEMORY IMPAIRMENT.** Intellectual and memory impairment can be observed after even relatively modest chronic consumption of ethanol (75 g or 5 drinks per day or more), although the severity is a function of the level of ethanol consumption. The impairment is correlated with an enlargement of cerebral ventricles, evidence of cerebral atrophy. After a period of abstinence, a partial reversal of both the cognitive deficit and the ventricular enlargement is observed.

• **DEPRESSION.** Depressive disorders and alcoholism are conditions that are found to coexist in many individuals. Although one disorder is as likely to precede as the other, depression is two to three times more prevalent among alcoholics than among nonalcoholics. Also, although alcoholics are at greater risk of suicide than nonalcoholics, major depression is a comorbid condition in two thirds of alcoholic suicides.

• **EPILEPSY.** Alcoholic intoxication is frequently responsible for falls. Head injuries resulting from such falls can lead to the development of epilepsy, although the grand-mal seizures seen in alcohol withdrawal are not of epileptic origin and do not respond to anticonvulsant therapy.

• **PSYCHIATRIC CONDITIONS.** Chronic alcohol consumption is associated with exacerbations of anxiety, schizophrenia, and bipolar depression. Personality disorders, especially antisocial personality disorder, are common comorbid conditions with heavy drinking.

• **WERNICKE'S ENCEPHALOPATHY.** Wernicke's encephalopathy is a condition that includes paralysis of ocular and facial muscles, nystagmus, loss of appetite, vomiting, and disorientation. It is a manifestation of thiamine deficiency, caused in part by the heavy drinker's diet being vitamin-deficient and also by ethanol's inhibition of thiamine absorption and increased excretion. It is readily prevented or reversed by the administration of thiamine.

• **KORSAKOFF'S PSYCHOSIS.** Korsakoff's psychosis is an irreversible condition, the chief characteristic of which is an inability to convert short-term to long-term memory. This results in a compensatory tendency of the subject to confabulate. The condition is thought to be brought about by thiamine deficiency.

• **PERIPHERAL NEURALGIAS.** Alcoholics commonly suffer from peripheral neuralgias. They have also been attributed to the thiamine avitaminosis.

• **CEREBELLAR DEGENERATION.** Initially, cerebellar degeneration manifests itself as a loss of proprioception in the lower extremities. It progresses to the point that individuals cannot walk or even get up unaided. The varied chronic neurological effects of alcohol are likely to be caused by the combination of the direct neurotoxic effects of ethanol plus the nutritional derangements.

• **OTHER NEUROLOGICAL SEQUELAE.** Optic neuropathy, locked-in syndromes, necrosis of the corpus callosum, paresis, dysarthria, central pontine myelinolysis, and cerebellar degeneration are also associated with chronic alcohol consumption.

Teratogenicity

Ethanol is a human teratogen. It increases the incidence of spontaneous abortions, low-birth-weight babies (although only if the mother also smokes), and congenital abnormalities.

• **FETAL ALCOHOL SYNDROME.** Fetal alcohol syndrome is a triad of congenital abnormalities first observed among Washington state residents, mostly Pacific Coast Native Americans. It involves

> Facial dysmorphology involving the eyes, which have short palpebral fissures (*ie*, small eyeballs); the nose, which is short and upturned and lacks a bridge; and the

mouth, which has a hypoplastic upper lip with a thinned upper vermilion and a diminished to absent philtrum

Growth deficiencies, both prenatal and postnatal

CNS involvement, which includes mild to moderate mental retardation; the involvement can include microcephaly, hypotonia, irritability in infancy, and hyperactivity in childhood

How prevalent the syndrome is in other venues or how large an intake of ethanol with which it is correlated is not clear, but a woman who drinks heavily during pregnancy places her unborn child at substantial risk (see Chapter 59).

Organ Toxicities

• **LIVER CIRRHOSIS.** Mortality from liver cirrhosis is very closely correlated with ethanol consumption (Fig. 48-5). Although liver cirrhosis can have a number of etiologies, in the absence of ethanol consumption per capita mortality from this condition is quite low. It rises rapidly, however, when ethanol consumption reaches a certain level. The prognosis of individuals with alcoholic liver cirrhosis is guarded at best, but it is particularly poor in those unable to cease their ethanol consumption (Fig. 48-6). The natural history of the condition includes

Fibrous tissue deposition, which represents tissue repair consequent to focal necrosis; such fibrous tissue, however, impedes hepatic blood flow.

Portal hypertension: the liver is supplied with blood through the hepatic artery and the portal vein. Hepatic resistance to blood flow results in a retrograde increase in blood pressure throughout the portal system.

Ascites results from portal hypertension-induced transudation of fluid into the peritoneal cavity.

Esophageal varices are another consequence of portal hypertension; internal hemorrhages from such varicose veins are frequently the cause of death in alcoholics.

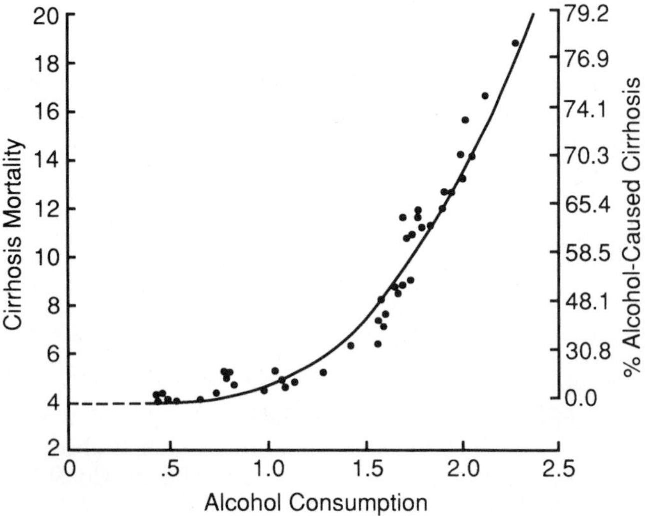

FIGURE 48-5. Incidence of yearly liver cirrhosis mortality as a function of per capita ethanol consumption in discrete geographical locations in Ontario, Canada. (From Schmidt W, Popham RE: Alcohol Problems and Their Prevention: A Public Health Perspective. Toronto: Addiction Research Foundation, 1977.)

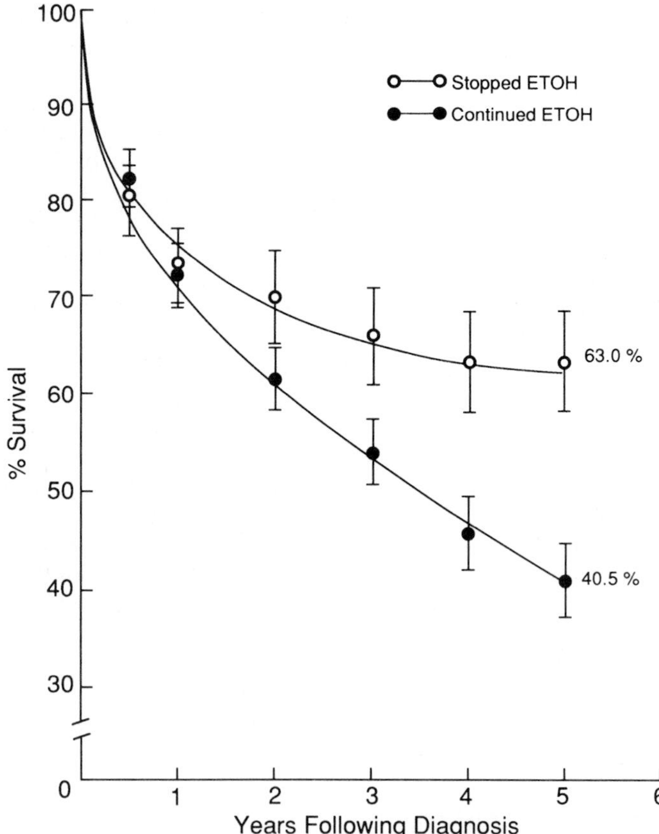

FIGURE 48-6. Percentage survival following diagnosis of alcoholic liver cirrhosis as a function of time and abstinence from ethanol. (From Powell WJ Jr, Klatskin G: Duration of survival in patients with Laënnec's cirrhosis. Influence of alcohol withdrawal, and possible effects of recent changes in general management of the disease. Am J Med 44:406-420, 1968; reprinted with permission from the American Journal of Medicine.)

Hepatic coma is caused by the inability of the cirrhosed liver to remove toxic metabolic products from the blood; this is another frequent cause of death in alcoholics.

Hepatomas represent yet another fatal complication observed in about one fifth of the patients with alcoholic liver cirrhosis.

• **CARDIOVASCULAR.** Chronic heavy ethanol consumption (more than four to six drinks per day on average) results in a significant increase in the incidence of **hypertension**, although moderate drinkers have hypertension rates no different from those of abstainers. Acutely, ethanol increases both systolic and diastolic pressures as well as pulse rate, although it has only sight effects of blood catecholamine levels. Additionally, alcoholics are found to have a longer QT interval on electrocardiography, a condition associated with a higher risk of lethal arrhythmias and sudden cardiac death.

Cardiomyopathy is seen in individuals with very high and prolonged alcohol consumption; it results in a lowering of the ejection fraction and in an increased left ventricular mass. Electron microscopic analysis of biopsy specimens reveals increased endometrial thickness, interstitial fibrosis, and loss of myofibrils. An abnormally low ejection fraction has been found in about 43% of individuals with a daily consumption of the ethanol present in 12 or more drinks for approximately 16 years.

• **PANCREATITIS.** Pancreatitis is a condition induced by heavy ethanol consumption. Compared with idiopathic pancreatitis, alcoholic pancreatitis has a higher incidence of severe pain, pancreatic calcification, overt diabetes, and a higher death rate (26%) in the 5 years following initial diagnosis. With abstinence, the severe pain either partially or completely disappears within a year in 90% of such patients, but it persists in about half of those who continue to drink.

• **MYOPATHY.** Myopathy occurs in individuals with a lifetime ethanol consumption of the equivalent of 12 drinks per day for a 70-kg man for 20 years. It is functionally evident as proximal muscle weakness and atrophy; patients with myopathy have elevated serum creatinine levels. Electron microscopic examination of biopsy specimens shows nonspecific but definite ultrastructural changes.

• **IMMUNOSUPPRESSION.** Heavy ethanol consumption lowers circulating T lymphocyte counts and results in nonspecific B lymphocyte activation. These effects on cell-mediated immunity may contribute to the high incidence of tuberculosis and other infections among alcoholics.

Therapy for Alcoholism

Treatment Goals

• **LIFELONG ABSTINENCE.** For many years, abstinence was considered the only appropriate goal of alcoholism therapy based on the rationale that a permanent "loss of control" over drinking was a concomitant of alcoholism.

• **CONTROLLED DRINKING.** Controlled drinking began to be discussed as an alternate treatment goal following the publication of two large Rand Corporation follow-up studies of patients who had received abstinence-oriented therapy 18 months and 4 years earlier, respectively. The 4-year study in particular documented that a significant proportion of those treated had apparently returned to stable moderate ethanol consumption (Fig. 48–7).

Since then it has become apparent that whatever the treatment goals are, some of those treated embrace long-term abstinence whereas others return successfully to relatively stable moderate drinking. This is also true of those in the community who recover without treatment (Fig. 48–8).

Matching Severity With Treatment Goal

From the Rand studies it is apparent that the controlled drinking outcome is much more frequently observed in those whose alcohol consumption at the time of entry into therapy is not very high.

- **Alcohol abusers**, *ie*, individuals with moderate alcohol problems, find the goal of lifelong abstinence and the necessary restructuring of their whole social life unacceptable and fail to remain in treatment. For those who have not progressed beyond problem drinking, achievement of stable moderate drinking appears to be a more realistic goal (Fig. 48–9).

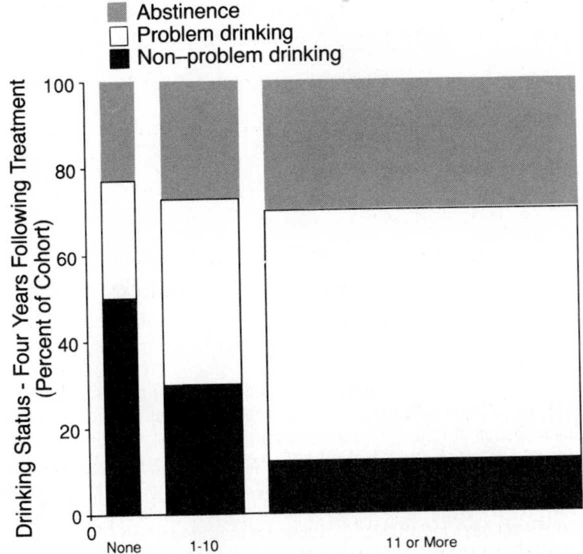

FIGURE 48–7. Long-term outcome of abstinence-oriented treatment of alcoholism as a function of the severity of the alcohol dependence at entry into treatment. Entry status: the treatment population (n = 508) was divided into three cohorts depending on the incidence of alcohol-dependence symptoms (continuous drinking for 12 or more hours, missing meals because of drinking, memory lapses, blackouts, loss of control, drinking first thing in the morning, having "the shakes," severe tremor) experienced in the 30 days preceding entry into treatment. The relative size of the three cohorts is given by the width of the respective columns. (Among those who reported no dependence symptoms, many sought treatment because of other adverse consequences.) Outcome status: the individuals in each cohort were classified at 4 years following entry into treatment according to whether their drinking behavior corresponded to abstinence—no consumption of ethanol in the last 6 months (*color*); problem drinking—consumption of ethanol resulting in either dependence symptoms during the preceding 30 days or adverse consequences in the previous 6 months (*white*); or nonproblem drinking—consumption of ethanol without any dependence symptoms or adverse consequences in the stated periods (*black*). At entry into treatment, the average ethanol consumption of individuals in the none, 1–10, and ≥11 dependency symptom-cohorts was 7, 14, and 23 drinks per day, respectively. At 4 years, the average ethanol consumption by the individuals in the problem and nonproblem drinking groups was 13.5 and 5 drinks per day, respectively. (Data from Polich JM, Armor DJ, Braiker HP: The Course of Alcoholism: Four Years after Treatment. Santa Monica, CA: Rand Corp, 1980.)

- **Alcohol-dependent individuals** find learning to drink in a controlled fashion very difficult. Lifelong abstinence may be the more realistic goal for those who have progressed to alcohol dependence.
- **Interim abstinence** is a treatment goal that is acceptable to alcohol abusers based on the rationale that a great deal of learning is required to achieve stable moderate drinking and that alcohol abuse induces an impairment of cognitive function. In fact, one of the best predictors of treatment outcome is the degree of cognitive impairment patients present. With abstinence, the impairment is to a large extent reversed. Disulfiram therapy can be used to achieve such interim abstinence.

Disulfiram

The primary problem in alcoholism is the consumption of large amounts of ethanol. Preventing ethanol ingestion is an obvious therapeutic strategy. This can be achieved by the ad-

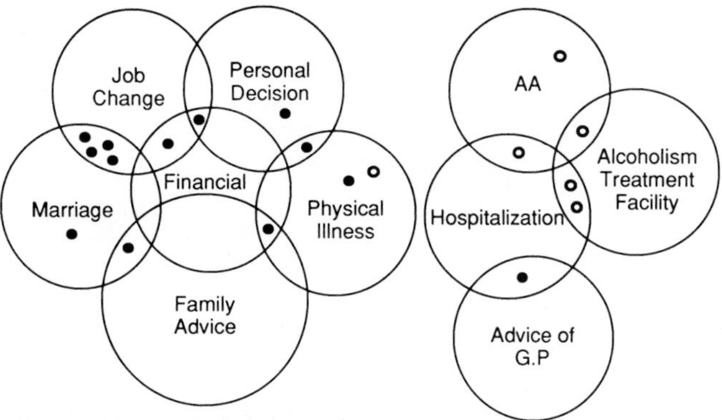

FIGURE 48–8. Previously alcoholic individuals (*small circles*) and the reasons they gave (*large circles*) for ceasing to abuse alcohol. Subsample of 3600 individuals chosen at random from those on the electoral register; mean duration of the recovery: 6.5 years, range 1–25 years. *Small open circles:* individuals who had become abstinent; *small closed circles:* individuals who had become moderate drinkers (mean consumption, two and a half drinks per day, range zero to five drinks per day). Individuals positioned at the intersection of more than one circle gave more than one reason for ceasing alcohol abuse. Individuals in the group of circles on the right received professional help; those in the group on the left recovered without seeking or receiving such help. (Data from Saunders WM, Kershaw PW: Spontaneous remission from alcohol—A community study. Br J Addict 74:251–265, 1979.)

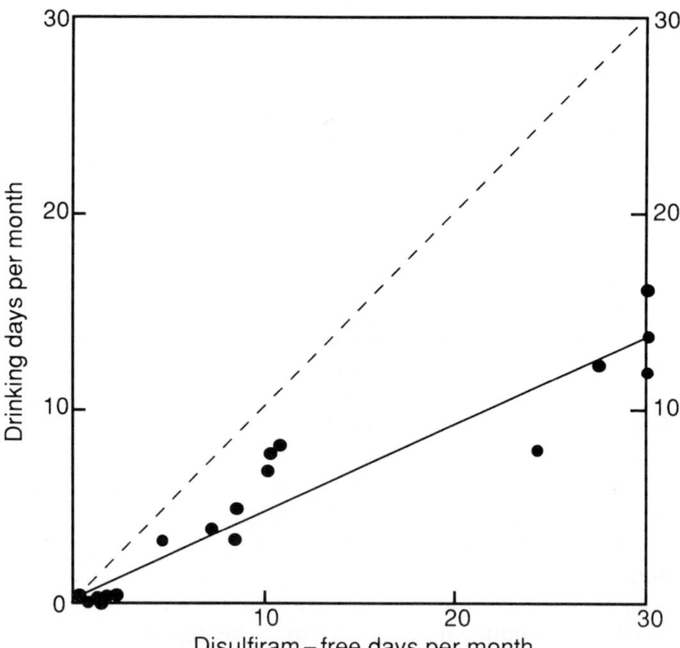

FIGURE 48–10. Correlation between the mean number of days on which disulfiram was not taken (disulfiram-free days) and the mean number of drinking days per 30-day months in groups of alcoholics being treated for alcoholism. (Data from Azrin NH, Sisson RW, Meyers R, Godley M: Alcoholism treatment by disulfiram and community reinforcement therapy. J Behav Ther Exp Psychiatry 13:105–112, 1982.)

ministration of disulfiram (ANTABUSE), an agent that in the doses used produces no evident pharmacological effect of its own, yet causes subsequent ingestion of ethanol to result in an unpleasant reaction, the disulfiram-ethanol reaction (DER).

• **Effectiveness.** Disulfiram therapy is very effective if adhered to. It results in virtually complete abstinence. A very high correlation is observed between the number of days in a month on which disulfiram is taken by alcoholics in a 250-mg dose and the number of days on which they consume alcohol (Fig. 48–10). Because disulfiram is long-acting, it can be given as a 400- to 500-mg dose every other day (or 3 days a week) with similar results. Two factors stand out as contributing to abstinence in disulfiram therapy: ascertaining compliance and creation of a behavioral contingency to help motivate the patient to remain compliant. If compliance is not assured, it tends to be marginal and the therapy ineffective.

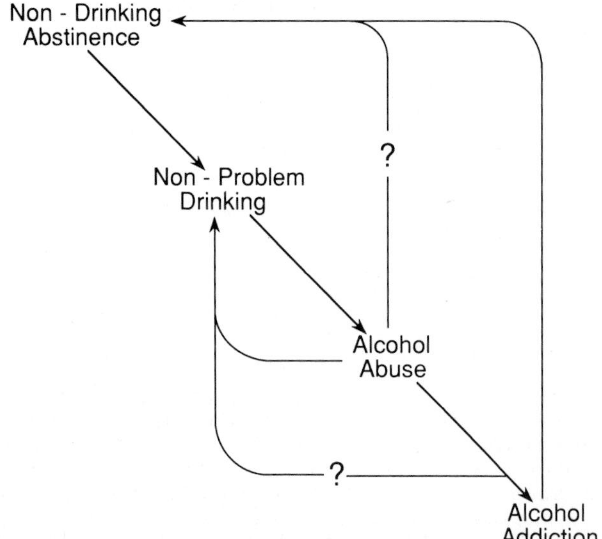

FIGURE 48–9. Progression of drinking behaviors and the range of advocated treatment goals.

• **Assuring Compliance.** Assuring compliance requires the participation in the treatment of a second individual, either a significant other (usually the spouse) or in an outpatient setting, a health care professional who helps the patient remain sober by monitoring the scheduled ingestion of the drug—daily in the home setting and 3 times per week in the outpatient setting.

• **Behavioral Contingency.** Compliance by the patient with the therapy can be the condition for such incentives as continuation of reinforcements by the family, continued treatment by the clinic, or positive progress reports to the employer. Because the benefits of the drug therapy are not evident on a day-to-day basis, such additional motivation is essential for the patient to remain compliant.

• **Side Effects.** In the now commonly prescribed doses (250 mg/day or 400 mg every other day), disulfiram is very safe. Several double-blind placebo-controlled studies have found either no side effects attributable to disulfiram or at most a higher incidence of drowsiness and abdominal discomfort. Encephalopathies and neuropathies, both reversible, have been reported when higher doses were used.

• **Duration of Therapy.** Therapy should continue for 2 years. When disulfiram therapy is terminated at the end of this period, the vast majority of patients do not resume drinking.

• **Mechanism.** The primary effect of disulfiram ingestion is the inhibition of the aldehyde dehydrogenase present in hepatic mitochondria, which is the enzyme responsible for acetaldehyde metabolism *in vivo.* Disulfiram does not inhibit this enzyme *in vitro* and must therefore act through a metabolite.

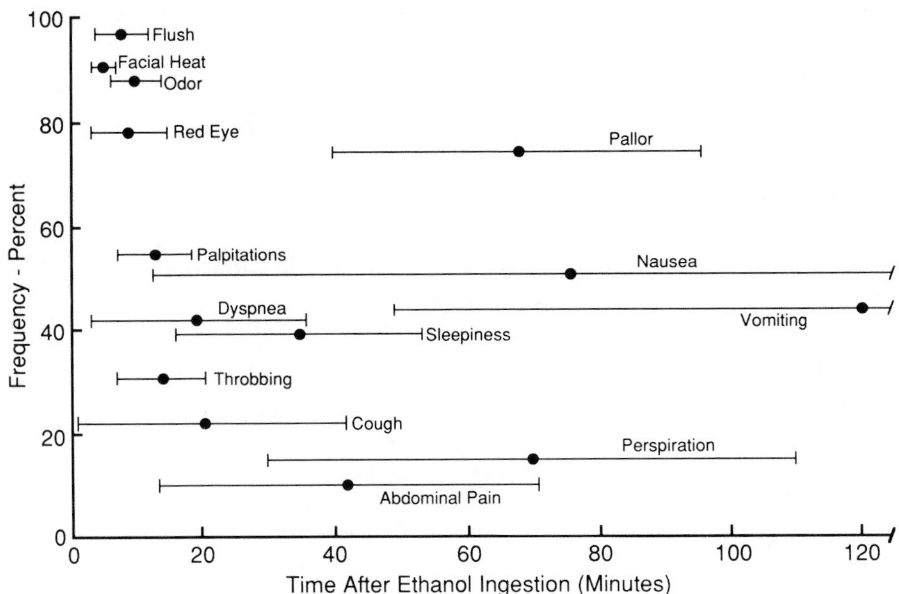

FIGURE 48–11. Incidence and mean onset time (*solid circle*) of symptoms and signs of the disulfiram-ethanol reaction. Horizontal bar represents ± 1 standard deviation of onset time. (Data from Hine CH, Burbridge TN, Macklin EA, et al: Some aspects of the human pharmacology of tetraethyl thiruam disulphide [Antabuse]-alcohol reactions. J Clin Invest 31:317–325, 1952; Raby K: Investigations on the disulfiram-alcohol reaction: Clinical observations. Q J Stud Alcohol 14:545–556, 1953.)

• **Disulfiram-Ethanol Reaction.** Elicitation of the DER does not form part of disulfiram therapy. Patients placed on disulfiram therapy are warned that if they drink, the DER will occur. Those who wish to test this for themselves usually do so gingerly, using small amounts of alcohol. The intensity of the DER correlates closely with the blood acetaldehyde level and is a function of the amount of alcohol consumed; Figure 48–11 features the main characteristics of the fully developed reaction with both their frequency and onset time. Components of the DER include

Dyspnea, an unpleasant subjective difficulty in breathing

Lowering of peripheral resistance by a direct action of acetaldehyde on blood vessels

Drop in diastolic and systolic blood pressures secondary to the decrease in peripheral resistance (Fig. 48–12)

Tachycardia, a response to the fall in blood pressure

The lowering of systolic blood pressure is not fully compensated because administration of disulfiram also results in inhibition of dopamine β-hydroxylase, the enzyme responsible for the synthesis of norepinephrine. This can lead to a partial depletion of the cardiac stores of norepinephrine, so that less is available to release when the sympathetic nerves are reflexly stimulated by the lowered blood pressure.

• **Treatment.** Cases of DER that call for medical intervention are extremely rare. Should one occur, the simplest way to counteract the drop in peripheral resistance is first to have the patient lie down and second to tilt the bed to a head-down position. Blocking ethanol oxidation and thereby acetaldehyde formation by administering 4-methylpyrazole is the best antidotal therapy.

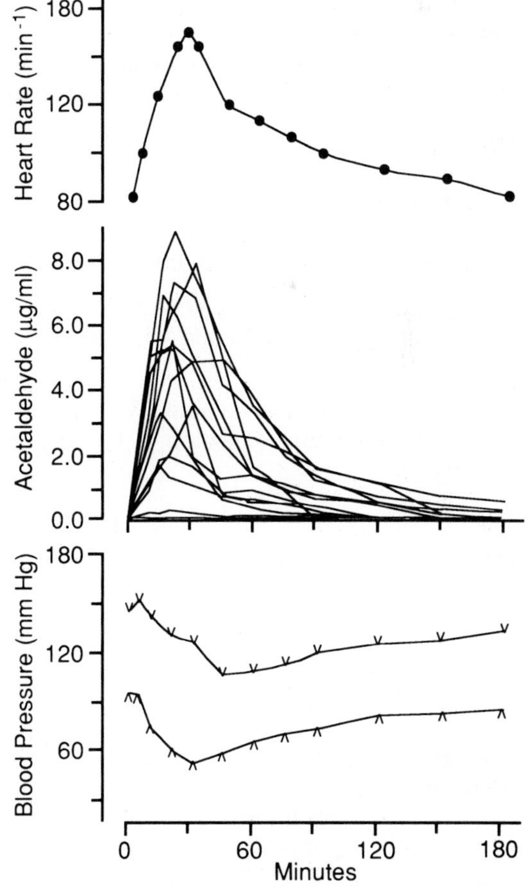

FIGURE 48–12. Time course of blood acetaldehyde levels and cardiovascular changes during the course of the disulfiram-ethanol reaction. Patients were administered 400 mg disulfiram daily for 3–6 days and were challenged with a 13.2-g dose of ethanol at zero time. (Data from Beyeler C, Fisch HU, Preisig R: The disulfiram-alcohol reaction: Factors determining and potential tests predicting severity. Alcoholism (NY) 9:118–124, 1985; Beyeler C, Fisch HU, Preisig R: Kardiovaskulare und metabolische Veranderungen wahrend der Antabus-Alkohol-Reaktion: Grundlagen zur Erfassung des Schweregrades. Schweiz Med Wochenschr 117:52–60, 1987.)

Naltrexone

Experimental data from animal studies suggest that alcohol drinking is influenced by opiate receptor activity. Naltrexone, a long-lasting blocker of opiate receptors, has been found, when used in relatively short-term (12-week) abstinence-oriented treatment of alcoholism, to decrease alcohol craving, to increase the duration of abstinence while the patient is in treatment, and to decrease incidence of relapse in those who sample alcohol while in treatment. The long-term effectiveness of naltrexone in the treatment of alcoholism remains to be demonstrated.

Serotonergic Agents

Serotonergic drugs are found to decrease alcohol consumption in animals. A number of such agents (fluoxetine, citalopram, zimeldine, and viqualine) have been found to bring about a modest (10 – 20%) decrease in alcohol consumption in nondependent drinkers. Additionally, another serotonergic drug, buspirone, has been found in a 24-week study to reduce anxiety and depression among recovering alcoholics and to be associated with longer continuation in treatment.

METHANOL

Sources

- **Wood**, when heated in the absence of air, produces wood spirits (*ie*, methanol) that distill over
- **Antifreeze** and windshield-washing fluid component
- **Ethanol diluent** and adulterant in products such as shellacs and varnishes

Metabolism and Excretion

Main routes of methanol elimination are

- **Oxidation** to formaldehyde via alcohol dehydrogenase with subsequent formation of formic acid; the oxidation is inhibited by

  Ethanol, which is an effective competitive inhibitor, completely blocking methanol oxidation at blood levels of 100 – 200 mg/dL

  4-Methylpyrazole

- **Excretion** in breath eliminates as much as 30% of the dose

Toxic Effects

The course of the intoxication is frequently insidious: symptoms, although delayed for many hours, develop rapidly once they begin to appear. The presence of ethanol in the material ingested impedes the oxidation of methanol to its toxic metabolites for as long as blood ethanol levels remain elevated.

- **CNS intoxication:** mild and transient
- **Headache, clammy skin, nausea, and vomiting:** symptoms that appear with a characteristic delay of several hours
- **Blurring of vision:** a characteristic toxic effect of formaldehyde, which progresses to irreversible blindness if untreated
- **Severe lower abdominal pain** due to the development of formate acidosis

Treatment of Intoxication

Three approaches need to be utilized for the successful treatment of this condition

- **Ethanol or 4-methylpyrazole administration** to inhibit formaldehyde formation
- **5% Bicarbonate infusion** to correct the acidosis caused by formic acid formation
- **Hemodialysis** if blurring of vision indicates significant blood levels of formaldehyde; note, however, that even if the blurring of vision clears as a result, it can return after the hemodialysis is stopped because hemodialysis is less effective in clearing methanol than formaldehyde, and additional formaldehyde can be formed from the methanol left behind

ETHYLENE GLYCOL

Metabolism, Intoxication, and Treatment

Ethylene glycol is a compound frequently used as a permanent antifreeze in car radiators. Its metabolism (Fig. 48 – 13) involves the formation of

- **Glycolaldehyde** via alcohol dehydrogenase
- **Glycine** as a nontoxic end product via a pathway of limited capacity
- **Oxalic acid**, which is an overflow pathway that is not utilized unless the rate of oxidation of ethylene glycol is high; oxalic acid is toxic by virtue of the formation of insoluble calcium oxalate crystals: deposition of such crystals occurs in

  Renal tubules; this causes their necrosis and leads to renal failure

  Cerebral capillaries if the dose of ethylene glycol is sufficiently high

The patient suffering from ethylene glycol poisoning can present with

- **Hematemesis, tachycardia, and coma**
- **Calcium oxalate crystals** in the urine and proteinuria

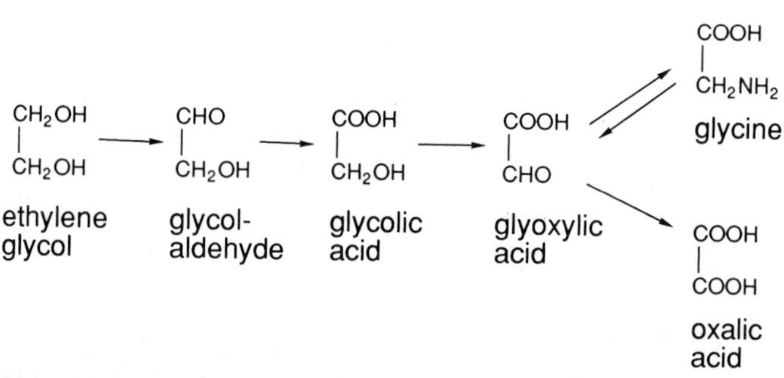

FIGURE 48 – 13. Scheme of the biotransformation reactions involving ethylene glycol metabolism.

Treatment components include

- **Alcohol dehydrogenase inhibition** by ethanol or 4-methylpyrazole; the treatment strategy is to slow down the oxidation of ethylene glycol so that it does not exceed the capacity of the glycine pathway
- **5% Bicarbonate infusion** to correct acidosis
- **Hemodialysis** for the removal of glycolic aldehyde, glycolic acid, and glyoxylic acid, all potential oxalic acid precursors

REFERENCES

Babor TF, Hesselbrock V, Meyer RE, Shoemaker W (eds): Types of alcoholics: Evidence from clinical, experimental, genetic research. Ann NY Acad Sci 708:1-258, 1994.

Brewer C: Supervised disulfiram in alcoholism. Br J Hosp Med 35:116-119, 1986.

Chan AWK: Treatment of alcohol withdrawal seizures with benzodiazepines: Neurochemical basis. *In* Porter R, Mattson R, Cramer J, Jr, and Diamond I (eds): Alcohol and Seizures. Philadelphia, FA Davis, 1990.

Chan AWK, Welte JW, Whitney RB: Identification of alcoholism in young adults by blood chemistries. Alcohol 4:175-179, 1987.

Charness ME: Brain lesions in alcoholics. Alcohol Clin Exp Res 17:2-11, 1993.

Deitrich RA, Dunwiddie TV, Harris RA, Erwin VG: Mechanism of action of ethanol: Initial central nervous system actions. Pharmacol Rev 41:489-537, 1989.

Eighth Special Report to the US Congress on Alcohol and Health. Washington DC: US Department of Health and Human Services, NIH Publication No. 94-3699, National Institutes of Health. September, 1993.

Gessner PK: Drug therapy of the alcohol withdrawal syndrome. *In* Majchrowicz E, Noble EP (eds): Biochemistry and Pharmacology of Ethanol, 375-435, Vol 2. New York: Plenum Medical Book Co, 1979.

Gessner PK, Gessner T: Disulfiram and Its Metabolite, Dithiocarb: Pharmacology and Status in the Therapy of Alcoholism, HIV Infections, and Heavy Metal Intoxication. London: Chapman & Hall, 1993.

Jacobsen D, Hewlett TP, Webb R, et al: Ethylene glycol intoxication: Evaluation of kinetics and crystalluria. Am J Med 84:145-152, 1988.

Johlin FC, Fortman CS, Nghiem DD, Tephly TR: Studies on the role of folic and folate dependent enzyme in human methanol poisoning. Pharmacology 31:557-561, 1987.

Lieber CS: Biochemical and molecular basis of alcohol-induced injury to liver and other tissues. N Engl J Med 319:1639-1650, 1988.

Martin PR, McCool BA, Singleton CK: Genetic sensitivity to thiamine deficiency and development of alcoholic organic brain disease. Alcohol Clin Exp Res 17:31-37, 1993.

Orrego H, Blake JE, Blendis LM, et al: Long-term treatment of alcoholic liver disease with propylthiouracil. N Engl J Med 317:1421-1427, 1987.

Peele S: The Meaning of Addiction: Compulsive Experience and Its Interpretation. Lexington, MA: Lexington Books, 1985.

Pristach CA, Smith CM, Whitney RB: Alcohol withdrawal syndromes—prediction from detailed medical and drinking histories. Drug Alcohol Depend 11:177-199, 1983.

Smith CM: The pharmacology of sedative/hypnotics, alcohol, and anesthetics: Sites and mechanisms of action. *In* Martin WR (ed): Handbook of Experimental Pharmacology, Vol. 45/1, Drug Addiction I. Heidelberg, Springer-Verlag, 1977, pp 413-587.

Smith CM, Barnes GM: Signs and symptoms of hangover: Prevalence and relationship to alcohol use. Drug Alcohol Depend 11:249-269, 1983.

Wilkinson PK: Pharmacokinetics of ethanol: A review. Alcoholism (Baltimore) 4:6-21, 1980.

49 Substance Abuse

Peter K. Gessner

DEFINITIONS

Substance abuse is a sociomedical problem. Its discussion by society at large involves not only medical and scientific considerations but also social and political ones. This is reflected in the terms employed, some of which refer to scientifically quantifiable phenomena associated with substance abuse, whereas others represent societal identification of behavior that is judged to be deviant. Any inquiry into the nature and characteristics of substance abuse requires not only that terms be clearly defined but that the two types of terms be clearly differentiated. In the context of the present chapter, these are identified below as category I and II terms, respectively.

Category I Terms: Scientifically Quantifiable Phenomena

- **Tolerance:** a phenomenon whereby an organism chronically exposed to a substance becomes progressively less sensitive to it. Tolerance develops to many but not all abused drugs. Users of narcotics can develop very high levels of tolerance. That developed by abusers of sedative-hypnotics (including ethanol) is not as high.
- **Cross-tolerance:** the phenomenon whereby an organism tolerant to one substance will also show tolerance to a second substance that has similar pharmacological effects.

- **Withdrawal syndrome:** an illness-like syndrome that develops when an organism habituated to a drug is suddenly deprived of it. The characteristics of the syndrome vary with the pharmacological class of the abused substance. With some drugs no syndrome is seen. A pathognomonic trait of the withdrawal syndrome is that it is both alleviated and terminated by administration of the substance of which the organism was deprived.
- **Physical dependence:** the condition of habituation defined by the occurrence of a withdrawal syndrome upon cessation of use of the substance.
- **Cross-physical dependence:** the phenomenon whereby different substances of the same pharmacological class will terminate each other's withdrawal syndrome.
- **Craving:** an intense drive that causes an organism to emit work in order to obtain and self-administer the craved substance.
- **Detoxication:** treatment designed first to alleviate, if present, the withdrawal syndrome of those physically dependent on a substance. Once that has been achieved, the second goal of the treatment is to wean the individual from the substance without again precipitating the withdrawal syndrome.

Category II Terms: Adjudicative of Behavioral Deviation from Societal Norms

- **Abuse:** a societal term applied to any use of a proscribed substance. In the case of legal substances, the term refers to their use in quantities or settings that result in medical, occupational, economic, family, or legal problems for the individual.
- **Addiction:** persistent drug abuse that continues in spite of significant problems it is causing.
- **Dependence:** a term synonymous with addiction when used alone or modified adjectivally by the name of an abused substance or a class thereof (as in alcohol dependence or narcotic dependence). Note the distinction from physical dependence.
- **Addictive behavior:** conduct that is continued in spite of the significant problems it is causing for the individual. The term encompasses behavior defined as addiction but also such phenomena as compulsive gambling.

ABUSED SUBSTANCES

In discussing abused substances, it is helpful to group them into sets or classes of pharmacologically similar agents. This is so because of the similarity of many of the phenomena attendant upon abuse of agents of the same pharmacological class. Accordingly, several classes of abused substances are listed below. All except the last two are subjects of more extensive discussion in the body of this chapter.

- Opiates (narcotics)—heroin, morphine, methadone, . . .
- Cocaine, amphetamines, . . .(stimulants)
- Depressants—ethanol, nitrous oxide, barbiturates, . . .
- Tobacco—nicotine . . .
- Phencyclidine
- Hallucinogens—lysergic acid diethylamide (LSD), . . .
- Ecstasy
- Deliriants—scopolamine, atropine
- Marijuana
- Anabolic steroids

(Reference is made to related diagnostic categorizations, eg, the DSM-IV [Diagnostic and Statistical Manual of Mental Disorders—Version IV].)

CONTINGENCIES REQUIRING MEDICAL INTERVENTION

The types of medical assistance required by individuals involved in substance abuse need to be focused upon prior to any detailed consideration of the pharmacology of the abused substances.

- **Overdose toxicity:** Self-administration can lead to dosing errors and hence acute overdose toxicity (*eg*, severe respiratory depression due to opiates). Many substances available on the illicit market are diluted by varying amounts of inert ingredients, which renders self-dosing all the more difficult. Acute medical intervention is frequently necessary to prevent death or serious sequelae.
- **Untoward effects:** The effects experienced acutely, even in the absence of an overdose, can be unanticipated by the user and quite alarming (*eg*, LSD-induced panic reaction), causing the user to seek medical assistance.
- **Incidental pathologies:** Parenteral self-administration frequently results in the introduction of vectors of infection (*eg*, human immunodeficiency virus [HIV] through the sharing of needles) or other foreign matter.
- **Organ pathologies:** Used in appropriately large quantities, many abused substances are inherently toxic and, in the long run, cause organ toxicities (*eg*, heart disease in cigarette smokers).
- **Acute withdrawal:** Many abused substances can induce physical dependence in users. Such users, if they stop the use of the substance, will experience a withdrawal that may be unpleasant or life-threatening and may need medical management.
- **Dependence:** Persistence in substance abuse or the recurrence of such abuse in the face of negative consequences and in spite of the declared intent of the user to abandon the abuse is viewed as an addiction, a negative. Medical management is considered one of the prime ways of dealing with the problem. Such management can take several forms, namely:
- **Maintenance**—whereby the user is switched to a pharmacologically analogous drug that, however, can be administered in a less hazardous and more controlled fashion (namely, methadone maintenance of opiate-dependent individuals) and that removes the need for the

user to resort to illegal activity to procure the abused substance or funds for its purchase.

Aversion—whereby the user is prescribed a drug that will make the use of the abuse substance either aversive (namely, disulfiram therapy of alcoholics) or ineffective (namely, naltrexone therapy of the opiate dependent).

Craving suppression—whereby the user is prescribed a drug that will lessen the craving felt for the abused substance (namely, desipramine therapy of cocaine dependence).

PRIMARY AND SECONDARY PREVENTION

In addition to the treatment of the above sequelae of substance abuse, physicians have an important role in the primary and secondary prevention of substance abuse. This role involves educating patients regarding substance abuse. The physicians can fulfill these functions by:

- **History taking:** ascertaining whenever taking a medical history from a patient whether substance abuse is present or absent, and sharing with the patient, in this context, information regarding the health consequences of substance abuse.
- **Professional advice:** providing any patients detected as developing or continuing substance abuse with a convincing exposition regarding such overt or incipient pathophysiology as the abuse is inducing in the patient.

ETIOLOGY OF SUBSTANCE ABUSE

No one factor drives substance abuse. It is a behavior that, though potentially injurious to the user, is nonetheless engaged in because the user experiences many stimuli that reinforce the personal use of abused substances. The user is likely to stop the abuse when the number and strength of negative stimuli or consequences outweigh those reinforcing it. In Figure 49–1 an effort has been made to present schematically many of the factors that play a role in determining whether an individual will engage in substance abuse or not. The most salient among these are:

- **Use in the microenvironment.** The extent to which individuals known to the subject (parents, family, friends) use or abuse substances, that is, the extent to which the substance is used in the subject's microenvironment (Fig. 49–2). The greater the number of such individuals, the greater the probability that the subject will be offered the abused substance and encouraged to try it.
- **Overall use in society.** The extent to which the substance is used by the population as a whole. The more the substance is used in the population, the higher will be its status, which in turn will enhance the probability that it will be used in the subject's microenvironment.
- **Pleasure.** The high that the subject experiences when using the substance. It is a characteristic of all abused substances that they can enter the brain and act on it. In the search for novel experiences, almost any effect on con-

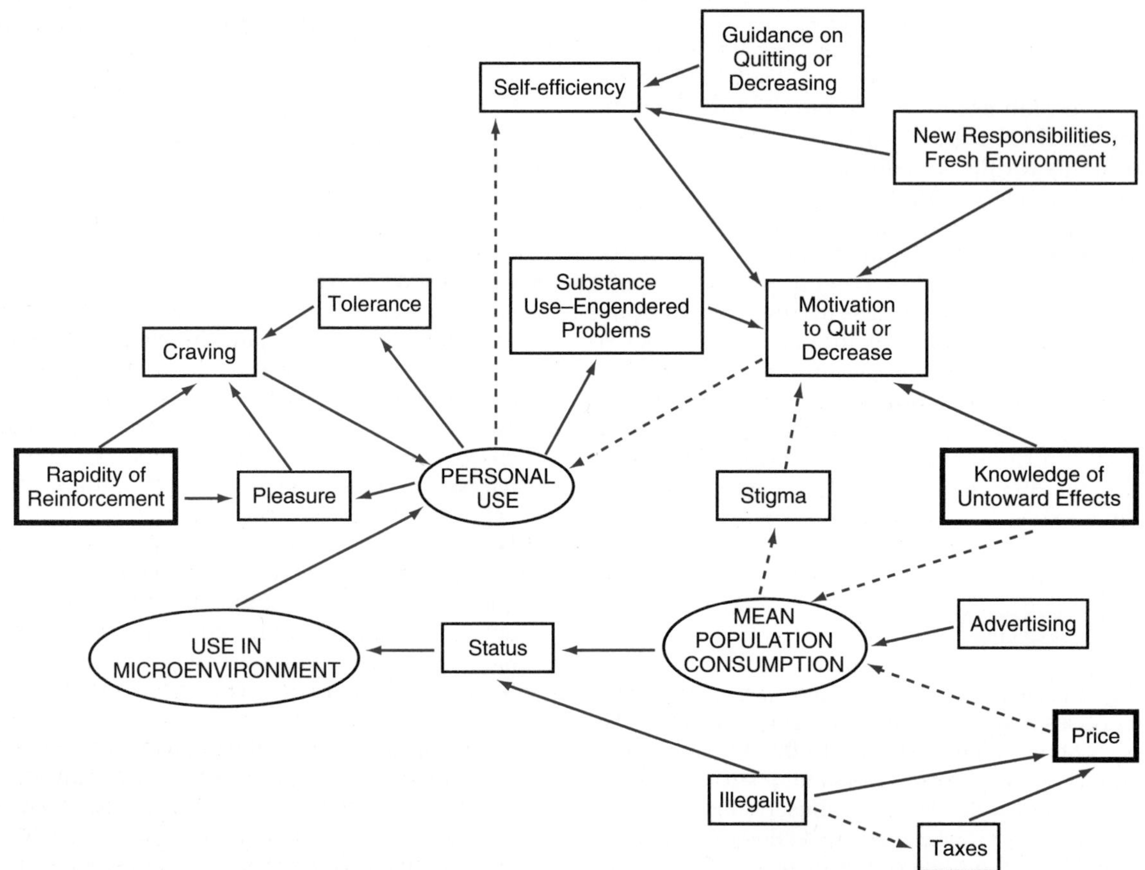

FIGURE 49–1. Substance abuse dynamics. *Solid arrows* represent positive effects, and *broken arrows* represent negative effects.

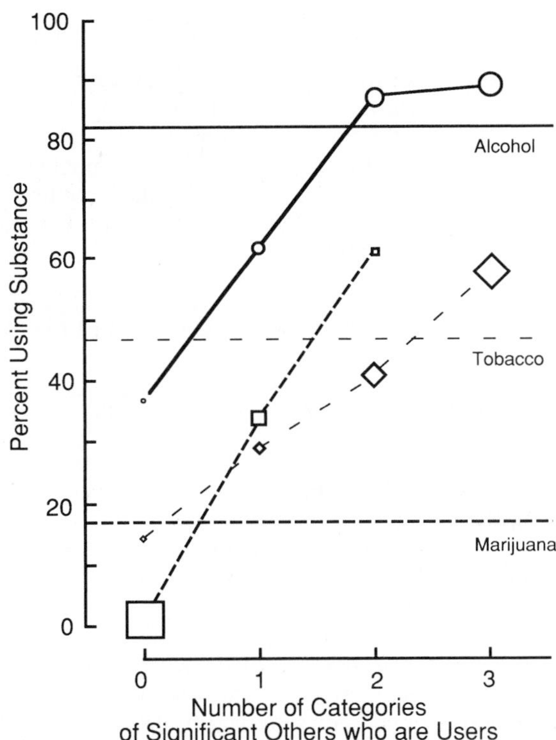

FIGURE 49–2. Substance use by adults as a function of its use by significant others. Census track respondents were asked for each of the three substances whether they were using it and whether any or all of three categories of their significant others, namely, their parents, their past friends, and their current friends, had used or were using the substance. The percentage of use of the substance by the respondents was then plotted as a function of the number of categories of significant others they reported to be using it. The area of each point is proportional to the number of respondents that cluster on it. The overall mean percentage of use of each substance by the respondents as a group is given by a *horizontal line*. (Data from Apsler R, Blackman C: Adults' drug use: Relationship to perceived drug use of parents, friends while growing up, and present friends. Am J Drug Alcohol Abuse 6:291–300, 1979.)

sciousness proves rewarding to some individuals. Substances that make the subject feel masterful or indifferent to the vicissitudes of life are particularly reinforcing.

- **Speed of onset.** The rapidity with which the abused substance acts. The more immediately the sought-after effect occurs, the more reinforcing it is. The speed of onset is a function of how quickly the substance enters the brain. This occurs sooner following parenteral than oral administration (Table 49–1), and more rapidly if administered via inhalation than intravenously. Two other factors contribute to the increased abuse potential of rapidly acting substances:
- **Ease of self-titration.** Self-administration requires careful dosing. Too low a dose results in a less than optimal experience whereas too large an amount leads to overdose. The optimal dose has relatively narrow limits. As a rule, abusers engage in self-titration using the effects they experience as end-points. Clearly, the task is much easier if the effects are elicited promptly. Because the active content of substances sold illegally varies, self-titration is more of a necessity than a choice.
- **Frequency of reinforcement.** The pleasure that is derived from the effects of a substance is highly reinforcing. The more times it is experienced, the more powerful the link between the abuse and the pleasure. Rapidly acting substances tend to be also short-acting, thereby providing ample opportunity for frequent reinforcement.
- **Tolerance.** The greater the tolerance that develops to the effects of the substance and the greater the amount of substance the subject has to use, the greater the subject's involvement with the abuse of the substance, the greater the adaptation of the subject's physiology to the substance, and the greater the craving for it.
- **Craving.** This is enhanced by the pleasure associated with the use of the substance, the rapidity of its effects, and the tolerance the subject develops to it. Upon chronic use, the administration of the substance and the pleasure derived from it become more and more associated with the circumstances (places, people, type of event, *etc*) or stimuli attendant upon its use. Subsequent exposure to these stimuli elicits intense craving sensations and can result in the substance being sought out and self-administered even though it may not have been used for an extended period of time.

TABLE 49–1. Oral Availability and Half-Lives

Drug	Oral Availability (%)	Half-Life (Hours)	References‡
Morphine	24	2	3
Codeine	50	3	7,8
Meperidine	56	5	1
Methadone	90	23	4,9
Buprenorphine	14*	7	2,5
Naloxone	Minimal	1	6
Naltrexone	High†	10	10

*Sublingual: 58%

†If calculated in terms of its active metabolite.

‡References

1. Edwards DJ, Svensson CK, Visco JP, Lalka D: Clinical pharmacokinetics of pethidine [meperidine]. Clin Pharmacokinet 7:421–433, 1982.
2. Hand CW, Sear JW, Uppington J, et al: Buprenorphine disposition in patients with renal impairment: Single and continuous dosing, with special reference to metabolites. Br J Anaesth 64:276–282, 1990.
3. Hoskin PJ, Hanks GW, Aherne GW, et al: The bioavailability and pharmacokinetics of morphine after intravenous, oral and buccal administration in healthy volunteers. Br J Clin Pharmacol 27:499–505, 1989.
4. Inturrisi CE, Colburn WA, Kaiko RF, et al: Pharmacokinetics and pharmacodynamics of methadone in patients with chronic pain. Clin Pharmacol 41:392–401, 1987.
5. McQuay H, Moore RA, Bullingham RES: Buprenorphine kinetics. *In* Foley KM, Inturrisi CE (eds:) Advances in Pain Research and Therapy, vol 6, 271–278, New York, Raven Press, 1986.
6. Ngai SH, Berkowitz BA, Yang JC, et al: Pharmacokinetics of naloxone in rats and in man: Basis for its potency and short duration of action. Anesthesiology 44:398–401, 1976.
7. Quinding H, Anderson P, Bondesson U, et al: Plasma concentrations of codeine and its metabolite, morphine, after single and repeated oral administration. Eur J Clin Pharmacol 30:673–677, 1986.
8. Rogers JF, Findley JWA, Hull JH, et al: Codeine disposition in smokers and nonsmokers. Clin Pharmacol Ther 32:218–227, 1982.
9. Sawe J: High-dose morphine and methadone in cancer patients. Clinical pharmacokinetics considerations of oral treatment. Clin Pharmacokinet 11:87–106, 1986.
10. Wall ME, Brine DR, Perez-Reyes M: Metabolism and disposition of naltrexone in man after oral and intravenous administration. Clin Pharmacol Ther 46:226–233, 1981.

- **Acute physical dependence.** This can develop to some substances. The phenomenon plays a limited part, however, in causing substance abusing behavior to continue. While it is true that high level users of such substances cannot discontinue their use abruptly without suffering withdrawal phenomena, yet such users, freed from the physical dependence by detoxication, tend, as a rule, to revert to use of the substance. Many abusers of substances that can induce physical dependence, use them intermittently and in doses so small that physical dependence does not result.
- **Protracted abstinence syndrome.** The chronic use of some substances can lead to subtle but prolonged changes in physiological functioning. In the case of opiate dependence, for instance, the syndrome, which can last many months, includes subclinical increases in respiratory rate, lowering of body temperature, and decreases in pupillary diameter (Fig. 49 - 3). These phenomena are accompanied by chronic fatigue, dysphoria and increased liability to stress. The phenomenon may well lessen the resolve of former users to remain abstinent.

A number of factors determine the overall level of use of abused substances in the population and thereby, indirectly, that of the individual. Among these, the most important are:

- **Price.** Substances of abuse comply with market forces. The higher the price, the smaller the consumption; to put it in economic terms, the demand is elastic. Illegality, if enforced, and taxes both cause prices to increase. Among some segments of the population, illegality adds adventure and excitement to abuse and can raise its status.
- **Advertising.** Although manufacturers of legal but frequently abused substances insist that their advertising is designed to bring about brand switching, the more powerful effect is on overall consumption and recruitment of new users.
- **Knowledge of untoward effects.** The general population is quite sensitive to any fresh findings regarding harmful effects of substances; if unchallenged, such information lowers overall consumption. Hence manufacturers have created of "Research Institutes" that routinely challenge any resulting conclusion as "unwarranted and requiring further research."

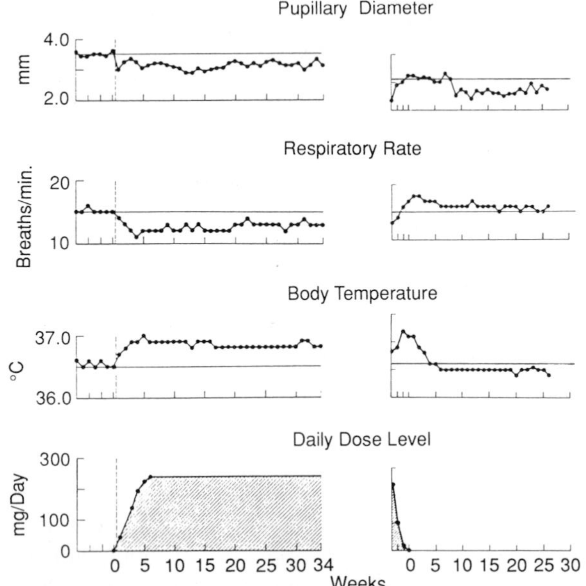

FIGURE 49-3. Effects of morphine on some physiological parameters when administered for a prolonged time. Data in the *left-hand column* are based on seven subjects and those in the *right-hand column* on six subjects, one subject having developed cholecystitis. (From Martin WR, Jasinski DR: Physiological parameters of morphine dependence in man—Tolerance, early abstinence, protracted abstinence. J Psychiat Res 7:9-17, 1969.)

SUBSTANCE ABUSE CESSATION

Substance abuse is an over-learned, partially conditioned behavior. Its cessation may require the coming together of many factors.

- **Awareness of the range of toxicities.** In considering the toxic effects of substance abuse, the public and abusers alike tend to focus on conditions that, because of their rarity in the absence of abuse, stand out as being induced by the abuse; for example, lung cancer as a consequence of cigarette smoking. The health professional can provide a better perspective by drawing attention to conditions that, though not uncommon in the absence of substance abuse, occur with significantly greater frequency in those who abuse a substance. Thus, in the instance of cigarette smoking, the professional can point out that smoking-induced mortality from heart disease is several-fold greater than that due to lung cancer (Fig. 49 - 4), and that lung cancer is but one of a long list of neoplams the incidence of which is significantly increased by smoking.
- **Calculus of consequences.** Cessation of substance abuse occurs when, in the user's mind, the reinforcements derived from using the substance are outweighed by the negative consequences of doing so. Coming to this conclusion is rendered difficult for the user by the fact that while most of the negative consequences are long-range whereas the positive reinforcements derived from substance abuse are immediate.
- **Triggering events.** Substance abusers internalize knowledge regarding the long-term negative consequences of substance abuse and contemplate its cessation. Usually, however, they fail to act on it until some immediate negative consequences, possibly trivial but more often serious, materialize. Health professionals can take advantage of such occurrences to recruit the abuser into treatment.
- **Self-confidence.** For abusers to cease or moderate their substance use, they must be convinced that it is in their power to be successful in this regard. The task is not an easy one regardless of the substance being abused. For instance, in many programs the rates of failure to remain abstinent are high (~70% at 6 months) and relatively similar regardless whether the starting point is alcohol abuse, opiate dependence, or cigarette smoking (Fig. 49 - 5). It is important, therefore, both to assure abusers that successful cessation is in their power and to appraise them of the methods, techniques, and treatments that maximize the probability of their success.
- **Craving control.** Abusers who cease abuse of a substance may experience intense cravings for it. Such cravings ebb and wane throughout the day and resisting them can be quite fatiguing. In some instances, drug therapy

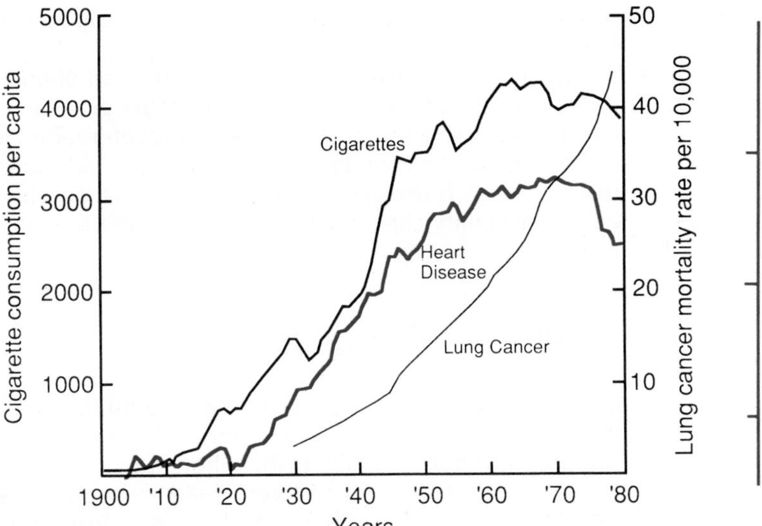

FIGURE 49–4. Historical trends in cigarette smoking and mortality from lung cancer and from cardiac disease in the United States from 1900 to 1980.

that will reduce the craving is available (desipramine, for example, is used to reduce the craving for cocaine). Alternatively, agents are available that prevent the abuser from being able to relieve the cravings by resort to the abused substance. For example, twice-weekly naltrexone will block all effects of opiates and thrice-weekly disulfiram will render the ingestion of alcohol highly aversive. While continuing with these therapies, abusers can more readily resist the moment-to-moment obsessive impulses to resume abuse.

- **Antecedent identification.** Very few substance abusers succeed immediately in remaining permanently abstinent. Most tend to resume the abuse, even if briefly. Such resumptions should not be viewed as failures, rather only as temporary setbacks and as learning experiences. Analysis of the antecedents of any given resumption should be undertaken so as to reveal factors that precipitated it. Subsequent conscious avoidance of such factors can help prevent further resumptions of the abuse. By becoming aware of the antecedents and avoiding them, the abuser experiences feelings of self-sufficiency; these are powerfully reinforcing.

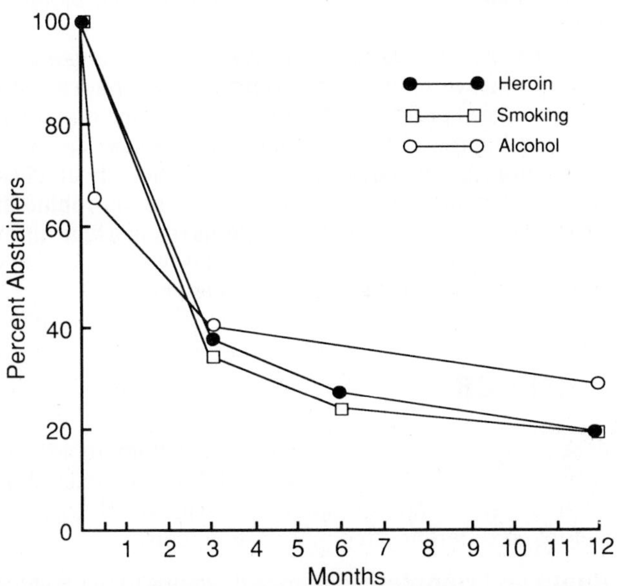

FIGURE 49–5. Comparison of the percentage of patients enrolled in three treatment programs (for ethanol, heroin, and cigarette smoking, respectively) who relapsed as a function of time. (From Hunt WA, Barnett LW, Branch LG: Relapse rates in addiction programs. J Clin Psychol 27P:455–456, 1971. Reprinted with permission of Clinical Psychology Publishing Co., Inc. Brandon, VT 05733.)

OPIATES

Heroin

Opioid structure-activity relationships

Buprenorphine

Naloxone

Illustration continued on following page

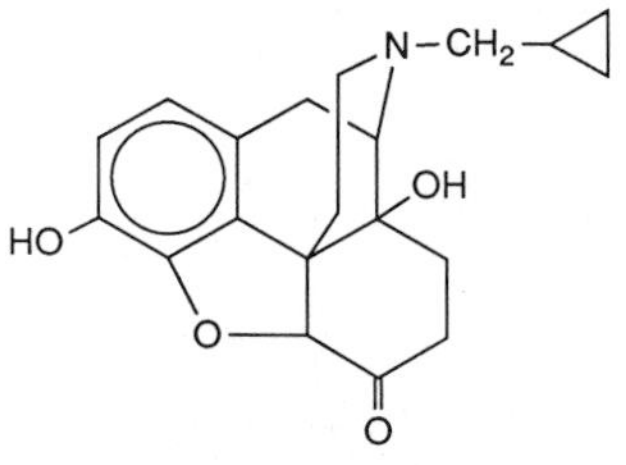

Naltrexone

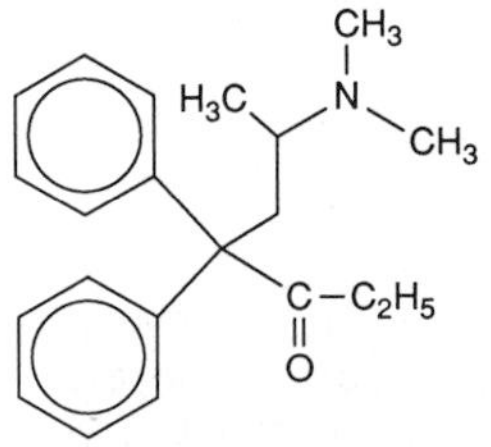

Methadone

For millennia, people have known that the seed pod of the poppy, particularly the opium variety, contains a narcotic and that incision of the seed pod while still green will result in an exudate that when dried can be ingested or smoked. This material is called *opium* (Chapter 14). *Morphine* and *codeine*, among many other substances, can be extracted

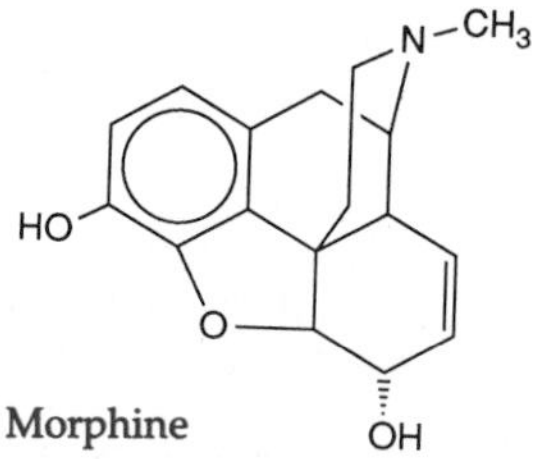

Morphine

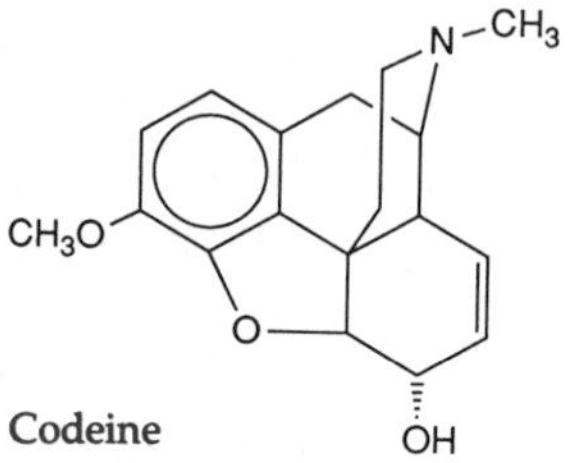

Codeine

from opium. *Heroin* (morphine diacetate) is formed by treating morphine with acetic acid. Administered intravenously, it both is more potent and acts faster than morphine and it has therefore become the staple of the illegal trade in narcotics. Unlike morphine and codeine, heroin is not available for medicinal use in the United States. Many drugs with morphine-like properties are manufactured synthetically. Opiate abuse constitutes a major social problem.

Definitions

- **Opiates:** a term applied to morphine and codeine, and to compounds derived from them.
- **Opioids:** synthetic compounds with morphine or codeine actions but with a different structure. At the present time, the term *opiates* is loosely applied to these compounds also.
- **Narcotics:** Pharmacologically, this term is applied to all agents with morphine-like actions. More generally, it has been used at various times with reference to agents that induce sleep or benumb and, at other times, to identify drugs subject to certain laws. This has led to ambiguity regarding the exact meaning of the term.

Reinforcing Properties

- **Mood elevation:** feelings of repose, tranquillity, and unconcern. As described by Homer: "Those who partook of it did not shed a tear the whole day long even though their father or mother were dead, even though a brother or beloved son had been killed before their eyes." The effect is longer lasting than the analgesic action of these compounds.
- **Orgasmic "high":** an immediate, thrill-like transient "high" experienced following intravenous administration. Although complete tolerance to many effects of opiates develops, tolerance does not completely prevent the occurrence of this effect.

Mechanism of Action

The reinforcing effects of opiates are mediated by their action on μ receptors, particularly those in the ventral tegmental and nucleus accumbens areas. To have high affinity for the receptor, opioids must possess a phenolic ring and a piperidine nitrogen. The substituents on the nitrogen determine the intrinsic activity of the agent.

- **High intrinsic activity** is characteristic of compounds with aliphatic chain substituents on the piperidine nitrogen.
- **Low or absent intrinsic activity** is characteristic of compounds with allyl or cyclopropyl side chain substituents on the piperidine nitrogen. If the intrinsic activity is low (*eg*, buprenorphine) the agent has limited morphine-like action. If the agent has no intrinsic activity at all (*eg*, naloxone, naltrexone), it also possesses no morphine-like properties. Because all of these agents retain a high affinity for the receptor, their occupation of it blocks the actions of opiates. They are thus opiate antagonists.

Tolerance

Tolerance to many effects of opiates develops rapidly and can be marked (Fig. 49-6). Large differences exist, however, in the speed and completeness with which tolerance develops to different effects of these agents.

- **Rapid and complete** tolerance develops to the ability of morphine to induce vomiting. It is readily lost during abstinence from opiate use.
- **Rapid but not complete** tolerance develops initially to the respiratory depression, pupillary constriction, and

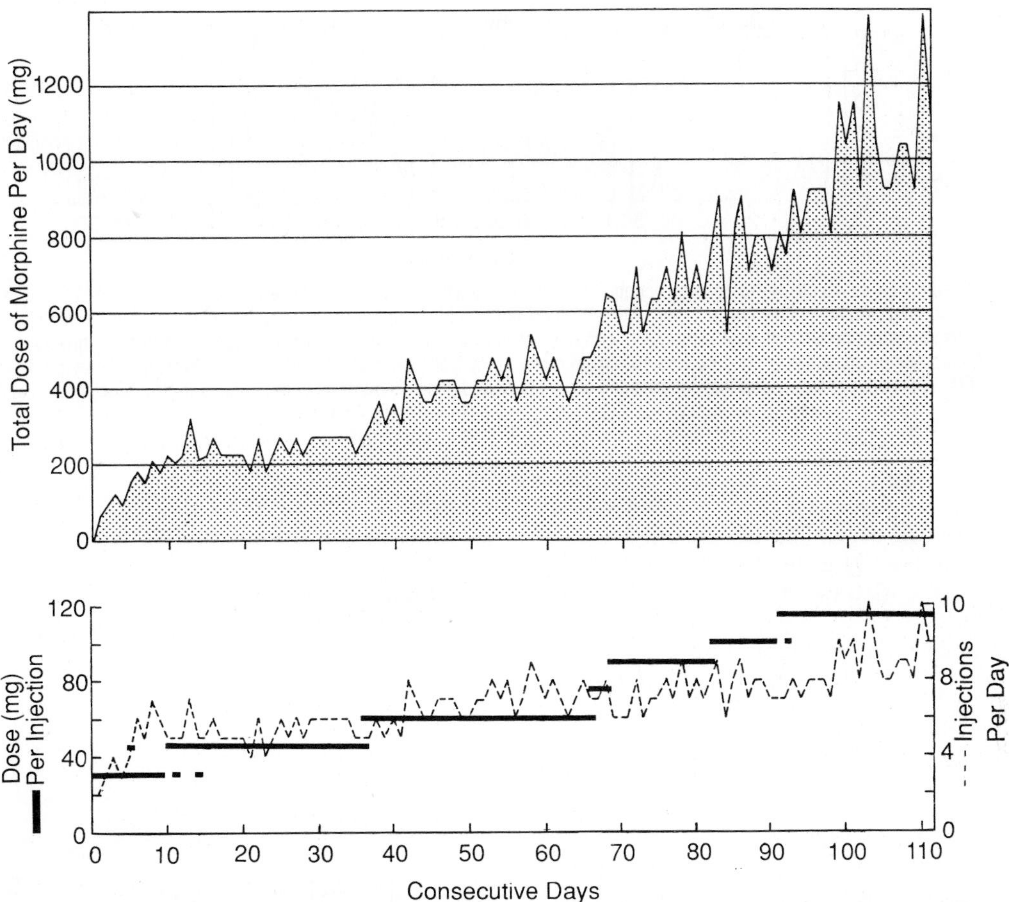

FIGURE 49–6. The subject, a previously narcotic-dependent individual who volunteered for the experiment, was advised that for an unspecified period of time (the duration of which would be communicated to him a month before its end), he could have any drug, in any amount, by any route, and as often as he liked. He was also told that he would not be required to work during this period and that he need not become physically dependent unless he wanted to. He appeared elated and asked for and received 30 mg of morphine intravenously. Immediately after the injection, his skin was flushed and he rubbed his nose and appeared very happy. The flush subsided in a few seconds. On interrogation, he said the sensation was comparable with sexual orgasm. This lasted only a few seconds and was followed by a feeling similar to that he would have experienced if he had had one or two drinks of whiskey but better because it lasted for hours. A few hours later, he was much more loquacious. He said he now had "pep" and could do anything he wanted—go to a show, go for a walk, or go to sleep. Over the period of the next 3 months the patient increased his daily consumption of morphine to as much as 1400 mg *(top panel)*. He spontaneously compared the feeling, before the next "shot" was due, with hunger, and the satisfaction afterward to satiation of hunger. He gradually increased the dose per injection to 115 mg *(lower panel)* because he was not getting the "hold" long enough. On the other hand, since he developed tolerance, he was able to get 6 to 8, and on occasion as many as 10, orgasmlike "thrills" a day. In this respect, being physically dependent was an advantage. He recalled that in the past after he had become physically dependent, he always felt as if some dear friend were missing during periods when he was not taking drugs at all. (Data from Wikler A: Psychodynamic study of patient during experimental self-regulated re-addiction to morphine. Psychiatric Quart 26:270–293, 1952.)

body temperature; thereafter tolerance continues to increase more slowly but never becomes complete.

- **Slow and never complete** tolerance develops to the analgesic actions of opiates and to the constipation they induce.

Physical Dependence

Physical dependence is not a prerequisite for chronic abuse of opiates (Fig. 49–7) but is a frequent concomitant of it. It is rendered evident by the appearance of a withdrawal syndrome upon abstinence or the test administration of an opioid antagonist (*eg*, naloxone).

- **Mechanism:** most clearly involved in the phenomenon are the noradrenergic cells of the locus ceruleus. Opiates act as antagonists at the inhibitory μ receptors of these cells, thereby decreasing presynaptic norepinephrine release by the cells. Over time this results in an up-regulation of postsynaptic norepinephrine receptors. Concurrently, morphine down-regulates the synthesis of β-endorphin, which normally acts at the inhibitory μ receptors. When the opiate is withdrawn, the cell—no longer being inhibited—releases norepinephrine presynaptically. At the same time, the postsynaptic supersensitivity, which results from the increase in norepinephrine receptors, leads to an amplification of the response and an adrenergic storm ensues.

Withdrawal Syndrome

- **Characteristics:** Yawning, rhinorrhea, and lacrimation are early symptoms. Sweating, chills and flushes, gooseflesh, nausea and vomiting, abdominal cramps, anorexia, and bone and muscle pains render the syn-

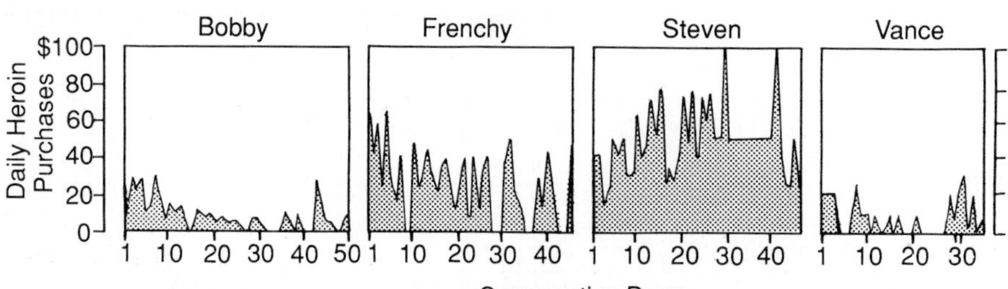

FIGURE 49–7. The subjects were residents of the Harlem section of New York City who considered themselves to be narcotic addicts. For a daily monetary reward ($5–$10) they agreed to report daily on their activities, including their purchases of heroin. Their heroin use is recorded in dollar units. With the exception of Steven, all the other 30 subjects in the study had heroin-free days alternating with days of heroin use. None reported withdrawal syndromes, however, implying an absence of physical dependence. The source of the subjects' income was 46% from crime, 11% from the drug business, and 14% from employment. (Data from Johnson BD, Goldstein PJ, Duchaine MA: What is an addict? Empirical patterns and concepts of addiction. Paper read at the Society for the Study of Social Problems, Boston, MA, August 1979.)

drome similar to a bad case of influenza, only more unpleasant and intense. Muscle spasms and kicking movements occur and have given rise to the term "kicking the habit."

- **Intensity:** proportional to habit size (Fig. 49–8). Many addicts use quantities so small that no withdrawal syndrome follows when they stop using the opiate.
- **Duration:** Acute phase lasts for 2 weeks (Fig. 49–9). See above for discussion of the protracted abstinence syndrome.

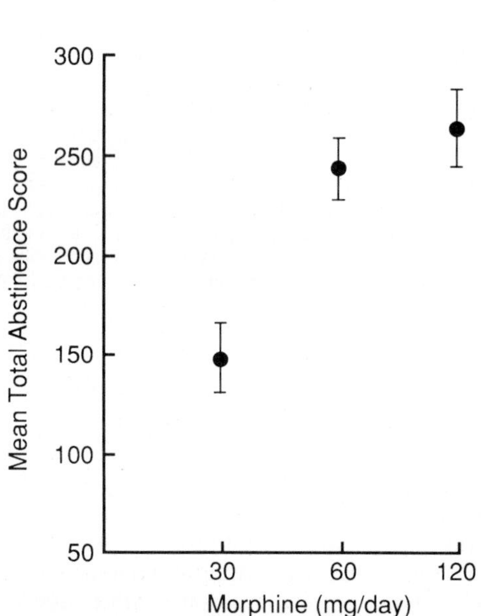

FIGURE 49–8. Intensity of morphine withdrawal in subjects dependent on different doses of morphine per day. The points represent mean total responses for 11 hourly observations from the 14th through the 24th hours of withdrawal. The abstinence score is based on deviations of blood pressure, rectal temperature, pulse rate, respiratory rate, and pupil size from the values obtained when the subjects were stabilized on morphine and on the presence of lacrimation, rhinorrhea, perspiration, yawning, tremor, piloerection, restlessness, and emesis. (From Jasinski DR: Assessment of the abuse potential of morphinelike drugs [methods used in man]. *In* Martin WR [ed]: Drug Addiction I: Morphine, Sedative/Hypnotic and Alcohol Dependence, 197–258. Berlin: Springer-Verlag, 1977.)

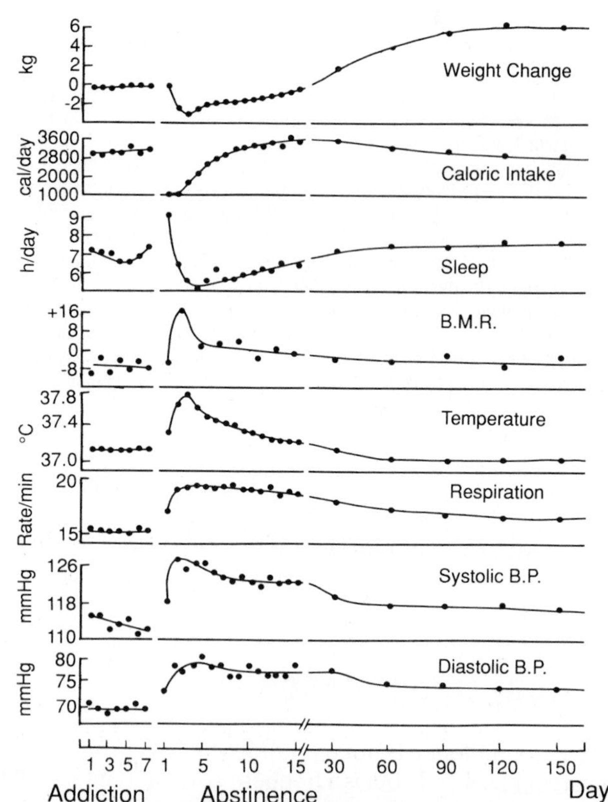

FIGURE 49–9. Abstinence correlates in opiate-dependent patients stabilized on morphine (N = 11) or morphine congeners (N = 10) and then withdrawn from it. *Abscissa:* Patients stabilized on opiate for 8 days, then withdrawn from it and followed daily for 150 days. *Ordinate:* Changes in a number of physiological variables. (BMR = basal metabolic rate; BP = blood pressure.) (From Himmelsbach CK: Clinical studies of drug addiction: Physical dependence, withdrawal and recovery. Arch Intern Med 69:766–772, 1942.)

BOX 49–1

TREATMENT OF THE OPIATE/OPIOID WITHDRAWAL SYNDROME

Though opiate withdrawal, if untreated, does not present danger to life or limb, it is highly unpleasant and it is considered appropriate to alleviate or eliminate its symptoms through treatment. It can be readily terminated by re-administration of an opiate. The next step is to render the individual opiate-free without again precipitating the withdrawal. Three pharmacological approaches are available. Each is predicated on inhibiting, in some way, the norepinephrinergic neurons of the locus ceruleus long enough for β-endorphin synthesis to be up-regulated.

- **Methadone detoxication:** Opiate administration is reinstated using a long-acting (half-life: 23 hours), orally available opioid to terminate withdrawal and the dose of methadone is thereafter gradually decreased to zero over a 2-week period (Table 49–1).
- **Clonidine detoxication:** Advantage is taken of the fact that the locus ceruleus noradrenergic neurons have a secondary inhibitory receptor, namely an α_2-adrenergic receptor. Administration of clonidine, a centrally active α_2-adrenergic receptor agonist (half-life: 12 hours), blocks the manifestations of the withdrawal. The therapy is continued for 2 weeks to allow for up-regulation of β-endorphin synthesis to take place, after which the clonidine administration is discontinued. Because clonidine can cause hypotension, the procedure requires medical supervision.
- **Combined clonidine-naltrexone detoxication:** Naltrexone is a long-lasting μ-receptor antagonist. Normally, it would precipitate withdrawal in a opiate-dependent individual. Pretreatment with clonidine prevents this. Because another action of naltrexone is to stimulate up-regulation of β-endorphin synthesis, co-administration of it with clonidine shortens the period during which the latter has to be administered to 3–5 days. The procedure calls for a fully protective dose of clonidine to be initially combined with a low dose of naltrexone, which is then increased while the clonidine dose is decreased. The two agents are, in effect, titrated against each other.

Opioid Dependence

Opioid dependence is a condition characterized by continued abuse of opioids despite the various manifest problems, be these medical, social, or other, that the abuse is engendering for the abuser. The abuse of the opioid may be intermittent and the therapeutic challenge is not the achievement of abstinence but rather its maintenance. The vast majority of detoxicated opioid-dependent persons return rapidly to opioid use. In a period when detoxication was the only treatment offered, the average half-life of opioid dependence was 24 years.

BOX 49–2

TREATMENT OF OPIATE/OPIOID DEPENDENCE

Two main strategies are currently employed in the treatment of opiate dependence. These are, respectively, opiate- and abstinence-oriented.

- **Methadone maintenance:** Opiate-dependent individuals are maintained on methadone, an institutionally dispensed, orally available, long-acting opiate. The individuals involved thus continue in their opiate dependence. The treatment strategy is predicated on the premise that, given the apparent great difficulty opiate-dependent individuals have in remaining abstinent, it is better to maintain them on methadone than to have them rely on illegal sources for their opiate and on criminal activity for the funds necessary for its acquisition. The treatment strategy is further based on the premise that, freed of the need to procure opiates, the dependent individual is more accessible to rehabilitation and that this will permit the opiate to be withdrawn after a period of social stabilization. Diversion of methadone into the illicit trade for use as an intravenous opiate (given intravenously, it produces a high comparable to that of morphine) has led to the drug being dispensed in a mixture with naloxone, an opiate antagonist. The latter is not absorbed following oral administration and is therefore without effect if the methadone is taken *per os*, but it antagonizes the effect of the methadone if the mixture is administered intravenously.
- **Naltrexone maintenance:** Detoxified individuals are prescribed naltrexone, a potent, orally effective, long-lasting μ-receptor blocking agent (duration of action 72 hours) requiring twice-weekly administration. In individuals thus blocked, opiate administration has no effect. Such individuals, if they continue with the naltrexone therapy, stop seeking opiates. In professionals and others for whom abstinence is very important in terms of regaining licenses or the like, naloxone therapy has proved effective. More generally, however, the fact that taking naloxone is not in itself rewarding and that the drug does not block opiate craving leads to very low acceptability and compliance rates.
- **Buprenorphine maintenance:** A prototypical therapy with a partial μ-receptor agonist that shows promise but has not been widely implemented. Because it is a partial agonist, this type of compound has some slight reinforcing properties and its acceptability by the opiate-dependent individual is high, as is compliance. At the same time, because it has high affinity for the μ receptor, it blocks the effects of opiates and causes the opiate-dependent individual to stop seeking them. Compounds of this type have a considerable market potential as nonaddictive analgesics, and manufacturers are reluctant to having such drugs identified with the treatment of opiate dependence.

COCAINE AND AMPHETAMINES

Cocaine

Amphetamine

Methamphetamine

Cocaine is an alkaloid ester present in the leaves of a shrub that grows at elevations of 2000 to 8000 feet in the Andes Mountains. It can be liberated therefrom by maceration with alkali. From time immemorial this has been accomplished in the Andes by chewing the leaves with lime (calcium carbonate) or ash (source of potassium hydroxide). Cocaine is now produced on an industrial scale in the Andean region of South America and imported illegally into the United States, where its wide use constitutes a major social problem. *Amphetamines* are synthetic phenylamines with an unsubstituted phenyl ring and ethylamine side chain that has an alkyl substituent on the α carbon, that is, the carbon next to the amine nitrogen. At one time, large-scale diversion of amphetamines to the illicit trade created a widespread abuse problem. This has now been all but supplanted by cocaine abuse. Some of the better known amphetamines include D-amphetamine, methamphetamine, methylphenidate (RITALIN), and diethylpropion (TENUATE) (see also Chapter 26).

Methylphenidate

Definitions

- **Cocaine hydrochloride**, the product of industrial scale cocaine extraction, is a crystalline powder ("*crystal*" or "*snow*") that can be snuffed and that is soluble in water and therefore can be injected intravenously. When heated, it decomposes before it is vaporized, *ie*, before its boiling point is reached. It does not lend itself, therefore, to smoking.
- **Cocaine base** is obtained from the hydrochloride by using alkali. The "*free basing*" method involves extraction with ether and evaporation of the latter; "*crack*" cocaine, on the other hand, is obtained by heating the hydrochloride with bicarbonate. Because the base boils if heated (boiling point: 250°C) it can be inhaled in smoke and absorbed via the lungs.
- **Stimulants or psychostimulants** are names at one time applied to drugs of the cocaine-amphetamine class. These terms are ambiguous and hence better not used.

Pharmacokinetics

Both cocaine and amphetamine have high oral availability, although this route of administration results in a 30-minute delay in the onset of action. Accordingly, cocaine abusers resort to intranasal, intravenous, or inhalation routes. The biological half-life of cocaine is short, 0.7 – 1.5 hours; its action is mostly terminated by metabolism. The half-life of amphetamine is much longer, 4 – 20 hours; it is mostly eliminated by urinary excretion. Because it is a strong base, its half-life is therefore a function of urinary pH (Fig. 49 – 10). Methamphetamine is more lipid-soluble and enters the brain more rapidly than D-amphetamine, to which it is demethylated.

Reinforcing Properties

The reinforcing effects of cocaine and D-amphetamine are very intense and quite similar; users are unable to distinguish intravenous injections of D-amphetamine from those of cocaine. The intensity and nature of the effects of these agents are very much a function of dose.

- **Low doses** make the user feel energetic, clearheaded, and effective as well as wide awake and anorexic; according to Sigmund Freud, "Long-lasting, intensive mental or physical work can be performed without any fatigue; it is as though the need for food and sleep were completely banished."
- **Larger doses** cause the user to experience a sense of exhilaration, self-confidence and power. Athletic performance can be objectively shown to be enhanced. As the

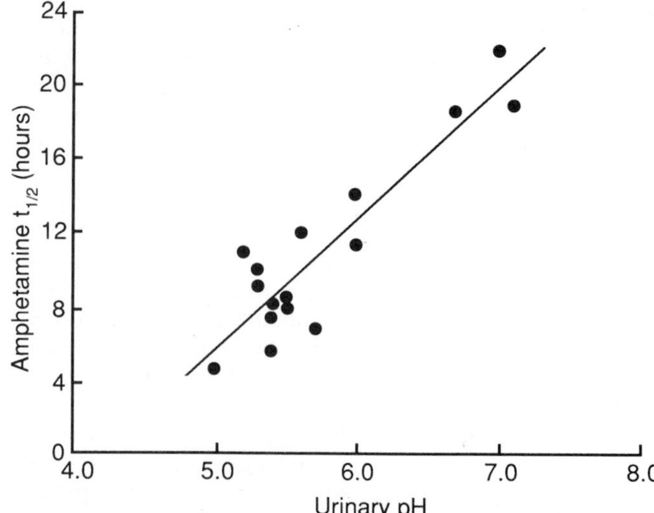

FIGURE 49 – 10. Half-life of amphetamine ($t_{1/2}$) as a function of urinary pH. (From Änggärd E, Gunne LM, Jönsson LE, Niklasson F: Pharmacokinetic and clinical studies on amphetamine-dependent subjects. Eur J Clin Pharmacol 3:3 – 11, 1970.)

dose is increased, the subject comes into a frame of mind dismissive of calamity and danger.

- **Intravenous** administration induces a rush, an intense, orgasm-like sensation.

Mechanism of Action

Cocaine and amphetamine have multiple actions on central nervous system (CNS) monoamine neurotransmitters, namely norepinephrine, dopamine, and serotonin. The reinforcing properties of cocaine are specifically mediated by inhibition of the re-uptake of dopamine. Those of amphetamine are mediated primarily by its enhancement of the release of dopamine from its storage sites. In both instances this results in higher concentration of dopamine at its postsynaptic receptor as well as at the site of its enzymatic deactivation. Although this leads to an enhanced response to dopaminergic stimulation, it also causes depletion of dopamine stores.

Toxicology

- **Vasoconstriction:** Both cocaine and the amphetamines potentiate the peripheral effects of sympathomimetic innervation, causing vasoconstriction. Applied to the nasal mucosa, these agents are therefore effective decongestants. If the vasoconstriction is severe enough, however, ischemia and necrosis follow, resulting in a perforated nasal septum; at least one instance of a nasal drip of cerebrospinal fluid secondary to a perforation has been reported. Intestinal ischemia secondary to intense mesenteric vasoconstriction can follow ingestion of large doses of cocaine: untreated, it can lead to gangrene.
- **Extreme surges in blood pressure,** caused by large parenteral doses, lead to myocardial infarctions, cerebrovascular accidents, ruptured aortas, and abruptio placentae in pregnant women.
- **Other adrenergic effects** include marked tachycardia, hyperpyrexia, anxiety, paranoia, and generalized convulsions.
- **Arrhythmias** are seen following not only intravenous and inhalation dosing but also intranasal administration in young adults with no pre-existing conditions. Postmortem examination of heart sections indicates the presence of contraction bands. Such bands are known to occur as a consequence of catecholamine-induced cardiac damage and represent a disruption of intracellular calcium homeostasis.
- **Teratological effects:** Maternal cocaine use can lead to smaller than normal fetal birth weight and length for gestational period and smaller head circumference. Maternal cocaine use is associated with a fourfold greater incidence of congenital malformations, and an 8% stillbirth rate owing to abruptio placentae.
- **Paranoia:** Chronic cocaine or amphetamine abuse is correlated with toxic paranoid schizophrenia – like reaction characterized by vivid hallucinations (visual, auditory, tactile), paranoid ideation, and changes in affect. All these symptoms occur with a clear sensorium and, if the abuse of the agent is discontinued, resolve in a week or so.

Tolerance

Cocaine and amphetamine use are associated with atypical tolerance phenomena. High-level use is characterized by episodes ("runs") of repetitive self-administration that may last many hours or days. During such periods the user remains continually awake. During a run, the reinforcing effects of the substance become increasingly attenuated. Some chronic tolerance does build up in time to the euphoric, cardiovascular, and hyperthermic effects, but so does kindling, a phenomenon whereby the threshold for seizures is lowered following repeated cocaine exposure.

Physical Dependence

Physical dependence to these agents is not as dramatic or self-evident as in the case of narcotics or depressants. Yet, abrupt cessation of use is followed by symptoms that are reversed when use resumes. Also, typically the run is continued until supplies are exhausted. Monkeys allowed to self-administer cocaine at will continue to do so until they die.

Withdrawal Syndrome

The cessation of amphetamine or cocaine use is followed, first, by increased hunger and prolonged sleep and, second, by depression, general fatigue, and a marked increase in rapid eye movement (REM) sleep. These effects are reversed by administration of either cocaine or amphetamine and thus have the characteristics of a withdrawal syndrome. On the other hand, the withdrawal does not result in major, grossly observable physiological disruption.

Abstinence Symptomatology

Naturalistic evaluation of psychic symptoms that follow cocaine runs has led to conceptualization of a three-phase sequence of post – cocaine abuse abstinence symptoms. The three phases are:

- **Crash** phase, which begins within 15 – 30 minutes following the last dose of cocaine and lasts from 3 to 6 days. It is heralded by rapidly mounting depression and characterized by anhedonia, insomnia, irritability, anxiety, and suicidal ideation. The craving for cocaine diminishes, and after 2 – 5 hours the individual refuses cocaine even if offered. Gradually, lethargy and somnolence become apparent and eventually lead to a long sleep, occasionally interrupted by bouts of eating.
- **A second phase** can last from 1 to 10 weeks. It begins with negligible cocaine craving and near-normal mood and functioning. In due course dysphoria, joylessness, and a perception of intense boredom develop and are accompanied by increasing craving for cocaine, by memories of the reinforcing effects of the drug, by increasing anxiety, and by efforts to arrange for supplies.
- **The third phase** follows. The affective state returns to near-normal levels and craving is episodic, but extreme

when triggered by environmental clues such as friends who previously shared in cocaine use or the sight of venipuncture. Such episodes suggest conditioned tolerance as the responsible mechanism. This phase can last for months.

BOX 49-3
TREATMENT OF COCAINE DEPENDENCE

Efforts to treat cocaine-dependent individuals with dopamine agonists have been disappointing. Greater success has been achieved by using antidepressants, which are dopamine receptor blockers. Such agents are thought to reverse the supersensitivity induced by stimulant use in a dopaminergic inhibitory autoreceptor. The agents most effective in this respect are:

- **Desipramine:** Administered to cocaine abusers, it significantly reduces both cocaine use and cocaine craving and has been found to remain effective for at least 6 weeks. Its main disadvantage is that the reduction in craving develops slowly over 7–14 days. The long delay in the onset of craving reduction by desipramine poses a problem because, among outpatients, resumption of cocaine use in the interim is frequent.
- **Flupenthixol,** a neuroleptic agent administered in a depot form, has been reported to decrease cocaine craving and increase retention of patients in treatment. In low doses it has a rapid antidepressant activity that lasts for 2–4 weeks, and it is considered to act by blocking the inhibitory dopamine autoreceptors.

DEPRESSANTS

Ethanol, barbiturates, and other nonbenzodiazepine *sedative-hypnotic drugs*—namely, chloral hydrate, paraldehyde, glutethimide, meprobamate, methyprylon, ethinamate, and ethchlorvynol—have similar pharmacological effects. A marked similarity also exists with respect to the tolerance, dependence, and withdrawal phenomena seen when ethanol or these other agents are abused. Pharmacologically all these agents are classified, therefore, as belonging to the same category of substances, namely CNS depressants of the alcohol-barbiturate type. The *benzodiazepine* antianxiety agents share many but not all the properties and problems of these substances. Accordingly, the focus of this section is on the similarities and differences between the abuse characteristics of these various agents and those of ethanol.

Reinforcing Properties

Those of barbiturates, benzodiazepines, and other CNS depressants of this type are qualitatively similar to those of ethanol. The abuse potential of such agents tends to be determined primarily by how rapid is the onset of their action, this in turn being a function of the lipid solubility and route of administration of these drugs.

Tolerance

Tolerance of both the functional and metabolic type develops to the agents in this class, the former predominating. It is observed even when only small amounts of barbiturates or other nonbenzodiazepine sedative-hypnotics are used.

Physical Dependence

Physical dependence to depressants of the alcohol-barbiturate type develops only if the dose used is increased above that initially necessary to induce significant pharmacological effects. This is not necessarily the case with diazepam and alprazolam, however; physical dependence has been observed in some individuals who had used only therapeutic doses of these agents. (See Chapter 25.)

Withdrawal Syndrome

In the withdrawal syndrome from depressants of the alcohol-barbiturate type, the rapidity with which symptoms of withdrawal appear is a function of the half-life of the drug. The withdrawal syndrome from barbiturates of intermediate duration (*eg*, pentobarbital, secobarbital) bears a striking similarity to that from ethanol (Table 49-2). The withdrawal syndrome from other nonbenzodiazepine sedative-hypnotics is quite similar. That from longer acting barbiturates such as phenobarbital is milder and more prolonged. Generally, as with ethanol, the severity of the withdrawal is correlated with the dose to which the individual is dependent. The symptoms and signs can be subdivided by severity:

- **Minor signs and symptoms:** coarse tremor, progressive weakness, insomnia, anorexia, nausea, and vomiting
- **More serious symptoms:** Hallucinations and grand mal-type seizures
- **Hyperthermia and delirium** analogous to those of delirium tremens can develop, in absence of treatment, in individuals dependent on the highest doses of these agents.

In the withdrawal syndrome from benzodiazepines, severity is not necessarily proportional to the size of the dose employed and, in the case of diazepam, is usually seen only after use of the agent for long periods of time, stretching into many months.

- **Signs and symptoms** seen in alcohol/barbiturate withdrawal have all been seen also in diazepam and alprazolam withdrawal. In addition, however, signs and symptoms that are unique to the benzodiazepines also occur. These include paranoia, blurring of vision, headache, and for diazepam also facial numbness and cramps.
- **Onset:** for alprazolam the onset of the withdrawal syndrome is 18-48 hours. For diazepam it is much delayed and its course is prolonged. Seizures, if these occur, are typically seen on the eighth to tenth day. The inability of diazepam to control, in a number of instances, the alpra-

TABLE 49–2. Withdrawal Reaction Severity as a Function of Preceding Exposure

Period of Maximal Exposure			Incidence of Withdrawal Signs and Symptoms					
			Minor		Major			
Daily Amount	Duration	Number	TREMOR (%)	OTHER (%)	HALLUCINATIONS (%)	SEIZURES (%)	DELIRIUM TREMENS (%)	FEVER (%)
Ethanol								
Drinks*	Days							
30	52	6	100	100	60	33	33	100
23	23	10	80	80	50	0	0	10
26	10	4	100	100	0	0	0	0
19	3	8	100	†	0	0	0	0
Barbiturate								
Doses*	Days							
9–22	90	18	100	100	67	78	39	†
8	90	8	†	100	26	13	0	†
6	90	18	†	50	0	14	0	†
4	90	18	†	6	0	0	0	†

From Gessner PK: Drug therapy of the alcohol withdrawal syndrome. *In* Majchrowicz E, Noble EP (eds): Biochemistry and Pharmacology of Ethanol, vol 2, 375–435. New York, Plenum Press, 1979.
*Dose units: ethanol drinks—15 ml ethanol; barbiturate—100 mg secobarbital or phenobarbital.
†Data not available.

zolam withdrawal syndrome suggests that these agents may be acting on different populations of receptors (see Chapter 25).

NICOTINE AND TOBACCO

Nicotine is an alkaloid present exclusively in the tobacco plant indigenous to the American continent. Both the plant products and the methodology for self-administration by smoking were brought back to Europe in the 1600s by the early explorers. Tobacco met there both enthusiastic adoption and fervent opposition. The alkaline nature of the smoke derived from air-dried pipe and cigar tobacco generally prevents its inhalation, delays the onset of action of the nicotine in the smoke, and curbs the extent of its use. The discovery at the turn of the nineteenth century that flue-dried tobacco gives a less irritating acidic smoke that can be readily inhaled led to the introduction of cigarettes and a marked escalation in the proportion of the population using tobacco.

Reinforcing Properties

The smoking habit is so old, so commonplace, and currently enjoys such low status that appreciation of its considerable reinforcing properties is jaded. These are nonetheless considerable.

Tolerance

In naive subjects, nicotine induces nausea and vomiting, but tolerance to this and its other effects develops rapidly. Both functional and metabolic tolerance are observed.

Physical Dependence

Smokers seek to maintain certain nicotine blood levels but are usually consciously unaware of relative levels. Administration of ammonium chloride, which leads to acidification of the urine and more rapid nicotine elimination, results in an increase in the number of cigarettes smoked.

Withdrawal Syndrome

Upon sudden cessation of smoking, individuals who smoke 20 or more cigarettes a day develop an abstinence syndrome. This includes a lower diastolic blood pressure, bradycardia, palpitations, gastric disorders, irritability, difficulties in concentrating, anxiety, and restlessness.

Nicotine Dependence

The craving for cigarettes may be intense and persistent during withdrawal. It can also last many months. As a consequence, over half of the cigarette smokers who seek treatment for alcohol and drug dependence identify quitting cigarette smoking as harder than stopping the use of the substance for which they seek treatment. Before cigarettes were widely used, individuals smoking pipes or cigars also found quitting very hard. Freud, for instance, continued his cigar habit (20/day) until death, in spite of an endless series of operations for mouth and jaw cancer (the jaw was eventually totally removed), persistent heart problems that were exacerbated by smoking, and numerous attempts at quitting.

> **BOX 49–4**
> **THERAPY OF NICOTINE DEPENDENCE**
>
> Craving for cigarettes can be reduced by one of two methods, that is by using:
>
> - **Nicotine**-containing devices designed to provide nicotine release gradually and at a rate calculated to decrease the probability of dependence. Of these the best known are nicotine chewing gum and nicotine skin patches.
> - **Clonidine** administration in a low dose (200 mg/day). This reduces withdrawal symptoms and craving in heavy cigarette smokers and doubles (from 30 to 60%) the number who remain abstinent for 6 months or more. Individuals with a history of major depression (although no current symptoms) are only half as likely to succeed in quitting smoking. Although individuals with such a history do have a higher quitting rate if receiving clonidine rather than placebo, in both groups the rate is lower than among individuals with no such history.

Toxicity

Cigarette smoking is a major cause of mortality and morbidity. It results in:

- **Cancers** of the lung (Fig. 49–11), the larynx, and the oral cavity, and is a factor in the genesis of numerous other neoplasms, including cancers of the bladder, kidney, esophagus, pancreas, stomach, uterus, and prostate.
- **Cardiovascular disease:** Smoking causes coronary heart disease, and is a significant factor in sudden cardiac death and stroke.
- **Chronic obstructive lung disease**, thus chronic bronchitis and emphysema.
- **Teratogenic effects:** Babies born to women smokers are small for their gestational age. At age 11, children of mothers who smoked during pregnancy are found to be significantly shorter in stature and lower in mathematical ability and reading comprehension than children of nonsmokers.

PHENCYCLIDINE

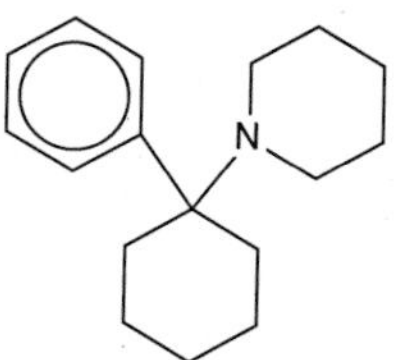

Phencyclidine

Phencyclidine, commonly called PCP, is an agent that was developed in 1957 by Parke-Davis, a pharmaceutical company, as a dissociative anesthetic. Its chemical structure is similar to the anesthetic ketamine (see Chapter 11). The vivid dreams experienced by patients, particularly young males, during emergence from PCP anesthesia and the confused and irrational behavior manifested by them led the company to restrict the use of the agent after 1962 to veterinary medicine. Early illicit experimentation with PCP use was hampered by the difficulties abusers experienced with dosing. After 1972, when users realized that the substance could be inhaled in smoke, its abuse spread rapidly (see also Chapter 50).

Reinforcing Properties

The effects of PCP are such that it was not thought anyone would consider them rewarding, yet users apparently find them worth evoking. PCP produces spatial distortions and a

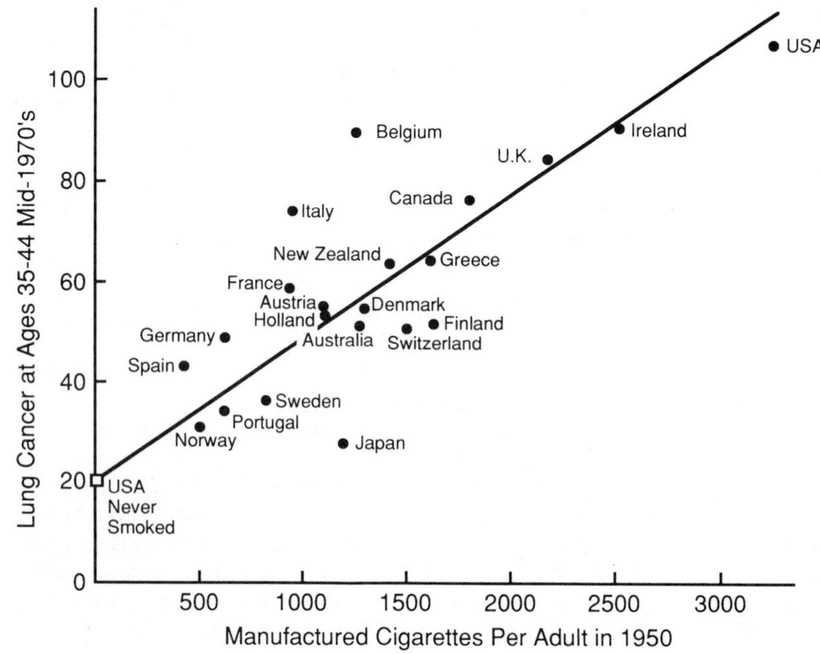

FIGURE 49–11. International correlation between per capita manufactured cigarette consumption among adults and the lung cancer rates in the mid-1970s among those who were entering adulthood around 1950. (From Doll R, Peto R: The causes of cancer: Quantitative estimates of avoidable risks of cancer in the United States today. J Natl Cancer Inst 66:1191–1308, 1981.)

dissociation from current concerns, from the environment, and from the body. It causes decreased touch (two-point discrimination), pain, and position sense. Also, thresholds to audiometry and visual perimetry are increased, causing a dissociation between sensory and motor functioning.

Mechanism of Action

PCP has been shown to have affinity for two receptors in the CNS. One of these is what used to be termed the σ opiate receptor, but it is now referred to simply as the σ receptor because opiate antagonists such as naloxone do not displace agonists from it, although haloperidol does. The other is referred to as the PCP receptor, and haloperidol does not displace agonists from it. The respective role of these receptors in mediating the effects of PCP is not yet clear.

Pharmacokinetics

The lipid solubility of phencyclidine is high (the brain/plasma ratio is between 6 and 9) and so it has a rapid onset. Thus, following its inhalation in smoke, the effects are evident in 1-5 minutes. Following ingestion the onset occurs in 15-30 minutes, with peak blood levels being observed at 2 hours. The duration of action is 4-6 hours, but it can be much longer depending on dose. The high lipid solubility renders redistribution an important mechanism in the termination of its action. The half-life of the compound is 21 hours. Because about 10% of the substance is excreted unchanged in the urine, the half-life is dependent on urinary pH.

Tolerance

Chronic PCP users report that gradual tolerance develops to the psychic effects of low doses. This forces users to take larger amounts, but that, in turn, is correlated with increasingly dysphoric experiences. Such experiences are reported by three quarters of the users, and many feel trapped by the drug. In animals, tolerance to the anesthetic effects of PCP is observed following repeated administration over a period of weeks or months.

Physical Dependence

Animals will maintain themselves on PCP. Withdrawal in monkeys after 10 days on the drug produces a syndrome marked by emesis, anorexia, tremors, and contact avoidance, fighting, and restlessness. No description of a well-characterized withdrawal syndrome in humans is available.

Toxicity

The acute effects of PCP change, as the dose is increased, from a mild euphoria and stimulation (which does not interfere with normal functioning) to a body-wide anesthetic effect (legs and feet especially) that makes coordination difficult, produces slurred speech, and may involve an out-of-body experience. This can lead to bizarre behavior, unresponsiveness, combativeness, and with higher doses, to catatonia as the individual becomes incoherent and immobile, although conscious. With further increases in dose, convulsions (diazepam has been used for these) and coma ensue.

- **Clinical signs and symptoms:** The intoxication is characterized by nystagmus, which in 90% of patients is both horizontal and vertical, by ataxia, and by hyperreflexia. Other clinical correlates of the intoxication are an elevation of systolic and diastolic pressure (potentially controlled by diazoxide), hyperthermia (potentially controlled by naloxone), and oliguria. The last is accompanied by elevated serum creatinine phosphokinase activity and serum uric acid, as well as myoglobinuria. It is indicative of rhabdomyolysis. The possibility of the latter renders acidification of the urine, which would speed the renal elimination of PCP, hazardous because myoglobin is more likely to cause renal damage under such circumstances.
- **Effects on the psyche:** include unique and profound alterations of thought, gross changes in body image, loss of ego boundary, depersonalization, estrangement, and isolation. Patients may have religious ideation, feelings of God-like power, perceptions of superhuman strength (local anesthetic effects permit behavior that would otherwise be too painful) and invulnerability, as well as a pathological preoccupation with death (*meditatio mortis*). Behavior is extremely unpredictable, the patients being cooperative one minute and violently assaultive the next. Patients present an immediate danger to others merely on the basis of their misperceptions, paranoia, and hostility. This threat is compounded by their confusion and their inability to cooperate. Patients are ambivalent and unpredictable even toward their close friends and relatives.
- **Schizophrenic episodes:** Following PCP self-administration, patients may present with psychoses indistinguishable clinically from schizophrenia. Haloperidol may be useful in alleviating the symptoms. As the body burdens of PCP are cleared, the psychoses resolve in most patients. In some, however, they persist for weeks or months. In schizophrenic patients, PCP brings about a rapid and extreme exacerbation of psychoses.
- **Chronic effects:** Following prolonged use of PCP, users develop persistent speech difficulties (stuttering, blocking), an inability to think clearly, problems with recent memory, incoherence, and unreliability. They also appear to undergo personality changes and to develop severe depression and social withdrawal. Recovery is slow, the effects lasting 6 months to a year. (Clonidine has been reported to alleviate the depression.)

HALLUCINOGENS

Although knowledge of hallucinogenic substances is ancient, the abuse of such substances first became widespread in the 1960s when taking LSD became a fashionable component of the hippie lifestyle and LSD was used by some with considerable frequency. Although the actions of the other agents in this group are similar to those of LSD, these latter hallucinogens never achieved widespread use (see also Chapter 50).

Classification

Briefly, the agents in this class include the following:

- **LSD** was discovered, in the early 1940s, by Hofmann, a chemist with the Swiss pharmaceutical company Sandoz, while he was trying to develop an analeptic. Noting that he was experiencing marked mental changes after handling the drug. Hofmann concluded that this was likely to be due to his having inhaled or ingested some of the substance accidentally. To confirm this, he deliberately self-administered a very small quantity of LSD and experienced rather dramatic effects.
- **Mescaline** (3,4,5-trimethoxphenyl-ethylamine) is found in a Mexican cactus, the dried top of which is called peyote or mescal and is used by some Native Americans in their religious ceremonies.
- **N,N-dimethyltryptamine** and **5-methoxy-N,N-dimethyltryptamine** are both present in snuffs of plant origin used by natives of the Caribbean and Amazon basin areas, respectively. These agents have a very rapid onset and very short duration of action.
- **Psilocin** (4-hydroxytryptamine) and its phosphate ester, *psilocybin.* These compounds are found in the psilocybe mushrooms, which are native to Mexico.
- **Synthetic substituted amphetamines**, including 2,5-dimethoxy-4-methylamphetamine (MDA, STP) and 2,5-dimethoxyamphetamine (DMA).

Reinforcing Properties

Perception and interpretation of both external and internal sensory stimuli are altered by LSD. Although visual perception is the modality most obviously affected (objects assume great plasticity: walls, faces, and so on recede, advance, change shape and color, and acquire halos and new qualities), other senses are also affected (*eg*, touch: clothes may feel velvety one moment, gritty the next). So is proprioception, with resulting distortions of body image, out-of-body sensations, and depersonalization. Fragments of the perceptual field are perceived out of context with the usual frame of reference. Background stimuli, normally ignored (the sound of a breeze, the drip of a tap), compel attention. Unusual associations come to mind and stimulate each other. The drug is a potent enhancer of suggestibility, exceeding in this respect the effects of hypnosis. It has major effects on mood. Objects seen and events occurring are felt to have great portentousness. Feelings of insight and unity with the universe, with humankind, and so on may be experienced. Chains of thought are less subject to critical review and appear to take command, resulting in thinking that is more innovative, but also more tangential. LSD-induced feelings of greatly enhanced creativity, insight, and so on cannot be either verbalized or otherwise documented.

Course of Action

The onset of central effects of LSD is relatively slow — during the first 30 minutes only somatic effects (weakness, tremor, occasionally paresthesias, sometimes muscle cramps, and nausea) are perceived. Thereafter the central effects become rapidly manifest and reach a peak at about 3 hours. The following day the individual feels fatigued and depressed. The other hallucinogens act more rapidly and for a shorter time.

Tolerance

Tolerance develops if LSD is taken repeatedly in a short period of time: the effects become less and less. Also there is cross-tolerance to other hallucinogens (*eg*, psilocybin). On the other hand, no withdrawal phenomena from LSD have been observed in humans or animals.

Toxicity

Knowledge of the toxic and other properties of this group of substances derives primarily from the clinical experience with LSD. Users of LSD usually retain enough insight to know that the mental changes and hallucinations being experienced are consequences of ingestion of the hallucinogen and are self-limiting. Individuals may seek medical attention because of:

- **Panic reaction:** Anxiety, fear of the unknown, perhaps of losing one's mind, can become intense enough that frank panic occurs, requiring hospitalization. In individuals unaware of having ingested a hallucinogen, such fears have resulted in suicide.
- **"Bad trips":** Some fraction of the LSD-induced experiences are sufficiently dysphoric for users to seek medical assistance. The user's expectations regarding the effects of the drug (the "set"), the "setting," and the presence of an experienced user, or "sitter," who can lead and reassure the neophyte, decrease, to a degree, the probability of a dysphoric experience, but even seasoned users have some occasionally.
- **Flashbacks:** Some LSD users may seek medical assistance because of the recurrence of the hallucinogenic experience at a later date and in the absence of the ingestion of a hallucinogen. To some, this can be extremely distressing.
- **Psychoses:** Although relatively rare, these constitute the most serious toxic effect of LSD. They can occur in previously normal individuals. Such psychoses do not always respond to treatment and can be long-lasting (weeks, months).

BOX 49–5

TREATMENT

Chlorpromazine decreases the intensity of the effects of LSD and has been used in the treatment of dysphoric experiences. Diazepam can be used to relieve anxiety. Additionally, the patient needs continued reassurance or "talking down."

ECSTASY AND EVE

3,4-Methylenedioxymethamphetamine (MDMA, Ecstasy, Adam) and its homologue, 3,4-methylenedioxyethamphetamine (MDEA, Eve) are ring-substituted amphetamines that became popular on college campuses in the 1980s as recreational drugs. During this period, MDMA was also used as an adjunct to psychotherapy by some psychiatrists. The drug causes irreversible neurotoxicity in experimental animals, and the possibility that it may do so also in humans has led the drug to be placed on the list of Schedule I substances by the United States Food and Drug Administration. MDEA is said to have effects similar to those of MDMA, although they are milder.

Reinforcing Properties

Upon first-time use, most MDMA users experience a pleasant mood change without hallucinations. The effects range from a lowering of interpersonal anxiety and defenses, a sense of greater closeness with others, and increased communication and sociability to a visionary experience of a mystical nature inducing a sense of wholeness, connectedness, or enlightenment.

Course of Action

Onset occurs in about 30 minutes following oral ingestion. Somatic effects include some tingling and spasmodic jerking as well as a sensation of coldness. The acute effects peak after a couple of hours and wane by 6 hours.

Toxic Effects

Jaw clenching, teeth grinding, muscle aches, difficulty concentrating, fatigue, and depression are reported in the days immediately following MDMA use. Upon repeated use of the drug, the pleasurable effects are much diminished and the side effects enhanced; this is true even when long periods of time elapse in the interim.

Destruction of Serotoninergic Neurons

In the rat, both racemic MDMA (the substance in illicit trade) and each of the enantiomers cause an acute depletion of brain 5-hydroxytryptamine (serotonin, 5-HT), with recovery to control levels within 12 hours. Animals given either the racemic MDMA or the (+) enantiomer suffer a secondary depletion of 5-HT 7 days later, although this is not seen with the (−) enantiomer. Repeated injections of MDMA destroy serotoninergic neurons in rats and monkeys, the latter species being much more sensitive. Such monkeys become extremely passive and insomniac. The increase in serum prolactin concentrations seen following L-tryptophan infusion appears to be blunted in human MDMA users. Because the rise in serum prolactin is a response mediated by 5-HT synthesis and release, this finding has raised concerns that MDMA may cause long-term loss of 5-HT neurons in human users also.

ATROPINE-TYPE DELIRIANTS

The belladonna alkaloids—atropine, scopolamine, and hyoscine—as well as plant materials containing them (*eg, Datura stramonium*, jimsonweed) have a long history of use to induce mental effects. This history includes application of salves containing them to skin or mucosal surfaces by witches in the Middle Ages. Although these agents were never widely used as recreational substances in this century, isolated instances of such use continue to be encountered.

Toxic Properties

These substances are classic muscarinic cholinergic-blocking agents. They cause dry mouth, inability to swallow, dilated pupils and blurred vision, hyperthermia, tachycardia, and urinary retention. Toxic manifestations include disorientation, irrationality, amnesia, and a delirium characterized by hallucinations and loss of insight (see also Chapter 50).

> **BOX 49-6**
> **TREATMENT**
>
> Physostigmine, infused slowly, reverses the delirium; in its absence, diazepam can be used to control the excitement and alcohol or sponge baths to lower body temperature.

REFERENCE

Diagnostic and Statistical Manual of Mental Disorders: DSM-IV, 4th ed. Washington DC, American Psychiatric Association, 1994.

50 Adverse Drug Reactions and Interactions

Cedric M. Smith, Katherine R. Bonson, Jerrold C. Winter, and Roger K. Cunningham

ADVERSE DRUG REACTIONS

Relevance to All Drug Use

Although estimates vary, more than 2 – 5% of all hospitalizations in the United States are due to adverse drug reactions, and 0.2% were severe, life-threatening reactions. As many as 30% or more of hospitalized patients experience an adverse drug event! Even the studies probably underestimate the prevalence. In response to the increase in reactions, the United States Pharmacopeia (USP), the Food and Drug Administration (FDA), and the American Medical Association (AMA) collaborated in 1993 with the launching of MEDWATCH, a system designed to improve the as-yet voluntary reporting of possible serious adverse events. *The most current investigation (Johnson and Bootman, 1995) documents an annual cost in the United States of the astounding figure of 76 billion dollars from the failure to monitor and manage effectively drug therapy.*

Although serious reactions receive the most attention, among the most common adverse drug reactions are gastrointestinal upsets with nausea, vomiting, or diarrhea or cutaneous reactions. Such symptoms are not only troublesome but also a major cause of nonadherence to therapeutic regimens. *The ready availability of compendia of drug reactions and computer-based tabulations of symptoms that may be of drug origin behooves all health professionals, when presented with a new symptom, to rule out a possible drug interaction with another drug or food as the cause! (For some techniques for the use of these computer-based systems, see Chapter 62.)*

Drug Intolerance

Unfortunately, the mechanisms of many adverse reactions are not known with certainty; allergic reactions appear to explain a minority of these; these are discussed in a separate section, below. The majority of reactions are thus nonimmunologic reactions and are variously referred to and defined. *Drug intolerance* to a given drug occurs when side effects occur at doses tolerated by most individuals. In other words, there is a *quantitative* difference in the response to the drug. The condition is sometimes referred to as *metareaction.* An example would be severe respiratory depression occurring in a patient given a fraction of the usual analgesic dose of morphine. The underlying basis for intolerance is poorly understood, but probably reflects one extreme of a gaussian distribution of responses in the population.

Idiosyncrasy

Idiosyncrasy, in contrast, is used most often to describe a state of altered response or altered drug metabolism. An example would be the development of hemolytic anemia in individuals deficient in glucose-6-phosphate dehydrogenase who are given primaquine. The underlying basis for this state is clearly genetic, and the nature of the untoward response is *qualitatively* different.

Overdose or side effects reactions clearly imply a predictable reaction in most normal individuals.

Drug allergy or teratogenetic reactions are usually among the unpredictable adverse reactions.

The adverse reactions can also be classified under two other rubrics: (1) the specific organ or physiological system involved, such as the nervous, psychiatric, skin, cardiovascular system, respiratory system, hematological, liver, *etc*; and (2) the drug class and specific drug. For example, in some studies antibiotics have been implicated in 40 – 50% of reactions, nonsteroidal anti-inflammatory agents in 14 – 27%, and central nervous system (CNS) depressants in 10 – 12% of all reactions. A more useful analysis addresses the specific type of reaction in relation to the number of patients receiving the drug. For some examples, Bigby and associates (1989) reported that in a large group of medical inpatients, 12.8% of those receiving cimetidine had a skin reaction, compared with 51.4% of those receiving amoxicillin, and only 0.4% of those receiving diazepam.

Drug interactions with adverse consequences also can be viewed along similar categories.

Because of their importance and frequency we present as examples selected groups of drugs that cause some specific diseases and symptoms — psychiatric and renal, as well as some unique and unusual reactions that serve as examples of the concerns in accurate diagnosis and management. (Drugs causing sensory disturbances are discussed in Chapter 13.)

Psychiatric Symptoms Produced by Drugs

Many drugs can produce effects on the CNS, including those drugs that are primarily used for their peripheral effects. Medically, agents that rely on a central action for therapeutic benefit are prescribed most often by psychiatrists in an attempt to alleviate mental disturbances. However, in obvious contrast to this practice, millions of people consume or inject chemical substances (drugs). Such effects are not only dependent on the nature of the substance but also are related to the magnitude of the dose and the biological state of the individual. For example, a relatively small increase in the dose of any drug may result in a marked increase in central nervous stimulation or depression.

Delirium and Hallucination

The essential feature of delirium is a clouded state of consciousness — a reduction in the clarity of awareness of the environment. This is manifested by a difficulty in sustaining attention to either external or internal stimuli because of sensory misperception or disordered stream of thought. In addition, disturbances of sleep-wakefulness and psychomotor activity are commonly present.

Agitation and disorientation are characteristic of delirious patients; these patients often do not know where they are or what day it is. In the case study, the man had suffered a delirium after a woman had secretly put *scopolamine*, an anticholinergic drug, into his drink (see Box 50 - 1 and Chapters 8 and 49).

> **BOX 50 - 1**
>
> **CASE: SCOPOLAMINE**
>
> *A 42-year-old man was brought to the emergency room by police after he was found apparently intoxicated, wandering the streets dressed only from the waist up. On admission, the patient was extremely agitated and was disoriented to time, place and person (Goldfrank et al, 1982).*

Hallucination is different from delirium in that people who are hallucinating have a false sensory perception that occurs in the absence of relevant or adequate stimuli. Although the hallucination may have a compelling sense of reality, people sometimes may be able to identify that it is in fact not a real occurrence.

The visual hallucinations described by the French poet Gautier occurred to him following ingestion of *hashish*, material derived from the cannabis plant. Such vivid hallucinations are possible without the loss of a clear sensorium or confusion about who one is or where one lives. However, the effect of a drug is influenced not only by the chemical itself but by the mind/brain upon which it is acting. The frame of mind and situation a person is in when taking a drug is commonly referred to as the effect of "set" and "setting." For example, when ministers were given a hallucinogen in a church on Good Friday, there was a preponderance of religious hallucinations among them. Conversely, when convicts with hostile personalities were administered the same drug while in prison, they tended to become very violent. The complexity of the brain accounts for the vast differences in behavior and thought among individuals that can result from a single agent.

Clinical lore has it that drug-induced hallucinations tend to be visual, whereas those that occur in schizophrenia are generally auditory. This conclusion is not based on strong evidence, however, so it is not a good basis for an accurate diagnosis of the source of a hallucination. In addition, hallucinations and delirium may present together and should be noted as distinct conditions.

> **BOX 50 - 2**
>
> **CASE: HASHISH**
>
> *My eyelashes grew to infinity and like golden threads wound around little wiry spindles that spun by themselves with dazzling speed. About me were rivers, many torrents of gems of all colors, with endlessly changing floral patterns that I can only compare with kaleidoscopic patterns . . . One of the guests addressed me in Italian, which the drug in its omnipotence changed into Spanish. The questions and answers were almost reasonable and touched upon such important subjects as literature or the theatre (Gautier, as cited in Moreau, 1845, 1973).*

Indole and Phenethylamine Hallucinogens; Lysergic Acid Diethylamide

It is useful to distinguish "true" hallucinogenic substances from agents that can produce hallucinations as a side effect. The classic example of a true hallucinogen is lysergic acid diethylamide (LSD), which produces profound behavioral manifestations including sensory distortions and hallucination. Table 50 - 1 lists some of the true hallucinogens. These can be contrasted with other drugs that induce hallucinations secondarily to their main effect, or only upon chronic administration, or on abrupt withdrawal after chronic exposure.

LSD is capable of causing its intense effects at the minute dose of 50 μg or greater. It was discovered serendipi-

TABLE 50-1. True Hallucinogens: Some Drugs Whose Primary Known Effect is the Production of Hallucinations

Indoles

- N,N-dimethyltryptamine (DMT)
- (4-phosphoryloxy-DMT) psilocybin (phosphorylated psilocin; *Psilocybe mexicana* Heim)
- Lysergic acid diethylamide (LSD)

Phenethylamines

- Mescaline (3,4,5-trimethoxyphenylethyl-amine; *Lophophora williamsii*; peyote)
- DOM (2,5-dimethoxy-4-methylamphetamine)

Tetrahydrocannabinols

tously by Albert Hofmann, a Swiss medicinal chemist who was working in the field of obstetric pharmacology (see Chapter 49).

LSD is one of many hallucinogens that contain an indole ring in its chemical structure. This ring structure was not developed in a laboratory; this ring is found naturally in the form of dimethyltryptamine in many Central and South American plants. People in these regions have used hallucinogenic plants for thousands of years, often in conjunction with religious ceremonies. Another drug with dimethyltryptamine as its base is the 4-phosphoryloxy derivative psilocybin, a compound found in hallucinogenic mushrooms. The mechanism of action of these drugs in the brain is thought to be very similar, involving certain serotonin receptors.

In addition to indole compounds, hallucinogens are also derived from phenethylamines. Mescaline, the active agent in the peyote cactus, is a phenethylamine with methoxy substitutions at three positions. Mescaline has been used for centuries by native people throughout the Americas in peyote cults. These cults have even incorporated the side effects of nausea and vomiting into the ceremony as a cleansing ritual. Mescaline is the only hallucinogen that has been legal in the United States for religious purposes—but only if one belongs to the Native American Church.

When the basic phenethylamine structure is substituted at the position with a methyl group, it becomes amphetamine. There are many hallucinogenic derivatives of amphetamine, including DOM (2,5-dimethoxy-4-methamphetamine, also known at one time as "STP"). The presence of the α-methyl group delays deamination in the body, giving compounds a longer half-life and therefore more time to act in the brain. Another phenethylamine recently popular "on the street" is MDMA (methylenedioxymethamphetamine, "ecstasy"). In addition, MDMA is one of a variety of psychoactive substances that have been tested for their potential as "nonlethal" disorienting chemical weapons. There is currently some scientific concern that MDMA may be neurotoxic in serotonergic systems (see Chapter 49).

Generally, indolamines and phenethylamines produce strikingly similar perceptual and subjective effects despite their structural differences. Pharmacological research with both classes of hallucinogens suggest that these drugs act at a specific subtype of serotonergic receptor (5-HT_2) in the brain, with possible interaction at dopamine sites. The neurochemical model of schizophrenia proposes similar receptor stimulation, based on initial studies of hallucinogens in humans that showed effects thought to resemble psychosis. In fact, the term psychotomimetic was coined by the French psychiatrist J. J. Moreau de Tours in the nineteenth century as a classification for drugs that produce hallucinations.

Tetrahydrocannabinol (THC), the active ingredient in marijuana, is now being made available as a Schedule II drug for use in lessening the nausea resulting from cancer chemotherapy. It has also been experimentally tested for use in reducing intraocular pressure in glaucoma. As with indole and phenethylamine hallucinogens, there are no reports of directly fatal effects due to marijuana; it should be kept in mind that adequate doses of THC can be hallucinogenic, as described above.

Nonhallucinogenic Drugs That Induce Hallucinations

Many drugs can produce hallucinations as a secondary effect. Often these agents have also been classified as psychotomimetic, but as with the true hallucinogens the behavioral changes do not faithfully replicate clinical psychosis. Drugs that cause hallucination as a side effect often produce delirium as an additional component of the intoxication. This is especially true of the first category of drugs to be discussed, the anticholinergics.

ANTICHOLINERGICS. Antagonists of the neurotransmitter acetylcholine are found in many members of the plant family Solanaceae, which includes deadly nightshade, jimsonweed, and the eyes of the common potato. The active substances are alkaloids such as atropine (hyoscyamine), scopolamine (hyoscine), and a number of related substances.

Varieties of the genus *Datura* contain these alkaloids in their leaves, flowers, stems, and seeds. *Datura stramonium* (the common jimsonweed or thorn apple) can be smoked or brewed as a tea. Its effects are described in this account.

BOX 50-3
CASE: ANTICHOLINERGIC

A 16-year-old girl was admitted with a six-hour history of bizarre behavior. She was seen by the casualty officer, a neurosurgeon, and by a psychiatrist before the possibility of poisoning was considered on the clinical presentation of an acute psychosis with disorientation. She was agitated, talking incoherently and plucking at the bed clothes. The skin and mucous membranes were dry, the pulse was 100/min. and the bladder was slightly distended. The pupils were dilated and reacted sluggishly to light, rotary nystagmus was present, and the tendon reflexes were hyperactive with flexor plantar responses. Her agitation was controlled with diazepam and within 24 hours of admission she was rational and admitted eating two Surama cigarettes. She described vivid frightening hallucinations of dead babies in a satanic black mass (Ballantyne et al, 1976).

The clues that these symptoms were not the result of indole or phenethylamine hallucinogens are the classic signs of dry mucous membranes and urinary retention typical of parasympathetic blockade.

Another case illustrates why it is important to consider anticholinergic intoxication when delirium and hallucinations are the presenting behavior.

BOX 50–4
CASE: SCOPOLAMINE

Recently we were asked to see a 71-year-old woman admitted for evaluation of her long-standing problem of dizziness. Although she exhibited normal behavior on admission, within 24 hours she became psychotic, displayed agitation and paranoid behavior and complained of visual hallucinations. Her transfer medications were listed as propranolol hydrochloride, 40 mg twice daily; isosorbide dinitrate, 10 mg four times daily; digoxin, 0.125 mg four times daily; furosemide, 40 mg four times daily; and meclizine hydrochloride, 15 mg/day.

The patient was not clinically hypoxic and on physical examination her condition was essentially normal except for a tachycardia of 100 beats per minute, a BP of 220/111 mmHg, widely dilated pupils, and aberrant behavior that did not seem to be altered by the intramuscular administration of 2 mg of haloperidol.

Although not listed on her transfer medications, the patient finally admitted on further questioning to have had "some medicine stuck behind my ear three days ago." A Transderm-V disk (containing scopolamine) was removed and physostigmine salicylate, 1 mg intramuscularly, was administered with complete resolution of her psychotic features, tachycardia and cycloplegia within three hours (Osterholm and Camoriano, 1982. Copyright 1982, American Medical Association).

Because older people tend to be more sensitive to the behavioral effects of drugs, as seen in this case with a scopolamine patch (see Chapters 8 and 58), dosages should be monitored. Medications as diverse as over-the-counter allergy remedies (antihistamines), phenothiazine-type antipsychotics, and tricyclic antidepressants produce anticholinergic effects; frequently overlooked as a source of anticholinergic toxicity are bladder and urinary anti-spasmodics. The wide spectrum of such anticholinergic effects have been summarized:

> *The symptoms and signs of toxicity develop promptly after ingestion of the drug. The mouth becomes dry and burns, swallowing and talking become difficult or impossible, and there is marked thirst. The vision is blurred and photophobia is prominent; the pupils are dilated. The skin is hot, dry and flushed. The body temperature tends to rise. The pulse is weak and rapid. Palpitations may occur and the blood pressure is elevated. Urinary urgency and difficulty in micturition occurs especially in older men. The behavior and mental symptoms may suggest an acute organic psychosis. Memory is disturbed, orientation is faulty, hallucinations (especially visual) are common, the sensorium is clouded and mania and delirium are not unusual.*
>
> *The patient may be restless, excited and confused, and exhibit muscular incoordination. Gait and speech are disturbed. The diagnosis of an acute schizophrenic episode or alcoholic delirium has been mistakenly made (Weiner, 1980, p 127).*

These symptoms have given rise to various aphorisms summarizing the side effects:

- Dry as a bone (blockade of salivation and sweating)
- Blind as a bat (mydriasis and paralysis of accommodation)
- Hot as a hen (hyperthermia and peripheral vasodilation)
- Red as a beet (no sweat and peripheral vasodilation)
- Mad as a hatter (delirious; reference from insanity seen in hat makers in nineteenth-century England who were chronically exposed to mercury)

The treatment for anticholinergic overdose is as for atropine poisoning and includes gastric lavage, control of body temperature, and maintenance of urine flow. Because anticholinergics act as competitive antagonists at acetylcholine receptors, their effects may be overcome by the careful use of physostigmine. If sedation is required, a barbiturate or benzodiazepine may be given.

PHENCYCLIDINE. Phencyclidine, known also as PCP or "angel dust," was developed in the 1950s as a potential anesthetic-analgesic (see Chapter 49). PCP is generally termed a dissociative anesthetic as is the close chemical congener, ketamine (see Chapter 11). Some of the common features of PCP intoxication are illustrated in these case reports:

BOX 50–5
CASE: PHENCYCLIDINE (PCP)

A 22-year-old male was traveling at approximately 5 mph at 4:15 p.m. on a busy highway. He was pulled over by police who described the subject as sitting behind the wheel, staring straight ahead, clenching and unclenching his fists and foaming at the mouth. There was no response to questions. The attending physician described the patient as non-responsive to verbal commands, eyes open but unable to follow moving objects and nonresponsive to painful stimuli (Clardy et al, 1979).

BOX 50–6
CASE: PHENCYCLIDINE

A 29-year-old man . . . became floridly psychotic after . . . having smoked a marijuana cigarette laced with [PCP]. He suffered from auditory hallucinations that told how his hands had offended him, and commanded punishment by biting both his arms. It is possible the phencyclidine serves as the trigger in the development of a long-lasting psychosis (Grove, 1979).

Other symptoms and treatment of PCP intoxication are discussed in Chapter 49.

STIMULANTS. CNS stimulants include such drugs as amphetamine, cocaine, and methylphenidate. Although many stimulants share a structure that resembles amphetamine, this is not always the case. Hence, although there are many pharmacological similarities among the various compounds, each stimulant also has effects that are unique.

Chronic use of relatively low levels of a stimulant, as well as large acute doses, can result in a syndrome resembling psychosis. This was first noted in individuals who were using amphetamines for their anorexic effects as appetite suppressants (Connell, 1958), although related behavior has been seen in people using cocaine. Agitation and paranoia are characteristic, and these may be accompanied by tactile hallucinations of bugs crawling underneath the skin. This syndrome is often seen in people who take stimulants to maintain adequate work performance.

BOX 50–7

CASE: AMPHETAMINE

A 27-year-old truck driver shot his boss in the back of the head because he thought the boss was trying to release a poison gas into the back seat of the car in which he was riding:

"I thought they had gassed me. My boss kept reaching down beside him and pulling on something. I rolled the window down to let the gas out. I got nauseated and passed out due to the gas. I then got up on my elbow and shot my boss, who was driving."

Over the previous 20 hours, in order to make a nonstop 1,600 mile trip, Mr. A had ingested 180 mg of amphetamine; he had not slept for 48 hours (Ellingwood, 1970).

Acute high-dose intoxication has been encountered from what has been called the cocaine body-packer syndrome. This results from the rupture of condoms filled with cocaine that had been swallowed to smuggle cocaine through customs at border checks. It is clear that cocaine can be lethal. The causes of death appear to include fatal cardiac arrhythmias and cerebrovascular accidents as well as uncontrollable seizures.

BOX 50–8

CASE: COCAINE

A 44-year-old was admitted after having been arrested for suspicion of cocaine smuggling. He admitted to having hidden 14 rubber condoms filled with cocaine in his rectum before departure from a South American country.

Initially, the patient appeared well. On the day of admission the patient was given oral laxatives and subsequently passed 11 rubber condoms, each containing approximately 20 g of a white powder substance identified as cocaine on toxicologic study. The patient remained asymptomatic that day. In an attempt to induce elimination of the remaining balloons, a tap-water enema was given the next morning. An hour later, agitation, diaphoresis and tachycardia suddenly developed in the patient, followed by a generalized seizure, after which he was apneic with a rapid feeble pulse and hypotension (systolic blood pressure of 90 mmHg; condensed from Jonsson et al, 1983).

With the rising popularity of smokable forms of cocaine ("crack") and amphetamines ("ice"), the possibility of overdose from stimulants increases because users often administer these drugs repeatedly within a short period of time.

Experimental evidence shows that all stimulants acutely block the re-uptake of the monoamine neurotransmitters, and some also cause the release of these chemicals. With prolonged use, there is depletion of neurotransmitters and compensatory up-regulation of receptor numbers, making the systems more sensitive. Treatment of stimulant intoxication with antipsychotics has been suggested, based on neurochemical changes in the brain, but it is preferable to give clinical support and protection. Acidification of the urine is theoretically of value but has not been practically useful in increasing stimulant elimination.

Selected Therapeutic Agents

The following are but a few examples of other drugs that can produce mental disturbances when given in sufficient quantity or to a sensitive person. A more extensive list of agents that cause psychiatric symptoms is found in Table 50–2; note that this list is undoubtedly incomplete, but it can serve as a checklist when a patient presents with psychiatric symptoms.

Digitalis glycosides are one of the very common but frequently overlooked causes of peculiar behavior in elderly adults. The ability of digitalis to induce clouded perception was recognized in 1874 by Duroziez, who called it *delire digitalique*. This case history is but one from hundreds in the literature.

BOX 50–9

CASE: DIGOXIN

A 56-year-old white male . . . [had] an aortic valve replacement. He was discharged 24 days after the operation feeling well, apyrexial, with no evidence of cardiac failure, and mentally normal. Therapy at the time of discharge was digoxin, furosemide, potassium, and coumarin. Two weeks after returning home he became progressively more confused and disoriented, particularly at night, with hallucinations typical of . . . a toxic delirious state. He was restless, paranoid and extremely agitated and there was marked intellectual deterioration. He was readmitted. In view of the absence of congestive cardiac failure, his digoxin and diuretic were stopped . . . Within 24–48 hours his agitation and confusion lessened and he developed insight into his abnormal behavior . . . After one week he had returned to complete normality (Sagel and Matisonn, 1972).

Propranolol has been repeatedly linked to behavioral changes as a result of withdrawal as illustrated by this case.

BOX 50–10

CASE: PROPRANOLOL

A 52-year-old man with no previous history of psychiatric illness was admitted to our inpatient service for evaluation of acute mental status changes. Four days earlier, he had become confused and disoriented. He refused to speak to anyone and began to stare blankly into space. He began to mutter to himself about "going to jail, going to jump in the river." His family described apparent paranoic ideation; the patient talked to them about "someone coming to burn my house down," and despite their reassurances, he was convinced that he would no longer be able to live with them.

The patient's family reported that he had been taking 80 mg/day of propranolol for many weeks until a few days before the change in his behavior, when he abruptly discontinued the medication after "running out of pills."

Upon admisstion, the patient reported seeing bugs crawling over him and the examining physician. His mood was suspicious, hostile and perplexed. Physical examination was remarkable for mildly elevated blood pressure (144/100). The neurology consultation team . . . did not feel that CT scan findings could account for the patient's acute symptomatology.

The patient's mental status began to improve dramatically approximately 12 hours after restarting the propranolol. By the tenth hospital day, the patient was completely back to his baseline (Golden et al, 1989).

TABLE 50–2. Psychiatric Symptoms Produced by Drugs, and a Partial List of the Drugs

Delirium: Ranging From Mild Confusion and Disorientation to Frank
Anticholinergic: antiasthmatic preparations; urinary tract antispasmodics; mydriatric agents; atropine, scopolamine, belladonna alkaloids, trihexyphenidyl, benztropine
Antiparkinsonian: levodopa, SINEMET, amantadine, bromocriptine
Antihistaminics
Phenothiazines
Antidepressants: tricyclic, atypical, and trazodone
Cardiovascular: digitalis glycosides, quinidine, captopril, propranolol, lidocaine, tocainide, clonidine, theophylline, calcium channel blockers, diuretics, atenolol, methyldopa
Opioids: meperidine, pentazocine, propoxyphene
Gastrointestinal: cimetidine, ranitidine, famotidine, metoclopramide
Antiepileptic: phenytoin, barbiturates
Chemotherapeutic: penicillins, cephalosporins, chlorambucil, amphotericin B, cisplatin, chloroquine, chloramphenicol, cycloserine, gentamicin, trimethoprim-sulfamethoxazole, tobramycin, acyclovir, asparaginase
Anti-inflammatory: indomethacin, naproxen, salicylates (chronic)
Miscellaneous: disulfiram, metrizamide, niridazole, podophyllin, folate deficiency, benzodiazepines

Depression
Corticosteroids
Oral contraceptives
Nonsteroidal anti-inflammatory drugs (NSAIDs): naproxen, ibuprofen, indomethacin, phenacetin
Cardiovascular: digitalis glycosides, timolol, methyldopa, propranolol, reserpine, clonidine, prazosin
Thiazide diuretics
Opioids: pentazocine, meperidine
Phenothiazines
Benzodiazepines: diazepam, alprazolam, others
Anti-parkinsonian: levodopa, SINEMET
Gastrointestinal: cimetidine
Others: amitriptyline, disulfiram, phenylephrine, fenfluramine, vinblastine, thyroid hormone deficiency, bromides, asparaginase, trichlormethiazide, folate deficiency, baclofen, cycloserine, isoniazide, theophylline, primaquine

Hallucinations
Those on the Delirium list, plus:
Hallucinogens: (See Table 50–1) lysergic acid diethylamide (LSD), cannabis (marijuana, hashish), ergotamine, phencyclidine (PCP)
Corticosteroids
Opioids: methadone, meperidine, propoxyphene, pentazocine
Benzodiazepines: triazolam, diazepam, clonazepam (and withdrawal therefrom), and related zolpidem
Anticonvulsants: ethosuximide, phenytoin, primidone
Miscellaneous: isocarboxazid, diphenidol, albuterol, dapsone, vincristine, trazodone, thiabendazole, cyclovir, caffeine, pseudoephedrine, phenylephrine, cyclosporine, cycloserine, prazosin

Schizophrenia-like Symptoms
Those on the Hallucinations list plus:
"Stimulants": amphetamines, cocaine
Antiparkinsonian: levodopa, SINEMET, bromocriptine, pergolide
Corticosteroids
Anticholinergic agents
Cardiovascular: reserpine, diuretics, digitalis glycosides
Antiepileptics: phenytoin, carbamazepine
Sedative/hypnotics/benzodiazepines
Miscellaneous: acyclovir, potassium deficiency

Paranoia
(Plus many more under Delirium)
"Stimulants": cocaine, phenylephrine, amphetamines
NSAIDs: ibuprofen, indomethacin, salicylates (chronic), sulindac, naproxen
Cardiovascular: propranolol, albuterol, methyldopa, procainamide, lidocaine
Gastrointestinal: cimetidine
Miscellaneous: baclofen, cycloserine, clonazepam, isoniazid

Quinidine is representative of a large group of agents that are infrequently associated with psychiatric disturbances. Nonetheless, in isolated instances, behavioral changes may be the first sign of toxicity:

BOX 50–11
CASE: QUINIDINE

A 72-year-old woman was hospitalized because of severe memory loss and chronic confusional state of several years' duration. She could not perform household tasks, cope with small amounts of money, remember a shopping list, find her way about indoors or along familiar streets or recall events.

Since suffering acute myocardial infarction 14 years previously, the patient had regularly taken 400 mg of quinidine sulfate and 50 mg of hydrochlorothiazide daily. The results of all laboratory studies—including urinalysis, lipid profile, thyroid profile, blood serologic test, skull x-ray, brain scan, cerebrospinal fluid exam, medial supraorbital telethermometry, serum vitamin B_{12} and magnesium levels and a computerized axial tomographic brain scan—were all normal. The EEG showed a mild and diffuse slowing. On admission the serum sodium level was 125 mEq/liter and the potassium level was 3.3 mEq/liter. Diuretic medication was discontinued on admission . . . and by the fourth day the serum sodium had risen to normal (138 mEq/liter) without any improvement in her mentation.

The patient remained severely confused and disoriented and had vivid nocturnal hallucinations. After the patient had been hospitalized for two weeks without evidencing any improvement, it was elected to discontinue the quinidine. The following day she was greatly improved; within 48 hours she was well oriented for time and place (Gilbert, 1977. Copyright 1977, American Medical Association).

Antihistamines can produce a variety of behavioral disturbances in different individuals. In some they cause drowsiness, in others stimulation, and in others very bizarre effects.

BOX 50–12
CASE: ANTIHISTAMINE

A 3-year-old girl received two 5 ml doses of Actifed (pseudoephedrine and triprolidine) during the night. The following day she suddenly developed episodes of uncontrollable terror, complaining of seeing spiders and insects. On examination she was intermittently pushing and brushing away invisible objects and also hitting out and stamping. The episodes continued intermittently for three days (Sankey et al, 1984).

To what extent the pseudoephedrine or the combination contributed to this response is not known.

Medications that produce orthostatic hypotension in therapeutic doses may also be the cause of any of the following behavioral symptoms: dizziness, confusion, visual difficulties, impotence, or fatigability (Lipsitz, 1989).

So-called "paradoxical drug effects" have been observed with a variety of benzodiazepines and antidepressants as well as with alcohol. Age may well be a critical determinant (Lanius et al, 1994).

Drug-Induced Anxiety

A variety of drugs can produce, precipitate, or aggravate anxiety (Table 50–3). As discussed in Chapter 25 on antianxiety agents, the symptom of anxiety is an almost universal affective and physiological response to threatened or real danger, or the anxiety may consist of unrealistic fears in the absence of apparent stimuli. It is also a common component of such psychiatric syndromes as schizophrenia, paranoia, depression, mania, and many personality disorders. The diagnostic work-up of an individual with symptoms of anxiety mandates that all potential sources of the anxiety be explored, including any drugs the person may be taking. CNS stimulants in particular should be assessed in detail, especially the daily levels of caffeine, because its use is so pervasive.

CAFFEINE. It is widely recognized that there are marked differences in the amounts of caffeine different individuals consume, the corresponding blood levels of caffeine obtained, and the magnitudes of the effects experienced. Some of the obvious factors involved are age, acquired functional and metabolic tolerance, differences in rates of metabolism, and physical dependence. Caffeine predictably produces increased alertness, decreased sleep and sleepiness, insomnia, and increased ability to work out mathematical and cognitive problems. At low doses there is usually an increased sense of well-being and mental capacity. With larger doses irritability may develop into what is commonly called coffee nerves. Physiological tremor is increased, and reflexes are hyperactive; there is also a modest bronchodilating effect.

In the absence of a decrease in caffeine intake, sleep will eventually occur from exhaustion in spite of large doses that may have kept a person awake for up to 24 hours. Overt seizures, however, have occurred only with massive overdoses in some people.

TABLE 50–3. Drugs That Induce Anxiety, Panic, and Central Nervous System Stimulation

Caffeine
Theophylline (*cf* interactions with the numerous drugs that can alter theophylline levels)
Cocaine
Amphetamines
- Amphetamine (formerly BENZEDRINE; now in BIPHETAMINE with dextroamphetamine)
- Dextroamphetamine (DEXEDRINE and others)
- Ephedrine (common ingredient in cold remedies/OTC stimulants, dietary supplements)

Methylphenidate (RITALIN)
Other appetite suppressants
- Diethylproprion
- Phenylpropanolamine (PPA)
- Fenfluramine (more often sedation)

Local anesthetic/antiarrhythmic: lidocaine, procaine, 2-chloroprocaine, tocainide, verapamil
Lactate intravenous infusion (experimental induction of anxiety)
CO_2 (by rebreathing, respiratory insufficiency, or drug-induced, such as with opioids or benzodiazepines
Camphor
Tricyclic antidepressants (jitteriness may be prominent; anxiety upon withdrawal)
Antipsychotics (phenothiazines, haloperidol)
Mianserin (panic anxiety increased after discontinuation)
Benzodiazepines (acute withdrawal after chronic use and acute paradoxical reaction)
Beta carbolines
Fluoxetine (acute vs withdrawal effect)

OTC = over-the-counter.

BOX 50–13
CASE: CAFFEINE

An ambitious 37-year-old Army lieutenant colonel was referred from a medical clinic to a psychiatric outpatient facility because of a two-year history of "chronic anxiety." The symptoms, which occurred almost daily, included dizziness, tremulousness, apprehension about job performance, "butterflies in the stomach," restlessness, frequent episodes of "diarrhea," and persistent difficulty in both falling and remaining asleep.

Three complete medical workups had been negative . . . In reply to questioning from the psychiatrist, he described consuming at least 8–14 cups of coffee a day . . . . he also frequently drank hot cocoa before bedtime . . . and his soft drink preference was exclusively colas (3–4 a day). Total caffeine intake thus approximated 1,200 mg a day.

He was initially unwilling to limit his intake of coffee, cocoa and colas. When symptoms persisted, however, he voluntarily reduced his daily intake of caffeine and four weeks after his initial visit, he reported distinct improvement of his long-standing tremulousness, loose stools and insomnia (Greden, 1974).

Although not well studied, older individuals appear to have an increased sensitivity to the sleep-disturbing effects of caffeine. Probably the major source of individual differences is related to the remarkable extremes in the rates of caffeine metabolism. For some the half-life is only 2 hours, whereas others may show a half-life for caffeine of greater than 15 hours. The longer half-lives are consistent with some individuals' observation that even a cup of coffee at noon or early afternoon may result in difficulty in falling asleep at night. On a population basis, the more rapid metabolizers are those who are the heaviest consumers; the slower metabolizers tend to consume much less.

The sources of caffeine are numerous, yet their intake is all too often not determined or recognized in medical diagnostic assessments. Besides the familiar sources of coffee, cola drinks, and teas, caffeine is found in over-the-counter preparations for pain, colds, asthma, and menstrual symptoms. Diet aids, sleep prevention aids, and noncola soft drinks also may contain significant amounts of caffeine. Caffeine is a primary ingredient in the mail-order "look-alike drugs" sold as energizers, stimulants, "cocaine-like" drugs, herbal remedies and dietary supplements such as "guarana," and enhancers of sexual prowess. Table 50–4 lists the caffeine content of some of the many sources of this substance.

Although caffeine is demonstrably a common cause of anxiety or other disturbances, its effects are often not fully appreciated by the individual outside of the fact that routine coffee drinkers know they need the beverage to get started in the morning. Even patients with extreme insomnia frequently deny that coffee or another caffeinated beverage plays a role in their troubles with sleeping. At least some of the failure to make a connection between caffeine and one's symptoms derives from the fact that as a young adult the person may not have experienced any disruption of mood or sleep from caffeine consumption. The apparent change in

TABLE 50–4. Caffeine Content of Certain Beverages and Drugs

Source	Approximate Amount of Caffeine per Unit (5 oz cup or tablet)
Beverages	
Brewed coffee	80–150 mg
Instant coffee	85–100 mg
Decaffeinated coffee	2–4 mg
Tea (bag or leaf)	30–75 mg
Cocoa	5–40 mg
Cola drinks	35–60 mg*
Nonprescription (OTC) Drugs	
Analgesics	
ANACIN, BROMO-SELTZER, COPE, EMPIRIN compound	32 mg
EXCEDRIN, others	60 mg
Stimulants	
NO DOZ	100 mg
VIVARIN	200 mg
CAFFEDRINE	250 mg
Many cold preparations, proprietary mail-order "look-alikes"	32 mg

From Oakley R: Drugs, Society and Human Behavior, 196. St Louis: CV Mosby Co, 1978.
*12 oz.

sensitivity is possibly related to changes in sleep physiology with age as well as the fact that young adults are often sleep-deprived.

Assessing the impact of caffeine on a person is complicated by the fact that its chronic consumption results not only in tolerance but in physical dependence. The omission of the usual 1 to 4 cups of coffee in the morning in a regular user results in mental sluggishness, feelings of depression, plus an inability to think, write, or carry out cognitive procedures in a coherent manner. A dull, generalized headache and increased irritability appear late in the morning or early afternoon. These symptoms are promptly relieved by ingestion of caffeine, indicating that this is a withdrawal syndrome from a substance the person was physically dependent on. An interesting aspect of caffeine is the occurrence of increased irritability and anxiety both as acute effects and as symptoms of withdrawal.

Caffeine augments and aggravates conditions of anxiety, depression, panic, and mania. In recognition of this, many psychiatric and substance-abuse treatment centers avoid serving any caffeine-containing beverages.

Chemically, caffeine is classified as a methylated xanthine. Another compound in this category is theophylline, which has similar excitatory actions on the CNS as caffeine yet is not as potent. Theophylline is found in various teas and is also used extensively in the clinical treatment of cardiorespiratory disease. Methylxanthines are antagonists of the sedative actions of adenosine. It is thought that the CNS excitation produced by methylxanthines is the consequence of their blockade of adenosine receptors.

OTHER ANXIETY-INDUCING DRUGS. As was previously discussed, cocaine and amphetamine-like drugs may cause anxious behavior and irritability; this can be true even when psychotic-like symptoms are not present. Other drugs that have been known to produce anxiety are shown in Table 50–3. Anxiety is a predictable effect for many of them, such as the local anesthetics, camphor, and the endogenously occurring carbolines. For a number of others, such as antipsychotics, antidepressants, and benzodiazepines, the appearance of anxiety may be unique to the individual, making this possibility easy to overlook in management of patients with psychiatric or chronic medical disease. The source of anxiety in patients with a chronic disease may be confounded by postural hypotension, hypokalemia, or CO_2 retention.

In addition to being an acute drug effect, anxiety is an extremely common component of the withdrawal syndrome for many agents, including benzodiazepines, antidepressants, and alcohol. Except for alcohol, withdrawal syndromes may be delayed for over a week after discontinuation of a drug, so the connection between the anxiety and the discontinuation of one or more drugs is infrequently appreciated. Moreover, withdrawal need not be absolute for anxiety to appear; a reduction in dose or an increase in drug metabolism might be sufficient to evoke such symptoms.

Drugs That Produce Aggression

Human aggression can be thought of as being either appropriate or inappropriate. For example, when people are under physical threat or attack, aggressive self-defense is considered a rational response. Organized sporting events are also situations in which violent behavior is often socially acceptable. On the other hand, when hostility is unprovoked, excessive, or directed at an inappropriate target, it is deemed of concern to society. Hence, the aggression that is produced as a side effect of certain drugs usually indicates inappropriate behavior.

ANABOLIC STEROIDS. During the 1980s, anabolic steroids were brought to the public eye as one class of agents that can produce a broad spectrum of psychological derangements, including aggression. These effects were first utilized by German soldiers during World War II but are experienced today by modern athletes who take these agents primarily to build up muscle strength and dimensions.

Anabolic steroids are chemically derived from the male sex hormone, testosterone. They were developed as drugs that would produce more anabolism than testosterone does yet with a lesser degree of androgenizing effects. Anabolic steroids are used clinically in male hypogonadism and hereditary angioneurotic edema, but it is their nonmedical use by athletes that has drawn attention to their negative side effects. A football player who had been taking massive doses of anabolic steroids reported:

BOX 50–14
CASE: STEROIDS

My aggression level was so high that I got into an argument and went to my locker, put my hand through the metal mesh and ripped the door off its hinges. Then I went back to [my room] and took a baseball bat and demolished my refrigerator, smashed it to pieces and then ripped the phone off the wall. My nerves were on edge like they'd never been before. At practice one day I got into a fight with a linebacker . . . I threw him down . . . and smashed his eye. As he got up, bleeding and humiliated, I felt sympathy for him. But then the steroids kicked in and I said to myself, "All right! You're a tough guy!" (Chaikin and Telander, 1988).

This behavior is widely recognized by users and is referred to as "'roid rage." Anabolic steroid abuse is not restricted to professional athletes; studies indicate that up to 7% of high school students may be using the drugs. In addition to aggression, anabolic steroids are reported to produce a psychotic-like syndrome that can include auditory hallucinations, paranoid delusions, and manic episodes. In addition, chronic users report not only episodes of mania, but depression as well far more commonly than control groups. Immediate discontinuation of the drug is called for should psychiatric symptoms occur, and violent behavior may require behavioral restraint or administration of antipsychotic medications.

CORTICOSTEROIDS. People taking corticosteroids frequently report behavioral changes that may include aggression as well as more severe psychotic symptoms.

BOX 50–15
CASE: CORTICOSTEROIDS

The accused had a congenital malformation of his maxilla for which an operation was necessary. He was given dexamethasone, 8 mg daily for three days from the day before his operation and 4 mg on the fourth day.

During the days [following the operation] he experienced rapid fluctuations of mood, expressed suicidal ideas and attempted to jump from a car . . . Eleven days after the operation . . . he rammed his head forcibly against a wall and attacked his fiancee with . . . a knife. After arrest he struggled violently with the police and repeatedly attempted to commit suicide. He responded to neuroleptics and his psychotic symptoms remitted within 3 days (D'Orban, 1989).

COMMENTS. These case reports and tables demonstrate that it is not possible for anyone to remember all the potential behavioral effects of all drugs. What is feasible is, first, to remember those agents that are the most common or most striking offenders and, second, to establish one's own principles and procedures to follow in evaluating and assessing every patient who presents with a psychiatric symptom.

Without doubt, drugs can produce (frequently unbeknownst to the individual or others) delirium, dementia, psychosis, anxiety, hallucinations, aggression, paranoia, or disturbance of sleep/wakefulness. *Such psychiatric effects of drugs can occur with usual therapeutic doses and blood levels as well as with overdoses; the effects can be acute or chronic.*

Renal Failure

A variety of renal lesions may be found in renal failure associated with drugs. Relatively few of these events have occurred after therapeutic doses for established indications; rather, most reports of drug-induced nephrotoxicity have resulted from overdoses from suicide attempts or self-medication (Table 50–5). Nevertheless, a wide variety of agents have been reported to be associated with renal failure; in addition to those listed in Table 50–5 are antineoplastic agents such as methotrexate and asparaginase, carbamazepine, allopurinol, and captopril as well as diuretic agents known to alter kidney function.

TABLE 50–5. Examples of Some Drugs Reported to Produce Renal Failure—When Used in Excessive Doses

Myoglobinuric Tubular Necrosis
Amphetamine, cocaine, strychnine
Alcohol, barbiturates, glutethimide, benzodiazepines
Heroin, methadone
Phencyclidine
Phenylpropanolamine
Amoxapine, doxepin
Chronic Interstitial Nephritis (Analgesic Nephropathy)
Acetaminophen
Nonsteroidal anti-inflammatory drugs
Thiazides
Sulfonamides
Ciprofloxacin
Acute Tubular Necrosis
Acetaminophen, aspirin
Boric acid
Bismuth salts
Colchicine
Lead
Hypercalcemia
Vitamin A
Vitamin D
Oxalosis
Intravenous Vitamin C

Adapted from Abuelo JG: Renal failure caused by chemicals, foods, plants, animal venoms, and misuse of drugs. Arch Intern Med 150:505–510, 1990, copyright 1990, American Medical Association.

Chronic interstitial nephritis can be produced by nonsteroidal anti-inflammatory drugs such as acetaminophen, as initially extensively studied in abusers of phenacetin (a precursor of acetaminophen).

A relatively common cause of acute renal failure associated with drug use is rhabdomyolysis. A variety of agents and conditions have been implicated including alcohol, cocaine, malignant hyperthermia, and malignant neuroleptic syndrome, and pressure necrosis from lying in one position during coma caused by alcohol, barbiturates, and other drugs. Excessive muscular activity associated with hazing, phencyclidine, amphetamine, and cocaine can result in hyperthermia as well as rhabdomyolysis.

Nephrotoxins also occur extensively in plants, herbal medicines, and some foods; a large number of chemical substances are known to have the potential to produce kidney damage.

General Comments Regarding Adverse Drug Reactions

This chapter has illustrated the therapeutic relevance of considering adverse drug reactions, not only by drug and drug class, but by the nature of the reaction, such as psychiatric symptoms or renal failure. Other classes of reactions could have been addressed with equal merit; for example, the serious unpredictable reaction of agranulocytosis (Young, 1994) and high blood pressure (Grossman and Messerli,

1995), as well as numerous other types of reactions and agents, such as the burgeoning use of "dietary supplements" of unknown composition.

DRUG INTERACTIONS

Drug interactions refer usually to adverse effects associated with more than one drug; these adverse reactions may occur with concomitant use and be associated with some prior exposure that results in an allergy.

Allergy and Drugs

Idiosyncrasy and genetic individuality in drug responses must be distinguished from allergy, or hypersensitivity. Allergy to a drug must be developed, in contrast to intolerance and idiosyncrasy which are both pre-existing states. The capacity to develop an allergy pre-exists, but for the allergic state to develop an individual must have prior exposure to the drug. Thus, to understand allergy, one must understand the underlying immunological principles that govern both the development of the condition and the production of symptoms.

Immune Response

Allergy or hypersensitivity is the result of an immune response to a drug or preparation. As in any immune response, the substance is recognized by the immune system as foreign. That is, the compound is seen as antigenic. Once this occurs, a portion of the drug becomes sequestered into the lymphatics of the host, is processed immunologically, and evokes the production of two types of effectors—specific antibodies will be produced against the antigen by B lymphocytes, and specifically sensitized effector cells (T lymphocytes) will be elaborated in large numbers. Both the B and the T lymphocytes are precommitted to the structure on the drug molecule with which they react. In the case of a large complex molecule, as many drugs are, several different structures may be recognized by different precommitted T and B cells. The point is that as many different structures as possible are detected as foreign, and hence the response is polyclonal. More than one precommitted precursor cell can respond to different parts of the molecule, each capable of reaction with one small portion of the foreign molecule. That is, a normal immune response has multiple specificities within it. The antigen, in turn, is a mosaic of different substructures that give rise to a spectrum of specificities. The word "epitope" has been coined to describe each individual structure that has been identified. The totality of the epitopes makes up the antigen.

During a normal immune response, both humoral (antibody-mediated) and cellular immunity are evoked. This is also the case with allergy. After exposure to the antigen (allergen), a period ensues during which an immune response is being mounted but no symptoms appear (the lag period). After this time, IgM antibodies begin to appear in the serum of the individual. These are soon replaced by antibodies of the same specificity but of different chain structure. *The cells producing antibody undergo what is known as a switch from IgM to the other classes of antibody: IgG, IgA, and IgE. It is the IgE that is involved in allergy for reasons that are described later.* None of the other antibody classes has been shown to be responsible for allergy.

Molecules below a certain size are generally not recognized by the immune system as foreign. For example, proteins with molecular weights below approximately 10,000 do not evoke an immune response. Yet many drugs are recognized as foreign even though their molecules are quite small. This phenomenon is due to what is known as the hapten effect; some drugs are haptens. Many drugs have the capacity to bind to constituents of the blood. For example, penicillin binds to human serum albumin and erythrocytes. By so binding, the penicillin, in some individuals, causes a distortion of the normal structure of albumin or the erythrocyte membrane, or both. The distorted albumin or membrane is now recognized by the recipient as foreign and no longer self. During the immune response that follows, the penicillin forms an epitope on the larger structure and antibodies are produced both to the penicillin and to the altered host component. The altered host component has become a carrier for the hapten penicillin. The important point here is that after antibody has once been formed, the carrier is not required for reaction of the antipenicillin antibodies with penicillin to occur.

Some drugs are antigenic by themselves. As might be expected, these are usually large molecules. In general, the more complex the molecule, the more readily it will evoke an immune response. In addition, although any drug can be responsible for evoking allergy, some drugs have a much higher propensity to produce hypersensitivity than others. Drugs that are chemically reactive are more likely to sensitize a person than those that are less reactive.

The Patient's Role in Hypersensitivity

The other side of hypersensitivity is the patient. Some individuals are much more likely to develop allergy than others. Such persons are said to be *atopic*, and their condition is termed *atopy*. As a rule, individuals with many known allergies are more likely to develop allergies to drugs than are those who have no such history. Such individuals can be detected only by a careful history. The importance of a thorough history cannot be overstated.

Nevertheless, in spite of careful questioning many patients deny exposure to a substance that is, in fact, responsible for the allergic attack. For example, a patient develops an untoward reaction to injected penicillin, yet denies ever having received the drug. Two possible explanations for this are: (1) The drug was administered at an early age and the person was not informed. (2) Many food animals are routinely fed rations containing prophylactic antibiotics. Milk that contains penicillin is produced by cows that are treated for mastitis with the drug.

Immediate and Delayed Hypersensitivity

Hypersensitivity is divided into two types: immediate and delayed. *Immediate hypersensitivity* is so called because the reaction occurs within a period of minutes to hours. The state is due to IgE antibodies that have been produced through prior exposure to the allergen. Immediate hypersensitivity can manifest itself in many forms. The most severe form is a complete collapse of a patient into shock within minutes of administration of the drug (anaphylaxis). This usually occurs with administration of the drug by a route that maximizes the uptake of the drug, such as intravenously or by inhalation. Fortunately, anaphylaxis is a relatively uncommon event. Hypersensitivity is manifested more generally in organ systems other than the vascular compartment. Rashes, urticaria (giant hives), wheezing, photosensitivity, and gastrointestinal symptoms are the more common manifestations of allergy. Fever may accompany the administration of an offending drug. The so-called drug fever is typically a low-grade fever that waxes and wanes in synchrony with taking the drug. The fever may not develop for several days, but when it appears it may increase incrementally as more drug is taken. Cessation of a low-grade fever following discontinuation of a drug is good evidence that allergy is involved.

The role of IgE antibodies in immediate hypersensitivity is certain. (The role of other antibodies is doubtful; although a role for some subclasses of IgG has been postulated, evidence is lacking.) IgE antibodies are known to bind to mast cells and circulating basophilic granulocytes. They do so by virtue of a receptor on these cells that specifically binds to the Fc portion of the IgE antibody molecule. This leaves each mast cell with a bound layer of IgE antibodies oriented with the Fc bound to the membrane and the Fab portion of the antibody free to react with allergen (epitope). Each mast cell carries IgE antibodies of all the specificities present in a given individual. That is, a statistical representation of antibodies to all the substances that an individual is allergic to is distributed among her or his mast cells.

The atopic individual, then, after becoming immunized, carries IgE antibodies bound to mast cells. At low concentrations of IgE, there is little problem, even when the allergen is introduced into the patient. However, as exposure to the allergen continues, the amount of IgE increases, just as in any other immune response. At a certain critical concentration, when an allergen encounters a mast cell, it is able to react with the Fab portion of two IgE molecules that are side by side on the cell surface, both having specificity for that particular allergen. When this occurs, a signal is transduced through the membrane, causing the mast cell to degranulate. Degranulation in turn leads to the release of pharmacologically active compounds that produce the symptoms of the allergic reaction.

The list of mediators released by mast cells is prodigious and continues to grow. The major mediators are histamine, eosinophil chemotactic factor (ECF), slow-reacting substance of anaphylaxis (SRS-A), platelet-activating factor (PAF), and heparin. Secondarily, serotonin, prostaglandins, and kinins of many specificities are elaborated. The net effect of these mediators is the induction of smooth muscle contraction, increased vascular permeability, hypersecretion of glands, and alterations in blood coagulability. Subsequently, physiological alterations that include hypoxia, necrosis, hemorrhage, and shock result. The exact symptoms exhibited by the patient depend on the organ in which the release has occurred. In humans, most organs are rich in mast cells; thus, the so-called shock organ can be almost any organ. The route of exposure often determines which organ will manifest allergic symptoms. The term shock organ simply refers to that organ in which the allergic reaction occurs for a given species of animal. For example, the bronchioles of the lung in a guinea pig are more richly endowed with mast cells than is any other organ of the animal. When challenged, an allergic guinea pig will exhibit pulmonary distress; a dog will show liver failure. Humans have rich accumulations of mast cells in virtually every major organ, and almost any one can be the shock organ.

Delayed hypersensitivity, sometimes referred to as cell-mediated hypersensitivity, is mediated by T lymphocytes and normally requires 36–48 hours to develop. The classic model for delayed hypersensitivity is the tuberculin response, which requires 2–3 days to develop a skin lesion after challenge with purified protein derivative (PPD). This limb of the immune response is due to T lymphocytes that are specific for the allergen. As in humoral hypersensitivity, precommitted T cells undergo a clonal expansion caused by exposure to the allergen. These cells are then distributed throughout the lymphatics. When allergen is introduced into a hypersensitized individual, the T cells, through a poorly understood signaling system, migrate to the area where the allergen is located. Here, they react with the allergen by means of a specific receptor and begin to secrete a series of mediators collectively known as lymphokines. The lymphokines have an effect on both tissue and circulating cells. As a result of their release, inflammation ensues. The delay in reaction is due to the time required for the T cells to migrate into the offending area of allergen. *In a given individual both immediate and delayed hypersensitivity may occur sequentially.*

Diagnosis

The diagnosis of allergy can be difficult. The concentration of IgE in an individual's serum can be helpful, but often is uninformative. More difficult still can be the identification of the offending substance. Patients may be taking more than one drug. They may be taking a drug that they do not report. There are a few testing methods: Skin testing by challenging is commonly used as a screening method. Weak dilutions of common or suspected allergens are placed on the skin, and a needle is used to scratch the skin beneath the drop of allergen solution. If IgE antibodies to the allergen are bound to the mast cells in the individual's skin, a wheal and flare reaction will occur within a few minutes. This is typically a reddening of the skin and induration at the site of challenge.

Tests for specific IgE are now available. The most widely used is the radioallergosorbent test (RAST). In this assay, the serum of the patient is mixed with allergen in a test tube. The allergen is usually bound to a particle or is otherwise made insoluble. If antibody is present, it will bind to the allergen. Note that both IgE and IgG are bound by this procedure. The bead is then washed to remove unbound protein, and the amount of IgE present is estimated by treating with a radiolabeled antibody to human IgE that does not cross-react with IgG. Such examinations are usually made against large panels of known allergens and require only small amounts of a patient's serum.

Treatment

What should be done if one suspects that a patient is allergic to a drug? If the patient is currently taking the drug, it should be immediately discontinued until evidence is available that the drug is not an allergen to this individual. If the history suggests that the person is allergic to a drug, change to a different drug. The use of any drug should be balanced against its potential for harm. Once a patient is hypersensitive, he or she should be considered hypersensitive for life. There is at present no method for reversing hypersensitivity in any individual. In general, the reactions begin as mild skin manifestations, but they grow progressively more severe with continued challenge.

In particular situations—for example, a construction worker who has become severely allergic to wasp venom—attempts can be made to *desensitize* the individual. This is done by repeated injections of venom into the individual, beginning with a highly diluted preparation that evokes no untoward reaction. Over time, the injections are continued using increasing concentrations of venom, until such time that an undiluted injection is tolerated, at least reasonably well. It might seem paradoxical that to extinguish an allergy, injections of the offending allergen are used, but some amount of success has been achieved with this method. Why the method works is difficult to explain. The commonest, and probably most accepted explanation maintains that the secondary IgE response is feeble and the bulk of antibodies produced are IgG. Thus, the idea is to take advantage of the brisk secondary production of IgG, which then competes for the allergen before it can reach the IgE bound to mast cells (see Chapter 17).

Hemolytic Anemia

Although hemolytic anemia is not strictly an allergic response, it is a manifestation of antibodies produced against a given drug. The antibodies in these cases are not IgE but rather IgG and IgM. The drug binds to the patient's erythrocytes and serum proteins as described previously. Antibodies that can react with the erythrocyte-bound drug are then evoked. Complement may be activated as well. In either case the presence of immunoglobulin or complement components causes a shortened lifespan of the antibody-coated cells, which are prematurely removed by the reticuloendothelial system. Antibodies specific for red cell antigens may also be evoked.

Only a proportion of patients with antibody to drugs will develop a hemolytic anemia severe enough to require treatment, and the condition may be entirely overlooked in the absence of symptoms. In fact, the majority of patients who develop a positive antiglobulin test do not have decreased red cell survival times. When the condition is suspected, however, the diagnostic test of choice is a direct Coombs (antiglobulin) test on the patient's erythrocytes. A positive direct Coombs test is highly correlated with hemolytic anemia caused by drugs but is not associated invariably with it. For example, methadone may cause the development of a positive Coombs test but is not associated with hemolytic anemia. Table 50-6 lists some drugs that cause positive direct antiglobulin tests and that are also associated with hemolytic anemia. This table lists only the most well-documented offenders.

Most cases of drug-induced, antibody-mediated hemolytic anemia can be resolved by merely discontinuing the drug. In some instances, however, when the drug is stopped, the hemolytic episode persists, even after the drug is undetectable.

More detailed information regarding specific drugs and the management of reported allergic manifestations can be found in Anderson (1992).

TABLE 50-6. Some Drugs That Cause Positive Direct Antiglobulin Tests and That Are Associated With Hemolytic Anemia

α-Methyldopa	*p*-Aminosalicylate
Cephalothin	Penicillin
Chlorpromazine	Phenacetin
Chlorpropamide	Aminopyrine
Dipyrone	Quinidine
Insulin	Quinine
Isoniazid	Stibophen
Mefenamic acid	Streptomycin
Melphalan	Sulfonamides

Drug-Drug Interactions

Drug-drug interactions may involve diagnostic, prophylactic, or therapeutic drugs. Moreover, some drugs may interfere with diagnostic tests. Although some drug interactions are deliberately sought by the physician because they are advantageous, such as in the use of antagonists in poisonings, the majority of drug interactions are unplanned, and most (but certainly not all) drug interactions are disadvantageous. When a disadvantageous, or adverse, drug interaction has occurred or is likely to occur, the physician may choose to (1) discontinue one (or both) of the drugs; (2) modify the dose of one (or both) of the drugs; or (3) continue without change, despite the potential for actual interaction, if the benefit clearly outweighs the risk.

Although an adverse drug interaction is potentially a problem whenever any two drugs are given in close time proximity, *situations in which the probability of important drug-drug or drug-food interactions are likely to occur or be unappreciated are:*

1. Whenever starting or changing therapy
2. Whenever a new physician takes over responsibility for a patient
3. Whenever a therapeutic regimen fails to have an expected beneficial effect or has resulted in an unexpected adverse effect.

Types and Mechanisms of Drug-Drug Interactions

Because the number of possible drug-drug and drug-food interactions is astronomical, the only practical way to deal with the potentially frequent problems is:

- Have immediately available for consultation a resource that lists all the known interactions (see Chapter 62).
- Possess an understanding of the main types and mechanisms of drug interactions.

The different types and mechanisms of interactions are presented in relation to the time course of events following the administration of a drug. Each of these types is illustrated by a few of many possible examples.

INCOMPATIBILITIES IN INTRAVENOUS SOLUTIONS. Examples: Mixing tetracyclines and sulfonamides may cause the latter to precipitate. Methicillin and ampicillin are easily degraded in the presence of drugs affecting the pH, whereas chloramphenicol and tetracyclines often inactivate other drugs in the intravenous (IV) solution. Carbenicillin and gentamicin interact in the IV solution with loss of activity (direct chemical reaction between the two drugs). Among the general caveats is the undesirability of mixing solutions containing proteins with other solutions. Therefore, before modifying any IV solutions, consult a definitive, up-to-date manual on IV solutions and compatibilities, such as the Handbook on Injectable Drugs.

INTERACTION IN THE GASTROINTESTINAL TRACT. Examples: Foods in the gastrointestinal tract may increase, decrease, or have no effect on the absorption of specific drugs (Table 50–7). A constipating or laxative drug may increase or decrease, respectively, absorption of another drug. Some antibiotics alter vitamin K synthesis by gut flora, which can result in an increase in the effect of oral anticoagulants (Table 50–8). Some antibiotics, especially erythromycin, alter the bacterial degradation of digoxin. Cholestyramine can bind a variety of acidic drugs and thus interfere with their absorption. A number of drugs may alter intestinal absorption of other drugs; for example the intestinal absorption of levothyroxine is impaired by aluminum hydroxide, sucralfate, lovastatin, and ferrous sulfate (reviewed by Watts and Blevins, 1994).

DIRECT INTERACTION IN THE BLOOD AND ADJACENT COMPARTMENTS. Examples: Neutralization of a venin by an antivenin; antagonism of heparin by protamine by direct chemical reaction; treatment of severe digitalis intoxication by use of a neutralizing antibody, or its Fab fragment.

INTERACTIONS INVOLVING PLASMA PROTEINS. Examples: Warfarin and phenylbutazone are both largely bound to albumin in the plasma. Phenylbutazone can therefore displace warfarin from its binding sites and increase warfarin's effect. Other examples of displacement reactions identify some important displa*cers*—phenylbutazone, indomethacin, tolbutamide, and amiodarone. Among important displa*cees* are warfarin, phenytoin, and tolbutamide.

INTERFERENCE WITH THE DISTRIBUTION OR STORAGE OF ONE DRUG BY ANOTHER. Examples: A decrease in uptake of ^{131}I by the thyroid gland in the presence of large doses of stable iodine or iodine-containing contrast media; quinidine-induced decreased binding of digoxin in peripheral tissues results in increased digoxin levels in plasma.

INTERACTION AT THE RECEPTOR. Examples: competitive and allosteric antagonism at the receptor, such as the antagonism of the effect of morphine by naloxone. Potassium depletion (corticosteroids, diuretics, amphotericin B, diarrhea, poor potassium intake, and so on) increases the reactivity to cardiac glycosides and to neuromuscular blocking agents, a result probably mediated by interactions at their

TABLE 50–7. Examples of Reported Food Effects on Absorption of Drugs From the Gastrointestinal Tract (Selected Drugs)*

Some Drugs Whose Absorption Is:			
Decreased by Food	***Increased by Food***	***Not Affected by Food***	***Increased or Decreased Depending on Preparation***
Alcohol	Carbamazepine	Prednisone	Theophylline
Aspirin	Phenytoin	Procainamide	Erythromycin
Ibuprofen	Diazepam	Verapamil	
Diclofenac	Dicoumarol		
Piroxicam	Diftalone		
Cimetidine	Erythromycin estolate		
Digoxin	Erythromycin ethyl succinate		
Hydrocortisone	Erythromycin stearate		
Levodopa	Nitrofurantoin		
Methyldopa	Griseofulvin		
Metronidazole	Hydralazine		
Nafcillin	8-Methoxsalen		
Penicillin G	Metoprolol		
Penicillin V	Labetalol		
Ampicillin	Propranolol		
Amoxicillin	Spironolactone		
Isoniazid	Chlorothiazide		
Rifampin	Itraconazole		
Cefaclor			
Cephalexin			
Ketoconazole			
Sulfonamides			
Tetracycline			
Doxycycline			
Erythromycin stearate (film-coated tablets)			
Sotalol			
Atenolol			
Tacrine			

*See also Winstanley PA, Orme ML. The effects of food on drug bioavailability. Br J Clin Pharmacol 28:621–628, 1989.

TABLE 50–8. Drug-Vitamin Interactions

Drug	Vitamin	Possible Mechanism	Possible Manifestation
Antibiotics, sulfa drugs, PABA	Vitamin K	Decreased vitamin K from intestinal bacterial metabolism	Hypoprothrombinemia
Anticonvulsants	Folic acid	Decreased absorption of folacin; competitive inhibition of dehydrofolate reductase; enzyme reduction	Megaloblastic anemia
	Vitamin D	Enzyme induction	Rickets; osteomalacia
	Vitamin K	Enzyme induction	Neonatal hemorrhage
Cholestyramine	Folic acid	Complexing of the vitamin	
	Vitamin B_{12}	Inhibition of intrinsic factor function	
	Vitamin A	Binding of bile salts	Osteomalacia
	Vitamin D	Binding of bile salts	Osteomalacia
	Vitamin K	Binding of bile salts	Osteomalacia
Colchicine	Vitamin B_{12}	Malabsorption of B_{12}	
Coumarin anticoagulants	Vitamin K	Antagonism	Hemorrhage
Estrogen-containing oral contraceptives	Folic acid	Inhibition of absorption of folic acid; increased synthesis of folate-binding macroglobulin	Megaloblastic anemia
	Vitamin B_{12}	Enzyme induction	
	Vitamin B_6	Pyridoxine deficiency; competition for vitamin-binding sites	Depression
	Riboflavin		Deficiency
	Thiamin		Deficiency
	Vitamin C	Decreased absorption	Scurvy symptoms
Hydralazine	Vitamin B_6	Increased excretion of vitamin-drug complex	Peripheral neuropathy
Irritant cathartics	Vitamin D	Increased peristalsis; damage to the intestinal wall	Osteomalacia
Isoniazid	Vitamin B_6	Increased excretion of vitamin-drug complex; clinically effective antagonist of isoniazid toxicity	Peripheral neuropathy; generalized convulsion (infants); anemia
	Niacin	Competitive inhibition of vitamin coenzymes; secondary to vitamin B_6 deficiency	Pellagra
Levodopa	Pyridoxine	Antagonism by increasing rate of amino acid decarboxylation; note that carbidopa, as in SINEMET, inhibits this action of pyridoxine	Levodopa ineffective
Methotrexate	Folate	Inhibition of dihydrofolate reductase enzyme	Megaloblastic anemia
Mineral oil	Vitamin A	Lipid solvent	Rickets; osteomalacia in elderly
	Vitamin D	Lipid solvent	
	Vitamin K	Lipid solvent	
Neomycin	Vitamin B_{12}	Damage to the intestinal wall; inhibition of intrinsic factor function	
	Vitamin A	Damage to the intestinal wall; inhibition of pancreatic lipase; binding of bile salts	
Nitrous oxide (chronic)	Vitamin B_{12}	Block of B_{12} action	Megaloblastic anemia, blood dyscrasias
Potassium chloride	Vitamin B_{12}	Decreased ileal pH	
Pyrimethamine	Folic acid	Inhibition of dihydrofolate reductase enzyme	Megaloblastic anemia
Salicylates	Folic acid	Decreased protein binding of folate	Deficiency
	Vitamin C	Decreased tissue uptake	Deficiency
	Vitamin K	Antagonism	Increased bleeding
Sulfasalazine	Folic acid	Decreased absorption of folic acid	
Tetracycline	Vitamin C	Decreased tissue levels of vitamin C	
	Niacin	Decreased absorption with deficiency of niacin	
Triamterene	Folic acid	Inhibition of dihydrofolate reductase	Megaloblastic anemia
Trimethoprim	Folic acid	Inhibition of dihydrofolate reductase	Megaloblastic anemia

PABA = para-aminobenzoic acid.

receptors. Halogenated hydrocarbon anesthetics may increase the cardiac arrhythmic effects of catecholamine.

MODIFICATION OF THE METABOLISM OF ONE DRUG BY ANOTHER

Inhibition of Metabolism. Examples: Isoniazid inhibits metabolism of phenytoin. Allopurinol inhibits metabolism of azathioprine and 6-mercaptopurine. Ethanol inhibits the metabolism of diazepam. Caffeine inhibits the metabolism of phenylpropanolamine (PPA). Cimetidine inhibits the metabolism of warfarin, diazepam, theophylline, and other drugs.

MAO inhibitors reduce the metabolism of serotonin, thus making any drug that acts via serotonin potentially toxic, such as dextromethorphan, clomipramine, fluoxetine, paroxetine, or meperidine (Nierenberg and Seniprebon, 1993), a serious interaction that can present weeks after the MAO inhibitor is discontinued; combinations of any in the latter group also cause the "serotonin syndrome." Other examples involving inhibition of metabolism are the alcohol-disulfiram (ANTABUSE) reaction. Disulfiram inhibits the metabolism of ethanol such that acetaldehyde levels rise to levels that cause a number of unpleasant and undesirable symptoms. (A variety of drugs other than disulfiram, including metronidazole and some cephalosporins, may cause this reaction.)

A special case of inhibition of *first-pass metabolism* is now being recognized. Such metabolism can take place in the intestines or in the liver. A recent chance finding lead to the discovery that grapefruit juice could produce a considerable increase in the bioavailability of a number of calcium channel blockers (felodipine, nitrendipine, nifedipine; Bailey et al, 1994; Table 50-9) as well as terfenadine, cyclosporine, caffeine, and probably a number of other substances as well. This interaction appears to be quite variable and unpredictable among different individuals. *Thus patients generally should be cautioned to avoid grapefruit juice while taking a variety of drugs.* Grapefruit juice appears to contain a substance that inhibits oxidative enzymes including 11-β-hydroxysteroid dehydrogenase. The effects of grapefruit juice on first-pass metabolism may parallel those of erythromycin.

Enzyme Induction. Examples: Barbiturates or a diet rich in Brussels sprouts increases the hepatic metabolism of warfarin. In addition many drugs are inducers of drug metabolism, and many drugs besides warfarin are affected.

MODIFICATION OF THE EXCRETION OF ONE DRUG BY ANOTHER. Examples: Excretion of phenobarbital is increased after administration of a systemic alkalinizing drug because of ionic trapping; probenecid competes with penicillin for renal excretion; cimetidine competes with procainamide for renal excretion; quinidine decreases renal clearance of digoxin.

ADDITION OF EFFECTS OR SIDE EFFECTS OF EACH DRUG; COMBINATION EFFECTS. Examples: Additive central nervous system depression results in a patient who takes a benzodiazepine while consuming alcohol. These additive effects can be illustrated by a number of drug effects, such as the additive effects on anticoagulation by aspirin plus warfarin; the potential heart block with verapamil plus a β-adrenergic blocking drug; hypotension produced by enalapril or captopril plus a vasodilating drug; the additional chemotherapeutic effects that may be achieved with penicillin plus an aminoglycoside against streptococcal infections; the increased neuromuscular block produced by a curarizing drug plus an aminoglycoside; the increased risk of ototoxicity with ethacrynic acid plus an aminoglycoside; increased cardiac work after methamphetamine and ethanol (Table 50-10).

SUBTRACTION IN DRUG EFFECTS. Examples: Normal serum potassium concentration is preserved in the presence of a potassium-losing diuretic by the simultaneous administration of a potassium-sparing diuretic; the anticoagulant effects with an oral contraceptive with warfarin; the decrease in the emetic effects of cisplatin by metoclopramide.

CROSS-REACTIONS

Allergic Cross-Reactions. These were discussed earlier in this chapter. Examples: Allergic cross-reactions to thiazide diuretics — furosemide or sulfonylureas — occur in a patient allergic to sulfonamides or a patient allergic to penicillin may have a cross-reaction to a chemically similar compound such as cephalosporin.

Pharmacological Cross-Reactions. Examples: A patient hyperreactive or intolerant to morphine is at risk of having a cross-reaction to a pharmacologically similar compound such as meperidine.

Cross-Tolerance. Examples: Tolerance to meperidine may occur in a patient tolerant to morphine or any morphine agonist; cross-tolerance among benzodiazepines and to benzodiazepines may be seen in those who consume large quantities of alcohol.

Drug antagonism is the basis for many of the treatments of poisonings and overdoses. These are covered in Chapters 46 and 47 on toxicology and poisoning.

Drug-Food Interactions

The effects of foods on drug absorption have been discussed briefly earlier (Table 50-7). Looked at from the other direction, drugs interact with foods and nutrition along analogous

TABLE 50-9. Some Selected Drug-Food Interactions

Drug	Food	Adverse Interaction
Calcium antagonists (felodipine, nifedipine, nitrendipine); terfenadine; caffeine	Grapefruit juice	Increased bioavailability; inhibition of first-pass metabolism; increased toxicity
MAO inhibitors	Foods containing tyramine (liver, pickled herring, cheese, bananas, avocados, soup, beer, wine, yogurt, sour cream, yeast, nuts)	Palpitations, headache, hypertensive crises
Digitalis	Licorice	Digitalis toxicity
Griseofulvin	Fatty foods	Increased blood levels of griseofulvin
Timed-release drug preparations	Alcoholic beverages	Increased rate of release for some
Lithium	Decreased sodium intake	Lithium toxicity
Quinidine	Antacids and alkaline diet (alkaline urine)	Quinidine toxicity
Thiazide diuretics	Carbohydrates	Elevated blood sugar
Tetracyclines	Dairy products high in calcium; ferrous sulfate; or antacids	Impaired absorption of tetracycline
Vitamin B_{12} (cyanocobalamin)	Vitamin C — large doses	Precipitate B_{12} deficiency
Fenfluramine	Vitamin C addition	Antagonism of antiobesity effect of fenfluramine
Thiamine	Blueberries, fish	Foods containing thiaminases
	Alcohol	Decreased intake, absorption, utilization
Benzodiazepines	Caffeine	Antagonism of antianxiety action

MAO = monoamine oxidase.

TABLE 50–10. Summary of Adverse Interactions of Drugs with Alcoholic Beverages

Drug	Adverse Effect With Alcohol
Anesthetics, antihistamines, barbiturates, benzodiazepines, chloral hydrate, meprobamate, narcotics, phenothiazines, tricyclic antidepressants	1. Increased central nervous system depression due to additive effects 2. Decreased sedative or anesthetic effects with chronic use due to tolerance
Phenothiazines	Increased extrapyramidal effects, drug-induced parkinsonism
Diazepam (VALIUM)	Increased diazepam blood levels, varying with beverage
Amphetamines and cocaine	Increased cardiac work; possible increase in probability of cerebrovascular accident
Calcium channel antagonists—felodipine, verapamil, nifedipine	Increased bioavailability; possible toxicity
Acetaminophen (TYLENOL), others	Hepatotoxicity
Anticoagulants	Chronic—decreased anticoagulant effect Acute—increased anticoagulant effect
Bromocriptine	Nausea, abdominal pain (due to increased dopamine-receptor sensitivity?)
Disulfiram (ANTABUSE), chloramphenicol, oral hypoglycemics, cephalosporins, metronidazole, quinacrine, moxalactam	Disulfiram-alcohol syndrome reactions
Cycloserine	Increased seizures with chronic use
Imipramine (see also above)	Lower blood level with chronic alcohol consumption
Isoniazid	Increased hepatitis incidence, decreased isoniazid effects in chronic alcohol use due to increased metabolism
Propranolol (INDERAL)	Decreased tremor of alcohol withdrawal; decreased propranolol blood levels
Sotalol	Increased sotalol blood levels
Phenytoin (DILANTIN)	Decreased metabolism with acute combination with alcohol; but increased metabolism with chronic alcohol consumption; increased risk of folate deficiency
Nonsteroidal anti-inflammatory agents (aspirin and related)	Increased gastrointestinal bleeding

dimensions to drug-drug interactions. In fact, many foods are also drugs, *eg*, fatty acids (Dannenberg and Reidenberg, 1994). In addition, drugs can alter the nutritional effects of a variety of foods including vitamins. Drugs also frequently alter food palatability, appetite, and consumption. Some drugs directly affect taste (see Chapter 13), whereas others appear to influence appetite and consumption—either to increase or to decrease (Table 50–11). These effects have been used in therapy, for example to induce anorexia in obesity (see Chapter 26). Note that some drugs appear to cause an increased appetite in some patients and a decreased appetite in others.

TABLE 50–11. Drugs That Modify Appetite and Food Intake

Suppress
Numerous drugs that evoke nausea or vomiting (approximately 75% of all oral agents)
Appetite suppressants:* amphetamines, diethylpropion, fenfluramine, mazindol, phenmetrazine, phentermine
Antiepileptics
Antineoplastic agents
Carbonic anhydrase inhibitors
Cardio-renal: digitalis glycosides, thiazides, procainamide
Endocrine: estrogens
Psychotropic: benzodiazepines, lithium, MAO inhibitors
NSAIDs: indomethacin
Antiparkinsonian: levodopa
Chemotherapeutic: metronidazole, tetracyclines
Oral hypoglycemic agents
Also, experimentally, opioids, inosine, cholecystokinin

Stimulate
Endocrine: androgens, corticosteroids, hypoglycemic agents, oral contraceptives
Antihistamines and antiserotoninergic agents
Psychotropic: benzodiazepines, lithium, phenothiazines and related agents, tricyclic antidepressants
Cannabinoids: marijuana, dronabinol

*Drugs that have had some use in the treatment of obesity (see Chapter 26).
MAO = monoamine oxidase; NSAIDs = nonsteroidal anti-inflammatory drugs.

The tables of numerous drug-food interactions illustrate the importance of a full dietary history; all diagnostic histories should include information about the previous few days as well as the intake in relation to medications. Such a diet history should include all intake—including multivitamins (Table 50–8), aspirin, laxatives, snacks of all kinds, all beverages including alcoholic beverages—as well as information regarding the pattern and variability in eating habits and dietary supplements.

The major useful generalization regarding the interactions of foods and drugs is that they do occur, that they can be clinically significant, and that individuals vary in terms of their responses to specific doses of specific drugs and in terms of the impact of food and its consumption on drug effects and conversely (Table 50–9). Careful attention to potential interactions among foods and drugs is especially warranted:

1. When consumption is characterized by any large excesses.
2. When there is a marked change in food intake.
3. When any nutrient or class of nutrients is absent from the diet.
4. Whenever starting or changing therapy.
5. Whenever a new physician takes over responsibility for a patient.
6. Whenever a therapeutic regimen fails to have an expected beneficial effect or has resulted in an unexpected adverse effect.

Some view alcoholic beverages as a food, others emphasize that alcohol is a drug. From either point of view, alcohol consumption has a number of important interactions with drugs (Table 50–10).

REFERENCES

For more specific references, see Chapters 59 and 62 in Smith CM and Reynard AM: Textbook of Pharmacology. Philadelphia: WB Saunders Co, 1992, and the reviews listed.

Abed RT, Clark PJ: Acute psychotic episode caused by the abuse of phensedyl. Br J Psychiatry 151:868, 1987.

Abuelo JG: Renal failure caused by chemicals, foods, plants, animal venoms, and misuse of drugs. Arch Intern Med 150:505-510, 1990.

Anderson JA: Allergic reactions to drugs and biological agents. JAMA 288:2845-2857, 1992.

Bailey DG, Malcolm OA, Spence JD: Grapefruit juice and drugs: How significant is the interaction? Clin Pharmacokinet 2:91-98, 1994.

Ballantyne A, Lippiette P, Park J: Herbal cigarettes for kicks. Brit Med J 2:1539-1540, 1976.

Bigby M, Stern RS, Arndt KA: Allergic cutaneous reactions to drugs. Primary Care Clin Office Pract 16:713-727, 1989.

Braunig P, Bleistein J, Rao ML: Suicidality and cortiscosteroid-induced psychosis. Biol Psychiatry 26:209-210, 1989.

Chaiken T, Telander R: The nightmare of steroids. Sports Illustrated Oct 24, 1988, 82-102.

Clardy DO, Cravey RH, MacDonald BJ, et al: Phencyclidine-intoxicated driver. J Anal Toxicol 3:238-241, 1979.

Connell PH: Amphetamine Psychosis. London: Oxford University Press, 1958.

Dannenberg AJ, Reidenberg MM: Dietary fatty acids are also drugs. Clin Pharmacol Ther 55:5-9, 1994.

D'Orban PT: Steroid-induced psychosis. Lancet 2(8664):694, 1989.

Drug Interactions and Side Effects Index. Oradell, NJ: Medical Economics Co, 1994.

Drugs that cause psychiatric symptoms. Med Lett Drugs Ther 35:65-70, 1993.

Ellingwood EH: Assault and homicide associated with amphetamine abuse. Am J Psychiatry 127:1170-1175, 1970.

Gautier. Cited in Moreau JJ: Hashish and Mental Illness, 12. 1845. Reprint, edited by Peters H, Nahas GG, translated by Barnett GJ. New York: Raven Press, 1973.

Gilbert GJ: Quinidine dementia. JAMA 237:2093-2094, 1977.

Golden RN, Hoffman J, Falk D, et al: Psychoses associated with propranolol withdrawal. Biol Psychiatry 25:351-354, 1989.

Goldfrank L, Flomenbaum N, Lewin N: Anticholinergic poisoning. J Toxicol Clin Toxicol 19:17-25, 1982.

Greden JF: Anxiety of caffeinism; A diagnostic dilemma. Am J Psychiatry 131:1089-1092, 1974.

Grossman E, Messerli FH: High blood pressure. A side effect of drugs, poisons, and food. Arch Intern Med 155:450-460, 1995.

Grove VE Jr: Phencyclidine (angel dust) invades Texas. Texas Med 75:64-65, 1979.

Hamberg O, Ovesen L, Dorfeldt A, et al: The effect of dietary energy and protein deficiency on drug metabolism. Eur J Clin Pharmacol 38:567-570, 1990.

Handbook on Injectable Drugs. Bethesda, MD: American Society of Hospital Pharmacists.

Hollister L: Drugs that mimic or exacerbate psychiatric disorders. *In* Melmon KL, Morrelli HF, Hoffman BB, Nierenberg DW (eds): Melmon and Morelli's Clinical Pharmacology, 3rd ed. New York: McGraw-Hill, 1992.

Johnson AG, Seidemann P, Day RO: NSAID-related adverse drug interactions with clinical relevance. Int J Clin Pharmacol 32:509-532, 1994.

Johnson JA, Bootman JL: Drug-related morbidity and mortality: A cost of illness model. Arch Intern Med, 1995, in press.

Jonsson S, O'Meara M, Young JB: Acute cocaine poisoning—Importance of treating seizures and acidosis. Am J Med 75:1061-1064, 1983.

Lanius RA, Pasqualotto BA, Shaw CA: Age-dependent expression, phosphorylation and function of neurotransmitter receptors: Pharmacological implications. Trends Pharmacol Sci 14:403-408, 1994.

Levitsky DA: Drugs, appetite, and body weight. *In* Roe DA, Campbell TC (eds): Drugs and Nutrients: The Interactive Effects, 375-400. New York: Marcel Dekker, 1984.

Lipsitz LA: Orthostatic hypotension in the elderly. N Engl J Med 321:952-957, 1989.

Mego DM, Omori DJM, Hanley JF: Transdermal scopolamine as a cause of transient psychosis in two elderly patients. South Med J 81:394-395, 1988.

Melander A, Lalka D, McLean A: Influence of food on the presystemic clearance of drugs. Pharmacol Ther 38:253-267, 1988.

Mendelson J, Upton R, Jacob P III, Jones T: Methamphetamine and ethanol interactions: Pharmacokinetics and dynamics. Clin Pharmacol Ther 55:132, 1994.

Nierenberg DW, Semprebon M: The central nervous system serotonin syndrome. Clin Pharm Ther 53:84-88, 1993.

Oakley R: Drugs, Society and Human Behavior. St Louis: CV Mosby Co, 1978.

Osterholm RK, Camoriano JK: Transdermal scopolamine psychosis. JAMA 247:3081, 1982.

Ovesen L, Lyduch S, Idorn ML: The effect of a diet rich in Brussels sprouts on warfarin pharmacokinetics. Eur J Clin Pharmacol 34:521-523, 1988.

Peterkin K, Black DV (eds): Directory of On-line Healthcare Databases, 5th ed. Oak Park, IL: Medical Data Exchange, Alpine Guild, 1990.

Pope HG, Katz DL: Psychiatric and medical effects of anabolic-androgenic steroid use. Arch Gen Psychiatry 51:375-382, 1994.

Rieder MJ: Immunopharmacology and adverse drug reactions. J Clin Pharmacol 33:316-323, 1995.

Rizach MA, Hillman CDM: The Medical Letter Handbook of Adverse Drug Interactions. New Rochelle, NY: The Medical Letter, 1989 and subsequent editions.

Roe DA: Geriatric nutrition. Clin Geriatr Med 6:319-334, 1990.

Roe DA: Handbook on Drug and Nutrient Interactions: A Problem-Oriented Reference Guide, 4th ed. Chicago: American Dietetic Association, 1989.

Sagel J, Matisonn R: Neuropsychiatric disturbances as the initial manifestation of digitalis toxicity. S Afr Med J 46:512-514, 1972.

Sankey RJ, Nunn AJ, Sills JA: Visual hallucinations in children receiving decongestants. Br Med J 288:1389, 1984.

Sun DK, Reiner D, Frishman W, Grossman M, Luftschein S: Adverse dermatologic reactions from antiarrhythmic drug therapy. J Clin Pharmacol 34:953-966, 1995.

Watts NB, Blevins LS: Endocrinology. Contempo, 1994; JAMA 271:1666-1668, 1994.

Weiner N: Atropine, scopolamine and related anti-muscarinic drugs. *In* Goodman AG, Goodman LS, Gilman A (eds): Goodman and Gilman's The Pharmacological Basis of Therapeutics, 6th ed, 127. New York: Macmillan Publishing Co, 1980.

Young NS: Agranulocytosis. Grand Rounds at the Clinical Center of the National Institutes of Health. JAMA 271:935-938, 1994.

PART X

ENDOCRINE PHARMACOLOGY

Thyroid Hormones and Drugs That Affect the Thyroid 51

Stephen W. Spaulding and Edward A. Carr, Jr.

THYROID HORMONES

Genesis and Fate of Thyroid Hormones

The concentration of iodide ions in the thyroid gland is normally about thirty times the concentration in the plasma. When acted upon by thyroid-stimulating hormone (TSH) or thyrotropin, the thyroid's "iodide pump" can raise the intrathyroidal level as much as 200 times that in the plasma. Iodide in the gland is oxidized by a peroxidase, permitting iodination of tyrosyl moieties in thyroglobulin to form monoiodotyrosyl and diiodotyrosyl residues ("organification of iodine").

Following this second step, some of the iodotyrosyl residues transfer their phenolic ring, "coupling" it to other iodotyrosine residues within the thyroglobulin molecule, to form diiodothyronine (T_2), triiodothyronine (T_3), or tetraiodothyronine (thyroxine, T_4) (Fig. 51 – 1). The iodinated thyroglobulin is stored in thyroid follicles as "colloid" awaiting the fourth step, in which colloid droplets fuse with lysosomes and hydrolyze thyroglobulin, releasing the two active hormones T_4 and T_3, along with reverse T_3 and T_2, which are inactive. Monoiodotyrosine and T_2 residues that escaped coupling do not go completely to waste, however, for a dehalogenase in the gland removes their iodine atoms, thus retaining the iodine in the thyroid for reuse. The normal thyroid produces 80 – 90 μg of T_4 and about 30 μg of T_3 (Refetoff and Larson, 1989), which represent about 70 μg of hormonal iodine daily (Riggs, 1952). In the course of secreting thyroid hormones, the thyroid also releases a small amount of thyroglobulin into the plasma: elevated levels occur in some pathological conditions.

If the serum level of T_4 rises, the secretion of TSH from the pituitary is suppressed. TSH acts via a specific receptor on the thyroid cell membrane to stimulate the formation and secretion of thyroid hormones. Many of the actions of TSH are mediated by its activating enzyme, adenylate cyclase. Patients suffering from Graves' disease, the common form of

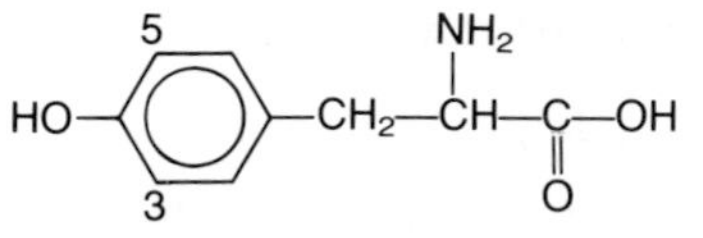

Tyrosine
Monoiodotyrosine
Diiodotyrosine

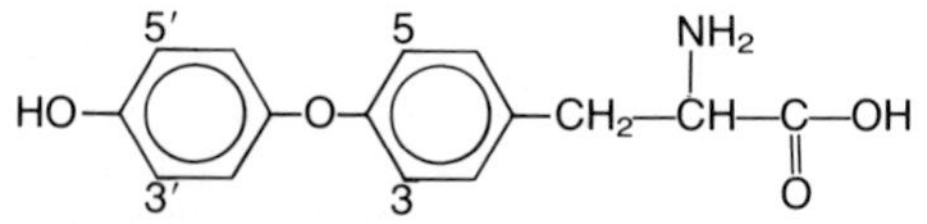

Thyronine
3,3′-diiodothyronine (T_2)
3′,3,5-triiodothyronine (T_3)
3′,5′,3-triiodothyronine ("reverse T_3")
Thyroxine (T_4)

FIGURE 51–1. Tyrosine, thyronine, and their iodinated derivatives.

hyperthyroidism, have a circulating antibody to the TSH receptor that stimulates thyroid hormone secretion and thyroid growth.

A common cause of goiter in some parts of the world is dietary deficiency in iodine, resulting in prolonged stimulation of the gland with TSH; however, the cause of most "nontoxic" goiters in the United States remains unclear.

The T_4 and T_3 in the plasma are tightly bound to a specific globulin, thyroxine-binding globulin (TBG); therefore, only a small fraction of the hormones circulates in the free form. The amount of TBG produced by the liver is increased if estrogen levels are raised, whereas androgens have the opposite effect. Hence, a woman who is given an estrogen-containing oral contraceptive produces more TBG, thus increasing the fraction of T_4 bound in her serum. Her hypothalamic-pituitary axis then responds to the fall in free hormone concentration by increasing hormone secretion from the thyroid, restoring her free T_4 to normal levels; however, the *total* serum T_4 concentration becomes higher than normal. If only the total serum T_4 were measured, a physician might conclude that the patient was hyperthyroid; however, the physician could avoid making this type of diagnostic error by directly measuring either the free T_4 or the TBG level, or (more commonly) by performing a test that estimates the degree of saturation of TBG, such as the T_3 resin uptake. The normal level of T_4 in serum is between 4 and 11 μg/dL (50–140 nmol/L), whereas only about $\frac{1}{3000}$ of the total is free (approximately 2 ng/dL or 25 pmol/L). The total normal level of T_3 in the plasma is between 100 and 150 ng/dL (1.5–2.3 nmol/L), of which about 0.4 ng/dL (6 pmol/L) is free (Committee on Nomenclature, 1987). Transthyretin (thyroxine-binding prealbumin, TBPA) and albumin provide additional thyroid hormone binding sites in blood. Certain drugs such as salicylate can compete with thyroid hormone for binding sites on serum binding proteins; therefore, if the serum level of these drugs is very high, the ratio of free-to-bound hormone is increased.

Thyroid hormones undergo extensive biotransformation once they enter the circulation. Most of the T_3 in the plasma actually is produced by deiodination of T_4 in peripheral tissues. Therefore, even if only T_4 is administered to a hypothyroid individual, the plasma T_3 concentration is restored to low normal levels. Deiodination of T_4 is a crucial step in metabolic regulation because two possible pathways exist. The first involves deiodination of the outer ring (5′-deiodination), producing T_3, which is about three times more potent than T_4. Conversely, the second involves deiodination of the inner ring (5-deiodination), which converts T_4 into the inactive substance, reverse T_3. In some tissues, T_4 and T_3 are conjugated to sulfate at their phenolic hydroxyl group. This enhances the rate of inner-ring deiodination, thus promoting the inactivating pathway. The deiodinating pathways can be affected by decreased caloric intake or by the administration of a variety of drugs (*eg*, propylthiouracil or glucocorticoids) and iodinated roentgenographic contrast media, such as iopanoate.

Although deiodinated metabolites represent the major pathway for eliminating thyroid hormones, some conjugated hormone is excreted in the bile and urine. Inhibitors of deiodination increase the amount of hormone eliminated via this route. Transplacental transfer of thyroid hormones is another, although limited, route of elimination in a pregnant woman (see Replacement Therapy).

Mechanism of Action of Thyroid Hormones

Thyroid hormone is critical for normal growth and development of the brain. The actions of thyroid hormone are complex because most of the processes it affects are also influenced by other hormones—particularly adrenergic agents. For example, thyroid hormone is required for expression of the uncoupling protein in brown fat that is regulated by norepinephrine in adaptation to cold. Thyroid hormone also affects several other pathways involving thermogenesis: it increases both lipogenesis and lipolysis and influences adenosine triphosphatase (ATPase) activities in a variety of tissues.

Actions of Thyroid Hormones at the Molecular Level

Nuclear thyroid hormone receptors are part of the superfamily of proteins that also includes receptors for the glucocorticoids, mineralocorticoids, vitamin D, and retinoic acid. Two genes encode thyroid hormone receptors, and each also has alternative splice products. The levels of receptor expression vary according to the tissue and to its stage of development. The level of thyroid hormone itself can modulate the amount of transcript formed; for example, the high-affinity form of thyroid hormone receptor that is found in the rat pituitary displays down-regulation in response to thyroid hormone.

Thyroid hormone plays a leading role in regulating the expression of a few tissue-specific genes, such as the TSH gene in the pituitary. Thyroid hormone also plays a supporting role in regulating the expression of numerous "housekeeping" genes that are required on a day-to-day basis. Thyroid hormone can modulate gene products via at least three mechanisms: (1) it can interact with the nuclear receptors that bind to 5′ upstream sequences (so-called thyroid response elements, TREs), which affects gene expression; (2) it can regulate the stability of specific messenger RNAs; and (3) it can affect mRNA transcript processing of some genes.

Clinical Manifestations of Hyperthyroidism (Thyrotoxicosis)

The typical thyrotoxic patient appears "hypermetabolic," reflecting the direct effects of the excessive level of thyroid hormone plus the responses of organs that are compensating for increased metabolic activity elsewhere in the body. The basal metabolism of many energy-producing substrates is increased, reflecting an increase in tissue functions in some instances and a decrease in efficiency in others. Flushed, hot skin reflects in part the patient's need to dissipate an increased production of heat. Most hyperthyroid patients lose weight, despite increased appetite, and defecate more frequently. Muscle weakness is a common complaint: bone and muscle turnover is increased. The muscle tremor that is also frequently observed can be ameliorated with β-adrenergic blocking drugs. Another common symptom, a bounding pulse, reflects an increase in cardiac output, due in part to the increased demand for oxygen in peripheral tissues and possibly to an increased responsiveness to catecholamines; however, circulating catecholamine levels actually tend to be low. Thyroid hormone levels affect the proportion of myosin isoforms in ventricular cells, and the basal contractility of cardiac muscles is increased in hyperthyroidism.

Clinical Manifestations of Hypothyroidism (Myxedema)

Hypothyroid patients are generally sluggish, reflecting the hypometabolic state of many organs. They often complain of feeling cold. It should be noted, however, that not all of the signs of hypothyroidism are simply the opposite of those observed in hyperthyroidism. For example, hypothyroid patients commonly have a puffy face and doughy skin. This myxedema reflects the mucinous infiltration of connective tissue and is caused by overproduction of glycosaminoglycans, which are suppressed by normal levels of thyroid hormone.

Preparations for the Treatment of Hypothyroidism

Levothyroxine sodium tablets (*eg*, SYNTHROID, LEVOTHROID) are the preferred drug and dosage form for the treatment of most patients with hypothyroidism. Levothyroxine sodium is also available in a lyophilized preparation that may be reconstituted for intravenous or intramuscular injection when oral therapy is impossible.

Liothyronine sodium tablets (*eg*, CYTOMEL) represent the oral dosage form of triiodothyronine. T_3 has approximately three times the potency of T_4. Because of its shorter half-life and high-peak free serum levels, T_3 is not generally used for therapy.

Desiccated thyroid and other "natural" preparations contain a variable amount of thyroid hormones and thus require chemical and biological standardization. They are no longer recommended.

Absorption and Elimination

When thyroid hormones are given orally for replacement therapy, bioavailability can vary somewhat among preparations but is approximately 70%. Absorption is reduced if certain other compounds are administered simultaneously (Table 51 - 1). After initiation of daily administration of T_4 to a severely hypothyroid patient, the onset of such clinically observable metabolic effects as increased body temperature, heart rate, and warmth of the skin is slow, and responses do not reach a maximum for 7 - 10 days after administration. Even intravenous administration does not substantially reduce the lag in these effects.

If maintenance T_4 therapy is abruptly discontinued, the hypometabolic state may reappear very gradually, a situation that can mislead a patient into thinking that his or her disease is "cured." T_4 disappears from the blood with a half-life of about 1 week, but the half-life of clinical effects, which reflect what is happening in the tissues, is closer to 2 weeks. The peak in biological effects of a single dose of T_3 occurs about 2 days after administration, and its effects generally disappear with a half-life of about 1 week.

Replacement Therapy

Treatment of severe long-standing hypothyroidism usually should be initiated with low doses of levothyroxine, *eg*, 25 μg by mouth daily, and gradually increased, with similar in-

TABLE 51 - 1. Drugs Interfering With Thyroid Hormone Synthesis or Affecting Its Absorption or Metabolism

Effect	Drug or Agent
Intrathyroidal	
Iodide transport	ClO_4^-, TcO_4^-, SCN^-, high iodide intake
Organification of iodide	Propylthiouracil, methimazole, some sulfonamides, SCN^-, phenylbutazone
Coupling of iodotyrosyls	Propylthiouracil, methimazole, some sulfonamides
Thyronine release	I, Li^+
Dehalogenase	Nitrotyrosines
Absorption and Peripheral Metabolism	
Inhibition of intestinal absorption	Cholestyramine, other resins, sucralfate, $AlOH_3$, soy flour, $FeSO_4$
Inhibition of peripheral deiodination	Propylthiouracil, iopanoate, glucocorticoids, other iodide-containing radiographic contrast agents
Induction of catabolic microsomal enzymes	Phenobarbital

crements being used every 2 – 3 weeks. The clinical symptoms and serum TSH levels should be carefully monitored until the proper maintenance dose is reached (usually in the range of 100 – 200 μg daily, but wide individual variability exists). A severely hypothyroid patient who is abruptly given a full replacement dose of hormone may suffer the onset of angina, worsening of heart failure, or even acute myocardial infarction. Furthermore, if certain coexisting disorders, *eg,* adrenal cortical insufficiency or angina, already exist in a patient, they may be partially alleviated by hypothyroidism. Thus, giving thyroid hormone replacement can actually exacerbate those disorders if they remain untreated. Adjustment of antianginal medications (or coronary artery intervention therapy) usually is necessary in the latter case. Giving thyroid hormone therapy *before* initiating adrenal cortical hormone replacement in a patient who is suffering from a combined deficiency of the adrenal and thyroid glands can precipitate a life-threatening crisis of adrenal insufficiency. In such patients, it is essential to treat the adrenal insufficiency first before initiating thyroid hormone replacement. Elderly patients may require very cautious initiation of therapy, *eg,* 12.5 μg daily, although, as with all hypothyroid patients, consideration also must be given to the dangers of undertreated hypothyroidism.

Replacement therapy generally needs to be lifelong, except for such cases as the transient hypothyroidism that can occur with subacute thyroiditis. The serum TSH level should be checked periodically in patients receiving replacement therapy (unless the hypothyroidism is secondary to pituitary disease) because the patient's requirement for thyroid hormone can change before clinical symptoms appear, and prompt adjustment in dosage will forestall complications.

Two special situations exist in which replacement therapy should be vigorous from the onset. The first is when a patient has congenital hypothyroidism (cretinism); such a patient is born already suffering from some intrauterine deprivation of thyroid hormone. The normal fetus depends on its own thyroid function during the latter part of gestation to maintain euthyroidism. Transplacental passage of thyroid hormone from a euthyroid mother can only partly compensate for a fetal thyroid defect, and this maternal supply of hormone is lost after birth (Vulma et al, 1989). It is therefore essential to diagnose hypothyroidism immediately after birth. Although neonatal hypothyroidism is fairly uncommon (1 in 4000), it represents a situation in which prompt neonatal therapy may prevent a serious lifelong problem. Screening of all newborns by measuring T_4 concentration in an eluate of blood spots on filter paper is emphatically recommended. If the T_4 concentration is below normal, further studies including TSH determinations should be performed. Therapy for neonatal hypothyroidism should be initiated at once, with frequent readjustment of the dose on the basis of careful clinical monitoring. Generally, a child should be receiving approximately half of the adult dose by the age of 1 year. Immediate postnatal therapy greatly increases the likelihood of satisfactory mental development. If treatment is delayed, normal physical development may still occur, but complete mental development may not be achieved; furthermore, belated replacement therapy can precipitate behavioral problems.

A second indication for rapid initial treatment is the rare condition of myxedema coma. In such cases, despite the attendant risk, initial intravenous therapy with a high dose of L-thyroxine or triiodothyronine is indicated (*eg,* 150 – 400 μg of sodium levothyroxine), together with therapy for accompanying problems such as infection and electrolyte disturbances. Because of its faster onset of effect, triiodothyronine might be theoretically preferable to T_4 in the treatment of myxedema coma; however, clear clinical evidence of such an advantage is lacking.

The use of thyroid hormone to treat obesity, sluggishness, and other ill-defined complaints in patients who are *not* hypothyroid is neither safe nor effective and should not be condoned.

Suppressive Therapy

Goiters can develop even when dietary iodine intake is adequate if an increased demand for thyroid hormone exists, such as during pregnancy or when mild thyroiditis or a mild intrathyroidal metabolic defect is present. If such a goiter has only been present for a short time, the gland usually returns to normal size if the patient is given exogenous thyroid hormone in doses adequate to suppress TSH secretion. Unfortunately, long-standing goiters and those with an element of non – TSH-dependent enlargement are not likely to return to normal size with suppressive therapy, particularly if they have developed fibrosis and calcification.

Suppressive therapy for euthyroid patients who have a thyroid nodule is controversial. Administration of thyroid hormone for 3 – 6 months may cause a benign nodule to regress, whereas a malignant nodule is less likely to do so; however, this test does not distinguish unequivocally between the two types of nodule.

Prophylactic Use

If a benign goiter has become so large that it requires subtotal thyroidectomy, the thyroid tissue remaining after surgery may still be subject to the same factors that initially caused the goiter to grow. To decrease the chance of recurrence due to TSH stimulation, thyroid replacement therapy is often prescribed.

Adverse Effects

Because most of the abnormalities observed in the hyperthyroid patient are the result of an endogenous "overdose" of thyroid hormone, the administration of excessive doses of exogenous thyroid hormone produces similar effects. Chronic overreplacement, even with a dose that causes no obvious thyrotoxic symptoms, is still hazardous because its long-term effects may include early epiphyseal closure in children and osteoporosis in adults.

DRUGS USED IN THE TREATMENT OF HYPERTHYROIDISM (ANTITHYROID DRUGS)

Thioureylene Drugs

The thioureylene drugs are the antithyroid drugs of choice (Fig. 51 – 2). Their most important mechanism of action is interference with the iodination of tyrosyl residues in thyroglobulin, a process catalyzed by thyroid peroxidase. The thioureylene drugs also interfere with the "coupling step" in thyroid hormone synthesis. In peripheral tissues, propylthiouracil has an additional antithyroid effect: it inhibits the conversion of thyroxine to triiodothyronine by inhibiting deiodinases. Methimazole does not have this effect. Thioureylenes also may affect certain immunological mechanisms, such as reducing the circulating level of TSH-receptor antibodies.

Propylthiouracil

Propylthiouracil is well absorbed after oral administration and is widely distributed in body tissues. Of special interest is its accumulation in the thyroid gland. Although the drug's half-life in the plasma is only about 1.5 hours, its effect on the thyroid gland lasts longer. The usual schedule of administration is three to four times per day. Propylthiouracil's metabolites, together with a small amount of the parent drug, are excreted in the urine. Propylthiouracil crosses the placenta and also appears in breast milk.

Methimazole (TAPAZOLE)

Methimazole also is well absorbed, is widely distributed in body tissues, and accumulates in the thyroid gland. Its plasma half-life is 4 – 9 hours, but its effect on the thyroid gland lasts longer. Nevertheless, methimazole is commonly administered on a schedule of three times per day. Metabolites of methimazole plus a small amount of parent drug appear in the urine. Like propylthiouracil, it crosses the placenta and also appears in breast milk.

Carbimazole

Carbimazole, which is commonly used abroad for the treatment of hyperthyroidism, is rapidly and almost completely converted to methimazole in humans; its subsequent fate in the body is the same as that of methimazole.

Therapeutic Strategies

Three possible therapeutic strategies for treating hyperthyroidism exist. The role of the thioureylene drug depends upon the strategy chosen.

Successful treatment of Graves' disease by any modality relieves those clinical features that result from excessive secretion of thyroid hormone (*eg*, nervousness, tachycardia, and heat intolerance). However, certain manifestations of Graves' disease, particularly some eye signs, are not the result of high tissue hormone levels but are independent immunological manifestations of the disease. Treatment of the hyperthyroidism does not have predictable effects on these other manifestations of Graves' disease; exophthalmos, for example, sometimes grows worse even when the patient is no longer hyperthyroid.

DRUG THERAPY. In the most common approach, the drug plays the central role. It is given in full doses (*eg*, 200 mg propylthiouracil three times daily) until euthyroidism is established, which usually takes a few months. Although propylthiouracil, but not methimazole, inhibits the conversion of T_4 to T_3 in the periphery and thus has a theoretical advantage of faster effect, no good evidence for a clinically significant difference between the two drugs exists in this respect. After euthryoidism is achieved, the dose of the drug needs to be adjusted (*eg*, to 50 – 100 mg propylthiouracil two to four times daily) to maintain the euthyroid state: if the initial dosage were to be continued, the patient would gradually become hypothyroid. Some physicians administer T_4 along with propylthiouracil to prevent the development of hypothyroidism. At the conclusion of treatment (generally after 1 – 2 years), the drug is discontinued and the patient observed at regular intervals. Such therapy avoids surgery and does not entail exposure to radiation; however, a significant number of patients relapse after drug therapy is discontinued. The reported percentage of patients achieving a permanent remission with this therapy varies widely in different published series, ranging from 14% (Wartofsky, 1973) to 76% (Slingerland and Burrows, 1979). If this type of therapy is elected, both patient and physician must be prepared to commit a considerable length of time to it, as most thyroidologists believe that shortening the course of therapy to only a few months increases the likelihood of relapse. Patients who relapse require re-treatment, either with the drug or, more commonly, by one of the other modalities.

Because the thioureylene drugs simply interfere with the formation and utilization of thyroid hormone, the intriguing question is not why some patients relapse after treatment stops, but rather why any patients remain in permanent remission. The answer seems to lie in the autoimmune nature of Graves' disease. One suggestion is that an organ-specific defect in suppressor T cells occurs in Graves'

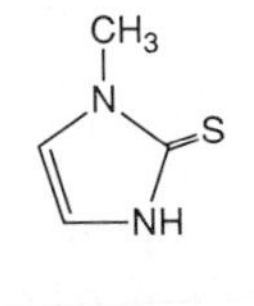

CH_3 N S NH — Methimazole

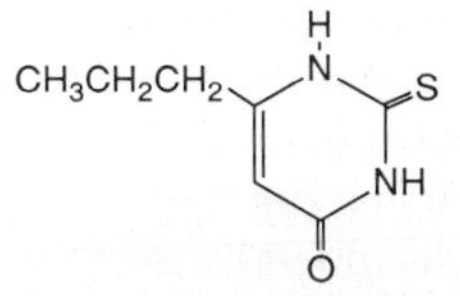

$CH_3CH_2CH_2$ H N S NH O — Propylthiouracil

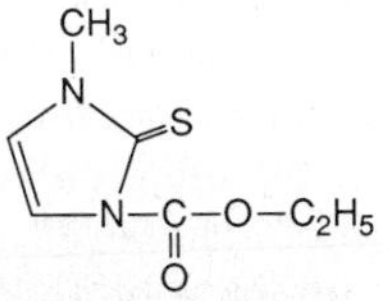

CH_3 N S N C O C_2H_5 O — Carbimazole

FIGURE 51–2. Thioureylene drugs in clinical use.

disease and that hyperthyroidism itself has an adverse effect on suppressor T-cell function, thus creating a vicious cycle that is broken by restoring euthyroidism. Another possible explanation is that gradual development of chronic thyroiditis may be a common spontaneous event in longstanding Graves' disease, leading not only to euthyroidism but often to eventual hypothyroidism.

SURGERY. If surgical removal of most of the hyperfunctioning thyroid is the treatment strategy chosen, the patient should still be rendered euthyroid with a thioureylene drug before the operation takes place. Any stress, especially the stress of surgery, in a hyperthyroid patient may precipitate an alarming and potentially fatal exacerbation of the hyperthyroid state, the so-called thyroid crisis or "thyroid storm" (see Clinical Use of "Stable" [*ie*, Nonradioactive] Iodine [Iodine 127] in Treatment of Hyperthyroidism). However, if a hyperthyroid patient develops a pressing indication for emergency surgery (*eg*, acute appendicitis) and it is impossible to wait until euthyroidism is achieved, the use of a β-adrenergic blocking drug and iodine (see Iodine) is a rational measure to decrease the risk of thyroid crisis. Corticosteroid drugs also may be useful. However, the availability of these drugs for the occasional emergency situation should not lure physicians away from the prudent course of delaying elective surgery until a hyperthyroid patient becomes euthyroid.

RADIOACTIVE IODINE THERAPY. If the primary treatment strategy is the use of radioactive iodine (RAI), it is not usually necessary to render the patient euthyroid with thioureylenes before treatment, although this approach has merit if a patient has significant cardiovascular disease because it will avoid the temporary exacerbation of thyrotoxicosis that sometimes follows administration of RAI (see Radioactive Iodine). The thioureylene drug must be discontinued several days before RAI, or else the RAI will not be incorporated into hormones in the gland and will leave the gland quickly; therefore, the usual RAI dose may prove insufficient. In contrast to surgical treatment of thyrotoxicosis, the antithyroid effect of the radiation on the thyroid gland is not immediate, and several months may elapse before a euthyroid state is reached.

Adverse Effects of Thioureylene Drugs and Contraindications

Allergic reactions, most commonly skin rash and pruritus, occur in 3–5% of patients. Less commonly, one or more components of the serum sickness syndrome, *ie*, fever, arthritis, lymphadenopathy, or peripheral neuropathy, may occur. Other serious disorders occasionally attributable to thioureylene drugs include thrombocytopenia, jaundice, polyarteritis nodosa, systemic lupus erythematosus, and very rarely, hypoprothrombinemia severe enough to cause dangerous bleeding.

The effect of these drugs on the white blood cells deserves special mention. A modest leukopenia, *eg*, to about 4000 white cells per mm^3 in the peripheral blood, is common. However, agranulocytosis, with a precipitous drop in the white blood count and virtual disappearance of all granulocytes, may occur without warning. Patients receiving thioureylene drugs should be instructed to report immediately to their physician the onset of severe pharyngitis or any other infection, which suggests a sudden loss of white cell defenses. Major adverse effects (chiefly but not exclusively agranulocytosis) have an incidence of approximately 0.3%.

A patient who is allergic to one thioureylene compound will not inevitably suffer a cross-reaction to another such compound; however, the chance of a cross-reaction is high enough to make the risk unacceptable, unless a pressing indication for continuing antithyroid drug treatment exists. In particular, it is dangerous to reinstitute any thioureylene therapy in a patient who has suffered an episode of agranulocytosis due to a thioureylene drug. In the treatment of a hyperthyroid pregnant woman, propylthiouracil is generally the preferred drug because it crosses the placenta less than methimazole. Care must be taken to use the lowest dose that maintains euthyroidism. To lessen the risk of hypothyroidism and goiter in the newborn infant still further, the thioureylene drug should be discontinued about 2 weeks before delivery. With this regimen, the risks of neonatal hypothyroidism or obstruction of the newborn's trachea by a goiter are low. Neonatal thyrotoxicosis may not become evident clinically or biochemically for some days after birth until the antithyroid medication but *not* the maternal thyroid-stimulating antibodies have disappeared from the infant's circulation. Neonatal hyperthyroidism must always be kept in mind as a possibility in an infant born of a mother who has ever had Graves' disease, because transplancental passage of thyroid-stimulating immunoglobulins can produce passive Graves' disease in the infant even if the maternal thyroid is in remission. Nursing mothers should not receive thioureylene drugs.

Iodine

Iodine, even if given orally in elemental form, is converted to iodide in the body; for simplicity, the term "iodine" is used here for both forms. Iodine can produce several markedly different effects on the thyroid gland. Depending on the circumstances it may

- **Prevent goiter and hypothyroidism in areas of dietary iodine deficiency.** Diets chronically deficient in iodine can lead to hypothyroidism, expressed in its most severe form as endemic cretinism. Supplementing the diet with iodized salt prevents the overworked thyroid gland from enlarging.
- **Precipitate hyperthyroidism in occasional euthyroid individuals.** Occasionally iodine produces hyperthyroidism in a previously euthyroid but iodine-deficient patient. The thyroid of such a patient has a defect, for the activity of the iodide pump normally should decrease after the iodine supply becomes plentiful. The normal thyroid also defends itself against excessive concentrations of iodine, blocking the formation and release of thyroid hormones; therefore, normal individuals remain euthyroid even after receiving large amounts of inorganic iodine (*eg*, in cough mixtures) or of organic iodine (*eg*, in contrast media used in radiography or in drugs such as amiodarone, which contains 49% iodine).
- **Cause goiter and even hypothyroidism in occasional euthyroid individuals.** The normal thyroid does not completely stop all hormone production in response

to an iodine overload. However, in some patients—especially those with thyroiditis, the thyroid cannot escape from the blocking effect of iodine, and it causes hypothyroidism.

- **Restore euthyroidism in hyperthyroid patients.** The inhibitory effect of iodine on thyroid hormone secretion is much more dramatic in hyperthyroid than in euthyroid individuals and occurs with much lower doses of iodine. Iodine may occasionally be used as adjunctive short-term therapy for hyperthyroidism in selected circumstances (see Clinical Uses of "Stable" [*ie*, Nonradioactive] Iodine [Iodine 127] in Treatment of Hyperthyroidism) but it is unsatisfactory for long-term therapy because the thyroid often "escapes" from its effect.

Preparations

Potassium iodide solution (saturated solution of potassium iodide [KI], SSKI) contains 1 g/mL of KI. Strong iodine solution (Lugol's solution) contains elemental iodine (5%) and KI (10%). Sodium iodide is available in bulk. In the treatment of a thyroid crisis, if the oral route is not available, sodium iodide may be dissolved, sterilized, and administered intravenously, starting 1 hour after thioureylene therapy has begun.

Clinical Use of "Stable" (*ie*, Nonradioactive) Iodine (Iodine 127) in Treatment of Hyperthyroidism

Iodine is not recommended as a sole treatment of thyrotoxicosis because the effect of iodine on thyrotoxic patients is usually transient and incomplete. If the thyroid escapes from its inhibitory effect, the large amount of iodine provides "fuel" to the overactive thyroid. In certain pressing circumstances, however, it is important to take advantage of the rapid effect of iodine on hormone release from the gland, an effect that usually begins within 24 hours and reaches its maximum in about 10–14 days. Iodine is primarily used to treat thyroid crisis, which is characterized by hyperthermia and cardiovascular collapse. This poorly understood phenomenon may be a consequence of various kinds of stress, such as an intercurrent illness, and is not simply caused by high levels of thyroid hormone *per se*. Thioureylene therapy should be instituted about an hour before the first dose of iodine is administered. Otherwise, the hyperthyroid gland would avidly incorporate additional iodine into thyroid hormones, as the gland is usually iodine-depleted. Once present in thyroglobulin, the iodine is beyond the reach of the thioureylene's blocking effect on hormone synthesis.

The action of iodine is not sufficiently rapid or complete to allow its use as the sole treatment of a thyroid crisis. Other adjunctive measures are commonly used, including a β-adrenergic blocking drug such as propranolol to control the tachycardia. Glucocorticoid drugs also may be used because they inhibit the peripheral conversion of T_4 to T_3, resembling propylthiouracil in this respect.

Neonatal thyrotoxicosis represents another emergency situation in which administration of propylthiouracil followed by iodine may be indicated. Adjunctive measures include the administration of propranolol and careful attention to nutrition and fluid balance, which are critical issues in these severely ill infants. Neonatal thyrotoxicosis is fortunately self-limited, and if death is prevented, the infant usually becomes euthyroid and requires no further treatment after the maternal thyroid-stimulating immunoglobulins have disappeared.

Iodine is sometimes used preoperatively to cause involution of the hyperplastic, highly vascular thyroid of Graves' disease. Administration of iodine for 7–10 days before subtotal thryoidectomy is therefore an important adjunct to thioureylene therapy; although the latter drug prevents iodine incorporation into hormone, it does not appear to prevent the iodine from decreasing the vascularity of the gland.

Nuclear reactor accidents can release variable amounts of radioactive iodine. If stable iodine is administered soon after such exposure, it lowers the specific activity of the iodide pool in the patient's body and decreases the net thyroidal uptake of radioactive iodine.

Adverse effects of inorganic iodine are not uncommon. Acute reactions include an acneiform eruption (ioderma), angioedema, vasculitis, and drug fever. The iodide ion is secreted into tears, saliva, gastric juice, and bronchial secretions, and it is sometimes employed as an expectorant. In some individuals, iodine provokes the syndrome termed *iodism*, with irritation of the eyes, nose, and throat and symptoms resembling a bad cold, as well as an unpleasant taste in the mouth; gastrointestinal and respiratory symptoms are also possible.

The levels of iodine in the current United States diet may actually be higher than necessary: some evidence suggests that this may promote thyroiditis.

Radioactive Iodine

A radioactive isotope of iodine (iodine 131, also called radioiodine, or RAI) is used therapeutically to treat hyperthyroidism and thyroid cancer. ^{131}I has a physical half-life of 8 days. It emits both beta particles and gamma rays; the beta particles provide about 90% of the absorbed radiation dose to the thyroid gland from this isotope. A different radioisotope, ^{123}I, has a half-life of 13 hours. It subjects the thyroid (and total body) to less radiation than ^{131}I and is the isotope of choice for clinical diagnostic tests of thyroidal iodine metabolism.

The primary treatment of thyroid carcinoma is as complete a thyroidectomy as is possible under the clinical circumstances. This produces a hypothyroid state, and the consequent increase in TSH secretion stimulates uptake of radioiodine by the remaining tissue, both normal and neoplastic, provided the latter is sufficiently differentiated to concentrate iodine. If a postoperative scan shows evidence of persisting thyroid malignancy or residual uptake in the normal thyroid bed after a "total" thyroidectomy, a high therapeutic dose of ^{131}I is given. After an appropriate interval to permit maximum uptake (*eg*, several days to a week), the patient's hypothyroid state is relieved by the administration of replacement doses of thyroid hormone. Immediate adverse effects of ^{131}I may include manifestations of acute radiation sickness, such as nausea, and transient marrow suppression as well as salivary and nonsalivary gland neck pain. It is important for the patient to void frequently: urine pooling due to cystocele or bladder outlet obstruction should be avoided to prevent radiation cystitis. Care must be taken in disposing of any vomitus because the radioactive iodine is also secreted by the salivary glands and the gastric mucosa. In those patients whose thyroid carcinoma takes up significant amounts of radioiodine, the benefit of treating the thyroid cancer outweighs the radiation risks because even distant metastases may be ablated in such patients. When extensive pulmonary metastases are treated repeatedly with high doses of ^{131}I, pulmonary fibrosis occasionally results.

The doses of radioiodine used for the treatment of hyperthyroidism are much lower than those for cancer, generally in the range of 10 – 20 mCi, depending upon the percentage of administered dose taken up by the individual patient's thyroid gland and the size of the gland. The patient should be given instructions so as to reduce the amount of radiation to which others are exposed. The patient should understand that radioiodine therapy is likely to cause hypothyroidism in the future, so periodic follow-up is necessary. If the first dose proves insufficient and re-treatment is necessary, the subsequent dosage must be readjusted because both the uptake of iodine and the gland's sensitivity to the radiation are likely to be lower than at the time of the first dose.

A temporary exacerbation of hyperthyroidism can follow the administration of the ^{131}I, caused by increased efflux of thyroid hormones from the radiation-damaged gland. Concurrent administration of a β-adrenergic blocking drug may lessen the risk of cardiac complications in patients with known coronary artery disease.

Graves' patients treated with ^{131}I show no significant increase in the incidence of leukemia above that occurring after other forms of therapy (Saenger et al, 1968). Similarly, no good evidence exists that the treatment of hyperthyroidism with ^{131}I significantly increases the risk of subsequent development of thyroid cancer. Nonetheless, ^{131}I therapy is less commonly administered to children or to those planning to become pregnant soon, in view of the small amount of data thus far available on its effects in such patients.

Over half the patients treated with ^{131}I are hypothyroid within 10 years of therapy. A suggested explanation for the steady increase in hypothyroidism occurring years after ^{131}I therapy is that subtle radiation effects on thyroid cells that eventually result in cell death may not become evident until cell divisions have occurred. In contrast, surgical damage to thyroid tissue is such that cells either succumb to it relatively soon or else escape it. About a third of patients treated surgically are hypothyroid 10 years later, whereas others have a recurrence of hyperthyroidism (Sridama et al, 1984).

In this country, radioiodine therapy is usually the treatment for adult hyperthyroid patients, for those who are poor surgical risks, and for those who have recurrent hyperthyroidism after previous surgical treatment. Radioiodine therapy is also indicated for hyperthyroid patients who have relapsed after antithyroid drug therapy, as well as for those who suffer a significant adverse effect from a thioureylene drug and have to discontinue the drug. Except for the obvious contraindication of pregnancy, some thyroidologists consider radioiodine the therapy of choice for most adult hyperthyroid patients.

Drug Interactions

Drugs commonly affecting thyroid hormone synthesis, absorption, or metabolism are listed in Table 51 – 1. Their interactions can be subtle. For example, when a euthyroid individual who is receiving lithium for a psychiatric disorder is also given iodine-containing medication, the combination may lead to goiter or even hypothyroidism.

The effects of several drugs can be modified by the thyroid status of the patient. For example, hypothyroid patients are very sensitive to central nervous system depressants, *eg*, narcotics. The responsiveness to digoxin may be increased in hypothyroidism and decreased in hyperthyroidism. Thus, heart failure in hyperthyroid patients may respond poorly to digoxin, but the drug may become more effective after euthyroidism is restored. In contrast, hyperthyroid patients are more responsive than normal individuals to oral anticoagulants. Thus, if a hypothyroid patient's condition is well controlled by a given dose of oral anticoagulant, restoration of euthyroidism makes the patient more sensitive to the anticoagulant, probably because of increased metabolism of some clotting factors; therefore, it may be necessary to reduce the dose of anticoagulant to avoid hemorrhage.

The clearance of theophylline and certain β-adrenergic blocking drugs such as propranolol and metoprolol is decreased in hypothyroidism. Requirements for insulin and oral hypoglycemic agents may be increased in hyperthyroid diabetic patients and decreased in hypothyroid diabetics. Hyperthyroid patients may be more sensitive to the effects of tricyclic antidepressant drugs than are euthyroid individuals.

REFERENCES

Committee on Nomenclature of the American Thyroid Association: Revised nomenclature for tests of thyroid hormones and thyroid related proteins in serum. J Clin Endocrinol Metab 64:1089 – 1094, 1987.

Refetoff S, Larson PR: Transport, cellular uptake and metabolism of thyroid hormone. *In* deGroot L, Besser GM, Cahill GF Jr, et al (eds): Endocrinology, 2nd ed, Philadelphia: WB Saunders Co, 1989.

Riggs DS: Quantitative aspects of iodine metabolism in man. Pharmacol Rev 4:284 – 370, 1952.

Saenger EI, Thoma GE, Tompkins EA: Incidence of leukemia following treatment of hyperthyroidism. JAMA 205:855 – 862, 1968.

Slingerland DW, Burrows BA: Long-term antithyroid treatment in hyperthyroidism. JAMA 242:2408 – 2410, 1979.

Sridama V, McCormick M, Kaplan EL, et al: Long-term follow-up study of compensated low-dose ^{131}I therapy for Graves' disease. N Engl J Med 311:426 – 432, 1984.

Vulma T, Gons MH, de Vijlder JJM: Maternal fetal transfer of thyroxine in congenital hypothyroidism due to a total organification defect on thyroid agenesis. N Engl J Med 32:13 – 16, 1989.

Wartofsky L: Low remission rate after therapy for Graves' disease. JAMA 226:1083 – 1088, 1973.

Pituitary Hormones 52

Steven M. Simasko

Six anterior pituitary hormones are of significant therapeutic interest in humans. These include two large single-chain polypeptide hormones (growth hormone, GH; and prolactin, PRL), three glycoproteins each consisting of a common α-subunit and a unique β-subunit (thyroid-stimulating hormone, TSH; follicle-stimulating hormone, FSH; and luteinizing hormone, LH), and the small single-chain polypeptide hormone, adrenocorticotropin (ACTH). The secretion of these hormones is controlled by hypothalamic factors released into the hypothalamic-hypophyseal portal circulation and by feedback effects from peripheral hormones. The physiological targets and regulators of these hormones are summarized in Table 52-1.

Both posterior pituitary hormones (vasopressin or antidiuretic hormone, ADH; and oxytocin, OXY) are of significant therapeutic interest. The physiological targets and regulators of these two hormones are summarized in Table 52-2.

THERAPEUTIC INTERVENTIONS INVOLVING PITUITARY HORMONES

Therapeutic interventions that utilize hypothalamic and pituitary hormones can be categorized into three general areas: (1) replacement; (2) control of excess secretion; and (3) diagnostic.

Growth Hormone Deficit

Children who lack GH do not suffer from a life-threatening condition. If GH is not replaced, these individuals grow into properly proportioned adults of short stature (dwarfs). GH is now produced biosynthetically (somatropin, HUMATROPE; and somatrem, PROTROPIN); thus supplies are virtually limitless. However, therapy is still extremely expensive.

A number of considerations arise in selection of patients for GH therapy:

1. There is a bias in our society for tall height. Because GH deficiency occurs on a continuum rather than absolutely, this bias causes a social pressure to be placed on selection of patients for GH therapy even though a pathological lack of GH is not present.
2. Proper diagnosis of a GH deficiency requires low circulating levels of GH and a negative response to a provocative challenge such as growth hormone-releasing hormone (GHRH), arginine infusion, or onset of sleep.
3. Care must be taken in the interpretations of basal levels of GH because the hormone is released in a pulsatile manner and plasma levels can fluctuate significantly. GH levels also fluctuate in a circadian rhythm with levels at their peak just after the onset of sleep. Exercise and stress also cause GH secretion to increase.
4. Serious side effects from GH treatments are rare; however, the expense and potential unknown effects that may appear years later support an argument for a conservative selection of patients.
5. GH therapy in adults has been shown to cause significant increases in lean body mass due to the metabolic actions of GH. The use of GH for this purpose, especially in patients who do not exhibit a GH deficit, remains controversial.

A number of therapeutic considerations also exist:

1. Somatropin (HUMATROPE) is identical to human GH whereas somatrem (PROTROPIN) has the addition of a methionine residue on its amino terminal end. The tendency to generate antibodies against these agents is slightly greater with somatrem. The presence of anti-growth hormone antibodies requires an increase in dosage to achieve the same therapeutic benefit.
2. Because of its protein nature, GH must be given by injection. Typically, GH is given intramuscularly or subcutaneously three times a week.
3. The half-life of intravenously injected GH is only

TABLE 52–1. Hormones of the Anterior Pituitary

Hormone	Structure	Pituitary Cell Type (% of Pituitary)	Hypothalamic-Releasing Hormone	Hypothalamic-Inhibiting Hormone	Target Tissue	Target Tissue Hormone
Growth hormone	Single chain, 191 amino acids	Somatotrophs (40–50)	GHRH	Somatostatin	Liver, muscle, fat	IGF-1
Prolactin	Single chain, 198 amino acids	Lactotrophs (10–25)	?PRF ?TRH	Dopamine ?PRIF	Mammary gland	
Thyrotropin	Two chains, glycoprotein	Thyrotrophs (3–5)	TRH		Thyroid	Thyroxine
Follicle-stimulating hormone	Two chains, glycoprotein	Gonadotrophs (10–15)	GnRH		Gonads (females—granulosa cells) (males—Sertoli cells)	Estradiol Inhibin
Luteinizing hormone	Two chains, glycoprotein	Gonadotrophs (10–15)	GnRH		Gonads (females—theca cells) (males—Leydig cells)	Androgens Testosterone
Adrenocorticotropin	Single chain, 39 amino acids	Corticotrophs (15–20)	CRH		Adrenal cortex	Cortisol

CRH = corticotropin-releasing hormone; GHRH = growth hormone-releasing hormone; GnRH = gonadotropin-releasing hormone; IGF-1 = insulin-like growth factor-1; PRF = prolactin-releasing factor; PRIF = prolactin release-inhibiting factor; TRH = thyrotropin-releasing hormone.

20–25 minutes, however the therapeutic actions last much longer due to the release of insulinlike growth factor-1 (IGF-1) from the liver. IGF-1 circulates bound to carrier proteins.

4. Frequently, a GH deficit is associated with a generalized hypopituitarism. These individuals are also hypothyroid due to the loss of TSH. Because adequate thyroid hormone levels are required for GH to work, in these individuals thyroid status must be normalized before GH therapy will be successful.

5. Hypothyroidism may also be induced by GH therapy. This is due to the suppression of TSH release from the pituitary caused by elevated somatostatin release from the hypothalamus in response to GH. Thus thyroid status should be monitored during the course of GH therapy.

6. Excess levels of glucocorticoids suppress GH action. Simultaneous treatment of patients with glucocorticoids or the presence of Cushing's syndrome may cause GH therapy to fail.

7. Because of the anti-insulin effects of GH, patients on GH therapy should be monitored for signs of diabetes mellitus.

8. A subset of growth-deficient individuals do not respond to GH therapy (Laron-type dwarfs). The defect in these individuals has been shown to be an inactive GH receptor.

Pituitary Tumors

Both hormone-secreting and nonsecreting pituitary tumors are encountered. Pituitary tumors that secrete hormones are usually discovered by the dysfunction caused by the inappropriate secretion of the particular hormone. Nonsecreting tumors are typically found as a result of symptoms related to the pressure caused by the growing mass of tumor cells. These symptoms frequently involve visual disturbances due to compression of the optic nerve or headache. Compromised function of normal pituitary tissue may also occur.

Definitive therapy for pituitary adenomas requires surgical removal of the tumor mass. However, recurrence of hypersecretion is frequently encountered after surgery. Treatment with hypothalamic hormones that inhibit release of pituitary hormones (somatostatin and dopamine) can ameliorate symptoms and cause shrinkage of the tumor mass. Use of pharmacological agents by themselves may be adequate to control the symptoms present. These agents can also be useful as a prelude to surgery to shrink the tumor

TABLE 52–2. Hormones of the Posterior Pituitary

Hormone	Structure	Location of Cell Body	Stimulus for Release	Target Tissue
Antidiuretic hormone or vasopressin	Single chain, 9 amino acids	Paraventricular nucleus, supraoptic nucleus	High plasma osmolarity, low plasma volume	Collecting ducts of kidney, small arterioles and venules
Oxytocin	Single chain, 9 amino acids	Paraventricular nucleus, supraoptic nucleus	Stimulation of nipple, parturition	Myoepithelial cells of breast, myometrium

mass or postsurgically to control recurrence of hypersecretion.

Acromegaly

Acromegaly is caused by excessive GH secretion in adults. This is typically caused by a pituitary adenoma; however, GHRH-secreting tumors have also been described. Acromegaly results in a progressive thickening of bones and the skin. This is especially apparent in the jaw and hands. Carbohydrate and lipid abnormalities are prevalent due to the anti-insulin effects of GH. Finally, heart and lung disease may also be present.

An 8-amino acid synthetic analog of somatostatin, octreotide (SANDOSTATIN), has been shown to be useful in the treatment of acromegaly. Octreotide reduces GH secretion and, in about 50% of cases, causes tumor shrinkage. Excessive GH secretion and tumor growth recur upon cessation of treatment. Octreotide has several advantages over native somatostatin. It has a longer half-life (50 versus 3 minutes), it is active when given subcutaneously, it preferentially suppresses GH secretion over insulin secretion, and it does not cause rebound hypersecretion upon cessation of treatment. This last effect is thought to be due to the long half-life of octreotide, which results in a slow decrease in plasma levels. Adverse reactions to prolonged octreotide therapy are similar to effects produced by somatostatin-secreting tumors. These include steatorrhea, diabetes mellitus, and cholelithiasis. These effects are a result of the well-characterized actions of somatostatin to decrease exocrine pancreas secretion, inhibit insulin release, and prevent gallbladder contraction, respectively. It has also been found that the dopamine agonist bromocriptine (PARLODEL) causes a decrease in GH secretion in acromegalics. The reasons for this are not yet apparent.

Prolactinomas

Prolactinomas are the most common type of pituitary tumor. The effects of excess prolactin secretion in females include amenorrhea, galactorrhea, infertility, and hypogonadism. In males excess prolactin causes infertility, impotence, and galactorrhea. Excessive prolactin secretion is one of the leading causes of infertility.

Bromocriptine (PARLODEL), an ergot alkaloid with agonist properties at postsynaptic D_2 dopamine receptors, has gained wide usage in the treatment of hyperprolactinemia due to PRL-secreting adenomas. Bromocriptine is successful in restoring menses and preventing galactorrhea in about 75% of patients. Relief of symptoms may be rapid (days) or may require many months. Reduction in tumor size has been noted. Tumor growth, galactorrhea, and amenorrhea usually return upon cessation of treatment. Adverse reactions to bromocriptine are quite common. These include nausea, headache, dizziness, fatigue, lightheadedness, vomiting, and diarrhea. Care should be taken when bromocriptine is given to those patients receiving antihypertensive medications because bromocriptine also lowers blood pressure. Because bromocriptine is given to restore fertility, it is present at the time of conception and during the first few weeks of pregnancy. Once pregnancy is established, bromocriptine therapy can be stopped. Incidences of spontaneous abortions or birth defects in mothers who have taken bromocriptine are no greater than expected in the general population.

Other Pituitary Tumors

Octreotide has also been reported to suppress secretion from TSH-secreting tumors, and in ectopic ACTH secretion. The use of octreotide in these situations has not been fully explored.

Stimulation of the Hypothalamic/Pituitary/Gonadal Axis

Pituitary gonadotropins (FSH and LH), the placental gonadotropin—human chorionic gonadotropin (hCG), and gonadotropin-releasing hormone (GnRH) can be used to stimulate the hypothalamic/pituitary/gonadal axis. These agents are used to treat infertility due to hypogonadotropic anovulation in females and hypogonadotropic hypogonadism in males, and may also be useful in cryptorchidism.

A number of preparations are available. These include:

1. Mentropin (PERGONAL) is a mixed preparation of purified FSH and LH isolated from the urine of postmenopausal women.
2. Urofollitropin (METRODIN) is a preparation of purified FSH from the urine of postmenopausal women.
3. Chorionic gonadotropin is prepared from human placenta (PREGNYL, PROFASI) or is isolated from the urine of pregnant women (A.P.L).
4. GnRH (gonadorelin), a 10-amino acid peptide, is made synthetically (LUTREPULSE, FACTREL). Because long-acting agonists of GnRH suppress pituitary function, the short duration of action of the endogenous compound is advantageous when stimulation of the hypothalamic/pituitary/gonadal axis is desirable.

Hypogonadotropic Anovulation

Before therapy with gonadotropins can be successful in hypogonadal females, it is important to determine that gonadal failure is secondary to pituitary or hypothalamic failure. This can be ascertained by low to nonexistent plasma estradiol levels concomitant with low to nonexistent plasma gonadotropin levels. The therapeutic regimen with gonadotropins is designed to mimic the natural menstrual cycle. Menotropin is given for 7 – 12 days to stimulate follicle development, followed by a single large dose of hCG to initiate ovulation. Major adverse reactions include ovarian enlargement, which may lead to ovarian hyperstimulation syndrome, pulmonary complications (atelectasis and acute respiratory distress syndrome), and cardiovascular complications (thrombosis and embolism). If gonadal failure is found to be tertiary to hypothalamic failure, gonadorelin can be used to stimulate the pituitary to produce gonadotropins.

Hypogonadotropic Hypogonadism in Males

Before therapy with gonadotropins can be successful in hypogonadal males, it is important to determine that gonadal failure is secondary to pituitary or hypothalamic failure. This can be ascertained by low to nonexistent plasma testosterone levels concomitant with low to nonexistent plasma gonadotropin levels. Treatment for 4–6 months with a preparation of hCG to elevate serum testosterone levels is recommended prior to combined menotropin/hCG therapy. Combined menotropin/hCG therapy should proceed for at least 3–4 months before examination of the ejaculate for spermatozoa, as it takes 74 days for the human male germ cell to develop into spermatozoa. Adverse reactions include fluid retention as a result of increased androgen production.

Cryptorchidism

Treatment with hCG of cryptorchidism not due to anatomical blockage is usually performed between ages 4 and 9. Although descent of the testes produced with hCG treatment is frequently temporary, a positive response is usually a good predictor of eventual descent during puberty. Use of hCG in prepubertal boys may result in the induction of precocious puberty. Therapy should be halted if any pubertal signs are observed.

Other Uses of Gonadotropins

Urofollitropin has been approved for use in the induction of follicle maturation in women with polycystic ovarian disease who have an elevated plasma LH/FSH ratio. Urofollitropin is also used for induction of multiple oocytes in women participating in *in vitro* fertilization programs.

Suppression of the Hypothalamic/Pituitary/Gonadal Axis

GnRH is released from the hypothalamus in pulses with a frequency of 1–2 hours. This pulsatile release of GnRH is important for the maintenance of gonadotroph responsiveness. If gonadotrophs are continuously exposed to high levels of GnRH they become desensitized and stop secreting LH and FSH. The loss of LH and FSH results in decreased sex steroid production in the gonads and suppression of germ cell maturation. This physiological phenomenon has been exploited to suppress the hypothalamic/pituitary/gonadal axis by the use of high-potency, long-acting GnRH agonists.

High-Potency Synthetic Analogs of GnRH

There are three preparations of high-potency synthetic analogs of GnRH. Histrelin (SUPPRELIN) is designed to be used by daily subcutaneous injections. Nafarelin (SYNAREL) is designed to be administered as a spray to the nasal mucosa. Leuprolide (LUPRON) comes in either an injectable form for use by daily subcutaneous injections, or as a depot suspension (LUPRON DEPOT) designed for use by monthly intramuscular injections.

BOX 52–1

THERAPEUTIC USES

Synthetic GnRH agonists are used:

1. In prostate cancer to suppress testosterone production when estrogen therapy or orchiectomy is either not tolerated or undesirable.
2. In endometriosis to suppress estrogen production.
3. To treat precocious puberty.

During the first week of use with a GnRH analog, sex steroid levels may become elevated. This may exacerbate some symptoms. However, this elevation is followed by a suppression that remains as long as the therapy is continued.

Synthetic GnRH agonists may also be used to suppress normal pituitary function during procedures designed to induce multiple oocyte release for *in vitro* fertilization.

Diabetes Insipidus

Diabetes insipidus is caused by the failure of antidiuretic hormone (ADH) to act on the kidney to concentrate urine. It may be of central origin as a result of genetic factors or head trauma (especially after pituitary surgery), in which replacement therapy is effective, or it can be of nephrogenic origin, in which replacement therapy is ineffective.

BOX 52–2

THERAPEUTIC USES

Therapeutic considerations in treatment of diabetes insipidus include:

1. Synthetic ADH (vasopressin, PITRESSIN) as well as synthetic analogs of ADH (desmopressin, DDAVP; and lypressin, DIAPID) are available. These agents may be given by subcutaneous or intramuscular injection, or intranasally on cotton pledgets, nasal spray, or dropper.
2. Overdosage results in water intoxication, of which the symptoms are drowsiness, listlessness, and headache that may eventually develop into coma and convulsions.
3. Other adverse reactions include abdominal cramps, nausea, vomiting, tremor, vertigo, headaches, and sweating. ADH must be used with caution in the presence of epilepsy, migraine, asthma, heart failure, or other conditions in which rapid expansion of vascular volume may precipitate an adverse reaction.

Labor and Delivery

Oxytocin (OXY) is a very potent inducer of uterine myometrial contractions. This action has led to the use of synthetic OXY preparations (OXYTOCIN, PITOCIN, and SYNTOCINON) in labor and delivery.

> **BOX 52-3**
> **THERAPEUTIC USES**
>
> Therapeutic considerations in labor and delivery include:
>
> 1. OXY preparations can be used in the induction of labor, in ongoing labor to aid in uterine contractions, and in the management of abortion to aid in the expulsion of the uterine contents.
> 2. OXY is given intravenously. During parturition, the patient is started on a relatively low dose of OXY, which is then steadily increased over time until the desired response is achieved.
> 3. At term, rates exceeding 9–10 mU/minute are rarely required; however, in preterm labor higher concentrations may be required as a result of lower uterine sensitivity to OXY.
> 4. Continuous monitoring of uterine responses and potential fetal distress is essential during OXY administration.
> 5. Adverse reactions of the mother include severe hypertensive episodes, subarachnoid hemorrhage, and rupture of the uterus. Prolonged administration at high concentrations may lead to significant water retention due to ADH-like effects.

Lactation

Proper functioning of lactation requires two pituitary hormones. PRL acts on the epithelial cells of the alveoli of the breast to increase milk production. OXY causes the myoepithelial cells of the breast to contract, thus expelling the contents from the lumen of the alveoli into the lobuloalveolar duct. Many lobuloalveolar ducts converge to form a single lactiferous duct, which carries the milk to the surface of the nipple.

> **BOX 52-4**
> **THERAPEUTIC USES**
>
> Therapeutic considerations include:
>
> 1. Synthetic OXY (SYNTOCINON) is available for use as a nasal spray. This can be used by lactating mothers in which the OXY release from the posterior pituitary is inadequate to produce a robust milk let-down response.
> 2. Bromocriptine (PARLODEL) can be used to inhibit PRL release in postpartum women who elect not to breast-feed. It is suggested that this use of bromocriptine be restricted to cases of significant engorgement because a rebound effect occurs in approximately 30% of women once therapy is halted.

DIAGNOSTIC PROCEDURES

Several of the hypothalamic-releasing hormones can be used in diagnostic tests to determine pituitary reserve or to differentially diagnose the origin of hormone hypersecretion or hyposecretion. ACTH can be used to assess adrenal function.

Thyrotropin-Releasing Hormone

Thyrotropin-releasing hormone (TRH, protirelin, RELEFACT TRH) stimulation test can provide useful information in the assessment of secondary (pituitary) versus tertiary (hypothalamic) hypothyroidism and in the evaluation of the effectiveness of thyroid therapy in patients with nodular or diffuse goiter and patients on thyroid replacement therapy. Patients with secondary hypothyroidism have normal to low basal TSH level and a blunted TSH response to a challenge with TRH. Patients with tertiary hypothyroidism have a normal to low basal TSH level and an exaggerated TSH response to a challenge with TRH. If thyroid hormone therapy for the suppression of TSH secretion in patients with nodular or diffuse goiter is adequate, basal TSH levels should be low and a TRH challenge should result in a blunted TSH response. If a hypothyroid patient is receiving adequate concentrations of synthetic thyroid hormone, a TRH challenge should result in a normal or slightly blunted TSH response. Adverse reactions occur in about 50% of patients tested with TRH. These reactions are usually minor and persist for only a few minutes. Significant changes in blood pressure (hypertension and hypotension) can occur as well as headache, lightheadedness, nausea, abdominal discomfort, and urge to urinate.

Gonadotropin-Releasing Hormone

Gonadotropin-releasing hormone (GnRH, gonadorelin, FACTREL, LUTREPULSE) can be used in hypogonadotropic hypogonadal individuals to determine if the failure of gonadotropin secretion is of pituitary origin or hypothalamic origin. For diagnostic purposes use of synthetic GnRH rather than high-potency analogs of GnRH is preferable due to its shorter duration of action.

Growth Hormone–Releasing Hormone

Growth hormone–releasing hormone (GHRH) can be used as a challenge for GH secretion to determine if an individual has a pathological loss of growth hormone secretion or merely has low physiological levels of GH secretion.

Corticotropin-Releasing Hormone

Cushing's disease of pituitary origin can be distinguished from that due to ectopic ACTH secretion by a corticotropin-releasing hormone (CRH) stimulation test. In Cushing's disease of pituitary origin, CRH produces an increase in ACTH, whereas ectopic production of ACTH does not respond to CRH.

Adrenocorticotropin

Purified ACTH (corticotropin, ACTHAR) and a synthetic analog of ACTH (1-24 corticotropin, CORTROSYN) are available for diagnostic purposes. Adrenal insufficiency can be determined by failure of an intravenous challenge of ACTH to produce an increase in plasma glucocorticoids. Separation of primary (adrenal) versus secondary (pituitary) can be made by determination of plasma ACTH levels (elevated in primary but suppressed in secondary). In secondary adrenal insufficiency, prolonged stimulation of the adrenal cortex with ACTH may be required before significant increases in plasma cortisol levels are achieved. Preparations of ACTH have been used therapeutically. The therapeutic profile is essentially that of glucocorticoids. Because ACTH must be injected and has a short half-life, use of glucocorticoids is the preferred mode of treatment.

MISCELLANEOUS USES OF HYPOTHALAMIC AND PITUITARY HORMONES

Many hypothalamic hormones are found in tissues other than the hypothalamus and have actions outside the pituitary. This has suggested use of these hormones in actions other than control of the hypothalamic-pituitary axis. In particular, somatostatin has been shown to inhibit hormone secretion from a variety of tissues. Of the posterior pituitary hormones, ADH has also been found to be therapeutically useful outside of its actions on the kidney.

There are a number of additional therapeutic uses of octreotide. The actions of octreotide can generally be described as inhibitory. Octreotide has been approved for use in the treatment of metastatic carcinoid, for which it has been shown effective in inhibiting the diarrhea and flushing associated with this disease. Octreotide has also been shown to be effective in reducing the diarrhea and restoring plasma electrolyte balance associated with vasoactive intestinal peptide secreting tumors.

There are also additional therapeutic uses of ADH. In addition to its actions on the kidney, ADH is the most potent vasoconstrictor known. This vasoconstriction leads to an increase in total vascular resistance; however, blood pressure usually does not change as a result of the baroreceptor reflex. ADH-induced constriction of small arterioles leads to a decrease in venous pressure. This has led to the use of ADH in the treatment of variceal hemorrhage, where the decrease in portal pressure is thought to help control bleeding. Additional uses of ADH include prevention and treatment of postoperative abdominal distention and in abdominal roentgenography to dispel interfering gas shadows.

Desmopressin (DDAVP) has been approved for use in hemophilia A and type I von Willebrand's disease, in which it has been shown to be effective in raising plasma levels of Factor VIII activity.

REFERENCES

Boepple PA, Manfield MJ, Wierman ME, et al: Use of a potent, long acting agonist of gonadotropin-releasing hormone in the treatment of precocious puberty. Endocrine Rev 7:24-33, 1986.

Burger HG, Baker HWB: The treatment of infertility. Annu Rev Med 38:29-40, 1987.

Cardozo L, Pearce JM: Oxytocin in active-phase abnormalities of labor: A randomized study. Obstet Gynecol 75:152-157, 1990.

Griffiths EC: Clinical applications of thyrotropin-releasing hormone. Clin Sci 73:449-457, 1987.

Katz MD, Erstad BL: Octreotide, a new somatostatin analogue. Clin Pharm 8:255-273, 1989.

Kaye TB, Crapo L: The Cushing syndrome: An update on diagnostic tests. Ann Intern Med 112:434-444, 1990.

Lamberts SWJ: The role of somatostatin in the regulation of anterior pituitary hormone secretion and the use of its analogs in the treatment of human pituitary tumors. Endocrine Rev 9:417-436, 1988.

Lantos J, Siegler M, Cuttler L: Ethical issues in growth hormone therapy. JAMA 261:1020-1024, 1989.

Lui L, Banks SM, Barnes KM, Sherins RJ: Two-year comparison of testicular responses to pulsatile gonadotropin-releasing hormone and exogenous gonadotropins from the inception of therapy in men with isolated hypogonadotropic hypogonadism. J Clin Endocrinol Metab 67:1140-1145, 1988.

Molitch ME: Management of prolactinomas. Annu Rev Med 40:225-232, 1989.

Stump DL, Hardin, TC: The use of vasopressin in the treatment of upper gastrointestinal haemorrhage. Drugs 39:38-53, 1990.

Androgens 53

Christina Wang and Ronald S. Swerdloff

ANDROGEN PHYSIOLOGY

Testosterone is the most important sex steroid in men. Over 95% of testosterone is secreted by the Leydig cells of the testes under the stimulation of luteinizing hormone (LH) from the pituitary gland. Approximately 7 mg/day of testosterone is produced by the testes in a young male. In addition, small amounts of the potent androgen 5α-dihydrotestosterone and the androgen precursor androstenedione are also secreted by the testes. Androgens circulate in women in much lower concentrations than those seen in men. The production rate of testosterone in women is 0.3 mg/day and that of androstenedione is 3.5 mg/day. Approximately 60% of androgen action in the female is the result of production of androgen or androgen precursors from the adrenal, and the remainder of the action comes from the ovary. Although the ovary in premenopausal women is not a major source of testosterone secretion, it does secrete large amounts of androstenedione, which is converted in the periphery to testosterone. The ovarian secretion of androgens comes from the theca and stromal cells of the ovary and is under the regulation of LH. The adrenal is the source of large amounts of androgen precursors, such as dehydroepiandrosterone, dehydroepiandrosterone sulfate, and androstenedione. The adrenal secretion of androgens and androgen precursors is under the regulation of pituitary corticotropin and possibly other putative pituitary hormones (corticoadrenal-stimulating hormone).

Testosterone is transported in blood bound to plasma proteins. It circulates tightly bound to a globulin, sex hormone–binding globulin (SHBG); loosely bound to albumin; or as a free (unbound) form. The free and albumin-bound forms of testosterone are available in target tissues for full biological activity. Adult women have about twice the plasma concentration of SHBG as adult men. This is because the liver production of SHBG is stimulated by estrogens and inhibited by androgens. In men, about 3% of testosterone is free, 67% bound to albumin, and 30% bound to SHBG. In contrast, in women about 2% of testosterone is free, 40% bound to albumin, and 58% bound to SHBG. Thus, the proportion of testosterone available for biological action at the target tissue is much higher in males than in females.

Testosterone exerts its androgenic effects directly on the target tissues or through the conversion to 5α-dihydrotestosterone by the enzyme 5α-reductase. In the skin, 5α-dihydrotestosterone is further metabolized to 3α-androstanediol and its glucuronide, which is a sensitive marker of peripheral androgen action. The actions of testosterone and 5α-dihydrotestosterone are mediated by specific androgen receptors present in the androgen target tissues. Androgen receptor contents vary in some tissues during different stages of development. For example, the androgen receptor is present in the penis during childhood but disappears in adulthood. Testosterone is also converted to estradiol by the aromatase enzyme, and some of the androgen effects (mammary gland, adipose tissue) are mediated by estradiol binding to the estrogen receptors.

The biological actions of androgens on target tissues are listed in Table 53–1. The action of testosterone on target tissues depends on the age and stage of development of the male. Testosterone is required during early fetal life for the differentiation of the wolffian ducts, the external genitalia, and the brain. As indicated in the table, masculinization of the external genitalia and stimulation of the accessory sex glands (*eg*, prostate) require the conversion of testosterone to dihydrotestosterone at the tissue site of action. During puberty and adolescence, testosterone together with growth hormone is responsible for the pubertal growth spurt. At puberty, testosterone stimulates epiphyseal closure, laryngeal enlargement, enlargement of the penis, rugation of the scrotum, and the appearance of sexual hair. During adulthood, androgens are required for maintenance of normal libido and potency, secondary sex characteristics, muscle mass, and prevention of loss of bone mass. One of the most important functions of testosterone is to initiate and maintain sper-

TABLE 53–1. Androgen Target Tissues and Biological Actions

Target Tissues	Biological Actions
Hypothalamus	Negative feedback on gonadotropin-releasing hormone secretion
Pituitary	Negative feedback on luteinizing hormone and follicle-stimulating hormone secretion
Reproductive tissues	
Seminiferous tubules, Seminal vesicles, Epididymis, Vas deferens (Testosterone-depenent)	Initiation and maintenance of spermatogenesis
Prostate, Penis, Scrotum (Dihydrotestosterone-dependent)	Differentiation and development of the male accessory ducts and external genitalia
Nonreproductive tissues	
Liver (enzymes/lipoprotein)	Stimulation or suppression of protein synthesis
Kidney	Stimulation of erythropoietin, which increases hematopoiesis
Hematopoietic system	Direct stimulation of growth of stem cells; indirect stimulation by erythropoietin
Central nervous system	Facilitation of libido and sexual function; male aggressive behavior
Muscle	Development of muscle mass and strength
Skin, sebaceous gland, and hair (dihydrotestosterone-dependent)	Stimulation of growth of beard, axillary, and pubic hair, increase in temporal hair recession and balding; increase in sebum secretion
Bone/cartilage	Promotion of epiphyseal fusion Maintenance of bone mass
Larynx and vocal cords	Enlargement of larynx and thickening of vocal cords; deepening of voice
Mammary glands (estrogen-dependent)	Development of gynecomastia affected by ratio of androgen to estrogen

matogenesis. It is important to note that very high levels of testosterone within the testis are required for its action. The administration of exogenous androgen does not have stimulatory effects on the germ cells but inhibits spermatogenesis and sperm production by the negative feedback action on LH secretion and intratesticular testosterone production.

The actions of androgens have traditionally been classified as androgenic or anabolic; all effects that cause growth of the male reproductive tract or development of secondary sex characteristics are termed androgenic, whereas the effects on nonreproductive tissue, *eg*, muscle, liver, bone, bone marrow, are termed anabolic. Although early studies suggested that two independent actions of the same class of androgens might exist, subsequent experiments showed that these are organ-specific responses and that all androgens act through the same molecular mechanisms. All androgens have both androgenic and anabolic actions. Most of the pharmacological anabolic androgens can be used for replacement therapy in hypogonadal men. The one exception may be danazol. This 17-alkylated testosterone is particularly effective in suppressing gonadotropin secretion but relatively ineffective in other anabolic or androgenic actions. However, if female infants are exposed to danazol *in utero*, masculinization can occur.

DISORDERS OF ANDROGEN SECRETION

Impaired testicular secretion of androgen leads to hypogonadism and infertility. Clinical features of androgen deficiency depend on the degree of deficiency, the age of onset of the dysfunction, and the relative sensitivity of the androgen-sensitive tissues (Table 53–1). Deficiency of androgens occurring in early fetal life leads to pseudohermaphroditism. The clinical spectrum ranges from mild hypospadias to female external genitalia. Androgen deficiency during late fetal development is associated with unambiguous male genitalia but a small phallus (micropenis). The development of hypogonadism during childhood results in failure of pubertal development and eunuchoidal proportions. Lack of androgens (and estrogens) causes delayed fusion of the epiphysis and continued long bone growth. This results in arm span being greater than height and the lower segment of the body being longer than the upper segment. Androgen deficiencies occurring after puberty result in decreases in facial, axillary, and pubic hair and in libido and potency, loss of muscle bulk, and a decrease in testis size. Gynecomastia occurs in some patients with androgen deficiency and reflects a decreased testosterone-estradiol ratio. In the assessment of body hair, the physician must take into account the patient's ethnic background. Asian, Native American, and black men frequently do not need to shave every day. White men usually have pectoral, back, and flank hair in addition to axillary and pubic hair.

Androgen excess occurs in boys with precocious puberty as a result of central (hypothalamic-pituitary) causes, testicular and adrenal tumors, and non–gonadotropin-mediated Leydig's cell hyperstimulation (familial testotoxicosis). The use of antiandrogens and androgen synthesis blockers in these conditions is discussed later in this chapter.

Androgen excess in females leading to hirsutism or virilism may be caused by ovarian or adrenal factors. As in the male, the ethnic background and the family history must be taken into consideration in a female patient with hirsutism. Most patients with hirsutism have an unexplained idiopathic increased androgen secretion or increased peripheral conversion of androstenedione and testosterone to dihydrotestosterone. The second most common cause of increased hair growth in the female is the polycystic ovary syndrome.

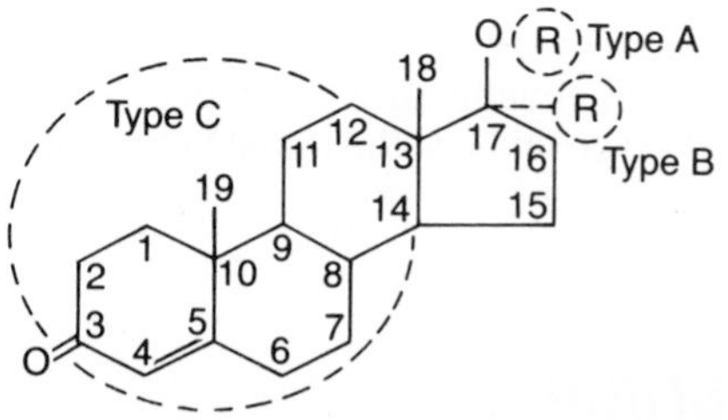

FIGURE 53-1. Categories of androgens commonly used pharmacologically. Type A, esterified androgens; type B, 17α-alkylated androgens; type C, androgens with alterations of the steroid nucleus. (Redrawn from Wilson JD: Androgen abuse by athletes. Endocr Rev 9[2]:181-189, 1988, © by The Endocrine Society.)

Other less common causes include Cushing's syndrome, adult-onset nonclassical congenital adrenal hyperplasia, androgen-producing tumors of the ovary or the adrenal, and ovarian hyperthecosis.

ANDROGEN PREPARATIONS AND THEIR PHARMACOLOGY

When unmodified testosterone is administered orally, it is rapidly absorbed into the portal blood, and after the first-pass degradation by the liver, very small amounts of testosterone reach the systemic circulation. Similarly, when testosterone is administered parenterally, it is absorbed from the injection site and rapidly degraded, preventing the effective androgen levels from being sustained in the plasma. To circumvent this problem, chemical modifications of testosterone are required to retard the rate of absorption and catabolism. The common modifications of the chemical structure of testosterone are (1) esterification of the 17-hydroxyl group (*eg*, testosterone enanthate); (2) alkylation at the 17 position (*eg*, methyltestosterone); and (3) changes in the ring structure of testosterone (*eg*, 19-norandrogen; nandrolone) (Fig. 53-1). Specific examples of available agents within these classes are shown in Table 53-2. More recent developments include the preparation of orally active micronized testosterone and testosterone cyclodextrins, the incorporation of testosterone into skin patches, and testosterone linked to polylactide-co-glycolide microspheres for intramuscular injections.

Oral

The alkylated derivatives of testosterone are effective when administered orally or buccally because they are slowly metabolized by the liver. They pass through the liver to reach the systemic circulation and produce effective plasma concentrations. Usually these drugs are administered on a daily basis. The alkyl groups are not removed, and most likely these 17-alkylated steroids act unmodified in the target tissue. These alkylated compounds are potentially hepatotoxic and cause more metabolic side effects than do testosterone esters; they should not be prescribed except for special indications such as hereditary angioneurotic edema.

Other alterations in the ring structure include alkylation at the 1 position. The resultant steroid mesterolone is a weak androgen that does not suppress gonadotropin secretion. Testosterone undecanoate ester is so nonpolar that it is absorbed into the lymphatics. As a result, it can maintain normal androgen levels after oral administration. The drug must be taken three times per day because of its short duration of action. The testosterone levels achieved tend to be variable within the same subject and between subjects. Although widely used in Europe and Asia, testosterone undecanoate is not available in the United States.

Orally active testosterone preparations under development include micronized testosterone and testosterone cyclodextrin preparation. When micronized testosterone is administered in large amounts, a small proportion of the

TABLE 53-2. Some Preparations of Androgens

Generic Name	Trade Name	Route of Administration	Dose	Supplier
α-Alkylated Androgens				
Methylestosterone	ANDROID	Oral	10, 25 mg/tablet	ICN
	METANDREN			CIBA
	TESTRED	Oral	10 mg/capsule	ICN
Fluoxymesterone	HALOTESTIN		2, 5, 10 mg/tablet	Upjohn
Oxymetholone	ANADROL	Oral	50 mg/tablet	Syntex
Oxandrolone	OXANDRIN	Oral	2.5 mg/tablet	BTG
Stanozolol	WINSTROL	Oral	2 mg/tablet	Sterling/Winthrop
Danazol	DANOCRINE	Oral	50, 100, 200 mg/tablet	Sterling/Winthrop
Testosterone Esters				
Testosterone undecanoate*	ANDRIOL	Oral	40 mg/tablet	Organon
Testosterone enanthate	DELATESTRYL	Intramuscular injection	200 mg/mL	BTG
Testosterone cypionate	DEPO-TESTOSTERONE	Intramuscular injection	100, 200 mg/mL	Upjohn
Modified Ring Structure				
Mesterolone*	PROVIRON	Oral	25 mg/day	Schering AG
Nandrolone phenpropionate	DURABOLIN	Intramuscular injection	25-50 mg/mL	Organon
Nandrolone decanoate	DECA-DURABOLIN	Injection	100-200 mg/mL	Organon

*Not available in the United States.

steroid escapes the first pass, and adequate blood levels can be obtained. Similarly, testosterone cyclodextrin preparations are rapidly absorbed orally and cleared quickly. Both preparations must be administered several times a day, and testosterone pulses occur after each dose.

Parenteral

The parenteral route of administration of testosterone is the one most commonly used for androgen replacement. Testosterone esters are lipophilic and are absorbed slowly when injected as an oil depot. These agents are of sufficient potency to achieve therapeutic effect without other significant side effects. The most commonly used testosterone ester is testosterone enanthate. After an intramuscular injection of 200 mg of testosterone enanthate in oil, peak supraphysiological levels of testosterone are reached rapidly within 1 – 3 days. The testosterone levels gradually decrease and reach baseline levels over the next 10 – 14 days (Fig. 53 – 2). Most hypogonadal men respond well to self-administration of intramuscular injections of testosterone enanthate 150 – 200 mg every 2 or 3 weeks. Occasionally, emotional lability and mood swings occur a few days prior to each injection. For these patients, 100 mg of testosterone enanthate can be administered every week. Testosterone cypionate has essentially the same pharmacokinetics and bioavailability as those of testosterone enanthate and can be used effectively as androgen replacement therapy.

Because of the occurrence of the initial peak of testosterone after each injection, long-acting esters of testosterone are currently under development for use in clinical medicine. One of these is testosterone-*trans*-4-*n*-butylcyclohexyl-carboxylate, which has a half-life of 63 days as opposed to 6 days for testosterone enanthate (in primates). Testosterone in polylactide-co-glycolide microspheres can be given intramuscularly and can sustain testosterone levels for over 70 days. These longer-acting testosterone preparations, capable of maintaining androgen levels within the physiological range without the initial burst, will probably be the agents of choice for androgen replacement in the near future.

Transdermal

Testosterone incorporated into transdermal delivery systems (40 or 60 cm^2) is worn as patches on the scrotum. These patches are changed daily. They can maintain normal testosterone levels when applied to hypogonadal men. Dihydrotestosterone levels are above the normal range, but the significance of a high dihydrotestosterone-testosterone ratio is unknown. These patches are now available in the United States for androgen replacement therapy.

Implants

Testosterone can be administered as subcutaneous implants. The pellets (400 – 600 mg of testosterone in four to six pellets) maintain testosterone levels within the physiological range for about 4 – 6 months. A minor surgical procedure involving local anesthesia is required to insert the pellets by a trained physician. Sometimes extrusion of the pellets can occur from the injection site, and fibroses around the pellets make removal difficult.

ANDROGEN REPLACEMENT THERAPY

The indications for androgen treatment are shown in Table 53 – 3. The primary use of androgens is for the treatment of hypogonadism. Patients with primary testicular failure must

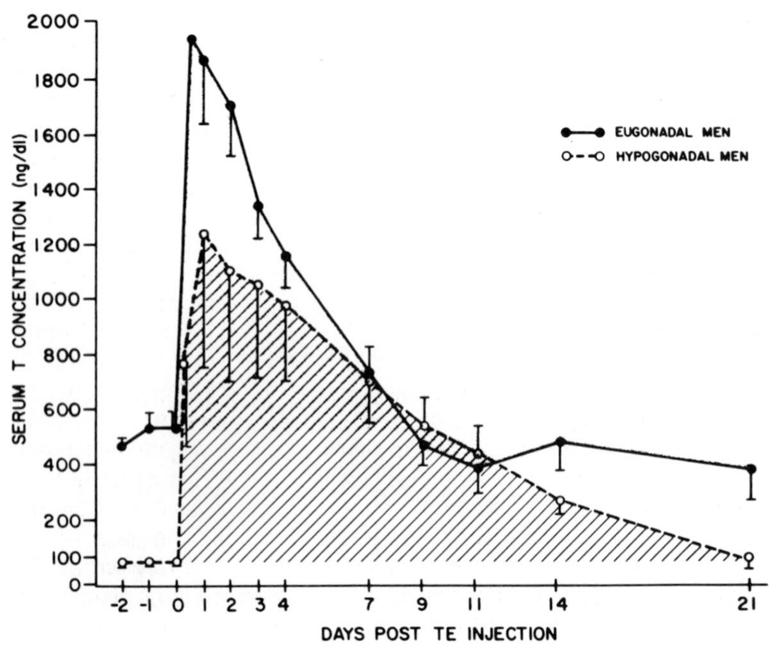

FIGURE 53 – 2. Mean and standard error of testosterone (T) levels in eugonadal and hypogonadal men before and at various time intervals after an intramuscular injection of 200 mg of testosterone enanthate (TE). (From Sokol RZ, Palacios A, Campfield LA, et al: Comparison of the kinetics of injectable testosterone in eugonadal and hypogonadal men. Fertil Steril 37:425, 1982. Reproduced with permission of the publisher, The American Fertility Society.)

TABLE 53 – 3. Indications for Androgen Therapy

Definite	Male hypogonadism
Probable or possible	Micropenis in children Constitutional delayed puberty Aging men (with evidence of androgen deficiency) Male contraception Hereditary angioneurotic edema
Dubious or controversial	Hematological disorders such as aplastic anemia, myelofibrosis with myeloid metaplasia, hemolytic anemia, autoimmune thrombocytopenia, and leukopenia Improvement of nitrogen balance in non-androgen-deficient catabolic state Improvement of libido in hypgonadal women
Not indicated	Anemia associated with renal failure Improvement of muscle strength and endurance in athletes and body builders

be treated with androgens to relieve their clinical symptoms and signs. Response to androgen replacement therapy is monitored by improvement in the clinical features of hypogonadism. Improvements in sexual function, frequency of shaving, secondary sexual characteristics, and general well-being occur rapidly after the initiation of treatment. It is often useful to monitor nadir and peak testosterone levels during the start of therapy and in patients who do not show adequate clinical response. Androgen treatment does not reverse their infertility. Patients with hypogonadotropic hypogonadism are also treated with androgens because of the ease of administration and low cost. If patients with hypogonadotropic hypogonadism desire fertility, human chorionic gonadotropin with human menopausal gonadotropin or pulsatile gonadotropin-releasing hormone (GnRH) injections or infusions may be given to induce spermatogenesis and fertility. Prior treatment with testosterone does not jeopardize the chances of fertility in these patients with hypogonadotropic hypogonadism.

In children with micropenis, a short course of low-dose androgen therapy is often tried. In adolescent boys with constitutional delay of puberty in whom the psychological effects of delayed puberty are significant, short-term treatment with testosterone enanthate for 3 – 4 months may be indicated.

Total and free testosterone levels decrease with age. A decrease in sexual function is often observed in older men. It has not been proved that androgen therapy in older men improves sexual function or prevents bone and muscle loss. At present, it is not known whether androgen replacement therapy improves the quality of life of aging men. The possible beneficial effect of androgens must be balanced against the possible adverse effects on lipids, prostate, and sleep-related breathing disorders.

In endocrine approaches to male contraception, when spermatogenesis is inhibited by suppression of hypothalamus and pituitary resulting in suppression of both LH and follicle-stimulating hormone (FSH), androgen supplementation is always required. Examples of experimental male contraceptives include androgens given alone or combined with progestogens or GnRH analogs. In these regimens, androgens function both to suppress sperm production by inhibiting gonadotropins and to provide physiological androgen replacement.

In hereditary angioneurotic edema, anabolic steroids such as stanozolol and danazol have been used to prevent attacks. These anabolic steroids increase the synthesis of complement 1 inhibitor, which is deficient in these patients. Because of the known side effects of these agents, they are not recommended for use in pregnant women and in children with this hereditary disorder.

The role of androgens in the treatment of hematological disorders remains controversial. Treatment of hypoplastic anemia with androgens may be tried for 3 – 6 months, but in responders treatment must be continued for a much longer period. The reader should refer to other chapters for information on the use of androgens in myelofibrosis, autoimmune thrombocytopenia, and hemolytic anemia (see Chapters 34 and 45). Because of the availability of recombinant human erythropoietin, with its more specific action and its lack of side effects, androgens should not be used for patients with anemia associated with chronic renal failure.

Androgens have been used in clinical situations, such as trauma or chronic illness, in which the patient is in a negative nitrogen balance. The long-term results are generally disappointing.

In postmenopausal women, low doses of androgens have been used together with estrogen-progestogen supplementation for improvement of libido. However, controlled trials showing a definite improvement in sexual drive after androgen therapy are lacking. Higher doses of androgens are associated with hirsutism and virilization in women.

An increasing trend toward the use of androgenic steroids by athletes and body builders can be seen. The pattern of androgen use by athletes involves the intermittent and cyclical administration of pharmacological doses of a combination of oral and parenteral agents. These unprescribed androgens may include huge doses of drugs, including veterinary agents that either are potentially toxic or have not been tested in humans. Androgens increase muscle mass and strength in women and prepubertal children. In normal adult men, it is not clear whether the administration of additional androgens enhances athletic performance. Most information is anecdotal; however, a number of studies have been performed. Double-blind studies either are in conflict or have not shown beneficial effects on athletic performance in postpubertal males. Even in those studies in which increased strength and performance was seen, the changes induced by these agents were small; thus documentation of clinically significant improvements in muscle strength and endurance may be difficult. Despite the controversy, some physicians have argued that changes in performance justify the use of these agents by some high-performance, competitive athletes. Most physicians, however, believe that the unsupervised use of androgens and high-dose androgen treatment impose some risk of undesired toxic effects. The toxic side effects of virilization in the female and premature bone closure in prepubertal children should preclude androgen use in athletes in these groups. In addition, the long-term abuse of supraphysiological doses of a combination of androgens in men may lead to gynecomastia, hepatic toxicity, polycythemia, lipid changes (lowering of high-density lipoprotein), and suppression of spermatogenesis. These toxic side effects are sufficient to discourage the use of androgens for nonmedical reasons in people of all ages, even adult men.

ADVERSE EFFECTS

In general, testosterone and its esters have fewer side effects than the 17-alkylated androgens. Acne and increased oiliness of skin are frequently experienced by patients at the initiation of androgen supplementation. Because testosterone is metabolized to estradiol, gynecomastia may develop. The gynecomastia is often mild, and treatment is unnecessary. Most patients gain weight when administered androgens. The weight gain is related to water retention, increased blood volume, and increased lean body mass. All patients given exogenous androgen therapy have suppression of spermatogenesis. Some patients notice a decrease in testicular size. The decreases in sperm production and seminiferous tubule volume are consequences of the suppression of LH and FSH. Androgens cause virilization in women and prepubertal children. In addition, androgens promote premature epiphyseal closure in children. For these reasons, androgens should not be used in women and in children of both sexes except for specific indications as discussed previously.

Hepatic Dysfunction

Changes in liver function and hepatic disorders are not observed with testosterone or its esters. The 17-alkylated androgens can produce liver dysfunction including cholestasis and elevation of plasma alkaline phosphatase and conjugated bilirubin. Methyltestosterone causes cholestatic jaundice with little parenchymal liver damage. Recovery is usually rapid after drug discontinuation. Peliosis hepatis or hepatic tumors occur rarely and only when high pharmacological doses of androgens are used to treat conditions such as refractory aplastic anemia. Because most of these reports involve conditions that are associated with increased incidence of neoplasms, the implications of such reports for the treatment of hypogonadal men remain controversial.

Lipid Changes

When a 17-alkylated androgen, stanozolol, is administered to normal men, high-density lipoprotein cholesterol and apolipoprotein A-I and A-II levels are decreased, and low-density lipoprotein cholesterol and apolipoprotein B levels are increased. These changes in lipid profiles have been identified as risk factors for coronary atherosclerosis. Such changes in lipid profile may not be associated with testosterone esters such as testosterone enanthate, perhaps because some of the testosterone is converted to estrogens that have effects on lipid profile opposite those of androgens. Another explanation for the difference on lipid profiles may be that the orally active anabolic steroids have a first-pass effect on the liver, leading to effects on lipids not apparent with the parenterally administered testosterone esters. More data are needed in larger groups of men to determine whether the testosterone esters are truly free of adverse effects on lipid profiles.

Hematopoiesis and Fibrinolysis

Androgens cause small increases in hemoglobin, hematocrit, and total red cell count when administered to normal or hypogonadal men. Androgens stimulate erythropoietin production by the kidneys. Androgens may also have a direct effect on the bone marrow stem cells. Clinically significant polycythemia is uncommon in hypogonadal men given androgen replacement except in patients who are likely to develop polycythemia, *eg*, those with chronic obstructive pulmonary disease or sleep apnea.

The 17-alkylated androgens, stanozolol and danazol, have been given to men with coagulation disorders. Although small increases of clotting factors have been recorded, these anabolic steroids increase fibrinolysis and antithrombin III levels (a natural anticoagulant). The net effect is that increased bleeding episodes occur. The increase in fibrinolysis may counterbalance the negative effects of lipid profiles on the risk of coronary heart disease.

Respiratory Problems

In hypogonadal men treated with androgen replacement, sleep-related breathing disorders have been reported. In obese patients and those with chronic obstructive airway disease, the physician should question the patient about sleep-related breathing disorders before the commencement of androgen replacement.

Carbohydrate Metabolism

Although reports of androgen-induced mild resistance to insulin action exist, the usual doses of testosterone esters, when given to normal men, are not associated with changes in glucose or insulin levels. Adverse effects on glucose control in diabetic patients given androgen replacement have been reported.

Prostate Problems

Benign prostatic hypertrophy (BPH) and prostate cancer rarely occur in men who developed androgen deficiency prior to puberty. Despite this fact, no clear evidence indicates that androgen replacement given to men who become hypogonadal after puberty increases the risk of prostatic disease. For all adult men, especially older men, on long-term androgen therapy, regular rectal examinations must be performed and prostate-specific antigen levels should be monitored. If a suspicion of prostatic enlargement exists, a transrectal prostatic ultrasound should be performed.

Psychosexual Problems

In prepubertal boys given testosterone replacement, changes in psychosexual behavior may occur. To avoid these problems, low dosages of testosterone enanthate (25 - 50 mg) every 3 - 4 weeks are administered at the initiation of androgen therapy. After 6 months or a year, the testosterone dosage can be increased to 50 - 100 mg every 3 - 4 weeks for the next 2 years and further increased to the adult replacement dosage as necessary. Frequent erections can occur at the start of androgen therapy. Priapism is uncommon. Psychosexual problems usually decrease with time.

ANTIANDROGENS

The antiandrogens exert their effect by interfering with the action of androgens at the target tissues. These include the mineralocorticoid antagonist spironolactone and the pure antiandrogens cyproterone and flutamide. The other groups of drugs are inhibitors of androgen biosynthesis including ketoconazole and the newly developed finasteride. The indications for antiandrogen therapy are listed in Table 53 - 4. The weak antiandrogen spironolactone has been used for the treatment of hirsutism (in women). Originally developed for male hypersexuality, cyproterone acetate, the antiandrogen with progestational activity, has been used extensively for the treatment of women with hirsutism and boys with precocious puberty. Flutamide has been tested in clinical studies alone or in combination with a potent GnRH agonist as hormonal therapy for metastatic advanced prostatic cancer. Finasteride has been shown to decrease prostate size in animals and humans and is potentially useful in the treatment of hirsutism, BPH, and carcinoma of the prostate.

Spironolactone

The aldosterone antagonist spironolactone has been found to have weak antiandrogenic properties. It inhibits the cytochrome P-450 enzyme system, which is required for the synthesis of androgens. It also interferes with the action of androgens by occupying the specific androgen receptors in the target tissues. Clinical studies have shown that spironolactone reduced the hair density and diameter in patients with hirsutism. The dose of spironolactone used is 100 mg/day orally. Although spironolactone is associated with menstrual disturbances when given to normal females, it can induce normal menstrual periods in patients with anovulatory hyperandrogenism.

TABLE 53 - 4. Indications for Antiandrogen Therapy

Hirsutism/virilism in females
Benign prostatic hypertrophy
Advanced prostatic cancer
Hypersexuality
Gonadotropin-independent precocious puberty in boys (familial testotoxicosis) (not recommended for control of precocious puberty in both girls and boys because of the availability of gonadotropin-releasing hormone analogs)

Cyproterone and Cyproterone Acetate

The pure antiandrogen cyproterone interferes with androgen binding to the nuclei receptor at the target tissue. Peripheral testosterone and gonadotropin levels are not suppressed but often elevated in patients given the drug. Its acetate derivative has both antiandrogen and strong progestational effects; the latter activity suppresses the secretion of gonadotropins, which secondarily decrease testosterone biosynthesis. Cyproterone acetate is widely used in Europe for the treatment of hirsutism. It is administered at an oral dose of 50 mg in combination with estrogens on days 5 - 25 of the menstrual cycle for the treatment of hirsutism. A much reduced dose of 2 mg of cyproterone acetate in combination with estrogens is available for the treatment of mild hirsutism and acne. Because of its suppressive effects on gonadotropins, cyproterone acetate has been used for the arrest of puberty in gonadotropin-dependent (central) precocious puberty. Although pubertal development is arrested, bone maturation usually continues, leading to a reduction in final height. GnRH agonist is more effective in the treatment of central precocious puberty, because its greater effectiveness in suppressing gonadotropin secretion results in arrest of secondary sexual development and skeletal maturation. The estimated final height of the children is, therefore, not compromised. Cyproterone acetate has also been used in Europe to treat advanced prostate cancer, although use of GnRH analogs with or without antiandrogens appears to be the preferred medical therapy. Cyproterone acetate sometimes causes hepatic dysfunction; despite its widespread use in other countries, the drug is not approved for use by the Food and Drug Administration in the United States.

Flutamide

Flutamide is a nonsteroidal antiandrogen that blocks androgen action at the target tissue. In humans, flutamide, like pure cyproterone, leads to elevated serum levels of testosterone and LH. It has been used as an investigational drug alone or in combination with GnRH agonists for the treatment of advanced prostatic cancer to achieve complete androgen blockade. The common side effect is gynecomastia. Very occasionally, flutamide may cause hematological disorders such as methemoglobinemia.

Ketoconazole

Ketoconazole, an orally administered imidazole used for treatment of fungal infections, blocks adrenal and testicular androgen biosynthesis. Keotoconazole directly inhibits the cytochrome system of steroidogenic enzyme, primarily on the enzyme C17-20 lyase and cholesterol side-chain cleavage enzymes. Ketoconazole has been shown to be effective in the treatment of gonadotropin-independent precocious puberty (familial testotoxicosis). The initial dose used for the suppression of precocious puberty is 3 mg/kg body weight per day. Ketoconazole has also been used for advanced prostatic cancer. The drug may cause some significant side effects when used in dosages in excess of 600 mg/day. These include transient adrenal suppression, nausea, vomiting, anemia, and elevated liver enzymes.

Finasteride

Finasteride is a specific inhibitor of 5α-reductase that converts testosterone to 5α-dihydrotestosterone. It has been shown to be effective in reducing prostate size in dogs and rats. In humans, finasteride causes dose-dependent decreases in serum 5α-dihydrotestosterone as well as its metabolites, 3α-androstanediol glucuronide and androsterone glucuronide. Preliminary studies demonstrated no decrease in serum levels of testosterone and little change in serum FSH and LH levels. Pilot studies of finasteride in patients with BPH demonstrated reductions in prostatic volume and increases in urinary flow. This drug is potentially useful in dihydrotestosterone-dependent disease conditions such as BPH, prostatic cancer, hirsutism, and virilism.

REFERENCES

ANDROGENS

Amuss SS: The role of androgens in the treatment of hematologic disorders. Adv Intern Med 34:191, 1989.

Cantrill JA, Dewis P, Large DM, et al: Which testosterone replacement therapy? Clin Endocrinol (Oxf) 21:97, 1984.

Mooradian AD, Morley JE, Korenman SG: Biological actions of androgens. Endocr Rev 9:181, 1984.

Snyder PJ, Lawrence DA: Treatment of male hypogonadism with testosterone enanthate. J Clin Endocrinol Metab 51:1335, 1980.

Sokol RZ, Palacios A, Campfield La, et al: Comparison of the kinetics of injectable testosterone in eugonadal and hypogonadal men. Fertil Steril 37:425, 1982.

Swerdloff RS, Sokol RZ: Manifestations of androgen deficiency and effects of androgen therapy. *In* Steinberger E, Frajese G, Steinberger A (eds): Reproductive Medicine, 39–53. New York: Raven Press, 1986.

Wilson JD: Androgen abuse by athletes. Endocr Rev 9:181, 1988.

ANTIANDROGENS

Ghormley GJ, Stoner C, Rittmester RS, et al: Effects of finasteride, a 5 alpha-reductase inhibitor on circulating androgens in male volunteers. J Clin Endocrinol Metab 70:1136, 1990.

Holland FJ, Fishman L, Bailey JD, Fazekas AT: Ketoconazole in the management of precocious puberty not responsive to LHRH-analogue therapy. N Engl J Med 312:1023–1028, 1985.

Neuman F: Pharmacology and potential use of cyproterone acetate. Horm Metab Res 9:1, 1977.

Shapiro G, Evron S: A novel use of spironolactone: Treatment of hirsutism. J Clin Endocrinol Metab 52:429, 1980.

Sogani P, Fair WR: Treatment of advanced prostatic cancer. Urol Clin North Am 14:2, 1987.

Estrogens and Progestins 54

Lynette K. Nieman

The cyclical secretion of estrogen and progesterone by the ovary is responsible for the development and maintenance of female sexual characteristics and function.

ESTROGENS

Chemistry

All natural estrogens are steroids, including estrone, estradiol, and estriol (Figs. 54 – 1 and 54 – 2), as well as preparations of conjugated estrogens derived from the urine of pregnant mares. Synthetic estrogens may be steroidal or nonsteroidal. All steroidal estrogens are derived from a C_{18} estrane skeleton, with an unsaturated A ring and a phenolic hydroxyl group at C3, a methyl group at C13, and an oxygen (ketone or hydroxyl) at C17. Structural changes at these positions can affect biological properties. Examples include the shift of the C17 hydroxyl group from β to α position, which eliminates nearly all biological activity, and the substitution of an ethinyl group at C17, which allows the compounds to be orally active.

Biosynthesis, Secretion, and Plasma Binding

Estradiol, the most potent and prevalent of the naturally occurring estrogens, is made by the gonads of both sexes, as is estrone. Estriol and estrone may be produced by the liver, and adrenal androgens may be converted to estrone by peripheral tissues. Aromatization of androstenedione to estrone occurs in fat, liver, skeletal muscles, hypothalamus, and hair follicles. This conversion is dependent on the availability of the substrate and increases with age and body mass.

In the menstruating woman, the dominant follicle and corpus luteum are the primary sources of both estradiol and estrone, whereas peripheral production contributes a small amount (approximately 25%) of circulating estrone. In men and postmenopausal women, peripheral aromatization of adrenal androstenedione to estrone is the major source of estrogen.

Little free estriol exists in the plasma (<10 pg/mL in nonpregnant women). Estrogen production increases dramatically during pregnancy. Nearly all of the androgenic precursors of estriol and about 50% of those for estradiol are derived from fetal adrenal precursors, dehydroepiandrosterone (DHA), and 16-hydroxy-DHA. These compounds are aromatized in the placenta, and the estrogens are secreted preferentially into the maternal blood stream.

Plasma estrogens are bound weakly to albumin and more tightly to sex hormone – binding globulin (SHBG). Estriol is less well bound than estradiol or estrone. About 50% of the estrogens in blood are conjugated.

Mechanism of Action

Estrogens, like other steroids, diffuse freely and rapidly into cells. Estrogen-sensitive organs contain specific high-affinity, low-capacity binding proteins called *receptors.* The hormone binds to the receptor, and the hormone-receptor complex binds to acceptor sites at or near DNA sites that initiate mRNA synthesis. Protein formation is one of the earliest measurable effects of estrogen on its target cell and occurs within the first 6 hours of exposure. DNA replication and cell division are promoted within 24 hours. Therefore, long-term exposure to estrogens results in tissue growth.

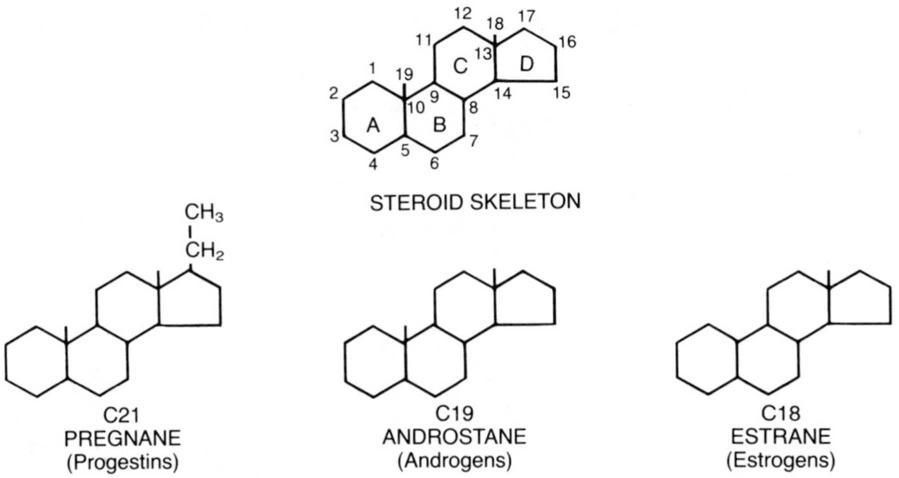

FIGURE 54–1. The basic steroidal structure. By convention, the carbon atoms are numbered and the rings are alphabetized as shown. The removal of successive carbons leads to the prototypic skeleton for the major classes of steroid hormones: C21 (pregnane, the progestins); C19 (androstane, the androgens); and C18 (estrane, the estrogens).

Estradiol receptors characterize hormonally dependent tumors. This has led to the use of hormones or hormone antagonists as chemotherapeutic agents. When compared with autonomous tumors, hormone-dependent breast carcinomas take up more estrogen, have more receptors, and respond better to hormonal chemotherapy. Therefore, the receptor content of the excised tumor has been used to predict the subsequent response to hormonal ablation therapy.

Absorption, Distribution, Metabolism, and Excretion

Estrogens are readily absorbed after oral, transdermal, intravenous, or transvaginal administration. The route of administration and the hepatic metabolism influence the biological effects.

After absorption through the gastrointestinal tract, estrogens are delivered to the portal system. In the liver, the natural unconjugated estrogens, estradiol and estriol, are converted primarily to estrone and then undergo conjugation and enterohepatic circulation, resulting in increased serum estrone levels. The conjugated estrogens, some synthetic derivatives of the natural estrogens, and the nonsteroidal estrogens are degraded more slowly and retain biological activity when given orally.

The rate of absorption through skin and mucous membranes is affected by the vehicle; vaginal administration of estradiol as a saline suspension or as a micronized tablet results in prompt absorption, whereas absorption of cream preparations is decreased. The enterohepatic circulation does not affect estrogens given by a nonoral route, and their subsequent biological action is related to their metabolism and intrinsic potency.

Estrogens are absorbed rapidly after injection as a crystalline aqueous suspension or as a solution in oil, leading to high peak plasma concentrations, a potential disadvantage. The rate of absorption can be decreased by esterification or polymerization of the estrogen.

The metabolism of exogenous and endogenous estrogens is similar. Estradiol and estrone are metabolized in the liver to more water-soluble, less protein-bound substances by hydroxylation (at the C16 and C2 positions) and by conjugation with sulfuric or glucuronic acid. These compounds are excreted by the kidney. Hepatic hydroxylation is catalyzed by microsomal enzymes and is affected by drugs that induce these enzymes. Estriol has little biliary excretion or metabolic transformation and is excreted more rapidly and quantitatively in the urine. Estrone sulfate, a major metabolite of estradiol, is cleared slowly because it is tightly bound to albumin.

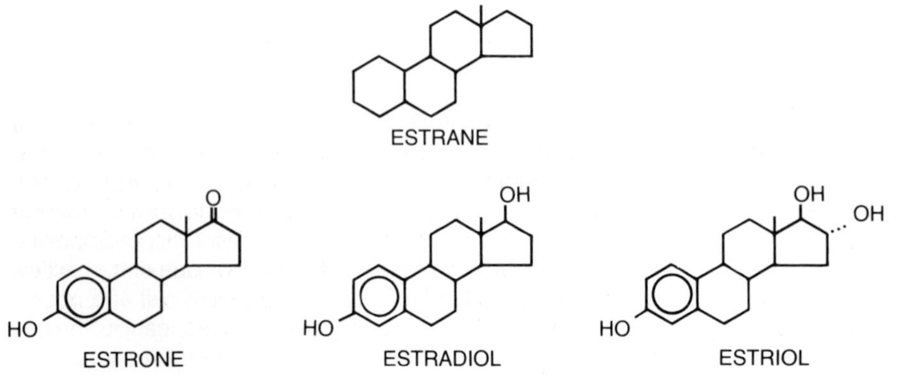

FIGURE 54–2. Structure of estrane, the prototypic estrogen, and the three major estrogens in women: estrone, estradiol, and estriol.

Biological Effects

Estrogen is necessary for the development and maintenance of normal secondary sexual characteristics in women (Table 54-1).

In men, estrogens antagonize the effects of androgens. They decrease the rate of prostatic growth, libido, and sebaceous gland activity. When estrogens are present in sufficient quantity, they cause gynecomastia.

Adverse Effects of Estrogen Replacement

The side effects differ according to the type and dosage of estrogen that is given and whether or not progestins are given concomitantly. The following sections report the effects seen with estrogen replacement therapy with conjugated estrogens, 0.625 or 1.25 mg/day (Table 54-2). A variety of side effects associated with contraceptive agents, including benign liver tumors and gallstones, are not seen with estrogen hormone replacement therapy, possibly because of the difference in estrogen dose. The side effects of combined contraceptive agents are discussed in the section Steroidal Contraceptive Agents.

TABLE 54-1. Estrogen Target Tissues and Biological Actions

Target Tissues	Biological Actions
Hypothalamus	Negative feedback on gonadotropin-releasing hormone secretion
Pituitary	Negative feedback on follicle-stimulating hormone secretion; inhibitory and stimulatory effects on luteinizing hormone
Reproductive Tissues	
External genitalia	Growth and maintenance
Vagina	Elongation, increased elasticity, rugation, distensibility Induction of fluid transudation, formation of cornified cell layer
Labia minora	Increase in size
Urogenital structures	Maintenance of elasticity and tone
Uterus	Increase in cell number and size
Nonreproductive Tissues	
Breast	Growth of mammary ducts
Fat	Female fat distribution
Skin	Maintenance of tone and elasticity
Hair	Promotion of growth of axillary and pubic hair
Bones	Stimulation of growth (low dose) Acceleration of epiphyseal fusion (high dose)
Fluid	Promotion of salt and fluid retention
Liver	
Lipids	Decrease total cholesterol and low-density lipoprotein Increase total triglycerides and high-density lipoprotein
Proteins	Stimulation of carrier proteins (CBG, TeBG, SHBG)

CBG = corticosteroid-binding globulin; SHBG = sex hormone-binding globulin; TeBG = testosterone-estradiol-binding globulin.

TABLE 54-2. Adverse Effects of Unopposed Estrogen

Effect	Confidence	Comments
Nausea	Definite	Dose-dependent
Breast		
Engorgement	Definite	
Cancer	Controversial	Relative risk perhaps slightly increased
Endometrium		
Hyperplasia	Definite	With unopposed estrogen
Bleeding	Definite	
Cancer	Definite	With unopposed estrogen; dose- and time-dependent
Genital abnormalities	Definite	Diethylstilbestrol in utero
Thromboembolism	Dubious	
Hypertension	Dubious	Both increases and decreases reported
Cholestatic jaundice	Definite	Uncommon; only occurs at high dose
Migraine headache	Probable	

Nausea

With conventional doses of estrogen, nausea may be worse in the morning, usually decreasing with continued administration of the drug and seldom causing weight loss. Nausea improves at lower doses of estrogen and may progress to anorexia and vomiting at higher doses.

Breast Neoplasia

The relationship between estrogen replacement therapy and the risk of developing breast cancer has not been resolved. Most well-designed studies either fail to show a relationship between estrogen replacement therapy and breast cancer or suggest a small increased relative risk that may not be significant. Certain aspects deserve further study. These include questions of the effects of the dose and duration of estrogen replacement therapy, history of oophorectomy, and the risk for older women with a family history of breast cancer.

Estrogen replacement therapy is contraindicated in women with estrogen-dependent malignancy.

Endometrial Cancer

Unopposed estrogen, from an endogenous or exogenous source, increases the risk of development of endometrial hyperplasia and carcinoma. The risk increases up to 12-fold as the dose and the duration of estrogen use increase. The addition of progesterone to estrogen replacement therapy reduces the risk of endometrial hyperplasia and endometrial cancer to equal to or below that seen in women receiving no hormonal treatment. The optimal regimen to prevent hyperplasia consists of 12-13 days of progestogen treatment each month.

Genital Abnormalities

Exposure to diethylstilbestrol (DES) *in utero* has caused urogenital tract abnormalities and reproductive problems in both males and females. Epithelial changes in the vagina and cervix occur in two thirds of the females exposed to DES, and a smaller proportion have structural abnormalities of the uterine cavity or fallopian tubes. Clear cell carcinoma of the vagina occurs in less than 0.1% of exposed females; incidence peaks at age 19 years and approaches baseline by age 30. Functional abnormalities include an increased incidence of first- and second-trimester miscarriages, ectopic pregnancies, and premature deliveries.

Data are not available for other estrogens given in pregnancy, but the presumption is that they would have similar effects. If a patient becomes pregnant while using estrogens or if estrogens are inadvertently prescribed to a pregnant patient, they should be discontinued and the woman should be informed of the potential hazards to the fetus.

Hepatic Effects

Estrogens enhance hepatic protein synthesis. Circulating levels of carrier proteins, including corticosteroid-binding globulin (CBG), SHBG, thyroid-binding globulin, transferrin, and ceruloplasmin, increase, allowing the quantity of the bound hormone and the total amount of hormone as measured by radioimmunoassay to increase; however, the unbound or free fraction of the hormone remains unchanged. A radioimmunoassay method that measures the total circulating hormone gives a result that may be increased above the normal range, perhaps giving the false impression that the free concentration of hormone is elevated as well. This effect is not counteracted by the addition of progestin to the treatment regimen. Estrogens also increase the hepatic synthesis of other proteins that may contribute to disease processes. These include clotting factors (especially VII and X) and angiotensinogen.

Central Nervous System Effects

Estrogens may precipitate headaches and should be stopped if migraine headaches begin or increase or if a new headache pattern emerges. Depression may occur with the use of conjugated estrogens.

Drug Interactions

Most drug interactions with estrogens are associated with the oral route of administration and a significant first-pass effect on the liver. Oral anticoagulant action may be decreased by estrogen therapy, an effect that may be mediated through an increase in vitamin K levels.

The action of estrogens may decrease when they are given with agents that increase activity of hepatic microsomal enzymes, probably because of accelerated metabolism of estrogens to less-active compounds. This effect is seen commonly with rifampin, phenylbutazone, phenytoin, primidone, carbamazepine, and the barbiturates.

BOX 54–1

THERAPEUTIC USES

Hormonal Replacement Therapy. In a young woman who has a failure to pubesce, estrogen alone may be used to induce puberty. If the epiphyses have not fused, low dosages of estrogen may be used (ethinyl estradiol, 100 ng/kg/day) to promote the growth of the long bones. The breasts and endometrium do not respond to this dose of estrogen. If the bones have fused, therapy can be initiated at a higher dosage (200–800 ng/kg/day) to promote breast development and feminization. Progestins should be added at the time of the first breakthrough bleeding episode to induce cyclical withdrawal bleeding.

In the castrated or climacteric woman, estrogen replacement therapy prevents or improves the symptoms of estrogen deficiency shown in Table 54–3. Vasomotor symptoms occur in as many as 85% of climacteric women and are common at night, resulting in sleep disturbance. Estrogens have not been shown to be useful in the treatment of menopausal depression and should not be used for that indication alone. Long-term estrogen replacement therapy may also be important for the prevention of osteoporosis and cardiovascular disease.

Postmenopausal osteoporosis may be retarded by the initiation of estrogen replacement therapy close to the onset of amenorrhea. Case-control and other retrospective studies suggest that the long-term use of estrogen in postmenopausal women may decrease the risk of fracture by up to 50%, especially if therapy is started within 5 years of the last menses. Prospective studies are necessary, however, to show that the eventual fracture rate is decreased by this approach.

Other risk factors for osteoporosis such as dietary intake of calcium, exercise, ethnic background, and weight should be factored into the decision to use estrogens.

Meta-analysis of descriptive retrospective studies of postmenopausal women receiving estrogen replacement therapy reveals a reduction in risk of cardiovascular disease by about 50%. The beneficial effect of estrogens is assumed to be related in part to a decrease in total and low-density lipoprotein (LDL) cholesterol and to an increase in high-density lipoprotein (HDL) cholesterol. Most of the patients in these series were taking conjugated estrogens and no progestin. The addition of progestins, especially of the 19-nor series, may reverse the beneficial effects on lipids seen with estrogen replacement.

Lipid levels change relatively little on average when medroxyprogesterone (5 mg/day for 10–12 days/cycle) is used. Few data are available to judge the effects on lipids of low-dose combined continuous estrogen and progesterone therapy.

Pros and Cons of Hormonal Replacement Therapy. The decision to recommend hormonal replacement therapy should be individualized for each woman, based on assessment of risks (Table 54–4) and benefits. Long-term use of estrogen in climacteric women ameliorates vasomotor and urogenital climacteric complaints and may yield a decreased risk of fracture and cardiovascular disease.

The major long-term risk of postmenopausal estrogen therapy is the development of endometrial cancer. The addition of a progestin appears to protect against the development of endometrial hyperplasia without having an adverse effect on bone density. The choice of progestin may overwhelm or negate the beneficial effects of estrogen on the serum lipid profile. The 19-norprogestin series has the most negative effect, and natural progesterone, the least negative effect on HDL levels. It seems prudent to advocate the use of the lowest dosage of progestin possible to adequately antagonize estrogen effects on the endometrium.

Chemotherapy. Estrogens such as DES have been used in the treatment of advanced metastatic tumors that have receptors for estrogen, including breast cancer in postmenopausal women and prostatic carcinoma in men.

Antiestrogens. Two weak estrogen agonists, tamoxifen and clomiphene, have found wide therapeutic use as estrogen antagonists. Tamoxifen is useful in the treatment of estrogen-receptor–positive breast cancer in postmenopausal women. Clomiphene is used to induce ovulation in anovulatory women.

Choice of Preparations and Dosages

Estrogens may be given as oral, intramuscular, and topical preparations. Oral administration is most common, and its effects are best understood. Intramuscular administration has the potential advantage of improved compliance, requiring only monthly administration with certain agents, and also avoids the hepatic side effects. However, the initial peak concentration of estrogen is high, and absorption may be variable. Topical routes such as transvaginal or transdermal administration may lead to a greater physiological estrone-to-estradiol ratio; however, vaginal absorption may be erratic.

TABLE 54–3. Symptoms of Estrogen Deficiency

Vasomotor Instability

- Hot flushes
- Dizziness
- Headaches
- Palpitations
- Diaphoresis
- Night sweats

Vagina, Bladder, Urethral Atrophy

- Dyspareunia
- Dysuria
- Frequency
- Urgency
- Nocturia
- Vaginitis

TABLE 54–4. Contraindications to Estrogen Therapy

Absolute Contraindications

Pregnancy
Estrogen-dependent tumor, such as breast, endometrium
Undiagnosed genital bleeding
Active liver disease

Relative Contraindications

Thromboembolic disease
Thrombophlebitis
Uterine leiomyomata
History of liver disease
Diabetes mellitus
Porphyria
Hypertension

The large number of estrogen preparations available may make the choice of a given preparation difficult (Table 54–5). The recommendations for specific therapeutic situations include regimens in common use as well as some of the more recent therapeutic options.

Hormonal replacement therapy for premenopausal women is generally chosen to mimic the normal cycle and to avoid deleterious side effects. Oral contraceptives containing the lowest dose of estrogen (20–35 μg ethinyl estradiol) and progestin (norethindrone acetate, 1 mg, or levonorgestrel in a triphasic pattern) are commonly used. These doses exceed the minimal replacement dosage of estrogen (about 20 μg/day of ethinyl estradiol) and have the disadvantages discussed under Steroidal Contraceptive Agents. The mnemonic packaging of these agents makes their use a convenient approach that can be recommended for women younger than 35 years of age. Other physiological regimens can be designed to mimic the menstrual cycle, using a low daily dosage of estrogen and a low dosage of progestin for the first 12 days of each calendar month. Micronized estradiol and progesterone given by mouth may best mimic normal hormone levels and physiological effects, but experience with this approach is limited.

Hormonal replacement regimens for postmenopausal women should maximize effects on urogenital organs and the bones and minimize undesirable side effects. Table 54–6 compares the effects of some of the more commonly used estrogen preparations given by the oral and topical routes without a progestin. The dose-response effects of a single preparation are different for different organs.

Strong consideration should be given to the addition of a progestin in women with an intact uterus (Table 54–7). Progesterone may be given intermittently for 10–13 consecutive days each month (often best remembered by starting on the first calendar day), or else daily. Although the addition of intermittent progesterone induces withdrawal bleed-

TABLE 54–5. Available Estrogen Preparations

Type of Estrogen	Doses Available			
	Oral (mg)	*Parenteral (mg/mL)*	*Vaginal (%)*	*Transdermal*
Steroidal				
ESTRADIOL				
Estradiol	1, 2	None	0.01*	0.05, 0.1*
Estradiol cypionate	None	1, 5	None	None
Ethinyl estradiol	0.02, 0.05, 0.5	None	None	None
Polyestradiol phosphate	None	20	None	None
ESTRONE	None	2, 5	None	None
Esterified estrogens	0.3, 0.625, 1.25, 2.5	None	None	None
Estropipate†	0.625, 1.25, 2.5, 5	None	0.15	None
Estrone	None	2, 5	None	None
CONJUGATED EQUINE Estrogens	0.3, 0.625, 0.9, 1.25, 2.5	25	0.0625	None
Nonsteroidal				
Chlorotrianisene	12, 25	None	None	None
Dienestrol	None	None	0.01	None
Diethylstilbestrol	1, 5	50	None	None
Quinestrol	0.1	None	None	None

*mg/24 hours.
†Equivalent dose of estrone sodium sulfate.

ing, combined continuous administration of both estrogen and progesterone eventually results in an atrophic endometrium and no bleeding. Until that state is achieved, usually after about 6 months, unpredictable intermittent bleeding requiring evaluation may occur.

Few studies have evaluated the dose-response effects of a combined estrogen-progestin preparation on gonadotropin levels, vaginal cytology, or the induction of (nonlipid) hepatic proteins. It appears that the addition of a progestin either enhances slightly or has no effect on bone density. The beneficial effect of oral estrogens on lipid metabolism may be negated or overwhelmed by the addition of progestin. This undesirable result depends on the type of progestin, with the 19-nor series having the most adverse effect, and micronized oral progesterone having the least adverse effect. More work is needed to define the optimal type and route of administration of estrogens and progestins in the postmenopausal woman.

TABLE 54–6. Dose-Response Effects of Commonly Used Estrogens

Estrogen Preparation	Bone Density Improvement*	Superficial Vaginal Cell Cytology*	Induction Hepatic Proteins*
Ethinyl estradiol oral (μg)	20	5–50	5
Conjugated estrogens			
Oral (mg)	0.625	1.25	0.625
Vaginal (mg)	ND	0.3	1.25
Estradiol transdermal (μg/day)	100	100	>200

*Minimal effective dose.
ND = no data.

PROGESTINS

Chemistry

Progestins, as implied by the name, are compounds capable of sustaining pregnancy. Progesterone is the only naturally occurring progestin, but many synthetic compounds have

TABLE 54–7. Daily Doses of Estrogens and Progestins Used for Hormonal Replacement Therapy for the Menopause*

Estrogen (mg)		Dose
Conjugated estrogens		0.625
Micronized estradiol		1.0
Transdermal estradiol		0.1
Progestin (mg)	**Intermittent Dose**	**Continuous Dose**
MPA	5	2.5
Norethindrone	1	0.35
Levonorgestrel	—	0.15

*The estradiol doses are roughly equivalent in terms of effects on bone density; the progestin doses, within each schedule (intermittent vs continuous), have similar effects on lipids and the endometrium. Thus, any of the estrogens could be paired with any of the progestins shown.
MPA = medroxyprogesterone acetate.

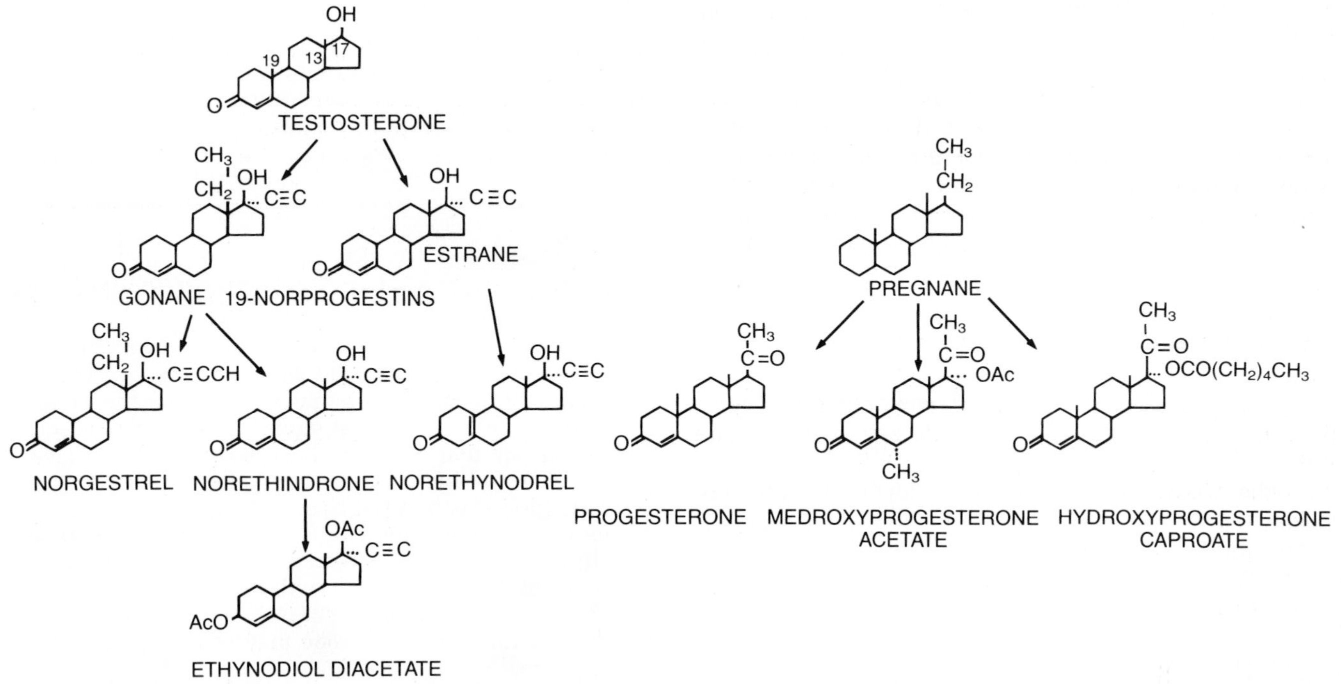

FIGURE 54–3. Structure of the gonane-, estrane-, and pregnane-derived progestins. The estranes are derived from testosterone by removal of the C19 methyl group and the addition of an ethinyl group at C17. The gonanes share this structure with an ethyl group at C13.

progestin activity. The synthetic progestins derive either from progesterone or from testosterone.

The progesterone derivatives (pregnanes) have properties most like native progesterone (Fig. 54–3). The testosterone derivatives (estranes and gonanes) have alterations at the C19 and C17 positions. The estranes lack a C19 methyl group and have an ethinyl group at C17. Removal of the C19 methyl group from testosterone yields a series of compounds called C19-norprogestins that have enhanced progestin and decreased androgenic activity. The addition of an ethinyl group at C17 further decreases androgenic activity and allows the compound to be orally active. Norethindrone (called norethisterone in Europe), 17-ethinyl-19-nortestosterone, is an example of this strategy. The estrane-derived progestins are converted to norethindrone in the liver.

The gonanes are estranes with an ethyl group at position 13. This addition yields one of the most active steroids parenterally, norgestrel, but at the cost of producing some androgenic side effects. The gonane-derived progestins do not require hepatic transformation for biological activity. Norgestimate, desogestrel, and gestodene are progestins with little androgenicity.

Biosynthesis, Secretion, and Plasma Binding

Progesterone is secreted from the dominant follicle beginning just before ovulation and from the corpus luteum once ovulation has occurred, reaching peak plasma concentrations of 10–30 ng/mL in the midluteal phase. When pregnancy does not occur, the corpus luteum regresses, progesterone levels decrease, and menses begin. In fertile cycles, human chorionic gonadotropin secretion by the trophoblast maintains corpus luteum progesterone production. The placenta begins to produce progesterone in amounts adequate to support pregnancy by the 2nd or 3rd month of gestation. After this, the corpus luteum is not essential.

Progesterone also is made by the adrenal cortex and testes. These sources account for the low plasma concentrations ($<$2 ng/mL) in men and in anovulatory and postmenopausal women.

Circulating plasma progesterone is bound largely to CBG. The pregnane-derived progestins show little binding to CBG or SHBG. The estrane derivatives, in contrast, bind strongly to SHBG.

Mechanism of Action

Unbound progesterone, like other steroids, diffuses into its target cell, where it binds to an intranuclear protein receptor that is specific for the progestins. The progestin-receptor complex binds to DNA and activates specific mRNA synthesis, resulting ultimately in the production of proteins. Progesterone action is modulated by the concentration of receptors in the cell. Estrogen secreted during the follicular phase increases the amount of progesterone receptor in the endometrium. Progesterone in turn inhibits the synthesis of both its own receptor and that of estradiol.

Absorption, Distribution, Metabolism, and Excretion

Micronized progesterone is well absorbed and has significant oral activity. The oral absorption of the synthetic progestins is variable and is subject to first-pass hepatic hydroxylation and conjugation. Progesterone is well absorbed from the vagina, rectum, and muscles. The long-acting parenteral preparations rely on the injection of a hydrophobic suspension or solution or on the incorporation of an active compound into a carrier substance and provide long-term steady-state levels of drug. Progesterone is metabolized primarily in the liver. The metabolites are conjugated with glucuronide or sulfate and excreted. The major urinary metabolite is pregnane-3, 20-diol-glucuronide (pregnanediol).

Biological Effects

Progesterone action at the primary target organs, the uterus and the breasts, is dependent on prior estrogen exposure (Table 54–8).

Other biological effects are seen with the synthetic progestins that bind to other steroid receptors and act as hormone agonists or antagonists. The 17-hydroxy or -acetoxy compounds are the most similar to progesterone. The 19-nor derivatives, on the other hand, exhibit some estrogenic or androgenic properties, including nitrogen retention, weight gain, exacerbation of acne, and impaired glucose tolerance.

Hepatic lipid metabolism also is affected by the administration of synthetic progestins, especially the 19-nor compounds. These agents tend to decrease the concentrations of very low density lipoprotein triglycerides and HDL, especially HDL_2. It remains unclear whether a dose of progestin that affects the endometrium but not lipid levels can be defined.

Contraindications to progestin use include a history of thrombophlebitis, thromboembolic disease, cancer of the breast, undiagnosed vaginal bleeding, a missed abortion, and active liver disease.

Adverse Effects of Progestin Treatment

The most common untoward effect of progestin treatment is abnormal menstrual bleeding, *ie*, breakthrough bleeding, spotting, changes in the amount of flow, or amenorrhea.

TABLE 54–8. Progesterone Target Tissues and Biological Actions

Target Tissues	Biological Actions
Hypothalamus	Increase in body temperature by 0.5–1°F
Pituitary	Negative feedback luteinizing hormone and follicle-stimulating hormone secretion
Reproductive Tissues	Differentiation
Uterus	Secretory changes in glands
	Differentiation of stroma
	Maintenance of pregnancy
	Increase in myometrial mass
Fallopian tube	Decrease in contractility
Cervical mucus	Decrease in amount; increase in thickness
Nonreproductive Tissues	
Breast	Growth of alveolar tissue
Fluid	Promotion of natriuresis

Synthetic progestins have been associated with masculinization of female fetuses and feminization of male fetuses and should not be given to pregnant women. Effects seen with combined estrogen-progestin contraceptives are discussed in Steroidal Contraceptive Agents.

BOX 54–2
THERAPEUTIC USES OF PROGESTINS

Dysfunctional uterine bleeding is common at the extremes of reproductive life when anovulatory cycles frequently occur. It probably results from the breakdown of an estrogen-stimulated hyperplastic endometrium that has not been exposed to progesterone. Active bleeding can be treated with progestins alone (5–10 mg norethindrone every 4–6 hours for 24 hours and then 5 mg twice daily for 1–2 weeks) or with an estrogen-progestin combination (ethinyl estradiol, 100 μg, or mestranol, with a progestin given daily). Once bleeding is controlled, the monthly administration of progesterone may normalize bleeding episodes.

Palliative treatment of recurrent metastatic endometrial carcinoma with progesterone (megestrol acetate or medroxyprogesterone acetate) may benefit as many as 50% of patients. This regimen, which should be continued for a few months to achieve full efficacy, works best in younger patients whose tumor contains progesterone or estradiol receptors.

Endometrial estrogen exposure can be inferred if withdrawal bleeding occurs after administration of natural progesterone (75–100 mg in oil intramuscularly) or medroxyprogesterone acetate (10 mg daily for 5 days by mouth). Intramuscular medroxyprogesterone acetate should not be used for this indication because it may cause prolonged suppression of gonadotropin secretion.

Contraceptive and postmenopausal indications: progesterone has been used alone (norethindrone, norgestrel) and in combination with estrogen for contraception (see Steroidal Contraceptive Agents) and may be used in conjunction with estrogen in the therapy of postmenopausal women (see Estrogens). Natural progesterone is used widely for the treatment of threatened abortion or inadequate luteal phase, but few controlled studies are available to evaluate its efficacy.

Preparation and dosages of the progestins are shown in Table 54–9.

TABLE 54–9. Currently Available Progestin Preparations

Progestin	Oral Dose (mg)	Parenteral Dose
Medroxyprogesterone acetate	2.5, 5, 10	100, 400 mg/mL
Hydroxyprogesterone caproate	NA	125, 250 mg/mL
Megestrol acetate	20, 40	10 mg/mL
Norethindrone	0.35, 0.5	
Micronized progesterone	100	
Norethindrone acetate	5	NA
Norgestrel	0.75	
Levonorgestrel (D-norgestrel)		

Drug Interactions

Concurrent use of rifampin may decrease the effectiveness of the progestins because of accelerated metabolism.

STEROIDAL CONTRACEPTIVE AGENTS

Chemistry and Mechanism of Action

Progestin-only contraceptives, available in oral, injectable (DEPO-PROVERA), and implantable (NORPLANT) formulations, prevent pregnancy by altering cervical mucus and endometrial receptivity in nearly all users and by decreasing ovulatory cycles in some users. These approaches avoid estrogenic side effects but are frequently associated with breakthrough bleeding. The intrauterine device can be used as a vehicle to deliver progesterone locally to the endometrium, creating a hostile environment for implantation. Estrogens alone have not been used as long-term contraceptive agents, but they can prevent implantation when given within 48 hours of unprotected intercourse.

Combined oral estrogen-progestin preparations (oral contraceptives or birth control pills) are highly effective (~99%) contraceptive agents that prevent pregnancy by suppression of ovulation and creation of a hostile cervical mucus and endometrium. The pills usually are taken continually for 21 of every 28 days. The many formulations differ primarily in the type and amount of synthetic progestin that they contain. Most combinations use 30 or 35 μg of ethinyl estradiol; one contains 20 μg. Higher daily doses of ethinyl estradiol (up to 100 μg) were used in earlier formulations and their use may underlie some of the complications reported at that time. Current preparations contain no more than 50 μg of ethinyl estradiol or a roughly equipotent amount of mestranol (80-100 mg). The progestin component is usually a 19-nortestosterone derivative. Of these, levonorgestrel and norgestrel are the most potent, and norethynodrel, the least potent. Levonorgestrel, norgestrel, and norethindrone have the greatest androgenic effects. Ethynodiol diacetate, a 17-hydroxyprogesterone derivative, also is used. Preparations containing the gonane-derived progestins with little androgenic activity, norgestimate and desogestrel, recently have become available.

Formulations with a fixed daily dosage of both estrogen and progestin are referred to as combination or monophasic preparations. Preparations with a variable dosage of hormone are designed to mimic the hormonal pattern of a normal cycle. These preparations are referred to as sequential or phasic formulations. Phasic preparations contain two (biphasic) or three (triphasic) different combinations of progestin and estrogen to be given sequentially during separate periods within the same cycle.

Absorption, Distribution, Metabolism, and Excretion

The oral contraceptive formulations in widespread use are well absorbed. As discussed in the respective sections Estrogens and Progestins, the compounds undergo hepatic metabolism and conjugation and then are excreted.

Biological Effects

The biological effects of estrogen-progestin combination pills represent, for the most part, the additive effects of each agent. The endometrium tends to regress, leading to decreased menstrual flow and, occasionally, amenorrhea. When birth control pills are discontinued, the pituitary recovers first, followed by the ovary (ovulation) and, finally, the endometrium.

Oral contraceptives induce a variety of both desirable and undesirable effects (Table 54-10). The beneficial effects of oral contraceptive use include a decreased incidence of ovarian cysts, menorrhagia, ovarian and endometrial carcinoma, endometriosis, iron deficiency, and dysmenorrhea.

Progestin-related effects include adverse changes in serum lipids, including increased total cholesterol, decreased HDL_2 cholesterol, and increased triglyceride levels. These actions appear related to relative androgenicity. Compounds with greater progestin/androgen ratio characteristics least antagonize the favorable estrogen effect on lipids (Table 54-11). The triphasic preparations and those containing desogestrel, norgestimate, or norethisterone (1000 μg/day) preserve the normal HDL-to-cholesterol and HDL-to-triglyceride ratios. A trend toward increased HDL levels is seen at a lower dosage of norethisterone (400 μg/day). Preparations containing levonorgestrel, 150-200 μg/day, have favorable or neutral effects on lipid metabolism.

Oral contraceptive use is associated with an increased risk of thrombosis. Studies including preparations with up to 50 μg ethinyl estradiol showed that the incidence of pulmonary thromboembolism and thrombotic stroke was increased fourfold. Although this may reflect a risk confined largely to higher estrogen doses, these agents should be used with caution in hypertensive patients and in those who smoke, as these factors increase the risk of thromboembolic disease.

Fatal and nonfatal myocardial infarctions are increased two to five times in contraceptive pill users. The risk in-

TABLE 54-10. Adverse Effects of Estrogen-Progestin Contraceptives

Effect	Contributing Factors
Weight gain	Frequent, diminishes with time or lower estrogen dose
Nausea	
Breast tenderness	
Migraine headaches	Estrogen component is implicated
Chloasma	
Impaired glucose tolerance	Progestin component is implicated
Altered lipids	Depends on progestin component
Hepatic adenoma	
Gallbladder disease	Estrogen component
Cholestatic jaundice	
Increased thrombosis	
Myocardial infarction	Increases with age, smoking
Hypertension	Increases with renal disease, duration of use
Acne	Progestin component

TABLE 54–11. Currently Available Estrogen-Progestin Oral Contraceptive Agents With 30–35 μg Ethinyl Estradiol, Listed in Order of Increasing Androgenicity

Agent	Progestin (mg dose/cycle)	Relative Androgenicity
Newer Progestins/ Low Doses		Lowest
ORTHO-CYCLEN	Norgestimate (5.25)	
DESOGEN	Desogestrel (3.15)	
OVCON 35	Norethindrone (8.4)	
BREVICON, MODICON	Norethindrone (10.5)	
Mono- to Triphasics		Middle
TRI-NORINYL	Norethindrone (15)	
ORTHO-NOVUM 7/7/7	Norethindrone (15.75)	
ORTHO-NOVUM 10/11	Norethindrone (15)	
TRIPHASIL, TRI-LEVLEN	Levonorgestrel (1.925)	
NORINYL, ORTHO-NOVUM 1/35	Norethindrone (21)	
Higher Dose		Highest
NORDETTE, LO/OVRAL	Levonorgestrel (3.15)	
LOESTRIN 1/20*	Norethindrone (21)	
LOESTRIN 1.5/30	Norethindrone (31.5)	

*20 μg ethinyl estradiol.

creases with the duration of oral contraceptive use, age, smoking (especially if more than 15 cigarettes are smoked daily), and coexisting hypertension. The risk of myocardial infarction decreases but is not eliminated at the lowest dosages of estrogen. The overall mortality is increased two- to fourfold, primarily as a result of fatal myocardial infarction or cerebrovascular accident. Thus, oral contraceptive use should be limited to nonsmoking women who have normal blood pressure.

Reversible hypertension develops in as many as 5% of women, possibly by stimulation of the renin-angiotensin system. Hypertension is usually gradual in onset but may be rapid and severe. The risk of hypertension increases with age, a family history of hypertension, a history of renal disease, and increasing duration of use.

Neither short-term nor long-term use of oral contraceptives appears to increase the risk of malignancy. The incidence of breast cancer is similar in users and nonusers.

Vitamin metabolism changes associated with oral contraceptives are as follows:

- Serum B_{12} levels may decrease.
- Pyridoxine deficiency secondary to impaired tryptophan metabolism has been reported.
- Estrogen may interfere with the absorption of dietary folate, leading to a deficiency.

High dosages of oral estrogens may elevate hepatocellular enzyme levels and, less commonly, cause cholestatic jaundice. The risk of gallstones increases. Oral contraceptive use is associated with the development of hepatocellular adenomas, benign liver tumors that are highly vascular and may hemorrhage, with serious consequences.

The estrogenic component of oral contraceptives stimulates hepatic synthesis of a variety of proteins, as noted above, which may affect the results of a number of laboratory tests. The response to metyrapone is decreased in women taking oral contraceptive agents. These agents also may cause false-positive results for lupus erythematosus cells or an antinuclear antibody titer.

BOX 54–3
THERAPEUTIC USES

Combined estrogen-progestin preparations are prescribed for contraceptive use. Preparations containing ethinyl estradiol at a daily dosage of 30 μg or less also may be used for steroid replacement therapy in hypogonadal women.

Contraindications

Table 54–12 lists relative and absolute contraindications to oral contraceptive use. These agents are contraindicated during pregnancy and should not be started until 1 month after parturition. Similarly, they should be discontinued 1 month before and not started until 1 month after elective surgery.

Drug Interactions

Oral contraceptives increase the metabolic clearance of coumarin, acetaminophen, and prednisolone. The dosages of these drugs may need to be increased. Oral contraceptives increase the bioavailable amounts of imipramine and theophylline.

Barbiturates, hydantoins, griseofulvin, and rifampin increase the hepatic metabolism of estrogens by mixed-func-

TABLE 54–12. Contraindications to Estrogen-Progestin Contraceptives

Absolute Contraindications
Estrogen-dependent tumor, such as breast, endometrium
Pregnancy
Undiagnosed genital bleeding
Cholestatic jaundice
Active liver disease
Thromboembolic disease
Thrombophlebitis
Cerebrovascular disease
Coronary artery disease
Relative Contraindications
Migraine headaches
Hyperlipidemia
Uterine leiomyomata
History of liver disease
Diabetes mellitus
Porphyria
Hypertension

tion oxidases. Antibiotics decrease the plasma concentrations and efficacy of estrogens and progestins, probably by killing the gut flora responsible for hydrolysis of hepatic conjugates and thereby interrupting the enterohepatic circulation.

Preparations and Dosages

The oral contraceptive chosen should contain the smallest quantity of steroid possible to minimize potential side effects (Table 54-12). High-dose estrogens (containing more than 50 μg ethinyl estradiol) have been taken off the market by the Food and Drug Administration.

REFERENCES

The Boston Collaborative Drug Surveillance Program: Surgically confirmed gallbladder disease, venous thromboembolism, and breast tumors in relation to postmenopausal estrogen therapy. N Engl J Med 290:15-19, 1974.

Barret-Connor E, Bush TL: Estrogen and coronary heart disease in women. JAMA 265:1861-1867, 1991.

The Centers for Disease Control: Cancer and steroid hormone study. Long-term oral contraceptive use and the risk of breast cancer. JAMA 249:1591-1595, 1983.

The Centers for Disease Control: Cancer and steroid hormone study. Long-term oral contraceptive use and the risk of ovarian cancer. JAMA 249:1596-1599, 1983.

The Centers for Disease Control: Cancer and steroid hormone study. Oral contraceptive use and the risk of endometrial cancer. JAMA 249: 1600-1604, 1983.

Chetkowski RJ, Meldrum DR, Steingold KA, et al: Biologic effects of transdermal estradiol. N Engl J Med 314:1615-1620, 1986.

Ettinger B, Genant HK, Cann CE: Long-term estrogen replacement therapy prevents bone loss and fractures. Ann Intern Med 102:319-324, 1985.

Fahraeus L, Larsson-Cohn U, Wallentin L: L-Norgestrel and progesterone have different influences on plasma lipoproteins. Eur J Clin Invest 13:447-453, 1983.

FDA: Labeling guidance text for combination oral contraceptives. Physician labeling. Contraception 37:434-455, 1988.

Gambrell RD: The role of hormones in the etiology and prevention of endometrial cancer. Clin Obstet Gynecol 13:695-723, 1986.

Gaspard UJ: Metabolic effects of oral contraceptives. Am J Obstet Gynecol 157:1029-1041, 1987.

Geola FL, Frumar AM, Tataryn IV, et al: Biological effects of various doses of conjugated equine estrogens in postmenopausal women. J Clin Endocrinol Metab 51:620-625, 1980.

Gordon T, Kannel WB, Hjortland MC, et al: Menopause and coronary heart disease: The Framingham Study. Ann Intern Med 89:157-161, 1978.

Hale RW: Phasic approach to oral contraceptives. Am J Obstet Gynecol 157:1052-1058, 1987.

Henderson BE, Ross RK, Paganini-Hill A: Estrogen use and cardiovascular disease. J Reprod Med 30(Suppl):814-820, 1985.

HEW recommends follow-up on DES patients. FDA Drug Bull 8:10-11, 1978.

Hunt K: Long-term effects of postmenopausal hormone therapy. Br J Hosp Med 38:450-459, 1987.

Hutchinson TA, Polansky JM, Feinstein AR: Postmenopausal oestrogens protect against fracture of hip and distal radius. Lancet 2:705-709, 1979.

Jensen J, Riis B, Strom V, et al: Long-term effects of percutaneous estrogens and oral progesterone on serum lipoproteins in postmenopausal women. Am J Obstet Gynecol 156:66-71, 1987.

Lindsay R, Hart DM, Clark DM: The minimum effective dose of estrogen for prevention of postmenopausal bone loss. Obstet Gynecol 63:759-763, 1984.

Mandel FP, Geola FL, Lu JKH, et al: Biologic effects of various doses of ethinyl estradiol in postmenopausal women. Obstet Gynecol 59:673-679, 1982.

Mandel FP, Geola FL, Meldrum DR, et al: Biological effects of various doses of vaginally administered conjugated equine estrogens in postmenopausal women. J Clin Endocrinol Metab 57:133-139, 1983.

Ross JL, Cassorla FG, Skerda MC, et al: A preliminary study of the effect of estrogen dose on growth in Turner's syndrome. N Engl J Med 309:1104-1106, 1983.

Sitruk-Ware R, Bricaire C, DeLignieres B, et al: Oral micronized progesterone. Contraception 36:373-403, 1987.

Stadel BV: Oral contraceptives and cardiovascular disease. N Engl J Med 305:612-618, 672-677, 1981.

Sturdee DW, Wade-Evans T, Paterson MEL, et al: Relationships between bleeding pattern, endometrial histology, and oestrogen treatment in menopausal women. Br Med J 1:1575-1577, 1978.

Sullivan JM, Vander Zwaag R, Lemp GF, et al: Postmenopausal estrogen use and coronary artherosclerosis. Ann Intern Med 108:358-363, 1988.

Wahl P, Walden C, Knopp R, et al: Effect of estrogen/progestin potency on lipid/lipoprotein cholesterol. N Engl J Med 308:862-867, 1983.

Weiss NS, Szekely DR, Austin DF: Increasing incidence of endometrial cancer in the United States. N Engl J Med 294:1259-1262, 1976.

Weiss NS, Ure CL, Ballard JH: Decreased risk of fractures of the hip and lower forearm with postmenopausal use of estrogen. N Engl J Med 303:1195-1198, 1980.

Whitehead MI, Townsend PT, Pryse-Davies J, et al: Effects of various types and dosages of progestagens on the postmenopausal endometrium. J Reprod Med 27(Suppl):539-548, 1982.

Wingo PA, Layde PM, Lee NC, et al: The risk of breast cancer in postmenopausal women who have used estrogen replacement therapy. JAMA 257:209-215, 1987.

55 Adrenal Cortex

Paul J. Davis, Kathleen M. Tornatore, and Alexander C. Brownie

The adrenal gland elaborates three types of steroids:

- Glucocorticoids, which, among other actions, regulate hepatic gluconeogenesis.
- Mineralocorticoids, which have important actions on sodium and potassium homeostasis.
- Adrenal androgens.

Cortisol and aldosterone are primary examples, respectively, of glucocorticoids and mineralocorticoids. The adrenal gland exhibits functional zonation, with aldosterone being biosynthesized and secreted by the outer zona glomerulosa, and cortisol and androgens by the zona fasciculata/reticularis.

Cholesterol, the precursor of all the adrenocortical steroid hormones, is derived from circulating low-density lipoproteins. Most of the reactions involved in cholesterol conversion to steroid hormones (Fig. 55–1) are catalyzed by a family of mixed-function oxidases that are specific cytochromes P-450. Corticotropin (ACTH) controls cortisol and androgen production through the activation of P-450scc in zona fasciculata/reticularis cells, whereas angiotensin II stimulates the same reaction and therefore aldosterone production in zona glomerulosa cells.

The spontaneous syndromes of hyperfunction of the adrenal cortex (hypercortisolism and hyperaldosteronism — each associated with either adrenocortical hyperplasia or adrenal adenoma), of hypoadrenocorticism, and of defects in adrenal steroidogenesis (congenital adrenal hyperplasia) that result in excess adrenal androgen production have been important historically in defining the nature of the pituitary-adrenal hormonal feedback loop and complex steps in steroidogenesis. Cushing's syndrome refers to the clinical picture of hypercortisolism regardless of pathogenesis, and includes ectopic (*ie*, nonpituitary) production of ACTH by cancers and the setting of therapeutic administration of high doses of synthetic anti-inflammatory glucocorticoids; Cushing's disease specifically refers to hypercortisolism that results from excess pituitary release of ACTH. The risk of iatrogenic Cushing's syndrome is appreciably greater than that of endogenous hypercortisolism: the prevalence of anti-inflammatory glucocorticoid administration in our teaching general hospital inpatient population is 6.1%. Conn's syndrome describes the clinical pattern of spontaneous excess of adrenal mineralocorticoid production (primary hyperaldosteronism). Although primary hyperaldosteronism is rare, clinical syndromes in which aldosterone production is increased

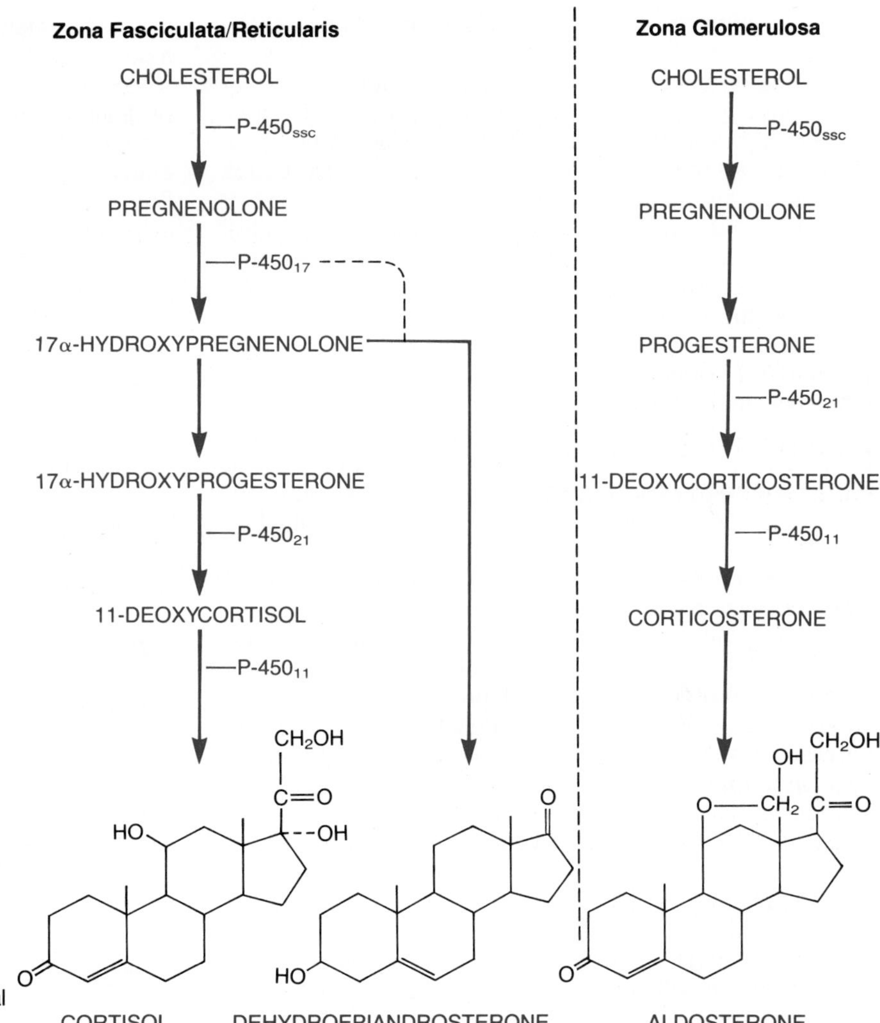

FIGURE 55–1. Biosynthetic pathway for adrenocortical steroids in the human adrenal cortex.

owing to heart failure or hepatic cirrhosis (secondary hyperaldosteronism) are frequent. An aldosterone inhibitor, spironolactone, may be employed in these settings, and the prevalence of inpatient spironolactone use in our teaching hospital is 1.7%. Primary failure of the adrenal cortex (Addison's disease) includes loss of both glucocorticoid and mineralocorticoid secretory capacity.

PITUITARY-ADRENAL CORTEX PHYSIOLOGY

The pituitary-adrenocortical axis is a classic hormonal feedback loop in which a target gland secretory product, cortisol, inhibits pituitary gland secretion of a trophic hormone, ACTH; ACTH in turn is responsible for regulation of cortisol biosynthesis and release by the adrenal cortex (Fig. 55–2). ACTH also controls the growth of the adrenal cortex and the synthesis of steroidogenic enzymes.

Corticotropin is part of a 26,000-d polypeptide, proopiomelanocortin (POMC), which is synthesized in the corticotrophs of the anterior pituitary. POMC also contains β-endorphin and melanocyte-stimulating hormone sequences. Production and secretion of ACTH by pituitary corticotrophs involve specific processing of POMC under the influence of the hypothalamic hormone, corticotropin-releasing hormone (CRH). Negative feedback inhibition of pituitary ACTH secretion by cortisol and by potent synthetic glucocorticoids such as prednisolone and dexamethasone

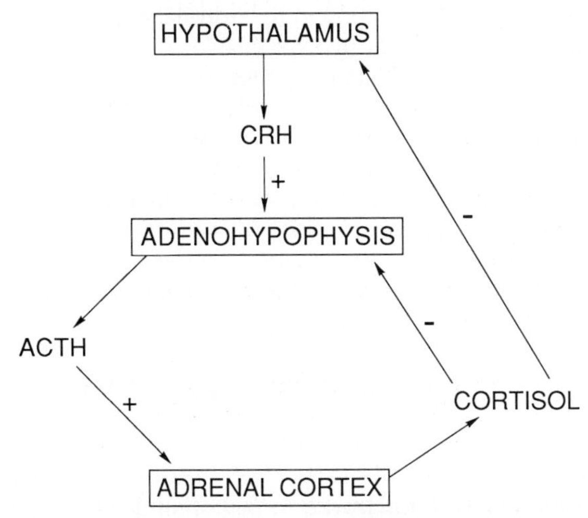

FIGURE 55–2. The hypothalamic-adenohypophyseal-adrenocortical axis. ACTH = corticotropin; CRH = corticotropin-releasing hormone.

occurs at both the pituitary and the hypothalamic (CRH) levels.

Corticotropin secretion is pulsatile, with a dozen or more principal pulses occurring through each 24 hours, conforming to a cycle that imposes a characteristic circadian (diurnal) rhythm of cortisol secretion (highest plasma concentrations at 5:00–7:00 A.M. in humans, lowest at 3:00–6:00 P.M., assuming a traditional wake-sleep cycle). The pulsatile nature of ACTH/cortisol secretion is generated by central nervous system (CNS) input to the hypothalamus. Stress on the organism, whether physical (including systemic (nonadrenal) disease), or emotional, significantly alters ACTH/cortisol secretion and metabolism. The major effects of stress on the pituitary-adrenocortical axis include (1) increased cortisol secretion, (2) enhanced degradation of cortisol (shortened $t_{1/2}$), (3) loss of circadian variation in ACTH/cortisol release, *eg*, absence of the afternoon nadir, and (4) reduced susceptibility of the hypothalamus/pituitary gland to inhibition by cortisol and dexamethasone.

Body habitus may affect cortisol secretion, in that obesity is associated with enhanced secretion but the response of the hypothalamic/pituitary unit to dexamethasone is intact. Also, evidence exists for alterations in the circadian rhythm of cortisol secretion in depression, apparently related to changes in the negative feedback inhibition of ACTH by cortisol in such patients. Alteration of the wake-sleep cycle in normal subjects is associated with a change in the circadian rhythm of cortisol secretion, so that the peak anticipates the new wake period. Two weeks of an altered wake-sleep cycle is required to achieve a new, stable cortisol secretion pattern.

In contrast to cortisol and despite the increase in their secretion by ACTH, aldosterone and adrenal androgens do not affect hypothalamic-pituitary control of ACTH release. Pharmacological suppression of endogenous ACTH is associated in humans with a 25% decline in circulating levels of aldosterone; the major regulators of aldosterone secretion, however, are the renin-angiotensin system and circulating levels of potassium. Adrenal androgen secretion is controlled by one or more POMC-derived peptides, the most well characterized being ACTH, and another, cortical androgen–stimulating hormone, being a product of the processing of the N-terminal portion of POMC. Interruption of normal cortisol production in the adrenal cortex, *eg*, in the setting of the 11- and 21-hydroxylase forms of congenital adrenal hyperplasia, results in excessive ACTH secretion (release of negative feedback inhibition), increased adrenal androgen release, and virilization in affected females. Administration of ACTH-suppressive doses of dexamethasone can reduce adrenal androgen secretion in this setting.

The system-specific actions of cortisol and aldosterone are reviewed later in this chapter, under "Specific Organ System Effects of Glucocorticoids and Mineralocorticoids."

ANGIOTENSIN-ALDOSTERONE AXIS

Aldosterone secretion by the zona glomerulosa of the adrenal cortex is regulated primarily by the products of the hydrolysis of a liver-derived protein, angiotensinogen (renin substrate). Renin, an enzyme secreted by renal juxtaglomerular cells, catalyzes the production from angiotensinogen of a decapeptide (angiotensin I) that has little or no biological role and is itself hydrolyzed rapidly in the lungs and in blood by angiotensin-converting enzyme to an octapeptide, angiotensin II. Angiotensin II is the principal stimulator of aldosterone synthesis, but it is also a pressor substance. Enzymatic removal of the N-terminal aspartic acid residue of angiotensin II results in angiotensin III, a peptide with less pressor activity but with aldosterone-stimulating ability comparable to that of angiotensin II. Renin release is provoked by decreased renal artery blood pressure or intravascular volume depletion, reflecting apparent baroreceptor function of the renal juxtaglomerular apparatus. β-adrenergic stimulation and lowered filtered sodium load, as well as potassium depletion, also act to enhance renin production.

In contrast to its damping effect on renin production, potassium is a potent stimulator of aldosterone production through a direct action on the adrenal cortex. Ambient plasma sodium concentration appears to have little effect on aldosterone synthesis.

CORTICOTROPIN PREPARATIONS

Chemistry

The NH_2-terminal 24 residues of the ACTH polypeptide make up the bioactive portion of the molecule. Residues 25–39 represent the immunogenic end of ACTH. Thus, a commercially available $ACTH_{1-24}$ peptide, cosyntropin, is minimally allergenic.

Mechanism of Action

Corticotropin interacts with specific receptors on the surfaces of adrenocortical cells, promoting adenylate cyclase activity and cyclic 3′,5′-adenosine monophosphate (second-messenger) generation with subsequent phosphorylation of adrenal proteins, a process related in some unknown way to the production of a polypeptide(s) and which facilitates the interaction of cholesterol with P-450scc. Another second-messenger system in adrenal plasma membranes, the phosphoinositide pathway, can also be activated by ACTH and appears to be the principal mechanism involved in the stimulation by angiotensin II of aldosterone secretion by adrenal zona glomerulosa cells.

Adverse Effects

Chronic ACTH administration results in excess adrenal steroid production (hypercortisolism), the consequences of which are reviewed later in this chapter.

ADRENAL CORTICOSTEROIDS

Absorption, Distribution, and Metabolism

The ultimate pharmacological effect of glucocorticoids is dependent on dose of the agent, type of disease to be treated, clinical status of patient (age, gender, renal and he-

BOX 55-1
USES OF CORTICOTROPIN PREPARATIONS

Corticotropin stimulation test. ACTH, specifically the 1–24 peptide (cosyntropin), is a diagnostic agent. The patient is given 0.25 mg of cosyntropin as an intravenous (IV) bolus or an intramuscular (IM) injection (1-hour test) or as an 8- or 24-hour infusion in patients with suspected adrenocortical insufficiency, with plasma cortisol determinations taken before either IV bolus or IM injection and 60 minutes after injection or before and at the conclusion of 8- or 24-hour infusion. Failure of plasma cortisol concentration to rise within 60 minutes of IV bolus or IM cosyntropin supports the diagnosis of primary adrenocortical insufficiency (Addison's disease) but does not exclude the diagnosis of secondary (hypopituitary) adrenocortical insufficiency. Very rarely, confirmation of the latter may require 8 or 24 hours of ACTH infusion.

Agent	Structure	Use
Cosyntropin	α_{1-24} ACTH peptide	Diagnostic agent
ACTH	Intact 39-amino acid molecule	Diagnostic agent
ACTH gel	Intact 39-amino acid molecule in gelatin	Diagnostic agent

Note: ACTH and ACTH gel offer no advantage as diagnostic agents over α_{1-24} ACTH.

Corticotropin therapy. The therapeutic advantages of the systemic use of ACTH (intact 39-amino acid molecule) or ACTH gel, rather than the use of glucocorticoid, is not established in the treatment of clinical states described later that respond to anti-inflammatory steroids. The utility of ACTH in other neuropathological states, such as demyelinating disorders, has not been established, but neurotoxicity associated with certain cancer chemotherapeutic agents, such as cisplatin, may be prevented by administration of an ACTH (4–9) analog.

patic function), and the interaction of these factors at the level of disposition of the specific steroid administered.

Cortisol and its analogs exhibit variable absorption from the gastrointestinal (GI) tract, *eg*, oral cortisol absorption ranges from 45% to 80%. It should also be understood that cortisone and prednisone are inactive analogs; the 11-ketone must undergo reduction to an 11-hydroxyl in order to achieve biological activity (Fig. 55 – 3). The bioavailability of oral prednisone formulations is more consistent than that of cortisol and ranges from 75% to 90%. Oral administration of mineralocorticoid is not practical because of poor GI absorption of desoxycorticosterone acetate and the short half-life (15 minutes; see later) of aldosterone.

It has become apparent that oxidation of the 11-hydroxyl of cortisol is of great importance in the context of the kidney, where failure to do so results in cortisol binding to Type I mineralocorticoid receptors. An indication of the importance of this inactivation reaction comes from the study of the apparent mineralocorticoid excess syndrome; patients with this syndrome lack the 11-hydroxysteroid dehydrogenase and develop severe hypertension caused by cortisol acting as a mineralocorticoid.

Cortisol and prednisolone are largely protein-bound (90%), but only the free fraction is biologically active. The principal corticosteroid transport protein, cortisol-binding globulin (CBG), is a low-binding capacity, high-affinity moiety. CBG synthesis is stimulated by estrogen and hyperestrogenemic clinical states (*eg*, pregnancy) elevate CBG and plasma cortisol levels. Albumin exhibits low-affinity binding of glucocorticoids. Mineralocorticoids are about 60% protein-bound at low-affinity sites; this largely determines the short-plasma half-life of aldosterone.

Metabolism of glucocorticoids to inactive byproducts includes reductions of the 4,5 double bond and of the 3-ketone or of the 20-ketone (Fig. 55 – 3), usually carried out in the liver. Reductions that occur in the A ring (3 or 4 – 5 positions) presage hepatic sulfoconjugation or glucuronidation of the steroid at the 3 position. These water-soluble metabolites are excreted by the kidney, together with small quantities of unconjugated (designated free) cortisol.

The pituitary-adrenal axis has a characteristic response to major medical and psychiatric stress. This includes increased ACTH secretion and a resultant rise in plasma cortisol concentration. Adrenal androgen response to exogenous ACTH administration in the setting of stress may be blunted. The diurnal rhythm of ACTH-cortisol secretion may be lost, and exogenous glucocorticoid, *eg*, dexamethasone, may not predictably suppress endogenous ACTH and cortisol secretion. Failure of the pituitary-adrenal axis to suppress normally after dexamethasone administration to psychiatric patients has been interpreted by a few observers to have psychiatric/diagnostic significance. Hyporeninemic hypoaldosteronism may also occur transiently in the setting of stress.

Glucocorticoids are absorbed through the skin, particularly erythematous or denuded skin. To alter the steroid molecule for topical administration, glucocorticoid is conjugated with a lipophilic ester, *eg*, an acetonide, that permits high topical steroid dosage but reduced systemic absorption. Applied over a large area, particularly occlusively, steroids may nonetheless be absorbed in sufficient quantities to suppress endogenous ACTH secretion. Corticosteroids are effective when applied topically to mucosal membranes, such as in the conjunctivae or airway. Mucosal administration offers the advantage of achieving high local concentrations with reduced systemic side effects and is effective in the management of asthma (by use of an aerosolized steroid) and ulcerative colitis, particularly that restricted to the rectosigmoid area (by use of a steroid enema).

Intra-articular administration of glucocorticoids can deliver temporary relief of inflammation in afflicted joints. The steroid molecule is modified with the substitution of a *tert*-butyl acetate (prednisolone tebutate) or a hexacetonide group (triamcinolone) that decreases the water solubility of these drugs' microcrystalline suspension. These microcrystalline suspensions result in delayed systemic absorption and prolonged exposure to the inflamed joint space.

To enable the parenteral (IV, IM) administration of glucocorticoids, manipulation of the water solubility of the steroid molecule is achieved through conjugation at carbon 21. Steroids (hydrocortisone, methylprednisolone, prednisolone, dexamethasone) that are formulated as sodium phosphate or sodium succinate salts exhibit a rapid rate of absorption because of increased water solubility. Parenteral

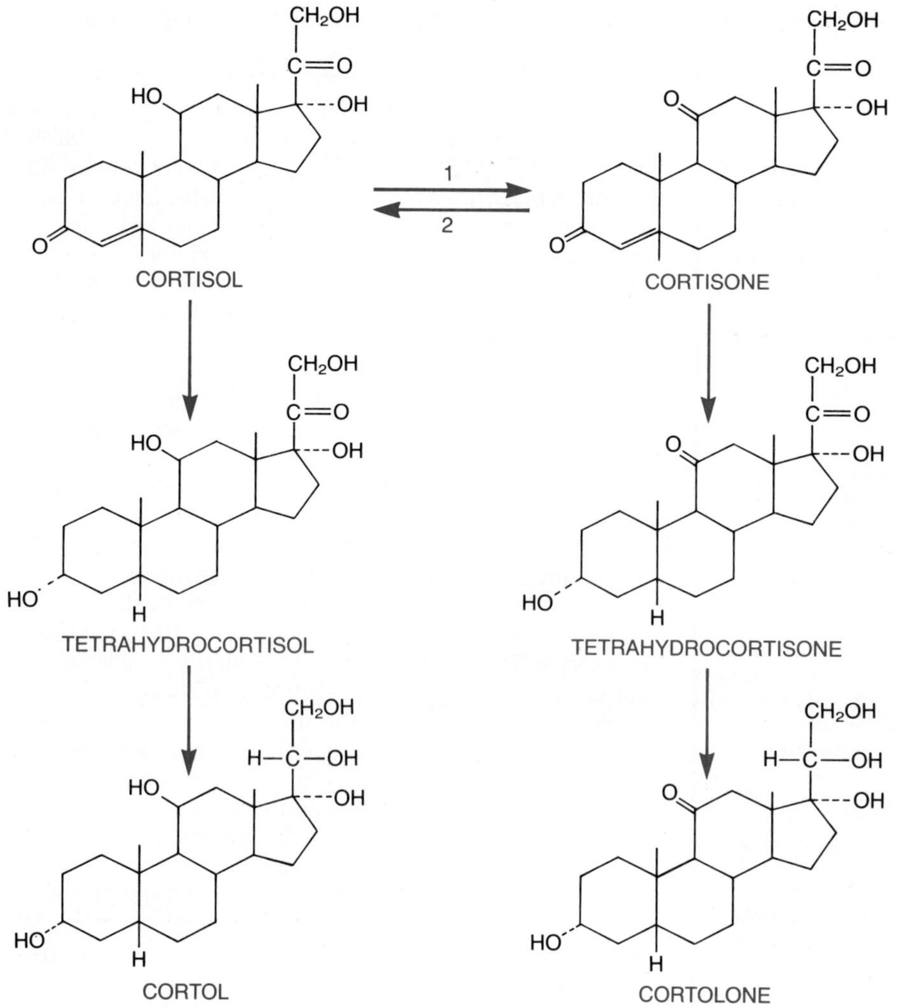

CORTISOL

CORTISONE

TETRAHYDROCORTISOL

TETRAHYDROCORTISONE

CORTOL

CORTOLONE

FIGURE 55–3. The catabolism of cortisol in the liver. Reaction 1 is catalyzed by 11β-hydroxysteroid dehydrogenase; reaction 2 by 11-ketosteroid reductase activity.

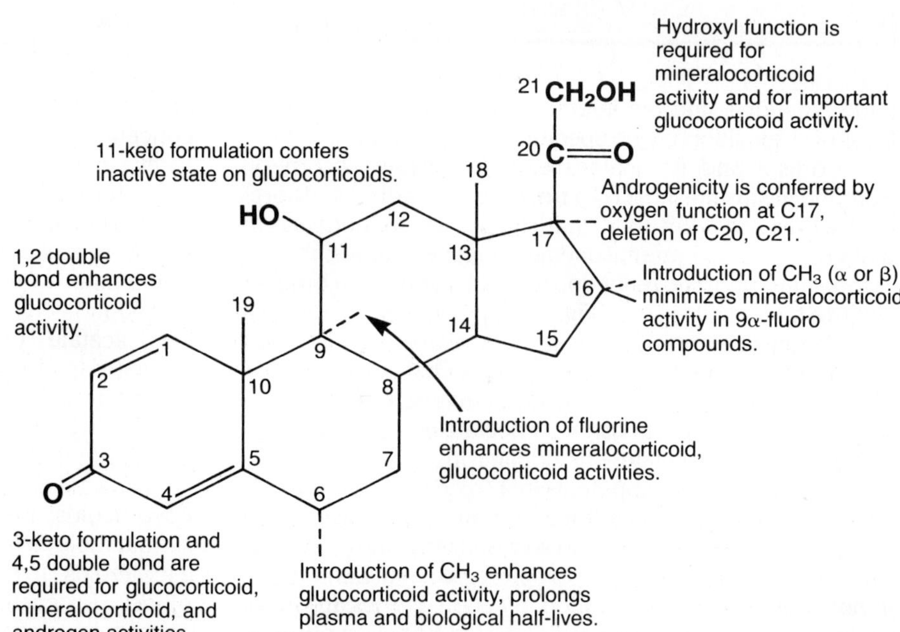
Hydroxyl function is required for mineralocorticoid activity and for important glucocorticoid activity.
21 CH2OH
20 C=O
11-keto formulation confers inactive state on glucocorticoids.
18
HO
Androgenicity is conferred by oxygen function at C17, deletion of C20, C21.
1,2 double bond enhances glucocorticoid activity.
Introduction of CH3 (α or β) minimizes mineralocorticoid activity in 9α-fluoro compounds.
19
Introduction of fluorine enhances mineralocorticoid, glucocorticoid activities.
3-keto formulation and 4,5 double bond are required for glucocorticoid, mineralocorticoid, and androgen activities.
Introduction of CH3 enhances glucocorticoid activity, prolongs plasma and biological half-lives.

FIGURE 55–4. Corticosteroid structure-activity relationships. *Dotted lines* reflect projection below the plane of the ring (α configuration); side chain bonds, represented by *intact lines*, project about the plane of the ring (β configuration). (Modified from Liddle GW: Clinical pharmacology of the anti-inflammatory steroids. Clin Pharmacol Ther 2:615–635, 1961.)

TABLE 55 – 1. Comparison of Pharmacokinetics and Potencies of Corticosteroids

Corticosteroid	Plasma $t_{1/2}$ (minutes)	Tissue $t_{1/2}$ (hours)	Relative Potency: *Glucocorticoid Activity*	Relative Potency: *Mineralocorticoid Activity*	Equivalent Dose* (mg)
Cortisol (hydrocortisone)	90	8–12	1	1	20
Cortisone (11-dehydrocortisol)	30	8–12	0.8	0.8	25
Prednisone (Δ^1-cortisone)	60	12–36	4	0.8	25
Prednisolone (Δ^1-cortisol)	200	12–36	4	0.8	5
6α-Methylprednisolone	180	12–36	5	0.5	4
Fludrocortisone (9α-fluorocortisol)	200	8–12	10	125	—
Triamcinolone (9α-fluoro-16α-hydroxyprednisolone)	300	12–36	5	0	4
Betamethasone (9α-fluoro-16β-methylprednisolone)	100–300	36–54	25	0	0.75
Dexamethasone (9α-fluoro-16α-methylprednisolone)	100–300	36–54	25	0	0.75

Modified from Truhan AP, Ahmed AR: Corticosteroids: A review with emphasis on complications of prolonged systemic therapy. Ann Allergy 62:375–390, 1989.
* Equivalent dosages are approximate and apply only to oral or intravenous administration. Potencies vary importantly when agents are administered intramuscularly or into the joint space.

administration of glucocorticoids is indicated when the oral/GI route is impractical. IV administration of drug is mandatory in acute adrenocortical insufficiency or when blood volume is reduced resulting in unpredictable absorption of IM or rectally administered agents.

A commonly utilized steroid for aerosolized inhalation is beclomethasone diproprionate, which has esterification of the hydroxyl groups at carbons 17 and 21, creating a potent local effect from a weak glucocorticoid.

Pharmacological Modification of Corticosteroid Structure

Introduction of a 1,2 double bond to the glucocorticoid nucleus (prednisolone and methylprednisolone) enhances glucocorticoid (anti-inflammatory) activity (Fig. 55 – 4) and reduces mineralocorticoid effect. Cortisone and prednisone are inactive agents until they are converted in the body from 11-keto formulations to 11β-hydroxyl compounds (cortisol and prednisolone, respectively). The introduction of a 6α-methyl group to prednisolone modestly enhances anti-inflammatory activity but also alters the pharmacokinetic properties. Introduction of fluorine at the 9α-position in the steroid B ring increases salt-retaining qualities (9α-fluorocortisol) and enhances anti-inflammatory properties. Modifications of the steroid nucleus are necessary to minimize the mineralocorticoid effects; however, the therapeutic action should be maintained as seen with betamethasone and dexamethasone, which are potent 9α-fluorinated anti-inflammatory agents with C16 modifications (α- or β-methyl group introductions). Potencies and biologic half-lives of various glucocorticoids and mineralocorticoids are compared in Table 55 – 1. These data are based upon limited, single-dose exposure studies.

Mechanisms of Action

Biological effects of glucocorticoids (cortisol and its natural and synthetic analogs) occur in target cells following the interaction of the steroid with a specific glucocorticoid receptor (GR). GRs are now recognized to be members of a superfamily of ligand-responsive DNA-binding proteins that have a zinc-finger structure that allows them to interact with the genome (Fig. 55 – 5). This family also includes mineralocor-

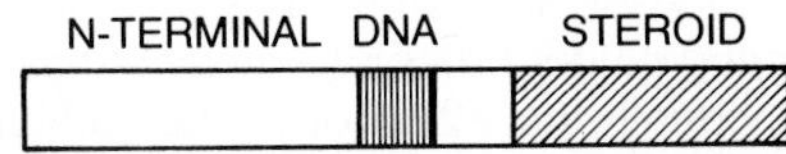

FIGURE 55 – 5. Schematic structure of steroid hormone receptors illustrating the steroid-binding and DNA-binding domains.

Steroid hormone-binding occurs at the C-terminal region of the receptor. This domain is preceded by two zinc-finger DNA-binding motifs. The N-terminal region is hypervariable but is thought to fine-tune the regulation of gene expression. Occupancy of the ligand-binding sites on the glucocorticoid receptor (GR) by cortisol or by dexamethasone has allosteric effects on the receptor protein that enable its interaction(s) with genes. Steroids appear to be critical to the nuclear action of the steroid receptor proteins *in vivo*, but they may not be necessary under certain experimental *in vitro* conditions. The nuclear effects of these steroid receptor proteins promote nucleus-direct synthesis of certain proteins and inhibit synthesis of other proteins. Aldosterone action is also cell nucleus–mediated through its binding to the mineralocorticoid receptor (MR) in target tissues. There is 94% homology between the DNA-binding domains of GR and of MR and, understandably, significantly less (57%) in the hormone-binding domain. Glucocorticoids have catabolic effects (increased protein degradation) as well, the biochemical mechanisms of which are not understood.

ticoids, thyroid hormone (c-*erb*-A), 1,25-dihydroxy-vitamin D_3, retinoic acid, estrogen, progesterone, and androgen receptors. As opposed to the receptors for progesterone, estrogen, and androgen, the GR is localized in the cytoplasm, and following binding of the glucocorticoid the complex moves to the nucleus. The steroid-binding domain is located at the C-terminal end of the receptor separate from the more centrally located DNA-binding domains (Fig. 55-4). Occupancy of the steroid-binding sites by cortisol or dexamethasone has allosteric effects on the receptor protein that enable its interaction with specific glucocorticoid-responsive elements in nuclear DNA.

Systemic Pharmacology of Adrenal Corticosteroids

The systemic and organ-specific effects of glucocorticoids are extensive (Table 55-2). They promote hepatic gluconeogenesis and also mobilize amino acids through muscle (and other tissue) protein catabolism to support gluconeogenesis. This action underlies cortisol's classification as a counterregulatory hormone, *ie*, defined in the intact organism against hypoglycemia, particularly insulin-induced hypoglycemia. Glucocorticoids also support or elevate blood glucose concentration by inhibiting glucose uptake/utilization in peripheral tissues, *eg*, fat cells. Supraphysiological doses of corticosteroids cause frank hyperglycemia. In addition to these effects on carbohydrate metabolism, corticosteroids importantly affect lipid metabolism by stimulating lipolysis (free fatty acid liberation from triglycerides); they also enhance the lipolytic effects of catecholamines on adipose tissue. Supraphysiological amounts of glucocorticoids, whether exogenous or endogenous (Cushing's syndrome), foster redistribution of body fat into a centripetal pattern (truncal obesity) characteristic of Cushing's syndrome.

Glucocorticoids are generally catabolic, resulting in loss of muscle mass (at least in part through enhanced proteolysis), bone mass (osteoporosis), and lymphoid tissue elements. Mineralocorticoids (aldosterone, corticosterone) are critical to body sodium and potassium homeostasis and enhance urinary potassium excretion and the reabsorption of sodium from renal tubular filtrate at Site 3 (distal tubule). Cortisol has modest sodium-retaining capacity, whereas certain synthetic glucocorticoids (dexamethasone) (Table 55-1) have virtually no effect on renal sodium handling. Mineralocorticoids enhance renal sodium reabsorption and cause expanded plasma volume.

Specific Organ System Effects of Glucocorticoids and Mineralocorticoids

Endocrine System

As indicated earlier, cortisol and its glucocorticoid analogs defend against hypoglycemia (counterregulation) and can, particularly when present in excess, exacerbate carbohydrate intolerance (Table 55-1).

TABLE 55-2. Principal Effects of Glucocorticoids

Metabolic Effects of Physiological Concentrations of Glucocorticoids

Effect	*Consequence*
FUEL HOMEOSTASIS	
Increased hepatic glycogenolysis*	Contribution to counterregulation (restoration of normoglycemia after hypoglycemia); promotion of hyperglycemia
Increased hepatic gluconeogenesis*	
Decreased uptake of glucose by peripheral tissues	
Increased protein degradation in striated muscle and adipose and lymphoid tissues†‡	Provision of amino acid substrates for gluconeogenesis; catabolic state
Decreased protein synthesis in striated muscle and adipose and lymphoid tissues‡	
Increased lipolysis*	Mobilization of free fatty acids and glycerol
METABOLIC ADAPTATION	
Increased myocardial contractility	Increased cardiac output
Increased sensitivity of myocardium to catecholamines	
Increased capacity for work of striated muscle§	

System-Specific Effects of Pharmacological Concentrations of Glucocorticoids

Host Defense/Inflammatory Response
- Decreased resistance to bacterial, viral, and fungal infections‖
- Decreased antibody formation
- Decreased phagocytic performance of granulocytes
- Decreased lymphocyte, thymocyte mass, with impairment of delayed hypersensitivity
- Decreased vascular permeability

Gastrointestinal Tract
- Decreased absorption of calcium

Endocrine System
- Decreased peripheral, *ie*, extrathyroidal, conversion of L-thyroxine to 3,5,3′-L-triiodothyronine
- Decreased pituitary thyrotropin secretion
- Increased pituitary corticotropin secretion

Musculoskeletal System
- Myopathy of proximal (limb girdle) striated muscles§
- Osteopenia
- Decreased growth of bone in immature skeleton

Connective Tissue
- Decreased collagen, glycosaminoglycan formation¶
- Decreased wound healing

Eye
- Posterior subcapsular cataract

Data from Loriaux DL, Cutler DB Jr: Diseases of the adrenal gland. *In* Kohler PO, Jordan RM (eds): Clinical Endocrinology, 167-238. New York: John Wiley & Sons, 1986. (Additional details of the side-effect profile of glucocorticoids are presented in Table 55-3.)

*Glucocorticoids are essential to endogenous epinephrine- and glucagon-stimulated gluconeogenesis, glycogenolysis, and lipolysis.

†Myocardium and diaphragm are spared, as may be exercise-hypertrophied striated muscle.

‡Protein (enzyme) synthesis in liver is enhanced by glucocorticoids and supports gluconeogenesis.

§Enhanced work capacity is a short-term effect of glucocorticoids. Long-term increases in endogenous cortisol secretion (Cushing's syndrome) or administration of pharmacological doses of glucocorticoids enhances striated muscle catabolism, chiefly of the proximal muscles.

‖Compromised host response to infectious agent, particularly opportunistic organisms, is characteristic of clinical settings in which pharmacological doses of glucocorticoids are administered as anti-inflammatory agent, but opportunistic infections may occur occasionally in states of endogenous hypercortisolism.

¶Physiological concentrations of glucocorticoids may also regulate glycosaminoglycan formation.

Cardiovascular System

Glucocorticoids appear to sensitize blood vessels to the actions of catecholamines and angiotensin on vasomotor tone. Excess glucocorticoids usually provoke hypertension.

Skeletal Muscle

Although muscle weakness is a hallmark of adrenocortical insufficiency, this manifestation very likely represents decreased plasma volume and cardiac output. Administered in pharmacological doses, cortisol and the glucocorticoid analogs produce profound muscle wasting, particularly of the proximal muscles of the shoulders and hip girdle.

Bone

In supraphysiological concentrations, glucocorticoids inhibit osteoblast activity or the proliferation of periosteal cells that give rise to osteoblasts.

Gastrointestinal Tract

Glucocorticoids decrease absorption of calcium by the GI tract. In part, this reflects glucocorticoid inhibition of vitamin D activation and removal of the stimulation by 1,25-dihydroxy-vitamin-D_3 of calcium absorption. This effect is observed at supraphysiological levels of cortisol. The reduction in plasma calcium levels that results from glucocorticoid action causes a homeostatic rise in circulating concentrations of parathyroid hormone. When clinical glucocorticoid use is prolonged, a new steady state of induced hyperparathyroidism is developed, associated with parathyroid hormone–induced osteoclast activation and loss of bone mass.

Bone Marrow and Lymphoid Tissues

Glucocorticoids are growth factors for cells cultured *in vitro*, and these agents may have modest trophic effects on erythroid precursors in bone marrow.

Administration of pharmacological doses of anti-inflammatory corticoids results in elevated peripheral white blood cell counts because of recruitment of mature granulocytes into the circulation. Eosinophils are reduced in this setting, and eosinophil counts are increased in patients with primary adrenocortical insufficiency, indicating that a cell-specific response of glucocorticoids of this cell line exists. Lymphoid tissue atrophies under the influence of supraphysiological levels of anti-inflammatory glucocorticoids, and peripheral lymphocytosis develops in the face of chronic adrenocortical insufficiency.

Immune System

Glucocorticoids in supraphysiological concentrations inhibit the proliferation of macrophages and lymphocytes, as well as that of antigen-presenting cells. They also block the production of interleukin-2, a lymphokine critical to the normal immune response. Thus, prolonged glucocorticoid use clinically induces an immunocompromised state in which opportunistic bacteria and fungi may establish tissue infections in the steroid-treated host. On the other hand, it is sometimes necessary to suppress the immune response, *eg*, in the settings of rejection of a transplanted (allograft) organ or a serious systemic allergic reaction; here, systemic glucocorticoid administration may be essential.

Inflammatory Response

Glucocorticoids suppress the features of local inflammatory response (erythema, warmth, edema) and a major systemic inflammatory response, fever. These suppressive actions are mediated by the ability of anti-inflammatory steroids to diminish cytokine production, including interleukins, prostaglandins, and leukocyte migration inhibition factor, and to inhibit the proliferation of various mononuclear cell types important to the inflammatory process. Suppression of inflammatory or immune responses may justify high-dose systemic glucocorticoid administration in the management of rheumatological disorders (collagen vascular diseases), sarcoidosis, or local edema associated with primary or metastatic tumors in closed spaces, specifically, in the CNS.

Nervous System

Although the efficacy of high-dose glucocorticoid administration has been established in localized tumor–related edema within the CNS, it is not established that glucocorticoids alter the course of trauma-induced brain edema. Dexamethasone alone, or with metoclopramide, may be effective as an antiemetic in patients who receive cancer chemotherapy with cisplatin.

Adverse Effects of Glucocorticoids

The side-effect profile of glucocorticoids presented in Table 55–3 largely represents exaggerations of Cushing's syndrome. All glucocorticoids can induce these effects, except that pharmacological doses of cortisol rarely induce mineralocorticoid side effects. Anti-inflammatory glucocorticoids administered for 3 weeks or more suppress the hypothalamic-pituitary-adrenal axis, and upon withdrawal of these drugs the pituitary-adrenal axis may be inadequately responsive to stress. The incidence of each of the major adverse effects from glucocorticoid administration is difficult to define (Table 55–3). Patients develop side effects of glucocorticoids at various rates, which may reflect interpatient variability in pharmacokinetics or, possibly, altered cellular sensitivity to steroids.

Diagnostic Use of Corticosteroids

The intactness of the normal relationship between the pituitary gland and the adrenal cortex may be assessed in the setting of suspected hyperadrenocorticism by administering an exogenous corticosteroid in amounts sufficient to suppress endogenous ACTH and measuring the latter or plasma corti-

TABLE 55–3. Principal Side Effects of Anti-inflammatory Corticosteroid

System-Specific Side Effects

Endocrine-Metabolic

Hyperglycemia, including hyperosmolar nonketotic stupor/coma and, rarely, diabetic ketoacidosis
Truncal obesity, enlargement of cervical, supraclavicular,and mediastinal fat pads
Retarded somatic growth (pediatric patient population)
Acne
Hirsutism
Negative nitrogen and calcium balances
Sodium retention (except with synthetic 16-substituted, 9α-fluorinated corticosteroids)

Cardiovascular System

Hypertension

Gastrointestinal Tract

Pancreatitis
Peptic ulcer disease*

Musculoskeletal System

Osteoporosis
Aseptic necrosis of femoral and humeral heads
Myopathy

Nervous System

Pseudotumor cerebri
Mood disorders, including both euphoria and depressive states
Psychosis

Host Defenses Against Infectious Agents

Increased susceptibility to opportunistic infections because of impaired cellular and humoral responses

Eye

Posterior subcapsular cataract

	Incidence of Major Side Effects			
Complication	***Incidence Range (%)***	***Duration of Therapy Prior to Appearance of Complication***	***Minimal Daily Dose Reported to Result In Complication (mg)***	***Reversibility***
Diabetes mellitus	2–28	Days to months	Prednisone, 7.5	Yes
Redistribution of body fat	13	<2 months	Triamcinolone, 4–12	Variable
Hypertension	4–25	2 weeks	Prednisone, 7.5	Yes
Peptic ulcer disease*	0–14	<1 month		Yes
Aseptic necrosis of bone	1–10	<6 weeks	Prednisone, 5–20	No
Myopathy	10	1 week	Prednisone, 10	Yes
Psychiatric disorders	1–18	Days	Hydrocortisone, 60	Yes
Cataract	4	2 months	Prednisone, 5	No

Adapted from Axelrod L: Glucocorticoid therapy. Medicine 55:39–65, 1976; and Truhan AP, Ahmed AR: Corticosteroids: A review with emphasis on complications of prolonged systemic therapy. Ann Allergy 62:375–390, 1989. (Duration and dosage requirements cited are estimates and highly dependent on concurrent clinical factors that may, in addition to glucocorticoid administration, promote some of the complications listed, such as diabetes mellitus, hypertension, and psychiatric disturbances.)

*The risk of peptic ulcer disease during glucocorticoid administration is controversial.

sol. Dexamethasone is usually utilized for this purpose; this glucocorticoid does not cross-react with cortisol antibodies in the cortisol radioimmunoassay and permits monitoring of endogenous cortisol levels while dexamethasone is administered.

The normal pituitary gland interrupts its ACTH release after administration of 0.75 mg of dexamethasone (overnight dexamethasone suppression test [DST]). The paradigm for further testing of the pituitary-adrenal axis is as follows: 0.5 mg of dexamethasone is administered orally every 6 hours for 48 hours ("low dose"), then 2 mg is administered orally every 6 hours ("high dose") for an additional 48 hours. Plasma cortisol concentration at 8:00 A.M. or 24-hour urine excretion of cortisol (or both) is measured during this sequence. Normal response is a reduction in plasma cortisol to <5 μg/dL with the low-dose test. Failure to suppress with the low-dose regimen usually indicates an abnormal hypothalamic-pituitary-adrenal axis. Patients who do not suppress at 2.0 mg/day but do at 8 mg/day have Cushing's disease (bilateral adrenocortical hyperplasia caused by excess pituitary ACTH or CRH-ACTH output). Patients who fail to suppress plasma cortisol to 55 μg/dL in the high-dose paradigm have adrenocortical adenoma, adrenal carcinoma, or ectopic ACTH syndrome.

It should be noted, however, that an abnormal DST may occur in patients with glucocorticoid-resistance syndrome or who are receiving phenytoin. A modified DST has been widely applied to patients with psychiatric syndromes in an effort to standardize diagnoses or predict responses to therapy. A DST has not yet proved to be reliable for either purpose. The regimen has been midnight administration of 0.75 or 1.0 mg of dexamethasone, with measurement of plasma cortisol concentration at 4:00 P.M. rather than at 8:00 A.M. the following day.

Therapeutic Uses of Corticosteroids

Adrenocortical Insufficiency

Inadequate function of the adrenal cortex in humans results from (1) primary destruction of the adrenal gland (Addison's disease), usually on an autoimmune basis; (2) loss of pituitary ACTH secretory capacity or hypothalamic CRH secretory capacity (secondary adrenal insufficiency); or (3) suppression of the hypothalamic-pituitary axis by sustained administration of exogenous glucocorticoid and subsequent withdrawal of the steroid.

The principal symptoms and signs of the state relate to loss of both glucocorticoids and aldosterone — asthenia, orthostatic dizziness, weight loss, GI tract dysfunction — although certain findings are caused by cortisol loss alone (hypoglycemia) or inadequate aldosterone secretion (hyperkalemia). Hyponatremia is usually present. The hyperpigmentation noted in previously fair-skinned patients who become addisonian reflects ACTH and β-lipotropin action on susceptible melanophores in skin creases, elbows, knees, mucocutaneous junctions, and mucosae. Freckling and moles also darken. Subjects with secondary adrenal insufficiency have minimal hyponatremia and lack hyperkalemia because the renin-angiotensin-aldosterone axis is intact. Asthenia or hypoglycemia may be a predominant finding, and signs of loss of other pituitary trophic hormones (hypothyroidism, hypogonadism) are frequently present. Excessive cutaneous pigmentation cannot develop.

Adrenocortical insufficiency resulting from anti-inflammatory steroid withdrawal after long-term steroid administration is usually manifested by weakness and hypotension. It may be subtle or, in the context of major physical stress (*eg*, surgery or systemic infection), dramatic. Hyperpigmentation is not encountered because of the chronic suppression of the hypothalamic-pituitary axis that exogenous steroid therapy causes. Daily anti-inflammatory steroid dosage equivalent to more than 60 mg of cortisol (*ie*, 15 mg of prednisone daily) is frequently sufficient to suppress the hypothalamic-pituitary axis when such therapy is continued for more than 3 weeks. High-dose steroid therapy of 40 - 60 mg of prednisone daily for 1 week or less has no consequence in terms of pituitary-adrenal suppression. Duration of therapy, size of dose, and periodicity of dosing are the critical factors in determining axis suppression.

Daily prednisone administration is a risk for hypothalamic-pituitary suppression, whereas alternate-day corticosteroid administration is not; *ie*, a regimen of 40 mg of prednisone daily when modified to one dose of 80 mg every second day has minimal impact on the ACTH axis. Because of the pharmacokinetics of prednisone, ACTH secretion is restored by 36 - 48 hours after a dose of the agent.

Glucocorticoid Replacement Therapy

Acute adrenocortical insufficiency (adrenal crisis, addisonian crisis) may be life-threatening; its management is to be conducted in the hospital and includes

- Restoration of intravascular volume with 0.9% saline solution, 1 L or more over minutes to several hours, titrating against (orthostatic) blood pressure and heart rate and taking cognizance of the age and possible intrinsic heart disease of affected patients
- Replacement IV bolus glucocorticoid, 100 mg of hydrocortisone, then 50 - 100 mg of hydrocortisone every 8 hours as a continuous infusion for 24 hours or more, according to clinical state, converting to oral glucocorticoid replacement (see later) at 24 - 72 hours
- Specific management of concomitant nonendocrine illness (stress), which may have incited acute adrenocortical insufficiency

Acute adrenocortical insufficiency is a potentially life-threatening state; when its presence is suspected, therapy, as described, should be introduced, even when a definitive diagnosis has not been made. Confirmatory studies (*eg*, ACTH stimulation test) may be carried out after replacement therapy has been initiated.

Chronic adrenocortical insufficiency is managed by replacement corticosteroid — cortisol (hydrocortisone), 20 mg, or cortisone (acetate), 25 mg, orally each morning and 10 or 12.5 mg, respectively, of each agent in midafternoon — mimicking the diurnal variation in plasma cortisol levels that occurs in intact subjects. Some mineralocorticoid activity is obtained with these agents. A significant minority of adrenocortical insufficiency patients may require adjunctive mineralocorticoid treatment with 0.05 - 0.10 mg of 9α-fluorocortisol (fludrocortisone) by mouth daily or on alternate days. Indications for mineralocorticoid replacement include evidence of plasma volume depletion, impaired sense of well-being, myalgia, or modest hyperkalemia.

An alternative regimen for hypoadrenocorticism is prednisone (5.0 mg in the morning, 2.5 mg in the afternoon) with mineralocorticoid. It should be noted that excessive mineralocorticoid therapy promotes hypertension and sodium retention with edema.

The fully replaced adrenocortically insufficient patient requires increased glucocorticoid dosage when she or he is subjected to the stress of acute or intermittent systemic illness. Steroid half-lives decrease under these circumstances. The daily dose of glucocorticoid is doubled for the duration of the illness. Profound illness, *eg*, acute myocardial infarction of bacteremia, should be treated with the equivalent of maximal endogenous corticoid output from the normal adrenal gland, 200 - 300 mg of hydrocortisone daily as an IV infusion. Mineralocorticoid is not used in this setting because, in such inpatients, volume and solute replacement are critically and selectively managed.

Mineralocorticoid Replacement Therapy: Hypoaldosteronism

Hypoaldosteronism may also occur independently of glucocorticoid insufficiency. This may be an isolated, idiopathic event; a consequence of dysfunction of the renin-angiotensin axis (hyporeninemic hypoaldosteronism); or a reversible biochemical action of high-dose IV heparin administration.

Isolated hypoaldosteronism is a very rare clinical syndrome associated with hyperkalemia. It is treated with 0.05 - 0.10 mg of fludrocortisone by mouth daily. Hyporeninemic hypoaldosteronism is occasionally encountered in patients with mild renal insufficiency (serum creatinine concentrations 1.5 – 2.5 mg/dL) and presents as hyperkalemia. The syndrome is seen with increased frequency in non–insulin-dependent diabetic patients. Hyperkalemia is sometimes alarming in these patients (>7.0 mEq/L) and may be managed with sodium polystyrene sulfonate (KAYEXALATE) chronically or with fludrocortisone. The dosage of the latter required to control serum potassium concentration ranges from 0.05 mg by mouth daily to 1.0 mg or more. Caution is to be exercised in the use of high doses of synthetic mineralocorticoid.

Mineralocorticoid may also be indicated in the management of idiopathic orthostatic hypotension or in other dysautonomic states in which hypotension is symptomatic.

Chronic Use of Glucocorticoids as Anti-inflammatory Agents

The goal of the anti-inflammatory use of glucocorticoids is to provide acceptable control of the inflammatory, immunological, or allergic state for which it is employed while minimizing, insofar as is possible, the unfavorable side-effect profile of glucocorticoids. The principles of anti-inflammatory steroid therapy include

- Continuation of steroid therapy only as long as the disease state for which steroid treatment is indicated is active
- Use of the lowest steroid dose effective against the disease treated and tapering of the glucocorticoid as the activity of the disease permits
- Use of local steroid where feasible (*eg*, airway, skin)
- Use of alternate-day systemic steroid administration when the disease under treatment permits such a regimen
- Anticipation of side effects
- Appreciation that withdrawal of chronic daily systemic steroid therapy leaves a pituitary-adrenal axis that may not be fully normal for months
- Understanding that 1 – 2 weeks of high-dose daily systemic glucocorticoid administration has no clinically significant effect on the hypothalamic-pituitary-adrenal axis.

The advantages of alternate-day therapy are well characterized in terms of reduced risk of corticosteroid side effects and of suppression of the hypothalamic-pituitary axis. Steroid-responsive disease states are frequently, but not invariably, controlled by alternate-day steroid administration.

When a disease process responsive to daily corticosteroid administration permits reduction or withdrawal of steroids, the strategy is to (1) taper dosage systematically and (2) convert, whenever feasible, to an alternate-day administration regimen. A conventional program is to convert to alternate-day; for example, for a patient receiving 40 mg prednisone daily, change to 80 mg every other day, then reduce prednisone dose by 5 mg weekly, monitoring the subject closely for appearance of activity of the underlying disease or symptoms of adrenal insufficiency. At 20 mg/dose, tapering may proceed at a reduced pace (2.5 mg/week or every other week), but the regimen should be individualized. Withdrawal of chronic anti-inflammatory corticosteroid therapy can result in adrenocortical insufficiency; exacerbation of the disease for which steroid therapy was indicated; or the steroid withdrawal syndrome, an occasional state of fever, asthenia, and myalgias. The latter appears not to be a hypocortisolemic state, but it responds to reinstitution of glucocorticoid treatment and slower tapering of dosage.

Replacement Therapy for Hypoadrenocorticism

Hydrocortisone

Hydrocortisone is available for oral administration in 5-, 10-, and 20-mg tablets. The 20-mg dosage should be used in the morning, and the 10-mg dosage in the evening.

Hydrocortisone is available for IV administration as the sodium phosphate (solution); a 100-mg IV dosage should be given every 8 hours for 24 hours or more for management of hypoadrenal (addisonian) crisis.

Cortisone

Cortisone is available for oral administration as the acetate in 5-, 10-, and 25-mg tablets. The 25-mg dosage should be given in the morning, and a 12.5-mg dosage in the evening.

Cortisone is available for IM administration as the acetate in 25 mg/mL and 50 mg/mL suspension in a dosage comparable to that for oral administration.

Fludrocortisone

Fludrocortisone is available for oral administration as the acetate in 0.1-mg tablets. Administration should be in conjunction with glucocorticoid in hypoadrenal patients as 0.05 mg – 0.1 mg daily or every other day. Higher doses may be required to treat salt-losing forms of congenital adrenal hyperplasia or the hyperkalemia of hyporeninemic hypoaldosteronism.

Anti-inflammatory Use

Hydrocortisone

Hydrocortisone is available as an enema, 100 mg/60 mL, for management of localized inflammatory bowel disease.

Cortisone

Cortisone is available as a rectal foam, 10%, for management of localized inflammatory bowel disease.

Prednisone

Prednisone is available for oral administration as 1-, 2.5-, 5-, 10-, 20-, 25-, and 50-mg tablets, prescribed in the dosage needed to control corticosteroid-responsive systemic illness. The initial dosage may be 5 – 80 mg/day or more. The lower-dose tablets may be useful in completing withdrawal of steroid therapy after control of systemic illness.

Prednisolone

Prednisolone is available for oral administration in 5-mg tablets, prescribed in the dosage required to control corticosteroid-responsive systemic illness. Oral solution and syrup are also available. The initial dosage may be 5 – 80 mg/day or more.

Prednisolone is also available as the acetate, 25 or 50 mg/mL, for intra-articular or soft tissue (not IV) administration.

Methylprednisolone

Methylprednisolone is available for oral administration in 2-, 8-, 16-, 24-, and 32-mg tablets for daily doses of 2 – 60 mg. It is also available as the acetate in sterile suspension (20, 40, or 80 mg/mL) for intra-articular or soft tissue injection.

Triamcinolone

Triamcinolone is available for oral administration as 1-, 2-, 4-, 8-, and 16-mg tablets and as syrups, prescribed in the dosage required to control corticosteroid-responsive illness.

Triamcinolone is also available as the diacetate in suspensions, 25 or 40 mg/mL, or as acetonide, 10 and 40 mg/mL, for intra-articular or skin (not IV) injection.

It is also available in various formulations for topical administration to patients with skin diseases.

Betamethasone

Betamethasone is available for oral administration as 0.6-mg tablets and as the sodium phosphate/acetate suspension, 3 mg of each form/mL, for local injection (intra-articular or soft-tissue administration).

Dexamethasone

Dexamethasone is available for oral administration as 0.25-, 0.5-, 0.75-, 1-, 1.5-, 2-, 4-, and 6-mg tablets to control corticosteroid-responsive illness or for diagnostic purposes (DST).

Dexamethasone is also available as acetate or sodium phosphate for systemic IM therapy (not IV) or for intra-articular or soft-tissue administration.

Beclomethasone

Beclomethasone is available as dipropionate aerosol for inhalant therapy, 42 μg delivered/puff to patient, for bronchial asthma.

Use of Inhibitors of Steroidogenesis or Steroid Action in Adrenocortical Hyperfunction

Excessive corticoid action may be the result of

- Increased pituitary secretion of ACTH, resulting in bilateral adrenocortical hyperplasia and usually a consequence of unregulated hypothalamic release of CRH into the pituitary-portal circulation
- Unilateral disease of an adrenal gland, *eg*, adenoma or carcinoma
- Nonpituitary (ectopic) production of ACTH, usually by a lung or GI tract carcinoma
- Prolonged administration of therapeutic glucocorticoid

The major signs and symptoms of hypothalamic-pituitary hypercortisolism (Cushing's disease) are centripetal fat distribution (truncal obesity), excess facial fat (moon face), hypertension, muscle weakness, and osteoporosis. Hypokalemia is observed in only about 20% of patients with Cushing's disease, reflecting the small effect of ACTH on the aldosterone secretory mechanism of the adrenal cortex. In hypothalamic-pituitary hypercortisolism, dexamethasone at 2 mg daily for 2 days does not suppress ACTH (or endogenous cortisol), whereas 8 mg for 2 days results in suppression.

Cushing's syndrome caused by adrenocortical adenoma produces a clinical pattern similar to that of hypothalamic-pituitary hypercortisolism. Dexamethasone administration at 2 or 8 mg daily for 2 days does not suppress circulating levels of endogenous cortisol.

Ectopic ACTH syndrome presents differently. Systemic levels of ACTH are very high, sufficient to promote aldosterone production and cortisol levels substantial enough to manifest mineralocorticoid activity. Thus, hypokalemia usually results. Hyperpigmentation may also be dramatic. The lung tumors (small cell carcinoma) associated with ACTH elaboration are extraordinarily aggressive, and patients usually to not survive long enough to manifest other classic signs of hypercortisolism.

High-dose anti-inflammatory steroid use leads to a side-effect profile of body fat redistribution, skin changes, hypertension, osteoporosis, and diabetes mellitus. Because the potency of the synthetic steroids far exceeds that of endogenous corticoids, immunological suppression may be achieved, and increased susceptibility to infection may be apparent. This latter state is rarely achieved with endogenous hypercortisolism. Infections may develop with conventional or opportunistic bacteria or with fungi or mycobacteria. Wound healing is also impaired.

Excessive endogenous aldosterone production without hypercortisolism results from either bilateral adrenocortical hyperplasia or an adrenocortical adenoma. Primary aldosteronism is manifested by hypertension and hypokalemia. Other occasional findings are neuromuscular irritability and hypomagnesemia. Renin levels are suppressed in this condition.

Pharmacological Interventions in Hyperadrenocorticism

A number of pharmacological agents have actions on the adrenal cortex that are clinically important.

Metyrapone (METOPIRONE) 11β-Hydroxylase Inhibitor

Administration of metyrapone inhibits cortisol production, leading to de-repression of endogenous ACTH production and increased circulating levels of 11-deoxycortisol. The latter has little bioactivity and does not suppress ACTH production. Metyrapone (single dose, 2 – 3 g by mouth at midnight, plasma cortisol levels at 8:00 A.M.) has been used to test for hypopituitary hypoadrenocorticism (failure of plasma 11-deoxycortisol levels to rise after drug administration supports hypopituitarism). Availability of other diagnostic approaches for hypopituitarism (radioimmunoassays for ACTH, thyrotropin, gonadotropins, and growth hormone) minimizes the diagnostic need for this agent. In addition, administration of the drug to patients with borderline (and untreated) primary adrenocortical insufficiency has provoked profound adrenocortical failure ("crisis") and, rarely, death.

Metyrapone (250 – 500 mg by mouth three times a day) has been used to palliate the syndromes of ectopic ACTH production and of excess cortisol production by adrenocortical carcinoma. Inhibition of 11β-hydroxylation inhibits both cortisol and aldosterone biosynthesis.

Aminoglutethimide

Aminoglutethimide inhibits cholesterol side-chain cleavage. Administered in a dosage of 250 – 500 mg by mouth four times a day, aminoglutethimide palliates the hypercortisolism of ectopic ACTH production and of adrenocortical carcinoma. Mineralocorticoid biosynthesis may be insufficient with this agent (in contrast to metyrapone), and clinically significant hypoadrenocorticism with hyperkalemia may result.

Ketoconazole

Ketoconazole inhibits steroid synthesis through enzyme blockage. Ketoconazole is an imidazole broad-spectrum antifungal agent that interferes with gonadal and adrenal steroid synthesis *in vivo* and *in vitro* by inhibition of adrenal P-450 – dependent enzymes, 11β-hydroxylase, and C17 – 20-lyase. The inhibition of cortisol synthesis is dose-dependent when 400 mg or more of ketoconazole is administered as single or multiple doses. Ketoconazole causes a diminished adrenocortical response to ACTH administration with reduction in serum and urinary cortisol concentrations and can produce acute adrenocortical insufficiency. The long-term efficacy and safety of the use of ketoconazole in hyperadrenocorticism have not yet been established.

Mitotane (*o,p'*-DDD)

Mitotane is a direct adrenocortical cytotoxic agent. Mitotane can cause primary degeneration in the zona fasciculata and the zona reticularis. This drug may also specifically inhibit cortisol and aldosterone synthesis by action at the 11β-hydroxylation step as well as depression of the adrenocortical response to ACTH. For treatment of Cushing's syndrome caused by adrenal carcinoma, this agent is initiated at doses of 3 – 6 mg daily in three or four divided doses, with maintenance doses ranging from 500 mg biweekly to 2 g daily. When mitotane is administered chronically, glucocorticoid (and mineralocorticoid) replacement therapy is usually necessary to avoid adrenocortical insufficiency. Side effects are relatively frequent with mitotane, including GI tract disturbances and CNS effects (lethargy and, less often, vertigo and depression).

Mifepristone (RU 486)

RU 486 is a glucocorticoid analog (17α-hydroxy-11β-(4-dimethylaminophenyl)-17β-(prop-1-ynyl)-estra-4,9-dien-3-one) with negligible agonist action and potent antiglucocorticoid, antiprogesterone, and antiestrogen activities. It has been shown to be effective in the treatment of Cushing's syndrome and may be effective in reversing the immunosuppressive actions of traditional glucocorticoids. The agent has not been approved by the United States Food and Drug Administration for clinical applications.

Other Agents that Affect Steroidogenesis or Steroid Action

It should be noted that several other agents may interfere with adrenal steroidogenesis to clinically significant degrees, but these are not used as antiadrenal drugs. The anticoagulant heparin selectively interferes with aldosterone synthesis and, when it is used in high-dose IV bolus regimens, may result in acute hypoaldosteronism and hyperkalemia. This biochemical effect is reversible with interruption of heparin therapy. Cyclosporine is a cyclic peptide of fungal origin (see Chapter 45) and induces hyperreninemic hypoaldosteronism in rats; however, it can result in hypertension and hypoaldosteronism in humans. Among its adrenocortical effects are acute blockage of induction by angiotensin II of aldosterone secretion by the zona glomerulosa. Phenytoin, rifampin, and barbiturates enhance hepatic microsomal metabolism of corticosteroids. Macrolide antibiotics, *eg*, erythromycin and troleandomycin, impair the elimination of methylprednisolone because of their inhibitory action on the cytochrome P-450 system.

Contraindications to and Precautions During Steroid Therapy

No contraindications exist to replacement glucocorticoid use in patients with adrenocortical insufficiency.

Relative contraindications to high-dose anti-inflammatory steroid use are the presence of systemic bacterial infection, poorly controlled diabetes mellitus, and advanced demineralizing bone disease. Mineralocorticoid use is relatively contraindicated in the setting of expanded intravascular volume, *eg*, congestive heart failure.

Patients receiving glucocorticoids as a component of chronic immunosuppressive therapy should be monitored closely for the appearance of secondary bacterial or viral infections.

Close pediatric patient observation is mandatory during high-dose glucocorticoid therapy because of the impact of steroids on growth and bone maturation in children. Alternate-day therapy in children results in less inhibition of growth as well as decreased cushingoid effects.

Glucocorticoids utilized in pharmacological doses during pregnancy may result in increased fetal deaths and congenital malformations, such as cleft palate. If possible, use of these drugs should be avoided in the first trimester, and they should be used in a discriminating manner throughout pregnancy. However, glucocorticoids should not be withheld in conditions that are considered life-threatening to the pregnant mother.

REFERENCES

Axelrod L: Glucocorticoid therapy. Medicine 55:39 – 65, 1976.

Bondy PK: The adrenal cortex. *In* Bondy PK, Rosenberg LE (eds): Metabolic Control and Disease, 8th ed, 1427 – 1499. Philadelphia: WB Saunders Co, 1980.

Bondy PK: Disorders of the adrenal cortex. *In* Wilson JD, Foster DW: Williams Textbook of Endocrinology, 7th ed, 825-826. Philadelphia: WB Saunders Co, 1985.

Dluhy RG, Newmark SR, Lauler DP, Thorn GW: Pharmacology and chemistry of adrenal glucocorticoids. *In* Azarnoff DL (ed): Steroid Therapy, 1. Philadelphia: WB Saunders Co, 1975.

Gelehrter TD: Glucocorticoids and the plasma membrane. Monogr Endocrinol 12:561-574, 1979.

Gifford RH: Corticosteroid therapy for rheumatoid arthritis. *In* Azarnoff DL (ed): Steroid Therapy, 78. Philadelphia: WB Saunders Co, 1975.

Hunder GG, Sheps S, Allen GL, Joyce JW: Daily and alternate-day corticosteroid regimens in treatment of giant cell arteritis: Comparison in a prospective study. Ann Int Med 82:613-618, 1975.

Intra-articular steroids [Editorial]. Lancet 1:38, 1984.

Ling MHM, Perry PJ, Tsuang MT: Side effects of corticosteroid therapy. Arch Gen Psychiatry 38:471-477, 1981.

Loriaux DL, Cutler DB Jr: Diseases of the adrenal gland. *In* Kohler PO, Jordan RM (eds): Clinical Endocrinology, 167-238. New York: John Wiley & Sons, 1986.

MacGregor RR, Sheagren JN, Lipsett MB, Wolff SM: Alternate-day prednisone therapy. Evaluation of delayed hypersensitivity responses, control of disease and steroid side effects. N Engl J Med 280:1427-1431, 1969.

Nieman LK, Loriaux DL: Corticotropin-releasing hormone: Clinical applications. Annu Rev Med 40:331-339, 1989.

Smith AI, Funder JW: Proopiomelanocortin processing in the pituitary, central nervous system, and peripheral tissues. Endocr Rev 9:159-179, 1988.

Szefler SJ: General pharmacology of glucocorticoids. *In* Schleimer RP, Claman HN, Oronsky A (eds): Anti-inflammatory Steroid Action: Basic and Clinical Action, 354-376. Toronto: Academic Press, 1989.

Tyrell JB, Baxter JD: Glucocorticoid therapy. *In* Felig P, Baxter JD, Broadus AE, Frohman LA (eds): Endocrinology and Metabolism, 2nd ed, 788-817. New York: McGraw-Hill, 1987.

56 Carbohydrate Metabolism, Insulin, and Oral Hypoglycemic Agents

Suzanne G. Laychock

CARBOHYDRATE METABOLISM

Ingested carbohydrates are reduced to the hexoses glucose, fructose, and galactose, which are absorbed in the intestine. Blood glucose levels are decreased by insulin and increased by glucagon, epinephrine, norepinephrine, cortisol, and growth hormone. Insulin is referred to as a regulatory hormone and the others are called counterregulatory hormones.

Figure 56–1 summarizes the mechanisms regulating blood glucose levels in humans. Glucose can be supplied to the body either from exogenous sources (ingestion) or from endogenous sources (liver and muscle) in response to the counterregulatory hormones (Table 56–1). After an overnight fast glucose is primarily derived from liver glycogenolysis (75%) and gluconeogenesis (25%).

Glucose is removed from the circulation for energy (catabolism), as well as during storage as glycogen and fat (Fig. 56–1). All animal cells can metabolize glucose, but the brain, blood cells, and muscle are the major consumers of glucose.

Glucose is the sole source of energy for the brain in humans except during prolonged starvation. The brain consumes 60–70% of endogenous glucose production. During starvation blood ketones increase and become an alternative source of energy for the brain. A diminished supply of glucose to the brain results in degrees of dysfunction, including coma and death if severe.

Whereas hypoglycemia is acutely life-threatening, the effects of hyperglycemia can be acute as well as chronic. Acute hyperglycemia may result in hyperosmolar coma if the water loss due to hyperglycemia is not compensated by water intake. The chronic effects of hyperglycemia are related to pathophysiological conditions of diabetes mellitus, which involve nerve, kidney, retina, and pancreatic beta cells among others.

DIABETES MELLITUS

Diabetes mellitus is characterized by a spectrum of organ disorders all linked to a common origin: relative or absolute deficiency of insulin or its metabolic action.

The acute effects of insulin deficiency are ketoacidosis and hyperosmolar coma. Chronic complications of insulin deficiency include:

- Microvascular disease and atherosclerosis involving medium and large vessels.
- Renal complications with microalbuminuria and renal failure; neuropathy with pain in the extremities.
- Predisposition to infection.

Criteria for the diagnosis of diabetes mellitus in the adult (nonpregnant) human are:

- Plasma glucose of 200 mg/dL or above, and symptoms of polyuria, polydipsia, polyphagia, and weight loss.
- Fasting plasma glucose level of 140 mg/dL or greater.
- Fasting plasma glucose levels less than 140 mg/dL plus a sustained elevated plasma glucose level (200 mg/dL or greater) within 2 hours after oral glucose (75 g).

In children, the criteria for diagnosing diabetes are based upon a glucose tolerance test correlated to the patient's weight. A fasting glucose of above 100 mg/dL, and

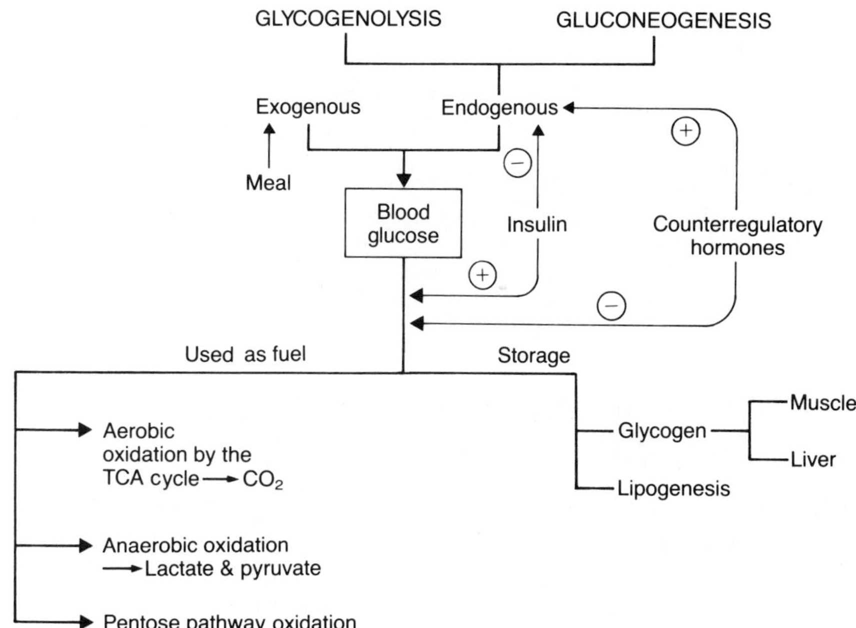

FIGURE 56–1. The mechanism of maintenance of blood glucose in humans. CO_2 = carbon dioxide; TCA = tricarboxylic acid cycle.

plasma glucose during the glucose tolerance test of 160 mg/dL (1 hour) and 140 mg/dL (2 hours) are characteristic of the disease. In pregnant women plasma glucose tends to fall and plasma glucose levels during fasting and a glucose tolerance test may be lower than normal.

Type I Diabetes Mellitus or Insulin-Dependent Diabetes Mellitus

Insulin-dependent diabetes mellitus (IDDM) was formerly known as juvenile diabetes; about 10–20% of diabetes is Type I. Patients are usually thin. There is an abrupt onset of symptoms (described above) with insulinopenia before the age of 40 years. Injected insulin is required to prevent ketosis and preserve life. Genetic and etiological factors, and islet cell antibodies to proteins such as glutamic acid decarboxylase (GAD) may contribute to the onset of the disease.

TABLE 56–1. Effects of Insulin and Glucose Counterregulatory Hormones on Glucose Metabolism

Hormones	Liver	Muscle
Insulin	Glycogen synthesis ↑ Glycogenolysis ↓ Gluconeogensis ↓	Glycogen synthesis ↑ Glycogenolysis ↓
Glucagon	Glycogenolysis ↑ Gluconeogenesis ↑	
Catecholamines	Glycogenolysis ↑ Gluconeogenesis ↑	Glucose uptake ↓ Glycogenolysis ↑
Cortisol	Gluconeogenesis ↑	Glucose uptake ↓
Growth hormone		Glucose uptake ↓

Type II Diabetes Mellitus or Non–Insulin-Dependent Diabetes Mellitus

Non–insulin-dependent diabetes mellitus (NIDDM) was formerly known as adult or maturity-onset diabetes; 80–90% of diabetes in the United States is Type II. Onset is insidious; it is diagnosed by blood or urinary glucose measurements. Insulin resistance as well as a loss of insulin secretion sensitivity to glucose contribute to the disease. About 60–90% of Type II diabetics are obese; weight reduction and exercise may correct hyperglycemia and will improve glycemic control in conjunction with oral hypoglycemic agents or insulin.

Secondary Diabetes Mellitus

Symptoms result from the following:

- Pancreatic dysfunction (pancreatitis, pancreatectomy)
- Hormonal imbalance (*eg*, acromegaly, pheochromocytoma, Cushing's syndrome, glucagonoma)
- Drug- or chemical-induced reactions (*eg*, glucocorticoids, anticancer agents streptozotocin or diazoxide, thiazide, some psychoactive agents)
- Insulin receptor abnormalities (expressed as acanthosis nigricans)
- Certain genetic syndromes (hyperlipidemia and muscular dystrophy)
- Malnutrition

Impaired Glucose Tolerance Test

Criteria for the impaired glucose tolerance test (IGT) are:

1. fasting plasma glucose of less than 140 mg/dL;
2. a 2-hour oral glucose tolerance test plasma glucose level between 140 and 200 mg/dL; and

3. an intervening oral glucose tolerance test plasma glucose value of 200 mg/dL or greater.

About 25% of patients with IGT become diabetic.

Gestational Diabetes Mellitus

Onset or discovery of glucose intolerance during second or third trimester of pregnancy. Early diagnosis and meticulous blood glucose control help prevent maternal and fetal complications.

INSULIN: CHEMISTRY, BIOSYNTHESIS, AND SECRETION

Insulin is a protein hormone secreted by the beta cells of the pancreatic islet of Langerhans (Fig. 56–2). Insulin is composed of two peptide chains (A and B) connected by two disulfide linkages; proinsulin also contains a C-peptide linkage between the chains. C-peptide is cleaved from insulin in the secretory granule of the beta cell. Insulin and zinc form aggregates in the secretory granule, which are released by exocytosis.

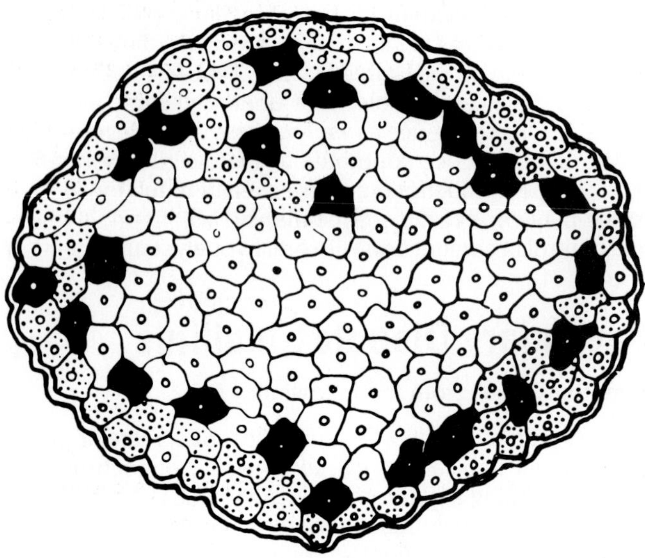

FIGURE 56–2. Schematic representation of a rat islet showing the topographical relationships of the major cell types. (Reprinted by permission of the publisher from Unger RH, Orci L: Glucagon. *In* Ellenberg M, Rifkin H [eds]: Diabetes Mellitus: Theory and Practice, 3rd ed, 203–224. New York: Medical Examination Publishing Co., 1983. Copyright 1983 by Elsevier Science Publishing Co., Inc.)

C-peptide and insulin are secreted in equimolar proportions into the blood. Thus, C-peptide quantitation is a reliable means of determining insulin secretion.

Stimuli affecting insulin secretion are:

- Glucose is the primary stimulus for insulin secretion. Secretion is initiated at a glucose concentration of about 90 mg/dL, and reaches a plateau at about 360 mg/dL.
- Amino acids (especially leucine and arginine), ketones, and fatty acids.
- Potentiators of glucose-induced insulin release include secretin, pancreozymin, acetylcholine, glucose-dependent insulinotropic peptide, glucagon and glucagonlike peptide (GLP), cholecystokinin, and other gastrointestinal hormones. Cyclic adenosine monophosphate (AMP) mediates many of these responses.
- Inhibitors of insulin secretion include norepinephrine and epinephrine (α_2-adrenoceptor agonists), and somatostatin. Cyclic AMP synthesis is inhibited by these agents, in addition to other actions.

Insulin Action

The action of insulin occurs in three principal tissues: liver, muscle, and adipose tissue. Insulin has metabolic and growth-promoting effects. Insulin:

- Increases glycogen synthesis in liver and muscle
- Decreases glycogenolysis and gluconeogenesis
- Inhibits lipolysis and stimulates lipogenesis
- Stimulates the synthesis of free fatty acids and their esterification into triglycerides
- Inhibits ketogenesis in liver

The growth-promoting effects of insulin are due to stimulation of DNA synthesis and stimulation of cell growth and differentiation. Insulin can also stimulate amino acid transport across membranes, stimulate protein synthesis and inhibit proteolysis, and stimulate RNA synthesis. The growth-promoting activities of insulin correlate with the activities of insulinlike growth factors (IGFs), which have more growth-promoting effects than metabolic effects in comparison with insulin.

Insulin binds to specific receptors on the plasma membrane of the cell. The receptor is a glycoprotein composed of two alpha and two beta subunits. The alpha subunits bind the hormone while the beta subunits are protein kinases that can autophosphorylate the protein on tyrosine residues and promote signal transduction within the cell (Fig. 56–3). Insulin binding promotes the mobilization of glucose transporters in the plasma membrane of cells and increases glucose uptake (Fig. 56–4). Insulin bound to receptors is also internalized and processed so that the insulin can interact with the nuclear chromatin to stimulate mRNA synthesis. Internalized (down-regulated) insulin receptors can be either degraded or recycled back to the plasma membrane.

Hyperinsulinemia results in insulin receptor down-regulation with a loss of cell sensitivity to insulin; a reduction in insulin levels restores insulin sensitivity.

Insulin resistance is characterized by a loss of sensitivity (receptor binding defect) and/or responsiveness (post-receptor binding defect) to insulin (Fig. 56–5). The causes

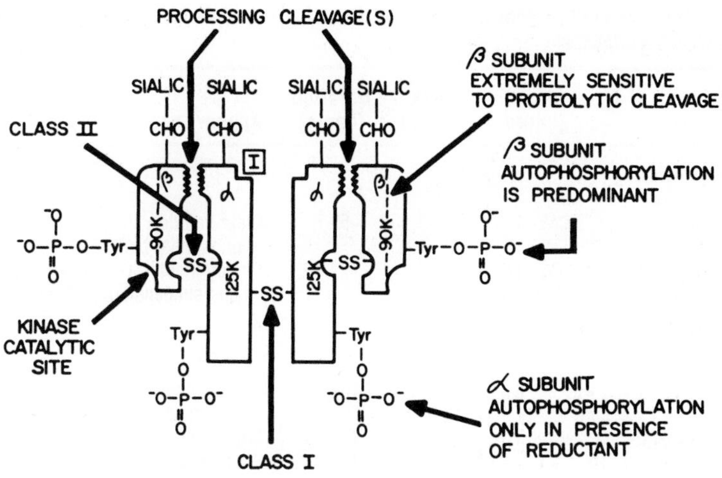

FIGURE 56–3. Several major features of the insulin receptor structure, as it is currently understood. The major form of the mature insulin receptor appears to be a heterotetrameric, disulfide-linked configuration of α and β subunits. The disulfide linkages are of two classes (class I and class II) that can be distinguished experimentally by their differential sensitivity to reduction by dithiothreitol and other reductants. Both α and β subunits contain oligosaccharide and sialic acid. The mature α and β subunits appear to be derived from a single precursor polypeptide chain by a proteolytic cleavage or cleavages. The β subunit exhibits a site at about the center of its amino acid sequence that is exquisitely sensitive to elastaselike proteases. Tyrosine-kinase catalytic sites are associated with the β subunits that are autophosphorylated *in vitro* in the presence or absence of reductant. Alpha subunits, which appear to bind insulin, are also autophosphorylated on tyrosine residues *in vitro* but only in the presence of millimolar concentrations of reductants. The insulin receptor tyrosine-kinase activity is markedly activated upon binding insulin. (See text for further details.) (From Czeck MP: The nature and regulation of the insulin receptor: Structure and function. Reproduced, with permission, from the Annual Review of Psychology, Vol. 47, © 1985 by Annual Reviews Inc.)

of insulin resistance may be prereceptor (*eg*, insulin degradation or insulin structural abnormality). Insulin antagonists can also contribute to resistance (*eg*, elevated levels of counterregulatory hormones, anti–insulin receptor antibodies, or anti-insulin antibodies). The insulin receptor may also be reduced in number, have reduced hormone-binding affinity, or have altered signal transduction activity, thus reducing the insulin sensitivity of cells. Postreceptor defects in metabolic pathways or pathways of insulin action also reduce cellular responsiveness to insulin. Some defects appear to be genetically linked.

Insulin Pharmacokinetics

Insulin is destroyed in the gastrointestinal (GI) tract and must be administered parenterally (subcutaneously or intramuscularly). The half-life of insulin in plasma is less than 9 minutes. Insulin is filtered at the glomerulus and reabsorbed in proximal tubules of the kidney; renal impairment affects the clearance of insulin and the appropriate dosage.

Insulin for injection is derived from beef or pork pancreas; or human insulin is prepared by recombinant DNA synthesis in *Escherichia coli.* Insulin for injection is prepared with the addition of zinc or protamine in a neutral buffer in

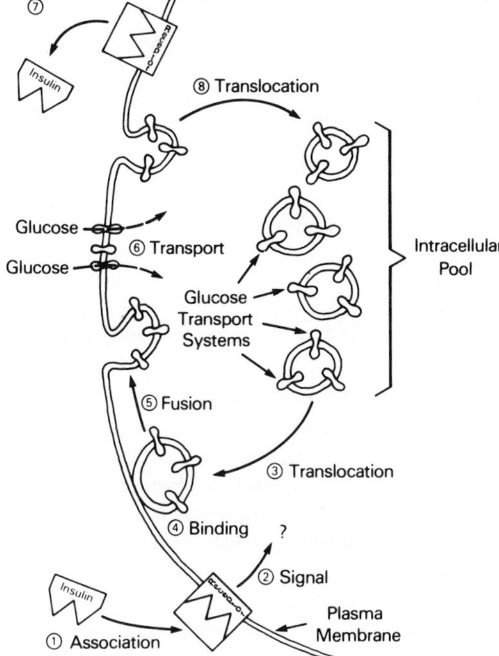

FIGURE 56–4. Hypothetical model of insulin's stimulatory action on glucose transport. According to this hypothesis, insulin binds to its specific cell surface receptor, inducing a signal. In response to this signal, intracellular vesicles containing the glucose transporter are translocated to the plasma membrane. Following fusion of these vesicles with the plasma membrane, glucose transporters are exposed to the extracellular medium, giving rise to the increase in glucose transport activity. On removal of insulin from its receptor, glucose transporters are retranslocated back to the intracellular fluid by a mechanism similar to receptor-mediated endocytosis. (From Karnieli E, Zarnowski MJ, Hissin PJ, et al: Insulin-stimulated translocation of glucose transport systems in the isolated rat adipose cell: Time course, reversal, insulin concentration, dependency and relationship of glucose transport activity. J Biol Chem 256:4772–4777, 1981.)

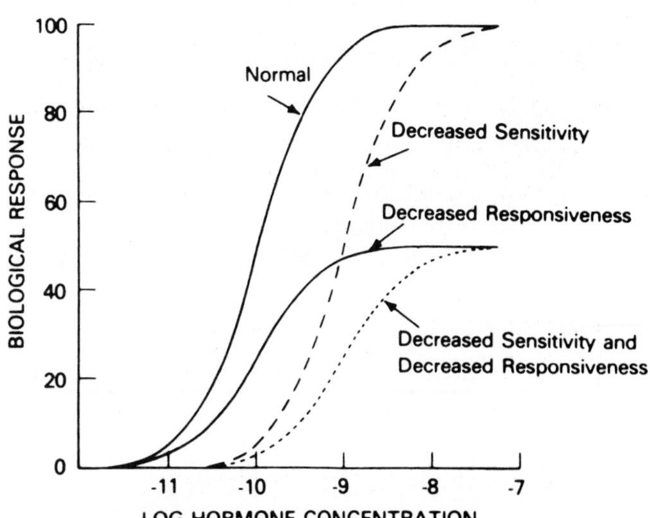

FIGURE 56–5. Classification of insulin-resistant states by the dose-response curve for insulin action. Decreased insulin sensitivity usually represents a receptor binding defect, whereas decreased responsiveness usually represents a postbinding defect. (From Kahn CR: The molecular mechanism of insulin action. Reproduced, with permission, from the Annual Review of Medicine, Vol 36, © 1985 by Annual Reviews Inc.)

TABLE 56–2. Pharmacokinetics of the Insulins

Types	Onset (hours)	Peak (hours)	Duration (hours)	Appearance
Short-Acting Insulins				
Regular	½–1	2–3	5–7	Clear solution phosphate buffer
Semilente	½–1	4–6	12–16	Cloudy insulin zinc suspension
Intermediate-Acting Insulins				
Lente	1–2	8–12	18–24	Cloudy insulin zinc suspension
Isophane (NPH)	1–2	8–12	18–24	Cloudy insulin protamine suspension
Long-Acting Insulins				
Ultralente	4–8	16–18	36	Cloudy insulin zinc suspension

order to delay the absorption of insulin and prolong its activity.

Except for regular insulin, which is soluble and prepared as a clear solution appropriate for intravenous (IV), subcutaneous (SC), or intramuscular (IM) injection, all of the other preparations are cloudy suspensions. The various insulin preparations differ in onset, peak, and duration of action (Table 56–2). They are classified as short-, intermediate-, and long-acting preparations, which may be used alone or in combination to attain the desired control of blood glucose levels at various times during the day and night. Insulin potency is expressed in USP units (*eg*, U-100).

BOX 56–1
INDICATIONS FOR INSULIN TREATMENT

Insulin therapy is indicated for the following reasons:

- All patients with Type I diabetes mellitus (IDDM)
- Patients with ketoacidosis or hyperosmolar coma
- Patients with Type II diabetes mellitus (NIDDM) when diet restriction, exercise, and oral hypoglycemic agents fail to maintain satisfactory blood glucose levels
- Patients with NIDDM in the presence of surgery, fever, infections, renal or hepatic dysfunction, pregnancy, or other metabolic disturbances

Methods of Insulin Delivery

Insulin is usually injected subcutaneously. This is achieved either by single bolus injections, or by continuous subcutaneous insulin infusion (*eg*, insulin pump). Insulin is delivered IV in acute conditions such as diabetic ketoacidosis and hyperosmolar coma. Small-dose, multiple injections IM may be used to treat ketoacidosis where an IV infusion is not possible. Jet injection of insulin is available.

The objective of insulin treatment is to correct the metabolic abnormalities resulting from insulin deficiency and prevent the acute and chronic complications of diabetes. The aim of insulin replacement is to normalize blood glucose levels.

Blood glucose measurements monitor diabetic control and index blood glucose levels at a particular time. Glycosylated hemoglobin levels are an index of long-term (10–14 weeks) blood glucose control.

Complications of Insulin Treatment

Hypoglycemia is the most serious and common complication of insulin therapy. Symptoms of hypoglycemia include sweating, weakness, hunger, tachycardia, tremor, headache, blurred vision, mental confusion, incoherent speech, coma, and convulsions. The oral administration of carbohydrates relieves mild hypoglycemia. Glucagon administration may be necessary in patients who are stuporous or unconscious.

Less common complications of insulin therapy include allergic reactions such as itching, redness, and swelling at the site of injection. Systemic allergic reactions are rare. Atrophy of subcutaneous fat at the site of injection may lead to scarring, but this is rare with the pure forms of insulin.

Resistance to insulin may occur in some patients and is manifested by requirements of a very high insulin dosage (more than 200 U/day). All patients on insulin therapy develop a low titer of circulating IgG anti-insulin antibodies. Switching to another insulin preparation may help decrease the insulin dosage requirement.

ORAL HYPOGLYCEMIC AGENTS

Patients with NIDDM often have insulin resistance as a major defect in insulin signalling. They may have a compensatory increase in insulin release resulting in hyperinsulinism; however, the beta cells of the pancreas eventually become desensitized to the glucose stimulus for insulin secretion and circulating plasma insulin levels fall. The defective insulin release (especially first-phase release) leads to hyperglycemia and the signs and symptoms of NIDDM. Obesity contributes to insulin resistance and diminished insulin sensitivity of tissues. Weight reduction by dietary restriction and exercise to improve glucose tolerance and insulin sensitivity may be sufficient to control blood glucose levels in NIDDM.

Defects at the major sites of insulin action—insulin molecular structure, hormone binding, glucose transport, and intracellular glucose metabolism—have been recognized in different forms of the disease.

The oral medications available in the United States for treating hyperglycemia in NIDDM are the sulfonylureas. The biguanides (metformin) are not approved in the United States because of risk factors, but they are used in Europe and other parts of the world.

TABLE 56–3. Pharmacokinetics of the Sulfonylureas

Drug	Duration of Action (hours)		Time to Peak Plasma Concentration (hours)	Half-Life (hours)	Doses per Day	Hepatic Metabolites
Tolbutamide	Short	6–8	3–5	—	2–3	Inactive
Chlorpropamide	Long	>40	2–4	36	1	Inactive
Acetoheximide	Intermediate	12–18	2*	1.5*	1–2	Active
Tolazamide	Long	~20	4–8	7	1	Active†
Glipizide	Intermediate	10–16	1–3	4	2	Inactive
Glyburide	Intermediate	24	—	10	1	Inactive

*Active metabolite (hydroxyhexamide) peaks at 4 hours; half-life is 6 hours.
†There are also inactive metabolites.

Oral hypoglycemic agents are indicated in NIDDM only when dietary restrictions and exercise fail to achieve adequate diabetic control.

Sulfonylureas

The first-generation sulfonylureas include tolbutamide, tolazamide, chlorpropamide, and acetohexamide. Second-generation sulfonylureas include glyburide and glipizide, which differ from the first-generation drugs in their increased potency and fewer drug-drug interactions due to reduced ionic binding to plasma proteins. The sulfonylureas all share a common molecular structure, and only the side chains change structure to define the different activities and metabolic profiles of these drugs.

The sulfonylureas lower blood glucose mainly by stimulating insulin release from the islet beta cells of the pancreas.

The sulfonylureas are largely ineffective in IDDM patients who lack functional beta cells and the capacity to secrete insulin. The cellular mechanism of action of the sulfonylureas is to block ATP-sensitive K^+ channels, leading to cell depolarization and increased Ca^{2+} entry through voltage-sensitive channels, thus stimulating insulin release through calcium-dependent mechanisms. The beta cells become refractory to prolonged sulfonylurea stimulation, and insulin release will then return to diabetic levels. Second-generation sulfonylureas are efficacious in cases of secondary failure to first-generation forms of the drugs.

Extrapancreatic effects of the sulfonylureas include an increase in insulin receptor number and receptor sensitivity, and reduced glucose output by the liver.

Pharmacokinetics

Sulfonylureas are oral agents readily absorbed from the GI tract. They are highly protein bound (92–99%). These drugs can be classified as short-, intermediate-, and long-acting forms. All these drugs are metabolized by the liver and excreted in the urine. Dosages must be adjusted in cases of renal impairment. Active metabolites may increase the duration of action of some of the sulfonylureas (Table 56–3).

Adverse Effects

Hypoglycemia is the major adverse reaction of sulfonylureas. The longer-acting sulfonylureas are more likely to result in hypoglycemia as an adverse reaction. Patients with impaired renal or hepatic functions are more likely to have hypoglycemic episodes.

Chlorpropamide can potentiate the action of antidiuretic hormone and may precipitate the syndrome of inappropriate antidiuretic hormone (SIADH) manifested by signs and symptoms of water intoxication. Chlorpropamide also causes a disulfiram-like reaction in patients ingesting alcohol.

Nausea, vomiting, and epigastric pain have occurred in patients receiving sulfonylurea drugs. Allergic skin reactions have been reported.

The University Group Diabetes Project (UGDP) also concluded that patients taking sulfonylureas may experience cardiac effects, such as ventricular fibrillation, triglyceride deposition, and an increase in automaticity.

Drug Interactions

Sulfonylureas are highly protein bound. The ionic binding of first-generation sulfonylureas may displace, or be displaced by, other protein-bound drugs such as oral anticoagulants, salicylates and other nonsteroidal anti-inflammatory agents, and sulfonamides. This interaction does not occur with the nonionic binding of the second-generation sulfonylureas.

TABLE 56–4. Interactions of Sulfonylureas With Other Drugs

Drug Name	Effect	Mechanism of Action
Anticoagulant (dicumarol)	Increased hypoglycemic effect	Inhibition of metabolism of sulfonylureas
Ethanol	Both hypoglycemia and hyperglycemia; acute alcohol intolerance may occur	Inhibition of hepatic gluconeogenesis and increased metabolism of drug
Monoamine oxidase inhibitors	Increased hypoglycemic effect	Probably direct effect on insulin release and interference with symptomatic response
Phenylbutazone	Increased hypoglycemic effect	Impaired metabolism
β blockers (nonspecific)	Possible increased hypoglycemic effect; blunting of symptoms of hypoglycemia	

Phenylbutazone enhances the hypoglycemic action of sulfonylureas by a combination of protein-binding displacement, inhibition of hepatic enzyme activity, and decreased renal excretion (Table 56-4).

Beta-adrenergic blocking agents may impair glucose tolerance, block hypoglycemia-induced tachycardia, and alter the hemodynamic response to hypoglycemia. Nonselective β-adrenergic blockers may mask the signs and symptoms of hypoglycemia and delay recovery.

Anticoagulants, ethanol, and monoamine oxidase inhibitors also affect the activity of sulfonylureas (Table 56-4). Corticosteroids, contraceptives, phenytoin, rifampin, isoniazid, calcium channel-blocking agents, and phenothiazines decrease the hypoglycemic effect of sulfonylureas.

Biguanides

Neither of the biguanides, metformin and phenoformin, is approved for use in the United States.

In the UGDP both biguanides were associated with increased risk of lactic acidosis; however, metformin has the lower risk of lactic acidosis and is used in other parts of the world.

Biguanides do not stimulate insulin secretion and they do not cause hypoglycemia. Metformin may enhance the actions of insulin on peripheral tissues, reduce glucose uptake in the GI tract, and have an anorexigenic effect. In addition, metformin stimulates anaerobic glycolysis, inhibits hepatic and renal gluconeogenesis, increases high-density lipoprotein (HDL) cholesterol, and reduces triglycerides and blood pressure, which may be beneficial in diabetic control. Other side effects associated with biguanides include GI upsets and diarrhea.

Metformin is not bound to plasma proteins. It is excreted primarily by the kidney. The bioavailability is 50% of the ingested dose. Therapeutic indications are indicated in NIDDM patients after other strategies fail to control blood glucose levels. The drug may be most beneficial in obese, hyperinsulinemic NIDDM patients. Metformin is administered three times a day, and may be combined with sulfonylurea therapy.

GLUCAGON

Glucagon is a polypeptide secreted by the alpha cells of the pancreatic islet (Fig. 56-2). A glucose counterregulatory hormone, glucagon secretion is responsive to hypoglycemia. Amino acids and proteins can also enhance release.

Glucagon stimulates its target tissues by binding to its receptor and increasing both adenylate cyclase activity and cyclic AMP formation. Glucagon stimulates glycogenolysis and ketogenesis.

Plasma glucagon levels are often elevated in IDDM and in other types of stress conditions. Rebound glucagon secretion may occur in response to hyperinsulinism and hypoglycemia, resulting in hyperglycemia. Glucagon's main therapeutic use is in the emergency treatment of hypoglycemia. It can be administered IV, IM, or SC.

Glucagon can cause nausea and vomiting and should be used cautiously in unconscious patients.

REFERENCES

Banerge MA, Lebowitz HE: Insulin-sensitive and insulin resistant variants in NIDDM. Diabetes 38:84-92, 1989.

Binder C, Lauritzen T, Faber O, Pramming S: Insulin pharmacokinetics. Diabetes Care 7:188-199, 1984.

Cryer PE, Gerich JE: Glucose counterregulation during intensive insulin therapy in diabetes mellitus. N Engl J Med 312:232-241, 1985.

Czeck MP: The nature and regulation of the insulin receptor: Structure and function. Annu Rev Physiol 47:357-381, 1985.

Kahn CB: Advances in insulin therapy of diabetes mellitus. *In* Brownlee M (ed): Handbook of Diabetes Mellitus, Current and Future Therapies, Vol 5, 75-94. New York: John Wiley & Sons, 1981.

Kahn CR: The molecular mechanism of insulin action. Annu Rev Med 36:429-451, 1985.

Khardori R, Soler NG: Hyperosmolar hyperglycemic nonketotic syndrome. Am J Med 77:899-904, 1984.

Lockwood DH, Ferick JE, Goldfine I: Effects of oral hypoglycemic agents on receptor and post receptor actions of insulin. Diabetes Care (Suppl) 7:1-2, 1984.

Melander A: Clinical pharmacology of sulfonylureas. Metabolism 36:12-16, 1987.

Nair KS, Halliday D, Matthews DE, Welle SL: Hyperglucagonemia during insulin deficiency accelerates protein catabolism. Am J Physiol 253:E208-213, 1987.

National Diabetes Data Group: Classification and diagnosis of diabetes mellitus and other categories of glucose intolerance. Diabetes 28:1039-1057, 1979.

Osei K: Concomitant insulin and sulfonylurea therapy in patients with type II diabetes — Effects on glucoregulation and lipid metabolism. Am J Med 77:1002-1009, 1984.

Owen OE, Den G: Insulin and sulfonylurea agents in noninsulin dependent diabetes mellitus. Arch Intern Med 146:673, 1986.

Reaven GM: Role of insulin resistance in human disease. Diabetes 37:1595-1607, 1988.

Skyler JS: Insulin pharmacology. Med Clin North Am 72:1337-1354, 1988.

PART XI

SPECIAL TOPICS IN PHARMACOLOGY

57 Vitamins

Peter J. Horvath

The science and research of vitamins is relatively new, but the therapeutic use of foods that are good sources of certain vitamins is ancient. Vitamins are organic compounds that cannot be synthesized by an organism and are required for proper functioning of the body. Humans have a wide range of individual requirements that change with age, state of health, types of activity, and many other factors. The requirements listed in Table 57-1 were developed to provide the vast majority of people with the amounts required to meet certain criteria. The daily values used on the new food labels are listed in Table 57-2. These are based on a 2000-kcal daily intake. The variability in human biochemistry must be kept in mind when considering the effectiveness of vitamin supplements or treatments.

OIL-SOLUBLE VITAMINS

Vitamin A: Retinoids and Carotenoids

There are ancient historical records in China and Egypt of the use of foods rich in vitamin A or its precursors to cure

TABLE 57–1. Food and Nutrition Board, National Academy of Sciences—National Research Council Recommended Dietary Allowances*
(Designed for the Maintenance of Good Nutrition of Practically All Healthy People in the United States)

							Fat-Soluble Vitamins				Water-Soluble Vitamins							Minerals						
Category or Condition	Age (Years)	Weight† (kg)	Weight† (lb)	Height† (cm)	Height† (in)	Protein (g)	Vitamin A (μg RE)‡	Vitamin D (μg)§	Vitamin E (mg α-TE)‖	Vitamin K (μg)	Vitamin C (mg)	Thiamin (mg)	Riboflavin (mg)	Niacin (mg NE)¶	Vitamin B_6 (mg)	Folate (μg)	Vitamin B_{12} (μg)	Calcium (mg)	Phosphorus (mg)	Magnesium (mg)	Iron (mg)	Zinc (mg)	Iodine (μg)	Selenium (μg)
Infants	0.0–0.5	6	13	60	24	13	375	7.5	3	5	30	0.3	0.4	5	0.3	25	0.3	400	300	40	6	5	40	10
	0.5–1.0	9	20	71	28	14	375	10	4	10	35	0.4	0.5	6	0.6	35	0.5	600	500	60	10	5	50	15
Children	1–3	13	29	90	35	16	400	10	6	15	40	0.7	0.8	9	1.0	50	0.7	800	800	80	10	10	70	20
	4–6	20	44	112	44	24	500	10	7	20	45	0.9	1.1	12	1.1	75	1.0	800	800	120	10	10	90	20
	7–10	28	62	132	52	28	700	10	7	30	45	1.0	1.2	13	1.4	100	1.4	800	800	170	10	10	120	30
Males	11–14	45	99	157	62	45	1000	10	10	45	50	1.3	1.5	17	1.7	150	2.0	1200	1200	270	12	15	150	40
	15–18	66	145	176	69	59	1000	10	10	65	60	1.5	1.8	20	2.0	200	2.0	1200	1200	400	12	15	150	50
	19–24	72	160	177	70	58	1000	10	10	70	60	1.5	1.7	19	2.0	200	2.0	1200	1200	350	10	15	150	70
	25–50	79	174	176	70	63	1000	5	10	80	60	1.5	1.7	19	2.0	200	2.0	800	800	350	10	15	150	70
	51+	77	170	173	68	63	1000	5	10	80	60	1.2	1.4	15	2.0	200	2.0	800	800	350	10	15	150	70
Females	11–14	46	101	157	62	46	800	10	8	45	50	1.1	1.3	15	1.4	150	2.0	1200	1200	280	15	12	150	45
	15–18	55	120	163	64	44	800	10	8	55	60	1.1	1.3	15	1.5	180	2.0	1200	1200	300	15	12	150	50
	19–24	58	128	164	65	46	800	10	8	60	60	1.1	1.3	15	1.6	180	2.0	1200	1200	280	15	12	150	55
	25–50	63	138	163	64	50	800	5	8	65	60	1.1	1.3	15	1.6	180	2.0	800	800	280	15	12	150	55
	51+	65	143	160	63	50	800	5	8	65	60	1.0	1.2	13	1.6	180	2.0	800	800	280	10	12	150	55
Pregnant						60	800	10	10	65	70	1.5	1.6	17	2.2	400	2.2	1200	1200	320	30	15	175	65
Lactating	1st 6 months					65	1300	10	12	65	95	1.6	1.8	20	2.1	280	2.6	1200	1200	355	15	19	200	75
	2nd 6 months					62	1200	10	11	65	90	1.6	1.7	20	2.1	260	2.6	1200	1200	340	15	16	200	75

From Food and Nutrition Board: Recommended Dietary Allowances. 10th ed. Washington, DC: National Academy of Sciences, National Research Council, 1989.

*The allowances, expressed as average daily intakes over time, are intended to provide for individual variations among most normal persons as they live in the United States under usual environmental stresses. Diets should be based on a variety of common foods to provide other nutrients for which human requirements have been less well defined. See text for detailed discussion of allowances and of nutrients not tabulated.

†Weights and heights of reference adults are actual medians for the US population; of the designated age, as reported by National Health and Nutrition Survey (NHANES) II. The median weights and heights of those under 19 years of age were taken from Hamill et al (1979) (see pp 16–17). The use of these figures does not imply that the height-to-weight ratios are ideal.

‡Retinol equivalents. 1 retinol equivalent = μg retinol or 6 μg β-carotene. See text for calculation of vitamin A activity of diets as retinol equivalents.

§As cholecalciferol. 10 μg cholecalciferol = 400 IU of vitamin D.

‖α-Tocopherol equivalents. 1 mg d-α tocopherol = 1 α-TE. See text for variation in allowances and calculation of vitamin E activity of the diet as α-tocopherol equivalents.

¶1 NE (niacin equivalent) is equal to 1 mg of niacin or 60 mg of dietary tryptophan.

TABLE 57–2. Reference Daily Intakes (RDIs)

Nutrient	Amount	Nutrient	Amount
Vitamin A	5,000 IU	Vitamin B_6	2.0 mg
		Folic acid	0.4 mg
Vitamin C	60 mg	Vitamin B_{12}	6 μg^f
Thiamin	1.5 mg	Phosphorus	1.0 g
Riboflavin	1.7 mg	Iodine	150 μg
Niacin	20 mg	Magnesium	400 mg
Calcium	1.0 g	Zinc	15 mg
Iron	18 mg	Copper	2 mg
Vitamin D	400 IU	Biotin	0.3 mg
Vitamin E	30 IU	Pantothenic acid	10 mg

Adapted from Kurtzweil R: "Daily Values" encourage healthy diet. FDA Consumer May: 40–45, 1993.

Based on 2000 calories a day for adults and for children over 4 years of age only.

night blindness. Vitamin A is actually a group of retinoids and carotenoids. One of the key features of the vitamin A group is the presence of conjugated double bonds.

Retinoids usually contain five trans-double bonds with different functional groups at carbon 15, usually either an alcohol, an aldehyde, or an acid. The retinol may be esterified with palmitate, acetate, or propionate. The unit of measurement is based on all-trans retinol, with 1 g equal to 1 RE (retinol equivalent). Retinoic acid itself has activity only for some functions, such as growth and some aspects of reproduction.

There are over 400 naturally occurring carotenoids, making them the most prevalent pigment in nature. Many of the carotenoids, termed provitamin A, have vitamin A activity. Some carotenoids have biological actions independent of their vitamin A activity. The carotenoids have widely varying activity, with carotene being the highest. Theoretically, carotene can be split into two retinols, but considering the variability of absorption and incomplete conversion, 1 mg of carotene is equivalent to 1/6 RE. Most other carotenoids are at most half as potent; moreover, some have no vitamin A activity.

Absorption

For absorption of the vitamin A group, fat must be present in the meal (except with the synthetic, watersoluble forms). In some cases, the vitamin has to be released from proteins by digestion. The fat is necessary for the release of bile and pancreatic enzymes, and bile acids and phospholipids are required for micelle formation. Provitamin A carotenoids, carotenoids, vitamin A, and esters remain in the micelle. The retinol esters are hydrolyzed by a specific esterase; the ester is poorly absorbed. Retinol may be absorbed by a carrier-mediated mechanism at low concentrations and by passive cellular diffusion at higher concentrations. The absorption of carotene is much lower than that of the retinoids. Before transport from intestine, some carotene may be cleaved by carotenoid 15-15′ dioxygenase to retinal. The retinal is reduced to retinol by alcohol dehydrogenases and esterified with palmitate. Chylomicrons carry mostly retinylester, with retinoic acid going into the portal vein.

In the liver, carotene cleavage is continued. ApoRBP (retinol-binding protein) made in the hepatocyte is combined one to one with retinol to form holoRBP. HoloRBP in plasma combines with prealbumin, thus avoiding excretion into the urine. There are holoRBP receptors in the intestine, in the Ito cells in the liver, in the retina, and in many other tissues; these receptors internalize the retinol and bind it to intracellular RBPs. The liver can further metabolize retinol to retinoic acid; this process is irreversible. The retinoic acid can be glycosylated to glucuronide and is secreted into bile and eventually to the feces; the glucuronide pathway may represent 67% of retinoic acid excretion, with the kidney excreting the remainder as retinoic acid and its metabolites. The Ito cells in the liver store most of the vitamin A in humans, whereas adipocytes are the primary storage area for carotenoids. The presence of the carotenoids provides a yellowish tint to fatty tissue. An excess of carotenoids may appear as jaundice, but the eyes do not change color.

Functions

The function of retinol and retinal in vision is well known. Retinoic acid cannot be used for this function. Vitamin A also plays a key role in differentiation and, in this case, retinoic acid may be the most important. The mechanism of the effect of vitamin A on gene expression involves retinoic acid and retinol binding to chromatin through the supersteroid receptor family. With a vitamin A deficiency, columnar epithelial and mucous cells change to a keratin type of cell. Vitamin A also causes differentiation of carcinoma cells.

The effects of a vitamin A deficiency on reproduction are not permanent and can be reversed. The deficiency syndrome is characterized by cornified tissue replacing the normally functioning columnar squamous cells, which are required for the maintenance of the placenta and spermatogenesis.

The importance of the vitamin A group and other carotenoids in immunological processes has come to the forefront of research. Vitamin A is necessary for lysosome production in saliva, tears, and sweat, having an important antibacterial function. Carotenoids may have their own effects by increasing natural killer cell activity, increasing T-cell and B-cell proliferation, and inhibiting the proliferation of neoplastic cells. Cancer risks may be decreased by an increase in differentiation and by the antioxidant function of carotene.

Deficiency

Deficiency can be caused by a low intake or by fat malabsorption due to cystic fibrosis, cholestasis, pancreatic insufficiency, or chronic diarrhea. Alcohol consumption may decrease the storage in liver by the Ito cells. Kidney disease can lead to a tubular reabsorption decrease. Total parenteral nutrition (TPN) solutions may also be low in vitamin A, which results from adsorption to intravenous (IV) tubing. Signs and symptoms of vitamin A deficiency may include xerophthalmia and keratomalacia, with the clinical signs being conjunctival xerosis, Bitot's spot. and corneal xerosis. Another important sign of vitamin A deficiency is night blindness. The health and integrity of the skin is also decreased with vitamin A deficiency.

There are two levels of vitamin A deficiency, defined by

plasma or liver levels. One is frank deficiency, and the other is termed marginal deficiency. Another good measure of vitamin A nutriture is based on the response to a supplement; plasma levels are measured before a dose and 5 hours after a 450-g dose.

Vitamin D

The history of vitamin D started in 1809 with Bardsley, who found that cod liver oil could cure rickets. Vitamin D is a sterol, with the two major vitamin D compounds being D_2 from ergosterol in plants, yeast, and fungi, and D_3 from 7-dehydrocholesterol from animal sources. Hydroxylation can occur at three positions: 1, 24, and 25 monohydroxy; 1,25 or 24,25 dihydroxy; or 1,24,25 trihydroxy (in terms of activity in rats, D_3 and D_2 are equal, but not in chickens, where D_2 is 10 times more potent). The 25 hydroxylated vitamin D is between two and five times as effective as the unhydroxylated form, and 1,25 $(OH)_2$ vitamin D is an order of magnitude more potent.

Sources

Aside from the dietary sources, UV light exposure can produce vitamin D. 7-Dehydrocholesterol is converted in the skin to previtamin D_3, producing adequate daily needs in 15 minutes with sun exposure of hands and face. Photobiogenesis is not controlled, but the production of melanin may act as a protective agent against vitamin D toxicity. Prolonged light exposure can result in the production of other metabolites, such as lumisterol. Previtamin D_3 is thermally converted to vitamin D_3.

Absorption

As with vitamin A, fat digestion products are required for optimal intestinal absorption of vitamin D. Absorption probably occurs in both the jejunum and ileum. It is transported then in chylomicrons to the liver and fat tissue and stored with DBP (vitamin D-binding protein) in the liver. Subsequent transport from the liver or skin uses DBP. Previtamin D_3 is not taken up by DBP, and this acts as a key control site. The first major step in vitamin D metabolism is 25 hydroxylation in the hepatocytes; it may also occur in the lung, kidney, and intestine. This may increase with deficiency. The second important step is 1 hydroxylation by the kidney and placenta, a step tightly regulated by hormones. Low serum calcium causes release of parathyroid hormone (PTH), which lowers intracellular phosphate and in turn stimulates 1 hydroxylation of 25 vitamin D. It is suppressed also by 1,25 $(OH)_2$ vitamin D and serum calcium. 24 Hydroxylation, which probably occurs in the kidney, is regulated also, but opposite to 1 hydroxylation in relation to 1,25 vitamin D levels. 24 Hydroxylation is a preliminary step to biliary excretion, which is the major pathway. Chronic alcohol consumption can cause an increased loss of 25 vitamin D into bile.

The active form of vitamin D is the metabolite 1,25 $(OH)_2$ vitamin D, which acts as a hormone that controls calcium and phosphorus homeostasis. Calcium absorption is increased by 1,25 vitamin D. 1,25 Vitamin D binds to a cytosol receptor protein (RP) that is similar to the other steroid receptors. RP with 1,25 vitamin D binds to DNA, causing mRNA transcription for calcium-binding protein (CaBP). This process is inhibited by glucocorticoids, which are therefore useful in the therapy for hypervitaminosis D. Phosphorus absorption is increased by 1,25 vitamin D also. Renal reabsorption of calcium by the distal kidney tubule and bone mobilization of calcium is stimulated by PTH with existing 1,25 vitamin D. Calcitonin from thyroid blocks the action of vitamin D and is useful also in the therapy for hypervitaminosis D (see Chapter 32).

Bone formation is another important function of 1,25 vitamin D, which can increase receptors for epidermal growth factor and stimulate transforming-growth factor (TGF). TGF stimulates bone resorption and cartilage induction. Vitamin D also affects differentiation of some cells; *ie*, myelocytes to monocytes or macrophages. It inhibits the growth of some carcinomas, especially breast cancer and malignant melanoma, exhibiting a biphasic effect, stimulating replication at low physiological levels, and inhibiting replication at higher levels.

Deficiency

Deficiency can be detected by using serum levels of 25 OH vitamin D. Infants (especially breast-fed) and the elderly are at risk. Breast-fed infants may have a dietary deficiency that may be exacerbated by lack of sunlight exposure. The elderly may be at risk for a vitamin D deficiency also because of a decreased 1,25 vitamin D synthesis, decreased milk intake, decreased light exposure (exposure during bad weather), and decreased 7-dehydrocholesterol in the skin. Renal failure can also result in a deficiency in 1,25 vitamin D due to a lack of synthesis that results in low serum calcium and high serum phosphorus; hypoparathyroidism and estrogen administration can result in decreased parathyroid hormone (PTH) levels and have similar effects. There is an inborn error of metabolism that affects 1,25 vitamin D status, familial hypophosphatemia. There are significant drug interactions with the anticonvulsive drugs phenytoin and phenobarbital. These drugs may induce hepatic 25 hydroxylation and renal 1 hydroxylation, which induces further metabolism and may increase inactive vitamin D metabolite excretion in the bile (possibly as 24,25 vitamin D). Finally, fat malabsorption and alcohol consumption may result in deficiency. Alcohol consumption may cause pancreatic and bile acid deficiency, and 25 hydroxylation may result from hepatocyte failure.

The classical deficiency syndromes of vitamin D are rickets and osteomalacia. The sequence of events are decreased calcium absorption — low calcium levels — hyperparathyroidism with PTH release — PTH elevates serum calcium from bones and causes phosphaturia — and finally, bone disease and lack of mineralization. The treatment consists of 1.25 – 2.5 mg of vitamin D weekly (50,000 IU/week). Osteoporosis may be caused by the result of estrogen-induced release of bone calcium, which decreases PTH release and 1,25 vitamin D synthesis; in the face of no increase in calcium absorption, there is subsequent bone loss. Hypocalcemic tetany can also be the result of vitamin D deficiency.

Vitamin K

In 1929, Dam and associates reported hemorrhages in chickens fed a low-fat diet in a study of cholesterol metabolism. They found a delay in coagulation due to an effect on prothrombin time. Vitamin K is a quinone derivative, labile to alkali and light. A key function of vitamin K involves its capacity to form a stable free radical. Vitamin K_1, phylloquinone, is from plants. K_2, menaquinone, with unsaturated side chains of various numbers of prenyl units (usually 7 through 13), is derived from bacterial sources. Menaquinone-4 is the most biologically active form; there is lessened activity observed with compounds with longer or shorter side chains, reaching a low with menaquinone (no side chain and 1/120 the activity). K_3, menadione, is a synthetic that can be elongated by alkylation with digeranyl pyrophosphate to form menaquinone-4.

Absorption

The absorption of vitamin K requires bile and pancreatic juices and probably occurs by a passive mechanism, but K_1 may also have an active transport process in the distal small intestine. Vitamin K is transported in chylomicrons, very low-density lipoprotein (VLDL), and low-density lipoprotein (LDL). Vitamin K has a short half-life, 2–3 hours, excreted primarily as lactones and glucuronides in the feces through bile, with a much smaller amount appearing in the urine. This reduces the toxicity of vitamin K.

Functions

The primary function of vitamin K is in the posttranslational modification of glutamate (Glu) to γ carboxyglutamate (Gla). This carboxylase-epoxidase system requires nicotinamide-adenine dinucleotide (NADH) or nicotinamide-adenine dinucleotide phosphate (NADPH). The vitamin K cycle is almost completely blocked by warfarin. Warfarin is used as an oral anticoagulant, for prevention of thrombosis, and as rat poison (see Chapter 34). Warfarin is also teratogenic. Coagulation occurs through the clotting factor cascade, with many factors involved with vitamin K. The major factor is prothrombin, which is synthesized in the liver with many Gla amino acids. In the clotting process, there are many other Gla proteins. Another Gla protein is found in the bone, Bone-Gla protein (BGP) or osteocalcin, which makes up 1% of total bone protein and is regulated by 1,25 vitamin D_3. Osteocalcin binds Ca_{2+} and hydroxyapatite. Other possible effects of vitamin K relate to anti-inflammatory actions and rheumatoid arthritis. Vitamin K inhibits the rise in intracellular calcium that stimulates leukocyte function. This may be through the reduction of glutathione, which is used to protect the macrophage from its own superoxide, which is stimulated by vitamin K.

Deficiency

Few people develop vitamin K deficiency because of its common occurrence and microbial production. However, drug therapy with anticoagulants (warfarin), anticonvulsants (hydantoins), and antibiotics (neomycin, moxalactam), especially when used in patients undergoing surgery and maintained on TPN, may result in a vitamin K deficiency. Adult TPN solutions do not contain vitamin K. Newborns, especially premature or home births, are at risk because of the low amount of vitamin K in breast milk and low intestinal synthesis. Fat malabsorption resulting from ingestion of mineral oil and other unabsorbed lipids, low fat intake, bile acid deficiency caused by biliary obstruction, cystic fibrosis, chronic liver disease, or megadoses of vitamin E can exacerbate marginal situations. The primary symptom of vitamin K deficiency is a lengthened prothrombin time (see Chapter 34).

Vitamin E: Tocopherols and Tocotrienols

The history of vitamin E and the tocopherols started with an observation that has yet to be made in humans: Evans and Bishop in 1922 showed that a fat-soluble substance prevented fetal death in rats when the diet contained rancid lard. There are many stereo isomers of vitamin E. All are labile to light (important in using TPN solutions), oxygen, peroxides (*eg*, as occurs in rancid fat), and heating at high temperature. Therefore, most vitamin E in oils and fried frozen foods is lost. Two thirds of that in the germ of grains can be lost in processing the oil, and most is lost in white bread with the removal of the germ and bleaching.

Absorption

The various tocopherols differ only in the methylation on the benzene ring, but they have different activities. All are alcohols that can be esterified; the acetate ester is the most watersoluble. All must be de-esterified to be biologically active. The reactive hydroxyl groups that can form free radicals are crucial to the functional action of vitamin E. Alpha-tocopherol is the most abundant with the d form — the one present in foods and the most potent. Synthetic α-tocopherol has eight epimers and is less potent. Beta-tocopherol with one less methyl is at least half as potent as the α-form and is found in high quantities in wheat. Gamma-tocopherol is much less potent than either, but is present in much higher concentrations in oils, especially corn and soybean, and also in margarines, depending on the oil used. Gamma-tocopherol also has one less methyl than the δ-tocopherol, which is high in some oils (safflower) and has two less methyls than α-tocopherol and has almost no biological activity. Another group of vitamin E compounds, the tocotrienols, have many double bonds, similar to vitamin K, with intermediate biological activities. Fat digestion products are important in the absorption of vitamin E, the amount absorbed being proportional to the amount of lipids in the diet. The percent of absorption can range from 10 to 70%. Absorption is also inversely proportional to the amount of vitamin E in the diet. The absorbed vitamin E is transported from intestine in chylomicrons; one of its storage sites is Ito cells in the liver. Further transport to most other tissues occurs by way of VLDL and LDL. The major excretory route is through the bile in the feces.

Functions

An important function of vitamin E is as a biological antioxidant that acts in concert with the enzymes glutathione peroxidase, superoxide dismutase, and catalase. Vitamin E prevents peroxidation by stopping a chain reaction between free radicals and other compounds (especially polyunsaturated fatty acids). Vitamin E also prevents the formation of ceroid pigments (lipofuscin), pigment granules in soft tissue that result from oxidized unmetabolizable lipids cross-linked with proteins. The amount of lipofuscin present appears to be a function of age.

The function of vitamin E in reproduction, which brought about its discovery, has not been demonstrated in humans. Other functions and properties include decreased fecal mutagens, decreased prostaglandin and thromboxane synthesis (PGI_2, which promotes platelet aggregation and is low in diabetics; this may be correctable with additional vitamin E), increased blood circulation in the elderly (300–600 mg/day for 3 months), increased esterification and decreased de-esterification of vitamin A in the liver, and protection of the lung from air pollutants such as nitrogen dioxide and ozone.

Deficiency

Deficiency of vitamin E can occur in humans with fat malabsorption from pancreatic disease, biliary obstruction, cystic fibrosis, cirrhosis of the liver, or enteritis. Premature infants are at risk of vitamin E deficiency because of the low storage of vitamin E that results from low transplacental delivery, low body fat, poor fat absorption, and rapid growth. Patients with abetalipoproteinemia, being unable to synthesize apoprotein B, may develop symptoms of vitamin E deficiency. Two good tests for low levels of vitamin E nutriture are peroxide hemolysis and blood analysis. It is important to express plasma levels in relationship to lipids. It may be useful also to do an isomer analysis. The symptoms of vitamin E deficiency include hemolysis, anemia, neural degeneration, and perhaps retrolental fibroplasia (neonatal infants with low vitamin E and oxygen toxicity) and abnormal lung development.

WATER-SOLUBLE VITAMINS

Vitamin C: Ascorbic Acid

Vitamin C deficiency states, like those of vitamin A, have a long history, with many folk remedies and a long history of treatments. Vitamin C became especially important when long sea voyages became common, with perhaps more sailors dying of scurvy than any other single cause. In the 1500s, Hawkins prescribed oranges and lemons for long sailing voyages. Possibly the first controlled clinical trial was done by Lind in 1742, who used citrus fruits as a preventive for scurvy.

Vitamin C exists as either L-ascorbic acid or dehydroascorbic acid; both forms are watersoluble. L-Ascorbic acid is oxidized easily in water with 0_2 to dehydroascorbic. L-Ascorbic acid has a half-life of less than 2 minutes in water at pH 6 and 158° F. It is sensitive to heat, with metals such as iron and copper acting as catalysts, and is unstable in TPN solutions because of the cupric ion and 0_2. In general, it is the most easily lost of all vitamins. There is a significant seasonal variation in the daily intake, with citrus juice and potatoes being the main sources in American diets. Of the ascorbic acid in orange juice, 75% may be lost in 3 weeks even when the juice is stored in the refrigerator in breathable paper containers. Potatoes retain 75% of the ascorbic acid after being fried, but within 1 to 2 hours of slicing, 30–50% of the vitamin C can be lost by oxidation.

Absorption, Metabolism, Excretion

Absorption occurs by two mechanisms. Both forms can be absorbed by passive diffusion, but only ascorbic acid is absorbed by a sodium-dependent, carrier-mediated mechanism. The percent of absorption decreases with increasing intake, ranging from 90 to 20%, with the maximal percent of absorption occurring at amounts below 180 mg and the lowest at levels at or above 2 g. Vitamin C is stored in all tissues, with the highest concentrations in the adrenal and pituitary glands, and lower levels in the liver, spleen, and brain. Humans have about 100 days of storage, but this can change with the season, being lower in the winter.

Ascorbic acid is reversibly converted to dehydroascorbic acid. There is irreversible oxidation to diketo-L-gulonic acid. Further metabolism results in oxalate and threonic acid; 5-keto acids, L-lyxonic, and L-xylonic acid are also formed. Ascorbic acid is not metabolized to CO_2 in humans (although this is a major pathway in guinea pigs). In humans, vitamin C can be excreted in the urine without being metabolized; renal reabsorption of L-ascorbic acid occurs using a sodium-dependent mechanism. The amount in the urine is usually less than 3 mg/day at low intakes (approximately 3–30 mg/day), but urinary levels increase with increasing intakes. Metabolites are excreted also in the urine, with oxalate being prominent at low intakes. At megadose levels (over 1000 mg), some ascorbic acid is excreted in the feces, and oxalate is not prominent. Thus, oxylate kidney stones with megadoses of vitamin C are unlikely to be a problem.

Functions

Vitamin C has many important functions. A crucial feature of vitamin C is its antioxidant properties. It can reduce ferrous iron to ferric iron with the promotion of nonheme iron absorption. Other aspects of iron metabolism are also related to vitamin C. It acts as a protective agent with enzyme reactions. As a hydroxylation enzyme cofactor, it is essential for collagen formation. Therefore, without vitamin C, wound healing and bone formation are impaired and capillary walls are weakened. This defect in collagen formation involves the enzymes proline prohydroxylase and lysyl hydroxylase. The carrier for activated fatty acid into mitochondria for β-oxidation, carnitine, can come from the diet or be synthesized. Its synthesis requires vitamin C, as do biogenic amines such as norepinephrine and epinephrine (see Chapter 9). Many hormones undergo amidation with the addition of an amide on the carboxyl end of the peptide, and this requires vitamin C. Hydroxylations also employ vitamin C for cholesterol degradation to bile acid synthesis and for drug metabolism.

At large doses of at least 1 g/day, there are effects on immunological functions and possibly cancer development. Vitamin C (50 mg/kg/day) can increase the chemotaxis of neutrophils in chronic granulomatous disease, a genetic disorder of leukocyte function, leading to a reduction in a number of infections in this condition. Cancer treatment with vitamin C is still controversial and is based on observations that vitamin C alters certain immunological functions. The type of cancer may be crucial; earlier studies examined vitamin C effects on cancer in general, whereas cancer in the stomach and uterus may be more responsive. Some of the possible actions in preventing cancer may be due to the effect of vitamin C on nitrosamine protection or a possible reduction in the occurrence of mutagens in feces that can occur with increases in vitamin E. Nitrosamines are powerful cancer-causing agents, especially in the stomach and colon. They can be produced by the conversion of nitrates to nitrites, with the nitrites reacting with amines or amides. Vitamin C reduces nitrite conversion. Nitrate intake can be quite high, 75 - 100 mg/day, with vegetarians taking in about 250 mg/day because of their higher consumption of vegetables. Nitrites, which are more potent than nitrates, are consumed usually in amounts less than 1 mg/day, but a high intake of cured meat intake can increase this up to 2 mg/day. The oral intake of vitamin C that has been demonstrated to reduce the conversion of nitrates to nitrosamine is rather large, some 4 g/day.

Other possible health effects of vitamin C in high doses include a lowering of hyperlipidemia and protection from heavy metal toxicity. The reduction in hexavalent chromium to trivalent chromium, which is much less toxic, may be helpful in those exposed. There is also a reduction in the toxicity of cadmium, vanadium, nickel, and lead.

Deficiency

The main cause for marginal vitamin C deficiency is an increased requirement combined with a low intake. Increased requirements may be due to many causes: disease (such as cancer and rheumatoid disease, which result in increased turnover), oral contraceptives (progesterones increase mixed-function oxidases), stress (such as burns and infection), and smoking. In addition, the elderly may have an increased requirement. Low intake can occur most easily in the winter, with a lower intake of fresh vegetables. Chronic heavy alcohol consumption may be associated with both a low intake and altered liver metabolism.

Early marginal deficiency is manifested by either normal or lowered plasma ascorbic acid levels, with the next stage exhibiting not only a decrease in plasma levels but also decreases in leukocyte and urine levels. There are also biochemical changes with vitamin C deficiency, with an increase in proline/hydroxyproline ratio and a decrease in serum carnitine. Diabetic retinopathy and periodontal disease are both associated with low vitamin C levels. In addition, marginal vitamin C deficiency might contribute also to general symptoms of ill health, including fatigue, poor wound healing, increased susceptibility to bruising, loss of appetite, and reduced immune responses.

Rebound deficiency can occur following one abrupt discontinuation of large doses taken chronically. Clinical (scorbutic) deficiency occurs when plasma levels are less than 0.2 mg/L plasma. Scurvy presents with red, swollen, and bleeding gums; perifolliculosis, increased capillary fragility; subcutaneous hemorrhages; and swollen joints. Long-term, untreated vitamin C deficiency can result in sudden death.

Vitamin B_1: Thiamin

The deficiency disease of thiamin (vitamin B_1) is an ancient disease that has become more apparent with the widespread consumption of polished rice. In the 1880s, Takaki used dietary supplements of meat and grains to cure sailors of the Japanese navy of shipboard beriberi. The factor that cured beriberi was found to be a water-soluble pyrimidyl with a thiazole ring existing either free, as hydrochloride, as the coenzyme thiamin diphosphate (TDP), or as thiamin triphosphate (TTP). The coenzyme is heat-stable; all the forms are destroyed by alkalis, including phenobarbital. Because they are water-soluble, they are lost in cooking water when it is thrown away. Some antinutrients to thiamin exist. The most important antithiamin is the enzyme thiaminase, which is found in some raw fish, tea, coffee, blueberries, brussels sprouts, and red cabbage. Tannins found in tea and red wine may also destroy thiamin.

Absorption

Thiamin can be absorbed passively in the small intestine and large intestine and by an active, carrier-mediated mechanism, probably in the jejunum. In the intestine, thiamin is phosphorylated by thiaminokinase to TDP and secreted into the portal blood. It is in this form (TDP) that most of the thiamin is stored, with about one half in muscle and one tenth in the brain (as TTP). The pool in the brain is slow to turn over, being metabolized to thiamin monophosphate (TMP). Most of the thiamin in the plasma is free as alcohol. Thiamin and many thiamin metabolites are excreted in the urine.

The primary function of thiamin is to act in the transfer of an aldehyde. There are three important enzymes in which it is a cofactor, the oxidative decarboxylases of α-keto acids and transketolase (TK) of the pentose phosphate shunt for synthesis of ribose and NADPH. It is also a cofactor for pyruvate decarboxylase for the tricarboxylic acid cycle (TCA) cycle and α-ketogluterate decarboxylase for branched-chain amino acid catabolism and the TCA cycle.

Deficiency

Thiamin deficiency can be determined by using urine measurements or the response of plasma TDP activity to additional TDP. Rice-eating populations are at risk of becoming deficient in thiamin, especially in Southeast Asia. Heavy alcohol consumption causes decreased absorption and increased excretion; renal disease (renal dialysis) can increase the risk for thiamin deficiency. The elderly are also at risk because of a low intake and low absorption. There are some inborn errors in metabolism that are associated with thiamin: lactic acidosis associated with low levels of pyruvate decarboxylase and branched-chain ketoaciduria.

Symptoms of thiamin deficiency include mental confusion, anorexia, and neuropathies. Beriberi can take two forms: dry beriberi (muscle wasting) with peripheral neuropathy, and wet beriberi (edema) with cardiovascular effects (frequently associated with a high carbohydrate diet or exercise that leads to a retention of sodium). Wernicke's encephalopathy and Korsakoff's psychosis (amnesic disorder) are examples of dry beriberi that may be the consequence of disturbed carbohydrate metabolism in the neurons with a lack of the triphosphate form. A dietary deficiency can be corrected with 10 – 20 mg/day oral (3 g/IU), given adequate intestinal absorption; the inborn errors can be alleviated with 10 – 200 mg/day.

The thiamin deficiency syndromes of Wernicke's encephalopathy and Korsakoff's psychosis are irreversible if not treated promptly. The most common occurrence of these serious syndromes is with individuals who are acutely hospitalized and given IV glucose, such as after an accident. (The presence of dietary deficiency or prior heavy alcohol consumption is frequently not clinically apparent.) The combination of marginal thiamin deficiency consequent to possible heavy alcohol consumption and the infusion of glucose *requires* parenteral administration (usually IM) of thiamin (*eg*, 100 mg or more daily); the susceptibility to Wernicke's encephalopathy may be associated with a genetic difference in the transketolase enzyme system.

Vitamin B_2: Riboflavin

Riboflavin as part of the complex antiberiberi factor was separated from thiamin by McCollum, based on its stability to heating. The name riboflavin is partially derived from the ribitol portion of the vitamin, which also contains an isoalloxazine ring. Riboflavin exists free but usually occurs as riboflavin-phosphoric acid, flavin mononucleotide (FMN), or flavin adenine dinucleotide (FAD). It is only slightly soluble in water. It is heat-stable, but is light-sensitive.

Absorption

Before absorption, riboflavin is removed from dietary protein by acidic gastric conditions, and phosphatases release it from the covalently linked forms. It is absorbed by a passive and active mechanism. There is little storage of riboflavin, and this occurs mainly in the plasma, which is complexed with proteins (for transport), and intracellularly with flavoprotein complexes and covalent flavoproteins. The amount of riboflavin excreted in the urine provides a fairly accurate measure of riboflavin intake.

Functions

The primary function of riboflavin is an oxidation/reduction reaction for metabolism and respiration (oxidative phosphorylation). It acts as a direct link between the TCA cycle and the respiratory chain. It is involved also in fatty acid synthesis and oxidation, amino acid oxidation, and many other reduction reactions. FAD, a stronger oxidizing agent than nicotinamide-adenine dinucleotide (NAD), is used by cytochrome C reductase for NAD^+ reduction.

Deficiency

The symptoms of riboflavin deficiency are vascularization of cornea, sore throat, fissures at the side of the mouth, and a magenta-colored tongue. It can be precipitated by general malnourishment and malabsorption associated with lactose malabsorption, diarrhea, and the irritable bowel syndrome. Increased requirement for riboflavin because of protein wasting or increased excretion associated with phenothiazine administration exacerbates a mild deficiency. Therapy for riboflavin deficiency is either 6 mg/day oral or 25 mg/day IM.

Niacin

Niacin deficiency was first described by Casal in 1735 as the *Mal de la Rosa* disease, sickness of the rose, because of the skin roughness and color. This disease was the result of the corn brought from the New World for the masses in Europe. The deficiency disease is now called pellagra. There are two active forms of niacin: nicotinic acid (niacin) and nicotinic acid amide (nicotinamide) and four derivatives: NMN (nicotinic acid mononucleotide), NaMN (nicotinic acid amide mononucleotide, a tryptophan metabolite), NAD, and NADP (phosphate on the ribose). Nicotinic acid is a pyridine-3-carboxylic acid; the reduced form is labile to acid, and the oxidized form is labile to alkali. Both are stable to heat and are stable as solids. Tryptophan can be converted to niacin with an efficiency of about 60 tryptophan molecules for 1 niacin molecule. This ratio varies with individuals and certain conditions (*eg*, estrogen administration increases the efficiency of conversion).

Absorption

Nicotinic acid is absorbed passively in the intestine, but nicotinamide is not readily absorbed. The total storage of niacin is low but occurs in all tissues. The usually storage forms are NAD or NADP, but some is stored in the liver as niacin. The liver is also the primary site of nicotinic acid formation from tryptophan. NaMN and NMN are metabolized eventually by different routes to NAD and then to NADP. With a normal intake of niacin, most of the metabolites are excreted in the urine as 1-methyl-nicotinamide (20 – 30%) and 1-methyl-3-caroxamido-6-pyridone (40 – 60%). These metabolites are made in the liver through a pathway that utilizes methionine. A high intake of nicotinic acid results in an increase in the 1-methyl and glycine conjugates, whereas a high intake of nicotinamide increases the excretion of unmetabolized nicotinamide.

Functions

As with riboflavin, the main function of niacin is in oxidation/reduction reactions using NAD or NADP. It is essential for many dehydrogenases in the Krebs cycle, for anaerobic carbohydrate metabolism, and lipid and protein metabolism. Electron transport also requires niacin. There are other less defined functions of niacin involved with ADPR transferase, as a treatment of hypercholesterolemia (see Chapter 31), and in association with chromium and the glucose tolerance factor.

Deficiency

At high risk for niacin deficiency are individuals with Hartnup's disease, which involves disturbed amino acid absorption that leads to a low absorption of tryptophan. The absorption of tryptophan is also lowered in certain foods, such as corn. Corn is also low in niacin. Therefore, the undernourished populations of the world, for whom corn is the major protein source, are at risk of developing niacin deficiency. Tryptophan can be released with alkali treatment of the corn, which is used traditionally in the Mexican diet; the corn for tortillas is soaked in lime water. Tryptophan metabolism is altered by carcinoid disease or a high intake of leucine, and both decrease the conversion of tryptophan to niacin. Therapy for Hartnup's or carcinoid disease involves 40 - 200 mg of niacin equivalent/day.

Symptoms of pellagra are the "three Ds": dermatitis, dementia, and diarrhea. The dermatitis is erythematous, especially on sun-exposed areas. The dementia involves fatigue, insomnia, apathy, with confusion that leads to psychoses. The diarrhea is due to inflammation of intestinal epithelium and may also include vomiting and dysphagia. A "fourth D" can occur — death. Laboratory signs of niacin deficiency include the development of a urinary pyridone : methyl metabolite ratio of less than one.

Vitamin B_6: Pyridoxine, Pyridoxamine, and Pyridoxal

Vitamin B_6 is basically a modified pyridine: pyridoxine is an alcohol, pyridoxamine an amine, and pyridoxal an aldehyde. Pyridoxal phosphate (PLP) is the most common coenzyme in animals; pyridoxamine phosphate (PMP) is used for transamination in animals; and pyridoxine phosphate (PNP) is used in plants. All are water-soluble and sensitive to light and alkali, and PLP is subject to thermal degradation. During pasteurization of milk, there is a 20 - 40% loss in vitamin B_6 activity.

Absorption

After ingestion, the unphosphorylated forms are absorbed by passive diffusion, and the phosphorylated forms after dephosphorylation by luminal phosphorylases. Pyridoxine is transported as the free vitamin bound to albumin and converted to pyridoxal in the liver. PLP can be formed by phosphorylation by pyridoxal kinase or from PMP and PNP by a riboflavin (FMN)-dependent oxidase. PLP is the active form that binds to enzymes. Most of the body's store of vitamin B_6 is as PLP with glycogen phosphorylase. Excretion of vitamin B_6 occurs through the urine as pyridoxic acid from pyridoxal oxidized with NAD.

Functions

Vitamin B_6 functions with at least 60 known enzymatic reactions: tryptophan metabolism to niacin; transamination; deamination; decarboxylation for the formation of biogenic amines; the formation of taurine; carbon side-chain transfer (involving folic acid); amine oxidation (histamine breakdown); desulfuration of amino acid; amino acid absorption; heme formation; glycogen phosphorylase in skeletal muscle for glycogen degradation; sphingolipid formation; and antibody production (which is reduced with a deficiency).

Deficiency

A common test for deficiency involves looking for xanthurenate in the urine after administration of a tryptophan load. However, this test may not have clinical significance and may only represent a stress response. Elevated levels of kynurenic acid (KN) and hydroxykynurenic acid can also be used, but KN levels increase with estrogen, pregnancy, and oral contraceptives because of the inhibition of kynureninase. Other measures involve urine measures of B_6 and pyridoxic acid, plasma PLP activity measured by tyrosine decarboxylation with apodecarboxylase, or increase in erythrocyte aminotransferases with PLP addition. Plasma levels by themselves are not useful because they may be elevated in a variety of diseases. Deficiency is uncommon all by itself, although the elderly and people with heavy alcohol consumption are at some risk.

There are some genetic disorders that may be responsive to additional vitamin B_6: homocystinuria, primary cystathioninuria, xanthurenic aciduria, and infant convulsions. Vitamin B_6 nutriture can also be affected by drug interactions with penicillamine (see Chapter 47, heavy metal poisoning antidote and Wilson's disease), isoniazid (see Chapter 40, a tuberculostatic), and oral contraceptives (see Chapter 54). Indicators of vitamin B_6 deficiency may include decreases in serum PLP, B_6 urinary metabolite levels, and transaminases. Convulsions can result from glutamate decarboxylase inactivity or aminobutyrate deficiency; dermatitis also can occur. Therapeutic dosages of 2 - 6 g/day may be useful for carpal tunnel syndrome and pre-eclampsic edema; paradoxically, long-term ingestion of excessive dosages of vitamin B_6 can result in peripheral neuritis.

Pantothenic Acid

Pantothenic acid is an acidic compound with widespread occurrence (hence its name, *pan*, found everywhere). It is made up of pantoic acid linked to alanine by an amide bond. It is water-soluble and labile to acid, alkali, and heat. Much of its activity is lost during cooking (33% in meat, especially if cooked hot and long, but much less in vegetables). Processing also removes pantothenate with milling of wheat. Absorption is almost complete with normal intakes, with subsequent transport as the free vitamin. Most of the pantothenic acid is stored as coenzyme A (CoA) (80%), with the highest levels found in the liver. Excretion in the urine is as pantothenate.

Functions

The active forms of pantothenic acid are CoA and acyl carrier protein (ACP), which is derived from CoA. CoA is a part of more than 70 enzymes, with its major function being the formation of thio esters of acyls with little energy lost during its formation. It is involved in condensation reactions to form citrate, acetylcholine, and acetoacetate. CoA is crucial for carbohydrates and ketogenic amino acid catabolism, especially branched chain amino acids and the TCA cycle with acetyl CoA. It is involved also in cholesterol and steroid synthesis and bile acid conjugation. Its importance is shown by the necrosis of the adrenal gland that occurs in deficient animals. Anemia is also common in deficient animals, because it is needed for heme synthesis. CoA is used also in xenobiotic metabolism for acetylation before excretion. ACP is used for lipid synthesis and catabolism.

Deficiency

A pantothenic acid deficiency has not been clinically recognized because pantothenic acid is so common in foods, but patients with liver disease and heavy drinkers may be at risk for developing a deficiency. A test for deficiency includes whole blood levels and urine excretion. Symptoms include irritability, hypotension, rapid heart rate with exertion, and numbing and tingling of feet and hands. Therapeutic dosages fall in the range of 10 – 100 mg/day.

Biotin

Biotin as an acid is only slightly soluble in water, but as a salt it is water-soluble. It is stable and oxidized in hot alkali. There are eight stereoisomers, but only d-biotin is biologically active. There are some biologically active analogs: oxybiotin, dethiobiotin, and the sulfoxide form, which is converted slowly to biotin. Biotin is linked through lysine to proteins, with a product of digestion being biocytin. Microflora in the intestine can provide enough biotin to meet the human requirement, with fecal output being many times greater than the usual intake. Avidin, the toxin in egg whites, forms a complex with biotin, inhibiting its digestion. Absorption is rapid and active in the upper small intestine and at least passive in the large intestine. There is little storage of biotin, mostly in the liver as carboxylases. It is excreted in the urine as biotin.

Functions

Biotin is involved in the functioning of only a few enzymes. It is most important with a carboxylase in the phosphorylation of bicarbonate to carbonylphosphate. It is involved in fatty acid synthesis via malonyl CoA. The odd-chain fatty acid catabolism, leucine catabolism, and succinyl formation use biotin also. The conversion of leucine to isovalerate to methylcrotonyl in the liver is crucial for branched-chain amino acid catabolism. Finally, it is used in the metabolism of pyruvate for gluconeogenesis. Brain function has been shown to be related to biotin, inasmuch as biotin-deficient rats learn more slowly. This may be due to the fact that glucose is important for brain metabolism and, therefore, it is the organ to show an effect of deficiency.

Deficiency

The major possible causes of biotin deficiency include long-term TPN and antibiotic treatment; infants and alcoholic patients are at the most risk. Deficiency has been observed with large doses of streptomycin for many days. The avidin in raw egg white can cause a deficiency if it is consumed in large amounts, especially in infants. There are some inborn errors of metabolism involving the carboxylases. Symptoms of deficiency include anorexia, nausea, vomiting, glossitis, pallor, depression, general lassitude, and a dry dermatitis. Therapy for a biotin deficiency requires 150 – 300 μg/day for 3 to 5 days. Larger dosages of 5 mg/day for 2 to 3 weeks may be useful for seborrheic dermatitis and Leiner's disease.

Vitamin B_{12}: Cobalamins

The history of vitamin B_{12} has long been intermingled with folic acid and the disease pernicious anemia. Minot and Murphy (1926) received a Nobel Prize for showing that injections of raw liver could cure pernicious anemia. This, combined with the work of Castle and associates in 1929 that showed that an "intrinsic factor" in gastric secretions combines with vitamin B_{12} in food, forms the basis of the understanding that pernicious anemia is due to the lack of the intrinsic factor.

The cobalamins are both a complex group and the most complex vitamin, but only a small part of the molecule varies from one analog to the next. The basic structure of vitamin B_{12} consists of a planar corrin nucleus linked to a nucleotide through a aminopropanol, with a cobalt bound to a nitrogen on the nucleotide and to four of the corrin nuclei. The synthetic cyanocobalamin is the oxidized form, with the last coordination site of the cobalt bound to the carbon of a cyano group. The cyanide (CN) is removed from cyanocobalamin enzymatically and converted to coenzymes in the epithelial cells. The vitamin B_{12} coenzyme form is methylcobalamin (methyl B_{12}), with a methyl group instead of CN; this is a common form for transportation in the body. It may also be the most active. Coenzyme B_{12} has a phosphorylated deoxyadenosyl instead of a methyl and is the storage form. Hydroxycobalamin is found in foods. There are also inactive analogs, such as pseudo B_{12}. The active enzyme form is reduced and conjugated with peptides. The different analogs have varying stability. Cyanocobalamin is labile to heavy metals and strong reducing/oxidizing agents (*eg*, vitamin C), forming new analogs (usually antivitamins). It is stable and soluble in water. The methyl and deoxyadenosyl forms are labile to light, but are fairly stable to heat at pH 4 – 5.

Absorption

The physiological absorption of vitamin B_{12} is a complicated process. Large oral doses of vitamin B_{12} are taken up by a passive mechanism that may account for 1% of the total absorption at normal intakes. Initially, if the vitamin is not linked to a protein, it is bound to a salivary protein. If it is attached to a protein, hydrolysis of the peptide linkages occur through acid denaturation and proteases, primarily pepsin, and then it is bound to the salivary protein. B_{12} is then freed from salivary protein by trypsin and the neutral pH of the small intestine, where it binds with intrinsic factor (IF). IF is released by the parietal cells in the fundus of the stomach; it has a higher affinity for true B_{12} than for some of the inactive analogs. This complex of vitamin B_{12} and IF then binds to receptors in the ileum and is taken into the cell.

Vitamin B_{12} is transported to other tissues from the intestine bound to transcobalamin II (TC II), a protein that is made in the liver. TC II is usually free for binding and may be elevated in autoimmune diseases. The total vitamin B_{12}-binding capacity (TBBC) of the plasma is between 1 and 1.8 ng/mL and is usually 60 – 75% saturated. The difference is unsaturated vitamin B_{12}-binding capacity (UBBC), which is mainly composed of unsaturated TC II. There is a 0.1 – 0.2% turnover, regardless of nutrient state. The storage of vitamin B_{12} is rather large in relationship to its requirement, being between 2 and 10 mg, mostly in the liver in the form of coenzyme B_{12}. This amount can last for up to 3 to 6 years, but with the efficient reabsorption of vitamin B_{12}, it may be decades before a deficiency develops with a sustained low intake of vitamin B_{12}. The bile is the main pathway for excretion of the unmetabolized vitamin B_{12}, which can be reabsorbed. Urine has significant amounts only when intakes are excessive.

Functions

There are only two known systems that use vitamin B_{12}: methymalonyl-CoA isomerase for the conversion of methylmalonate to succinate from propionate, and folate regeneration. The involvement of vitamin B_{12} with 1-C metabolism and its interaction with folate may explain how B_{12} deficiency is associated with impaired DNA synthesis. N5, 10 methylene tetrahydrofolic acid (THFA) is used for DNS synthesis. Methylene THFA has to be regenerated from N5 methyl THFA through THFA, and the major pathway utilizes B_{12}. Vitamin B_{12} may be involved with folate transport and storage. A yet-to-be-defined relationship between vitamin B_{12} and myelin synthesis may be the origin of the neurological effects of B_{12} deficiency.

Deficiency

Deficiency of vitamin B_{12} is associated with low plasma levels. However, these levels may vary greatly during the day. Excess urinary methylmalonic acid can be used also as a measure of vitamin B_{12} deficiency. Patients with achlorhydria, stomach, ileum, or pancreas dysfunction, or following gastrointestinal resection for problems associated with diseases such as Crohn's disease may become deficient because of a low absorption of vitamin B_{12}.

This can occur also with the genetic pernicious anemia, characterized by the lack of IF. Fish tapeworm infection and the use of H_2 blockers such as cimetidine at dosages of 1 g/day can also lead to a decreased absorption of vitamin B_{12}. Bacterial overgrowth due to the blind loop syndrome with bacterial utilization of vitamin B_{12} is another cause of deficiency. Furthermore, low intake because of a strict vegan diet without special sources of B_{12} can result, over time, in deficiency. This low intake of true vitamin B_{12} may be combined with the higher intake of analogs that can occur in special food sources. The use of nitrous oxide as an anesthetic can produce excessive analog formation, with the development of a functional B_{12} deficiency (see Chapters 11 and 34).

Symptoms of a B_{12} deficiency are pernicious anemia, numbness and tingling in the extremities, poor musculature coordination, ataxia, bilateral vision failure, and mental changes (moodiness, poor memory, depression, delusions, or psychosis). As discussed in Chapter 34, pernicious anemia can present as a psychiatric, neurological, or hematological disease, or as a combination, and is still frequently misdiagnosed.

The therapy for B_{12} deficiency differs if it results from nutritional causes or from impaired absorption: for a nutritional deficiency, 0.05 mg IM weekly for 2 weeks followed by 1 μg/day oral, for vegetarians or B_{12}-rich food; for deficiency caused by impaired absorption, 100 μg IM monthly, or at least every 3 months. Vitamin B_{12} has a large safety margin, so therapy can employ dosages beyond the recommended daily requirement. For many pernicious anemia patients, oral doses of vitamin B_{12} of 1000 μg/day avoid IM injections and are effective, as well as practical and inexpensive.

Folic Acid

Channing in 1824 identified an anemia associated with pregnancy and the puerperium that was fatal when combined with the nutritional stress of repeated pregnancies. Later, this was shown to be different than the one caused by B_{12} deficiency. The tropical macrocytic anemia was associated with pregnancy and a diet of primarily white rice and bread; this could be cured by a crude liver extract. The term folic acid was coined by Mitchell and associates in 1941, because this factor was obtained from more than 10 tons of spinach (Latin: *folium*, leaf). Folic acid (pteroylglutamic acid) as such is not found in foods; it is prepared synthetically. There are many forms of folic acid, mainly reduced forms such as THFA with four hydrogens; dihydrofolate; and with R groups, linkages occurring through N5 or 10, or both. The N-linked compounds include N5 formyl THFA, N10 formyl THFA, N5 formimino THFA, N5,10 methenyl, N5,10 methylene, and N5 methyl THFA. They may all have glutamate residues ranging from 1 to 11, with the average being 7 or 3. The THFAs are unstable in light, and THFA is labile to oxidation. Folic acid, the oxidized form, is more stable but is labile at a pH of less than 4. Because of the labile nature of folic acid, most of it is lost with long cooking or canning.

Absorption

There is a brush border conjugase that hydrolyzes the glutamate tail of folic acids in foods. The ileum is the primary site of absorption, being both passive and facilitated. The percentage absorbed with the diet can be high, up to 90%, but is usually lower, around 50%. Transport from the intestine, at low physiological levels, occurs after it is converted to N5 methyl THFA. At high levels of intake, it may get into blood as unmethylated THFA. With normal body stores, humans can last 3 – 6 months with no intake; about half of this storage is in the liver as polyglutamates. It is transported as the free acid, competitively bound to plasma proteins with a low affinity and on high affinity-binding proteins. Although these high affinity-binding proteins are present in low concentrations, they may have an important function in the transport of folic acid from cerebrospinal fluid. Further metabolism occurs after cellular uptake by active mechanisms, involving the glutamate tails, which may be related to activity and storage. The formation of THFA requires vitamin C and NADPH for both formation of DHFA and THFA. The interconversion of THFA and N5,10 methylene THFA requires vitamin B_6. N5 methyl THFA is a storage form that has to be converted to THFA and then to other forms for functioning; this requires B_{12}. Without vitamin B_{12}, THFA that enters the metabolic pool may not be regenerated and thus may explain some of the effects of B_{12} deficiency. Folic acid is excreted mainly in the bile, with 0.1 mg/day reabsorbed. The amount excreted is increased with liver disease. It is excreted also in the urine as acetamidobenzoylglutamate. Also filtered by the kidney is N5 methyl THFA, but most is reabsorbed.

Functions

The primary function of folic acid is as methyl group donor. One specific involvement is in the synthesis of thymidylate for DNA, using N5,10 methylene THFA. This process is the rate-limiting step in DNA formation. The result of folic acid deficiency is megaloblastosis (see Chapter 34) in association with bone-marrow pancytopenia (anemia and leukopenia). Megaloblastosis occurs also in the rest of the body, including the GI tract. Another key function of folic acid is for purine synthesis using N5,10 methenyl THFA to N10 formyl THFA. Folic acid is involved also in amino acid conversions (serine : glycine, cysteine : methionine, and histidine : glutamic acid). N10 formyl THFA incorporation into choline is crucial to initiation of protein synthesis and methylation of transfer RNA.

Deficiency

Deficiency can be detected using plasma and red cell measurements, tests for defective DNA synthesis, and by measuring urinary excretion of formiminoglutamate (FIGLU), urocanate, formate, or amino-imidazole carboxamhistidine (AIC, which may occur also with B_{12} deficiency). Pregnant women are likely to be deficient; in fact, up to one third of pregnant women may exhibit a deficiency. It has now been shown that prenatal supplements of folic acid can then be very useful in preventing neural tube defects. Alcoholic patients are also at risk of folic acid deficiency because of increased loss of folic acid metabolites in the bile; increased mean corpuscular value (MCV) is one of the common laboratory findings in alcoholism. Increased excretion of folic acid occurs with dialysis also. Diets high in glycine or methionine increase the need for folic acid. There are significant drug interactions with phenytoin, barbiturates, antimalarial drugs, methotrexate (an analog), aminopterin (an analog that interferes with dihydrofolic reductase), and oral contraceptives (which interfere with polyglutamate tail metabolism and decrease absorption by 50%; see Chapters 44 and 54).

BOX 57–1
RATIONAL USES OF VITAMINS AND DIETARY SUPPLEMENTS

Facts:

1. Vitamins are both drugs and foods; "dietary supplements" may be foods, drugs, or botanicals of established *or of unknown composition.*
2. Diseases both of excess and of deficiency of vitamins occur; dose is critical in therapy as well as in prevention.
3. Individuals differ markedly as to their optimal vitamin and nutrition intakes.
4. Many identifiable populations have unique nutritional, vitamin, and biochemical needs; at recognized risk are:
   - The pregnant mother and her fetus
   - Children
   - The poor
   - The elderly
   - Those with any disease condition (especially chronic)
   - Those receiving any drugs
   - The drinker
   - Anyone with an extreme diet

Know what/why/how vitamins should be prescribed:

1. For prevention or correction of dietary deficiencies—ask yourself what preparations really are appropriate for "prevention," and prevention of what?
   A complete medical history includes dietary, alcohol, caffeine, and vitamin intake. Try a brief diary approach or global assessment (Detsky et al, 1994).
2. Determine what interactions, possibly adverse, with other medications, drugs, and foods could be occurring or might occur?
3. Knowledge of the indications, uses, toxicity, and hazards of specific vitamins is essential.
4. Avoid abrupt discontinuation of a vitamin supplement because of the hazard of possible rebound relative deficiency (as documented for vitamin C).
5. Assume, until proven otherwise, that some type of nutritional disturbance probably exists in those at risk (see Facts 4.); deficiency is known to be common for D, C, thiamine, and folic acid.

Decide on the criteria for assessing benefits and risks of vitamin therapy:

1. Decide on your criteria for what is useful and valid information about vitamins and dietary supplements; what constitutes proof and how/when would you act on the information.
2. Decide on your criteria for "authority" on nutrition and vitamins, *eg*, what you read in newspapers or read in vitamin/nutrition promotions; your friends; dietitian; what you agree with; or only that tested with controlled clinical trial. When in any doubt, perhaps a consultation is in order.

Signs and symptoms of deficiency are wasting of body tissue, diarrhea, and macrocytic anemia. The deficiency associated with pregnancy can be prevented by folate supplements. Folate deficiency can be corrected with 15 mg IM, followed by 5 mg/day orally for a month with 100 μg/day for 1 - 4 months or one serving of fresh fruit or vegetable a day.

Note: "Dietary supplements," the new legal entity, are not drugs and not foods, and they are not covered by Food and Drug Administration regulations. Accurate labeling for content and composition, safe use, and efficacy does not currently exist. These substances present serious potential hazards of adverse effects and interactions with drugs and foods.

REFERENCES

Alhadeff LC, Gualtieri T, Lipton M: Toxic effects of water-soluble vitamins. Nutr Rev 42:33 - 40, 1984.

Briggs M (ed): Vitamins in Human Biology and Medicine. Boca Raton: CRC Press, 1981.

Brown ML (ed): Present Knowledge in Nutrition. 6th ed. Washington, DC: The Nutrition Foundation, 1990.

Combs GF: The Vitamins. New York: Academic Press, 1992.

Detsky AS, Smalley PS, Chang J: Is this patient malnourished? JAMA 271:54 - 58, 1994.

England S, Seiffer S: The biological functions of ascorbic acid. Annu Rev Nutr 6:365 - 406, 1986.

Food and Nutrition Board: Recommended Dietary Allowances, 10th ed. Washington, DC: National Academy of Sciences, National Research Council, 1989.

Hathcock JN, Torendle GJ: Oral cobalamin for treatment of pernicious anemia. JAMA 265:96 - 97, 1991.

Hunt SM, Groff JL: Advanced Nutrition and Human Metabolism. New York: West Publishing, 1990.

Kurtzweil R: "Daily Values" encourage healthy diet. FDA Consumer. May, 40 - 45, 1993.

Lederle FA: Oral cobalamin for pernicious anemia — Medicine's best-kept secret. JAMA 265:94 - 95, 1991.

Linder MC: Nutritional Biochemistry and Metabolism, 2nd ed. Norwalk, CT: Appleton & Lange, 1991.

Machlin LJ (ed): Handbook of Vitamins. New York: Marcel Dekker, 1990.

Plesofsky-Vig N, Brambl R: Pantothenic acid and coenzyme A in cellular modification of proteins. Annu Rev Nutr 8:461 - 482, 1988.

Sauberlich HE: Bioavailability of vitamins. Prog Food Nutr Sci 9:1 - 33, 1985.

Selhub J, Jacques PF, Wilson PWF, et al: Vitamin status and intake as primary determinants of homocysteinemia in an elderly population. JAMA 270:2693 - 2698, 1993.

Shane B, Stokstad ELR: Vitamin B12-folate interrelations. Annu Rev Nutr 5:115 - 141, 1985.

Shils ME, Olson JA, Shike M (eds): Modern Nutrition in Health and Disease, 8th ed. Philadelphia: Lea & Febiger, 1994.

Stampfer MJ, Willett WC: Homocysteine and marginal vitamin deficiency: The importance of adequate vitamin intake. JAMA 270:2726 - 2727, 1993.

Watts DT: Vitamin B_{12} replacement therapy: How much is enough? Wis Med J 93:203 - 205, 1994.

Winter J: True Nutrition, True Fitness. Clifton, NJ: Humana Press, 1991.

58 Principles of Prescribing: Drug Therapy in Pediatrics and Geriatrics

Cedric M. Smith

The **general prescribing and therapeutic principles** applicable to adults also apply to both geriatric and pediatric patients. This chapter examines the major principles and illustrates some important aspects of drug therapy in the very young and the very old, including how these populations may differ from the adult populations.

PRINCIPLES OF PRESCRIBING—THERAPY FOR ELDERLY PATIENTS

Healthy old people, in general, respond to drugs in the same way and to the same degree as younger adults. Yet, they frequently deserve special attention because

- *The elderly are more likely than young adults to have one or more chronic disease conditions; ie,* their drug responses are much more likely to be influenced by the presence of preexisting disease(s).
- *As a corollary, they are more likely to be receiving or to have received recently other drugs. Thus, drug-drug and drug-food interactions may be critical issues.*
- *Social and psychiatric problems may loom larger on average in the elderly because of the greater potential loss of social and economic supports.*

Following is a series of general principles of preventive medicine on how to improve prescribing and to avoid errors in prescribing.

Accurate Diagnoses and Understanding of the Patient

- Treating symptoms in the absence of a definitive diagnosis is not justified and can be hazardous.
- Prevention of disease is preferable over treatment after disease appears.
- Every patient needs and deserves a *decision* about treatment.
- The context of diagnosis and treatment is as critical as the treatment itself—age, sex, socioeconomic status, ethnic and cultural background, family history and situation, and developmental history are all important.

Appropriate Selection of Drug and Drug Dosage

- Patients deserve and should be encouraged to obtain adequate information on potential benefits and side effects of every drug, inasmuch as prescribed treatment is only carried out with the patient's (informed) consent.

- Prescribe from a limited number of useful drugs.
- Choose the least toxic drug.
- Choose the least expensive drug.
- Treatment of cause has priority over treatment of symptoms.

- *Before prescribing*, review previous and current drug regimens and previous adverse experiences with drugs, medicines, over-the-counter (OTC) medicines, and foods; listen to the patient and consult physicians prescribing other medications; take account of smoking, alcohol, and caffeine habits of the patient.
- Review special precautions, contraindications, and potential interactions for each drug, including pharmacogenetic variability (Chapter 59).
- Do not assume that patients are taking the drugs you prescribe or that you are the only one prescribing.
- Choose specific end-points of therapy so that dosage can be optimized, irrational combinations avoided, and side effects minimized.
- Start with a low dose and increase the dose slowly (*"start low; go slow"*).
- Monitoring of effects and side effects is essential.

- *Review medications regularly on an established schedule with respect to response to therapy, adverse reactions, and the necessity for continued treatment.*
- *Before changing a drug or adding a new drug*, consider changing the dose of the current medication.

Prescribe a Minimal Number of Drugs — Avoid Polypharmacy

- With any new sign or symptom, review all drugs prescribed or taken as a possible cause.
- Consult the literature and/or an expert whenever the patient's response is inadequate or inconsistent with expectations, an untoward response is obtained, or if you have any doubt regarding the wisest drug or drug dosage.

Look for Side Effects

Ensure that the patient's responses and side effects are assessed periodically throughout therapy.

Avoid Prescribing for the Wrong Reasons

Do **not** prescribe because

You want to try out a new medication

You have samples

The patient wants it

You want to give the patient something

"It's the drug to give"

The medication is what the patient has been taking

Staff/counselor/nurse/family wants you to

It will make you look good

You hope for an impressive solution to a difficult problem

Assess the Possible Physiological and Biochemical Changes That Occur With Aging

Certain changes that occur with aging might modify or alter specific drug actions, adverse effects, and time course and termination of action. *Note that the changes and implications for therapy are complex functions of the specific drug and drug class, mechanisms of action, and disposition.*

• Absorption

Few alterations in absorption occur simply because of advanced age, but some decrease in gastrointestinal (GI) motility or blood flow may occur.

• Distribution

Cardiovascular distribution is not specifically altered *per se* with aging. Lean muscle mass and total body water decrease, whereas total body fat tends to increase with age. Thus, drugs that are largely distributed in water tend to have higher concentrations with aging (with a given dose and a given body weight); those agents largely soluble in fat have a relatively larger volume of distribution and thus a lower blood level. These changes are of most importance with single doses; with chronic administration, age-related changes are of limited importance.

• Protein Binding

Plasma albumin levels decrease with age, resulting in potentially higher blood levels for those agents that are highly protein-bound, *eg*, benzodiazepines.

• Hepatic Metabolism and Clearance

The first-pass effect is largely a function of hepatic blood flow, and hepatic blood flow is decreased with age. The result is a relatively larger amount of a drug that is subject to appreciable first-pass metabolism, resulting in higher systemic blood levels in the geriatric patient; examples of this are the more intense sedative effects of triazolam, midazolam, tricyclic antidepressants, and neuroleptics. Of course, some drugs (*eg*, flurazepam [DALMANE]) are metabolized to one or more active derivatives; the final effect is the sum of actions of all of the active compounds.

• Capacity for Drug Oxidations

Capacity for drug oxidations via the hepatic cytochrome P-450 drug metabolizing systems decreases with age; elimination half-lives of extensively metabolized drugs may be increased by two to three times in older patients. An example of such drugs are the long-acting benzodiazepines such as diazepam, chlordiazepoxide, and most likely flurazepam. This is one reason why the recommended dose of flurazepam in the elderly, if it is to be used at all, is 15 mg, one half the more usual 30-mg dose for adults.

• Phase II Drug Metabolism

Aging has a relatively weak effect on phase II drug metabolism, such as glucuronidation and sulfation.

• Renal Clearance

Renal blood flow and glomerular filtration rate decrease with age. Congestive heart failure would be expected to further reduce renal clearance. *Therefore, because many drugs are taken chronically by elderly patients, for any given dose and dosing interval, the steady-state blood level is likely to be higher in older people. In addition, the differences among individuals are frequently greater than any average "age-related" differences.*

• Pharmacodynamics

Elderly patients are generally more susceptible to a number of drug effects, especially sedation, mental confusion, anticholinergic effects, and orthostatic hypotension (*ie*, altered organ response). These side effects occur with many, many drugs (see Chapters 50 and 62).

Ensure That Medications Are Taken as Directed

Assess the patient's compliance and adherence. Confusion and behavioral problems compromise compliance with taking medication and increase the likelihood of adverse drug interactions. For example, patients who are confused may take too many drugs or too much of one drug, or take a drug too often, too little, or erratically. They are also unlikely to remember or to be able to report all of the drugs they take. Moreover, when you ask a patient about what drugs he or she takes, keep in mind that the "usual" pills are frequently not considered "drugs" or "medications" by patients; specific inquiry is essential to find out about OTC vitamins or cold or hay fever medications, laxatives, antidiarrheals, headache medications, arthritis medications, herbal medicines, dietary supplements, or even sleep medications. All patients can benefit from education and insightful management of chronic medications.

- Try to use a once-a-day or twice-a-day regimen.
- Use a medication calendar or timed dispenser.
- Use drug information summaries.
- Encourage supervision of therapy by significant others.
- Label all drug containers clearly.

PEDIATRIC THERAPEUTICS

The topic of pharmacology in the developing individual is sufficiently large to warrant major reviews (*eg*, Berlin, 1993) and large comprehensive textbooks (*eg*, Yaffee and Aranda, 1992); particularly useful is the up-to-date neonatal and pediatric drug formulary included as an appendix (Johnson et al, 1992) in the latter textbook.

The principles listed for the geriatric population apply with almost equal force to the pediatric situation. The unique challenges of pediatric pharmacology lie largely in the rapid and marked age-related changes in physiology during the prenatal period, in the newborn, in the breast-feeding nursing infant, and continuing through childhood to puberty and adulthood. *Thus, children can be expected to differ from adults in terms of possible qualitative differences in drug effects, drug metabolism, and excretion and most certainly quantitatively in terms of absorption, peak levels, duration of action, and steady states.*

Other than the emphasis on possible differences, few other unique overarching principles of pediatric pharmacology can be enunciated. Rather, what is truly important are the specifics and the particular conditions, which are outlined as follows:

Accurate Diagnoses and Understanding of the Patient

- Treating symptoms in the absence of a definitive diagnosis is not justified and can be hazardous.
- Prevention of disease is preferable over treatment after disease appears.
- Every patient/family needs and deserves a *decision* about treatment.
- The context of diagnosis and treatment is as critical as the treatment itself—age, sex, socioeconomic status, ethnic and cultural background, family history and situation, and developmental history are all important.
- Identify the properties of the drug(s) that will probably be involved (for an example, see the section in Chapter 26 on the treatment of attention deficit disorder).
- Determine the routes of administration available.

Appropriate Selection of Drug and Drug Dosage

- *Before prescribing*, review previous and current drug regimens and previous adverse experiences with drugs, medicines, OTC medicines, and foods; listen to the patient and consult physicians prescribing other medications; take account of smoking, alcohol, and caffeine habits of the patient; assess potential adverse effects of drugs and chemicals in the breast milk consumed by nursing infants (Tables 58-1 and 58-2) or those in the environment, including cosmetics. Although only a few drugs pose a significant hazard to the nursing infant, be cautious and presume, until you have determined otherwise, that every

TABLE 58–1. Drugs Contraindicated During Breast-Feeding

Drug	Adverse Effect
Alcohol (large dose)	Drowsiness, diaphoresis, growth retardation, Cushing's syndrome, decreased milk ejection reflex
Amiodarone	Potential pulmonary toxicity
Amphetamines	Irritability, poor sleeping pattern
Bromocriptine	Suppressed lactation
Cannabis	Drowsiness
Chloramphenicol	Possible bone marrow suppression, refusal to eat, vomiting
Cimetidine	Suppressed gastric acidity in infant, inhibited drug metabolism, central nervous system stimulation
Cocaine	Signs of withdrawal, seizures, behavioral development abnormalities
Cyclophosphamide	Immune suppression
Cyclosporine	Potential nephrotoxicity
Doxorubicin	Cardiac toxicity and myleosuppression
Ergotamine	Vomiting, diarrhea, convulsions, suppressed lactation
Gold salts	Rash, inflammation of kidney and liver
Heroin	Neonatal narcotic dependence
Iodine^{131}	Thyroid suppression
Iodine^{125}	Risk of thyroid cancer
Isotretinoin	Potential tumorigenicity
Lithium	Central nervous system disturbances, cardiovascular dysfunction
Methadone	Signs of opiate withdrawal if rapidly withdrawn
Methimazole	Decreased thryoid function; use propylthiouracil as an alternate
Methotrexate	Immune suppression
Metronidazole	Secreted into milk to same level as plasma; thus mutagenic and carcinogenic adverse effects too risky
Morphine	Prolonged habituation
Phencyclidine	Tremors, generalized spasticity
Phenindione	Hemorrhage
Radiopharmaceutical agents (gallium 67)	Bone marrow suppression
Salicylates (aspirin)	Metabolic acidosis, rash (use acetaminophen as alternate)
Tinidazole	Secreted into milk to same level as plasma; thus high risk of mutagenic and carcinogenic effects

From Kacew S: Adverse effects of drugs and chemicals in breast milk on the nursing infant. J Clin Pharmacol 33:213–221, 1993.

agent to which a mother is exposed appears in the breast milk.

- Patients and their parents and caregivers deserve and should be encouraged to obtain adequate information on potential benefits and side effects of every drug.
- *Review medications regularly on an established schedule with respect to response to therapy, adverse reactions, and the necessity for continued treatment.*
- Choose specific end-points of therapy so that dosage can be optimized, irrational combinations avoided, and side effects minimized. In general, start with a low dose and increase the dose slowly (*"start low; go slow.*)
- Consider the possibility of "paradoxical" reactions and age-related qualitative differences in the actions to psychotoxic drugs (Lanius et al., 1993).
- In general, choose the least toxic, least expensive drug; treat causes in preference to symptoms; and review special precautions, contraindications, and potential interactions for each drug.
- Monitor effects and side effects.
- Use methods available for monitoring drug levels and effects. Pediatric patients have limited ability to communicate symptoms and perceived effects. Monitoring of therapeutic levels would appear to be especially useful for many drug classes, *eg*, for antiseizure, chemotherapeutic, theophylline, and digoxin medications. Nevertheless, serious limitations remain: for many drugs and conditions poor correlations between a single level and clinical effects exist; the blood level may not reflect drug concentrations at target tissue receptors; the timing of the blood samples may well miss the expected peak or trough times; and many reference therapeutic values lack appropriate validity (Tange et al, 1994). Therapeutic drug monitoring is uniquely useful when the effects of a drug cannot be measured directly or the drug has a very narrow margin of safety. Thus, most attention for pediatric drug monitoring has been focused on theophylline, chemotherapeutic agents, antiepileptic drugs, and cardioactive agents such as digoxin. Nevertheless, in view of the serious limitations on the available information about pediatric pharmacotherapy, perhaps the most important principle is that because *the differences from adult populations may only have been documented recently, it is critically important to consult literature reporting recent clinical trials.* It is widely recognized that the need for controlled clinical trials in pediatrics is only beginning to be addressed (Wil-

TABLE 58–2. Drugs to Be Used with Caution During Lactation

Drug	Adverse Effect
Aluminum antacids	Developmental retardation
Amantidine	Urinary retention, vomiting, skin rash
Atropine	Possible suppressed lactation, anticholinergic effects
Chlorpromazine	Drowsiness, lethargy, gynecomastia in males, galactorrhea in females
Diazepam	Sedation, accumulation in infant
Doxepin	Paleness, unresponsiveness
Estrogens	Feminization
Indomethacin	Convulsions
Isoniazid	Pyridoxine deficiency development, hepatotoxicity, neurotoxicity
Nalidixic acid	Hemolytic anemia
Nitrofurantoin	Hemolysis in glucose-6-phosphate dehydrogenase–deficient infant
Novobiocin	Hyperbilirubinemia
Oral anticoagulants (ethyl biscoumacetate)	Cephalohematoma, increased risk of bleeding problems
Oral contraceptives	Breast enlargement, decrease in milk production and protein content, feminization, decreased weight gain
Phenobarbital	Sedation, decreased responsiveness, methemoglobinemia, poor suck reflexes
Phenytoin	Methemoglobinemia
Prednisone	Growth suppression, adrenal suppression
Sulfonamides	Increased risk of kernicterus, allergic manifestations, neonatal jaundice
Tetracycline	Permanent staining of developing teeth
Theophylline	Irritability, fretful sleep: theobromines and caffeine cause a cumulative effect
Tolbutamide	Jaundice, hypoglycemia

From Kacew S: Adverse effects of drugs and chemicals in breast milk on the nursing infant. J Clin Pharmacol 33:213–221, 1993.

son, 1993). Even the reference standards for therapeutic levels still have major limitations. Table 58–3 lists some psychotropic agents for which the *Physicians' Desk Reference* provides indications and dose guidelines.

- As with adults, do not assume that patients are taking the drugs you prescribe or that you are the only one prescribing.
- Before changing a drug or adding a new drug, consider changing the dose of the current medication.
- Consider the possibility of "paradoxical" reactions and other age-related qualitative differences in the actions of psychotropic drugs.

Prescribe a Minimal Number of Drugs—Avoid Polypharmacy

- With any new sign or symptom, review all drugs prescribed or taken as a possible cause.
- Consult literature and/or an expert whenever a patient's response is inadequate or inconsistent with expectations, if an untoward response is obtained, or if you have any doubt regarding the wisest drug or drug dosage.

TABLE 58–3. Commonly Used Psychotropic Medications for Which Specific Indications and Dose Guidelines for Children Exist in *Physicians' Desk Reference*

Drug	Indication	Age
Methylphenidate (RITALIN)	Attention deficit-hyperactivity disorder (ADHD)	≥6 years
α-Amphetamine (DEXEDRINE)	ADHD	≥3 years
Pemoline (CYLERT)	ADHD	≤6 years
Haloperidol (HALDOL)	Tourette's disorder, severe explosive behaviors unresponsive to other treatments	≤3 years
Thioridazine (MELLARIL)	Severe explosive behaviors, short-term management of severe ADHD	≤2 years
Chlorpromazine (THORAZINE)	Severe explosive behaviors, short-term management of severe ADHD	≤6 months
Pimozide (ORAP)	Tourette's disorder	≤12 years
Imipramine (TOFRANIL)	Enuresis	≤6 years
Clomipramine (ANAFRANIL)	Obsessive-compulsive disorder	≤10 years

Commonly Used Psychotropic Medications for Which no Specific Indications for Children Exist ("Not Recommended Below Age 12 Since Safety and Efficacy Have Not Been Proven in This Age Group")

Desipramine (NORPRAMIN)
Nortriptyline (PAMELOR)
Fluoxetine (PROZAC)
Lithium
Thiothixene (NAVENE)
Fluphenazine (PROLIXIN)

From Jensen PS, Vitiello B, Leonard H, Laughren TP: Design and methodology issues for clinical treatment trials in children and adolescents. Psychopharmacol Bull 30:3–8, 1994.

Look for Side Effects

Ensure that patient's responses and side effects are assessed periodically throughout therapy.

Avoid Prescribing for the Wrong Reasons

Avoid prescribing because

You want to try out new medication

You have samples

You, the patient's parents, or the staff want the patient to be given something

"It's the drug to give"

The medication is what the patient has been receiving

Parent/patient/staff/counselor/nurse/family wants you to give a specific drug

It will make you look good

You hope for an impressive solution of a difficult problem

Assess the Possible Physiological and Biochemical Changes That Occur With Age or Developmental Stage

Certain changes that occur with age or development might modify or alter specific drug actions, adverse effects, and time course and termination of drug action. *Note that the changes and implications for therapy are complex functions of the specific drug and drug class, mechanisms of action, and disposition.* The following is an overview of such changes.

• Absorption

Lower and more erratic gastric emptying occurs in the newborn. Absorption after oral administration is affected by many factors, including malnutrition and GI motility alterations. Absorption from intramuscular administration effectively takes place for many drugs in children, with surface exposed and muscle activity playing some role. Absorption from other sources, such as from rectal and percutaneous sites, is not as well studied, but absorption after rectal administration for many drugs is equal to or not as rapid or complete as oral or intramuscular absorption. Time of day of administration may have significant influence on absorption.

• Distribution

Cardiovascular distribution is not specifically altered *per se* with aging. Total body water decreases slightly from 75% of body weight at term to 50–60% as an adult. The extracellular fluid volume decreases from around 40% at birth to 30% at 1 year and 20% in puberty and adulthood. Conversely, intracellular fluid volume increases from around 33% at birth to 40% at puberty.

• Protein Binding

Relative to adult values, plasma protein levels in the child are similar to those in the adult. However, in the neonate total plasma protein, albumin, and globulin are lower. Moreover, the affinity can change; for example, albumin affinity for acidic drugs increases from birth into early infancy. Clinically significant protein binding displacement reactions occur only when the binding is high, *ie,* 80–90%, as can occur with drugs such as diazepam or phenytoin. Bilirubin binding to albumin is a special case of interest in the neonate, because the lower the binding, the greater the potential for the development of kernicterus; a number of analgesics and antinflammatory agents are potent displacers, whereas a number of substances such as benzodiazepines and aminoglycosides are bound at sites different from bilirubin.

• Hepatic Metabolism and Clearance

Liver metabolic pathways mature at different rates; phase I reactions in newborns are generally slow; sulfation matures rapidly after birth, whereas glucoronidation and conjugation pathways require months to years before adult rates are established. For example, glucoronidation of acetaminophen does not reach adult rates until about 12 years of age. Even the kinetics of handling a water load differs markedly with age; the elimination half-life of water at 8 days of age is five times greater than it is for adults.

The first-pass effect in relation to hepatic blood flow has received relatively little research in pediatric populations. Drug-metabolizing systems are generally less active in the newborn but can increase markedly over a few days after birth. For example, the mean plasma half-life for phenytoin decreases from 80 hours at 0–2 days of age to 15 hours at 3–14 days to 6 hours (approximately the adult level) at 14–150 days of age; a similar pattern was observed for phenobarbital. However, the metabolism of other drugs by other pathways and reactions may differ markedly. Some have similar half-lives in adults and in children (*eg,* carbamazepine), whereas others have prolonged half-lives; unfortunately many agents and drug-metabolizing systems have not been adequately investigated.

• Renal Clearance

Glomerular filtration in the newborn is one third of the adult level and reaches nearly adult values by 3 months of age. Maximal tubular excretion capacity in the newborn approximates one half to one fourth the adult value; it reaches adult levels at 1 to 3 years of age.

These generalizations are inadequate because renal drug excretion has not been adequately studied in children; thus, predictions about age effects are difficult. Some of the known clinical implications of these pharmacokinetic differences are illustrated in Table 58–4.

Ensure that Medications Are Taken as Directed

Assess the patient's compliance and adherence. Confusion and behavioral problems compromise compliance with medication and increase the likelihood of adverse drug interactions. For example, patients or parents who are confused may take or administer too many drugs or too much of one drug, or take or administer a drug too often, too little, or erratically. Children are also unlikely to remember or to be able to report all of the drugs administered. Moreover, when you ask patients or their parents about what drugs are being taken, keep in mind that the "usual" pills are frequently not considered "drugs" or "medications" by patients; thus, specific inquiry is essential for OTC vitamins, dietary supplements, cold or hay fever medications, laxatives, antidiarrheals, weight-control diets or pills, or headache medications. All patients and their parents can benefit from education and insightful management of chronically taken medications.

- Try to use a once-a-day or twice-a-day regimen.
- Use a medication calendar or timed dispenser.
- Use drug information summaries.
- Therapy should be supervised by a parent or guardian.
- Label all drug containers clearly.

TABLE 58–4. Drug Disposition in Infants Compared With Adults: Potential Influence of Pharmacokinetics*

Disposition Parameter	Newborn Vs Adult	Possible Pharmacokinetic Result	Example Drug
Absorption	↓	↓AUC	Penicillins, sulfonamides
Volume of distribution	↑	↓Peak	Gentamicin, digoxin
% Protein binding	↓	↑Free fraction	Clindamycin, theophylline
Metabolism	↓	↓Clearance	Chloramphenicol, theophylline
Excretion	↓	↑AUC ↑$t_{½}$	Gentamicin, furosemide

From Brumer JL, Reed MD: Principles of neonatal pharamcology (*In* Yaffe SJ, Aranda JV (eds): Pediatric Pharmacology, 2nd ed, 164–177. Philadelphia: WB Saunders Co, 1992.)

AUC = area under the concentration versus time curve; *t*½ = elimination half-life.

* ↓ = less in newborns than in adults: ↑ = greater in newborns than in adults.

REFERENCES

See also the references for Chapters 50 and 62.

Berlin CM: Advances in pediatric pharmacology and toxicology. Adv Pediatr 40:405-439, 1993.

Bonson KR, Winter JC, Smith CM: Drug-induced psychiatric symptoms. *In* Smith CM, Reynard AL (eds): Textbook of Pharmacology, 380-398. Philadelphia: WB Saunders Co, 1992.

Brumer JL, Reed MD: Principles of neonatal pharmacology. *In* Yaffe SJ, Aranda JV (eds): Pediatric Pharmacology, 2nd ed, 164-177. Philadelphia: WB Saunders Co, 1992.

Bressler R, Katz MD (eds): Geriatric Pharmacology. New York: McGraw-Hill, Inc, 1993.

Calkins E, Ford AB, Katz PR (eds): Practice of Geriatric Medicine, 2nd ed. Philadelphia: WB Saunders Co, 1992.

Cooper JW: Drug-related problems in geriatric nursing home patients. Binghamton, NY: Haworth Press, 1991.

Guven H, Tuncok Y, Guneri S, Cavdar C, Fowler J: Age-related digoxin-alprazolam interaction. Clin Pharmacol Ther 545:42-44, 1994.

Jensen PS, Vitiello B, Leonard H, Laughren TP: Design and methodology issues for clinical treatment trials in children and adolescents. Psychopharmacol Bull 30:3-8, 1994.

Johnson KW, Yaffee SJ, Aranda JV: Neonatal and pediatric drug formulary [Appendix I]. *In* Yaffe SJ, Aranda JV, (eds): Pediatric Pharmacology, 2nd ed. Philadelphia: WB Saunders Co, 1992.

Lanius RA, Pasqualotto BA, Shaw CA: Age-dependent expression, phosphorylation and function of neurotransmitter receptors: pharmacological implications. Trends Pharmaceut Sci 14:403-408, 1993.

MacDonald JB: The role of drugs in falls in the elderly. Clin Geriatr Med 1:621-636, 1985.

Melmon KL, Morrelli HF, Hoffman BB, Nierenberg DW (eds): Clinical Pharmacology—Basic Principles in Therapeutics, 3rd ed. New York: McGraw-Hill, Inc, 1992.

Niems AM, Warner M, Loughnan PM, Aranda JV: Developmental aspects of the hepatic cytochrome P-450 mono-oxygenase system. Annu Rev Pharmacol Toxicol 16:427-445, 1976.

Piepho R, Whelton A, Mayor G, Neu H, Laddu A: Clinical Therapeutic Conference—Case Presentation and Discussion of Geriatric Nephrology. J Clin Pharmacol 32:310-316, 1992.

Reynard AM, Smith CM: Information and learning resources in pharmacology. *In* Smith CM, Reynard AM (eds): Textbook of Pharmacology, 1166-1182. Philadelphia: WB Saunders Co, 1992.

Salzman C: Clinical Geriatric Psychopharmacology, 2nd ed. Baltimore: Williams & Wilkins, 1992.

Snodgrass WR: Drugs in special patient groups: Neonates and children. *In* Melmon KL, Morelli HF, Hoffman BB, Nierenberg DW, (eds): Clinical Pharmacology—Basic Principles in Therapeutics, 3rd ed, 826-850. New York: McGraw-Hill, Inc, 1992.

Tange SM, Grey VL, Senecal PE: Therapeutic drug monitoring in pediatrics: A need for improvement. J Clin Pharmacol 34:200-214, 1994.

Vestal RE, Montamat SC, Nielson CP: Drugs in special groups: The elderly. *In* Melmon KL, Morrelli HF, Hoffman BB, Nierenberg DW (eds): Clinical Pharmacology—Basic Principles in Therapeutics, 3rd ed, 851-874. New York: McGraw-Hill, Inc, 1992.

Yaffe SJ, Aranda JV (eds): Pediatric Pharmacology, 2nd ed. Philadelphia: WB Saunders Co, 1992.

Drug Effects on the Fetus; Pharmacogenetic Principles 59

Luther K. Robinson and Laurie S. Sadler

Prior to the 1960s most congenital anomalies were considered intrinsic abnormalities in a genetically liable fetus. However, in 1961 McBride and Lenz independently recognized that the newly released sedative-hypnotic thalidomide could produce profoundly abnormal limbs in the offspring of women who ingested this drug during pregnancy. Thalidomide was removed from the market later in 1961 but thousands of affected infants were born. Although the drug was never released for general use in the United States, about 3500 women of childbearing age ingested this agent through investigational studies. Of these 624 were pregnant, and 10 affected infants were born (Schardein, 1993). Perhaps equally significant about the thalidomide tragedy was the observation that pregnant women showed few, if any, toxic effects of the drug. The observations of McBride and of Lenz brought to worldwide attention that extrinsic, intrauterine environmental factors could adversely affect fetal development. Such factors have been termed "teratogens" (Gr. *teratos*—"monster", *gen*—"to form") and refer to those agents, whether pharmacological, viral, or physical, or those maternal conditions that, **by acting during pregnancy**, increase the **risks** of structural or functional abnormalities in the fetus above the background 3–5% rate. Teratogenically induced abnormalities account for approximately 3% of congenital anomalies, and recognition and avoidance of these agents is one means of diminishing the incidence of birth defects associated with mental retardation.

Fortunately, not all exposed pregnancies culminate in the birth of an infant with structural defects. The purpose of this chapter is to set forth the principles and variables that affect the risk of teratogenically induced abnormalities, giving examples of each, and to delineate those pharmacological agents that are considered teratogenic in humans (Table 59–1). Neither the teratogenic effects of fetal infection nor physical agents such as hyperthermia or radiation will be examined in this chapter; the interested reader is encouraged to seek information on specific agents in comprehensive texts (Briggs et al, 1986; Shepard, 1989; Schardein, 1993).

PRINCIPLES OF TERATOGENESIS

Five of the important teratological principles that affect the risk of birth defects following fetal exposure are addressed in the following sections.

Susceptibility Depends on Fetal (and Possibly Maternal) Genotypes and the Manner in Which These Respond to Environmental Factors

Just as genetically determined forms (polymorphisms) of enzymes such as hepatic N-acetyl-transferase affect the metabolism of pharmacological agents such as isoniazid, maternal and/or fetal genotypes influence the metabolism of drugs and their potentially teratogenic effects. Some of these variables relate to interspecies differences, whereas others reflect genetic differences within a group, for example, data that show that glucocorticoids are teratogenic in rodents but not in humans (Wilson, 1977). Conversely, thalidomide and cis-retinoic acid, two powerful human teratogens, failed to produce teratogenic effects in many of the rodent models in which they were tested. With respect to intraspecies variation, Strickler and associates (1985) and Buehler and colleagues (1990) showed diminished activity of the genetically determined microsomal enzyme, epoxide hydralase, in human subjects with hydantoin-induced anomalies but not in controls. Unfortunately, few such genetic risk data exist

TABLE 59–1. Pharmacological Agents as Human Teratogens

Pharmacological Agent	Pattern of Malformation
Nonprescription drugs	
Alcohol	Growth/mental retardation Microcephaly Small eyes Craniofacial anomalies
Cocaine	Growth retardation Limb hypoplasia Genitourinary anomalies
Tobacco	Growth retardation
Prescription Drugs	
Androgenic hormones	Virilization
Aminoglycosides	Neurosensory deafness
Aminopterin/methotrexate	Craniofacial hypoplasia Limb hypoplasia
Angiotensin converting enzyme inhibitors	Oligohydramnios? Renal dysplasia?
Carbamazepine	Developmental delays Bifid uvula/cleft palate Hypoplastic fingernails
Lithium	Ebstein anomaly Macrosomia, mild
Penicillamine	Cutis laxa
Phenytoin	Growth/mental retardation Cleft lip/palate Digital hypoplasia
Primidone	Tetecanthus Short nose Cardiac defects
cis-Retinoic acid	Hydrocephalus Craniofacial anomalies Ear anomalies
Tetracycline	Dental staining
Thalidomide	Limb anomalies Ear anomalies
Trimethadione/paramethadione	Growth/mental retardation
Valproic acid	Midface hypoplasia Neural tube defects
Warfarin	Nasal hypoplasia Bony calcifications

for teratogenic effects of other pharmacological agents on humans. (See last section in this chapter.)

Susceptibility Depends on the Developmental Stage at Which an Exposure Occurs

In contrast to the controlled nature of laboratory experiments, exposures in human pregnancy often occur inadvertently over intervals of days or weeks prior to the recognition of pregnancy. In other instances exposures may occur throughout pregnancy. Therefore, teratogenic exposures in humans result in a **clinical spectrum** that ranges from miscarriage, through recognizable patterns of major and/or minor malformations, to normal, to increases in isolated (major) malformations such as cleft palate.

Human pregnancy is most vulnerable in the first and early second trimesters. During these periods the embryo and fetus are growing rapidly, and perturbations of metabolism and/or other insults have the greatest potential for adversely affecting structural development and/or tissue differentiation. Knowledge of the timing of exposure and correlating this with the concurrent developmental processes of the embryo might allow one to predict the risk of specific malformations as delineated below.

- **All-or-none period**—Exposures that occur before implantation of the blastocyst (about 9 days after conception) result in an "all-or-none" phenomenon. In cases of the former, an exposure results in such severe damage to the developing cell mass that the pregnancy culminates in miscarriage. With respect to the latter, exposure to pluripotential cells in early development allows for complete recovery with no increased risk of defects above the normal 3–5% risk observed in all human pregnancy. In either case, the risk of congenital malformations after exposures before implantation is not increased in the pregnancy carried to term.
- **Embryonic period**—The embryonic period begins with the formation of the primitive streak (about 15 days after conception) and ends at 9–10 weeks, after formation of the external genitalia. During this time arrests of morphogenesis result in major malformations such as cleft lip/palate. For example, one might speculate that a teratogenic exposure that occurs between 21 and 28 days' gestation, the time at which the neural tube closes, might increase the risk of a defect such as myelomeningocele. Similarly, an exposure at or prior to lip closure (35 days' gestation) might cause an increase in the risk of a cleft of the lip, with or without a cleft of the palate. The time at which an agent exerts the greatest potential for embryonic damage is termed the "critical period." In the case of thalidomide the human embryo was observed to be most vulnerable at 20–35 days after conception. It must be emphasized that exposures during critical periods **do not necessarily induce malformations**. Rather, the risk of a malformation may be increased such that techniques such as high-resolution ultrasound examination of the fetus may prove useful in the perinatal management regimen.
- **Fetal period**—The fetal period begins at 9–10 weeks after conception and signals a period of growth and differentiation. Teratogenic exposures during this period do not increase the risk of major malformations such as spina bifida, but rather increase the risks of alterations of growth or function. The clinical evidence of such may be found in minor malformations such as alterations of the palmar or digital flexion creases (Popich and Smith, 1970) or the location of the posterior parietal hair whorl (Smith and Gong, 1974). Nail hypoplasia and altered dermatoglyphic patterning observed in the fetal hydantoin syndrome are engendered at or prior to 18 weeks, the time at which the developing digital fat pads exert mechanical stretch on the overlying skin (fetal fingertips).

Exposures that occur later in pregnancy (*eg*, in the third trimester), while not causing malformation, may adversely affect fetal growth or function. For example, heavy alcohol use (Jones et al, 1973) and heavy maternal cigarette smoking (US Dept of HHS, 1989) impair fetal growth. On the other hand, fetal lithium exposure is associated with enhanced growth (Jacobson et al, 1992). Maternal hyperglycemia such as that observed in gestational diabetes may lead to fetal hyperglycemia and secondary hyperinsulinemia. The latter conditions contribute to structural problems such as macrosomia and asymmetrical cardiac septal hypertrophy and to such functional problems as neonatal hypoglycemia and deficient or delayed synthesis of pulmonary surfactant. Other examples of fetopathic effects of pharmacological agents include cocaine, which appears to cause vascular disruption of previously normal structure (Hoyme et al, 1990). Functional problems appear to reflect the fetal metabolism of the drug and include tachycardia and fetal hyperactivity. Withdrawal symptoms in the newborn period are a tragic example of fetal exposure. For example, fetal exposures to β-adrenergic antagonists such as propranolol or nadolol, while not causing structural defects, may increase the risk of bradycardia, hypotension, and hypothermia in the immediate newborn period (Rubin, 1982; Fox et al, 1985).

Teratogens Act in Specific Ways (Through Specific Mechanisms) on Developing Tissues to Alter Form and Function

Teratogens do not cause nonspecific increases in rates of congenital malformations (*eg,* Down syndrome, limb defects, other nonspecific "adverse outcomes of pregnancy"). Rather, such agents produce adverse fetal effects through their respective metabolic pathways or pharmacological mechanisms of action. Thus, the structural and behavioral manifestations of the fetal alcohol syndrome (microcephaly, central nervous system heteropias, mental retardation, small eyes, thin upper lip) are believed to reflect the toxic effects of alcohol or its byproducts on developing neural crest cells (Jones, 1974; Clarren et al, 1978; Sulik et al, 1981). On the other hand, the craniofacial defects that characterize the retinoic acid embryopathy are believed to reflect disturbances of homeogene expression or neural crest cell retinoid receptor interactions (Newell-Morris et al, 1980; Yip et al, 1980; Lammer et al, 1985, Murphy and Hill, 1991; Chisaka et al, 1992). As noted previously, the structural defects observed after fetal cocaine exposure are disruptive in nature, reflecting the vasoactive effects of this agent.

Susceptibility Depends on Dose

For obvious moral and ethical reasons no dose-response curve has been generated for any known or suspected human teratogen. Data from teratological experiments in other organisms, however, suggest that dose-response curves do in fact exist, with manifestations ranging from a no-effect level to that of malformation and/or fetal death. In the clinical arena the greatest risk of birth defects is posed to the offspring of women with the most severe exposure. In the case of alcohol, the rate of abnormality is greatest among the offspring of women who drink heavily throughout pregnancy (44%, Jones et al, 1973) in contrast to those who drink more moderately (11%, Hanson et al, 1978). It is important to recognize further that no dose-response curve for alcohol exists below which a fetal effect is not observed. Therefore, women who contemplate becoming pregnant should abstain from drinking alcohol before conception or when pregnancy is recognized.

Teratogens Cause a *Spectrum of Abnormalities* Ranging from Lethality (Pregnancy Loss) to Malformation, Growth Retardation, and Functional Disorder

As implied in principles 2 and 3 above, embryonic and fetal responses after exposure are variable. Therefore, one should expect to observe a variety of phenotypic effects following teratogenic exposure rather than observing specific, easily identified major malformations. For example, the outcomes of pregnancy complicated by poorly controlled maternal diabetes range from infertility to an increased rate of miscarriage to major malformations such as sacral agenesis to altered growth (macrosomia) and such functional problems as neonatal hypoglycemia and surfactant deficiency. Similarly, the clinical spectrum of fetal alcohol exposure ranges from impaired fertility and miscarriage to the full-blown fetal alcohol syndrome (FAS) and an increased rate of mental deficiency, even among those who are phenotypically normal.

RECOGNIZING SUSPECTED TERATOGENS

That the number of known human teratogens is small suggests that more research is needed in this area. Little is known about the mechanisms of action of known agents or the genetic variables that determine liability to their potentially teratogenic effects. Moreover, many agents appear not to alter structure so much as fetal or neonatal function. For example, data are emerging that angiotensin converting enzyme (ACE) inhibitors increase the risks of fetal renal dysfunction with resultant risks of oligohydramnios, pulmonary hypoplasia, intrauterine growth retardation and fetal/neonatal death (Pryde et al, 1993).

Unfortunately, no human teratogen has been **prospectively** identified by laboratory studies in lower organisms or by epidemiological methods. Most have been recognized by astute clinicians using their powers of observation. There are several reasons for this. As was noted previously, genetic differences between humans and laboratory animals are significant enough that metabolic or enzymatic pathways in one organism may not be present in another. It also is important to recognize that the organism with which humans have the greatest genetic similarity is the nonhuman primate. However, teratological experiments involving such organisms are relatively expensive and lengthy, owing to the long gestations and limited numbers of offspring produced. One should recognize further that the questions asked by the teratologist often are different from those of the clinician. Examples of the former include such problems as understanding mechanisms of dysmorphogenesis or fetal dose-response. These questions involve administering pharmacological doses of drugs that may exceed those experienced in the clinical situation. In contrast, the clinician is concerned with minimizing fetal exposure while maximizing maternal benefit.

Epidemiological studies may be adversely affected by recall bias or retrospective ascertainment such that conclusions derived therefrom may not identify a teratogenic agent or allow for a practical fetal risk assessment. For example, Safra and Oakley (1975), in a retrospective analysis of diazepam, showed a fourfold increase in the risk of facial clefts. However, this increased risk rose from 1 case per 1000 to 4 cases per 1000, relatively low risks for a surgically correctable defect.

BOX 59-1

One means of collecting and evaluating data on exposures in human pregnancy is by registry (Chernoff et al, 1985). Prospective ascertainment and follow-up with blinded examination of exposed and "control" subjects minimizes the shortcomings of the methods listed above. The registry method allows for accurate timing of exposure and a better delineation of fetal risk. Using this methodology Jones and colleagues (1989) identified the teratogenic effects of carbamazepine. Collaborations among registries such as the Organization of Teratology Information Services (OTIS, USA) or the European Teratology Information Service (ENTIS) enhance the data collecting capabilities of individual investigators and have allowed for the reevaluation of the teratogenic effects of lithium (Jacobson et al, 1992). Such collaborations also permit the ascertainment of cadres of exposed infants for future evaluations of cognitive performance.

CONCLUSION

As emphasized throughout this chapter, fetal exposures to drugs increase the **risk** of abnormality, the spectrum of which ranges from impaired fertility to malformation to normal. Research efforts at both the clinical and laboratory levels provide promise for recognizing previously unknown teratogens and for delineating the developmental and/or pharmacological mechanisms through which these agents act.

PHARMACOGENETICS

Pharmacogenetics is the study of the genetically based variability in the actions of drugs, the receptor systems with which they interact, and the biotransformations (metabolism) that they undergo. The variability among individuals and various groups frequently can account for both qualitative and quantitative differences in drug action. Some causes of this variability (*ie*, polymorphisms) identified to date are common and affect large populations; others are rare, and many others have yet to receive systematic investigation. Needless to say, this is a fast-moving research area with wide applications and implications for therapy, toxicity, and prevention. A recent book reviews in detail major portions of this research (Price Evans, 1993). Among the major concerns in therapeutics are:

- The wide individual differences in the rates of metabolism of many drugs can be attributed to polymorphisms in the metabolizing enzymes involved in both Phase I cytochrome P-450 systems and in Phase II conjugations. The Phase II N-acetyltransferase polymorphisms have been especially well studied.
- The clinical consequences of such polymorphisms will be dependent on the activities and effects of both the parent compound and the metabolite(s), as well as the possible interactions with differences in excretion functions (for example, age-related decreases in renal function). Some drugs exist as "pro-drugs" with active metabolite(s), whereas the activity of other drugs is terminated by biotransformations. Thus, some metabolites may have desirable pharmacological effects; for example, among the opioids is the morphine metabolite of codeine. By contrast, the metabolite may produce greater or different toxic effects, such as the normeperidine metabolite of meperidine.
- The potential clinical consequences of the large number of metabolic polymorphisms are only just beginning to become established and their implications understood. These genetically based individual differences clearly involve a number of genes with a complex interplay with environmental and hereditary factors. Among the many currently used drugs with proven clinical consequences of polymorphisms in their metabolism (with poor metabolizers, rapid metabolizers, and complex differences in metabolic products and their interactions) are: codeine, meperidine and its drug interactions, dextromethorphan, succinylcholine, ethanol, phenothiazines, haloperidol, tricyclic antidepressants, propranolol, antiarrhythmics encainide and flecainide, phenformin, chlorpropamide, quinidine, smoking/nicotine, erythromycin, cimetidine, theophylline, isoniazid, caffeine, procainamide, phenelzine, hydralazine, halothane, carbamazepine, glucocorticoids, chloramphenicol, lithium, chloroquine, dicumarol; others most certainly exist.
- Genetic polymorphisms also exist in receptor systems and drug response mechanisms.
- Genetic polymorphisms in metabolism are critically important as determinants in the interethnic differences in drug action and drug metabolism (for example, ethanol), the consequence of exposure to potential carcinogens, and as possible etiologies of some common disorders, such as drug-induced parkinsonism, agranulocytosis, drug-induced liver damage or lupus syndrome, to mention just a few.
- One of the practical corollaries of the knowledge of pharmacogenetic differences is that genetic differences should be considered in each of the following situations: whenever prescribing a new drug; when failure to obtain the expected drug effect occurs; and when the patient manifests an untoward or unexpected condition.

The appropriate initial response to such situations would be to consult an up-to-date database on drug side effects and potential interactions for the specific drug, the drug class, and the possible drug effect (Chapter 62), as well as a comprehensive reference source such as Price Evans (1993).

REFERENCES

Briggs GG, Freeman RK, Yaffe SJ: Drugs in Pregnancy and Lactation. A Reference Guide to Fetal and Neonatal Risk, 3rd edition. Baltimore: Williams and Wilkins, 1993.

Buehler BA, Delimont D, van Waes M, et al: Prenatal prediction of risk of the fetal hydantoin syndrome. N Engl J Med 322:1567, 1990.

Chernoff GF, Jones KL, Kelley CD: The California Teratogen Registry: Five and one-half years of operational experience. J Perinatol VI:44, 1985.

Chisaka O, Musci TS, Cappechi MR: Developmental defects of the ear, cranial nerves, and hindbrain resulting from targeted disruption of the mouse homeobox gene *Hox 1.6*. Nature 355:516, 1992.

Clarren SK, Alvord Jr EC, Sumi SM, et al: Brain malformations related to prenatal exposure to ethanol. J Pediatr 92:64, 1978.

Fox RE, Marx C, Stark AR: Neonatal effects of maternal nadolol therapy. Am J Obstet Gynecol 152:1045, 1985.

Hanson JW, Streissguth AP, Smith DW: The effects of moderate alcohol consumption during pregnancy on fetal growth and morphogenesis. J Pediatr 92:457, 1978.

Hoyme HE, Jones KL, Dixon SD, et al: Prenatal cocaine exposure and fetal vascular disruption. Pediatrics 85:743, 1990.

Jacobson SJ, Jones KL, Johnson K, et al: Prospective multi-centre study of pregnancy outcome after lithium exposure during first trimester. Lancet 1992;339:530–533.

Jones KL, Smith DW, Ulleland CN, et al: Pattern of malformation in offspring of chronic alcoholic mothers. Lancet 1:1267, 1973.

Jones KL: Aberrant neuronal migration in fetal alcohol syndrome. Birth Defects 11:131, 1974.

Jones KL, Lacro RV, Johnson KA, Adams J: Pattern of malformations in the children of women treated with carbamazepine during pregnancy. N Engl J Med 320:1661, 1989.

Jones KL, Lacro RV, Johnson KA, Adams J: Pattern of malformations in the children of women treated with carbamazepine during pregnancy. N Engl J Med 320:1661–1666, 1989.

Lammer EJ, Chen DT, Hoar RM, et al: Retinoic acid embryopathy. N Engl J Med 313:837, 1985.

Lenz W: Kindliche Missbildungen nach Medikament-Einnahme wahrend der Graviditat? Dtsch Med Wochenschr 86:2555, 1961.

McBride WG: Thalidomide and congenital abnormalities. Lancet 2:1358, 1961.

Murphy P, Hill RE: Expression of mouse *labial*-like homeobox-containing genes, *Hox 2.9* and *Hox 1.6* during segmentation of the hindbrain. Development 111:61, 1991.

Newell-Morris L, Sirianni JE, Shepard TH, et al: Teratogenic effects of retinoic acid in pigtail monkeys (Macaca nemistrina). II. Craniofacial features. Teratology 21:87, 1980.

Popich GA, Smith DW: The genesis and significance of digital and palmar hand creases: Preliminary report. J Pediatr 77:1017, 1970.

Price Evans DAP: Genetic Factors in Drug Therapy: Clinical and Molecular Pharmacogenetics. Cambridge: Cambridge University Press, 1993.

Pryde PG, Sedman AB, Nugent CE, Barr M Jr: Angiotensin converting enzyme inhibitor fetopathy. J Am Soc Nephrol 3:1575, 1993.

Rosa FW: Spina bifida in infants of women treated with carbamazepine during pregnancy. N Engl J Med 324:674, 1991.

Rubin PC: Beta blockers in pregnancy. N Engl J Med 305:1323, 1982.

Safra MJ, Oakley JP: Association between cleft lip with or without cleft palate and prenatal exposure to diazepam. Lancet 2:478–480, 1975.

Schardein JL: Chemically Induced Birth Defects, 2nd ed. New York: Marcel Dekker, 1993.

Seaver L, Hoyme HE: Teratology in pediatric practice. Pediatr Clin North Am 39:111, 1991.

Shepard TH: A Catalog of Teratogenic Agents, 6th ed. Baltimore: Johns Hopkins University Press, 1989.

Smith DW, Gong BT: Scalp-hair patterning: Its origin and significance relative to early brain and upper facial development. Teratology 9:17, 1974.

Strickler SM, Dansky LV, Miller MA, Seni M-H, et al: Genetic predisposition to phenytoin-induced birth defects. Lancet 2:746, 1985.

Sulik KK, Johnston MC, Webb MA: Fetal alcohol syndrome: embryogenesis in a mouse model. Science 214:936, 1981.

US Department of Health and Human Services: Reducing the Health Consequences of Smoking: 25 Years of Progress: A Report of the Surgeon General. Rockville, MD: Office on Smoking and Health, Centers for Disease Control, Public Health Service, 1989. US Department of Health and Human Services publication CDC 89-8411.

Wilson JG and Fraser FC: General Principles and Etiology, Handbook of Teratology, Vol 1, 49–62. New York and London: Plenum Press, 1979.

Yip JE, Kokich VG, Shepard TH: The effect of high doses of retinoic acid on prenatal craniofacial development in Macaca nemestrina. Teratology 21:29, 1980.

Thompson MW, McInnes RR, Willard HF (eds): Genetics in Medicine, 5th ed, 392–394. Philadelphia: WB Saunders Co, 1991.

PART XII

PRACTICAL ASPECTS OF DRUG DEVELOPMENT AND PRESCRIBING

60 Drug Development and the Regulatory Process

William Kennedy

INITIAL TESTING

REGULATION

SAFETY AND EFFICACY

DOSAGE FORM

TIME REQUIREMENTS

A critical aspect of pharmacology is the availability of compounds, whether these are compounds for research in animal laboratories or drugs for the treatment of patients in the clinics. These compounds come from a very complex and expensive drug research and development process. Since 1975, the majority of the new drugs that have become available to patients have been the product of innovation in the pharmaceutical industry. It is therefore important to understand the drug development process.

Several studies have attempted to define the time and cost required to bring a new chemical entity from the laboratory bench to the patient. No single figure exists upon which industry, academia, and government can agree. It is sufficient to say that drug development is a long (> 7 years) and expensive (> $200 million) process.

No single document, no matter how large, can address all of the complexities of the drug development process. What follows is necessarily a very superficial treatment of this process.

INITIAL TESTING

All drug research must start with the collaboration of chemists and pharmacologists. They collaborate to explore opportunities in specified therapeutic areas. As the pharmacologists test the compounds, they suggest refinements in the activity, which the chemists translate into refinements in the molecule. Computer modeling is becoming an increasingly valuable tool. When the desired pharmacological property is achieved, the team is expanded to include a toxicologist who studies the drug in some preliminary measure of toxicology.

Once evidence is found that the compound has the desired pharmacologic effect and lacks any measurable toxic effect in animals, it can be formally considered for development as a drug. With this decision, the team that is dedicated to researching and developing the compound and the activities that take place becomes greatly expanded. Additional pharmacological studies are conducted to more fully understand all of the drug's properties and to predict the activity that it will have in humans. Formal toxicological studies that will satisfy the most rigorous regulatory agencies begin. Animal pharmacokinetic studies also begin at this time to further define the parameters of the drug's properties.

It should be apparent that to perform these activities, more of the drug must be manufactured. The original compound for early studies would have been easily supplied by bench-top synthesis. The demand for an increase in the production of the drug places demands on the synthetic chemists to refine the process to produce larger quantities in a reasonable time and at a reasonable cost.

DOSAGE FORM

The drug development team must also begin addressing the dosage form of the drug that will be used in the remaining animal studies, the clinical development studies, and, eventually, the dosage form that will be made available to patients. Dosage form selection involves many disciplines, with heavy emphasis on the clinician's determination of the best practice of medicine. This is generally very specific to the drug class; for example, most would agree that an oral tablet is not the best dosage form for an antiemetic.

REGULATION

Each country has very specific data requirements that must be fulfilled before it will authorize the investigation of a new drug in humans. These requirements generally include the performance of basic pharmacological and toxicological studies; the latter include single-dose and multiple-dose studies in several species of animals that are predictive of the human response.

A requirement also exists to provide evidence that the new drug that will be administered to humans for the first time has been synthesized and manufactured in a reproducible manner.

TIME REQUIREMENTS

It is very difficult to provide accurate estimates of the amount of time needed to develop a drug. It should be obvious that time needed is dependent upon the number of times that a compound is recycled for refinement of activities by having its structure modified. It is generally agreed that from the point at which the basic pharmacology and toxicology have been established to the time that an initial dose is given to humans takes from 12 to 15 months.

Beginning with the initial introduction of a drug to humans, a very intense and regulated process begins. Using the United States as an example, a typical development program can be described. The initial protocol to study the safety of single doses of a drug in humans must be reviewed by professional medical staff at the Food and Drug Administration (FDA) before the protocol can be initiated. Following the initial study, multiple-dose studies take place. At the same time, additional animal toxicological and animal pharmacological studies are undertaken to expand the knowledge about the drug. The human safety studies constitute Phase I, and exploratory efficacy, safety, and dosage range studies compose Phase II. It is usually at the end of Phase II that the pharmaceutical company must determine whether the drug will continue in development or be dropped; the latter would occur either because of a lack of efficacy or because of toxicity issues. Phase I can involve up to 100 healthy human subjects and can take anywhere from several months to a year to complete. Phase II usually involves several hundred patients and can take up to 2 years to complete. The number of patients and the duration of dosing in Phase I and Phase II are dependent upon the drug and the disease.

Historically, of all drugs that enter into Phase I, only one of three continues to be developed beyond Phase II.

SAFETY AND EFFICACY

Phase III studies are conducted to demonstrate the pivotal safety and effectiveness data for a drug and are used to clearly establish the dosing regimen that will be recommended in clinical practice. Generally, several thousand patients are enrolled in exquisitely detailed, well-controlled studies involving up to 100 investigators from around the world. Investigators are generally world-recognized experts in the field of study. This phase of development can take from 2 to more than 4 years to complete. During the latter part of Phase III, additional studies are initiated that can involve several thousand more patients. These studies are designed to gather additional data, primarily regarding the safety of the drug.

At the completion of the Phase III studies, the data are assembled in a very structured format and presented to the FDA or to an equivalent foreign national health authority with a request for approval to market the drug. The review and approval process can take from 6 months to several years.

61 Legal Aspects of Drug Prescribing

Robert M. Cooper

This chapter is designed to provide the reader with a basic understanding of the legal aspects of drug prescribing. Because of the distribution of this text, this chapter deals primarily with federal law. The reader must keep in mind, however, that state law may at one extreme be stricter than federal law, and at the other, not even deal with a particular issue. Throughout the chapter, reference is made to examples of state requirements. *Remember that stricter law always applies and that practitioners need to know the law in the state in which they practice.*

CLASSIFICATION OF DRUGS

The 1951 Durham-Humphrey Amendment to the Federal Food, Drug and Cosmetic Act established two major drug classifications:

1. Drugs sold only by prescription, known as *legend* or prescription drugs
2. Drugs sold without prescription, otherwise known as nonlegend or over-the-counter (OTC) drugs

Prescription drugs may also be defined as hypnotic or habit-forming drugs; drugs not safe for self-medication; and drugs classified as "new drugs." They require the use of the Rx legend, "CAUTION: Federal Law Prohibits Dispensing Without Prescription" on the manufacturer's label. Hence the term *legend drug.* The legend status of a drug is determined by the United States Food and Drug Administration (FDA).

OTC drugs are those that the FDA has approved for specific uses and in specific dosage and determined to be safe for a layperson to use in self-medication. The drug must bear adequate directions for safe and effective use and provide warnings against misuse by the layperson.

WHO MAY LEGALLY PRESCRIBE?

It is up to the states to determine who may legally issue a prescription. States have indicated clearly that a licensed physician, dentist, and veterinarian may prescribe. Others also may be able to do so with full or qualified privileges (*eg,* no controlled substance prescriptions, special training, and so forth), including podiatrists, physician's assistants, and nurse practitioners. Throughout this chapter, the term *practitioner* is used to denote the persons authorized by a state to prescribe. Consult state law to determine who can prescribe and what qualifications might apply in your state.

When a practitioner is licensed by a state, it is done with regard to the areas of the practitioner's specific training and practice set forth in the States Practice Act. For example, a veterinarian cannot practice on humans. In addition, a practitioner may prescribe only in the specific area of licensure. For example, a podiatrist may only write prescriptions for drugs used in the treatment of problems associated with the human foot.

Whereas a practitioner may be licensed to practice and write prescriptions in a state, to prescribe controlled substances (narcotic, stimulant, depressant, and hallucinogenic substances), the practitioner must register and obtain a Federal Drug Enforcement Administration (DEA) registration number as well. The procedure is discussed later in this chapter.

PRESCRIPTION BLANKS

Although some states may require that a prescription blank be presented graphically in a certain way or that various statements be printed on the blank, usually in conjunction with state drug product selection laws, federal law does not require a particular form for the prescription. Some states do require special blanks (duplicate or triplicate prescription blanks) for some or all controlled substances.

Practitioners should use one prescription pad at a time and keep blanks in a safe place to reduce the possibility of the blanks being stolen. Blanks should be used only for writing prescription orders. Never sign prescription blanks in advance. Prior to printing blanks, consult state laws and consider practical considerations such as size of the blank, amount of space provided to clearly indicate the drug and amount prescribed, placement of refill instructions, and so forth.

WRITTEN PRESCRIPTIONS

The information that must be indicated by the prescriber on a written prescription depends on whether the drug prescribed is classified as a controlled or a noncontrolled prescription drug. Controlled drug status is established by federal and state law. Prescription regulations pertaining to controlled substances are stricter.

Although federal law does not clearly and unambiguously spell out what information must be written on a prescription for a noncontrolled prescription drug, labeling requirements identify the following information that should appear:

- *Name* of the *patient*
- *Date* prescription written
- *Name* of the *drug*
- *Strength* of drug, if applicable
- *Quantity* to be dispensed
- *Directions* for use
- *Prescriber's name*
- *Prescriber's signature*

Often state laws require additional information for a written prescription, including the patient's address and age and the prescriber's address, telephone number, profession, and so forth.

In addition, many states require that the pharmacist label the prescription "as to content" (*eg*, tetracycline hydrochloride, 250 mg) unless the practitioner indicates otherwise somewhere or in some way on the prescription. The procedure may be as simple as checking a box or may require the prescribers to indicate such in their own handwriting. Federal law does not require the automatic labeling of a prescription "as to content."

In the case of prescriptions for controlled drugs, federal law requires the practitioner to indicate the following information:

- *Name* of the *patient*
- *Address* of the *patient*
- *Date* prescription signed by practitioner
- *Name* of the *drug*
- *Strength* of drug, if applicable
- *Quantity* to be dispensed
- *Directions* for use
- *Name* of the *prescriber*
- *Prescriber's address*
- *DEA registration number* of the prescriber
- *Signature* of the *prescriber*

Furthermore, states may require the patient's age and sex, the practitioner's telephone number, specific directions for use, designation of the practitioner's profession, and instructions for labeling "as to content."

Prescribers must write prescriptions in ink or indelible pencil or they may be typewritten. Written prescriptions must be signed by the prescriber. A stamped signature is not valid. Federal law indicates that erasable pens may not be used to write and sign prescriptions for controlled substances. Because the ink in such pens does not become permanent for 3 days, prescription information could be altered without detection.

In some states, practitioners may write only one prescription per blank. Preprinted prescription blanks may be illegal also. A preprinted blank is one that has the name, strength, amount and directions for use of a drug, or some combination of same, preprinted on the blank.

Federal law allows a nurse or secretary to prepare prescription orders (including those for controlled substances) for the signature of the practitioner. The prescriber is responsible for making sure that the prescription conforms in all essential respects to the law and regulations. State law may not allow such a practice. Practitioners also should be aware that the pharmacist has an equal responsibility with the practitioner to make sure that the prescription meets all legal requirements.

When writing a prescription, practitioners should be sure to write clearly, avoid writing for a larger quantity of a drug than is necessary, provide for specific and clear directions for use, and meet all legal requirements.

ORAL PRESCRIPTIONS

The Durham-Humphrey Amendment to the Federal Food, Drug and Cosmetic Act established the legality of filling an oral order to dispense medication. Federal law provides that oral orders must be reduced promptly to writing and filed by the pharmacist. Oral prescriptions must indicate the same information described in the discussion under written prescriptions, except for the practitioner's signature.

However, not all drugs may be prescribed by giving an oral order. Certain controlled substances may be dispensed only pursuant to a written prescription. Exceptions may be made in some cases for an emergency situation, as discussed later. Requirements for controlled drugs vary from state to state.

ORAL AUTHORIZATION OF REFILLS

Federal law allows pharmacists to take oral authorization for refills for noncontrolled drugs and for some controlled substances, as noted later. The Durham-Humphrey Amendment specifies that refill instructions may be entered by the pharmacist on the oral instruction of the practitioner or a legally authorized representative.

A legally authorized representative may be an employee or agent of the practitioner, most likely a nurse or secretary. A patient is not recognized as an authorized representative. Because the practitioner may not delegate authority to make decisions to someone else, the agent may only *communicate* or transmit the prescriber's decision or instruction to the pharmacist. Agents may not issue prescriptions or authorize refills. Again, note that state law may not allow such a procedure.

Federal law also allows for the oral authorization of refills for Schedule III and IV controlled substance prescriptions. Refer to the section on controlled substances for details.

EXPIRATION OF PRESCRIPTIONS

Federal law does not establish any legal time by which a patient must have a prescription filled after having been written by a practitioner. Some states have established time limits, particularly for controlled drugs. New York, for example, only allows a controlled substance prescription to be filled by the pharmacist within 30 days of the date the prescription was written by the practitioner.

Although noncontrolled prescriptions do not have to be filled within any particular time limit, patients should present prescriptions within a reasonable period of time. The pharmacist should question and the practitioner should be concerned about patients presenting prescriptions written some time prior to the presentation. Pharmacists should consult with the practitioner in such cases. Of course, a good reason for such a prescription may exist, such as a chronic condition, being away from home, or the nature of the drug.

Prescriptions for controlled substances authorizing refills must be refilled within a specified period of time, which is discussed under Refill Instructions.

REFILL INSTRUCTIONS

The Durham-Humphrey Amendment legalized the refilling of written and oral prescriptions as long as the refilling was authorized by the prescriber, either in the original prescription or by oral order.

In the case of a written prescription, it is the practitioner's responsibility to indicate clearly whether or not the prescription is to be refilled. The best and clearest method is to indicate a specific number of times a prescription may be refilled. Most prescription blanks are printed with a space for the practitioner to indicate the number of refills. It can be as simple as

refill: ______ times,

or a series of numbers that can be circled, such as

refill: 0 1 2 3 4 5 times.

If no refills are to be allowed, the practitioner should indicate "none," "zero," or "0" in the refill space. The absence of any refill instruction on the prescription means that no refills are allowed.

Again, if refills are to be allowed, a specific number is desirable. However, some practitioners use the designation "prn" (*pro re nata*), which means to refill "as needed" or "as necessary." Over the years, the FDA has discouraged the use of the term prn, indicating that the physician cannot delegate his or her authority to someone else. In other words, it is not up to the pharmacist to decide the number of times the prescription should be refilled. In *The Rx Legend*, the FDA recommends that a pharmacist receiving a prn prescription

1. Use care and professional judgment in handling it
2. Refill it only with a frequency consistent with the directions for use
3. Check with the practitioner after a reasonable time to make sure that the medication is to be continued

Pharmacists are encouraged also to urge the prescriber to indicate the number of refills on the prescription.

Whereas the federal law reluctantly allows the practitioner to use prn, states may not allow the use of prn to indicate refills, claiming that it is not a specific instruction. At least one state indicates that using prn means that the prescription can be refilled only once.

A variation, prn with some time limit (*eg*, prn — 1 year), may be seen. In this case a limit to the number of refills exists. "Prn — 1 year" would mean refill this prescription for 1 year from the date of writing consistent with the directions for use. Controlled substance regulations do not allow the use of prn or any variation.

Lastly, instructions such as "refill for lifetime" are clearly unreasonable. Federal law limits the number of refills for Schedule III and IV controlled drugs to five times or 6 months, whichever comes first.

A question often asked is whether a prescription may be refilled if the practitioner who wrote the prescription dies. The FDA has stated that once a physician-patient relationship is broken, the prescription is no longer valid, because the physician is no longer available to that patient to oversee his or her use of the prescribed medication.

It is highly desirable for the practitioner to maintain an on-going tabular and graphic record for all medications prescribed or ordered, such as one of the computer-based medical record systems described in Chapter 62. Accurate records are especially needed when refills are prescribed.

PRESCRIPTION LABELING

Specific legal requirements affecting the labeling of prescription drugs have been established by the Federal Food, Drug and Cosmetic Act, the Federal Controlled Substances Act, and various state acts. Requirements are discussed for noncontrolled and controlled drugs.

For noncontrolled drugs, federal law requires that the pharmacist indicate the following information on a prescription label:

- *Name* and *address* of the pharmacy
- *Prescription number*
- *Name* of the *patient* (if stated in the prescription)
- *Name* of the *practitioner*
- *Date* the prescription was filled or refilled
- *Directions* for use
- *Caution/warning* statements

In addition, states may require such information as the patient's name and address; labeling "as to content;" the dispensing pharmacist's name or initials; lot numbers; expiration dates; the name of the drug manufacturer/distributor; and the telephone number of the pharmacy.

Federal law requires the following information on a controlled substance prescription label:

- *Name* and *address* of the pharmacy
- *Prescription number*
- *Name* of the *patient*
- *Name* of the prescribing *practitioner*
- *Date* the prescription was filled or refilled
- *Direction* for use
- *Caution/warning* statements
- *Federal warning* statement for Schedules I–IV controlled substances, which reads: "Caution: Federal law prohibits the transfer of this drug to any person other than the patient for whom it was prescribed"

In addition, states may require the items listed under noncontrolled prescription labeling as well as additional legends, the practitioner's DEA number, and the pharmacy's DEA number. Some states may require the label to be of a specific color. For example, New York requires an orange controlled substance label.

Practitioners dispensing medication to patients may be subject to any or all of the labeling requirements mentioned. Consult your state law.

DRUG PRODUCT SELECTION LAWS

Most states have enacted legislation that, under a specific set of circumstances, allows the pharmacist to substitute a different brand or a generic drug product for the drug product prescribed by the practitioner on the prescription.

The substitution must be authorized by the practitioner. Various mechanisms are employed by states to indicate authorization, including a designated signature line(s) or box that must be checked or the use of a specific statement or abbreviation.

The substituted drug must be of the same chemical entity and dosage form as the drug prescribed. Many states have established a formulary system to help professionals in the selection process. Some may be of the positive type, indicating drugs that may be substituted, whereas others are of the negative type, indicating drugs that may not be substituted. Consult your state law.

COPIES OF PRESCRIPTIONS

In general, a patient has a right to get a copy of a prescription from a pharmacy. However, some states may limit the patient's possession to noncontrolled prescriptions. In such a case, the patient may request that a copy of a controlled drug prescription be sent to the patient's practitioner.

Copies have no legal status as valid prescriptions; they cannot be filled or refilled. They are a source of information only and must be so worded. Some states require the pharmacist to indicate a specific statement, such as "COPY—FOR INFORMATION ONLY," on the copy of the prescription or to indicate "COPY" or a specified statement in a color (red for example). Other states do not require a specific statement.

The FDA has indicated that copies are not valid prescriptions because there is no assurance:

1. That it is an accurate or valid prescription
2. That other copies have not been delivered to other pharmacies
3. That the original prescription will not be recognized for the remaining refills

Pharmacists receiving such prescriptions must call the practitioner for authorization to refill (fill) the prescription.

Federal regulations allow for the transfer of original prescription information between pharmacies for the dispensing of refills or controlled substances in Schedules III, IV, and V. State law may not allow for such a procedure.

OUT-OF-STATE PRESCRIPTIONS

Practitioners may legally write prescriptions only in the states in which they are licensed to practice. In any other state that practitioner is considered a layperson. A practitioner who is a federal employee must be licensed in at least one state to have prescription-writing authority in any federal facility.

Can a pharmacist fill a prescription written by a practitioner licensed in another state? The answer depends on state law. Some do not address the problem. Others indicate a limited filling of such prescriptions, allowing them to be filled by practitioners of neighboring states or border communities. Some limit the filling to noncontrolled drugs.

The FDA has indicated that no federal requirement exists that a prescriber be licensed in the state where the prescription is filled, provided the prescription was valid where written. Consult your state law for particulars.

SAFETY PACKAGING

The Poison Prevention Packaging Act of 1970 was enacted to provide special packaging to protect children from serious personal injury and illness from ingesting, handling, or using household substances. The Act is administered by the Federal Consumer Product Safety Commission (CPSC).

Products covered by the Act include human prescription drugs in oral dosage forms, all controlled drugs (whether prescription or not), aspirin, acetaminophen, iron-containing drugs and dietary supplements, diphenhydramine hydrochloride, ibuprofen, loperamide, and a host of household products. Some prescription and OTC products are exempt from the Act. Examples include sublingual dosage forms of nitroglycerin and specific aspirin-containing products.

Normally it is the pharmacist who is responsible for making the appropriate decision as to whether or not a prescription must be dispensed using a child-resistant container. However, practitioners dispensing medication directly to the patient are also responsible for dispensing drugs in packaging that complies with the requirements of the Act. Child-resistant containers are available in a wide variety of formats.

The law makes provision for waiving the safety packaging requirements of the Act. For example, patients may request that a prescription medication be dispensed in a noncomplying container. Also, a patient may ask the pharmacy for a blanket waiver for all the medication that he or she has dispensed at a particular pharmacy. A practitioner may request a waiver for the patient on a single prescription-by-prescription basis. However, practitioners may not request blanket waivers for patients.

Whereas the federal law does not require that a request for noncomplying packaging be in writing, some states do require written documentation. Pharmacists and practitioners are encouraged to get the waiver in writing from the patient.

Practitioners should note that federal law indicates that the container cannot be reused, because the closure may lose its child-resistant properties after continued use. In the case in which a plastic container has been used, the cap and container must be replaced. When glass is used, only a new cap is required. State law may modify these requirements.

It should be noted that provisions of the Poison Prevention Packaging Act do not apply to inpatient situations.

SYRINGES AND NEEDLES

Federal law does not make any provision for the sale or prescribing of hypodermic syringes and needles. However, state laws may restrict sales to pharmacies or require that they be dispensed only by prescription. Consult your state law.

PRESCRIPTIONS FOR OVER-THE-COUNTER MEDICATION

A practitioner may decide that a medication normally available OTC without a prescription should be provided to the patient only on the basis of a prescription. This is likely to occur when the dosage regimen requires supervision or the possibility of a drug interaction exists. In this case the practitioner should provide the patient with a prescription that is legally complete (*eg*, name, address, and so forth). Simply writing the name of the medication on a prescription blank may not clearly convey the practitioner's intentions.

If refills have been indicated, they should be handled in the same manner as the original filling of the prescription.

CONTROLLED SUBSTANCES

Registration

Practitioners who wish to administer, prescribe, or dispense any controlled substance must be registered with the Federal DEA.

Practitioners are required to register with the Drug Enforcement Administration, Registration Unit, P.O. Box 28083, Central Station, Washington, D. C. 20005 by applying on Form DEA-224, available through the Unit or DEA Field Office.

Once an application is approved, a certificate of registration is issued to the practitioner. Valid for a period of 3 years, the certificate must be maintained at the registered location and be made available for official inspection. A practitioner who has more than one office in which controlled substances are administered or dispensed is required to register for each office.

According to the DEA, any physician who is an intern, resident, foreign physician, or physician on the staff of a Veterans Administration facility (exempted from registration) may dispense, administer, and prescribe controlled substances under the registration of the hospital or other institution in which he or she is employed, provided that

1. The dispensing, administering, or prescribing is in the usual course of professional practice
2. The physician is authorized or permitted to do so by the state where he or she is practicing
3. The hospital or institution has verified that the physician is permitted to dispense, administer, or prescribe drugs within the state
4. The physician acts only within the scope of employment in the hospital or institution
5. The hospital or other institution authorizes him or her to dispense or prescribe under its registration and assigns a specific internal code number for each physician so authorized (*eg*, BD1234567-08, where the "-08" represents the practitioner's hospital code number, and the other numbers represent the hospital DEA number—the code number must be included on all prescriptions issued by the physician)
6. A current list of internal codes and the corresponding individual practitioners is kept by the hospital or other institution and is made available at all times to other registrants and law enforcement agencies upon request for the purpose of verifying the authority of the prescribing physician

In addition, each written prescription must have the name of the physician stamped, typed, or handprinted on it, as well as the signature of the physician.

Schedules of Controlled Substances

The drugs and drug products covered under the Federal Controlled Substances Act are divided into five schedules. Schedules are indicated by roman numerals, with Schedule I having the strictest control and Schedule V having the least control. A definition and examples for each schedule are indicated in Table 61-1. A complete list of drugs covered under the Act can be obtained from the DEA.

The reader should keep in mind that states also have regulations governing controlled substances and may assign a drug to a different schedule than the federal law. In such a case, the strictest law applies. Check your state law.

Prescribing Requirements for Schedule I-V Drugs

Prescription orders must be prepared in the manner described for controlled substances earlier in this chapter. Prior to writing a prescription, a practitioner must understand the rules that apply to each drug.

Schedule I

Under normal circumstances, practitioners cannot write for, and pharmacists cannot fill, prescriptions for Schedule I drugs. Consult the DEA and your state agency with responsibility for controlled substances for specific requirements that must be met to prescribe and write prescriptions for drugs in Schedule I.

Schedule II

The Federal Controlled Substances Act requires a written prescription for the dispensing of substances listed in Schedule II. Such prescriptions may not be refilled. Several states require the use of a special triplicate prescription form to dispense Schedule II and sometimes other scheduled drugs.

The federal law makes a provision for an Emergency Telephone Prescription Order for Schedule II controlled substances. In such an emergency, a practitioner may telephone a prescription order for a Schedule II controlled substance to a pharmacist. An emergency means that the immediate administration of the drug is necessary for proper treatment, that no alternative treatment is available, and that it is not possible for the physician to provide a written prescription order for the drug at that time.

In such an emergency, the amount of drug furnished on the order is limited to that needed to treat the patient during the emergency period. Within 72 hours of the emergency order, the practitioner must furnish the pharmacy with a written, signed prescription for the controlled substance prescribed. The prescriber must have written on the face of the prescription the statement "Authorization for Emergency Dispensing," and the date of the oral order. If the pharmacist does not receive the written prescription within the 72-hour period, he or she is required by law to notify the DEA of that fact. States may have stricter requirements.

TABLE 61-1. Schedules and Examples of Controlled Substances

Schedule I
These drugs have no currently accepted medical use in treatment in the United States and have a high potential for abuse.
Examples: many opiates; opium derivatives, including heroin; hallucinogenic substances, including LSD (lysergic acid diethylamide) and marijuana; certain depressants, including methaqualone; and certain stimulants.

Schedule II
These drugs have a high potential for abuse and have a currently accepted medical use in treatment in the United States or a currently accepted medical use with severe restrictions.
Examples: opium derivatives, including extracts and tincture of opium; morphine; codeine; hydromorphone (DILAUDID); oxycodone (PERCODAN); cocaine; meperidine (DEMEROL); amphetamines; phenmetrazine (PRELUDIN); methylphenidate (RITALIN); amobarbital (AMYTAL); pentobarbital (NEMBUTAL); and secobarbital (SECONAL). Some forms of codeine and amo-, pento-, and secobarbital appear in other Schedules.

Schedule III
These drugs have a potential for abuse lower than that of the drugs in Schedules I and II and have a currently accepted medical use in the United States.
Examples: some derivatives of barbituric acid, BUTISOL; paregoric; APC (aspirin, phenacetin, and caffeine) with codeine; aspirin with codeine (EMPIRIN WITH CODEINE); codeine, aspirin, caffeine, and butalbital (FIORINAL WITH CODEINE); acetaminophen with codeine (TYLENOL WITH CODEINE); chlorpheniramine polistirex with hydrocodone polistirex (TUSSIONEX); and suppository forms of amo-, pento-, and secobarbital; substances classified as "anabolic steroids" under federal law, such as methyltestosterone and fluoxymesterone. See also Schedules II and IV for other codeine preparations.

Schedule IV
These drugs have a low potential for abuse relative to the drugs in Schedule III with a currently accepted medical use in the United States.
Examples: phenobarbital; chloral hydrate (NOCTEC); meprobamate; paraldehyde; pentazocine (TALWIN); dextropropoxyphene (DARVON); benzodiazepines, including alprazolam (XANAX), chlordiazepoxide (LIBRIUM), clorazepate (TRANXENE), diazepam (VALIUM), flurazepam (DALMANE), lorazepam (ATIVAN), oxazepam (SERAX), and triazolam (HALCION); diethylpropion (TENUATE); and phentermine (IONAMIN).

Schedule V
These drugs have a low potential for abuse relative to the drugs in Schedule IV with a currently accepted medical use in the United States.
Examples: codeine-containing cough preparations, such as elixir of terpin hydrate and codeine, ROBITUSSIN A-C, and TRIAMINIC EXPECTORANT WITH CODEINE; diphenoxylate hydrochloride with atropine sulfate (LOMOTIL); and attapulgite (PAREPECTOLIN).

Schedules III and IV

Prescription orders for substances in Schedules III and IV may be issued in writing or given orally to the pharmacist. If authorized on the prescription, orders may be refilled up to five times within 6 months of the date of issue. A new prescription would then be required.

Federal law allows for the oral authorization of *additional refills* to the original prescription for Schedules III and IV controlled substances, provided the following provisions are met:

1. The *total quantity* of the drug authorized (including the amount of the original prescription) does not exceed five refills or extend beyond 6 months from the date of issue of the original prescription
2. The quantity of each additional refill authorized is equal to or less than the quantity authorized for the initial filling of the original prescription

3. The prescribing practitioner must execute a new and separate prescription for any additional quantities beyond the five-refills, 6-months limitation

For example, the practitioner who had provided a written prescription for 100 tablets and two refills could telephone the pharmacist and authorize a maximum of three additional refills of the prescription of no more than 100 tablets per refill.

Schedule V

The Federal Controlled Substances Act does not require Schedule V drugs to be prescribed by prescription. Such drugs may only be purchased from a pharmacy by a person 18 years or older, in limited quantities (*eg*, 4 fl oz), and only after 48 hours has elapsed since a previous purchase. Pharmacists are required to indicate certain information about the sale in a register designated for the purpose. Some states require that Schedule V drugs be dispensed only on prescription.

Security Requirements

Practitioners who store controlled substances in their office must keep them in a securely locked, substantially constructed cabinet or safe. The DEA recommends that controlled substance stock be kept to a minimum. If larger quantities are needed, the DEA encourages practitioners to have a security system that exceeds the minimum requirements, such as a safe and alarm system. Access to controlled substance storage areas should be restricted to a minimum number of employees.

Practitioners must notify the nearest DEA field office and the local police department upon discovering any loss or theft of controlled substances.

ORDERING DRUGS

How do practitioners obtain drugs for office or medical use? The most appropriate method is to establish an account with a local wholesaler or by using direct-order privileges with a pharmaceutical manufacturer. Controlled substances may be ordered only from a pharmacy that is registered as a wholesaler.

Schedule II controlled substances must be obtained through the use of a federal order form (not to be confused with the duplicate or triplicate prescription blanks used in some states).

Order Forms for Schedules I and II Controlled Substances

Federal order forms are triplicate forms issued in mailing envelopes that contain either 7 or 14 forms. They may be obtained at the time of initial registration (by marking the appropriate space on form DEA-224) or by using a separate form (DEA-222) thereafter. No charge is made for the order forms. Directions for completing the forms are indicated on the reverse side of the purchaser's copy. Figure 61-1 indicates a sample order form.

RECORD-KEEPING REQUIREMENTS—CONTROLLED SUBSTANCES

The Federal Controlled Substances Act requires that certain practitioners keep records of drugs purchased, distributed, and dispensed. The scope of a practitioner's activities determines what records must be kept.

Prescribing

Practitioners involved in the prescribing of Schedules II, III, IV, and V controlled substances in the course of their professional practice are not required to keep records of the transactions. This provision should not be confused with any medical practice requirements regarding documentation in the patients' medical records.

Dispensing

Practitioners who dispense controlled substances as a part of their medical practice are required to keep a record of each transaction.

Administration

The DEA *Physician's Manual* indicates that a physician who regularly engages in the administration of controlled substances in Schedules II, III, IV, and V is required to keep records if patients are charged for drugs either separately or with other patient services. When a physician dispenses a controlled substance and administers this substance occasionally or regularly from the same inventory, he or she must keep a record of all transactions. A physician who occasionally administers a controlled substance and does not dispense the controlled substance from the same inventory is not required to keep records of these transactions.

Inventories

Practitioners who are required to maintain records must take an inventory of all stocks of the substance on hand every 2 years. An initial inventory must be taken on the date that the practitioner first engages in such activity. Specific requirements for taking the inventory may be found in the DEA *Physician's Manual* or from a DEA field office.

Narcotic Treatment

The DEA *Physician's Manual* indicates that records are required for controlled substances prescribed, dispensed, or

See Reverse of PURCHASER'S Copy for Instructions	No order form may be issued for Schedules I and II substances unless a completed application form has been received (21 CFR 1305.04).	OMB APPROVAL No. 1117-0010
TO: *(Name of Supplier)*	STREET ADDRESS	
CITY AND STATE	DATE	TO BE FILLED IN BY SUPPLIER SUPPLIER'S DEA REGISTRATION No.

LINE No	TO BE FILLED IN BY PURCHASER					
	No. of Packages	Size of Package	Name of Item	National Drug Code	Packages Shipped	Date Shipped
1						
2						
3						
4						
5						
6						
7						
8						
9						
10						

◀ NO. OF LINES COMPLETED	SIGNATURE OF PURCHASER OR HIS ATTORNEY OR AGENT	
Date Issued	DEA Registration No.	Name and Address of Registrant
Schedules		
Registered as a	No. of this Order Form	

DEA Form -222 (Jun. 1983)

U.S. OFFICIAL ORDER FORMS - SCHEDULES I & II
DRUG ENFORCEMENT ADMINISTRATION
SUPPLIER'S COPY 1

FIGURE 61–1. Sample order form for Drug Enforcement Administration (DEA) Schedules I and II drugs. (Courtesy of the United States Drug Enforcement Administration.)

administered for maintenance or detoxification treatment. A physician is required to be registered as providing a narcotic treatment program to conduct these activities.

All controlled substance records and inventories must be filed in a readily retrievable manner from all other business documents and retained for 2 years. Schedule II records must be maintained separately from all other records. Schedules III, IV, and V records must be maintained separately or be kept in such a way that they are readily retrievable from the ordinary professional and business records of the practitioner.

The DEA *Physician's Manual* indicates that all records, including controlled substance records maintained as part of a patient's file, shall be available for inspection and copying by duly authorized officials of the DEA.

DISPOSAL OF CONTROLLED SUBSTANCES

A practitioner who is registered with the DEA and wishes to dispose of excess or undesirable controlled substances should request DEA Form 41. The form should be completed as directed and submitted to the DEA regional director. State law may dictate disposal procedures also.

PACKAGE INSERTS

A question arises as to whether or not a practitioner or pharmacist may give a patient a drug product package insert. Such inserts are provided with the product as part of its labeling for use by professionals. The FDA has stated that no regulation prevents the practitioner or pharmacist from providing the patient with the package insert. However, practitioners should use caution because such inserts are written for professionals using language and providing information that may not be understood by the patient.

The FDA has required that the manufacturers of several drug products prepare and provide *patient* package inserts for dispensing to the patient whenever a prescription for the drug is filled by the pharmacist. Patient package inserts are written at a patient level of understanding and provide information regarding the appropriate use of the drug, methods of administration, and possible side effects. Current examples of drugs providing such inserts include oral contraceptives, estrogenic drug products, and intrauterine devices. Patient information is available in the USP-DI and in many computer-based drug information programs (see Chapter 62).

DRUG SAMPLES

The 1987 Prescription Drug Marketing Act amended the Federal Food, Drug and Cosmetic Act for various purposes, including the placing of restrictions on the distribution of drug samples. Specifically, the law defines a drug sample as a unit of a drug subject to the act that is not intended to be sold and is intended to promote the sale of the drug.

Licensed practitioners who desire drug samples must make a written request of a manufacturer or distributor on a form that provides the following information:

- Name
- Address
- Professional designation
- Signature of the practitioner making the request
- Identity of the drug sample requested
- Quantity requested
- Name of the manufacturer of the drug sample
- Date of the request

Once the sample is received, the practitioner must execute a written receipt and return it to the manufacturer or distributor of the sample drug.

INSTITUTIONAL REQUIREMENTS

Generally, the requirements listed in this chapter can be applied to institutions such as hospitals, nursing homes, and so forth. However, states may have established additional or substitute regulations that pertain specifically to institutions. Consult your state law.

REFERENCES

Approved Prescription Drug Products With Therapeutic Equivalence Evaluations, 8th ed. Washington DC: US Department of Health and Human Services, 1988.

Code of Federal Regulations, Title 21, 1300. Superintendent of Documents, US Government Printing Office, Washington DC 20402.

Drug Enforcement Administration: Physician's Manual. Washington DC: Drug Enforcement Administration.

The Rx Legend—An FDA Manual for Pharmacists. Rockville, MD: US Food and Drug Administration.

Information and Learning Resources in Pharmacology

62

Cedric M. Smith and Alan M. Reynard

THE NEED FOR KNOWLEDGE ABOUT DRUGS

The rapidly growing knowledge base about individual drugs creates the necessity of having available a variety of accurate, up-to-date sources of information. This is true not only for the medical student, but also for all health professionals, including the house officer, the experienced physician, pharmacist, and nurse practitioner. This chapter was prepared as a guide for students as a reference and learning resource and to provide some advice on the effective and rational utilization of these resources.

To assist the teachers of health science professionals, the Association for Medical School Pharmacology, composed of the chairpersons of all the departments of pharmacology in schools of medicine, has prepared a consensus document, *Medical Knowledge Objectives in Pharmacology* (Fisher, 1990). This has proved useful for the design of learning programs, for review, and for the development of questions for certification examinations. The editors used these knowledge objectives in the planning of the present book. Another expertly prepared overview of relevant knowledge in all areas of medicine, including pharmacology, is published by the National Boards of Medical Examiners.

There is a general problem in agreeing on the core of "minimal essential information." In trying to be succinct, there is the serious risk of misleading oversimplifications that is inherent in presenting limited, and therefore at least partially inaccurate, information. In view of the fact that no one can really know and apply all of the potentially relevant information about a drug, a disease, and a patient, *the more physicians know about the principles of drug actions and side effects, the more patients will be benefited and the fewer harmed. In truth, those who prescribe and receive medications can never know too much about medications' actions and possible harmful side effects.*

SOURCES OF PHARMACOLOGICAL INFORMATION

Table 62-1 presents suggestions for any doctor or practitioner's "compleat" reference and learning resources, listed by primary use, starting with readily accessible textbooks and reference sources familiar to most readers. To illustrate, our choices start with the classic Goodman & Gilman textbook or the newly announced Munson (1994), the comprehensive *Drug Evaluations* from the American Medical Association (AMA), *Facts and Comparisons* because it is comprehensive and arranged conveniently for selection of drugs, the America Society of Hospital Pharmacy compendia, and the USP Drug Information for prescribers and patients. These provide a wide variety of, albeit not exhaustive, choices, and they reflect the biases of the authors. The remainder of the chapter serves to elaborate and critique some of the major resources; extensive lists of citations are included in the tables, as well as in an earlier publication (Smith and Reynard, 1992), and in the References.

Resources for Sources of Drug Information

Books, Drug Indexes, and Computer-Based Databases

The single most comprehensive resource about drug information is the compact, yet exhaustive, compilation of Snow (1989) (a new edition is being prepared). Smaller but useful

TABLE 62–1. Drug Information—The Editors' Choices for the "Compleat Practitioner's Bookshelf" (See Comprehensive Reference List)

Resource Type with Some Selected Examples	
Comprehensive Textbooks	***Adverse Drug Reactions and Interactions***
Gilman et al, 1990, or DE Drug Evaluations (AMA)* (now being combined with USP-DI) Munson, 1994	Drug Interaction Facts* DRUG GUIDE† Drug Interactions Handbook from The Medical Letter Meyler's Side Effects of Drugs (Dukes MNG, ed) Drug Interactions Decision Support Tables (Hansten PD)* AskRx† Clinical Pharmacology† RxTRIAGE† MEDI-SPAN Drug Therapy Monitoring System (DTMS)† MEDICOM Drug Interaction Database (MEDICOM Clinical Laboratory Test Interference Database and Parenteral Admixture Incompatability Database, Drug to Food Interaction Module (DFIM)*
Shorter Textbooks	***Poisoning and Toxicology***
This book, Smith and Reynard, 1992, or Craig and Stitzel, 1994; Katzung, 1994; or Kalant and Roschlau, 1989	Amdur et al, 1990 Ellenhorn and Barceloux, 1988 Statox† Environtox†
General Principles of Drug Action	***Governmental and Hospital Formularies: Information for Patients***
Pratt and Taylor, 1990	USP Drug Information* USP-DI/AMA-DE AskRx† S-O-A-P Medical Information† RxTRIAGE† Clinical Pharmacology†
Comprehensive Information	**Computer-Assisted Instruction**
Package Inserts for each drug (Physicians' GenRx, many available in PDR) United States Pharmacopeia (USP) Drug Information (USP-DI)* Facts and Comparisons; Drug Interaction Facts* ASHP Drug Information and Handbooks PDR Side Effects and Drug Interactions* Nonprescription drug information such as the American Pharmaceutical Association Handbook Computer Databases such as AskRx, S-O-A-P Rx, Drug Interaction Facts, Clinical Pharmacology, Micromedex software programs, ASHP Drug Information†	HyperPharm† MacPharmacology† PharmAid† MICAL, PSYCAL, ENDOCAL, DERMCAL† MacDog Lab† Cardiolab† Clinical Pharmacology† MD Challenger†
Convenient Access to Medical Literature	
MEDLINE, TOXLINE online and many others via modem, or medical libraries* Current Contents* Citation Index*	
Clinical Pharmacology and Therapeutic Manuals	
Melmon et al, 1990 Textbooks of medicine such as Cecil Essentials of Medicine (Andreoli et al, 1993) or the comprehensive two-volume Cecil Textbook of Medicine (Wyngaarden et al, 1992); Scientific American Medicine* Washington Manual, 1994 Larson and Ramsey, 1994 Therapeutic manuals for medical specialties, for example, Janicek et al, 1993	

*Available in both software and print form.
†Available as software.

citation lists are available under other auspices (*eg*, Morgan and Raper, 1992). Comprehensive catalogs of books in print and the massive bibliographic listings of the National Library of Medicine (NLM), the Institute for Scientific Information (ISI), and Excerpta Medica form the backbone of accessible readible information about drugs.

The most comprehensive and useful reviews of available computer-based medical information and software is the new journal *Medical Software Reviews*. A number of journals review products; a detailed compilation appears in an annual issue of the journal *M.D. Computing*. Among the resources are journals devoted to drug information, *Drug Information Journal*, or *Medical Education, Journal of Medical Education Technologies*.

World Databases in Medicine (Armstrong, 1994) is a directory providing a detailed listing of the huge number of electronic databases—on-line, on CD-ROM, on magnetic tapes and diskettes, or via fax, wire, or data broadcast, both here and in foreign countries. The NLM's periodical compilations and their *Audiovisuals Catalog* and *AudioVisuals onLine* (*AVLINE*) provides bibliographical citations for all audiovisuals and software cataloged by NLM since 1975. Other examples of directories are the *Medical Disc Directory* and the *Medical and Health Information Directory*.

Information about drugs would appear to be ideally suited for computer-based databanks because of the huge amount of discrete pieces of data, much of which is neither intuitive nor capable of being deduced from general principles, even by experts. Much of the information about drugs, drug testing, and drugs in clinical trials is now retrievable.

A unique computer software program, CIMD, designed for the practitioner, is easy to use and provides a wealth of

BOX 62–1
NOTE

BEWARE: THE REFERENCE INFORMATION YOU OBTAIN IS MOST CERTAINLY INCOMPLETE AND IS LIKELY TO BE AT LEAST PARTIALLY INCORRECT!!!!!!

information focused on computer-based systems for use in medical practice, including drug programs and references to review articles. However, unless this program is periodically updated it will soon become obsolete.

Limitations Inherent in all Information Resources

Although many of the drug database software programs are quite helpful and many truly deserve much wider use, most of them have one or more serious limitations. One of the serious limitations inherent in all of the programs derives from the flaws and deficiences in the actual primary information used for the computer tabulations. Furthermore, a new hazard can now be identified — the all-too-frequent (erroneous) assumption on the part of the user that the data obtained are all the information that possibly can be known. The extensiveness of the information and the authority implied by the programs (in spite of cautions and qualifiers) tempts the user of the computer-based databases to think and behave as if the data obtained with a search query retrieve all of the relevant extant information. Like all of the software programs, this chapter comes with a caution that the programs and the contents are in the process of continual updating and modification. Thus, an opinion or observation provided now may not be accurate by the time this is published.

Given this important caveat to their use, it also should be emphasized that these drug information programs are not equivalent. Thus, it becomes critically important that users explicitly identify their purpose(s) in using an information program, as well as address the risks they inevitably incur when they act on the information obtained.

In addition, newer computer systems such as *Clinical Pharmacology*, have nested information, such that important cautions and warnings are presented only if the user searches for more detailed information. We have recently cautioned that all such programs should bring up the warnings or cautions immediately whenever a drug monograph or information is selected (Smith, 1994).

Based on his extensive experience in studying psychotropic drugs, Klein (1993) has concluded that much of the scientifically based knowledge necessary to decide on a proper course of treatment, supervise the treatment, monitor for both benefit and toxic effects, and change treatment as indicated is *not* presently available for most treatments. He defines in some detail what the clinician usually does *not* know about a drug at the time of its marketing. The fact is that applied clinical psychopharmacologic science falls far short of the wide range of clinically important — life and death, quality of life — factual information that is potentially available but seldom actually is. Thus, current medical practice is seriously limited both by (1) the inappropriate and insufficient use of current knowledge, and by (2) the lack of a scientific, rational basis for much of clinical practice.

Access to Medical Literature and Keeping Current

Keeping informed and aware of information pertinent to one's practice presents a continuing challenge to all professionals. Table 62-2 lists many of the more useful journals in the area of therapeutics and pharmacology.

TABLE 62-2. Selected List of Journals That Publish Articles That Evaluate Basic and Clinical Pharmacology and Therapeutics

Annals of Internal Medicine
Annual Review of Pharmacology and Toxicology
British Journal of Pharmacology
Archives of Internal Medicine
Biochemical Pharmacology
Clinical Pharmacology and Therapeutics
Drugs
JAMA
Journal of Clinical Pharmacology
Journal of Pharmacology and Experimental Therapeutics
Journal of Clinical Psychopharmacology
Lancet
Nature
The Medical Letter on Drugs and Therapeutics
Molecular Pharmacology
New England Journal of Medicine
Pharmacological Reviews
Postgraduate Medicine
Science
Toxicology and Applied Pharmacology
Toxicon
Trends in Pharmacological Sciences, including toxicological sciences
Yearbook of Drug Therapy

There are literally thousands of medical journals that publish reputable articles that have received rigorous peer review. Each specialty has its own journal(s); major journals are found among the national and international medical organizations — for example, the *New England Journal of Medicine*, *Journal of the American Medical Association* (JAMA), *British Medical Journal*, and *Lancet*. In relation specifically to therapeutics, the *Medical Letter on Drugs and Therapeutics* is among the more accessible sources of consistently high quality; this newsletter also includes a continuing medical education (CME) program (Table 62-3). The regular perusing of the *Medical Letter* and following the CME program are effective ways to learn and keep up-to-date with important drug use and toxicity.

Almost as important as having these references is knowing where and how to obtain answers to new questions regarding drug uses or effects. To obtain answers to this class of question, the most generally available useful resource is MEDLINE, the NLM's on-line index of medical articles and journals — available directly or through GRATEFUL MED, Silver-Platter, or other computer/modem connections, such as DIALOG or BRS. An abbreviated version of MEDLINE is available in many institutions, sometimes designated as MINIMEDLINE, but such abbreviated programs should be avoided if possible. For all patient-related and research-related questions, the full search capability of MEDLINE should be used.

It is not generally appreciated that there is a very large world of potentially relevant medical information that is not accessible via MEDLINE. For example, although MEDLINE does contain citations to reviews of computer software in a number of the indexed journals, it does not yet index *Medical Software Reviews*, perhaps the single most comprehensive source of reviews of available medical and drug information software useful to the practitioner. Some of this

TABLE 62–3. Utilizing Computer-Based Drug Information Programs — Some of the Reviewers' Current Choices

1. To determine if a condition or symptom is possibly/probably caused (or could be produced) by one or more drugs. (For any old or new symptom, the differential diagnosis appropriately asks "could this be due to a drug or drugs?")
   AskRx, S-O-A-P Rx, Clinical Pharmacology, DRUG GUIDE, and Micromedex are much more useful than the PDR (but if one only wants to know what is in package inserts as listed in the PDR, the computer-based PDR or Physicians GenRx are easy to use.)
2. To determine if a condition or symptom is possibly/probably caused (or could be produced) by an interaction among drugs
   Drug Interaction Facts; AskRx; S-O-A-P Rx; PDR Side Effects
   Consultation of original literature with medical information specialists and with such databases as MEDLINE
3. To check for, and possibly avoid in advance, possible interactions between drugs a patient will be prescribed or receive (see above)
4. Compare/select drugs and drug regimens for specific indication/disease condition/symptom/drug (re: what is available, efficacy and potential side effects, matching dosage schedule to desired blood/tissue level pattern, etc.)
   Monographs such as those in the USP DI, DE Drug Evaluations, textbooks and reference books, Medical Letter and specialty newsletters, comprehensive multitopic databases on-line or on CD-ROM such as STAT!Ref
5. Rapid access to current data on all aspects of a drug's pharmacology—such as names, chemical structure, actions, side effects, indications and uses, mechanisms of action, dose and preparations, available preparations, pharmacokinetic parameters, drug regulations or litigations
   Consult Medical Librarian or Medical Information Specialist.
   No single computer-based source appears to be all-around best; choice depends on needs or objectives inasmuch as many of the programs are quite different from others; all appear to have some major limitations on the comprehensiveness of information—breadth of topics covered and with drugs especially the low frequency events, OTC preparations, and foods (review reference citations)
6. To obtain reference citations for specific drug effects, side effects, and drug interactions
   Drug Interaction Facts; Handbook of Adverse Drug Interactions 1992
7. For patients to obtain information monograph and directions of a specific drug or drug class
   AskRx (for USP-DI); DRUG GUIDE; S-O-A-P Rx; RxTriage

drug-related 'missing' information is indexed under other rubrics (*eg*, TOXLINE), as well as a variety of other databases; nevertheless, much of this information is very likely to be overlooked and thus not used for everyone's potential benefit. At the very least, it is recommended for the protection of the public health and for scientific accuracy that all of the comprehensive drug databases (cited in references and products), and especially medical library searches such as MEDLINE, caution users with every inquiry that it has specific major deficiencies in its database. As Nierenberg and Seprebon (1994) emphasize, *many serious drug interactions are underreported and often go unrecognized.* They recommend that "reference sources should be revised so that they are more useful to prescribers, pharmacists, and patients alike." This will require long-term repeated efforts by all professionals, including practitioners.

In another example, Kleijnen and Knipschild (1992) compared the comprehensiveness of MEDLINE and EMBASE computer searches for controlled trials of homeopathy, ascorbic acid, and a natural product, ginkgo biloba, against what they knew had been published. They reported that some 20% of the articles located were not correctly indexed. MEDLINE found from 17 to 25% of the actual articles; EMBASE found 13 to 58%. The utility of searches could be improved by searching the references of each of the articles they did find, bringing their total to between 44 and 93%, depending on the topic. Thus, in actual practice MEDLINE and EMBASE alone provided only an impression of the actual drug-related information available, but only if the references in the actual articles were followed up. Even different software programs for searching MEDLINE fail to retrieve the same references (Bleich, 1994).

Although the latest scientific news is desirable, the latest report is not always the best or most accurate. Accurate and important information on many topics was reported prior to 1966, the initial year of the MEDLINE database! (*eg*, see von Lichtenberg, 1994).

In addition to much greater attention to the primary data, and its indexing and searching strategies, the user and practitioner direly need more reviews by users and information specialists of available software for accuracy and appropriateness of content. Few who consider use or purchase have the time or experience needed to locate or compare available products. All too often, current reviews have some general problems: they tend to focus on technical aspects of ease of use, learning curves, and applications, whereas accuracy and comprehensiveness of the data are less easily determined and frequently given short shrift. Moreover, the task of preparing a judicious review can be daunting, inasmuch as it can be a major, time-consuming project to critically and accurately compare the content of one or more large programs. In addition, a useful review frequently requires a period of use and experience, yet few users have either the time or the inclination; almost no one would use two similar programs simultaneously. Techniques for assessing the quality of drug studies are currently being proposed (Cho and Bero, 1994).

Networks — The Internet

The Internet offers a myriad of resources for the health professional. Most of the software tools available for use with the Internet are called clients; the client software runs on the machine that you are logged onto (your PC, a mini, a mainframe, a local area network) and allows you to interact with the many host computers attached to the net. The host has to run the equivalent software, so that if you are using gopher, you will log onto a host computer that is also running gopher. There are a variety of clients, including WWW, WAIS, gopher, telnet, FTP, news, and mail.

MAIL. Many people have mail, even if they do not have the newer clients, and mail is useful because it allows you to join lists. A list is run by software that takes each message sent to the list and forwards the message to everyone else who has joined the list. There is a rapidly growing number of lists devoted to healthcare topics. To get a list of all lists managed by listserv, send the message LISTS GLOBAL to a listserv host near you. To get the address of a listserv host near you, ask the e-mail postmaster at the nearest university.

FTP. FTP (file transfer protocol) allows you to transfer a file from a host computer to your computer. There is a limited amount of written material about healthcare available by FTP. However, there is a collection of medical software available at dean.med.uth.tmc.edu/ and more general information at sunsite.unc.edu/pub/academic/medicine.

NEWS. News (Usenet news) is similar to mail lists in that a message that is sent to news is seen by all others who are signed up. An additional similarity is that news is divided into newsgroups, about 3000 of them, each of which covers a specific topic. You may sign up for any number of the newsgroups, as many as you have time to read. There are relatively few newsgroups devoted to healthcare. The two currently most active ones are sci.med.telemedicine and sci.med.informatics.

GOPHER. Gopher is a newer technology. There are many gopher servers around the world; most universities and many government agencies have one. Use a gopher client to log onto a gopher server. The server presents you with a series of menus that you access sequentially until you find what you want. Gopher is very easy to use. A number of gopher servers are dedicated to healthcare, including gopher.nih.gov and caldmed.med. miami.edu. A way to find out about new gopher sites, some of which are healthcare-related, is to subscribe to a list (gopherjewels at listserv@einet.net).

WWW. WWW (world wide web) is the newest technology. When you log onto a WWW client, you see text or graphics or both. There will be hotspots in the text and graphics where a click of a mouse button will take you to another part of the text or to another document; the other document may even be on a different server. Similar to gopher's menus, you click on hotspots until you find what you want. There are WWW sites at http://vh.radiology.uiowa.edu/ and http://golgi.harvard.edu/biopages/medicine.html.

Some gopher and WWW client software permits you to transfer files, thereby eliminating the need for FTP. As network systems evolve, they are likely to become a major source of comparative information and experience (*Pharmacy Case Review*; Glowniak and Bushway, 1994; Yasnoff, 1992; Jones et al., 1994; Pharmline).

The Package Insert—The Product Label

The package insert is included with every available drug. It is the legally required labeling information for all drugs mandated by the Food and Drug laws. The variety of extent and format of the package inserts stems from the fact that *the text of the package insert is agreed upon after negotiation between the manufacturer and staff of the United States Food and Drug Administration (FDA), at the time the drug was accepted, or by mandated revisions.* They contain "indications" that range from medicines that are truly indicated for a given disease state (for example, penicillin for streptococcal infections), to medicines that might possibly have some efficacy in treatment (for example, a benzodiazepine for mild insomnia). Thus, the indications section is misleading and ambiguous. Moreover, it fails to include clinically justified uses beyond those in the label, so-called off-label uses.

More important than the indications section is the list of potential side effects and adverse drug interactions. Inasmuch as the benefit/risk decision of taking or not taking a drug belongs not only to the physician, but also to the patient and the patient's significant others, the prescriber is obliged, both ethically and legally, to inform the patient not only of the benefits, but also of the risks.

Many, but not nearly all, of the package inserts for currently approved drugs are included in the *Physicians' Desk Reference* (PDR), which is published each year by the Medical Economics Company from material provided by pharmaceutical manufacturers. *Physicians GenRx* contains a conveniently edited compilation of prescribing information for all FDA-approved prescription drugs (available as a book or on CD-ROM). *It is incumbent on all prescribers to review, at the very least, the package insert,* Physicians GenRx, *or a current PDR (also available on CD-ROM and hand-held computer)* ***before*** *prescribing any drug.*

DETECTION AND PREVENTION OF ADVERSE DRUG REACTIONS AND INTERACTIONS

A major use of both reference books and computer databases is for the prediction or detection of adverse drug actions and interactions. Much prevention is still in order, in view of the fact that some 2–10% of all hospitalizations are the result of a serious adverse drug- and device-induced diseases (for example, Nightingale, 1993), and this does not count those not identified as such. Of the many products listed at the end of the chapter, the AskRx, S-O-A-P Rx, the *Medical Letter,* RxTriage, and *Clinical Pharmacology* systems are recommended not only for their comprehensive and useable information, but for the fact that they facilitate keeping essential records of drugs that individual patients are, or have been, receiving. AskRx, S-O-A-P Rx, RxTriage, *Clinical Pharmacology,* and the PDR on CD-ROM also provide ready access to monographs on each drug, as well as patient information sheets. RxTriage limits its interactions to those that are well-established or of serious impact and thus will identify fewer potential interactions than other systems, such as Interaction Facts.

One of the most difficult aspects of searching for possible drug causes of specific symptoms is the absence of an established vocabulary, glossary, and thesaurus of symptoms (Gnassi and Barnett, 1993; Wang, 1993; Letimeyer and Gillum, 1993). For example, to identify a drug that may cause yellow vision as a side effect—as an occurrence or as possible drug effect—requires searching under yellow vision, disturbed vision, visual disturbances, and xanthopsia just for starters. Falls and falling are not a commonly cited side effect, whereas dizziness, faintness, or syncope might be. Moreover, it is not commonly appreciated that even for the package inserts, the tabulations and frequencies are only a relatively recent inclusion (in the past 5 or so years); thus, with older drugs the frequencies of side effects in clinical trials or in actual experience is rarely ever known, and even relatively common side effects may not be identified or only included at the bottom of list labeled "incidence unknown."

Most practitioners are not adequately aware of how frequently they make egregious and potentially harmful errors of commitment or omission. A study of one university-affiliated teaching hospital documented significant risks to patients with errors in prescribing at a rate of more than three per 1000 prescriptions, with almost two out of three judged as being significantly hazardous (Lesar et al, 1990); not included were errors of omission, diagnosis, and work-up, or errors actually detected and corrected by other staff. Moreover, a large percentage of all the medical staff were responsible for the errors; of 580 detected errors in a series, 170 different prescribers were responsible, ranging from first-year house officers to attending physicians, with one to 12 errors per prescriber.

That improvement in detection and awareness can be accomplished has been demonstrated (Scott et al, 1990). One practical way to keep abreast of all the new reports on such adverse reactions is to subscribe to an adverse drug reaction and interaction database. It should now be obvious that every practitioner should be aware of all drugs a patient is, or potentially could be, receiving. And the only way of being aware of all the potential interactions is to keep up to date with medical literature searches or receive the frequent updates of such programs as Drug Interactions Facts.

Inherent in all programs searching for drugs that could cause a given disease state or that cause a potentially adverse drug interaction is the problem of how fine should be the mesh of the search screen. Too fine, and one detects only a few, usually fairly obvious drugs; too wide open a search mesh, the list of drugs becomes huge and unmanageable. Again, which search system is most helpful lies in the purpose of the inquiry. For one searching for the most likely possibilities, the fine screen is appropriate; however, in a patient presenting with unexplained symptoms, the search needs to include not only the probable causes, but the improbable ones as well, because only a comprehensive search strategy is likely to be successful. Moreover, the unlikely drug causes are the very ones that will have had the least research and confirmation, and the ones most important for a given patient, as well as for general medical interest.

Among the case studies we have used in medical teaching was a patient with possible toxic effects of digoxin, benzodiazepines, and other agents. Digoxin was among the drugs listed for a symptom of fatigue; Drug Guide cited it, but AskRx and PDR did not. AskRx cited digoxin as cause of confusion, whereas Drug Guide and the PDR failed to do so. All three programs did identify digoxin as a cause of xanthopsia (yellow vision) when entered as xanthopsia, but not when listed as a disturbance of vision. And perhaps most instructive, dementia was not listed as a side or toxic effect of digoxin (LANOXIN) or digitalis glycosides, by any of these compilations, yet that possibility is well-documented in textbooks and literature, and is of continuing clinical importance. (Of course, the PDR could only search under the product name of LANOXIN.)

Adverse Food Reactions

Adverse food reactions are now available for computer access, such as Well-Aware: Food Sensitivity (see Smith and Reynard, 1992). Programs such as this provide a computer-based method of recording and cataloging every item a patient ingests and then correlating foods, ingredients, and symptoms. This program is useful for physicians, dieticians, and other health providers, as well as for patients, to keep track of all possible symptoms related to an allergic response to foods. Another example is Nutri-Calc HD (1990), a nutritional food database and nutritional values from the 10th edition of *Recommended Dietary Allowances*; it will prepare weight gain/loss dietary plans based on food intake and activity.

Adverse Drug-Food Interactions

As a class of interactions, adverse drug-food interactions are woefully inadequately documented (see Chapter 50), largely because of both the paucity of controlled studies and the absence of systematic analyses of the data.

SELECTION OF DRUGS FOR SPECIFIC DISEASE OR SYMPTOM

As noted previously, the "Indications" section of the package insert is, at best, an inadequate source of information for the selection of a drug, other than to know what the government agency, the FDA, has approved. More rational sources of guidance for therapy are specialty journals and newsletters such as *The Medical Letter*, the USP Drug information monographs, *DE Drug Evaluations* of the AMA, comprehensive multitopic databases on-line or on CD-ROM such as STAT! Ref or the MAXX "electronic library of medicine."

Formularies

Much of medical practice takes place in group clinics, health maintenance organizations, or hospital settings, and these usually have associated pharmacies with formularies that include only a limited number of drugs, frequently selected by a formulary committee. In some states, such as New York, the Department of Health mandates the prescribing and filling of prescriptions with generic agents unless otherwise specifically requested by the doctor in writing on each prescription.

Poisoning and Toxicology

Useful information is available from poison control centers. POISINDEX and TOXLINE are two extensive computer-accessible toxicology databases that cover medicinal, commercial, industrial, and botanical sources.

Prescribing Principles and Management Systems

A number of systems are now available for recording of patient data, clinical laboratory findings, diagnosis, progress notes, medication, and treatment records. These range from the primitive to the very complete. For management of patients' medication, we have found the AskRx, *Clinical Pharmacology*, and the S-O-A-P Rx systems comprehensive, accurate, and very easy to use. Other examples are Dr. Smartkey, a macro-writing program and macro editor designed for use with WordPerfect for progress notes, using templates for illnesses or drugs frequently encountered, as well as patient data, telephone dialers, and the like. A number of systems are now available, and many more will be appearing in the near future. Some available materials are listed in the References, and a detailed compilation appears in an annual issue of *M.D. Computing* magazine.

A major defect of most hospital patient records is the absence of a coherent, time-line based record of all medications, as described in the original problem-oriented medical record (Weed, 1969; Bleich and Lawrence, 1993; Litt and Loonsk, 1992), in analogy with temperature and vital signs records. Widespread interest in computer-based medical records has existed for some time; the issues and strategies to accomplish such systems has been presented in *Computer-based Patient Record* (Dick and Steen, 1991). A number of organizations are now working on developing practical systems (*eg*, Computer-based Patient Record Institute; four such hospital systems were featured at the Fourth National Conference on Clinical Computing in Patient Care: Evolving Computer-Based Patient Records, Harvard Medical School Department of Continuing Education, September, 1994; and Niebuhr and Marion, 1994). According to Lieff (1994), time-line clinical databases are now operational and available, and bare-bones practical systems are being utilized (Zupko, 1994).

Although noteworthy exceptions exist, many hospital records still have the handwritten order sheets for all orders, including drugs, and nurses' notes that may include medications given, or a separate chart of medications, listed by medication. The pharmacy records are usually not an integral part of the patient medical record. Thus, any chart review for medications requires the time-consuming generation *de novo* of a time-line and medications given, stopped, resumed, changes in dose, etc. It is no wonder that too many patients receive drugs to which they are allergic, and receive polypharmacy inadvertently, by ignorance, laziness in record review, or failure to communicate (Clements, 1994). A cost-of-illness model recently has documented the potentially enormous costs of inappropriate medication (Johnson and Bootman, 1995).

Patient Information

The United States Pharmacopeia (USP) and the AMA have pioneered the preparation and use of printed materials on specific drugs or drug classes that are written in a language suitable for the general public. The databases for USP-DI (Drug Information) and the AMA's Drug Evaluations (DE) are currently being combined. Both provide spaces for the physician to insert specific information for a given patient.

Such patient information materials are now available on a number of personal computer programs, as well as networks, for direct use by patients or as templates that can be edited by the physician for individual patients. In addition, some medical specialties, such as psychiatry, have developed videotapes for viewing by patients that explain the uses, side effects, and precautions for psychotropic agents.

The major important limitation to essentially all of the available patient drug information is the absence of an explicit benefit-risk assessment for that patient, or for that disease condition. This is not only an important issue, it is a complex one. Many practitioners truly do not want to alarm patients or have patients neglect taking their medicine out of fear of side effects; conversely, keeping information from the patient inherently denies them informed consent, as well as the ability to detect potentially serious side effects. The difficulty in assessing such information, for example, for the serious risk of death related to the common use of β-adrenergic blocking agents in asthma, even when it has been identified and the relevant articles read and evaluated, is evident in Levine et al (1994). The current patient information materials (*eg*, USP DI) frequently side-step the issue, and it remains for the practitioner and the institution to make the assessment and carry out the communication. Nevertheless, failure to communicate such risks and involve patients in decisions about their treatment is one the major sources of malpractice and medical liability claims and suits (Clements, 1994). Some techniques for generating patient handouts are presented by Kahn (1993a, b); current publications are cited in Macura and Macura (1994).

Medical Informatics

Medical informatics is a discipline emerging in medical school, health care institutions, and libraries; it focuses on the management of information used to support education and decision making in patient diagnosis and management, research, and communication. The establishment in medical institutions of academic and service units that deal with medical informatics is being implemented in a number of schools. Among the interests of this field are medical education, patient management, coping with new technology, and development and utilization of electronic knowledge resources (*eg*, hypertext, hypermedia, on-line textbooks, bibliographical databases, computer programs as adjuncts to lectures and laboratories, clinical case simulations, educational testing, and clinical medical record systems and decision aids).

Learning Resources

Question Banks

A number of computer-based question banks are available on computer disk, some of which are devoted to pharmacology. Since the 1950s, the editors' department, like many departments of pharmacology, have used examinations as much for learning exercises as for student evaluations (Smith, 1995). We routinely make available copies of current and old examinations to students as learning aids. The students are encouraged to use these questions in planning their studying, for review, and to test their knowledge.

Computer-based versions of question banks have an appreciably greater potential for learning, as well as for testing. Prime among these question banks have been the pioneering efforts of Walaszek and colleagues. Their system involves 240 lessons of four different types: review questions, self-study, case histories, and laboratory exercises. Examinations are drawn from a question bank of 14,000 items (Walaszek and Doull, 1985, 1990). Others are listed in the References (*eg*, Katzung, 1987; Hyperpharm — Aranow and Moore, 1990; MacPharmacology — Eisenberg, 1992; Elliott, 1987). Most of these contain at least some programs or text that comments on the reasons why a particular item selected is either correct or incorrect. One of the textbooks in pharmacology, Bevan and Thompson, unfortunately now out of print, included questions at the end of each chapter plus advice on how to use the book for self-study.

Almost uniformly, these pharmacology question banks are limited by the fact that they use, almost exclusively, the standard multiple-choice formats that stress recognition (or at least potentially can be answered using straight recall or recognition) as opposed to the "real world" context that requires uncued recall, synthesis of diverse pieces of information, or problem-solving. Even case management questions designed as "problems" are often trivial or can be answered correctly using some simple recall strategies and recognition knowledge.

In contrast, the more open-ended questions, such as those used in the Nierenberg and Smith book (1989), are at the same time more similar to the clinical situation as well as encouraging (or least permitting) more detailed recall and reconstruction of existing knowledge to address the problems presented by the clinical cases.

Problem-based learning and case-based learning systems are both currently used in numerous schools. Both of these learning strategies can be augmented by comprehensive information resources, such as MEDLINE, and various computer-based drug information (Aronow, 1994). The authors have adapted one of the patient-oriented problem sessions (POPS)-like case histories for use in conjunction with computer-based programs for the identification of drugs and drug-interactions as causes of disease (Smith, 1993a,b, 1994a,b).

With the current emphasis on case- and problem-based learning systems, an increasing number of individuals and institutions are authoring computer-based programs. One of the largest of these is the Health Sciences Consortium, with offices at the University of North Carolina. The Consortium is a nonprofit publishing cooperative dedicated to sharing instructional software and instructional materials in health sciences. Among materials pertinent to pharmacology is the first of a new series, *Case Studies in Essential Hypertension*, which has only recently been available. Members of the Consortium can obtain such programs for review in advance of any purchase.

Patient-Oriented Problem Sessions

The patient-oriented problem session (POPS) units in pharmacology have been developed to encourage and stimulate problem-solving by groups of students, with a focus on the patient, disease process, and specific drug classes (Burford et al, 1990; Ingenito, 1994). Experiences with these POP sessions in a basic pharmacology course for medical and graduate students found that some students use them enthusiastically, whereas others participate only reluctantly (Lathers and Smith, 1993). The POPS provide efficient learning of relevant material. However, it is necessary to update certain sections in light of new information. Currently available are sessions on pharmacokinetics, theophylline, antidepressant drugs, drug prescribing in the elderly, psychopharmacology, diabetes, drug therapy of hypertension and congestive heart failure, antiarrhythmic drugs, toxicity of analgesic agents, and treatment of poisoning.

Programmed and Case-Related Texts

A unique review text by Neal (1987) has a number of interesting summaries and presentations. Case-related, problem-oriented textbooks can be quite useful, especially for review. Among the more useful, in our opinion, are Nierenberg and Smith (1989) and Sweeney (1990). Both of these use selected cases to illustrate basic drug actions, uses, and principles of drug therapy.

Computer-Assisted Instruction

Computer-based systems are uniquely useful in the management, storage, and ready retrieval of vast amounts of information on medical topics, including drugs. A few of these resources have been discussed. Under development are practical and feasible use of computers for clinical decision-making in addition to more useful and readily available computer-accessible databases and knowledge databases. The drug interaction databases (such as those in *Interaction Facts* and the *Medical Letter* programs) are good examples of a functionally operational systems that are relatively inexpensive, readily available, and clinically extremely important.

To date there are no comprehensive, interactive computer-assisted instruction (CAI) programs focusing on medical students learning pharmacology for the first time. There are, nevertheless, programs available that feature limited aspects of pharmacology (Macura and Macura, 1994). For all of them, it appears that students use them only to the extent that the CAI is integrated with other components of the course and curriculum (Smith, 1994a,b; Aronow, 1990, 1994; Keith Killam, personal communication). In addition to education itself, computer systems are being implemented for curricular tracking, scheduling, and a variety of testing and evaluations.

PHARMACOKINETICS. One area of pharmacology, pharmacokinetics, lends itself to computer-based instruction, as well as practical application in designing drug-dosing regimens (Feldman et al, 1989; MacFadyen et al, 1993). Among the many programs available are PCNONLIN, PHARMKIN (Neubig, 1987), MINSQ, MacKinetics (Aronow and Moore, 1990), and Basic Principles of Therapeutic Drug Monitoring. Each of these seeks to assist the user to develop practical (and intuitive) knowledge of therapeutics by providing hands-on exposure to dosage selection and monitoring, using simulation of plasma concentrations as a function of dosing and time. Most of these programs are relatively rudimentary, although suitable for sophomore medical students; however, some provide a detailed simulation potential and regime design (*eg*, Washington et al, 1990); others include pharmacokinetics (*eg*, USC PC-PACK by Jelliffe and colleagues).

OTHER CAI PROGRAMS. *Gas Man*: Understanding Anesthesia Uptake and Distribution is a computer simulation program that illustrates the principles of anesthetic gas uptake and distribution. The program displays the information for several anesthetics graphically. It permits reviewing of current clinical situations, as well as testing theories by simulation. This program has a superb reputation for learning by residents in anesthesia and could be employed in the pharmacology curriculum.

MICAL (Upjohn) presents a series of patients and questions regarding choice of diagnosis of an infection, initial choice of an antibiotic, and how the medication should be managed. We have observed that medical students find the cases and program interesting, a glimpse of the practical and useful for review and learning.

PSYCAL (Upjohn), although focused on psychiatric diagnosis and not therapy, is well-edited and contains pertinent information. It has been judged by a small group of students as one of the best of a number of software programs; this series was characterized as providing more feedback and control than most (Xakellis and Gjerde, 1990).

ENDOCAL (Upjohn) is another in a series that provides good user control and feedback. The focus is on endocrinology rather than therapeutics.

MD Challenger is a PC computer-based software for review in emergency and primary care. This program is interesting and potentially useful as a learning tool in therapeutics. The program is formatted as both a rapid clinical reference and an interactive testing/educational program designed for use by emergency and acute care physicians. Approximately 4000 screens or "pages" of questions are accessible; most of the alternative answers are correct and make important points. The factual information is coupled with rapid response, easy-to-use indexes accessible by any topic covered including drug, disease, symptom, side effect, general area of content, as well as individual scores. As such, it contains extensive information about commonly used drugs presented in practical clinical settings. We found the program fun to explore, and look forward to the database expansion promised by the publisher.

Clinical Pharmacology includes a unique Quiz program that generates de novo questions or indications, interactions, and side effects by drug or by other topic. Some are interesting, but it requires some knowledge of the relevance of question or answer to use intelligently.

CAI programs in a number of other medical areas related to pharmacology are now being developed. The report of Hutcheon and El-Gawly (1991) illustrates how microcomputer technology can provide new ways of incorporating problem-based learning procedures by using both analog and digital systems. They describe a model system of four problem-oriented exercises that require the student to interpret electrocardiograms (ECGs) and the drug-induced changes in cardiac rhythm. Students obtain an understanding of the electrophysiological basis for managing cardiac arrhythmias in clinical practice that supplements and expands laboratory and conference sessions. In practice, the exercise can be run as an individual student or group activity.

Many other general medical programs contain major drug information; however, many diagnostic programs do not. The popular QMR is seriously deficient by its failure to include drugs as a possible source of illness or symptoms.

Interactive Video

Interactive video is considered the best computer-based method currently available to deliver didactic information to students. An interactive video system is one that can deliver images (and text) to an individual who can interact with the system to evoke responses. This can be accomplished in several ways. Currently, the most popular way is to combine a video disk player with a computer, so that images from the player appear on the screen, sometimes overlayed with text or graphics from the computer. The presentation of the images is controlled by a program running on the computer. The user can interact with the system with a keyboard, a mouse, a light pen, or by touching a touch-sensitive screen.

There is much effort under way to find efficient ways to store the images digitally on a computer's hard disk, rather than on a video disk. A few such systems currently are in development, but not yet commercially available. In summary, this type of delivery system consists of a computer, a method of delivering images such as a disk player, a disk, and a computer program. A video disk can hold 54,000 still images, 30 minutes of motion video, or a combination of both. An example of its use is the presentation of the image of a cell on the screen, with an arrow pointing to a structure in the cell and a corner of the screen devoted to a multiple-choice question that the user can answer. The computer program determines which image and question are put on the screen, monitors the user's response, and provides feedback to the user.

To our knowledge, there are no interactive video programs available exclusively for pharmacology, clinical pharmacology, or therapeutics. However, several programs/disks involve pharmacology while dealing with other areas of medicine; most of the pharmacology relates to treatment. The DxTER series of disks on emergency medicine was developed by Intelligent Images. In these, the student manages a patient in real time, using images displayed from the video disk. The computer program tracks decisions made by the student and calculates care costs. CBT, computer-based examinations produced by the National Board of Medical Examiners, use images from a video disk. These programs are currently being tested in a number of medical schools.

Other

The CYBERLOG system from Cardinal Health Systems is a hybrid system that covers nearly 20 topics dealing with clinical management. Some are concerned in detail with pharmacological matters; one focuses on clinical pharmacology and pharmacokinetics; others focus on specific clinical syndromes—hypertension, diabetes, coronary artery disease, arthritis, infectious diseases, cardiac arrhythmias, thyroid diseases, and gastrointestinal diseases. Each of these programs includes a general text, explicit objectives, tutorials, sample clinical case studies, and reference "tools," such as tables of established values, nomograms, and drug formularies. An illustrated text and computer disks are provided. For the most part, this system is programmed learning with some question-and-answer format. The didactic material is accessible by computer read-out or printed text.

Continuing Medical Education

There is a wealth of educational materials and programs available under continuing medical education (CME) auspices. Each medical school and most major medical institutions have ongoing medical education programs. Of more general accessibility are the many television video presentations. Many of these present focused clinical pharmacology instruction. As just one example, an AMA Videoclinic presented "Common Arrhythmias: New Concepts for the Selection of Antiarrhythmic Agents," including illustrated ECGs and current approaches to therapy. A tremendously important limitation to CME programs, including the video clinics, is the fact that most, if not all, receive major support from pharmaceutical and medical industries. Granted, some of the programs are exemplary in the balance of their discussions; however, drug industry expenditures are based on a variety of potential benefits to the industry involved. Those interests or industry objectives may not be readily apparent, and thus an industry's influence may not even be recognized, let alone compensated for, by the physician or student participant.

REFERENCES

(See also the extensive reference citations in Smith and Reynard, 1992)

Amdur MO, Doull J, Klaassen CD (eds): Casarett and Doull's Toxicology: The Basic Science of Poisons, 4th ed. New York: Pergamon Press, 1991.

Andreoli TE, Carpenter CCJ, Plum F, Smith LH Jr: Cecil Essentials of Medicine, 3rd ed. Philadelphia: W.B. Saunders, 1993.

Aronow L, Moore K: Q/Bank — A Macintosh-based question review system. FASEB J 4:A1237, 1990.

Aronow L: Drug Information Problem Set. Presented at The Workshop on Teaching Pharmacology to Medical Students. Association of Medical School Pharmacology. Sea Island, GA, February, 2-3, 1994.

Baselt RC: Disposition of Toxic Drugs and Chemicals in Man, 3rd ed. Chicago: Year Book Medical, 1990.

Bevan JA, Thomson JH: Essentials of Pharmacology, 3rd ed. Philadelphia: Harper & Row, 1983.

Bleich HL: Critique of an evaluation of software for searching MEDLINE. American Medical Informatics Association Proceedings of Seventeenth Annual Symposium on Computer Applications in Medical Care, October 30-November, 1994, pp 591-595.

Bleich HL, Lawrence L: Weed and the problem-oriented medical record. M.D. Computing 10:70-71, 1993.

Burford HJ, Balfour DJ, Stevenson IH: Development of PharmTest: A unique personal computer-mediated tool for assessment of pharmacology. J Clin Pharmacol 33:400-404, 1993.

Burford HJ, Ingenito AJ, Williams PB: Development and evaluation of patient-oriented problem solving materials in pharmacology. Acad Med 65:689, 1990.

Caravati EM, McElwee NE: Use of clinical toxicology resources by emergency physicians and its impact on poison control centers. Ann Emerg Med 20:147-150, 1991.

Cardiolab: Cardiovascular pharmacology simulation by I. Hughes. BIOSOFT, Cambridge, United Kingdom and Milltown, NJ.

Charles SC: Malpractice: Book review of Edwards (1989). JAMA 264:528, 1990.

Cho MK, Bero LA: Instruments for assessing the quality of drug studies published in the medical literature. JAMA 272:101-104, 1994.

Clark WG, Brater DC, Johanson AR (eds): Goth's Medical Pharmacology, 12th ed. St. Louis: C.V. Mosby, 1988.

Clayman CB: Medical CD-ROMS [reviews of CD-ROM programs]. JAMA 270:1613-1616, 1993.

Clements B: Don't get sued. 2: The most common causes of lawsuits and how you can protect yourself: Problems with prescribing. American Medical News, July 18, 1994: 17-19.

Conn PM, Gebhart GF (eds): Essentials of Pharmacology. Philadelphia: F.A. Davis, 1989.

Craig CR, Stitzel RE (eds): Modern Pharmacology, 4th ed. Boston: Little, Brown, 1994.

Cushing M Jr: SilverPlatter literature searches. MD Computing 9:178-180, 1992.

Davant C III: Review of Drug Guide 1.0. Medical Software Reviews 3:7-8, 1994.

DE Drug Evaluations: Subscription published quarterly by American Medical Association, Chicago.

Dick RS, Steen EB (eds): Computer-based Medical Record. Washington DC: National Academy Press, 1991.

Edward FJ: Medical Malpractice: Solving the Crisis. New York: Henry Holt, 1989.

Eisenberg R: MacPharmacology: A series of computerized study and review programs. J Clin Pharmacol 32:10-17, 1992.

Elliott HL: Self-assessment in Clinical Pharmacology. Oxford: Blackwell Scientific Publications, 1987.

Feldman RD, Schoenwald R, Kane J: Development of a computer-based instructional system in pharmacokinetics: Efficacy in clinical pharmacology teaching for senior medical students. J Clin Pharmacol 29:158-161, 1989.

Felitti VJ: Software. JAMA 264:529, 1990.

Fisher JW, Gourley DRH, Greenbaum LM: Knowledge objectives in medical pharmacology. Pharmacologist 27:73-78, 1985.

Fox GN: Review of USHEALTHLINK. Journal of Family Practice 36:572-573, 1993.

Fraser PJ (ed): Microcomputers in Physiology — A Practical Approach. Oxford and Washington DC: IRL Press, 1989.

Gilman AB, Goodman LS, Rall TW, Murad F (eds): Goodman and Gilman's Pharmacological Basis of Therapeutics, 8th ed. New York: Macmillan, 1990.

Gnassi JA, Barnett GO: A survey of electronic drug information resources and identification of problems associated with the differing vocabularies used to key them. Proceedings of the Annual Symposium on Computer Applications in Medical Care, 631-635, 1993.

Gnassi JA, Barnett GO: A survey of electronic drug information resources and identification of problems associated with differing vocabularies used to key them. American Medical Informatics Association Proceedings of Seventeenth Annual Symposium on Computer Applications in Medical Care, October 30-November, 1994, pp 631-635.

Glowniak JV, Bushway MK: Computer networks as a medical resource: Assessing and using the internet. JAMA 271:1934-1939, 1994.

Gorback MS: Anesthesia Simulator Consultant 1.0 AnesSoft. Medical Software Reviews 2:6-7, 1993.

Gorman P: Does the medical literature contain the evidence to answer questions of primary care physicians? Preliminary findings of a study. American Medical Informatics Association Proceedings of Seventeenth Annual Symposium on Computer Applications in Medical Care, October 30-November, 1994, pp 571-575.

Graham GK: Can safety labeling be harmonized? Drug Information Journal 27:437-446, 1993.

Greco P: Review of AskRx. Medical Software Reviews 3:4-5, 1993.

Greenes RA, Shortliffe EH: Medical informatics — An emgerging academic discipline and institutional priority. JAMA 263:1114-1120, 1990.

Hoffer EP: Review of Drug Interactions Facts. Medical Software Reviews 2:5-6, 1993.

Hoffer EP: Drug Interactions Software. Medical Software Reviews 1:1-3, 1992.

Hutcheon DE, Ed-Gawly HW: A computer-based, problem-solving system of instruction in clinical pharmacology. J Clin Pharmacol 31:198-204, 1991.

Ingenito AJ: Update on the POPS program. Workshop on the Teaching of Pharmacology to Medical Students, Association of Medical School Pharmacology, The Cloister, Sea Island, GA, February 2-3, 1994.

Ingenito AJ, Nobel BG, Wooles WR: The case conference approach to teaching clinical pharmacology. J Clin Pharmacol 32:502-510, 1992.

Janicek PG, Davis JM, Preskorn SH, Ayd FJ Jr: Principles and Practice of Psychopharmacology. Baltimore: Williams & Wilkins, 1993.

Jankel CA, Martin BC: Evaluation of six computerized drug interaction screening programs. Am J Hosp Pharm 49:1430-1435, 1992.

Jones RB, McGhee SM, McGhee D: Patient on-line access to medical records in general practice. Health Bull (EH) 50:1423-150, 1994.

Kahn G: Computer-based patient education: A progress report. M.D. Computing 10:93-100, 1993.

Kahn G: Computer-generated patient handouts. M.D. Computing 10:157-164, 1993.

Kalant H, Roschlau HE: Principles of Medical Pharmacology. Philadelphia: BC Decker, 1989.

Katzung BG (ed): Basic and Clinical Pharmacology, 3rd ed. Norwalk, CT, Appleton and Lange, 1987.

Kelly RB: Review of On Line:US Health Link. J Fam Pract 36P:574-575, 1993.

Kleijnen J, Knipschild P: The comprehensiveness of Medline and Embase computer searches: Searches for controlled trials of homeopathy, ascorbic acid from common cold and gingko biloba for cerbral insufficiency and intermittent claudication. Pharm Weekly [Sci] 14:316-320, 1992.

Klein DF: Clinical psychopharmacologic practice: The need for developing a research base. Arch Gen Psychiatry 50:491-494, 1993.

Lathers CM, Smith CM: Teaching clinical pharmacology: Coordination with medical pharmacology courses. J Clin Pharmacol 29:581-597, 1989.

Lathers CM, Smith CM (co-chairs): Second Annual Clinical Pharmacology Teaching Clinic. American College of Clinical Pharmacology, November 3, 1993.

Leitmeyer J, Gillum T: Consistency in adverse event terminology: Merck's modified Clinterm. Drug Information Journal 27:431-436, 1993.

Lesar TS, Briceland LL, Delcoure K, et al: Medication prescribing errors in a teaching hospital. JAMA 263:2329-2334, 1990.

Levine M, Walter S, Lee H, et al, for the Evidence-Based Medicine Working Group: Users' guides to the medical literature. IV: How to use an article about harm. JAMA 271:1615-1619, 1994.

Lieff JD: Clinical databases. Psychiatric Annals 24:33-36, 1994.

Litt HI, Loonsk JW: Digital patient records and the medical desktop: An integrated physician workstation for medical informatics training. Proceedings of the 16th Annual Symposium SCAMC, 555-559, 1992.

Litt H, Loonsk J: Graphical representation of medical information in the visual chart. Seventh Annual IEEE Symposium on Computer-Based Medical Systems in Winston-Salem, NC, June 11-12, 1994. Los Alamitos, CA: IEEE Computer Society Press.

MacFadyen JC, Brown JE, Schoenwald R, Feldman RD: The effectiveness of teaching clinical pharmacokinetics by computer. Clin Pharmacol Ther 53:617-621, 1993.

Macura RT, Macura KJ: Computer-assigned instruction in medicine. 1993-1994 Overview. MEDLINE citations listing. J Med Educ Technol 5:17-30, 1994.

Madoff SA, Pristach CA, Smith CM: Computerized medication instruction for acute psychiatric inpatients. Student Research Forum, School of Medicine and Biomedical Sciences, State University of New York at Buffalo. December 8, 1992; also presented as Poster at the 44th Institute on Hospital and Community Psychiatry, Baltimore: October 8-12, 1993.

Mandell GL, Douglas RG, Bennett JE, Dolin R: Principles and Practice of Infectious Diseases: Antimicrobial Therapy 1993/1994. New York: Churchill Livingstone, 1993.

McCullough LB, Chervenak FA: Ethics in Obstetrics and Gynecology, 142-147. New York: Oxford University Press, 1994.

McLeod P, Cuello C, Capek R, Collier B: A tutorial/essay project to expand the learning experiences in undergraduate medical pharmacology. Med Teach 14:343-346, 1992.

MEDWATCH, the new FDA adverse effects reporting system. J Clin Psychopharmacol 10:303-304, 1993.

Mennin SP, Waterman RE: 1994 Problem-Based Teaching in Clinical Pharmacology: A Training Workshop. New Orleans: American Society Clinical Pharmacology and Therapeutics, April 2, 1994.

MICAL: Microbiology Computer-Assisted Learning software on chemotherapy. Educational Services, The Upjohn Company, Kalamazoo, MI 49001. (Also available: PSYCAL, dealing with psychiatry, DERMCAL, dermatology, ENDOCAL, dealing with endocrinology, 1988.)

Moore L, Waechter D, Aronow L: Asssessing the effectiveness of computer-assisted instruction in a pharmacology course. Academic Medicine 66:194-196, 1991.

Morgan LK, Raper JE Jr: Selective guide to current reference sources on topics discussed in this issue. Cocaine:Physiological and physiological effects. J Addict Dis 11:111-123, 1992.

Munson P (ed-in-chief): Principles of Pharmacology—Basic Concepts and Clinical Applications. New York: Chapman and Hall, 1994.

Neal MJ: Medical Pharmacology at a Glance. Boston: Blackwell Scientific, 1987.

Neubig RR: PHARMKIN: A Pharmacokinetics Teaching Demonstration. San Diego, GraphPAD Software, 1987.

Niebuhr BR, Marion R: An idealized computer-based patient record for teaching diagnosis and treatment planning. American Medical Informatics Association Proceedings of Seventeenth Annual Symposium on Computer Applications in Medical Care, October 30-November, 1994, p 959.

Nierenberg DW, Seprebon M: The central nervous system serotonin syndrome. Clin Pharmacol Ther 53:84-88, 1994.

Nierenberg DW, Smith RP: Clinical Problems in Basic Pharmacology. St. Louis, C.V. Mosby, 1989.

Nightingale S: MedWATCH conference cosponsored by the FDA and AMA. JAMA 270:2669, 1993.

On Line: US Health Link, an On-Line Information Service for Health Professionals, IEI Network, Inc. Wheaton, IL. Includes EMPIRES (Excerpta Medica), MEDLINE, Comtex Medical News Service, and a variety of services (Reviewed by Kelly, 1993).

Pierzchajlo R: Review of CIMD. Medical Software Reviews 2:5-6, 1993.

Pies R: Response to "This Prescription May Be Hazardous to your Health: Who is Accountable to the Patient." J Clin Psychopharmacol 13:457, 1993.

Poirier TI, Giudici RA: Drug interaction microcomputer software evaluation: Drug interaction facts on disk. Hosp Pharm 27:334-335, 1992.

Pratt WB, Taylor P: Principles of Drug Action. The Basis of Pharmacology, 3rd ed. (Update of Goldstein, Kalman, Aronow, 2nd ed.) New York: Churchill Livingstone, 1990.

Reynard AM, Smith CM: Information and learning resources in pharmacology. *In* Textbook of Pharmacology. Philadelphia: W.B. Saunders, 1992, pp 1166-1182.

Rogers AS: Adverse drug events: Identification and attribution. Drug Intell Clin Pharm 21:915-920, 1987.

Rovers JP, Janosik JE, Souney PF: Crossover comparison of drug information online database vendors: Dialog and MEDLARS. Ann Pharmacother 27:634-639, 1993.

Satya-Murti S: STAT! Ref CD ROM Medical Reference Library [review]. JAMA 270:1616, 1993.

Scott HD, Thacher-Renshaw A, Rosenbaum SE, et al: Physician reporting of adverse drug reactions. JAMA 263:1785-1788, 1990.

Seifert S: Review of MD-Challenger 1.6. Medical Software Reviews 2:6-7, 1993.

Shumway JM, Abate MA, Jacknowitz AI: Development of a computer program to teach critical evaluation of drug studies. American Medical Informatics Association Proceedings of Seventeenth Annual Symposium on Computer Applications in Medical Care, October 30-November, 1994, p 967.

Smith CM: Computer based drug information. Annual Meeting, American College of Clinical Pharmacology, Boston: November 1-3, 1993a.

Smith CM: Drug data bases in the teaching of clinical pharmacology. Poster at the Teaching Clinic, Annual Meeting, American College of Clinical Pharmacology, Boston: November 1-3, 1993b.

Smith CM: Drug data bases in the teaching of pharmacology. Presented at the Workshop on the Teaching of Pharmacology to Medical Students, Association of Medical School Pharmacology, The Cloister, Sea Island, GA: February 2-3, 1994a.

Smith CM: Clinical pharmacology [Review of the computer-based software program]. Medical Software Reviews. 3:4, 5, 1994b.

Smith CM: Improving both assessment and teaching functions of examinations: Results of a challenge feed-back system used over 10 years, in preparation, 1995.

Snow B: Drug Information: A Guide to Current Resources. Chicago: Medical Library Association, 1989 (new edition in preparation).

Steiner JC: Software review of Finelli PF: Nervline: Microcomputer Information Retrieval System in the Clinical Neuro-sciences (version 1.3, by Pasquale F. Finelli, 3 floppy disks for the IBM PC/KT AT, or MS-DOS compatible; Stoneham, MA: Butterworths [distributor], 1988). JAMA 263:1572-1573, 1990.

Sweeney G: Clinical Pharmacology—A Conceptual Approach. New York: Churchill Livingstone, 1990.

Tallarida RJ, Raffa RB, McGonigle P: Principles in General Pharmacology. New York: Springer-Verlag, 1988.

Tallarida RJ, Murray RB: Manual of Pharmacologic Calculations with Computer Programs, 2nd ed. New York: Springer-Verlag, 1987.

von Lichtenberg F: Omega yes, alpha no. JAMA 272:1412, 1994.

Walaszek ED, Doull J: Use of computers in the teaching of pharmacology. FASEB J 4:A1236, 1990.

Walaszek ED, Doull J: Use of computers in the teaching of pharmacology, toxicology and therapeutics. Physiologist 28:419–421, 1985.

Wang P: Janssen Research Foundation's Adverse Experience Literature Database: A user-centered design for human/computer interaction. Drug Information Journal 27:437–446, 1993.

Washington C, Washington W, Wilson CG: Pharmacokinetic modeling using STELLA on the Apple MacIntosh. New York: Prentice Hall, 1990.

Waterman RE, Duban SL, Mennin SP, et al: Clinical Problem-Based Learning: A Workbook for Integrating Basic and Clinical Science. Albuquerque: University of New Mexico Press, 1988. (Reviewed by Verghese A: JAMA 261:3036–3037, 1989.)

Weed LL: Knowledge Coupling: New Premises and New Tools for Medical Care and Education. New York: Springer-Verlag, 1991.

Weed LL: Medical Records, Medical Education, and Patient Care. Cleveland: Case Western Reserve University Press, 1969.

Weintraub M: Multiple medication assessment form: Guidelines for use in elderly patients. DE MONITOR, Division of Drugs and Toxicology. American Medical Association, Summer 1992.

Wood MS (ed): Reference and Information Services in Health Science Libraries.

Wyngaarden JB, Smith LH Jr (eds): Cecil Textbook of Medicine, vols. 1 and 2, 18th ed. Philadelphia: WB Saunders, 1988.

Xakellis GC, Gjerde C: Evaluation by second-year medical students of their computer-aided instruction. Acad Med 65:23–26, 1990.

Yaffe SJ, Aranda JV (eds): Pediatric Pharmacology: Therapeutic Principles in Practice, 2nd ed. Philadelphia: W. B. Saunders, 1992.

Yasnoff WA: US HEALTHLINK: A national information resource for health care professionals. J Med Syst 16:95–100, 1992.

Zupko KA: The very best way to organize patient records. Medical Economics July 25:75–85, 1994.

INDEXES, DATABASES, AND PRODUCTS

Computer-based refers to products useful on personal computers or CD-ROM; many of the on-line items are indicated by an asterisk.

Alpha Media Catalog. Maryland Heights, MO: American Psychiatric Electronic Library. Washington DC American Psychiatric Press.

*ANALYTICAL ABSTRACTS: Royal Society of Chemistry, Nottingham, England; available on DIALOG, DATA-STAR, ORBIT. Anesthesia Simulator Consultant 1.0. AnesSoft, Bellevue, WA (reviewed by Gorback, 1993)

Anonymous: The tenth annual directory of medical hardware and software companies. M.D. Computing 10:231–267, 1993.

Armstrong CJ (ed): World Databases in Medicine, Vol. 2. London: Bowker-Suar, 1993. Drugs and Pharmacy, Chapter 14.

*ASHP (American Society of Hospital Pharmacists), Bethesda, MD; CD-ROM Drug Information, AHFS Drug Information, Handbook on Injectable Drugs, International Pharmaceutical Abstracts.

AskRx. Camdat Corporation, Warrendale, PA (See Greco, 1993).

*Biological Abstracts/BIOSIS PREVIEWS: BioSciences Information Service, Philadelphia, PA; available on DIALOG. Cambridge Scientific Abstracts

Cardiolab: Simulation of cardiovascular pharmacology dog lab. Biosoft, Milltown, NJ.

*Chemical Abstracts/CA SEARCH: Chemical Abstracts Service, Columbus, OH; available on BRS and DIALOG. American Chemical Society, Columbus, OH.

CD-ROM — Medical CD-ROM catalog from CMEA — Continuing Medical Education Associates, Chicago, IL.

CD-ROM medical programs: See Clayman, 1993, and Satya-Murti, 1993.

CD-ROM Guides and Catalogs. Some examples are: Medical CD-ROM Catalog from CMEA (Continuing Medical Education Associates, San Diego, CA), Catalogs from Dialog, Updata Publications, BIOSIS (Biological Abstracts), Silver Platter, Right on Programs (Computer software for libraries, offices, schools, Huntington, NY 11743), CMC ReSearch, Inc, Portland, OR.

CIMD: Computer Insight, MSD, 1st ed. Resource Systems Management, Inc., P.O. Box 20190, Boulder, CO. Information for Medicine - Software Package (Formerly Ciba-Geigy Medical Computing Resource Guide).

Clinical Pharmacology — An electronic drug reference and teaching guide. Gainesville, FL: Gold Standard Multimedia, Inc. Reents S and Seymour J [Authors], 1994. (See Smith, 1994b.)

CMEA Inc. Continuing Medical Education Associates, Chicago, IL.

Computer-Based Patient Record Institute, Inc., 1000 East Woodfield Rd, Suite 102, Schaumburg, IL 60173.

*Current Contents/Clinical Medicine/Life Science/Social and Behavioral Science Citation Index/SCISEARCH. Institute for Scientific Information, Philadelphia, PA.

CYBERLOG: The Library of Applied Medical Software: Perspectives in Rational Management. Diskettes, documentation, and manuals. Cardinal Health Systems, Edina, MN, 1989.

*DE HAEN DRUG DATA: Paul De Haen International, Englewood, CO; available on DIALOG.

*DIALOG: Provides via modem on-line or CD-ROM information from more than 320 databases, including all major medical and health care reference sources. Dialog Information Services, Inc.

*Directory of Online Databases. Cuadra/Elsevier (quarterly), New York.

*Drug Information Fulltext (DIF) — American Society of Hospital Pharmacists. Contains AHFS Drug Information and the Handbook on Injectable Drugs monographs. Available in bound format with supplements and online BRS, DIALOG, Knowledge Index, Mead Data Central.

Drug Interaction Facts; Drug Interaction Facts on Disk. Facts and Comparisons Division, J.R. Lippincott Co., St. Louis, Missouri, Tatro, DS (ed) 1988. Use current edition. (Reviewed by Hoffer, 1993.)

Drug Interactions and Side Effects Index. Medical Economics Company, Oradell, NJ. Annual. Also on PC disk and CD-ROM DRUG THERAPY SCREENING SYSTEM (DTSS): A variety of drug therapy monitoring and reporting databases, including drug-drug, drug-food, and adverse reactions. Med-Span, Indianapolis.

Electronic Drug Reference, Version 3.0. Computer-based information on 3500 drugs, extracted from the USP DI, Facts and Comparisons, Facts and Comparisons Drug Newsletter, Drug Interaction Facts, Medical Newsletter, PDR, and other sources. Clinical Reference Systems, Ltd., Englewood, CO.

*Excerpta Medica. Amsterdam, The Netherlands. Available on line as EMBASE.

GUIDE, Drug Guide 1.0: Computerized Prescription and Nhinon-prescription Drug Guide for Interactions and Side Effects. Patient Medical Records, Inc., Brownfield, TX. Program derived from the S-O-A-P Patient Medical Records System (For a review see Davant, 1994).

Handbook of Adverse Drug Interactions. Published by The Medical Letter Inc, 1000 Main Street, New Rochelle, NY 10801.

Health Sciences Consortium, 201 Silver Cedar Court, Chapel Hill, NC 27514–1517.

*Index Medicus. National Library of Medicine.

*INTERNATIONAL PHARMACEUTICAL ABSTRACTS, American Society of Hospital Pharmacists, Bethesda, MD. Available on BRS and DIALOG International Pharmaceutical Abstracts. Washington DC, American Society of Hospital Pharmacists.

MacDogLab: Simulation of mammalian pharmacology laboratory. Dr. Donald Barnes, (919) 551-2747.

MacPharmacology. Minnesota Medical Edu-Ware, Inc., Duluth, MN (See Eisenberg, 1992, above).

MAXX: An electronic library of medicine. Boston, MA: Little, Brown and Company.

MD-Challenger. Interactive training and rapid clinical reference (for emergency/outpatient medicine). Challenger Corporation, Belle Meade Cove, Eads, TN.

MD Computing. Springer-Verlag, New York, NY.

Medical Drug Reference (Data from FIRST DATABANK). Parsons Technology, Heawatha, IA.

Medical Software Reviews: Monthly publication that includes reviews of software and citations to objective appraisals of software appearing in other publications (volume 1 — 1992; volume 2 — 1993; volume 3 — 1994). Healthcare Computing Publications Inc., 462 Second Street, Brooklyn, NY 11215-2503.

*MEDLINE:National Library of Medicine, Bethesda, MD (See Index Medicus); available on-line or on CD-ROM or via on-line services such as DIALOG, BRS.

*MICROMEDEX, INC. publishes large, extensive medicine and toxicological databases, readily accessible for drugs as causes of symptoms/signs, side effects, adverse drug reactions, drug monographs, poisoning and treatment (the programs installed at a given institution could include: POISINDEX, DRUGDEX, EMERGINDEX, TOMES, IDENTIDEX, TOME Plus, SI*calc*, and CCIS information systems and AfterCare instructions, and also includes the PDR and the Martindale text. The MICROMEDEX program is available on CD-ROM or on networks.

Morgan LK, Raper JE: Selective guide to current reference sources on topics discussed in a given issue of J. Addictive Diseases; for example, 13:107–118, 1994.

MUST: Medication Use Studies. Database in excess of 10,000 records of the world literature on the use of medications. School of Pharmacy, The University of Mississippi, University, MS.

Nightingale SL: From the Food and Drug Administration. JAMA 272:1814, 1994; JAMA 270:2669, 1993.

Pharmacology Textstack:Theoharides TC. Keyboard Publishing, Blue Bell, PA.

PharmAid: Hypercard stack for basic and clinical pharmacology; pharmacokinetic examples. MedEd Software, Inc, Natick, MA.

*Pharmacy Case Review: A peer reviewed electronic journal available on Internet. Idaho State University College of Pharmacy, Pocatello, ID.

Pharmline: A pharmacy network on Internet (1-800-247-4276).

Physicians' Desk Reference (PDR). Medical Economics Company. New edition available each year, plus supplements during the year. Also available on CD-ROM, and portions for personal computers.

Physicians GenRx, Data Pharmaceutica, Inc., Smithtown, NY. Available each year as book or on CD-ROM, such as from CMEA, Inc., Chicago, IL.

RxTriage, Drug Interactions database with patient record system and monographs. First Data Bank, San Bruno, CA (Reviewed by Hoffer, 1992).

*Science Citation Index. Institute for Scientific Information, Philadelphia, PA.

S-O-A-P Drug Interaction Program for drug-, food-, disease-drug interactions and side effects of 2500 drugs. Brownfield, TX: Patient Medical Records, 1990, and updates.

Statox and Environtox: Toxicologic reference data bases. EM Alternatives, Inc., reviewed in Medical Software Reviews 3(9):6–7, 1994.

STAT!Ref Comprehensive software reference library on CD-ROM; available in customized groups depending on specialty and medical interests. (See Clayman, 1993.)

*TOXLINE/TOXLIT. National Library of Medicine, Bethesda, MD.

USC*PACK programs from the USC Laboratory of Applied Pharmacokinetics. Jelliffe, RW, Professor of Medicine, University of Southern California.

*US HEALTHLINK: On-line information service for health professionals; includes MEDLINE, Excerpta Medica EMPIRES, Comtex Medical News Service. IEI Network, Inc., Wheaton, IL 60187 (reviewed by Fox, 1992; Yasnoff, 1992).

USP DI: USP Dispensing Information; volume I—Drug Information for the Health Care Professional; volume II—Advice for the Patient; volume III—Approved Drug Products and Legal Requirements. United States Pharmacopeial Convention, Inc. Database used in a number of computer-based programs; *eg,* AskRx.

Washington Manual on CD-ROM: Manual of Medical Therapeutics. Department of Medicine, Washington University School of Medicine. St. Louis, MO. Boston: Little, Brown and Company.

INDEX

Note: Page numbers in *italics* refer to illustrations; page numbers followed by t refer to tables.

B

D

H

J

K

L

M

N

O

Q

R

S

T